GRABB AND SMITH'S
*Plastic Surgery*

GRABB AND SMITH'S

# *Plastic Surgery*

## FOURTH EDITION

EDITED BY

**James W. Smith, M.D.**
Associate Professor of Surgery (Plastic),
Cornell University Medical College; Associate
Attending Surgeon in Plastic Surgery, The New
York Hospital-Cornell Medical Center,
New York, New York

**Sherrell J. Aston, M.D.**
Associate Professor of Surgery, Institute of
Reconstructive Plastic Surgery, New York
University School of Medicine; Attending
Surgeon in Plastic Surgery, Manhattan Eye, Ear
and Throat Hospital, New York, New York

*Little, Brown and Company*
BOSTON/TORONTO/LONDON

*To Dr. William C. Grabb and all in the medical community who are committed to his standards of academic excellence and exert an inspirational influence on the development and teaching of plastic and reconstructive surgery*

# Contents

## III
### Skin and Adnexa

# Editor's Note

As William C. Grabb and I began to discuss our fourth edition of this text, Dr. Grabb suddenly had a cardiac arrest and died at the age of 53. I am still saddened by this loss of such an outstanding educator and dear personal friend at an early age. I am sure Bill would have wanted us to proceed for him in the preparation of the fourth edition. I am sure that his guiding spirit and enthusiasm for this textbook are as strong and vibrant as ever.

It is with love and respect for Bill and his wife, Cozette, that Dr. Aston, Little, Brown and Company, our publishers, and I have agreed to preserve the original title and editors' names in this, our fourth edition. By extending us this courtesy, neither Little, Brown nor I wish to lessen in any way our appreciation and thanks to Dr. Sherrell J. Aston for agreeing to serve as my co-editor. I thank him for his tremendous effort and help on our behalf.

J.W.S.

# *Preface*

The first edition of *Plastic Surgery: A Concise Guide to Clinical Practice* was published in 1968 with two specific objectives. The first was to provide a current and succinct guide to clinical practice in the field of plastic surgery. The second was to make available an inexpensive but comprehensive text for the student, medical house officer, and practicing physician. During the intervening 22 years since that first edition, the editors, through the publishing of a second edition (1973) and a third edition (1979) strived to keep those with an interest in plastic surgery aware of the more important changes, developments, and new ideas affecting our specialty.

The fourth edition of this book has been compiled to include some information from all aspects of plastic surgery, keeping the same two main objectives: to confine its contents to one volume and to keep its cost within an economic range that will fit the budget of most of our readers.

Of necessity the book has grown, and keeping it in one volume has been difficult. Ninety-three colleagues have contributed to this edition. We have tried to maintain a basic concise format but have remained flex-ible enough for each author to present material in his or her style. We thank the authors whose chapters are included in this fourth edition and appreciate their great loyalty and dedication. We also acknowledge the authors of all the articles included in the chapter references and the suggested reading lists.

We thank Little, Brown for preserving the color of the cover. For nearly a quarter of a century, our readers have referred to this text unofficially as the "Blue Book." It seems to have gained this designation from those plastic surgeons who, after completing their training in plastic surgery, packed their bags, took their "Blue Books," and went to take the examination for board certification by the American Board of Plastic Surgery.

Although we suspect it is probably just an old wives' tale, many board members who passed their exams the first time say they were superstitious about using the "Blue Book" in preparation. They say, "If you know your Blue Book, you're sure to pass!" Other candidates say they were advised by their predecessors to "take it along because it brings good luck." We hope this book continues to bring our readers good luck and at

**H. S. Byrd, M.D.**
Associate Professor and Vice Chairman of
Plastic and Reconstructive Surgery, University
of Texas Southwestern Medical School, Dallas;
Director of Service, Department of Plastic
Surgery, Children's Medical Center, Dallas,
Texas

**Alberto G. Camargos, M.D.**
Postgraduate Fellow, Division of Plastic Surgery,
University of Alabama at Birmingham School of
Medicine, Birmingham, Alabama; Director,
Department of Reconstructive Microsurgery,
Mater Dei Hospital, and Director of Plastic and
Reconstructive Surgery, Afonso Pena Clinic,
Belo Horizonte, Brazil

**Eric C. Carlson, M.D.**
Assistant Professor, Department of Orthopaedic
Surgery, Columbia University College of
Physicians and Surgeons; Assistant Attending
Surgeon, Department of Orthopaedic Surgery,
Presbyterian Hospital, New York, New York

**James H. Carraway, M.D.**
Professor and Chairman, Department of Plastic
Surgery, Eastern Virginia Medical School of the
Medical College of Hampton Roads, Norfolk,
Virginia

**I. Kelman Cohen, M.D.**
Professor and Chairman, Division of Plastic
Surgery, Virginia Commonwealth University
Medical College of Virginia, Richmond, Virginia

**Mark B. Constantian, M.D.**
Clinical Instructor in Surgery, Harvard Medical
School, Boston, Massachusetts; Attending
Plastic Surgeon, Memorial Hospital, Nashua,
New Hampshire

**Ralph Coonrad, M.D.**
Associate Clinical Professor of Orthopedic
Surgery, Duke University School of Medicine,
Durham, North Carolina

**Albert E. Cram, M.D.**
Associate Professor of Surgery, University of
Iowa College of Medicine; Director, Division of
Plastic and Reconstructive Surgery, University
of Iowa Hospitals, Iowa City, Iowa

**Christopher P. Demas, M.D.**
Clinical Lecturer in Plastic Surgery, University
of Arizona College of Medicine; Attending
Surgeon, Tucson Medical Center, University
Medical Center, St. Joseph's Medical Center, and
El Dorado Medical Center, Tucson, Arizona

**Charles J. Devine, Jr., M.D.**
Professor of Urology, Eastern Virginia Medical
School of the Medical College of Hampton
Roads; Sentara Norfolk General Hospital and
Children's Hospital of the King's Daughters,
Norfolk, Virginia

**Harold M. Dick, M.D.**
Frank E. Stinchfield Professor, and Chairman of
Orthopaedic Surgery, Columbia University
College of Physicians and Surgeons; Attending
Orthopaedic Surgeon, and Director of
Orthopaedic Surgery, Presbyterian Hospital,
New York, New York

**Richard G. Eaton, M.D.**
Professor of Clinical Surgery, Columbia
University College of Physicians and Surgeons;
Director, Hand Surgery Center, St. Luke's-
Roosevelt Hospital, New York, New York

**Deborah Ekstrom, M.D.**
Teaching Associate, University of
Massachusetts Medical Center; Plastic Surgeon,
St. Vincent Hospital, Worcester City Hospital,
and Medical Center of Central Massachusetts,
Worcester, Massachusetts

**Earl J. Fleegler, M.D.**
Assistant Clinical Professor of Plastic Surgery,
Case Western Reserve University School of
Medicine; Head, Section of Hand Surgery,
Cleveland Clinic Foundation, Cleveland, Ohio

**William C. Grabb, M.D.\***
Professor of Surgery (Plastic Surgery) and Head,
Section of Plastic Surgery, University of
Michigan Medical School; Staff Surgeon,
University of Michigan Hospital, Ann Arbor,
Michigan

*Deceased

*Jeffrey P. Groner, M.D.*
Assistant Professor of Plastic and
Reconstructive Surgery, Washington University
School of Medicine; Attending Surgeon,
Division of Plastic Surgery, Barnes Hospital,
St. Louis, Missouri

*Ulrich T. Hinderer, M.D.*
Professor of Plastic Surgery, Universitas
Complutensis; Director, Clinica Mirasierra de
Cirugia Plastica-Estetica, Madrid, Spain

*Charles E. Horton, M.D.*
Professor of Plastic Surgery, Eastern Virginia
Medical School of the Medical College of
Hampton Roads, Norfolk, Virginia

*Norman E. Hugo, M.D.*
Professor of Surgery (Plastic), Columbia
University College of Physicians and Surgeons;
Attending Surgeon and Chief, Division of Plastic
Surgery, Presbyterian Hospital, New York, New
York

*David H. Humphreys, M.D.*
Attending Surgeon and Chief, Plastic Surgery
Section, Memorial Mission Hospital and St.
Joseph's Hospital, Asheville, North Carolina

*Ian T. Jackson, M.D., F.R.C.S., F.A.C.S.,
F.R.A.C.S. (Hon.)*
Director, Institute for Craniofacial and
Reconstructive Surgery (Affiliated with
Providence Hospital), Southfield, Michigan

*Jonathan S. Jacobs, D.M.D., M.D.*
Assistant Professor of Plastic Surgery, Eastern
Virginia Medical School of the Medical College
of Hampton Roads; Chief, Department of Plastic
Surgery, Medical Center Hospitals, Norfolk,
Virginia

*Saulius Jankauskas, M.D.*
Attending Physician, Florida Hospitals, Navy
Hospital, and Winter Park Memorial Hospital,
Orlando, Florida

*José Juri, M.D.*
Professor of Plastic Surgery, National
University; Director, Clinica Juri de Cirugia
Plastica, Buenos Aires, Argentina

*Henry K. Kawamoto, Jr., M.D., D.D.S.*
Associate Clinical Professor of Plastic Surgery,
University of California, Los Angeles, School of
Medicine; Senior Attending in Plastic Surgery,
St. John's Hospital, Santa Monica, California

*Roger K. Khouri, M.D.*
Assistant Professor of Surgery (Plastic and
Reconstructive), Washington University School
of Medicine; Director, Microsurgery Service,
Barnes Hospital, St. Louis, Missouri

*Abdul-Ghani Kibbi, M.D.*
Research Fellow in Dermatopathology, Harvard
Medical School; Research Fellow in
Dermatopathology and Laser Pathology,
Massachusetts General Hospital and Wellman
Research Laboratories, Boston, Massachusetts

*L. Andrew Koman, M.D.*
Associate Professor of Orthopedic Surgery,
Bowman Gray School of Medicine of Wake
Forest University; Attending Surgeon,
Department of Orthopedics and Pediatrics,
North Carolina Baptist Hospital, Winston-
Salem, North Carolina

*Thomas J. Krizek, M.D.*
Professor and Chairman, Department of Surgery,
University of Chicago Pritzker School of
Medicine, Chicago, Illinois

*Don LaRossa, M.D.*
Associate Professor of Surgery (Plastic),
University of Pennsylvania School of Medicine;
Director, Cleft Lip and Palate Program,
Children's Hospital of Philadelphia,
Philadelphia, Pennsylvania

*Harvey Lash, D.D.S., M.D.*
Clinical Assistant Professor of Surgery, Stanford
University School of Medicine, Stanford;
Chairman, Department of Plastic and
Reconstructive Surgery, Palo Alto Medical
Foundation, Palo Alto, California

*Gregory S. LaTrenta, M.D.*
Assistant Professor of Surgery (Plastic), Cornell
University Medical College; Attending Surgeon,
New York Hospital and Manhattan Eye, Ear and
Throat Hospital, New York, New York

**Donald R. Laub, M.D.**
Clinical Associate Professor of Surgery, Stanford University School of Medicine; Department of Surgery/Plastic Surgery, Stanford University Hospital, Stanford, California

**Donald R. Laub, Jr., M.D.**
Resident in General Surgery, Oregon Health Sciences University, Portland, Oregon

**Victor L. Lewis, Jr., M.D.**
Associate Professor of Clinical Surgery, Northwestern University Medical School; Attending Surgeon, Northwestern Memorial Hospital, Chicago, Illinois

**Graham D. Lister, M.B., Ch.B.**
Professor of Surgery and Chief, Division of Plastic Surgery, University of Utah School of Medicine, Salt Lake City, Utah

**John W. Little III, M.D.**
Professor of Surgery, Georgetown University School of Medicine; Director, Division of Plastic and Reconstructive Surgery, Georgetown University Hospital, Washington, D.C.

**Nicholas J. Lowe, M.D.**
Clinical Professor of Dermatology, University of California, Los Angeles, School of Medicine; Director, Southern California Dermatology and Psoriasis Center, Santa Monica, California

**M. Vincent Makhlouf, M.D.**
Attending Surgeon, Illinois Masonic Medical Center, Chicago, Illinois

**Paul Manson, M.D.**
Professor of Surgery, Johns Hopkins University School of Medicine; Director of Plastic Surgery, Maryland Institute of Emergency Medical Services Systems, Baltimore, Maryland

**Morton R. Maser, M.D.**
Assistant Clinical Professor of Plastic Surgery, Stanford University School of Medicine, Stanford; Department of Plastic Surgery, Palo Alto Medical Foundation, Palo Alto, California

**G. Patrick Maxwell, M.D.**
Assistant Clinical Professor of Plastic Surgery, Vanderbilt University School of Medicine; Director, Institute of Aesthetic and Reconstructive Surgery, Baptist Hospital, Nashville, Tennessee

**Joseph G. McCarthy, M.D.**
Lawrence D. Bell Professor of Plastic Surgery, New York University School of Medicine; Director, Institute of Reconstructive Plastic Surgery, New York University Medical Center, New York, New York

**John B. McCraw, M.D.**
Professor of Plastic Surgery, Eastern Virginia Medical School of the Medical College of Hampton Roads; Attending Surgeon, Department of Plastic Surgery, Norfolk General Hospital, Norfolk, Virginia

**Peter McKinney, M.D.**
Professor of Clinical Surgery (Plastic), Northwestern University Medical School; Attending Surgeon, Northwestern Memorial Hospital, Chicago, Illinois

**Martin C. Mihm, Jr., M.D.**
Professor of Pathology and Chief of Dermatopathology, Harvard Medical School; Pathologist and Chief of Dermatopathology, Massachusetts General Hospital, Boston, Massachusetts

**Timothy A. Miller, M.D.**
Professor of Surgery, University of California, Los Angeles, School of Medicine; Chief of Plastic Surgery, Wadsworth Veterans Administration Medical Center and University of California, Los Angeles, Medical Center, Los Angeles, California

**Hanno Millesi, M.D.**
Professor of Plastic Surgery and Head, Department of Plastic and Reconstructive Surgery, First Surgical Clinic, University of Vienna Medical School; Director, Ludwig-Boltzmann Institute for Experimental Plastic Surgery, Vienna, Austria

**Ralph P. Pennino, M.D.**
Clinical Assistant Professor of Surgery,
University of Rochester School of Medicine
and Dentistry; Attending Surgeon, Division
of Plastic Surgery, Rochester General
Hospital and St. Mary's Hospital, Rochester,
New York

**Gary G. Poehling, M.D.**
Professor and Chairman of Orthopedic Surgery,
Bowman Gray School of Medicine of Wake
Forest University; Department of Orthopedic
Surgery, North Carolina Baptist Hospital,
Winston-Salem, North Carolina

**Barry Press, M.D.**
Assistant Professor of Surgery (Plastic), Stanford
University School of Medicine, Stanford;
Associate Chief of Plastic Surgery and Director,
Burn Center, Santa Clara Valley Medical Center,
San Jose, California

**Peter Randall, M.D.**
Professor of Plastic Surgery, University of
Pennsylvania School of Medicine; Chief,
Division of Plastic Surgery, Hospital of the
University of Pennsylvania, and Senior Surgeon,
Children's Hospital of Philadelphia,
Philadelphia, Pennsylvania

**Julien Reich, M.D.Sc., F.R.A.C.S.**
Director, Kooyong Clinic for Plastic Surgery, and
Freemasons Hospital, Melbourne, Australia

**Sharon Romm, M.D.**
Assistant Professor of Plastic Surgery,
Georgetown University School of Medicine and
Georgetown University Hospital, Washington,
D.C.

**Richard Sadove, M.D.**
Assistant Professor of Plastic Surgery, University
of Kentucky College of Medicine; Attending
Surgeon, Division of Plastic Surgery, Chandler
Medical Center and Chief of Plastic Surgery,
Lexington Veterans Hospital, Lexington,
Kentucky

**Gordon H. Sasaki, M.D.**
Clinical Associate Professor of Plastic Surgery,
University of Southern California School of
Medicine, Los Angeles; Attending Surgeon,
Department of Plastic Surgery, Huntington
Memorial Hospital, Pasadena, California

**Richard C. Schultz, M.D., F.A.C.S.**
Professor of Plastic Surgery, University of
Illinois College of Medicine, Chicago; Attending
Physician, Division of Plastic Surgery, Lutheran
General Hospital, Park Ridge, Illinois

**Donald Serafin, M.D.**
Professor of Plastic Surgery, Duke University
School of Medicine; Chief, Division of Plastic
Surgery, Duke University Medical Center,
Durham, North Carolina

**William W. Shaw, M.D.**
Associate Professor of Surgery (Plastic),
New York University School of Medicine,
New York, New York

**Jack H. Sheen, M.D.**
Clinical Professor of Surgery, Section of Plastic
and Reconstructive Surgery, University of
Southern California School of Medicine;
Associate Clinical Professor, Division of Plastic
Surgery, University of California, Los Angeles,
School of Medicine, Los Angeles, California

**John E. Sherman, M.D.**
Assistant Clinical Professor of Surgery, Mount
Sinai School of Medicine of the City University
of New York; Attending Surgeon, Doctors
Hospital and Beth Israel Medical Center, New
York, New York

**James W. Smith, M.D.**
Associate Professor of Surgery (Plastic), Cornell
University Medical College; Associate
Attending Surgeon in Plastic Surgery, The New
York Hospital-Cornell Medical Center, New
York, New York

**Arthur J. Sober, M.D.**
Associate Professor of Dermatology, Harvard
Medical School; Associate Chief of
Dermatology, Massachusetts General Hospital,
Boston, Massachusetts

**Scott L. Spear, M.D.**
Associate Professor of Plastic Surgery,
Georgetown University School of Medicine;
Attending Surgeon and Deputy Director,
Division of Plastic Surgery, Georgetown
University Hospital, Washington, D.C.

**Melvin Spira, M.D.**
Professor and Head, Division of Plastic Surgery,
Baylor College of Medicine; Chief, Plastic
Surgery Service, Methodist Hospital, Houston,
Texas

**Samuel Stal, M.D.**
Associate Professor of Plastic Surgery, Baylor
College of Medicine; Chief of Plastic Surgery
and Co-Director, Cleft Palate and Craniofacial
Center, Texas Children's Hospital, Houston,
Texas

**James M. Stuzin, M.D.**
Clinical Instructor in Plastic Surgery, University
of Miami School of Medicine; Attending
Physician, Department of Plastic Surgery, Mercy
Hospital and Cedars Medical Center, Miami,
Florida

**Kwan Chul Tark, M.D., Ph.D.**
Assistant Professor of Plastic Surgery, Yonsei
University College of Medicine, Seoul, Korea;
Research Fellow in Microsurgery and Clinical
Instructor in Plastic Surgery, Institute of
Reconstructive Plastic Surgery, New York
University Medical Center, New York, New
York

**Charles H. M. Thorne, M.D.**
Assistant Professor of Surgery and Associate
Director, Craniofacial Unit, New York
University School of Medicine; Attending
Surgeon, Institute of Reconstructive Plastic
Surgery, New York University Medical Center,
and Manhattan Eye, Ear and Throat Hospital,
New York, New York

**Andrew E. Turk, M.D.**
Resident in Surgery and Research Fellow in
Plastic and Reconstructive Surgery, University
of California, Los Angeles, School of Medicine,
University of California, Los Angeles, Medical
Center, and Wadsworth Veterans Administration
Medical Center, Los Angeles, California

**Mark A. Urban, M.D.**
Assistant Instructor in Orthopedic Surgery,
Hospital of the University of Pennsylvania,
Philadelphia, Pennsylvania

**Judy Van Maasdam, M.A.**
Coordinator, Gender Dysphoria Program, Inc.,
Palo Alto, California

**Luis O. Vásconez, M.D.**
Professor of Surgery, University of Alabama at
Birmingham School of Medicine; Chief, Plastic
Surgery, University of Alabama Hospitals,
Birmingham, Alabama

**Bert Vorstman, M.B.Ch.B., M.Ch.,
F.R.A.C.S., F.A.A.P., F.A.C.S.**
Clinical Assistant Professor of Urology,
University of Miami School of Medicine,
Miami; Attending Urologist, Coral Springs
Medical Center, Coral Springs, Florida

**H. Kirk Watson, M.D.**
Associate Professor, University of Connecticut
School of Medicine, Farmington; Yale
University School of Medicine, New Haven; and
University of Massachusetts Medical School,
Worcester; Chief, Connecticut Combined Hand
Surgery Service, Hartford Hospital, Hartford,
Connecticut

**Paul M. Weeks, M.D.**
Professor and Chief, Division of Plastic Surgery,
Washington University School of Medicine;
Attending Surgeon and Chief, Division of Plastic
Surgery, Barnes Hospital, St. Louis, Missouri

**David N. White, M.D.**
Physician Specialist, Department of Hand and
Upper Extremity Surgery, Stanford University
Medical Center, Stanford; Palo Alto Medical
Foundation, Palo Alto, California

**E. F. Shaw Wilgis, M.D.**
Associate Professor of Plastic and Orthopedic
Surgery, Johns Hopkins University School of
Medicine; Chief, Division of Hand Surgery,
Union Memorial Hospital, Baltimore, Maryland

*Jeffrey Wisnicki, M.D.*
Chief, Division of Plastic Surgery, John F. Kennedy Memorial Hospital, West Palm Beach, Florida

*S. Anthony Wolfe, M.D., F.A.C.S.*
Clinical Professor of Plastic and Reconstructive Surgery, University of Miami School of Medicine; Chief, Plastic Surgery, Victoria Hospital and Miami Children's Hospital, Miami, Florida

*John E. Woods, M.D., Ph.D.*
Vice Chairman and Stuart W. Harrington Professor, Department of Surgery, Mayo Medical School; Plastic Surgeon, Methodist Hospital, Rochester, Minnesota

*Harvey A. Zarem, M.D.*
Professor Emeritus, University of California, Los Angeles, School of Medicine, Los Angeles, California

*Barry M. Zide, M.D., D.M.D.*
Assistant Professor of Plastic Surgery, New York University School of Medicine; Attending Surgeon, New York Eye and Ear Infirmary, Bellevue Hospital Center, Manhattan Veterans Administration Hospital, and Manhattan Eye, Ear, and Throat Hospital, New York, New York

# 1

# Basic Technique of Plastic Surgery

Saulius Jankauskas
I. Kelman Cohen
William C. Grabb*

The techniques of plastic surgery are most often applied to the skin and soft tissues. In their most basic form they relate to the excision of skin lesions, closure of skin wounds, skin grafts, flaps, and Z-plasty. However, the concepts learned from these techniques provide the basic principles of all surgical care, from nerve repair to coronary artery bypass grafts. These basic techniques and the principles derived from them should be mastered by all surgeons.

## Excision of Skin Lesions
### OBTAINING A FINE LINE SCAR
The final appearance of a scar after lesion excision depends on many factors. Of importance are the use of atraumatic technique, eversion of the wound edges, and placement of the scar in the same direction as skin lines. Factors over which we have no control include the age of the patient, the region of the body, the type of skin, and such complicating factors as skin disorders, infection, and the individual's healing mechanism.

### Atraumatic Technique
Careful handling of tissues is essential to obtain a fine linear scar. Skin and the subcu-

taneous tissues that have been crushed, dried by exposure to the air, damaged with hot sponges, or strangled by a suture under too much tension undergo different degrees of necrosis. The necrotic cells may then serve as a culture medium for infection, which increases inflammation and could result in more collagen deposition (scar).

The concept of care for skin and subcutaneous tissue is a histologic one [46]. All cells are served by a network of blood vessels, lymphatics, and nerves. Any source of trauma, including the simple crushing effect of a forceps or hemostat, may cause an appreciable amount of damage to both cells and vessels, resulting in a loss of blood and lymph into the interstitial spaces. The destroyed or damaged cells provide the substance on which organisms can multiply, create infection, and destroy more tissue. An atraumatic technique aids in minimizing this trauma. Sharp knives, scissors, needles, and skin hooks, as well as sutures of the proper size, swaged to a needle, are all important to this end.

Even the normal tremor of the surgeon's hand can be detrimental. Both operator and assistant should brace their elbows against their bodies (or the arm board during hand surgery) or brace their hands on the patient whenever possible to reduce this tremor.

*Deceased

3

This maneuver is similar to the bracing we do every day when we write at a desk.

Hot sponges have no place in atraumatic surgery. They not only increase capillary bleeding [351] but also, as the applied heat approaches 66°C (the temperature produced by electric sponge basin warmers), the incidence of wound infection increases [211]. Such infections may be the result of an increase in tissue necrosis caused by heat.

*Skin Lines*

Mature, fine linear scars result from excisions or incisions planned so that the final scar lies in, or parallel to, the adjacent skin lines. Borges [35] has written extensively about skin lines and has listed 36 descriptive terms from the literature, including Langer lines and relaxed skin tension lines. Clearly, scars are less conspicuous if they follow any skin line. If there are conflicting directions of two or more lines, it is preferable to follow the relaxed skin tension line. An example of this line can be seen on the volar surface of the forearm, where the skin lines formed between a wide pinch with thumb and forefinger are longitudinal when the elbow is extended but horizontal with the elbow flexed and the skin released. In areas without skin lines, such as the open plane of the cheek of a young person, scars can be especially noticeable. They are best placed by planning the incisions in the wrinkle lines one would find on an older person (Fig. 1-1). As a practical matter, scars are least conspicuous when the following factors are considered.

WRINKLE LINES (INCLUDING LINES OF FACIAL EXPRESSION AND RELAXED SKIN TENSION LINES). The wrinkle lines of the skin generally lie perpendicular to the long axis of the underlying muscles and are caused by the wrinkling that accompanies muscular contraction [175]. Wrinkle lines of the face, known as the line of expression [162] (Fig. 1-1), develop in a rather predictable pattern and are frequently used as a criterion for judging a person's age. The lines of facial expression are accentuated with smiling, grimacing, frowning, pursing the lips, and closing the eyes tightly. If for some reason these active responses are not possible, the skin can be approximated passively with a wide pinch of the thumb and index finger in various directions (relaxed skin tension lines). In this way the most prominent ridges and furrows are produced in the natural wrinkle lines of the skin. In most instances, these relaxed skin tension lines are the same as the lines of facial expression. Wrinkle lines in many parts of the body can best be seen by having the patient flex or extend the part.

CONTOUR LINES. Contour lines are the lines of division at the juncture of body planes [315]. Examples are found at the juncture of the cheek with the nose, the cheek with the ear, the scalp with the ear, the skin of the lips with the vermilion (vermilion-cutaneous line), the cheek and neck skin in the submandibular region, and the juncture of the inferior aspect of the breast with the chest wall (inframammary fold). For example, a favorite place to hide a scar during a facelift is in the horizontal wrinkle line just under the chin, where it is usually out of sight, or at the ear–cheek junction.

LINES OF DEPENDENCY. The lines of dependency occur in older people owing to the effect of gravity on loose skin and fatty tissue. The "turkey gobbler fold" in the submental region and the more laterally located jowl lines of the mandibular region are typical lines of dependency. The cross-hatching pattern of lines on the facial skin of elderly persons is partly due to the intersection of lines of dependency and lines of facial expression [315].

*Age of the Patient*

Infant's scars (1 to 3 months) are often fine lines. In contrast, children's scars can remain erythematous and hypertrophic for prolonged periods, and the final result may be less satisfactory than those in adults. In general, scars on persons of middle age and

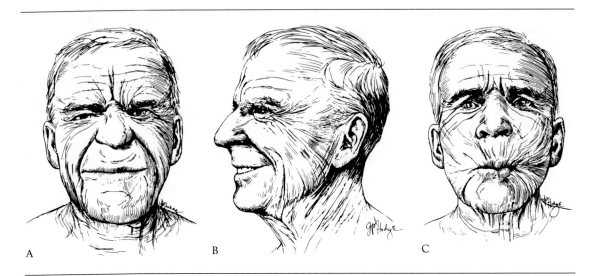

A        B        C

**Figure 1-1** *Skin lines: the lines of facial expression (A), contour lines (B), and lines of dependency (C).*

older are least conspicuous. *A time lapse of 2 years or more is important to allow the normal process of maturation to alter the raised, red scar into a flat, white one.* This time requirement must be stressed to patients, their families, and their attorneys.

*Regions of the Body*
Scars resulting from excisions or incisions in the eyelids, palms, soles, vermilion, or mucous membranes are usually finer and less conspicuous than those seen elsewhere [70], especially when contrasted with areas such as the sternum, shoulder, and back. Before incisions are made in these high risk areas, the patient is warned that the scar will probably become hypertrophic. Particularly disappointing are scars of the sternal region in women, where a butterfly-shaped keloid often develops. When a keloid in this region is excised, a new and larger one may recur in its place. A further discussion of scars and keloids can be found in Chapter 30.

*Length of Scar*
In general, the smaller the wound, the less disfiguring the scar. However, placement of

a longer scar in a wrinkle line may be preferable because the added length may make it less conspicuous. A long, straight scar may contract, producing bowstringing and hypertrophy that would not occur with multiple small scars or a long scar composed of small segments running in different directions in an accordion-like fashion [35]. However, the only time one must be cautious of this practice is when placing the incision on flexion surfaces and *especially* across crease lines.

U-*Shaped Scar*
The U-shaped scar is notorious in that it contracts to become a depressed groove circumscribing a bulging convex circle of skin. The appearance is not due to trapped edema fluid but to contracture.

*Angle of Wound to Skin Surface*
According to Borges, the more oblique the incision to the skin surface, the greater is the width of the scar in the dermis. This dermal scar then contracts, causing the overlying skin to bulge. The thicker the skin, the greater is the deformity, so that although the scar is significant in the forehead it is not a problem in the eyelid [35]. Borges' observations have never been clearly validated.

## Type of Skin

Some patients have thick, oily skin that contains hypertrophied and overactive sebaceous glands. Wounds in this type of skin may heal with a noticeable, depressed scar. Skin with these characteristics may be present over the distal half of the nose, the middle portion of cheeks, and the forehead. Single-layer closure in such circumstances is often preferable to avoid suture splitting and epithelial inclusion cysts.

## Skin Disorders

Patients who have abnormalities of fibrous and elastic tissue biosynthesis often develop wide scars. Patients with these fibroelastic diatheses can usually be detected preoperatively by looking for hyperextensibility of the fingers or by pinching and elevating the skin over the back of the hand to demonstrate increased elasticity. In certain forms of the Ehlers-Danlos syndrome, the skin heals slowly and with wide scars [217].

### METHODS OF EXCISION

Lesions of the skin can be removed by elliptical, wedge, or circular excision. The width of skin that can be excised and the type of excision varies enormously between young and old, between thin and corpulent, and of course in different regions of the body. The experienced plastic surgeon continually, almost automatically, estimates this factor by noting the wrinkling and aging characteristics of the skin, picking up the skin between thumb and index finger, and looking for the skin tension lines.

## Simple Elliptical Excision

Simple elliptical excision is the technique most often used for removing skin lesions. Ideally, an ellipse (i.e., a "surgeon's ellipse" or lenticular configuration, as a true ellipse is rounded at each end rather than angular) is planned so its long axis parallels a wrinkle line, contour line, or line of dependency (Fig. 1-2); ideally the long axis is about four times as great as the short axis. If the long axis be-

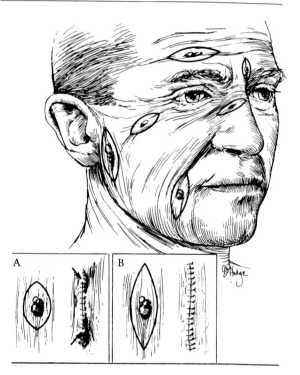

**Figure 1-2** *Elliptical excision. A. If the ellipse is too short, dog ears (arrows) form at the ends of the closed wound. B. Correct method.*

comes too short, its sides form too great an angle with one another, and excess bunching of skin, known as a "dog ear," results when the wound is closed (Figs. 1-2A and 1-3A). A dog ear can also result if one side of the ellipse is much longer than the other, i.e., one side approaching a semicircle and the other side a straight line (Fig. 1-3B). Dog ears tend to flatten over a period of several months but are excised if they persist. Suction lipectomy may be used secondarily to correct some dog ears.

The dog ear resulting from the short, broad ellipse can be corrected simply by extending the ellipse to include the excess tissue (Fig. 1-3A). When it is due to one side of the incision being longer than the other, it can be corrected by making a short, right-angled incision at the end of the ellipse. The excess skin overlaps at the wound edge and can be

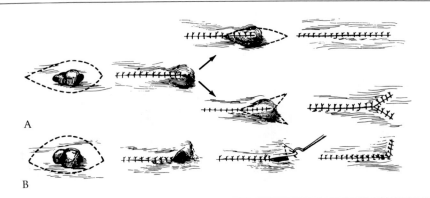

A

B

**Figure 1-3** *A. Two methods of removing a dog ear caused by making the elliptical excision too short. B. Method of removing dog ear caused by making one side of the ellipse longer than the other.*

trimmed away, permitting wound closure in the shape of an L (Fig. 1-3B).

*Multiple Excision Technique*
Although now frequently replaced by tissue expansion (discussed later in the chapter), the technique of multiple excisions can be employed for excising certain large skin lesions. The theory behind it is that skin that has been placed on tension (i.e., following elliptical excision and wound closure) stretches over a period of months. This relaxation permits the remaining part of the lesion to be excised in multiple stages [233, 304].

The technique of multiple excision can be used for excising non-hair-bearing areas (i.e., skin grafts or scars, male pattern baldness) of the scalp (Fig. 1-4). A well planned procedure is necessary to avoid excising such a wide ellipse of tissue that the wound cannot be closed. When incising a large burn scar, for example, the initial incision can be made along one side, between the scar and normal tissue. The normal skin can then be undermined extensively in a subcutaneous plane and pulled over the portion of the lesion that can be excised. The scar is marked along this line of normal skin, and an appropriate por-

tion of the scar is then excised. Several months are allowed to pass to permit the tissue to loosen up enough before further excision. Several operations may be required to resolve the defect. One must always compare the benefits and risks of serial excision with tissue expansion to select the appropriate procedure.

The multiple excision technique has a limited application for large lesions of the facial skin because distortion of the eyebrows, eyelids, nostrils, and lips may result from the tension placed on these structures [316]. The lateral deviation of the nose where a lesion has been excised in multiple stages is not an uncommon sequela in children and young adults. In children, excessive serial excisions of skin overlying the malar prominence, nose, or chin may even retard the growth of bone in these regions. The lateral aspect of the cheek is the most favorable area of the face for employing the technique of multiple excision, as it is well away from eyelids, nose, and lips. However, many of these problems can now be obviated by using tissue expansion techniques.

The use of the Z-plasty, rotation skin flaps, and skin grafts increase the effectiveness of multiple excisions. The Z-plasty can be used to transpose normal tissue to a critical area, such as the lip, nose, or eyelid, and at the same time move pathologic tissue to a position where it can be more easily excised at a subsequent stage. The Z-plasty can also be

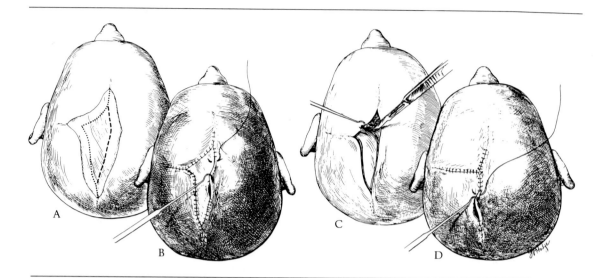

used to break up contracted lines of scar (see pages 71–77). Skin flaps may be rotated in from an adjacent area, e.g., the neck (platysma myocutaneous flap), to supplement serial excision. Again, all multiple excisions and local flaps must be weighed against the efficacy of tissue expansion before a final operative plan is formulated.

*Wedge Excision*

Lesions on or adjacent to such free margins of skin as the lips, nostril rim, eyelids, and ears can be excised in the shape of a wedge (Fig. 1-5). There is so much excess tissue in the lower lip that *one-third* of its length can be removed by a wedge incision and the wound closed primarily. The upper lip is not as full as the lower lip, but primary closure is still possible when *one-fourth* or less has been excised. One option for large defects of the upper lip can be reconstruction with a wedge-shaped Abbé flap from the lower lip [47]. When the lesion of the lip margin is a squamous cell carcinoma, it is usually advisable to execute a block V excision (Fig. 1-5) to remove additional tissue in the path of lymphatic drainage. Closure of these wounds requires careful realignment of the vermilion-cutaneous border. Tattoo of these

**Figure 1-4** *Multiple excision technique. A,B. First-stage excision. C, D. Second-stage excision several months later.*

**Figure 1-5** *Wedge excision. On the eyelid it may be possible to incise just below the lash line, removing only skin, though some lesions require removal of the full eyelid thickness. On the ear, notching of the helical rim can be prevented by stepping the limbs of the V at the helix. One-fourth the width of an eyelid or lower lip can be excised completely and simply closed without requiring elaborate reconstruction.*

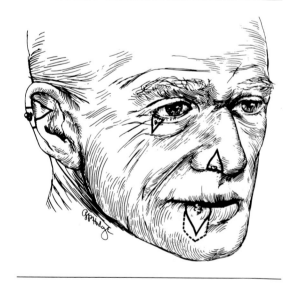

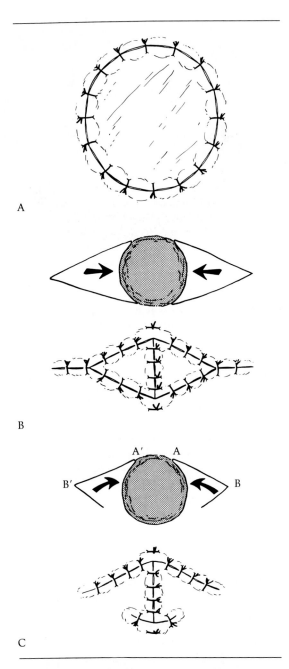

A

B

C

*Figure 1-6* *Closure of wounds following circular excision. A. The most common way of closing a circular defect is with a skin graft. B. Sliding triangular subcutaneous pedicle flaps can be advanced to close the circular defect; the triangular defect is closed in a V-Y fashion. C. Transposition flaps based on a skin pedicle and rotated toward each other can also be used.*

margins prior to incision often makes re-alignment easier.

The wedge excision of lesions of the nostril rim, if too large for primary closure, can be closed with a composite graft of similar size from the rim of the ear. Composite grafts usually survive if all parts of the graft are within 1 cm of the blood supply at the margins of the alar defect.

Lesions near the rim of the ear can be excised in the shape of a simple V or with the line of the V stopped at the helix to minimize the effect of scar contracture and to prevent notching at the helical rim following primary closure (Fig. 1-5). An Antia flap (for large lesions of the ear), which is a chondral cutaneous flap, allows smooth restoration of the normal helical rim at the expense of shortening the lobule and some diminution of auricle height [8]. Auricular reconstruction is further discussed in Chapter 15.

*Circular Excision*

When the facial skin is closely applied to underlying cartilage, such as over the nasal tip or anterior surface of the auricle, lesions can be excised in a circular fashion and the defect closed with a full-thickness skin graft (Fig. 1-6A). The graft maintains its size because it is splinted by the firm underlying cartilage. This technique is also employed following removal of some large skin lesions on other parts of the body.

Local skin flaps can also be used to close the defect following a circular excision. One ingenious method of closing a circular wound (e.g., up to 5 cm diameter in mobile skin and up to 2.5 cm diameter on the lower leg) involves sliding subcutaneous pedicle skin flaps (Fig. 1-6B) [323, 336]. Typically, two triangular subcutaneous flaps are planned in the direction of the skin lines on either side of the circular defect, giving the appearance of a large ellipse until the triangular flaps are advanced and sutured to each other, closing the circular defect. The triangular defects are each closed in a V-Y fashion. (Further information on subcutaneous skin flaps is provided in this chapter under the heading Flaps.) Another local skin flap for this same purpose involves local transposition flaps, one on either side of the circular defect, which are based on a skin pedicle and rotated toward each other to meet and close the defect (Fig. 1-6C). Caution is used when selecting such flaps for the face because the aesthetic results may be poor. Tissue expansion or rotation flaps may be more useful for placing scars in normal, less apparent folds.

When there is some doubt as to the direction of the skin lines, the circular excision may be helpful when planning an elliptical excision. Then, by noting the longer axis of the defect created by adjacent skin tensions, the long axis of the ellipse can be determined and an appropriate ellipse in the lines of relaxation accomplished [80].

### Concealing Scars in the Hair of the Scalp or Eyebrow

Concealing scars in the hair of the scalp or eyebrow is an excellent way to camouflage a scar. Incisions in the lateral aspect of an eyebrow can be used for removing dermoid cysts from the lateral supraorbital rim and for internal wiring of fractures of the zygomaticofrontal suture line. The skin in this region is mobile, a factor that aids exposure even if the operative area does not lie exactly underneath the incision.

Scars located at the juncture of the scalp and facial skin are often poorly concealed because the fine hairs in this region are short and sparse. However, in women it is not as much of a problem, as the hair usually can be arranged to hide such scars. Scalp scars in men are sometimes uncovered by progressing degrees of baldness. Using a W-plasty scar revision (discussed more at length later in this chapter) allows intermingling of the hairy scalp with the nonhairy forehead skin, thereby attaining a camouflage effect [36].

In many areas of the body scars can be covered by clothing. It is particularly true for men, in whom scars on the lower neck, supraclavicular region, and extremities are covered by collars, shirts with sleeves, and trousers.

### OPERATIVE TECHNIQUES OF EXCISING SKIN LESIONS

#### Instruments

Fine, sharp, single- and double-pronged skin hooks, sharp scissors, detachable knife blades (Nos. 11 and 15), and fine, sharp needles with the suture swaged on are the basic instruments needed for performing excisions and closure with minimal trauma. A sturdy but light needle-holder with smooth jaws and beveled joints is excellent for suturing and instrument tying. A small, fine-toothed tissue forceps, e.g., Brown-Adson forceps, must also be available. A skin hook can be made at any time by bending a hypodermic needle and pressing the cotton end of a swab stick in the needle hub.

#### Techniques of Excision

ELLIPTICAL EXCISION. The ellipse is outlined with a suitable marking material. Prior to excision, tension is placed on the surrounding skin. This stretching prevents false cuts and aids in following the lines of excision (Fig. 1-7). The No. 15 blade is used to cut through the skin at right angles to its surface so that vertical margins can be approximated in the closure. The X-shaped "over cuts" at the ends of the ellipse can be prevented by starting the incision at the end of the ellipse. Undermining the wound edges is usually advisable to facilitate wound closure without tension. With skin hooks at each end of the ellipse, undermining is carried out with a single sweep of the No. 15 blade in the superficial subcutaneous tissue. Usually, a two-layer closure is then carried out: The deep layer is approximated with inverted sutures of fine catgut, polyglycolic acid, or clear nylon. This deep dermal closure approximates the skin edges, taking all the tension off the skin. The skin sutures must serve *only* to approximate and adjust the skin margins so they are slightly everted.

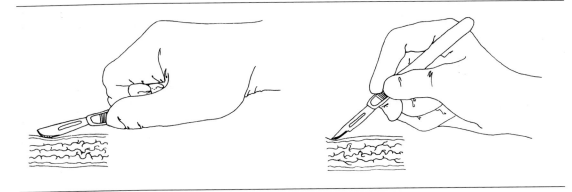

**Figure 1-7** *Proper use of the No. 10 and No. 15 blades.*

If the line of closure is within a natural wrinkle line or crease, two-layer closure may not be necessary to obtain a thin fine line scar.

WEDGE EXCISION. After outlining the wedge with marking solution, a No. 15 blade is used to incise through the skin surface. The tissue is then held firmly on either side of the wedge so the blade can be passed completely through the tissues. The wound can be closed in three layers: the two surfaces and deep tissue. If muscle is present it is restored.

*Methods of Hemostasis*

ELECTROCAUTERY. An electrical current of high frequency (2 million to 18 million cycles per second), relatively high amperage, and low voltage coagulates the wall of a blood vessel to produce hemostasis, coagulation being caused by the heat of the current. Although a small amount of tissue is charred by the electrical current, there is no evidence that wound healing is more impaired by this technique than by the use of ligatures.

Electrocautery techniques probably provide the most rapid, effective method for obtaining hemostasis of medium and small blood vessels. Trauma can be minimized and coagulation made more effective by bringing the active electrode of the electrosurgical unit into contact with a small hemostat or fine-tipped forceps that is accurately gripping the vessel. A fine-tipped electrode itself can also be used to touch the vessel. The latter method is especially helpful for obtaining the nearly absolute degree of hemostasis necessary in the recipient bed for a skin graft. Suction or frequent sponging aids in obtaining the dry field essential for effective cauterization. The assistant blots, not wipes, the fluid, as wiping tends to reopen vessels that have been electrocoagulated.

An electrosurgical unit may be either monoterminal or biterminal. A monoterminal unit, e.g., Hyfercator, makes use of only an active electrode, with the patient being in circuit through the surrounding environment. Electrical currents from monoterminal units are adequate for obtaining hemostasis. The large biterminal devices, e.g., Bovie units, have both an active electrode and a broad inactive electrode, with the patient being placed in the circuit between them.

Self-contained coagulation units have been developed; equipped with a waterproof, enclosed battery, they can be sterilized and used at the operating table as any other unit. Because of the explosion hazard, an electrosurgical unit is not used in the presence of explosive anesthetic gases.

The Shaw hemostatic scapel utilizes a

sharp blade for cutting that can also be heated to produce simultaneous hemostasis. Its temperature can be set from 0° to 180°C.

Millay et al. [221], in animal experiments, compared the tensile strength of wounds created by a regular scalpel and the Shaw scalpel at varying temperatures and times. They found that when tensile strength was compared the only significant difference was at day 14, when the regular scalpel had the advantage. However, the strengths later evened out. Keenan et al. [163] showed that wounds created with the Shaw scalpel and inoculated with bacteria had less resistance to infection.

LIGATURE. The ligation of blood vessels with fine suture materials is another way of effecting hemostasis. Bleeding vessels are clamped accurately with fine-pointed hemostats. A suture can be either simply tied about the vessel or, for more secure ligation, passed on a needle through the immediately adjacent tissue before being tied.

Chromic catgut or polyglycolic acid sutures of sizes 4-0 and 5-0 are suitable for ligating small and medium vessels. Large vessels are tied with nonabsorbable sutures. Absorbable sutures are preferred by many for ligating blood vessels and approximating deep layers of tissue because their absorption minimizes the possibility of a late, prolonged reaction and extrusion of permanent buried sutures.

PRESSURE AND TIME. Sustained pressure on the wound can effectively control capillary oozing. The pressure probably acts to occlude the capillaries until coagulation occurs. It is best to apply pressure for 5 minutes by the clock because there is usually a tendency to underestimate the time elapsed. If the recipient bed for a skin graft continues to bleed uncontrollably, a pressure dressing may be applied for 24 to 48 hours before the skin is placed on the wound. This procedure is termed *delayed skin grafting*.

Remember that aspirin (salicylic acid) and aspirin-containing medications inhibit platelet function and cause bleeding. Be sure that patients undergoing elective surgical procedures do not ingest these agents for at least a month prior to surgery.

CLAMPING AND TWISTING SMALL BLOOD VESSELS. Although clamping and twisting small blood vessels avoids introducing foreign material into the wound, the method is not reliable for hemostasis.

VASOCONSTRICTORS. Epinephrine continues to be the best vasoconstrictor for surgical procedures. Injection of epinephrine in a solution as dilute as 1:500,000 has been shown to provide excellent hemostasis if the surgeon is patient enough to wait approximately 7 minutes until the first vasoconstrictive effect is manifest [223, 297]. Epinephrine solutions of 1:100,000 and 1:200,000 are commercially available in combination with local anesthetic agents, but more dilute solutions must be made up fresh because they are sensitive to oxidative degradation and a pH over 5.5. Epinephrine 1:500,000 can be prepared at the time of operation by adding a 1-ml ampule of 1:1000 epinephrine to 500 ml of 5% dextrose in water (pH 4.0). Large volumes of epinephrine solution are especially helpful for operations requiring wide dissection of tissue. For example, we use 75 to 100 ml of epinephrine 1:500,000 per breast when performing a reduction mammoplasty, and 50 to 75 ml per side when performing a facelift. Topical epinephrine (1:100,000) can be applied to an open wound on a moistened sponge to diminish bleeding from small vessels.

In the constant search for better pharmacologic vasoconstrictors, phenylephrine, a pure α-agonist has been studied by Canepa et al. [50]. It differs from epinephrine only by missing one hydroxyl group on the benzene ring, which almost completely eliminates any beta activity. When used with lidocaine in rat experiments and compared to epinephrine and lidocaine, there is a highly significant delay in absorption of the lidocaine.

When using any vasoconstrictors, it is important to remember that they all reduce nutrient flow and produce a degree of ischemia.

The longer such vasoconstrictors act, the more extensive is the ischemic injury.

FIBRIN FOAM, GELATIN FOAM, TOPICAL THROMBIN, AND MICROCRYSTALLINE COLLAGEN. Several coagulative materials can be used as hemostatic agents, especially for packing a small cavity from which there is a constant oozing of blood. Fibrin foam is prepared from human fibrinogen and thrombin, and gelatin foam is prepared from an absorbable gelatin. Small pieces of these foams are readily absorbed in the tissues with minimal reaction. Microcrystalline collagen is a white flour-like substance with remarkable hemostatic properties [1].

Thrombin is a protein substance derived from bovine plasma. It can be used alone, in powder form or in solution, for hemostasis. In solution it can be used in conjunction with absorbable gelatin sponges. Thrombin USP appears to be nonantigenic when used topically [123].

## Closure of Skin Wounds

Wounds can be closed with sutures, skin tapes, skin clips, staples, or wound adhesives. These foreign materials act to hold the wound edges in approximation until the wound's tensile strength is increased to a degree sufficient to maintain wound closure without assistance.

### SUTURES

*Type of Suture Material*

Sutures are generally considered to be either absorbable (catgut-polyglycolic acid, polydioxanone) or nonabsorbable (nylon, Dacron, polypropylene, silk, cotton, stainless steel). They can also be judged in regard to their tensile strength, tissue reaction, pliability, knot-holding ability, capillary (or wick) action, and economy.

Sutures may be monofilament or have multiple filaments that are braided or twisted to form the suture. Nonabsorbable sutures may be coated with a medical grade of silicone (on silk), Teflon (on braided Dacron), or other synthetic materials to make them smoother or less reactive. The suture may have a cutting or noncutting needle swaged on one end, or it may have to be threaded through the eye of a needle in order to be used for wound closure.

With such a wide variation of suture materials, there is bound to be a difference of opinion as to which is the best. Usually the choice of suture material is of far less importance than many of the other concepts discussed in this chapter. Suture selection is often given much more discussion than it deserves [106].

ABSORBABLE SUTURES. Sutures made of collagen, polyglycolic acid, or polydioxanone are capable of being digested by body enzymes. They are frequently used as buried sutures to close the subcutaneous tissue layer or to repair mucous membranes. Because it is advantageous in children to be able to avoid the mechanical removal of skin sutures, fine absorbable sutures have also been used to suture skin grafts in place or to close skin wounds.

Catgut, the most common absorbable suture, is made from collagen of the submucosal layer of the small intestine of sheep and the serosal layer of the small intestine of cattle. An extruded collagen suture has been developed by dispersing the collagen from flexor tendons of cattle and then extruding it to form a much more uniform, more pliable, and stronger suture [222].

A plain catgut suture is absorbed faster than one that has been hardened by chromicization (chromic catgut). Chromic catgut retains its tensile strength for 30 days and is totally absorbed by 90 days. Plain catgut retains tensile strength for 15 days and is totally absorbed by 60 days. Both are absorbed by proteolytic enzymes [43]. The smaller the caliber of the catgut, the faster it is absorbed. Because sutures in certain tissues (e.g., serous and mucous membranes) are absorbed substantially faster than those in other tissues (e.g., muscle), it is difficult to specify an exact time for complete absorption [156].

Polyglycolic acid (Dexon) and polyglactin-910 (Vicryl) are absorbable sutures made by polymerization of the amino acid glycolic acid, which is extruded and stretched to form fibers that are then braided to form the suture. These sutures are stronger than catgut of comparable size, have greater knot security, and have an improved "feel" that closely resembles linen. Dexon loses all tensile strength in 30 days and is absorbed by 90 days, closely followed by Vicryl, whose tensile strength is gone by 32 days and is absorbed by 70 days. Whereas catgut is absorbed by phagocytosis as a part of the inflammatory response, Dexon and Vicryl undergo enzymatic degradation by hydrolysis, with little accompanying tissue reaction [4, 43, 139].

Polydioxanone (PDS) has several advantages. It loses its tensile strength by 56 days and is absorbed by 180 days. PDS is likewise absorbed by hydrolysis [43]. Because it is a monofilament it is less prone to harbor bacteria, as there are no interstices.

NONABSORBABLE SUTURES. Synthetic sutures (nylon, Dacron, or polypropylene), metallic sutures (stainless steel), or stainless steel staples can be used to close the skin. These sutures are stronger and less reactive to the tissues than any absorbable sutures. Polypropylene and stainless steel are excellent materials for a subcuticular suture because of their tensile strength, low frictional coefficient, and stiffness. When used as a running dermal "pull-out" suture, they can produce superb skin closure without the risk of suture marks. Polypropylene in particular is easy to remove because of its smooth surface. Other materials, e.g., nylon, tend to bind to surrounding tissues when one attempts removal. In addition, because the material is relatively nonreactive, it can remain in place for 3 weeks or longer. By this time, wound strength is sufficient to withstand most forces. Silk and cotton consistently produce more tissue reaction than the synthetic sutures [99, 264]. Multifilament sutures are more reactive than the same material in a monofilament suture and are more likely to develop a discharging sinus in the skin wound [196, 264].

Silk can be used to close the skin adjacent to the eye, as its pliability allows the suture ends to lie flat after the knot is tied, avoiding corneal injury. For tie-over dressings, silk is the suture material that is easiest to manage.

### Avoiding Suture Marks in the Skin

Suture marks are the permanently imprinted scars of suture material on the skin surface. The studies of Crikelair [70] on this subject are outstanding. Some of the factors that determine the severity of suture marks are the length of time a skin suture is left in place, tension, relation of the suture to the wound edge, region of the body, infection, and a propensity for keloid formation.

LENGTH OF TIME A SKIN SUTURE IS LEFT IN PLACE. Crikelair [70] found that the largest suture marks invariably occurred when skin sutures were left in place for about 14 days. The size of the suture and the needles used to insert them proved unimportant. In contrast, sutures removed within 7 days produced almost no permanent scar.

In the face, it is advisable to remove alternate skin sutures on the third to fifth postoperative day depending on the location and layers of closure. Skin tape can be used to support the area for several more days. On the extremities and anterior aspect of the trunk, sutures are left in place for about 7 days to prevent wound disruption. On the knee, the back, and the feet, it is almost imperative that some sutures be retained for 10 to 14 days or even longer. For this reason, permanent suture marks may remain in the skin. Whenever possible, closure with a running dermal pull-out suture avoids completely the problems of suture marks without interfering with the development of tensile strength. In all cases, individual judgment must be used.

TENSION. Skin suture marks are frequently caused by sutures tied too tightly or pulling laterally on the wound [70, 242]. It is important to learn to tie a suture just tight enough to approximate the wound edges but no tighter. During the early postoperative period, edema causes tissues to swell, creating additional tension within the circle of each suture. Wound edges not quite in contact become further approximated in this way. Edges already in contact and under tension are further strangulated by postoperative swelling. The selected suture material must be just a little stronger than necessary to maintain closure of the wound. Fine sutures (4-0, 5-0, 6-0) encourage closures with less tension than do heavy ones.

Lateral pull on the wound results when a large segment of skin has been excised or when muscles are pulling at right angles to the wound. Much of this lateral pull can be eliminated by using subcutaneous sutures to take the tension off the skin and by placing the long axis of the excision parallel to the skin lines.

### Relation of Suture to Wound Edge

When large bites of tissue are taken with the suture, large suture marks can result because a large segment of tissue is subjected to the constricting effect of the suture. These marks can be avoided by keeping the sutures closer to the wound edge.

### Region of the Body

Suture marks are fortunately not common on the face unless basic principles are violated or the skin is heavy with sebaceous glands. Skin suture marks almost never occur on the thin skin of the eyelids and mucous membranes. In contrast, the sternal area, trunk, and extremities (with the exception of the hands and soles of the feet) are common sites for these scars unless the most precise operative techniques are followed.

### Infection

Infection about a skin suture can lead to formation of a suture mark. When such an infec-

tion develops, it is best treated by removing the suture and applying warm, moist dressings to the wound. This method eliminates any constricting effect, removes the foreign body, increases circulation, and improves drainage. In a study of infection around sutures in experimental wounds (contaminated with *Staphylococcus aureus*), monofilament steel and nylon sutures have demonstrated minimal reaction. In this study there was reaction around other sutures in the following increasing order: silk, Mersilene, Dexon, and catgut. Monofilament sutures induced less infection than braided sutures [339].

There is little doubt that the less foreign material (i.e., smallest size and fewest number of sutures) left in a wound, the more readily and soundly the wound heals. One of the reasons was demonstrated by Elek and Conen [95], who found in human volunteers that to produce a pustule required the intradermal injection of at least 2 million organisms of *Streptococcus pyogenes*, whereas in the presence of a buried suture only 100 of these organisms were needed to produce a purulent lesion the size of an orange and a reaction so severe the researchers had great difficulty finding further volunteers. In contaminated experimental wounds, even buried monofilament nylon is associated with a significant potentiation of infection compared to no suture at all [82].

### Keloid Formation

In individuals susceptible to the formation of keloids, such a lesion may form at the site where a skin suture is placed. Additional information on this subject can be found in Chapter 30.

### Buried Sutures

In a clean wound, the subcutaneous tissue and dermis are sutured to remove tension from the site of skin repair [92]. There is no solid evidence that buried dermal sutures of absorbable versus nonabsorbable sutures make any difference on the final width of a scar. However, work by Nordström and Nordström [246] suggests that permanent sutures may decrease the final scar width.

*Eversion of Skin Edges*
Skin edges that have been everted gradually flatten to produce a level wound surface (Fig. 1-8). By comparison, a wound with an inverted edge persists as a valley-like scar, trapping the shadows as light is cast across its surface. These shadows make the depressed scar even more noticeable.

Use of the vertical mattress suture (Fig. 1-9B) is one effective method for everting the wound edges. Placement of buried sutures in the subcutaneous tissue is also important because it provides a firm foundation on which to evert the skin edges. Occasionally one or more Z-plasties (see Fig. 1-40) break up a long, linear, depressed scar to permit eversion of its edges.

Scars crossing areas such as the inferior border of the mandible tend to become inverted. This tendency can sometimes be corrected by making an elliptical incision around the scar, denuding it of surface epithelium, undermining the wound edges, and then advancing and closing the edges over the central buttress of the denuded scar. The central island of dermis helps raise the depressed scar, and the newly created margins tend to evert.

*Closure of Wound Edges of Unequal Thickness*
Occasionally, wounds whose edges are of unequal thickness must be sutured. To equalize the two sides, a flap of subcutaneous tissue from the thicker side can be turned under the thinner side. It is best first to undermine both wound edges at the same depth in the superficial subcutaneous tissue. Then a subcutaneous tissue flap of the desired thickness can be advanced from the thicker side across and under the thinner side, where it is sutured. Vertical mattress sutures may also help to compensate for these unequal thicknesses.

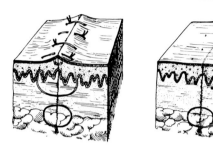

**Figure 1-8** *Skin edges that are everted gradually flatten to produce a level wound surface.*

*Operative Technique for Suturing Skin Wounds*
METHODS OF WOUND SUTURE. Buried sutures aid in closing a wound in layers. The periosteum or perichondrium and the muscular fascia are each closed by suture. "Subcutaneous tissue" usually does not require closure and may add to the risk of infection. Dermal or subcuticular sutures may help relieve tension and hence help to provide a fine line scar. It is wise to invert the suture in the dermal layer so that the knot is tied deeply, away from the skin surface.

Another method sometimes used for closing the dermal tissue is the continuous running dermal suture. The ends of this suture can be left permanently in the subcutaneous tissue or passed to the surface so that the suture can be removed after 2 to 3 weeks.

Skin sutures are of several types.

**1.** The *simple interrupted suture* (see Fig. 1-9A) is inserted so that the needle enters the skin of the first side at an angle of 90 degrees or more. Sufficient subcutaneous tissue is included to aid in eversion of the raw interface. As the needle passes through a comparable amount of subcutaneous tissue on the second side, it begins to angle back toward the wound edge. Ideally, the angle of exit for the needle is the same as its angle of entrance. If the same angle has been achieved, an identical volume of tissue is

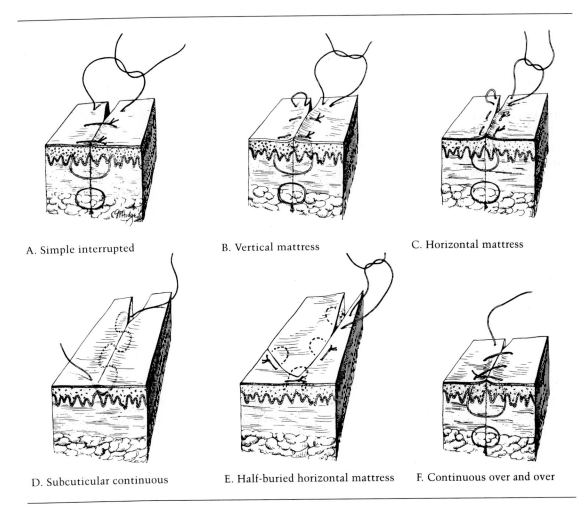

A. Simple interrupted

B. Vertical mattress

C. Horizontal mattress

D. Subcuticular continuous

E. Half-buried horizontal mattress

F. Continuous over and over

***Figure 1-9*** *Methods of skin suture (see text).*

present within the suture on each side of the wound, and the result is an exact approximation of the margins. The more accomplished a surgeon becomes in gaining equal amounts of skin and subcutaneous tissue from each side and in angling the needle, the less often are mattress sutures needed to gain symmetry. The number of sutures used for closing any wound vary with the case, location of the repair, and degree of accuracy required by the physician and the patient. In an area such as the face, sutures are probably placed 1 to 3 mm apart and 1 to 2 mm from the wound edge.

**2.** The *vertical mattress suture* (see Fig. 1-9B) is used principally to ensure eversion of skin edges and is unsurpassed for this purpose. A common technique for wound closure is to alternate a vertical mattress suture with a simple interrupted suture along the length of the wound.

**3.** The *horizontal mattress suture* (see Fig. 1-9C) provides close approximation of the skin edges with some eversion. This method can be helpful for closing skin wounds on the hand that are under tension. It causes more skin ischemia than either the simple interrupted or vertical mattress suture.

**4.** The *half-buried horizontal mattress suture* (see Fig. 1-9E) is effective for closing the point of a V-shaped wound. The use of this suture often prevents necrosis of the tip of the V, which may follow use of a simple interrupted suture. The suture is also advantageous for suturing a skin flap into place. The buried portion of the suture lies within the flap so that it effectively holds the flap in place, and yet the danger of damaging the skin by inserting sutures through it is avoided.

**5.** The *subcuticular (intradermal) continuous suture* (see Fig. 1-9D) is a practical, useful method of skin closure. The needle passes horizontally through the dermis, small bites being taken alternately on one side and then the other. As the suture is continued, care must be taken that it is maintained at the same level and that the entrance of each bite is backed up a little to prevent the entrance and exit on opposite sides from being opposite one another. When long wounds are closed by this method, it is well to pass the suture through the skin every 5 to 8 cm to facilitate its removal. This suture can usually be left in place for 2 to 3 weeks. Polypropylene is especially suitable for a subcuticular closure because of the ease of removal. A running subcuticular closure may obviate the need for any interrupted skin sutures, avoiding the risks of suture marks on the skin.

**6.** The *continuous over-and-over suture* (see Fig. 1-9F) is occasionally used for skin closure. It can be done rapidly and is hemostatic. Because it is hemostatic it has been used for closing scalp wounds. Although suture mark scars from the tension of this suture are covered by hair, it is well to remember that young men may eventually become bald in later years (i.e., be careful!).

KNOTS. Many of the sutures utilized for skin closure have needles that have been swaged onto the suture. Hence this discussion is primarily concerned with using a needle holder to tie knots. It is best to have a smooth-jawed, lightweight needle holder with beveled joints so that sutures do not catch in it during the process of tying.

The knot most commonly used during surgery is the square knot with an added half-knot [104]. Great care must be taken when placing the first portion of the square knot because if the pull on each end of the suture is not equal the knot does not lie flat but, instead, forms a half hitch, which has no holding power. During the second phase of tying a square knot, the free ends must lie in opposite directions to prevent the knot from disrupting when the suture is cut. To avoid disruption it is wise to place an added half-knot on top of the square knot. Thus even if the third knot were to come undone when the ends of the suture were held together, the underlying square knot remains secure.

Catgut and polyglycolic acid sutures are notorious for coming untied when located on the oral mucosa and tongue because of movement and licking. One way to avoid this problem is to tie at least five knots. When tying prolene or other smooth synthetic material, a "surgeon's knot" tied first may be helpful for obtaining accurate tension. (A surgeon's knot entails tying the first two throws of the knot in the same direction rather than as a square knot. This method allows the knot to slip for tension adjustment, which is impossible with the standard square knot.)

SKIN TAPE. Tapes that adhere to the skin surface across a wound are satisfactory for closure of skin wounds [97, 105, 116, 298, 346]. Although this tape holds the skin edges together without difficulty, buried sutures are often necessary to approximate deeper layers of tissue and to prevent inversion of the skin edges (Fig. 1-10).

Brunius [41, 42] has shown in the rat that skin incisions healed more rapidly when a nonsuture technique (skin tapes alone) was used or when skin sutures were removed after 3 days of healing. It was thought to result from the more optimal tension across the wound, in addition to a lessened inflammatory reaction.

Ellenberg [96] noted that microporous tape

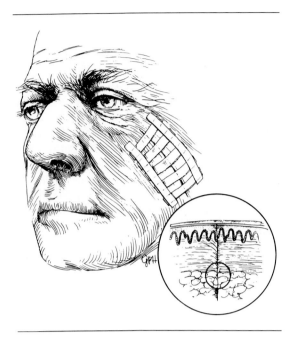

*Figure 1-10* Skin tapes. A buried suture is
usually necessary to approximate the deeper
layers of tissue.

is pervious to sweat but does not permit
blood or purulent material to pass through
it. This tape is more commonly used than
solid tapes for skin closure.

The technique of applying these tapes is
simple. For extensive wounds, the deeper
layers are first closed in layers by suture.
The skin can then be cleaned and dried, acetone or alcohol being used to remove oily secretions from its surface if necessary. The
tapes are applied perpendicular to the wound
edge, first on one side and then on the other,
so the edges can be pulled together. These
skin tapes usually stay firmly in place for 1
to 2 weeks, except on hirsute or oily skin.
On loose skin areas (e.g., eyelids, scrotum) or
areas in constant motion (e.g., lips, anterior neck, antecubital and popliteal regions),
these tapes frequently become loose. Although tapes were popular for attaching skin
grafts to convex surfaces, skin staples are
usually preferable because they can be applied more quickly and in a wet field.

Some of the advantages of skin tape are as
follows: It saves time during application and
removal, causes little or no skin reaction,
and avoids the possibility of skin suture
marks; moreover, tape can be left in place for
long periods underneath dressings or casts
and can be applied without an anesthetic.
Microporous surgical adhesive tapes have
the following disadvantages: They do not
produce eversion of the skin edges, do not
adhere to wet skin, come off in about two-
thirds of patients when bathing, and can be
removed prematurely by children or uncoop-
erative patients. Patients may also be allergic to the adhesive backing and may
develop skin reactions with blistering. However, such reactions are usually superficial,
and local wound care allows the blisters to
heal [96].

SKIN STAPLES AND SKIN CLIPS. The skin stapler has been used by some surgeons to close
skin wounds after procedures such as facelift, mammoplasty, abdominoplasty, and
skin grafts [330]. They are particularly helpful and time-saving when used temporarily
for adjusting skin position for simple wound
closure or flap positioning. If used for final closure in visible areas, they must be
removed early to avoid permanent staple
marks in the skin.

TISSUE ADHESIVE. Although tissue adhesives have been available since 1956, they
have still not been approved for general use
in humans by the Food and Drug Administration. The restriction on cyanoacrylates in
the United States is due to the development
of fibrosarcomas in animals after massive
amounts were injected. Many other studies,
however, have failed to show evidence of
malignancy. In addition, many surgeons in
Europe and Asia are using cyanoacrylates,
e.g., methyl-2-cyanoacrylate and isobutyl-2-
cyanoacrylate, for sealing vascular aneurysms, intestinal repairs, gynecologic surgery, skin wound closure, and skin graft
adhesion to the skin around an open wound
[103]. Cartilage or bone grafts may be layered
using this technique of tissue adhesives [337].

Animal studies by Edlich et al. [92] have suggested that tissue adhesives should *not* be used for skin closure for two reasons: (1) The polymer acts as a barrier between the wound edges and delays or prevents healing; and (2) the infection rate, especially in contaminated wounds compared to taped wounds, was significantly higher. However, we predict that the cyanoacrylates under development will play an important part in the management of surgical wounds. Painting or spraying the cyanoacrylate adhesive on either a recipient bed or the raw surface of a graft causes loss of the graft by preventing nutrients and capillary buds from entering the graft to nourish it [11, 158].

Fibrin glue has been used by various authors for fixing split-thickness skin grafts to irregular surfaces by taking advantage of the normal reaction of fibrinogen to fibrin. It has the advantage over the histoacrylic glues in that it is homologous, is not toxic to tissues, and is phagocytized within 2 to 3 weeks [132]. Fibrinogen is a human pooled blood product and carries the usual risks of blood-transmissible diseases, i.e., hepatitis and human immunodeficiency virus.

## Skin Grafts

When a wound deficient in surface covering is encountered, a systematic process for evaluating the wound is needed. The size, depth, vital structures exposed, and location of the defect must be taken into account before a plan for reconstruction is outlined. Always remember to begin your plan with the simplest of concepts and proceed to the more complex: (1) primarily close the wound using undermining; (2) allow the wound to heal by secondary intention; (3) apply skin grafts; (4) apply local, rotational advancement skin flaps; (5) apply local, rotational muscle, or musculocutaneous flaps; (6) apply pedicled, island, skin, muscle, fascial flaps; and lastly (7) use free-tissue transfer. Skin grafting is discussed in this section and the use of skin flaps in the following sec-

tion. Always remember the adage "The great plastic surgeon can enumerate on elegant flaps and free tissue transfers but usually does a skin graft" [329].

A skin graft is a segment of dermis and epidermis that has been completely separated from its blood supply and donor-site attachment before being transplanted to another area of the body, its recipient site. Skin grafts consist of the epidermis and a portion of the dermis if they are of the partial-thickness type (split-thickness skin graft). The complete thickness type (full-thickness skin graft) contains the epidermis and all of the dermis. All such grafts contain varying portions of the sweat glands, sebaceous glands, hair follicles, and capillaries of the skin, depending on their thickness (Fig. 1-11). Rudolph and Klein [281] have prepared a comprehensive review of the healing processes in skin grafts.

### SKIN GRAFT TYPES

Skin grafts can be classified as autografts, allografts (homografts), or xenografts (heterografts) (see below under Split-Thickness Skin Grafts and Full-Thickness Skin Grafts).

### Split-Thickness Skin Grafts

Autografts of skin, cut at the split-thickness level, are the most popular and useful of all skin grafts. They contain the epidermis and a portion of the dermis. The split-thickness graft is further subclassified, depending on the amount of dermis included: thin split-thickness skin grafts (Thiersch or Ollier-Thiersch grafts), intermediate (medium) split-thickness skin grafts, and thick split-thickness skin grafts (three-quarter thickness grafts) (Fig. 1-11).

The actual thickness of the graft is variable, as the thickness of the skin varies with the age, sex, and the region of the body [312]. Skin tends to be thinner in infants than in adults, with adult skin being 3.5 times thicker than that of the newborn. By the age of 5 years, though, the skin thickness of the child is essentially the same as that of the

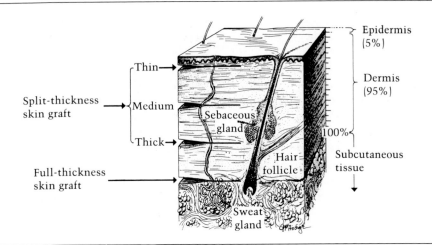

Thin →
Medium
Thick →

Split-thickness skin graft →

Full-thickness skin graft →

Epidermis (5%)

Dermis (95%)

Sebaceous gland

100%

Hair follicle

Subcutaneous tissue

Sweat gland

*Figure 1-11* Skin graft thickness. The thickness of the epidermis and dermis varies in different areas of the body. This drawing is characteristic of the lateral thigh skin of the adult.

adult [161]. The skin is thinner in women, especially in the dermal layer, than in men. Measurements by Southwood [312] of epidermal and dermal thickness in various age groups, sexes, and sites indicate that the skin varies from about 17 thousandths to 150 thousandths of an inch in thickness. It is thickest on the soles of the feet and palms of the hands and thinnest over the eyelids and in the postauricular area. To impart some idea of the much greater contribution of the dermis to the thickness of the skin, the dermis is calculated to be 20 times thicker than the epidermis on the lateral thigh of a male adult.

Surgeons tend to refer to split-thickness skin grafts as being either thin, intermediate, or thick, depending on the setting of the dermatome (10 thousandths to 25 thousandths of an inch), the translucency of the graft, and the bleeding pattern of the donor site. The setting of a dermatome or skin graft knife is always checked by sighting the distance between the blade and the drum of the dermatome that comes in contact with

the skin surface as the graft is cut. The translucency of a skin graft varies from the thin split-thickness graft, with its translucent tissue-paper appearance, to that of the thick split-thickness graft, which is nearly opaque. The pattern of bleeding at the donor site also varies from fine bleeding points with the thin graft to large bleeding points from the thick split-thickness skin graft [214].

The thinner a skin graft, the more is the contraction that occurs at the recipient site during the first few months after transplantation. The thick split-thickness skin graft contracts less than an intermediate-thickness graft, whereas the full-thickness graft contracts hardly at all [281].

Skin grafts taken from different parts of the body often have various color differences. The donor skin from the abdomen, buttock, and thigh often shows pigment gain, whereas a graft to the face from the postauricular, supraclavicular areas generally has a good color match. Exposure to sunlight may markedly darken grafts [281].

A thin split-thickness skin graft is more likely to survive on its recipient site because it can survive well during the phase of plasmatic absorption and can wait longer for vascularization. Note also that skin from a more vascular donor site becomes vascularized more rapidly [302].

The thin split-thickness skin graft taken from a hirsute donor site does not have hair growing in it after transplantation, whereas the thick split-thickness and full-thickness graft usually contains some hair follicles to permit the growth of hair. The donor site of a thin split-thickness skin graft reepithelializes more rapidly than that of a thick split-thickness skin graft. The donor site of a full-thickness skin graft does not reepithelialize because no accessory skin structures remain.

*Tissue-Cultured Skin Grafts*
In the extensively burned individual, obtaining enough skin grafts from remaining donor sites may be impossible. Although repeat harvesting of donor sites [53] and expansion by meshing the grafts are technically possible, they may not provide the needed skin. Allografts and synthetic skin are also available, but they can serve only as temporary coverage [154].

During the 1950s Billingham and Reynolds [26], Grillo and McKhann [127], and Najarian et al. [243] experimented with pure epithelial grafts. This early work on pure epithelial grafting was not satisfactory over the long term. However, the experiments were done on loose-skinned animals, where contraction is the dominant mode of healing and may not be applicable to human wound healing. Since 1975 Green and colleagues [274] and Burke's group [354] have been experimenting with culturing human epithelial cells. Yannas, Burke, and colleagues [354] developed a bilayer polymeric membrane to serve as a template for the formation of a neodermis. They contended that a skin substitute must have dermis to prevent contraction and epithelium to restore the integrity of the host's surface.

In 1984 Gallico et al. [113] used autologous cultured epithelium, with no dermis, to resurface burn wounds. These grafts adhered and formed a permanent epidermis much like a split-thickness skin graft.

*Full-Thickness Skin Grafts*
A full-thickness skin graft (Wolfe graft) contains the epidermis and entire thickness of dermis from the site of origin (see Fig. 1-11). After transplantation this free graft more closely resembles normal skin (in terms of color, texture, hair growth, and failure to contract) than split-thickness skin. Hence it is often selected for resurfacing the face. The usual full-thickness skin graft is relatively small, so its donor site can be closed by undermining and approximating the wound edges. Common donor sites include the groin, postauricular area, and clavicular region (Fig. 1-12).

USES OF SKIN GRAFTS
Skin grafts can be used to close any wound in the body that has a blood supply sufficient to support the viability of the graft. The most notable exceptions are cortical bone denuded of its periosteum, cartilage denuded of its perichondrium, tendon denuded of its paratenon, and nerve denuded of perineurium. Irradiated tissue is usually not a good recipient bed.

Most skin grafts are used to serve as permanent coverage for a wound, although in some instances a split-thickness skin graft is applied temporarily to a wound to aid in controlling bacterial growth or to cover some vital structure. Later, when bacteria are controlled and the wound has become smaller because the split-thickness graft has contracted, it may be replaced with a skin flap or full-thickness graft to provide more stable and cosmetically acceptable coverage. Overgrafting may also be used in such cases. Split-thickness skin grafts are durable if they have a good blood supply and good padding of subcutaneous tissue or muscle between the skin and bony pressure points.

*Facial Wounds*
Full-thickness skin grafts obtained from the preauricular, postauricular, or supraclavicular regions are commonly used to close intermediate-size defects because these grafts most closely resemble facial skin. Moder-

Composite grafts often are the best for closing defects of the alar rim. The ear is an ideal donor site for composite grafts, containing a piece of cartilage sandwiched between two pieces of skin [21].

For surfacing large areas on the face, such as that damaged by burns, it is frequently necessary to use split-thickness skin grafts and accept a cosmetically poor result. The shiny, stiff, scarred skin that results invariably imparts a mask-like appearance to the face. Skin expansion for secondary reconstruction offers new hope for improving these results.

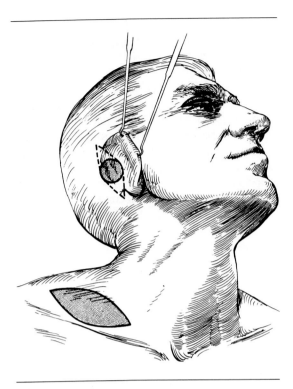

**Figure 1-12** *Common donor sites for full-thickness skin grafts to the face are the postauricular, upper eyelid, and supraclavicular regions. The entire area of postauricular skin from the helical rim to the hairline over the mastoid can also be excised and resurfaced with a split-thickness skin graft.*

ately thick split-thickness skin grafts from the scalp also provide a good color match for facial skin replacement [24, 53].

The large wounds that follow orbital exenteration or maxillectomy are most often closed with split-thickness skin grafts from the thigh or abdominal wall. Deficiencies of skin in the lower eyelid can be repaired well with full-thickness skin grafts of postauricular origin. However, split-thickness skin grafts are used for the upper eyelid because this skin must be sufficiently pliable and thin to permit folding and unfolding as the lids open and close. One excellent donor site for split-thickness skin that fills these requirements is the medial aspect of the upper arm, but this area must be used with caution because of scar visibility.

### Flexor Surfaces

When skin grafts must be applied to the flexor surfaces of the neck, fingers, palms, wrists, elbows, axilla, toes, ankles, or knees, they may require special care to prevent the development of late contracture. When these sites lie adjacent to such major joints as the shoulder or knee, it may be necessary to splint the part in extension for about 2 to 3 months, although for the anterior portion of the neck 6 months of splinting is probably best to prevent contracture [71]. During the period of splinting, the strong contracting forces subside. Extension splints on the extremities are removed at least once a day in order to put the joints through their full range of motion, thereby minimizing joint stiffness.

### Treatment of Burns

Split-thickness skin autografts are preferred for replacing the skin lost from burned surfaces. When thin split-thickness skin grafts are used, a new "crop" of skin can be taken from the same donor site about every 2 to 3 weeks.

Stored viable allografts of split-thickness skin have been a good second choice for closure of burn wounds when a sufficient amount of skin autograft is not available. These grafts provide only temporary covering and are rejected within a few weeks.

When possible, it is best to excise and replace them with autografts before the onset of rejection necrosis with its bacterial contamination and infection.

Because of the great depth of destruction caused by some electrical and radiation burns, skin grafts often are not sufficient for resurfacing the wound, and a skin flap must be utilized. For additional information regarding thermal and electrical burns, see Chapter 24.

### Closure of Skin Flap and Full-Thickness Skin Graft Donor Sites

A split-thickness skin graft may be necessary to close the donor site of a large skin flap or a large full-thickness skin graft when the wound margins cannot be approximated sufficiently to gain primary closure.

### Mucosal Replacement

Split-thickness skin grafts serve well as replacements for the mucosa of the mouth, pharynx, nose, vagina, and urinary bladder when there has been a large loss of lining. However, split-thickness skin so utilized tends to contract during the first 3 to 6 months, so unyielding molds or prostheses must be used during this period. Skin grafts used for mucosal replacement are altered somewhat in their characteristics, but they do not undergo metaplasia to become mucosa, as skin is too highly differentiated. Because hair follicles transplanted with skin continue to grow hair, grafts used for a mucosal replacement are ideally either of medium thickness or from a non-hair-bearing area.

Conjunctiva of the eyelids and nasal mucosa are best replaced with a split-thickness graft of oral mucosa. Mucosa is preferable to skin for conjunctival replacement, as the keratinized layers of the latter often cause corneal irritation. Full-thickness palate grafts are excellent for replacement of the tarsal plate and conjunctiva. Either mucosa or skin can be used for reconstruction of the nasal lining, but many prefer the latter because of its stability and resistance to trauma.

### Closure of Exposed Dura, Pericardium, Pleura, and Peritoneum

Split-thickness skin grafts survive on dura, pericardium, pleura, and peritoneum and can be used for either temporary or permanent wound closure. Skin grafts also grow on areas in the abdominal cavity denuded of peritoneum and on liver, spleen, and kidney [145]. Wounds that contain a large blood vessel, especially if it has been stripped of its surrounding adventitia, are more safely closed with a muscle or myocutaneous flap.

Split-thickness skin graft coverage usually is not sufficient to support an underlying bone graft at a later date. For example, if skin grafting is performed over dura, it would be folly to consider a bone graft between the dura and skin. In general, operations on deeper structures covered only with a skin graft are delayed until the graft has been replaced with a skin muscle or myocutaneous flap. Delay is necessary because there is a high risk of necrosis and failure to heal in an incised and undermined skin graft.

### Overgrafting Unstable Scars, Tattoos, and Nonhairy Pigmented Nevi

Hynes [153] introduced the technique of overgrafting. The epidermis is removed with either a knife or a dermabrader, following which the skin graft is applied to the resulting vascular dermal bed. In this way, layer after layer of dermis can be built up over such unstable scars as are found over the anterior tibia and other bony prominences. For best results, the scar is allowed to mature each time for 3 to 6 months before another layer is added. By using this overgrafting technique, the skin flap can be avoided.

According to Thompson [331] the donor sites of thick split-thickness skin grafts heal more rapidly and with less scarring when they are overgrafted with thin split-thickness skin grafts. Clinically, we have not found the technique to be particularly useful nor is the donor site more aesthetically pleasing.

DONOR SITES

The color, texture, vascularity, thickness, and hair-bearing nature of skin varies markedly from one area of the body to another. In general, the nearer the donor site is to the recipient site, the closer is the skin match. Skin grafts to the face from above the clavicle retain their natural blush state, whereas those from below the clavicle take on a yellowish or brownish hue [91].

*Postauricular Skin*

The postauricular surface of the ear and adjoining mastoid area (see Fig. 1-12) serve as excellent sources for grafts of full-thickness skin that match the skin of the face. Its color and texture are similar to that of facial skin.

Grafts as large as $2 \times 2$ cm can be removed with primary donor site closure by obliterating the depths of the postauricular sulcus. The entire area of postauricular skin from the helical rim to the hairline over the mastoid can be utilized for a full-thickness skin graft, and this large donor site can be closed with a split-thickness skin graft. When reconstruction of a nasal defect requires skin and cartilage, it is possible to include a portion of the conchal cartilage along with the full-thickness graft or to take skin, cartilage, and skin through the entire thickness of the external ear, then split the cartilage into two layers to provide a "banana split" for use as lining of the nasal alae [72]. Postauricular skin sometimes has a vascular "pinkish" appearance for 3 to 6 months postoperatively that usually subsides.

*Supraclavicular Skin*

The supraclavicular region (see Fig. 1-12) serves as a larger donor area for either full-thickness or split-thickness grafts of skin for the face. The color match and texture of this skin are nearly as good as those of the postauricular skin. Sufficient skin can be removed from this donor site to cover such units as an entire forehead, nose, cheek, upper lip, or chin. When grafting is performed in such units, the junctures can be hidden in the hair margins or along contour lines of the face (aesthetic unit borders).

The supraclavicular donor area may prove objectional as a source of split-thickness skin grafts because of the permanent changes found in the character of the skin in this exposed area. For this reason, many surgeons select other donor sites. Moreover, tissue expansion, various myocutaneous flaps, and free tissue transfers have lessened dramatically the need for this visible donor site.

*Upper Eyelid Skin*

The upper eyelid (see Fig. 1-12) is occasionally used as a donor site when a small, thin graft of full-thickness skin is needed for another lid. Underlying orbicularis muscle may be taken with such a graft, and care must be exercised not to deform the donor eyelid. In older patients the skin is looser and a wider graft can be obtained. These grafts are particularly helpful for correcting deformities of other lids.

*Antecubital and Inguinal Region Skin*

The antecubital flexor crease serves as a popular donor site for grafts of full-thickness skin for the finger, hand, or face. Although only a relatively small ellipse of skin can be removed if the wound is to be closed primarily, the proximity of this area to the fingertip makes it a common donor site for skin grafts to the finger. Before using, be sure the patient is aware of the visible scarring that results from taking the graft from this area. There are many other nonvisible donor areas.

The flexor crease of the inguinal region is usually hidden and therefore a much better donor area for full-thickness grafts. For example, it has been used in children as a source of full-thickness skin for denuded areas between the fingers following the division of a syndactylism. It has many uses in adults as well.

## Scalp

Split-thickness skin grafts can be taken from the scalp with the freehand knife or an electric dermatome. This area is an especially welcome source of skin in an extensively burned patient. Because of its thick dermis, deep and dense hair follicles, and excellent blood supply, one can harvest thin split-thickness grafts repeatedly within a period of 5 to 7 days [24, 53]. Five to six harvestings can be taken from the same site. Crawford [69] reported that little hair growth was noted in the grafted skin, even though hair growth in the scalp donor site was essentially normal. The skin also has a good color match to facial skin [328].

## Prepuce and Labia Majora

The preputial skin, removed by circumcision, is occasionally used when a graft of thin full-thickness skin is needed. Use of the labia majora for areolar reconstruction is usually discouraged because it is too dark and may be a painful donor site.

## Areola

The areola can be partially removed from one breast and grafted to a reconstructed breast by a variety of areola-sharing operations, as described in Chapter 48. The full thickness of the nipple has also been used as a graft. However, most areolar reconstructions are now performed by various flap methods [38, 60, 133, 190].

## ABDOMINAL WALL, BUTTOCK, AND THIGH

The abdominal wall, buttock, and thigh are the most common donor sites for split-thickness skin grafts. The grafts from these large donor areas often become yellowish, light brown, or dark brown. Thinner grafts tend to be darker than those of greater thickness [263, 281]. The pigmentation of a skin graft is increased even more by its exposure to the ultraviolet rays of the sun, and it persists for much longer periods than the usual suntan. Control of grafted skin pigmentation is one of the challenges in plastic surgery.

When possible, grafts are removed from the abdomen, buttock, or high posterior aspect of the thigh, where any permanent change in the skin of the donor site can be hidden by a bathing suit or shorts. Care is taken to not include the hair-bearing areas of the pubis. Bony prominences are avoided because it is difficult to remove grafts of split-thickness skin from these areas with any of the instruments currently available. With severe burns, where large amounts of skin may be required, any area of skin on the body, including the scalp, can be used as a donor site. Only such specific areas as the areola and nipples are avoided.

## DONOR SITE BLOOD LOSS

The average blood loss from the donor site after a $10 \times 20$ cm split-thickness skin graft has been removed was determined by Robinson [276] to be 46 ml. This amount can be reduced appreciably if either topical thrombin or a vasoconstrictor in low concentration is applied to the raw surface of the donor area.

## REQUIREMENTS FOR SURVIVAL OF A SKIN GRAFT

For a skin graft to take, it must have a vascular recipient bed, there must be contact of skin graft and recipient bed, and there must be proper preparation of any granulation tissue. The experimental work of Clemmesen [57] on the healing of skin grafts was outstanding.

## Vascular Recipient Bed

A skin graft requires enough blood supply in its recipient site for survival. Blood supply ample enough to support the growth of granulation tissue usually supports a skin graft. This fact does not imply that the skin graft has to be placed on granulation tissue but, rather, that it must be placed on a vascular bed. The only exception to this rule is the bridging phenomenon [214], whereby that portion of a skin graft overlying a small avascular area may survive. This phenomenon is based on the fact that collateral vessels connect the skin graft in the avascular area to the vascularized graft and serve as a network for transporting both an initial plasmatic circulation and a later ingrowth of capillary buds to nourish this area. In ideal circumstances this collateral circulation bridges a gap of 0.5 cm from any one margin.

It is sometimes possible to apply the principle of the bridging phenomenon for successfully covering a denuded tendon or nerve with a skin graft. If the tendon or nerve has a diameter of 1 cm or less and the recipient bed for the skin graft on either side is good, it may be possible to cover the area with a single, continuous skin graft carefully fitted to the contour of the area. This method ensures maximal contact between the skin graft and the recipient bed adjacent to the less vascular area. Also worthy of emphasis is the fact that the area being bridged through this indirect process requires a longer period to regain vascularity than areas overlying good recipient beds. Covering exposed tendons and nerves with skin grafts protects them from the detrimental effects of exposure and can for long periods prevent them from undergoing autolysis and death. However, in most cases, flap coverage of exposed tendons offers a greater chance for tendon survival and function. Another example of the bridging phenomenon is found in the vascularization of composite grafts (skin, cartilage, skin) such as those used for the reconstruction of nasal alae (see Chapter 16) [119]. Composite grafts of skin-cartilage-skin of the monkey's external ear have been demonstrated to have a greatly increased survival (88 percent complete survival compared to 22 percent complete survival in unprepared controls) by preparing the recipient wound 10 or 11 days in advance. Preparation involves simply excising the epithelium from the recipient wound, which leads to an increased number of vessels in the wound margin for inosculation with the graft vessels [86, 87, 206].

Smahel [300] demonstrated in the rat that the recipient bed could be "prepared" by first creating the wound and covering it temporarily with a skin graft. Two days later the permanent graft is placed on the wound. This skin graft becomes revascularized and heals at a definitely faster rate than normal, which is thought due to a reduction of the stage of plasmatic imbibition.

COMPARATIVE VASCULARITY OF RECIPIENT BEDS. Cortical bone denuded of periosteum, cartilage denuded of perichondrium, and tendon denuded of paratenon are avascular on their external surfaces and *cannot* be expected to nourish a skin graft placed in contact with them. Neither can any of the body's stratified squamous epithelial surfaces support the growth of a skin graft.

Heavily irradiated tissue is a relatively poor recipient bed for skin grafts because it has a poor blood supply. Fat has fewer blood vessels than dermis, fascia, and most other tissues and thus is considered among the less desirable recipient beds. Long-standing granulation tissue such as that seen in the exposed surface of chronic ulcers also serves as a poor bed for skin grafts because it becomes fibrotic, is less vascular, and usually has high bacterial counts. Arteriosclerotic changes in the blood vessels of the foot and ankle in older patients and diabetic patients make these regions poor recipient beds. Recurrent infections can be followed by massive amounts of fibrosis and ischemia. In general, recipient beds having limited circulation require a long period for the completion of vascularization of a skin graft and consequently require longer periods of immobilization and aftercare than do grafts placed on beds of greater vascularity.

COMPARATIVE VASCULARITY OF SKIN GRAFTS. Thin split-thickness skin grafts have a more abundant network of capillaries on their undersurface than do thick split-thickness or full-thickness grafts. This fine network of terminal vessels is located in the superficial dermis, whereas slightly larger vessels are located in the deep dermis.

Smahel [301] and Rudolph and Klein [281] have written extensively on the vascularization of skin grafts. Vascularization occurs as follows.

*1. Plasmatic imbibition.* Almost immediately after a skin graft comes into contact with the underlying bed it begins to absorb a plasma-like fluid from it. This fluid is absorbed into the sponge-like structure of the capillary network by capillary action, providing a state of in vivo tissue culture [28, 29, 55, 64, 290]. On microscopic examination it can be observed that this fluid lying in the endothelium-lined spaces of the graft contains a few erythrocytes. While this process continues, a fibrin network is being formed between the graft and the recipient bed to hold the graft in place. The plasma-like fluid appears to be absorbed into the graft (plasmatic imbibition) over the first 48 hours, causing its weight to gradually increase (20 percent increased weight in 24 hours and 30 percent increased weight in 48 hours) [56]. At 48 hours blood flow begins in the graft, and the plasma-like fluid is carried away. The pink color that some grafts attain during the first 12 hours after transplantation probably results from the accumulation of red blood cells drawn into the capillaries of the graft by the plasmatic circulation [63].

*2. Inosculation and growth of blood vessels.* During the first 48 hours after grafting, vascular buds grow in the intervening fibrin network that binds the skin graft to its recipient site [56, 61, 279, 306]. There are two views as to what happens next. One view is that there is random inosculation of the vascular buds from the bed with both arteries and veins in the graft, following which the blood enters the graft vessels moving to and fro in a sluggish manner until the fourth to seventh day, when true circulation occurs in the graft. The other view is that the vascular buds grow into the graft, even inside some of the old graft vessels, forming an entirely new vascular network [301]. There is a great deal of evidence supporting the first viewpoint. Haller and Billingham [128], for example, found the vascular pattern in the healed grafts in the hamster cheek pouch to be the same as before grafting. They also observed that blockage of the graft vessels by injecting them with silicone rubber solution prior to grafting was followed by necrosis of the graft.

The development of anastomoses between bed and graft and the flow of blood into the vessels of the graft have an inhibiting effect on further proliferation of the vascular buds [301]. Concurrent with these events in the hemic circulation is restoration of the continuity of the lymphatic systems in the bed and graft. Scothorne [289], Psillakis [265], and Oden [249] have shown that lymphatic drainage from the graft is established by the fourth or fifth postoperative day, when graft lymphatics connect with recipient bed lymphatics.

*Contact of the Skin Graft and the Recipient Bed*
Good contact between a skin graft and its recipient bed is essential for vascularization of a graft and its survival. The thin fibrin network that begins to form almost immediately between the graft and its bed seems to serve as glue to hold the surfaces together and prevent one from slipping on the other [326, 327].

Several factors prevent proper contact between the graft and its recipient bed, including improper tension on the graft, a collection of fluid underneath it, and movement between the graft and its bed. It is important that a proper degree of tension exists in a skin graft once it has been sutured into place. If the tension is insufficient, wrinkles result that never become revascularized because of a failure to be in proper contact with the recipient bed. This same lack of contact results when a graft is stretched too tightly: Acting like a drum head, the graft does not dip properly into the recesses of the recipient bed.

Blood, serum, and purulent material may separate the skin graft from its bed, prevent vascularization, and thus cause loss of the graft. The chance of a hematoma underneath a graft can be greatly decreased by careful hemostasis of even the smallest bleeding

points. Much of the bleeding stops spontaneously over a period of 5 to 10 minutes, so
the stages of the operation are planned in
such a way that this time can be consumed
in obtaining the skin graft. The use of fine-
tipped electrocautery is unexcelled for obtaining absolute hemostasis.

A delay of 24 to 48 hours before applying
the skin graft is definitely indicated when
oozing of blood from the bed persists. The
wound can simply be dressed with a pressure
dressing that is not removed until the time
of delayed grafting. This decision to delay
application of a skin graft is often a difficult
one to make, but it is usually a wise one.

Capillary buds must revascularize the graft
before the cells die. When a hematoma only
0.5 mm thick is present, the time required
for capillary buds to grow through the added
thickness of the clot might be only 12 hours;
if the maximal allowable time for vascularization has not been exceeded, the graft survives in these areas, even though it is vascularized 12 hours later than other areas.
When the clot is 5 mm thick, however, the
vascularization process is delayed by 120
hours. At body temperature, most grafts do
not survive this long a delay before revascularization, and so when the maximal allowable time for vascularization has been
exceeded, autolysis begins [326, 327]. Separation from the vascular bed not only delays
vascularization but, as Littlewood [191] has
demonstrated, a split-thickness skin graft
elevated from its bed by a seroma becomes
epithelialized on its dermal surface by the
fourth day after grafting.

The graft is inspected on the second postoperative day in most instances, except
when a tie-over dressing is used. At this
time the skin graft over any fluid collection
can be incised and the fluid expressed, a procedure that is repeated at least daily until
there is no further fluid collection. This simple technique of expressing any fluid collections has saved many grafts that would otherwise be lost. Perforating or meshing the
graft allows the inevitable wound exudate to

drain to the surface without lifting the graft
from its bed. When a tie-over dressing is
used, Randall [268] suggested inserting all
sutures around the margin of a graft but
tying only one of the two long ends of each
suture over a stent. Then 2 to 3 days postoperatively, the stent is removed and any
fluid collections evacuated. The graft is then
pressed back against its bed and the remaining sutures tied over a new stent. The moistened cotton-tipped applicator can be useful
for removing a small, discrete hematoma
lying away from the graft margin. Alternatively, we use rubber bands stapled to the
graft-skin margin and umbilical tape woven
through it for use in the tie-over dressing.
This method allows easy inspection, which
is done by removing the umbilical tape, inspecting the graft, and then simply reapply-
ing the dressing and reweaving the umbilical
tape through the rubber bands.

Movement between the graft and its bed
damages the capillaries growing into a
graft and prevents proper revascularization.
Therefore when a skin graft is applied to the
extremities, splinting is used to immobilize
the adjacent joints. Skin grafts on the trunk
can best be protected by keeping the patient
at bed rest and in a position that prevents
distortion or tension on the graft. Either a
tie-over dressing technique or complete exposure of the graft is the most satisfactory
way to treat the graft itself. It is especially
difficult to immobilize skin grafts on the
face because of the movement of the facial
muscles. A tie-over dressing that immobi-
lizes the graft in its bed as a unit is an effective way of handling the problem.

*Preparation of the Open Wound*
A sharp distinction must be made between
the recipient bed created just before a graft
is applied and one that has been an open
wound for a number of days. The important
aspects in the evaluation of an open wound
are its blood supply and quantitative bacteriology.

BLOOD SUPPLY. Almost all open wounds

have sufficient blood supply to give nourishment to connective tissue and to provide the capillaries that combine to make up granulation tissue. Even irradiated tissues produce granulations, though at a much slower rate than normal. Only bare bone and bare cartilage do not produce granulation tissue.

QUANTITATIVE BACTERIOLOGY. Robson and Krizek [176, 277] have written extensively on the subject of quantitative bacteriology. They demonstrated that all wounds containing more than 100,000 ($10^5$) bacteria per gram of tissue are infected to such a degree that a skin graft does not take on that surface. The source of these bacteria may be exogenous or endogenous. Endogenous sources include (1) direct contact of bacteria from within the body with the edges of the incision, and (2) bacteria present at a distant site in the body entering the wound through the bloodstream that localize at the site of injury.

A rapid (30 minute) slide technique has been used clinically for several years to determine the number of bacteria in tissue taken by a skin punch or scalpel from the open wound [176, 277]. Most wounds with fewer than $10^5$ bacteria per gram of tissue and a good blood supply support the growth of a skin graft.

The former designation of bacteria as pathogenic or saprophytic can be discontinued in light of our present knowledge that any bacteria present in sufficient numbers cause a clinical infection. The group A beta-hemolytic streptococcus is an exception to the rule using $10^5$ bacteria per gram of tissue as a dividing line, as this organism causes a clinically significant infection in much lower numbers. The presence of this organism causes dissolution of a skin graft, and it is therefore a contraindication to skin grafting.

There are $10^3$ staphylococci, streptococci, and other bacteria per gram of tissue deep in the skin of each of us, but so long as there is a normal balance between host resistance and the bacteria there is no clinical infection. In an open wound, time is an important factor. The "golden period" comprises the hours it takes for the initial inoculum in the wound to reach $10^5$ bacteria per gram of tissue. Foreign bodies in the wound enhance wound sepsis [92].

Removal of bacteria from a fresh wound is best accomplished by mechanical débridement and pulsating jet lavage [348]. For older wounds, some have advocated removing granulation tissue by scraping the wound with the back of a knife handle prior to applying a skin graft. However, this method may leave a bacterial colony count of more than $10^5$. The major problem is knowing when it is safe to apply a graft. Clearly, it is often impossible to make this decision by simple inspection of the wound. Hence quantitative bacteriology is the best assessment available. The wound may also be tested with allographs or xenographs. If the bacterial count is less than $10^5$, graft take is unlikely.

Biologic dressings (e.g., skin allografts and fresh amniotic membranes) placed on the granulating wound and changed every 24 hours have been shown to achieve marked reduction of the bacterial flora in an open granulating wound [3, 176, 283]. In wounds where skin allografts or autografts take, biopsies of the underlying tissue obtained 24 hours after placing the graft on the wound reveal no organisms, whereas prior to grafting there were large numbers of bacteria [296]. Systemic antibiotics fail to alter the quantitative level of bacteria in the granulating wound [15]. There is also abundant evidence to indicate that systemic antibiotics begun more than 3 to 4 hours after wounding are of no value. The mechanism for this bacterial "escape" has been postulated by Rodeheaver et al. [278] to be the fibrous coagulum that accumulates on the wound. This coagulum surrounds the bacteria and protects them from the antibiotic. These authors compared a proteolytic enzyme to a saline dressing change. They showed that by using topical proteolytic

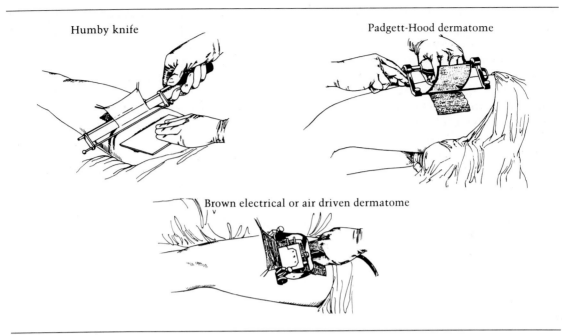

Humby knife

Padgett-Hood dermatome

Brown electrical or air driven dermatome

**Figure 1-13** *Instruments for cutting split-thickness skin grafts.*

enzymes the level of antibiotics, given intravenously, increased significantly at the wound surface. With this proteolytic treatment, the "golden period" (1 to 3 hours) can be prolonged indefinitely. Topical antibiotics have been shown to decrease bacterial growth in the open wound [232].

CUTTING THE SKIN GRAFT
*Split-Thickness Skin Graft*
Three basic types of instrument have been designed for removing a graft of split-thickness skin from its donor site: knife, drum-type dermatome, and electrical or air-driven dermatome (Fig. 1-13). The choice of instrument usually depends on the surgeon's experience. The principle on which all of these instruments are based is that a sharp blade moves back and forth to cut a piece of skin whose thickness is controlled by a calibrated setting on the instrument or by the surgeon.

KNIVES. Some knives (e.g., the Humby knife) have an adjustable roller that controls the thickness of the skin graft, whereas others (e.g., the Blair knife and Ferris-Smith knife) are simply long cutting blades with a handle at one end and no adjustable roller to control graft thickness. A Weck blade or even an ordinary razor blade can be used to take narrower skin grafts.

With the Humby knife (Fig. 1-13), modified by Bodenham, Braithwaite, and Marcks, the thickness can be measured with shims, which are included in the set, or the surgeon can learn to set the desired thickness by sighting between the blade and the roller. The thickness of a graft can also be checked from time to time as it is being cut by observing its translucency and the bleeding pattern of the donor site.

Long, narrow grafts of split-thickness skin can be obtained more easily from the thigh if they are cut in a longitudinal direction. The buttock or arm can serve in a similar fashion as donor sites. The abdomen is less satisfactory as a donor site for skin grafts cut with a knife because there is no underlying bony or cartilaginous framework to support it. Probably one of the most important prerequisites for successful cutting of a freehand graft is experience and a sense of self-assurance on the part of the surgeon.

Knives that have been fitted with an adjustable roller are used in the same way as the Ferris-Smith knife. The roller attachment has the important advantage of ensuring that the depth of the knife blade does not change significantly from its predetermined setting during the cutting of the skin graft.

Snow [309] has described the use of an unmodified Schick injector razor and blade for taking a split-thickness skin graft 0.012 to 0.014 inch in thickness and 1.25 inches wide. Shoul [295] modified a Gillette safety razor by simply filling out the central strut of the safety guard and using another blade with the cutting edge broken off as a shim. Each shim increases the space between the cutting blade and the safety guard, so that with three shims a graft 0.012 inch thick and 1.25 inches wide can be cut. Goulian [125] has modified the Weck straight razor by adding a fixed handle, removing two struts from the blade protector, and modifying the blade protector so that the razor can be preset at the factor to cut at 0.008, 0.001, or 0.012 inch in thickness and 1.25 inches wide. It is a handy portable instrument most suitable for emergency room work.

DRUM-TYPE DERMATOME. The drum-type dermatome is best for cutting a skin graft of uniform thickness. The Padgett-Hood dermatome (see Fig. 1-13), which is the prototype of the drum dermatomes, comes in three sizes: the baby model, which cuts 3 × 8 inch grafts; the standard model, which cuts 4 × 8 inch grafts; and the giant size, which can cut a graft as large as 4 × 16 inches. It works on the principle of fixing the outer surface of the skin to one-half of a metal drum and then moving a rotating blade back and fourth close enough to the surface of the drum to cut off a partial thickness of skin at the desired level. The knife blade, which is disposable, can be adjusted with a calibrated dial so that its cutting edge lies at any desired level between 0.005 and 0.050 inch from the surface of the drum. All settings are checked either by eye or with a measuring shim to be certain that the blade is the desired distance away from the drum before the graft is taken. Before inserting the disposable blade into the carrier arm, it is necessary to insert a thin metal strip (adapter) to keep the blade far enough from the drum. The original blades for this instrument were thicker and thus did not require the addition of a metal adapter strip.

The Padgett-Hood dermatome requires either a dermatome cement (Padgett-Hood dermatome cement, Reese compound, or Evo-stik "impact" household adhesive) or a removable dermatome tape to make the skin adhere to the drum. The donor site is best prepared by cleansing the donor site with acetone. While the dermatome is still resting on its special stand, either a thin layer of cement is applied to the surface of the drum or dermatome tape is placed on the drum. Petrolatum or mineral oil can be applied to the metal axis on which the blade moves back and forth as well as to the surface of the blade, which comes into contact with the skin.

Skin grafts can be cut more readily with the Padgett-Hood dermatome in a circumferential direction around the thigh. The drum can be pressed down firmly onto the skin to obtain the desired degree of adherence before gently rotating it to draw the skin up so it can be incised with the blade. The blade swings back and forth as the drum is rotated. Care must be taken to press the drum against the skin as it is rotated to maintain a constant degree of thickness and width. If the blade cuts into the skin beyond the edge of the drum, the skin can be gently retracted away with a hemostat. When necessary, the thickness of the graft can be changed during cutting simply by moving the calibrated dial. When the graft is completely cut, it can be removed from the drum by attaching small hemostats to each of its corners. The adhesive can be rubbed off with a gauze sponge. Care must be taken to avoid injury to the operator's hands. Surgeons have sustained significant wounds from this instrument when a guard is not attached.

A drum-type dermatome makes it possible to cut skin grafts to fit an exact pattern. An outline of the graft required can be drawn on the skin and then dermatome cement applied within the boundaries. Petrolatum or mineral oil is applied to the skin outside the pattern to be certain it does not adhere to the drum. Thus only the skin within the pattern adheres to the drum and is removed. Another technique for obtaining a graft of a given configuration is to apply the pattern upside down to the cut surface of a skin graft before the graft is removed from the drum. The skin can then be cut to this pattern with a knife.

Two other drum-type dermatomes were designed by Reese and Schuchardt. The Reese dermatome is more elaborate and precise than the Padgett-Hood dermatome. The distance between the blade and the drum is adjusted by inserting a shim of the desired thickness adjacent to the blade in its carrying arm. A tape containing an adhesive on its surface is fixed to the drum. A guard is present that prevents injury to the operator. The Schuchardt dermatome adheres to the skin without adhesives. The graft is removed by a to-and-fro motion of a knife blade, which is adjusted with thumbscrews to give the desired thickness.

ELECTRICAL OR AIR-DRIVEN DERMATOME. Motor-driven dermatomes allow the surgeon to rapidly remove long strips of skin, 8 cm or less in width, from almost any site on the trunk or extremities. This procedure saves a great deal of time during the grafting of patients with extensive burns. Another advantage of the motor-driven unit is that satisfactory grafts can be cut even by the less experienced surgeon.

The Brown electrical or air-driven dermatome (see Fig. 1-13) is equipped with a disposable knife blade that moves back and forth like the blade of a hair-cutter. A long, sterile cable, serving as the drive shaft, runs between the dermatome and its unsterile motor, which is taped to a stool or table adjacent to the donor site. A foot pedal activates the motor.

The thickness of the skin graft can be controlled by adjusting two calibrated knobs on either side of the instrument, which alters the pitch of the blade. Because the instrument can fall out of proper alignment, it is important to close the knobs down completely and use this reading as the zero point on each side. Once both sides are set, it is best to double-check by holding the instrument up to the light to see that the aperture between the blade and the instrument is the same on either side. The desired width of the graft can then be obtained by making an inward or outward adjustment of the shoe-like attachment on either side of the dermatome.

Sterile mineral oil, applied to the donor site, lubricates it so the instrument can move forward smoothly. After the skin has been steadied, the dermatome blade is set in motion and the instrument placed on the donor site so its flat undersurface lies at a slightly downward angle. A moderate, constant pressure is required as the dermatome moves steadily forward to keep it from jumping or skipping over the skin. As the graft begins to appear on the upper surface of the blade, the graft can be lifted by an assistant to ensure that it is of the proper thickness and to prevent it from bunching near the blade. After this initial maneuver, it is not usually necessary to continue to withdraw the skin cut by the dermatome.

Skin grafts are usually taken from the extremities in a longitudinal direction. Because multiple grafts of uniform thickness can be taken from a limb without wasting any space between adjoining donor sites, it is possible to "strip" an extremity of nearly its entire potential donor capability and yet know that it will heal with uniformity.

One disadvantage of the electrical dermatomes is that they can break down and require factory adjustment. For this reason, it is wise to have a second instrument available. It must also be emphasized that these instruments are not calibrated as accurately as the drum dermatomes and therefore do not cut grafts of a desired thickness as precisely. Thus for cutting thick split-thickness skin for such important areas as the face, when the graft must be wide and of an exact and consistent thickness, a drum-type dermatome is commonly used.

Other electrical dermatome devices include the Padgett, Stryker, and Castroviejo dermatomes. The Padgett electrical dermatome has its motor in the handle of the instrument. The Stryker dermatome is similar to the Brown dermatome and uses a cable to connect it to the motor. The Castroviejo dermatome was designed primarily for cutting split-thickness grafts of mucosa from the inner surfaces of the lips and cheeks with a small razor blade. Shims are used to regulate the thickness of the grafts.

Anesthesia of the skin graft donor site can be enhanced by cooling [146]. Local infiltration or regional blocks are also appropriate.

*Full-Thickness Skin Graft*
Full-thickness grafts contract so little that it is important to cut them to fit the recipient site as exactly as possible. When such lesions as a hemangioma, nevus, or foreign body tattoo are to be removed, the size of the defect and its contour are evident before the operation. Thus it is practical to prepare an exact pattern for the full-thickness graft before the excision. Such preparation eliminates the possibility of making the pattern too large, an error that almost invariably accompanies the making of an imprint of the defect after the excision has been carried out. This problem occurs because the skin edges around the margin of the defect retract as soon as the opposing skin tension is gone. The specimen, of course, is not suitable for a pattern, as it contracts as soon as it is removed.

In many instances, it is impossible to ascertain the size of the defect before surgery, either because the extent of the excision could not be determined beforehand, as in the case of malignancy, or because scar contracture disguises the true size of the defect. Under these circumstances, it is far better to carry out the excisional surgery before attempting to determine the size of the full-thickness graft that is needed.

Many materials have been suggested for patterning the defect: exposed x-ray film, Vinylite, lead sheet, silk, cloth toweling, rubber dam, and aluminum sheets. Transparent pliable substances that do not stretch and yet can be sterilized by either autoclaving or soaking in a solution without distorting their outline are the best. An outline of the defect can be made with methylene blue and either imprinted on the patterning material with pressure or cut to the desired size and shape. If the area is irregular, it is best to maintain proper orientation of both the pattern and the graft to the defect by marking each with corresponding symbols or dots. It is also important to identify which side of the pattern corresponds to the epidermal surface of the graft and which represents the dermal side. Without sufficient attention to this point, the pattern can be mistakenly turned over and a useless mirror image of the defect obtained.

Full-thickness skin grafts are cut with either a No. 15 or No. 10 knife blade. If the skin of the donor site has an irregular surface contour, it is helpful to distend the skin by injecting either saline or an anesthetic solution underneath the dermal layer. This step aids in obliterating the irregularities, allowing the surgical separation of the dermis from the underlying fat. If epinephrine (Adrenalin) is added to the solution, the line of incision between dermis and subcutaneous tissue can be visualized even more clearly.

The skin is incised just to the depths of the dermis (Fig. 1-14). Fine sutures of atraumatic silk can be inserted into the margins of the graft at the points where the identifying marks are located. Skin hooks may be used for countertraction. The graft, under tension, is turned back over the operator's index finger and removed under direct vi-

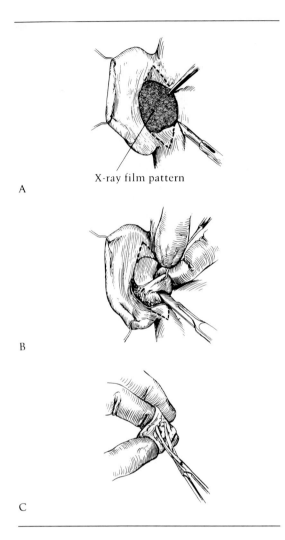

X-ray film pattern

A

B

C

**Figure 1-14** *Technique for cutting a full-thickness skin graft. Excess fat is trimmed away as shown in C.*

sion, with care to minimize the amount of fat left on it. Another method is to tense the graft in a plane almost parallel to the wound surface and cut blindly with an oscillating gesture in the plane immediately underneath the dermis. Seeing or feeling the tip of the blade through the thickness of the skin serves as a guide to keep the proper level.

After the graft has been cut, the epidermal surface of the graft is stretched over the surgeon's index finger, and the residual fat is usually removed with small, curved sharp scissors (Fig. 1-14C). However, the graft can survive with some fat left in place. The donor area is closed in most instances by converting the defect to an elliptical shape, undermining the wound edges, and approximating them by suture. If the defect is too large to permit primary suture, a split-thickness graft can be applied.

All of the postauricular skin and the adjacent non-hair-bearing mastoid skin can be used as a full-thickness skin graft and this large donor area covered with a split-thickness skin graft. Usually, grafting is unnecessary. The same is true for the inguinal area, which is another popular donor site.

APPLICATION AND CARE
OF SKIN GRAFTS
The basic techniques for applying split-thickness and full-thickness skin grafts are the same. It is important to remove any clot from the recipient bed before applying the graft. As the graft is being sutured into place, a cotton applicator stick can be twisted underneath the graft to remove any remaining clots that can be seen through the translucent graft. If there is significant bleeding, it must be controlled with fine tip electrocoagulation or ligatures before graft application is complete.

If a tourniquet has been used during preparation of the graft recipient site, it is released. Hemostasis is then obtained and the tourniquet reapplied until the graft and dressing have been completed.

When it is impossible to obtain absolute hemostasis of the recipient bed—a common occurrence following excision of a burn scar—it is sometimes worthwhile to delay applying the skin graft. The wound is simply covered with a pressure dressing that contains a layer of nonadherent material on the wound surface. The dressing is removed 24 to 48 hours later, and coagulated blood is removed from the recipient bed, which should now be dry. Skin grafts obtained at the initial operation can be stored by placing them back on the donor site temporarily or by re-frigeration at 4°C; they can then later be applied without anesthesia if they are simply laid on the wound without fixation or fixed to the surrounding skin with skin tape. Delayed grafting more than compensates for the additional time involved because it usually ensures success and a better functional and cosmetic result.

When the defect to be closed with a skin graft has been created by excising a nevus, scar, or other closed wound, the skin graft is usually applied in a sheet. When the wound has been open, however, and thus is at least contaminated with bacteria, it is usually wise to allow drainage through the skin graft, which is accomplished with a graft meshing device. The use of postage stamp grafts is rarely indicated. The Tanner-Van-deput cutting machine, the Michigan Research Corporation mesh expander, and the Concept mesh expander are designed to produce multiple uniform slits in the graft approximately 1 mm apart [196]. When the graft is pulled on the bias, numerous dia-mond-shaped openings appear. These openings eventually epithelialize, but the aesthetic appearance is usually not as good as that obtained with a sheet graft.

For skin grafting of concave defects, there must be sufficient skin to cover completely the depths of the wound, rather than only enough to bridge the skin like a drum head from the wound margins. A tie-over dressing is often helpful. Occasionally, it is useful for covering concave defects to cut a pie-shaped triangle out of a circular piece of skin and then close the triangle so as to form the skin into a cone.

### Fixation of Skin Grafts

SUTURES. Suturing probably remains the method most often used for approximating a skin graft to the margins of a wound. The sutures may be interrupted, continuous, or both. The interrupted sutures, if their ends are left long, may be tied over a bulky cotton dressing to aid in immobilizing the graft

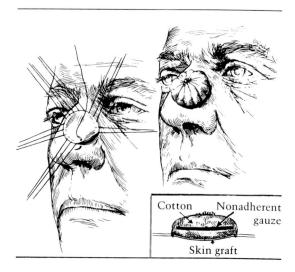

**Figure 1-15** *Tie-over dressing for skin grafts.*

(Fig. 1-15). Nonabsorbable sutures are preferred, although in children absorbable material is worthwhile to avoid the need for removing the sutures.

A three-point suture is often helpful for attaching the skin graft to a thick-edged wound. This suture is placed through the graft about 4 or 5 mm from its edge; it is then woven in and out of the subcutaneous tissue of the wound margin and finally through the skin, where it is tied. If the margin is a skin flap, it is wise to anchor the graft to the recipient bed as well. In this way, any blood underneath the flap is less likely to extend underneath the skin graft.

SKIN TAPES AND ADHESIVES. The use of microporous surgical adhesive tape or a single thickness of fine mesh gauze fixed with collodion adhesive can be used to secure a skin graft to the margin around the bed. The tapes are usually positioned across the wound margin in a radial fashion. This method, however, requires a completely dry graft and surrounding area for the adhesive strips to adhere. If there is oozing from the recipient site, the adhesives do not hold the graft in place.

Dermatome cement or methyl-2-cyanoac-rylate can also be used to hold the graft to the skin margins. The adhesive is applied to the skin surrounding the recipient wound. The undersurface of the graft is dried before it is applied, so the portion that comes into contact with the glue remains adherent. The overlapping wound edge does not survive and can be débrided away later. The methyl-2-cyanoacrylate is applied only in droplet size between the graft and the recipient bed because nutrients cannot penetrate this adhesive barrier, and the graft will fail. At present cyanoacrylates have not received Food and Drug Administration approval.

By far the most popular method of graft fixation is with stainless steel staples. They can be applied rapidly and precisely with good eversion of the graft and wound bed edges.

NO EXTERNAL FIXATION. The fibrin that normally forms between the skin graft and its recipient site rapidly binds the two surfaces together. Within a few minutes of application, most grafts have become adherent to the bed. Although this bond is not strong enough to withstand significant trauma, it is effective enough to hold either large, thin grafts or thick ones the size of a postage stamp to the wound. The tendency for large, thick, split-thickness skin grafts to retract makes this technique less satisfactory for their application to granulating wounds. The easiest way to eliminate this problem is to suture the graft at its four corners under its normal tension to the skin beyond the margin.

*Dressing of Skin Grafts*

TIE-OVER DRESSING. The tie-over dressing is one of the most satisfactory methods for immobilizing skin grafts (see Fig. 1-15). It is especially useful on the face and neck, where the movements of the muscles of facial expression can make graft immobilization difficult.

The tie-over dressing contains a nonadherent gauze next to the graft surface. Over this gauze is placed a bolus of saline-soaked cotton, and the sutures are then tied to hold firm pressure on the graft. Another modification we have found helpful is to staple on the graft and incorporate a heavy silk suture in the staple, then use these silks for the tie-over dressing. This method is a great time saver.

If the margin around the recipient bed remains dry and odorless, the tie-over dressing can be left in place 5 to 7 days or longer. If there is any question about whether fluid will collect underneath the graft, one of the tie-over sutures can be left untied initially but then tied after inspection of the graft at 1 to 2 days [268]. The edges of the tie-over dressing are inspected daily for evidence of infection underneath the graft. If any is found, the dressing is removed, the wound cultured, and saline dressings begun.

EPITHELIAL INLAY (STENT). The epithelial inlay technique is used less frequently today because of the increased efficacy of flaps [111]. The technique is good for applying a skin graft to the labial or buccal sulcus, orbital cavity, external auditory canal, inner surface of the nose, and vagina. Contact with the recipient bed is maintained by wrapping the graft about a preformed mold of acrylic, dental modeling compound, silicone, or similar material (Fig. 1-16). After the recipient bed has been created, an impression of it can be taken with acrylic or similar material. The mold or stent is allowed to harden before the skin graft is wrapped around it, with the raw surface to the outside. The graft can be trimmed and sutured to itself. It may be advisable to form a second mold or stent before tying the one covered with the skin graft into place. The second mold can serve as a model for making a more permanent splint of lighter weight that can be substituted when the skin graft is first inspected about 7 days later. Any extra skin beyond the edge of the defect that was not revascularized is dry and tissue-paper thin, and it can be easily trimmed at this time. It is important not to leave these grafts unsplinted for more than short periods because the cavity quickly becomes obliterated

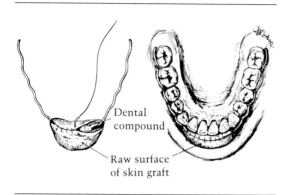

**Figure 1-16** *Epithelial inlay mold of dental compound to hold a split-thickness skin graft in the labial sulcus.*

as the graft contracts. Permanent units can be hollowed out to make them lighter. In the nose, an airway can be placed through the center of the mold for the patient's comfort.

In the mouth it may be advantageous to fix the epithelial inlay mold to the teeth to permit prolonged splinting of the graft during the period of graft contracture (see Fig. 1-16). Often the molds can be fashioned preoperatively to the approximate size and then altered to fit exactly at the time of operation. Skin grafts applied to mucosal areas seem to have an especially marked propensity to contract, so splinting must often be maintained for 3 to 6 months. Skin grafts applied to the periosteum of the maxilla or mandible, in contrast, do not contract.

PRESSURE DRESSING. Pressure dressings are often useful for immobilizing grafts on an extremity. After the nonadherent dressing and flattened gauze pads have been applied to a graft, padding of gauze, cotton waste, or cotton is applied on top of the graft and held in place by an elastic tape (Elastoplast) or an Ace bandage. The graft as well as the joints on either side of it are immobilized with a plaster or aluminum splint. Care must be taken, as excessive pressure could cause neurologic or vascular damage and even loss of the extremity.

OPEN METHOD. Leaving the graft open or exposed can be especially useful in such areas as the face, neck, and trunk, where the movement of muscles in the base of the wound might shear the graft from its bed if a pressure dressing were used. Contact from clothing and bed coverings can be prevented by keeping a wire cage or a cardboard box over the exposed grafts. This measure facilitates inspection of the graft and permits removal of any fluid that has collected underneath it. The open technique of skin grafting is not used in any patient (child or adult) whose willingness or ability to cooperate is in doubt.

## POSTOPERATIVE CARE OF SKIN GRAFTS
### Removal of Hematomas and Seromas

As a rule, any skin graft suspected of harboring a collection of fluid underneath it is inspected on the second postoperative day and the fluid, if present, evacuated. This treatment must be repeated every day until there is no further fluid underneath the graft. The exception to this rule can be found in sterile wounds where a tie-over dressing has been applied to an absolutely dry recipient bed under ideal circumstances. If neither odor nor fever is present and a sense of confidence prevails, the dressing change can be delayed for 5 to 7 days. Early dressing change just for curiosity may be harmful. Therefore it is a matter of judgment and no hard, fast rule can be set.

It is easy to recognize a hematoma or seroma underneath skin grafts because of the translucency of the graft. The No. 11 knife blade is good for incising the graft, the fluid being removed by either the pressure of a gauze sponge or the use of a sterile cotton applicator stick. Blood clots not expressed with pressure alone can be removed by twirling the cotton applicator and wrapping the clot around it. The term "roll the graft" is often used to describe removal of clot from underneath the graft. It is a confusing misnomer. Indeed, if the graft is "rolled" to remove the clot, the entire adherence between graft and bed may be disrupted. The clot *must* be removed directly from its specific location under the graft.

Skin grafts adhere strongly to a proper recipient site. The most rapid gain in adherent strength during the first 8 hours after grafting and then continue to gain in adherent strength more slowly with each subsequent 24 hours [262, 326, 327]. Careful dressing changes do not dislodge them. However, keep in mind the warning that more grafts are lost because of the first dressing change.

### Care of the Infected Skin Graft

Most infections arising underneath the graft usually do not cause temperature elevations during the first 24 hours after operation. The high temperature spike that appears this soon is usually caused by pulmonary pathology. Low-grade fever, odor, or redness around the margins of the graft between the second and fourth postoperative day support the diagnosis of infection.

When a patient complains of increased pain in the grafted site a few days after operation, it may indicate that there is a wound infection. The opposite is also true: A daily decrease of soreness in a grafted wound indicates that the graft has taken.

Local wound care to the site of infection includes debridement of any necrotic tissue in the wound and frequent moist saline soaks. Mechanical cleanliness is essential to good wound care.

When the predominant bacteria are group A beta-hemolytic streptococci *(S. pyogenes)*, the skin graft may be totally lost. To prevent a further loss of grafts, additional skin is not applied until this organism has been eradicated with appropriate topical and, if necessary, systemic antibiotic. When cellulitis is present, systemic antibiotics are clearly indicated. If there is a local wound infection with partial graft loss, topical antimicrobials (i.e., silver sulfadiazine, mafenide acetate, silver nitrate) control the local flora. Infections with *Pseudomonas aeruginosa (P. pyocyanea)* may be less deleterious to grafts.

Silver sulfadiazine and mafenide acetate as topical antimicrobials control most *Pseudomonas* graft infections, although some strains are resistant to these agents. A new topical antimicrobial, norfloxacin (a quinoline carboxylic acid compound) has been found to be 100 percent effective against *Pseudomonas.* In vivo studies are now being conducted [142].

### Hyperbaric Oxygen

Hyperbaric oxygen is *not* indicated for normal skin grafts or flaps. It can be used preoperatively to prepare the granulating base by promoting capillary proliferation in poorly granulating wounds. Kivisaari and Niinikoski showed in rats that twice-daily treatments at 2 atmospheres for 2 hours had no effect on wounds and flaps with circulation intact. However, with locally interrupted circulation, there was a significant increase in survival of flaps and healing of wounds in the group treated with hyperbaric oxygen compared to controls [77, 170, 245].

### Immobilization Period for Skin Grafts

Although it appears that skin grafts contract to varying degrees, it is usually the recipient bed that contracts, giving the appearance that the graft has contracted. This process begins about 10 days after the graft is applied and may continue for as long as 6 months [71, 212, 216]. There is less contraction associated with full-thickness skin grafts.

SPLINTING THE GRAFTED AREA. Skin graft areas are known to contract more rapidly and to a greater degree on certain areas on the body than at other locations. For example, the anterior aspect of the neck, oral mucosa, nasal lining, and vagina require splinting for periods up to 6 months; the axilla, flexor surface of fingers, and popliteal, antecubital, and postauricular regions must be splinted for periods of 2 to 3 months. The splint may need to be applied only intermittently during the day or at night during the last 1 to 2 months. Lightweight splints for all of these regions can be made and applied at the time of operation. When joints are involved, it may be advisable to remove the splints daily and put the part through a full range of motion. Grafts splinted at the time of application for several days contract less than the nonsplinted graft.

IMMOBILIZATION OF SKIN GRAFTS ON THE LOWER EXTREMITY. Skin grafts on the lower extremity or in relatively avascular areas (e.g., irradiated tissue) may require a longer time than usual before becoming completely revascularized and stable [268]. The many factors present in these cases do not allow any hard-and-fast rules regarding either the period of immobilization or the rapidity with which mobilization can be accomplished once it has been started.

One fundamental point to observe following skin grafting of lower-extremity ulcers is that the process that causes the ulcer must be eliminated, if possible, before ambulation has begun. Otherwise, the repair that might seem satisfactory with the extremity elevated and at rest is likely to fail. Venous disorders are common in the area of the malleoli. When perforating veins become incompetent, this area can be subjected to the entire weight of the column of blood within the vena caval system. Prolonged immobilization and elevation allows graft take without edema fluid separating the graft from its bed. Even after the graft has taken, if dependent edema remains untreated, decreased circulation and oxygen tension can cause the graft to slough. Patients must wear compression stockings for an extended period. Arterial disorders can have a similar deleterious effect on the local circulation.

Traditionally, patients with skin grafts on the lower extremity have been kept at bed rest for 1 to 2 weeks before being allowed to dangle their legs and then ambulate. Bodenham and Watson [32] have successfully ambulated 25 patients with lower limb grafts by 48 hours postoperatively. Their program is to suture the skin edge to the deep fascia with a continuous catgut suture, suture the graft in place with a few sutures, dress the wound, including a 2.5-cm foam pad over the graft, and wrap the leg with an elastic bandage. Ambulation is started 24 to 48 hours postoperatively, beginning with a 15-meter walk and progressing by 1 week to walking freely about the ward. Dressings are left in place until the third to fifth day, at which time the graft is inspected, any hematomas removed, and the complete dressing reapplied. When the graft is over a joint, immobilization of this joint with plaster is advised. Patients are discharged at 2 to 3 weeks postoperatively.

## STORAGE OF SKIN GRAFTS

A simple, effective way to store a split-thickness skin graft is to replace it on the donor site. The graft can then be removed easily and without anesthesia for up to 10 days; at 10 to 14 days it can be removed but with increasing difficulty and pain. Such grafts have been removed from their storage site on the thigh up to 24 days later. Split-thickness skin grafts stored in this manner have been "prepared" so they remain pink when placed on their new recipient site. They have a definitely higher rate of take than grafts stored in saline at 4°C [294].

Split-thickness skin can be refrigerated as long as 21 days and still be used for grafting. Sterile conditions must be maintained while the graft is being covered with a gauze sponge moistened with saline or Ringer's solution and placed in a sterile jar or rubber glove. It is refrigerated at 4°C, a temperature provided by any standard household refrigeration unit. No additional steps are necessary to prepare the graft for use. Several other points are worth mentioning: (1) Immersion of the skin in solution during the period of storage is not advisable because it tends to macerate the skin. (2) The longer a graft is stored, the less likely are its chances of being successfully revascularized when applied to the recipient area. (3) The viability of a skin graft can be maintained for longer periods when it is stored in Hank's tissue culture fluid, which contains plasma and neomycin [94, 100].

CARE OF THE DONOR SITE

After the split-thickness skin graft has been removed from a donor site, it heals by a process of reepithelialization. Epithelial cells from the remains of pilosebaceous units (hair follicles and sebaceous glands) and the sweat glands migrate across the surface until they unite with one another. Anatomically, pilosebaceous units do not extend into the subcutaneous tissue, whereas the sweat glands do. A donor site from which a thick split-thickness skin graft has been removed heals more slowly than one from which a thin graft has been removed. On the average, the donor site of a thin split-thickness skin graft heals within 10 days, whereas that of a medium-thick skin graft heals in 10 to 21 days. The donor area of a thick graft requires 21 to 56 days for healing [62]. The dermis itself is inactive and shows no evidence of regeneration. Thus the portion of the dermis removed with the graft is a net loss to the skin [287].

Donor sites require a proper amount of attention to gain early healing and to prevent them from becoming infected. When an open draining area is to be grafted, it may be advisable to prepare the donor site, remove the graft from it, and dress the area before exposing the infected or contaminated recipient site. The donor site may be cared for in various ways. Rayon cloth, xeroform, adaptic, and Opsite have been used to cover the donor site. The main principle is to protect the area from further mechanical trauma and dehydration. A study performed using several types of gauze, impregnated or not, compared to no dressing revealed that the nondressed site healed at the slowest rate [114, 355]. Hence moist donor areas heal more rapidly than dry areas.

The use of a semipermeable polyurethane membrane such as Opsite has been used to dress the donor sites of split-thickness skin grafts. Its use has been reported to be asso-ciated with almost complete absence of pain and discomfort [84]. With either method, as epithelialization continues the dressing comes away from the donor site in about 2 weeks. Once it is completely exposed, the donor site can be lubricated with either lanolin or cocoa butter.

Split-thickness skin allografts have been shown to be detrimental as a skin graft donor site dressing in that they produce a rejection reaction, which can lead to a full-thickness wound rather than the healed wound that was intended [224]. The nonsemipermeable dressing (i.e., rayon cloth, Xeroform gauze) on the donor site dries on exposure to air for a day or two. Although drying can be hastened with a heat lamp or an electric hair dryer, such maneuvers theoretically would retard epithelialization. Moreover, drying may cause donor site pain and discomfort as the dried dressing cracks on motion.

Delayed healing of the skin graft donor site may be due to infection or to removal of an excessively thick split-thickness skin graft. When the delayed healing is due to removal of a thick graft, it may be best to graft the donor site with a thin split-thickness skin graft from another site. When infection is the major factor in a donor site's failure to heal, it usually requires treatment with moist saline dressings or appropriate topical antibiotic therapy. These dressings are changed frequently (at least every 4 hours).

CHARACTERISTICS OF GRAFTED SKIN

Skin that has been transplanted from one region to another maintains most of its original characteristics, with the exception that sensation and sweating in the graft more closely resemble those of the recipient site.

*Contraction of Grafted Skin*

Skin grafts undergo two types of contraction: primary and secondary.

GRAFT ELASTICITY (PRIMARY CONTRACTION). The elastic fibers of a skin graft cause it to diminish in size as soon as it has been cut.

This process is *not* the biologic process of contraction. This problem can easily be overcome by stretching the graft as it is sutured into place. Because elastic fibers are located in the dermis, thick grafts with a thick dermis contract more than thin grafts. Davis and Kitlowski [79] found that full-thickness skin grafts shrank primarily 41 percent in surface area, whereas thin split-thickness grafts shrank only 9 percent.

CONTRACTION (SECONDARY CONTRACTION). The recipient bed, not the skin graft, is usually the site of contraction. The skin graft simply wrinkles on the contracting bed, permanently decreasing its surface area [267]. This true contracture is what plagues surgeon and patient. It is influenced by the following factors.

1. The thicker a skin graft, the less its tendency to undergo secondary contraction; full-thickness skin grafts show little or no evidence of contracture.
2. The more rigid the recipient bed, the less a skin graft contracts; grafts on the periosteum of bone contract less than grafts on more mobile areas and flexor surfaces.
3. Complete take of a skin graft also decreases its degree of contracture; areas of partial loss of a skin graft heal by contraction and epithelialization from the surrounding skin.

Bed contraction begins about the tenth day after grafting and continues up to 6 months [25, 27, 66, 71, 216]. The contracting force exerts a steady, unrelenting pull on the wound and can easily overcome even the efforts of strong muscles to prevent it. Occasionally, the surface of the skin graft becomes wrinkled because of the contraction of the underlying bed. Splinting of the skin grafted area is a principal means of preventing contraction.

Not all skin contraction is detrimental. In some areas, e.g., the fingertip, a skin graft for replacement of avulsed skin shrinks up to 50 percent, thus pulling normal tactile skin over the area.

## Color of Grafted Skin

Skin grafts and flaps from above the clavicles tend to retain their natural blush shade, whereas those from below the clavicle take on a yellow or brownish hue with no vestige of red coloration. Full-thickness skin grafts from the eyelid and postauricular and supraclavicular regions have a good color and texture match with the skin of the face. Although these grafts are initially redder than the facial skin, they usually pale over a period of months.

A major disadvantage of split-thickness skin grafts from the thigh or abdomen is their yellow, pale brown, and dark brown colors, which match poorly on the face and other exposed areas. Ponten [263] reported that thin split-thickness skin grafts from the same donor site are usually darker than thick ones, making them even less desirable.

Hyperpigmentation of skin grafts is due to the stimulation of melanocytes by both hormones and the ultraviolet rays from the sun. Mir y Mir [229] has demonstrated that dermabrasion lightens the color of hyperpigmented skin grafts. This lightening of the dermabraded skin graft is more permanent if enough time has passed for the graft to become reinnervated. Lopez-Mas et al. [194] found that by taking a split-thickness skin graft from a previously used skin graft donor site, the color match of the previously decolorized skin was retained. No severe hyperpigmentation was observed even on prolonged sun exposure.

Prevention of hyperpigmentation by keeping the grafted skin out of direct sunlight and by applying sunscreen creams that filter out the ultraviolet rays are of assistance. It is more difficult to apply cosmetics to the smooth, shiny surface of a split-thickness skin graft than to normal skin. Tattooing may be used to improve areas of hypopigmentation.

## Accessory Skin Structures in Grafted Skin

Any accessory skin structures (i.e., hair follicles, sebaceous glands, sweat glands) transplanted with a skin graft continue to function, but if not included in the graft, these accessory structures do not regenerate. For practical purposes, only in full-thickness and thick split-thickness skin grafts are hair growth, sebaceous gland function, and sweating retained. These grafts are the only ones thick enough to include the pilosebaceous apparatus and sweat glands [65, 193, 263].

Hair growth can be preserved in full-thickness skin grafts containing functioning hair follicles, and the technique is useful for eyebrow reconstruction and covering bald areas of the scalp with hair [162, 169, 252]. Hair-bearing scalp also can be transplanted successfully with skin punches as large as 12 mm in diameter or strips of scalp up to 5 mm in width. Some of the fat that contains hair follicles is left attached. Characteristically, the transplanted hairs are shed within 3 weeks, and a new growth of hair begins in 8 to 10 weeks.

Sebaceous secretion is destroyed by transplantation except in full-thickness and some thick split-thickness skin grafts, where function returns after several months. Thus skin grafts must be lubricated with lanolin, cocoa butter, or other creams to prevent dryness and crusting during the early postoperative period. Lacking normal lubricants, skin grafts are more prone to develop late infections than normal skin. Patients must be alert to the fact that erythema and tenderness at the site of an old skin graft may represent a beta-streptococcal or other type of infection.

Sweating is destroyed by transplantation except in grafts of full-thickness and some thick split-thickness skin. Its eventual return somewhat parallels that of sensory innervation, which is a prerequisite to sweat gland activity [263]. On the palms, soles of the feet, and axillae sweating is stimulated by emotion, whereas over the rest of the body (including the axillae) it is related to body temperature. After transplantation the sweating pattern of a graft is determined by where it is located. Thus a thick skin graft taken from the abdominal wall and transplanted to the palm is controlled by emotional, rather than thermal, stimuli [263, 315].

## Sensation of Grafted Skin

Nerves regenerate into the graft from both the margins and the graft bed when placed on a sufficiently innervated bed. These growing nerves are distributed randomly throughout the graft. However, in the areas of epidermal appendages, these nerves show a more oriented distribution. Reinnervation of hair follicles, sweat glands, and erector pili muscles has been demonstrated by Waris and colleagues [343, 344]. It is most likely secondary to a chemotactic influence from the target tissues on the regenerating nerves in the immediate vicinity.

When there is no dense scarring in the bed to prevent nerve fibers from penetrating the graft, its final sensation approximates that of the surrounding skin [150, 263, 320]. On the fingertip, Sturman and Duran [320] demonstrated that two-point discrimination in a split-thickness skin graft averaged 5 mm, whereas on the corresponding finger of the opposite normal hand it was 3 mm. The skin graft donor site area on the forearm averaged 33 mm. In a cross-finger flap the two-point discrimination is similar to that of a split-thickness skin graft.

The final return of sensibility in skin grafts placed on a scarred recipient bed, in granulation tissue from bone, or in an area of deep tissue destruction (e.g., full-thickness burns) is always less than in those skin grafts overlying more favorable recipient sites [343, 344]. The four sensory modalities (i.e., pain, touch, heat, and cold), if they return, follow the pattern of the recipient site.

Sensation begins to return 3 weeks after grafting and must be considered to have reached its maximum after 1.5 to 2.0 years [150]. At first there is hyperalgesia, but over a period of months a more normal sensation returns.

*Durability of Grafted Skin*
In general, thick split-thickness skin grafts that have regained sensation are durable. They function well on the palms of the hands and soles of the feet when there is sufficient soft tissue between the graft and the underlying bone for padding. Clearly, protective sensation is required on any weight-bearing surface.

*Growth of Grafted Skin*
Skin grafts grow in a manner paralleling the growth of the total body surface. Both split-thickness and full-thickness skin graft growth has been studied in growing rats. Grafts were placed on 300 sq mm defects and measured over a 3-month period. Following an initial stage of graft shrinkage, there was a secondary phase of growth at the same rate as the growth of the total body surface [173]. Tension was shown to be the greatest influence on growth. Similar growth was shown to occur in skin flaps.

## Flaps

Our choices for reconstruction of external body parts have greatly increased. To our 450-year heritage of skin flaps have been added the (1) muscle flap plus a skin graft, (2) omental flap plus a skin graft, (3) myocutaneous flap, and (4) fascial and fasciocutaneous flaps. These newer types of flap have in common the fact that they are arterialized tissues possessing a longitudinal artery and thus survive to a greater length than the earlier flaps (Fig. 1-17).

Wounds too extensive to permit primary repair by suturing can be closed by a skin graft or flap. Although the skin graft is often the simpler of the two methods and is con-sidered first, there are cases where a flap is required or may be more desirable. Flaps are usually required for covering recipient beds with poor vascularity; reconstructing the full thickness of the eyelids, lips, ears, nose, and cheeks; and padding body prominences (i.e., for bulk and contour); flaps are also used when it is necessary to operate through the wound at a later date to repair underlying structures. In addition, muscle flaps may provide a functional motor unit or a means of controlling infection in the recipient area. In an experimental study, Mathes and colleagues [205] compared musculocutaneous flaps with random flaps to determine the bacterial clearance and oxygen tension of each. Placement of $10^7$ *Staphylococcus aureus* underneath random flaps in dogs resulted in 100 percent necrosis of the flaps within 48 hours; however, the musculocutaneous flaps demonstrated long-term survival. Looking at the quantity of viable bacteria placed in wound cylinders under these flaps showed an immediate reduction of bacteria under the musculocutaneous flap. Oxygen tension was measured at the distal end of the random flap and compared to that underneath the muscle of the distal portion of musculocutaneous flap as well as in its subcutaneous area. It was found that the oxygen tension in the distal random flap was significantly less than in distal muscular and cutaneous portions of the musculocutaneous flap. Flaps, however, have some disadvantages in that they are bulky in appearance, may carry hair into non-hair-bearing areas, and may require multiple operations with long periods of hospitalization. Expressions usually conveyed by the facial muscles can be masked by the thickness and bulkiness of skin flaps used for facial reconstruction.

There are various types of flaps available: skin, muscle, omental, myocutaneous, and free flaps.

SKIN FLAPS
A skin flap consists of skin and subcutaneous tissue that is moved from one part of the body to another with a vascular pedicle

Axial pattern
skin flap

Muscle flap plus
skin graft

Omental flap plus
skin graft

Myocutaneous flap

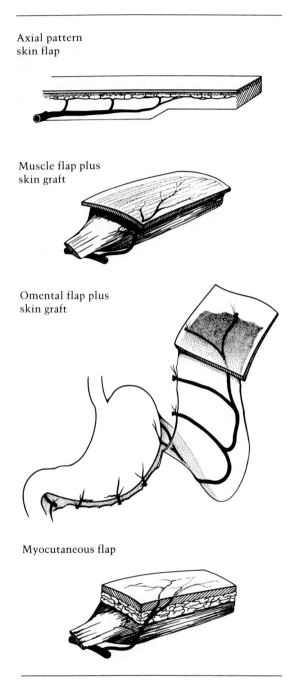

**Figure 1-17** *Arterialized flaps survive to a greater length than flaps that do not include a longitudinal artery. For example, an axial pattern skin flap survives to about 50 percent greater length than a random pattern skin flap.*

or attachment to the body being maintained for nourishment. This vascular attachment can be changed from one part of the flap to another as the flap is transplanted to a new area and can even be changed from one supplying segmental vessel to another by microvascular anastomosis. The word *flap* is used to denote a tongue of tissue, whereas *pedicle* is used to denote its base or stem. Thus the term "pedicle flap" is redundant.

FUNDAMENTAL PRINCIPLES
Although the principles for planning, developing, and transferring skin flaps have grown empirically over a period of centuries, during the past few years these principles have been altered and strengthened by experimental studies. The investigations of Milton [225, 227], Myers and Cherry [240, 241], and Daniel and Williams [75] are especially outstanding. The principles are as follows.

**1.** Think of using a skin graft first. The progression when choosing the type of skin coverage is from skin graft, to local skin flap, to distant skin flap, i.e., *from the simple to the most complex.*

**2.** Plan skin flaps carefully: begin at the recipient site to outline the tissue requirements; make a pattern of them and carry out, in an assimilated fashion, the steps required for transferring the needed tissue from the donor area to the recipient site; and be sure to add extra length on the pattern to allow for the thickness of casts and bandages and for tissue contraction.

**3.** The length of a rectangular single-pedicle or bipedicle skin flap depends on the perfusion pressure in the blood vessels of the flap. In general, it has been demonstrated experimentally that flaps made under similar conditions of blood supply survive to the same length regardless of width [226]. Increasing the width of a flap does not increase the surviving length (Fig. 1-18). The design of a skin flap of safe dimensions must take into account knowledge of the anatomy of the arteries and veins supplying the skin, and the perfusion pressure through these vessels to nourish the tissue. Favorable factors, learned by experience, that permit us to make a longer flap are the following.

*a.* The presence of large blood vessels (direct cutaneous artery and vein) coursing in the longitudinal axis of the flap (i.e., an *axial pattern flap*) are advantageous. Such arterial skin flaps survive to 50 percent greater length than flaps based on the musculocutaneous artery–perforator artery–dermal-subdermal plexi of vessels alone (i.e., a random pattern skin flap) [75, 227]. Thus an arterialized flap has the advantage of providing a great length of skin for immediate coverage, in contrast to a delayed random pattern flap (Fig. 1-19A).

*b.* The location of the flap is on the head and neck, where the vascularity is excellent.

*c.* Transfer of the flap may be delayed. Skin flaps that are delayed survive to somewhere between 60 percent [225] and 100 percent [137] greater length than undelayed flaps based on the musculocutaneous artery–perforator artery–dermal-subdermal vascular plexi [225].

*d.* The flap is designed as a bipedicle rather than a single-pedicle flap.

*e.* Young patients and those without diabetes and arteriosclerosis probably exhibit flap survival to a greater length.

4. Transfer of the flap is delayed when there is a question of its viability; most of these flaps are delayed about 1.0 to 1.5 weeks before being transferred.

5. When dividing the base of a cross-leg flap, one base of a bipedicle flap, or the third side of a delayed flap that was initially delayed by two parallel incisions and undermining, it is best done in two to three stages, each 2 to 3 days apart.

6. When planning flaps below the knee and in areas of scar or radiation therapy, especially in elderly patients, caution is advised because diminished vascularity is a frequent finding. Experimentally, it has been shown that pig skin that recently underwent

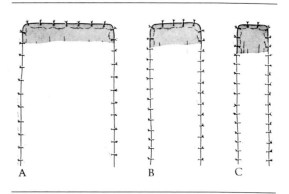

**Figure 1-18** *Experimental skin flaps of varying width. Note that the flaps survive to approximately the same length, regardless of width.*

intensive x-irradiation continues to support a skin flap of almost the same length as that in a control, but at 5 to 6 weeks after irradiation there is a definite reduction in the surviving length of the flap [256].

7. In most regions, the blood supply to the skin flap is via the dermal-subdermal plexus of blood vessels (random pattern skin flap).

8. Excessive tension, kinking, pressure, hematoma, and infection in the flap must be avoided, but if present they are treated promptly.

9. Cigarette smoking has been shown to diminish the rate of wound healing and cause peripheral vasoconstriction. It is also associated in almost a three times greater chance of skin slough after skin flap procedures, i.e., rhytidectomy [269].

## BLOOD SUPPLY OF THE SKIN
### Anatomy

Daniel and Williams [75] and others have underlined the importance of the skin's blood supply when planning a skin flap. The anatomy of the skin's blood supply tells us within reason how we may design and move a specific area of tissue as a flap. The major vessels from the aorta are segmental, anastomotic, or axial arteries. They then give off perforator-musculocutaneous or perforator-

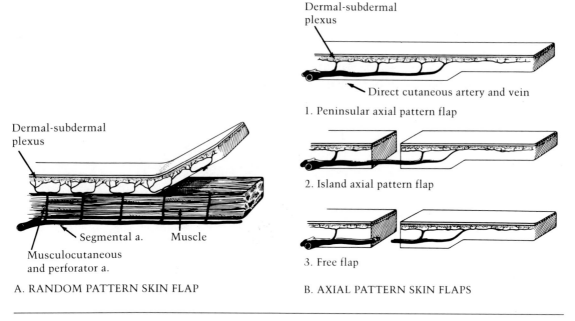

Dermal-subdermal plexus

Direct cutaneous artery and vein

1. Peninsular axial pattern flap

2. Island axial pattern flap

3. Free flap

B. AXIAL PATTERN SKIN FLAPS

Dermal-subdermal plexus

Segmental a.        Muscle

Musculocutaneous and perforator a.

A. RANDOM PATTERN SKIN FLAP

*Figure 1-19 Classification of skin flaps according to their anatomic blood supply. A. Random pattern flaps. These flaps have a segmental, anastomotic, or axial artery and vein coursing deep to the muscle and giving off perforator-musculocutaneous vessels to the dermal-subdermal plexus of the skin. These perforator-musculocutaneous vessels enter the base of the flap, supplying the blood to the plexus in a relatively small area of skin. The dermal-subdermal plexus, however, has a vast interconnection of different-size vessels in the dermal and perifollicular layers, which carry the blood supply to the random pattern flap. B. Axial pattern flaps. These flaps have direct cutaneous vessels, lying subcutaneously just above the muscular fascia, that supply the dermal-subdermal plexus. There is adequate perfusion pressure to support not only the arterial pedicle but also an additional random pattern portion of the flap. The* peninsular flap *has an artery, a vein, and skin in continuity at its base, whereas an* island flap *is connected to the body by only an artery and a vein. The* free flap *is an island flap with the vessels divided prior to being moved so that the vessels can be joined by microvascular techniques to segmental vessels.*

direct cutaneous arteries that supply the dermal-subdermal plexus of the skin. There are two main anatomic patterns of blood supply to the skin of importance to a surgeon planning a skin flap.

The first pattern is one in which the large artery from the aorta or major vessel lies deep to the muscle and sends up *perforator-musculocutaneous branches* to the dermal-subdermal plexus in the skin (most of the skin is supplied by this pattern of vessels). McCraw, Nibbell, and colleagues [208–210] experimentally and clinically have shown that from the perforator-musculocutaneous branches there are hundreds of minute vessels passing to the skin through the deep fascia. There is a dense lateral arborization of vessels at this fascia, and from this subcutaneous location the vessels pass perpendicularly outward to the skin. The second pattern is one in which a *direct cutaneous artery* comes off the large artery by way of a short perforator artery to lie superficial to the muscle and supply the dermal-subdermal plexus. Because the long direct cutaneous arteries are in the lower portion of the

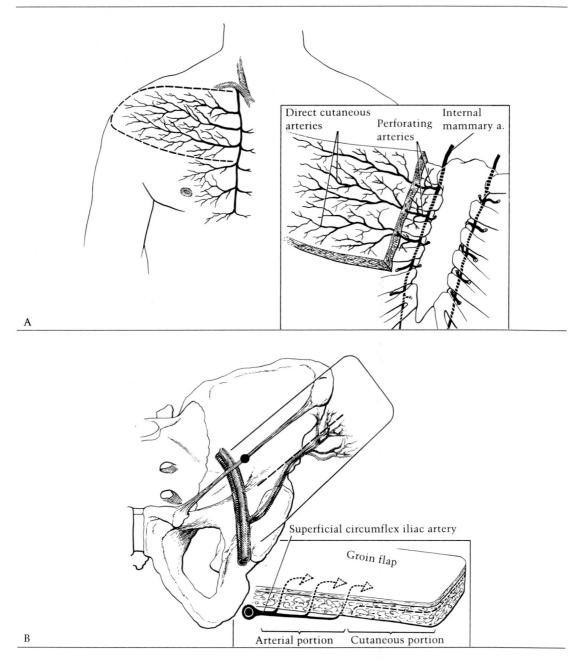

**Figure 1-20** *Examples of axial pattern skin flaps based on direct cutaneous arteries and veins that take advantage of the fact that flaps based on such vessels survive to a 50 percent or more greater length than flaps based on the musculocutaneous–perforator–dermal-subdermal plexus of vessels. A. The* deltopectoral (Bakamjian) flap *is based medially* on the second, third, and fourth anterior perforator arteries of the internal mammary artery. The second perforator is the largest and most important. The superior margin of the flap follows the underlying clavicle, whereas the inferior margin runs laterally at a level approximately three fingerbreadths above the nipple (in the recumbent male), and the lateral

subcutaneous tissue, a skin flap that can be designed to include such an artery survives to a greater length than a randomly based flap.

SEGMENTAL, ANASTOMOTIC, AND AXIAL ARTERIES. The large vessels in the trunk and extremities course deep to the muscles and give off a number of vessels, including those to the skin. Embryologically, there are some 30 rows of dorsal segmental branches from the aorta whose dorsal rami supply the spinal cord and whose ventral rami become the intercostal and lumbar arteries. A longitudinal ventral anastomosis exists between these parallel rows and develops into the internal mammary and epigastric arteries. Axial arteries to the extremities (e.g., brachial and femoral arteries) come off the aorta or major branches of the aorta and lie deep to the muscles proximally and more superficially distally [75].

In general, these segmental, anastomotic, and axial arteries have the following characteristics: (1) They are major arteries that are in continuity with the aorta in regard to perfusion pressure; (2) they course deep to the muscle; and (3) they are accompanied by

a single large vein and often a peripheral nerve [75].

PERFORATOR-MUSCULOCUTANEOUS AND PERFORATOR-DIRECT CUTANEOUS ARTERIES. These vessels arise from a segmental, anastomotic, or axial vessel and carry the blood to the skin. They can be described as follows.

*1. Perforator-musculocutaneous arteries* (providing blood supply for random pattern skin flaps) arise from segmental, anastomotic, and axial vessels, with the perforator portion passing perpendicularly through muscle to exit in the subcutaneous tissue, where its name changes to the musculocutaneous artery. This musculocutaneous artery then terminates in the spider-like dermal-subdermal plexus of the skin. Thus a random pattern flap after being elevated is supplied by perpendicular musculocutaneous arteries at its base and then longitudinally via the dermal-subdermal plexus. Venous drainage is via the same route plus the readily visible subdermal venous network. These vessels comprise the predominant blood supply to the skin of the human body [75].

*2. Perforator-direct cutaneous arteries* (providing blood supply for axial pattern flaps) parallel the skin for long distances [75, 213]. These arteries, which supply the dermal-subdermal plexus directly, lie in the subcutaneous tissue close to the muscle fascia. Venous drainage is by way of the associated named subdermal vein, the paired venae comitantes, and the dermal venous plexus. A listing of the named direct cutaneous arteries in the body include (1) superficial temporal artery (the vascular supply for a variety of forehead and scalp flaps); (2) posterior articular artery; (3) occipital artery; (4) supraorbital artery; (5) supratrochlear artery; (6) facial artery; (7) a grouping consisting of the anterior perforators of the internal mammary artery (arteries of the deltopectoral flap) (Fig. 1-20); (8) perforating branches of the deep epigastric arcade (the arteries of the transverse abdominal flap) [40]; (9) lateral

---

**Figure 1-20** *(continued)*
*margin can extend to the lateral or even posterolateral aspect of the shoulder without being delayed.*
*B. The* groin flap *is based medially, and the outline of the flap has a central axis that lies between a mark made 2.5 cm below the midpoint (solid black circle) of a line connecting the pubic tubercle and the anterior superior iliac spine and 2.5 cm below the anterior superior iliac spine. The flap is then made 7.5 to 10.0 cm wide and can extend 2.5 to 5.0 cm lateral to the anterior superior iliac spine [220]. All axial pattern skin flaps have an arterial and a cutaneous (random pattern) portion. The level of undermining of the arterial portion includes all the subcutaneous tissue so as to include the artery, whereas in the cutaneous portion only enough subcutaneous tissue to protect the subdermal plexus need be retained.*

(long) thoracic artery; (10) superior thoracic arteries (providing blood to the upper end of a thoracoepigastric flap); (11) superficial inferior epigastric artery (providing blood to the lower end of a thoracoepigastric flap); (12) superficial circumflex iliac artery (artery of the groin flap) (Fig. 1-20); (13) superficial external pudendal artery; (14) dorsal artery of the penis [75]; and (15) dorsalis pedis artery.

Hill and colleagues [140] have pointed out that the subdermal vascular plexus extends uninterrupted across the midline as in other areas of the body. Therefore the midline need no longer be considered a barrier to the design of flaps, as demonstrated by the fact that the transverse abdominal flap, the lumbodorsal rotation flap, and the transverse lumbosacral back flap are safe.

*Classification of Skin Flaps According to Their Blood Supply*

**1.** *Random pattern skin flaps* (cutaneous flaps). These flaps receive their blood supply from segmental, anastomotic, or axial arteries that lie deep to the muscle sending perpendicular perforator-musculocutaneous arteries at the flap's base to the interconnecting dermal-subdermal plexus of the skin. Thus they derive their blood supply through the cutaneous dermal-subdermal plexus (see Fig. 1-19). The surviving length of such a flap is related to the vessels' perfusion pressure [75]. Thinning of these flaps is safe so long as a small amount of fat remains to protect the dermal-subdermal plexus. These flaps can be made longer (50 to 100 percent) by the delay procedure, as is discussed subsequently. Most skin flaps are of this type.

**2.** *Axial pattern flaps* (arterial or arterialized flaps). These flaps receive their blood supply through a direct cutaneous artery that arises from a segmental, anastomotic, or axial artery, often by way of a short perforator artery. The length of such a flap is related to the length of the direct cutaneous artery included in the flap plus additional distal skin supplied by the dermal-subdermal plexus (see Fig. 1-19). Thus an arterial flap consists of a proximal arterial pedicle and a more distal cutaneous portion [75]. The arterial pedicle must include the full thickness of subcutaneous tissue because the direct cutaneous artery courses close to the underlying muscular fascia, but the cutaneous portion can be thinned, leaving only a little fat to protect the dermal-subdermal plexus (see Fig. 1-19B). Axial pattern flaps can be made even longer by the delay procedure. These arterialized skin flaps (see Fig. 1-19) can be further subdivided into the following.

a. *Peninsular flaps.* These flaps have a direct cutaneous artery and vein and a bridge of skin and subcutaneous tissue at their base. Examples are the deltopectoral (see Fig. 1-20A) and groin (see Fig. 1-20B) flaps.

b. *Island flaps.* Such flaps are connected to their base by a direct cutaneous artery and vein, with no skin bridge. Examples are the neurovascular island flap of the finger and the superficial temporal artery island flap. Converting a peninsular flap to an island flap provides greater flexibility when rotating the flap about its pivot point [75]. Another variation is to place a split-thickness skin graft directly on the direct cutaneous artery and vein such as has been done by dissecting out the superficial temporoparietal fascia from the scalp with its superficial temporal artery and vein pedicle. This vascularized flap is used to cover a cartilage framework for an external ear reconstruction. A split-thickness skin graft is then placed on the fascia, which is directly supplied by a direct cutaneous artery. This technique transforms a thin, hairless graft into a vascularized flap.

c. *Free flaps.* The perfection of microvascular surgery has enabled the transfer of free axial pattern skin, muscle, and musculocutaneous flaps from a distant site in one operation (see Fig. 1-19). The anatomy of muscle and musculocutaneous flaps that can be used as free flaps have been detailed by Mathes and Nahai [203, 204] and McCraw and Arnold [207]. Donor sites for free skin flaps include the ileofemoral island flap [73], lateral forehead island flap [248], deltopectoral island flap, a scalp flap nourished by the superficial temporal vessels [129, 130], and a neurovascular free flap from the medial arm [74]. Recipient sites are any areas that can supply a donor artery and vein.

Use of free arterialized skin flaps for lower extremity reconstruction has virtually replaced the cross-leg flap or jump flaps. Free flaps have the advantage of decreasing the total time of immobilization and hospitalization as well as the number of operations and cost.

## REQUIREMENTS FOR SURVIVAL OF A SKIN FLAP

When designing and transferring skin flaps, one's preoccupation must always be with the survival of the flap, with care taken that it has a sufficient inflow of arterial blood and outflow of venous blood to remain viable. Among matters that must be considered are the size and location of the flap that can be supported by the available blood supply, delaying the flap to increase its blood supply, and maintaining the blood supply present in the flap.

### Size and Location of the Flap

*There is no rule, no formula, and no proportion of length to width for the safe design of a skin flap.* When designing a skin flap the following information can be helpful: (1) The presence of large blood vessels (direct cutaneous arteries and veins) coursing in the longitudinal axis of the flap permits construction of a longer flap. (2) A flap designed in the head and neck region where the vascularity is greatest can be of more precarious design than in less vascular regions. (3) Delaying a skin flap increases its blood supply and thus its surviving length. (4) A bipedicle

skin flap survives to a greater length than a single-pedicle skin flap. (5) Young patients have a better blood supply to their tissues and thus probably have safe flaps of greater length than elderly patients.

Milton [226] has demonstrated experimentally in the pig the fallacy of the concept that the viable length of a skin flap depends on the width of its pedicle. Rather, he showed that flaps made under similar conditions of blood supply survive to the same length regardless of the width (see Fig. 1-18). Snell [308] has challenged this conclusion by showing in the pig that random pattern flaps with a narrower base (less than 3.0 cm) have a surviving length that increases with their width.

Planning a skin flap so that a large artery and vein enter through the base of the flap definitely increases its surviving length. Milton [227] demonstrated in the pig that the surviving length of skin flaps based on a direct cutaneous artery and vein is 50 percent greater than that of a skin flap based on the musculocutaneous artery–perforator artery–dermal-subdermal plexus.

The vascular supply within a segment of skin varies from area to area, but in general it decreases from the head down to the foot. Single-pedicle flaps of greater length can be designed with greater safety in the head and neck region than around the ankle, where it is usually necessary to delay the flap.

Decisions on the location of a flap or its dimensions must take into account other variables in blood supply. Arteriosclerotic changes decrease the arterial supply of blood to the skin. Such pathologic alterations in circulation must be considered in the design and execution of flaps in older patients [67]. If trauma, infection, or irradiation has resulted in scarring or extensive fibrosis of the skin and subcutaneous tissue, it can also alter the blood supply of a region and the efficiency of its collateral circulation. Several studies suggest that smoking contributes to flap necrosis [12, 30, 58, 68, 179, 234, 269, 273, 346].

*Delaying the Flap*

The term *delaying a flap* is frequently used in the field of reconstructive surgery to indicate that the flap is being developed and transferred in more than a single stage to ensure its safety. Although we understand the basic mechanism of skin flap delay, there is a lack of agreement on the details. There are two schools of thought that were summed up by the demonstrations of Finseth et al. in 1978 [101, 102]. They showed that devascularization (i.e., ligation of arterial or venous vessels to an island flap) and sympathectomy without devascularization produce the delay phenomenon. Thus delay (1) conditions the tissue to survive on less nutrient flow and (2) increases the size and number of functioning vessels partly through sympathectomy.

Hooper [144] reviewed the mechanism of delay and listed five possible mechanisms: (1) sympathectomy; (2) vascular reorganization; (3) reactive hyperemia; and (4) acclimatization to hypoxia. Initial work on sympathectomy and arteriovenous shunts carried out by Reinisch [270] was later disproved by Kenigan [164]. Pharmacologic delay [101, 271] has also been shown to be effective in delaying a skin flap.

Goetz [120, 121] studied by plethysmography the amount of blood flowing through normal skin under various circumstances. During rest the flow is 15 ml per minute for 100 cc of tissue, and with full vascular dilatation it is 90 ml per minute; however, the skin needs a flow of only 1 to 2 ml per minute to provide nutrition for 100 cc of tissue. Burton [49] has emphasized that the primary purpose of the blood supply to the skin is for thermoregulation (90 to 97 percent), not nutrition (3 to 10 percent). It is fortunate that such a low rate of flow sustains the skin, as Hoffmeister has shown that there is a profound drop in the circulatory efficiency of a flap immediately following incision and undermining [141].

Jonsson et al. [160], in an excellent study, measured tissue oxygen in skin flaps to re-evaluate the delay phenomenon. After the initial delay incision blood flow was re-routed parallel to the incision, a finding also shown by Velander [341]. The blood flow initially is increased by vasodilatation and then by angiogenesis. The vasodilatation is due to the release of acute inflammatory mediators, and the angiogenesis is probably due to a chemoattractant from macrophages in hypoxic areas [149, 172]. Jonsson et al. concluded that: "[t]here may be nothing particularly unique about surgical flap delay. It seems to be a useful sequence of inflammation, hemodynamic flow changes and angiogenesis in the wound of elevation that provides a temporarily improved collateral circulation to surrounding tissue" [160].

Clinically, most surgeons prefer delaying the skin flap by incision on the two parallel sides and undermining (Fig. 1-21), then dividing the third side in two or three stages, 2 or 3 days apart, beginning 7 days after the initial procedure. Such staging can usually be carried out under local anesthesia on an outpatient basis. Often the first incision across the end of the flap consists in dividing one-half of the remaining intact skin and resuturing it, and the second stage consists in division of the one-fourth or even the remaining one-half of intact skin. Although time-consuming, these staged incisions give us assurance that when the flap is finally moved it remains viable.

When one end of the flap is divided and transplanted, it usually takes 4 to 5 days before venous connections can be demonstrated (by microangiography) to have developed between the flap and the recipient site. Arterial anastomoses are not seen for 7 days. The number of arterial and venous connections increases rapidly during the second week [341]. Myers and Cherry [241] showed in the rabbit that the maximal surviving length of experimental skin flaps occurred at 8 to 10 days after delay. There was even a definitely increased survival at 4 days, reaching a maximum at 8 to 10 days, and then falling off. There was still a definitely

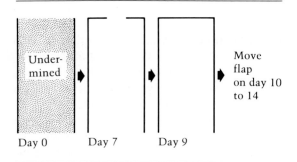

**Figure 1-21** *Delay of a random pattern skin flap. Initially the flap is incised on its two parallel sides, and the area of the flap is undermined. Seven days after this initial procedure, division of the third side is begun and is continued in stages usually 2 or 3 days apart. The flap is then moved 2 or 3 days after completion of this division of the third side.*

increased survival up to 21 days, the longest delay time studied. Hoffmeister [141], after studying the rates of radioactive sodium ($^{24}$Na) clearance, suggested that a flap that had been delayed by incising on three sides and then undermined could best be transferred about 2 to 4 weeks after being developed. Most flaps can be divided at 10 days to 3 weeks [113].

The use of a tourniquet or rubber-shod clamp across the base of a flap in an attempt to increase its vascular supply is not as effective as incising and undermining. Temporarily clamping the flap produces only a transient reactive hyperemia.

EXPANSION AS A FORM OF DELAYING A SKIN FLAP OR MYOCUTANEOUS FLAP. Tissue expansion provides donor tissue for reconstruction by increasing the surface area of the skin. Cherry et al. [52] compared the surviving lengths of random patterned skin flaps elevated on expanded tissue to nonexpanded bipedicled flaps delayed for 5 weeks. There was a trend toward increased survival length in the expanded flaps over the classically delayed flaps (14.3 ± 0.9 for expanded flaps, 11.4 ± 1.7 for delayed flaps). However, there was no statistically significant difference

between the two. Cherry et al. [52] and subsequently Sasaki and Pang [285] noted an increase in the vascularity of the flap associated with tissue expansion.

Barnhill and Ryan [19] demonstrated that simple mechanical force applied to vessels leads to an increase in vascularity. Although the mechanism for increased vascularity of expanded tissue is not known, the physical forces of expansion may act as a stimulus for angiogenesis.

Forte et al. [107], through experiments on pigs, demonstrated the feasibility of expanding musculocutaneous flaps. They reported a mean increase of 32 percent axial length and 51 percent width compared with nonexpanded controls. Using angiography, they noted an increase in nonspecific vessels supplying the flaps. Thorton et al. [334] clinically expanded and free transferred two musculocutaneous flaps.

The next logical progression in expansion research was reported by Stark et al. [314]. They showed experimentally that elongation of arteries and veins through tissue expansion is possible. In histologic, postexpanded sections, there was no reduction in vessel wall diameter or loss of intimal integrity. Microvascular anastomoses were performed with the elongated vessel with patency equal to that of nonelongated vessels.

TESTS OF CIRCULATION. Various tests of the circulation in a skin flap have been developed to aid in determining when the pedicle of a direct flap can be divided, if a flap that has been elevated can survive, and the earliest time a delayed flap can be moved safely. Harrison et al. [131] have reviewed elsewhere their experiences with monitoring the circulation of flaps.

There has been a trend toward earlier division of the pedicle of direct flaps. For example, the vermilion-bordered lip flap (Abbé flap) can be divided at 8 days [305] and the cross finger flap at 12 to 14 days [171].

The intravenous fluorescein test, a measure of the perfusion of tissues, is considered by many to be the best clinical test to predict skin flap viability *at the time of operation* [335]. However, it is far from ideal, and many experienced reconstructive surgeons do not rely on it. For this test, 20 ml of 5% sodium fluorescein is injected rapidly intravenously about 20 minutes after the flap has been raised. The almost immediate yellow fluorescence of the patient's epithelial surfaces is noted with an ultraviolet light in a darkened room. Areas of spotty fluorescence can be stroked with a hemostat, and if a yellow line appears where the flap was stroked the skin usually survives. Myers [237–239] has used this method for predicting the adequacy of blood supply to the skin of anterior chest skin flaps for closure after radical mastectomy. In some 65 cases there was a definite correlation of fluorescence (yellowish-green in ultraviolet light) with skin survival and of nonfluorescence (purplish-blue) with skin necrosis, but these correlations were not universal. Areas of nonfluorescence have an impaired blood supply and go on to necrosis; such areas must be excised. Goode and Linehan [122] reported a similar finding in 20 patients with irradiated neck skin who had a Y incision for radical neck dissection. These surgeons were successful for predicting skin viability in irradiated necks. However, they were not as successful for predicting skin viability in nonirradiated neck flaps, as there were false negatives due to the distal end of the flap not taking up the dye but remaining viable. At least one anaphylactic reaction to intravenous fluorescein has been reported with pruritus and partial respiratory obstruction [177].

The Doppler flowmeter can be used to monitor flow in even the small arteries of an arterialized flap. This instrument can also be used to map out the course of vessels in the axial pattern skin flap.

Other tests of circulatory efficiency include the following:

1. The histamine wheal test is a simple method of evaluating circulation in a skin flap. The rate of skin wheal formation in the flap is compared to wheal formation in a control area of skin [262].
2. A radioisotope can be injected into the flap and its rate of disappearance from the flap compared with that from a control area on the opposite side of the body [20, 135, 141, 325].
3. The absorption of atropine from the flap is noted as evidenced by tachycardia, inability to focus on newsprint, and dryness of the mouth [151].
4. The photoplethysmograph, which utilizes changes in the amount of light reflected by tissues to normal pulsatile blood flow, has been used successfully to determine the proper time for moving a delayed or distant skin flap [2, 137, 333].
5. The temperature of the flap is determined by thermography using an infrared scanner in a controlled environment [31, 332].
6. The saline wheal test, which has the disadvantage of requiring an hour to execute, has an indistinct endpoint [318].
7. A thermocouple may be used to measure skin temperature, a method that is probably too imprecise for clinical use [89, 352].
8. Tissue $PO_2/PCO_2$ may be measured.

### MAINTAINING THE BLOOD SUPPLY OF THE FLAP

Once a skin flap with an adequate blood flow has been moved to its recipient site, it can survive unless there is tension, kinking, pressure, hematoma, or infection in the flap or systemic changes such as hypotension or severe hypoxia. Each of these conditions must be treated.

Tension may develop in a local flap if it is stretched tightly in order to reach the furthest extent of the wound. Blanching of the skin along the line of greatest tension (the line between the pivot point and that part of the flap most distant to it) may be seen in rotation, transposition, and interpolation of flaps if they are stretched too tightly (Fig. 1-22; see also Figs. 1-24 and 1-27). Sundell [321] showed that a small tensile force (25

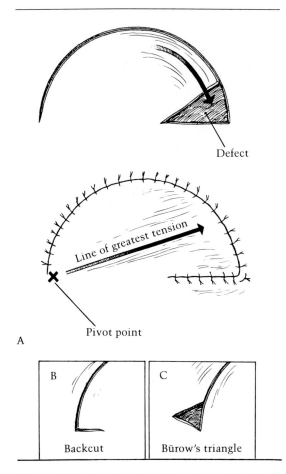

*Figure 1-22 Rotation flap. The edge of the flap is four to five times the length of the base of the defect triangle. A back-cut or a Burow's triangle can be used if the flap is under too much tension, although proper planning makes this measure unnecessary.*

gm) was sufficient to lead to venous congestion and partial flap necrosis unless the tension was released within 4 hours.

Kinking is most likely to occur in tubed pedicle flaps. It can be corrected by proper repositioning or immobilization, so there is no acute angulation of the flap.

Pressure may be either external or internal in origin. External pressure from too tight a dressing or compression of the flap by the patient's position can be easily corrected. Internal pressure, by contrast, is usually more

difficult to correct if it results from including too much fatty tissue in a tubed pedicle. Milton [225] studied the problems of enclosing enough fat in the tubed arterial flap to preserve the vessels without strangling the circulation by too much tension. It has been calculated that edema causes flaps to increase in weight by 35 percent during the first 24 hours. Allowing for this percentage of swelling, Milton calculated that the width must be at least 17 times the thickness of the tubed flap to prevent pressure necrosis.

Hematoma in a flap is treated by returning the patient to the operating room, evacuating the clotted blood, and obtaining absolute hemostasis. Initially, it was thought that the internal pressure caused by a hematoma can cause necrosis of the flap, but it was shown by Mulliken and Healey [235] to be untrue. By instilling different solutions and even silicone implants underneath raised flaps, they were able to show that "internal pressure" was not the cause of flap loss. Instead, it was something in the red blood cells (RBCs) or RBC hemolysate. Manson et al. [199] brought up the idea that skin flap necrosis involved superoxide radicals. Indeed, it is the hemoglobin in the RBCs that supplies the needed iron to help catalyze the superoxide–free radical reaction:

$$O_2^- + H_2O_2 \xrightarrow[\text{Fe}^{+2}]{M_A} OH \cdot OH^- + O_2$$

Angel et al. [6, 7], in a review of the density and pathophysiology of free radicals, showed how this free radical mechanism plays a major role in hematoma-induced necrosis [312].

Infection in a skin flap during the early postoperative period may be disastrous. Because of its decreased blood flow, a recently elevated flap may be capable of supplying or supporting only its basic metabolic needs [121] and is unable to provide the increased flow needed for an inflammatory reaction. Thus an infection that might be of little consequence in normal tissue can readily destroy the poorly vascularized tissue of a skin flap. Treatment consists in proper drainage, frequent wet dressing changes, and antibiotics.

Epinephrine is not detrimental to flaps raised primarily. However, the surviving length of a delayed flap is impaired by epinephrine [271].

Special consideration must be given to the effects of smoking. Studies in animals have provided evidence to support the hypothesis that smoking adversely effects wound healing. Rees et al. [269] showed that a significant number of skin sloughs after a facelift were due to patients smoking cigarettes. The effects are secondary to nicotine, which has been implicated in impairing the inflammatory phase and epithelialization of wound healing. Nicotine has also been shown to liberate catecholamines from sympathetic nerve endings and other sites and in this way produces sustained peripheral vasoconstriction [234, 273, 347]. It is currently thought that continued smoking, approximately 2 weeks preoperatively and postoperatively, leads to significant morbidity in any flap procedure.

DESPERATION MEASURES TO IMPROVE THE CIRCULATION IN A FLAP
A great deal of effort has been devoted to finding ways in which a flap with vascular insufficiency can be salvaged. Unfortunately, most of the methods described are of limited clinical value for improving the compromised circulation of a flap. *They never serve as a substitute for proper planning.*

Postural assistance to venous outflow from the flap may be of some benefit. It has been observed that if the base of a tubed flap is placed in a dependent position gravity may aid the flow of venous blood from the flap [152, 162]. Returning the flap to its recipient site probably has its most sound application when there is tension on the flap. Most of these measures have not been properly evaluated with suitable controls and are clinical observations.

Cooling the flap to a surface temperature between 0° and 20°C within 4 hours of operation reduces the severity of necrosis in experimental skin flaps but does not prevent it [110]. Such extreme cooling of flaps has not been adopted clinically.

The use of leeches *(Hirudo medicinalis)* have again become popular for relieving venous congestion in flaps of reattached digits [83, 182]. Leeches feed on mammalian blood, and their ingestion of blood can be up to 900 percent of their body weight. The saliva of *H. medicinalis* contains (1) hirudin, the most powerful anticoagulant known; (2) eglin, a leukocyte elastase inhibitor that inhibits superoxide radical production by neutrophils; (3) hyaluronidase; and (4) collagenase. Because of the hirudin, the wound continues to bleed for several hours after the leech detaches, which is good for a blood-engorged flap or digit. After the leech has ingested its meal, it falls off the subject. Because leeches have no proteolytic enzymes in the gut, they depend on a bacterium, *Aeromonas hydrophila,* to digest the blood. This situation has led to infections with *Aeromonas* in about 20 percent of patients. Therefore all patients who have leech therapy must be treated prophylactially with a β-lactamase-resistant antibiotic (i.e., Augmentin or cephalosporin) [219, 275].

*Low-Molecular-Weight Dextran*
Low-molecular-weight dextran (LMWD) is commonly used to alter pharmacologically the clotting mechanism during flap and microvascular surgery. Evidence shows that dextran reduces platelet adhesiveness, increases blood flow, and changes the fibrin structure of a clot to make it more amenable to fibrinolysis [88, 167, 254]. LMWD is given before the donor flap is harvested and is continued for approximately 3 days.

Eklöf et al. [93] investigated incomplete ischemia of the legs caused by aortic clamping. They suggested that LMWD prevents rheologic changes impairing the microcirculation during and after the ischemic period.

*Hyperbaric Oxygen Therapy*

The use of hyperbaric oxygen therapy to enhance flap or even skin graft survival remains equivocal. Both success and failure have been reported [10, 51, 165]. Davis [77], reviewing the place of hyperbaric oxygen therapy for skin grafts or flaps, concluded that it is *not* indicated for normal viable skin grafts or flaps. However, for skin flaps where the circulation has been interrupted or poor, there was an increase in flap length viability compared to controls not treated with hyperbaric oxygen.

*Fluorocarbons*

Fluorocarbons in the presence of a high oxygen environment for approximately 48 hours has been shown to significantly enhance flap survival in rats [54]. When a portion of a skin flap has definitely become necrotic, it is best to excise that portion immediately. Infection in necrotic tissue that is left in place acts to spread the extent of tissue loss.

PLANNING A SKIN FLAP

Proper planning of a flap is essential to the success of the operation. All possible sites and orientations for the flap must be considered to be certain that the most suitable one is selected.

Planning the flap in reverse is probably the most important part of the operation. A pattern of the defect is transferred onto a piece of cloth toweling (Fig. 1-23). The steps in the operative procedure are carried out in reverse order, using this pattern until the donor site is reached. If the flap is pedicled, it is important that the pattern is cut to in-

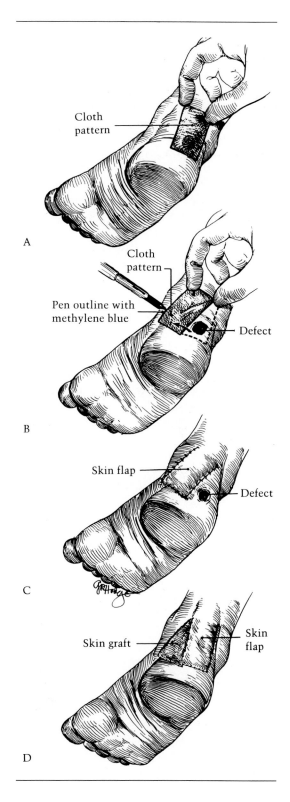

**Figure 1-23** *Planning a skin flap in reverse to cover a defect over the Achilles tendon.*
*A, B. With a cloth pattern the steps of the flap transposition are carried out; the base of the flap is held firmly in place. C. The flap is delayed because of the relatively poor blood supply of the foot and the excessive length-to-width ratio of this flap. D. Three weeks later the flap is transposed.*

clude the base of the flap and that it is made a little longer and wider than needed. The pattern is then tried again, being certain each time it is shifted that the base is held in a fixed position and not allowed to shift with the flap. The final pattern must be larger than needed, particularly its length, to avoid undue tension and kinking. It is easier to trim a flap that is slightly large than to add to one that is too small.

Planning a transposition or rotation flap requires special attention to ensure that the line of greatest tension from the pivot point to the most distal part of the flap is of sufficient length (Figs. 1-22 and 1-24). Flaps to be transferred from a distance are outlined with an additional margin of reserve in length, so the pedicle is not kinked or under tension during transfer.

All planning is done prior to operation when all of the possible sites and orientations of the flap can be considered adequately. The final pattern can then be sterilized for use in the operating room.

### Classification of Skin Flaps and Operative Technique

The use of many "skin flaps" has now been superceded by the use of myocutaneous and free flaps. However, many skin flap principles are helpful, especially for facial and extremity defects. Always remember to plan a skin flap that gives the best functional and aesthetic result. Too often the neophyte plastic surgeon becomes enamored of a flap discovered in a text such as this one. Although there may be great pleasure in surgical execution, the results may fall far short of the aesthetic possibilities that a much simpler procedure, which considers aesthetic units and lines of tension/relaxation, can accomplish.

Skin flaps can be classified as to their anatomic blood supply: *random pattern skin flaps*, supplied by a perforating musculocutaneous artery(s)–dermal-subdermal plexus, and *axial pattern skin flaps*, supplied by direct cutaneous arteries to the dermal-sub-

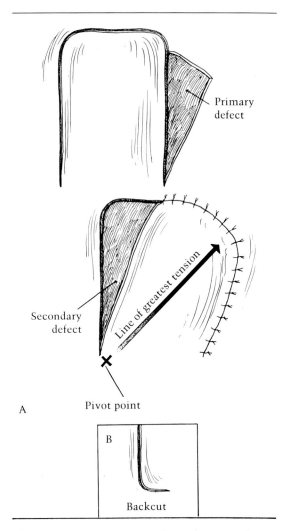

**Figure 1-24** *Transposition flap. The secondary defect is often closed by a skin graft. A back-cut can be used if the flap is under too much tension.*

dermal plexus. Skin flaps can also be classified as to where they are moved. The latter classification includes local skin flaps, distant skin flaps, and variations on this theme: free flaps, Crane principle flaps, and composite flaps.

LOCAL SKIN FLAPS. Local flaps contain tissues lying adjacent to the defect, which usually match the skin at the recipient site in color, texture, hair, and thickness. Such flaps require fewer operative stages and a shorter period of hospitalization than flaps from a distance. Atraumatic technique is important to the success of these flaps, and skin hooks are used for handling and rotating the flap to its new site. Half-buried horizontal mattress sutures or simple interrupted sutures can be used for approximating the skin margins. Large flaps are drained with a catheter connected to suction if there is reason to believe that fluid might accumulate underneath the flap. Pressure must be kept off the flap.

Local flaps are usually applied directly to the recipient site without leaving the subcutaneous surface of the pedicle exposed. These flaps may be closed or lined by applying a split-thickness skin graft to the undersurface of the flap or by folding the flap on itself.

Local skin flaps are of two types: (1) flaps that rotate about a pivot point (rotation, transposition, and interpolation flaps); and (2) advancement flaps (single pedicle advancement, V-Y advancement, Y-V advancement, and bipedicle advancement flaps). It bears mention that all of these local flaps are more easily executed in the older patient, whose skin is looser and adapts to a change in location more easily.

*Flaps Rotating About a Pivot Point.* Rotation, transposition, and interpolation flaps have in common a pivot point and an arc through which the flap is rotated. The radius of this arc is the line of greatest tension of the flap. The realization that these flaps can be rotated only about the pivot point is important to their planning.

The rotation flap is a semicircular flap of skin and subcutaneous tissue that rotates about a pivot point into the defect to be closed (see Figs. 1-22 and 1-24). Its donor site can be closed by a skin graft or by direct suture of the wound.

The line of greatest tension in a rotation flap extends from the pivot point outward in the direction indicated in Figures 1-22 and 1-24. Careful preoperative planning in reverse ensures that rotation of the flap into

the defect can be accomplished without excessive tension.

When the donor site is closed with a split-thickness skin graft, a tie-over dressing may prove advantageous; it permits pressure to be maintained on the skin graft without putting pressure on the skin flap. Sutures for the tie-over dressing are not placed in the flap but, rather, through the bed for the skin graft adjacent to the flap. These sutures are placed through the graft so that the edge of the graft can be approximated to the edge of the flap (Fig. 1-25). The donor site sometimes cannot be closed by primary suture because often this method places excessive tension on the flap itself.

A flap that is too tight along its radius can be released by making a short back-cut from the pivot point along the base of the flap (see Fig. 1-24B). Because this back-cut decreases the blood supply to the flap, its use requires some degree of caution. With some flaps it is possible to back-cut only the tissue responsible for the tension, without reducing the blood supply to the flap. Examples of this selective cutting are found in the galea aponeurotica of the scalp and in areas over the trunk where the fascia within the thick subcutaneous layer can be divided. The necessity for a back-cut may be an indication of poor planning.

A triangle of skin (Burow's triangle [48]) can be removed from the area adjacent to the

**Figure 1-25** *The skin flap donor site can be closed with a split-thickness skin graft that is held in place with a tie-over dressing. The tie-over sutures are inserted through the base of the wound, rather than at the edge of the flap.*

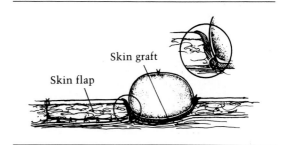

Skin graft

Skin flap

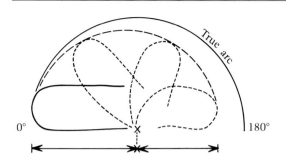

**Figure 1-26** *A skin flap rotated about a pivot point becomes shorter in effective length the farther it is rotated. Planning with a cloth pattern is most helpful when designing such a flap.*

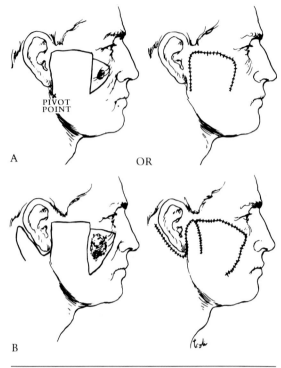

**Figure 1-27** *Transposition flap that can be used to close defects on the anterior cheek. A. Small defects can be closed by a single transposition cheek flap that follows the skin lines. B. Large defects can be closed by a double transposition flap that uses a flap of postauricular skin to close the cheek flap donor site.*

pivot point of the flap to aid its advancement and rotation (see Fig. 1-22C). This method is of only modest benefit in decreasing tension along the radius of the flap.

Gibson and Kenedi [117] have shown that the initial pull to stretch skin permits considerable stretching with little force. With continued force the stretching decreases rapidly, and then finally little stretching is produced by markedly increased force. This increased force produces blanching of the skin along the line of greatest tension, which Gibson and Kenedi were able to relieve by a tiny incision through the skin at right angles to, and in the center of, the blanched zone. Such a maneuver may be necessary when flap planning is inadequate.

The transposition flap is a rectangle or square of skin and subcutaneous tissue that also is rotated about a pivot point into an immediately adjacent defect (see Fig. 1-24). This fact necessitates that the end of the flap adjacent to the defect be designated to extend beyond it (Figs. 1-26 and 1-27). Then, as the flap is rotated, with the line of greatest tension as the radius of the rotation arc, the advancing tip of the flap is sufficiently long.

The flap donor site can be closed by skin grafting, direct suture of the wound, or a sec-

ondary flap from the most lax skin at right angles to the primary flap. An example of the last technique is the *bilobed flap* (Fig. 1-28) [81]. The key to a successful bilobed flap is an area of loose skin to permit direct closure of the secondary flap defect [81]. Pinching the skin between the examiner's fingers helps find the loosest skin, e.g., in the glabellar area and lateral to the eyelids. Care must be taken when selecting this theoretical maneuver because the aesthetic result may be disastrous.

The Z-plasty is another example of the transposition flap. Each of two adjacent triangular skin flaps is rotated into the defect left by the other flap (see Fig. 1-36). The Z-

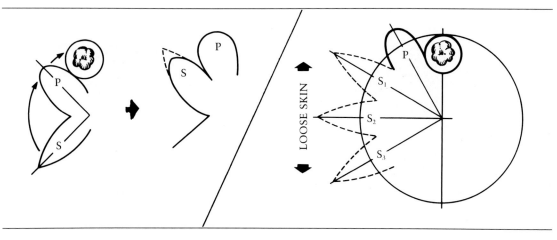

**Figure 1-28** *Bilobed flap. After the lesion at the top is excised, the primary flap (P) is transposed into the initial defect. The secondary flap (S) is then transposed into the defect left after the primary flap has been moved. The primary flap is slightly narrower than the defect caused by excision of the initial lesion, and the secondary flap is half the diameter of the primary flap. For the bilobed flap to be successful, the secondary flap must come from an area of loose skin, so the defect remaining after moving this secondary flap can be closed by approximation of the wound edges. Three possible choices for the secondary flap ($S_1$, $S_2$, $S_3$) are depicted.*

plasty is discussed extensively later in the chapter.

The *Limberg flap* is another transposition flap. This flap, like the bilobed flap and the Z-plasty, depends on the looseness of adjacent skin, which can be located by pinching various areas of skin between thumb and forefinger. Fortunately, most patients requiring local skin flaps are in the older age group and therefore have looser skin. A Limberg flap is suitable only for closure of rhomboid defects with angles of 60 and 120 degrees [157, 186, 188]. With the Limberg flap, the sides are of the same length as the short axis of the rhomboid defect. The planning of such a flap is illustrated in Figures 1-29 and 1-30.

The *Dufourmentel flap* is similar, except that it can be used for rhomboids with an-

gles up to 90 degrees [157, 186] and its planning is more complex. Because a rhomboid with an angle of 90 degrees can be converted to one with angles of 60 and 120 degrees by additional skin excision, we prefer to use the Limberg flap. Results are variable with both flaps, however [157].

An *interpolation flap* consists of skin and subcutaneous tissue rotated in an arc about a pivot point into a nearby, but not immediately adjacent, defect. The pedicle of this flap must therefore pass over or under the intervening tissue. The deltopectoral (Bakamjian) flap (see Fig. 1-20A), probably the most common interpolation flap still used, is a useful interpolation flap for head and neck reconstruction. In these examples of interpolated flaps, the pedicle of the flap passes across the surface of the intervening skin. The exposed portion of the pedicle may be closed with a skin graft, but it is usually unnecessary.

By definition, an *island flap* is another type of interpolation flap in which an island of skin with its neurovascular pedicle (in the hand) or an arteriovenous pedicle (in the face) is transferred through a tunnel underneath the skin and sutured into its new position.

*Advancement Flaps.* All advancement flaps are moved directly forward into a defect

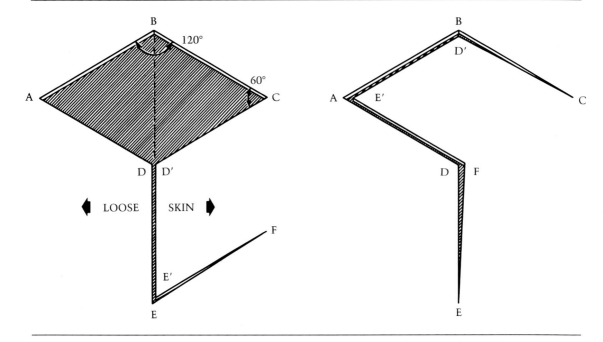

without any rotation or lateral movement. Modifications are the single pedicle advancement, the **V-Y** advancement, and the bipedicle advancement flaps.

The single pedicle advancement flap is a rectangular or square flap of skin and subcutaneous tissue that is stretched forward. Advancement is accomplished by taking advantage of the elasticity of the skin (Fig. 1-31A) and by excising Burow's triangles lateral to the flap (Fig. 1-31B). These triangular excisions help to equalize the length between the sides of the flap and adjacent wound margins.

The V-Y advancement technique has numerous applications. It is not an advancement in the same sense as the forward movement of a skin flap just described. Rather, a V-shaped incision is made in the skin, after which the skin on each side of the V is advanced and the incision closed as a Y (Fig. 1-32). This V-Y technique can be used to lengthen such structures as the nasal columella, eliminate minor notches of the lip, and in certain instances close the donor site of a skin flap.

**Figure 1-29** *Planning a rhomboid (Limberg) flap. The rhomboid defect must have 60- and 120-degree angles. The flap is planned in an area of loose skin so that direct closure of the wound edges is possible. The short diagonal BD (which is the same length as each side) is extended by its own length to point E. The line EF is drawn parallel to CD and is of the same length. After the flap margins have been incised, the flap is transposed into the rhomboid defect.*

Y-V advancement flap is just the opposite to the V-Y advancement flap. Y-V flaps are usually used in a serial arrangement to release skin scar contractures, such as occur with Dupuytren's contracture. The advancement is obtained in a direction perpendicular to the axis of the scar contracture (Fig. 1-33). For multiple Y-V flaps (Fig. 1-34), there are usually four flaps, the advancing angle is about 90 degrees, and the maximum length of the straight limb of the Y is determined by the amount of lateral give but does not exceed one-third the length of the side [18]. The theoretical gain is 1.4 times the straight limb of the Y. This procedure, however, is rarely used because of the good lengthening one can obtain with Z-plasties.

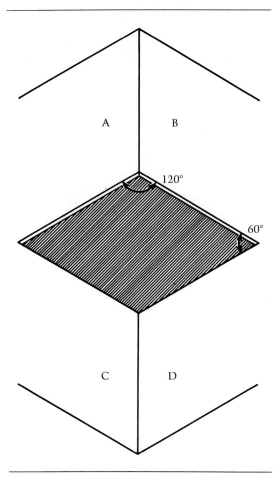

**Figure 1-30** *There are four Limberg flaps available for any rhomboid defect with 60- and 120-degree angles.*

Advancement flaps have the limitation of aiding closure only of defects of short length because tension decreases the flow of blood in the flap. Patients in the older age groups have looser skin, which increases the extent to which these flaps can be advanced.

DISTANT SKIN FLAPS. Flaps can be constructed at a distance from the defect and then transferred to it, either directly (e.g., by raising a skin flap on the chest wall and positioning the defect on a hand under the flap) or indirectly (e.g., by raising a skin flap on the anterior aspect of the trunk and then using the wrist as a carrier to transfer it to surface a large defect on the face). Of course, the

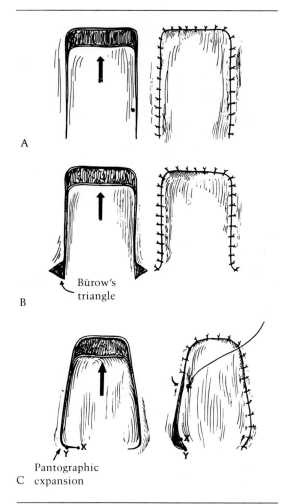

**Figure 1-31** *Single pedicle advancement flaps. A. Advancement by taking advantage of the skin's elasticity. B. Advancement by excising Burow's triangles of skin laterally to equalize the length of the flap and the adjacent wound edge. C. Pantographic expansion.*

**Figure 1-32** *V-Y advancement. It is the skin on each side of the V that is actually advanced.*

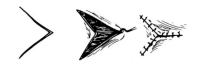

use of the latter is rare, having been supplanted by free flaps with microvascular anastomoses.

*Direct Flaps from a Distance.* Direct flaps are usually of the open type and can be constructed and transferred in a single stage.

*Direct flaps from the trunk* are usually transferred to the upper extremity. White [349] has described a V-shaped flap from the relatively hairless area on the lower anterior chest wall, a site that has a relatively thin subcutaneous layer (Fig. 1-35). The base of the flap, if placed laterally, takes advantage of the better blood supply but does not cross the midline medially. If the upper or lower limb of the V incision is extended for a distance equal to the width of the flap's base, the flap can be rotated 180 degrees to facilitate primary closure of the donor site. The flap is sutured directly into the defect on the upper extremity. The arm is held to the side, and the area between the arm and the chest must be padded carefully. After 10 to 14 days the immobilizing dressing may be discontinued. At 2½ weeks after the initial operation, the base of the pedicle can be divided under local anesthesia.

Large rectangular flaps can be elevated from the anterior aspect of the trunk and transferred directly to the upper limb. The donor site is usually closed with a skin graft and a tie-over dressing. In these cases the base of the pedicle also can be divided after 2½ weeks in two or three stages, a few days apart.

*Direct flaps from an upper extremity* are most often used for repairing the contralat-

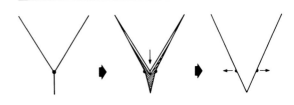

*Figure 1-33* Y-V advancement flap.

eral upper extremity (cross-arm flap) or the face (Tagliacozzi flap). The cross-arm flap is advantageous for closing defects on the hand and fingers because it provides thin skin with a minimum of subcutaneous tissue. A flap with either a single pedicle or a bipedicle is raised from the relatively hairless area on the flexor surface of the forearm or the anterior surface of the upper arm. Single-pedicle flaps are based proximally. Although the injured hand is joined to the opposite forearm or upper arm, the free hand can still be moved through a range of positions from the head to the perineum with little difficulty. The flap can be divided at its base in one or two stages beginning at 2 to 2½ weeks. The major disadvantage of this procedure is the long period of immobilization and resultant stiffness of the elbow and shoulder. Its use is *not* recommended for patients over age 40.

For small defects on the fingers, a cross-finger flap is often satisfactory.

The use of a skin flap from the upper arm for nasal reconstruction was first described

*Figure 1-34* Multiple Y-V advancement flaps.

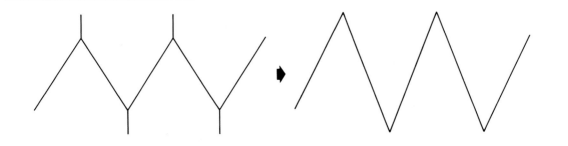

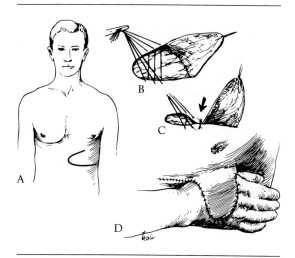

**Figure 1-35** *Direct skin flap from the lower anterior chest wall to an upper extremity. The lateral incisions are staggered at the base of the flap to permit rotation of the flap 180 degrees and primary closure of the flap donor site. The length of the longest side of the flap is designed to be longer than the shorter side by the same distance as the width of the base of the flap, as measured directly across from the end of the shorter limb.*

by Tagliacozzi in 1597 [324]. Proximally based flaps can be elevated and transferred in a single stage. When there is enough nasal skin available, it is turned down as an inner lining for the flap.

*Direct flaps from a lower extremity* are most often used on the opposite leg to provide stable coverage of exposed tendon or bone on the foot, ankle, lower leg, or knee. The calf is used most frequently as the donor site. When planned with a wide base, this flap can be transferred directly to the opposite extremity.

In children the lower extremity may be limber enough to permit a skin flap to be applied directly to the foot from the dorsum of the upper thigh or buttock [231]. Sharp flexion of the knee is required to permit use of this direct flap from a distance. Again, a major disadvantage is the prolonged immobilization period and resultant joint stiffness.

Further information on direct flaps to the lower extremity is included in Chapter 50. With the advent of muscle flaps, myocutaneous flaps, and free flaps, the cross-leg flap is becoming of only historical interest.

*Indirect Flaps from a Distance.* Indirect flaps from a distance, which are rather seldom used, are transferred to a distant site by a carrier (e.g., the wrist) or by migration. Such flaps are almost always tubed and are usually transferred to their new site using the wrist as a carrier. If they are moved by the technique of migration, they travel only a distance equal to the length of the flap at each stage; the disadvantage to this technique is that each operation causes further scarring of the end of the flap. Methods of migration include (1) waltzing (i.e., the ends of the flap are alternatively moved laterally one step at a time); (2) *caterpillar method* (i.e., one end of the flap is moved close to the other so the flap is doubled on itself at the first stage, following which the other end is moved forward as far as possible to migrate the flap); and (3) tumbling (i.e., the flap is moved in the same fashion as an athlete tumbles head over heels). Their interest is mainly historical.

Indirect flaps from the neck, however, can be used for reconstructing defects of the nose, lips, or auricle. This donor site has much in its favor because the color and texture of the skin are satisfactory, and the flap can be migrated without need of a carrier. In men a portion of the resulting scar can be covered by a shirt collar. Most of these flaps are bipedicle tubed flaps on the neck that are developed with their long axis in the direction of the flexion creases [317]. The donor site can be closed by direct suture when the defect is not too wide. Neck flaps of this type are either transferred directly or waltzed up to the face in one step or two steps about 3 weeks apart, depending on the case. Because of the excellent vascularity of this skin, the end of the flap to be transferred the first time can be divided and moved in one operation. Subsequent moves often require staged cutting of the end of the flap.

MUSCLE AND MYOCUTANEOUS FLAPS

Man's ingenuity has added a variety of composite tissues to the list of body parts that can be moved as free flaps. These tissues include the following: muscle flaps, myocutaneous flaps, omental free flaps, and free osteocutaneous flaps [22, 37, 39, 45, 76, 90, 203, 204, 207].

*Uses of Flaps*

The following four categories include many of the indications for using flaps of any nature: (1) closure of wounds with a poor vascular bed (e.g., bare bone, irradiated tissue); (2) provide bulk, as for reconstruction of facial features (eyelids, eyebrows, lips, ears, nose, and cheeks); (3) provide padding over bony prominences; and (4) permit operation through the flap on underlying structures.

CLOSURE OF WOUNDS WITH A POOR VASCULAR BED. *Wounds Overlying the Tibia.* Wounds of the lower extremity often have poor circulation and may require a skin flap, muscle flap, or myocutaneous flap for closure. When cortical bone is exposed in the bed of a wound and lacks periosteal covering, a permanent pedicle blood-carrying flap is considered. It adds an additional supply of blood to the poorly vascularized recipient site because the original pedicle is preserved. When local tissues do not provide a satisfactory donor source for this type of flap and more distant tissues are to be transferred (i.e., free flaps), it is important to excise sufficient surrounding scar so that the margins of the flap can be sutured to healthy tissues (to obtain satisfactory healing).

When the cortical surface of the tibia is removed, it may be possible for a skin graft to survive on the cancellous bone or on the granulations that form. Because these grafts often are not stable enough to ensure against recurrent ulceration, a flap is almost always the procedure of choice.

Muscle and myocutaneous flaps have a major role in lower extremity reconstruction. Mathis et al. have demonstrated clearly their role in the control of osteomyelitis [205].

*Wounds Overlying Bare Bone, Cartilage, Tendon, or Nerve.* Bone, cartilage, tendon, and nerve do not have sufficient circulation of their own to support a skin graft unless they are covered by the vascular envelope of periosteum, perichondrium, paratenon, or epineurium. Therefore a flap usually is necessary to obtain a closed wound of sufficient stability. Even on healthy periosteum, skin grafts often cannot withstand repeated trauma and must be replaced by a flap. Nerves must be covered by muscle, fat, or subcutaneous tissue to protect them from trauma.

*Open Cavities.* Open wounds of the chest, skull, or maxilla can be closed by a local permanent blood-carrying pedicle flap. A skin graft can be applied to the undersurface of the flap in any region where it bridges a cavity.

RECONSTRUCTION OF FACIAL FEATURES. Chapters 13 to 17 are concerned with reconstruction of the scalp, forehead, eyebrows, eyelids, ears, nose, lips, and cheeks. Flaps play an essential role in the reconstruction of these facial structures.

PADDING OVER BONY PROMINENCES. Flaps play an important role in the treatment of pressure sores and fingertip injuries in which all soft tissues have been lost. The principles of treating pressure sores are discussed in Chapter 51.

An injury of the fingertip with loss of skin and tactile pad may be treated with a skin flap to maintain finger length and restore proper padding. Treatment of fingertip injuries is discussed more fully in Chapter 31.

OPERATIONS THROUGH A FLAP ON UNDERLYING STRUCTURES. A skin graft can withstand only minimal degrees of undermining, manipulation, and wound retraction, and it has always been taught that it is not sufficiently stable for secondary operations on underlying nerve, tendon, artery, bone, or cartilage. Therefore some wounds are first closed with a flap and allowed to mature before operation on underlying structures. However, there are many instances where repair of underlying structures is done at the same time as flap coverage.

When avulsion of overlying skin is accompanied by the division of deeper structures, e.g., blood vessels, nerves, or tendons, the underlying structures can be repaired and the wound closed immediately with a local or free flap. These flaps are usually muscle or musculocutaneous.

OTHER USES OF FLAPS. The island flap, if transferred with its nerve supply intact, restores sensation to an area where it is needed. This technique has been particularly useful for providing sensation to anesthetic areas such as the ulnar aspect of the tip of the thumb or radial aspect of the index finger. An island of skin from the area of the tactile pad on the ulnar side of either the middle or the ring finger and based on one neurovascular bundle is utilized for this purpose [258]. Similarly, the sacrum can be reinervated in spinal cord injury patients with the intercostal flap described by Little et al. [189].

Composite flaps containing bone or cartilage are sometimes used for reconstruction. In addition, bone or cartilage can be inserted underneath a flap a few weeks before the flap is to be transferred, or the flap can be developed to include the clavicle or iliac bone. The choice of free composite flaps have all but eliminated these methods, which are mainly of historic interest.

*Skin Flap Utilizing Expansion of Adjacent Skin, the Crane Principle, and Compound Flaps*

EXPANSION OF ADJACENT SKIN BY AN INFLATABLE SUBCUTANEOUS SILICONE BAG AND TISSUE EXPANDERS. Supplying local tissue for reconstruction has distinct advantages because of color and texture match and the decreased need for distant donor sites. Since the last edition of this book, tissue expansion is a major advance and is used in a wide variety of reconstructive and aesthetic procedures.

Neumann [244] in 1957 first described placement of a rubber balloon underneath temporal skin in an attempt to reconstruct an ear. He originated the term "expansion of skin." Radovan [266], however, was the first surgeon to gain wide clinical experience in tissue expansion.

Tissue expansion is performed by first placing the empty expander in the subcutaneous tissue. Saline is then injected into the expander through a buried or externalized injection port connected to the expander via a connecting tube. Injections are made every 3 to 7 days over a 3- to 4-week period (depending on the desired end result). As the expander enlarges, it stretches the overlying tissue and skin. Once the tissue is sufficiently stretched, the expander can then be removed. The tissue may be spread to the adjacent recipient site, as for a defect left after tattoo removal, or it can be replaced with a permanent prosthesis, as for reconstruction of the breast after mastectomy [23, 59, 342]. A self-inflating expander has also been devised [14]. This device contains sodium chloride crystals in the collapsed bag, so that when it is placed subcutaneously the osmotic pressure differential on either side of the silicone membrane draws fluid into the bag, thus self-inflating. It is not clinically available, however, because of reports of skin necrosis with implant rupture.

Tissue expansion is used for solving a wide array of problems: breast reconstruction, burn reconstruction [201], male-pattern baldness [5, 197], alopecia [44, 183], reconstruction of upper extremities [338], and head and neck reconstruction [9], for example. The ever creative mind is now exploring the possibilities of flap/island flap expansion and axial vessel, peripheral nerve, and visceral elongation [107, 143, 197, 198, 288, 314, 334].

Hong and colleagues [143] expanded the saphenous neurovascular bundle of rats. The increase in length of elongated vessels ranged from 30 to 140 percent. They reported an 83 percent patency during the expansion period. The maintenance of patency is the limiting factor to the rate of expansion. As common sense dictates, gradual expansion is the best method for maintaining patency. One week after expansion they severed and reanastomosed these vessels. Patency rates 7 weeks postoperatively were 90 percent in both the expanded and the nonexpanded vessels.

Saxby [288] investigated island flaps after expansion. In microangiographic studies on the expanded pig buttock flap, other than the already known increase in random vessels (as discussed on page 53) there was a suggestion of an increase in diameter of the axial artery after expansion. Further work in pretransfer expansion of free flap donor sites with successful clinical application was performed by Leighton et al. [180, 181]. More detailed discussions of tissue expansion in specific cases are presented in other chapters [291].

TISSUE EXPANSION: HISTOPATHOLOGY. Since its clinical popularity during the 1970s tissue expansion has been criticized. Some accused it of thinning the skin and that use over implants or grafts would be less optimal. This suggestion has been disproved.

Johnson et al. [159] evaluated the dermal and epidermal response to tissue expansion in the pig. Expanders were placed subcutaneously and expanded over 6 weeks. Histologic changes and collagen content were evaluated at 6-week intervals up to 36 weeks. Their results showed that the epidermis thickens and the dermis and subcutaneous tissue thin in response to expansion. Histologically, there was no change in collagen distribution up to 36 weeks after expansion.

The next step, obviously, was to take this quantitative analysis to human tissue. Pasyk et al. [255] histologically compared postexpansion thickness of epidermis, dermis, and subcutaneous tissue to nonexpanded skin in the same patients. They found a significant increase in the thickness of epidermis in expanded skin compared to that in nonexpanded skin. Human dermis and subcutaneous tissue, on the other hand, showed significant thinning. There was no relation between epidermal thickness or dermal, subcutaneous thinness and time of expansion, volume of expansion, location of expander, or age of patient. Capsule formation was present and was thickest at 2.0 to 2.5 months of expansion. However, in the one patient biopsied 2 years after expansion, the capsule could not be identified, and both epidermis and dermis were of normal thickness.

CRANE PRINCIPLE. Although rarely used because of newer technologies, the Crane principle should be understood by the reconstructive surgeon. With this method subcutaneous tissue can be carried by a flap to cover bare bone, tendon, cartilage, or other structures. Then, the skin and a thin layer of subcutaneous tissue are returned to the flap donor site after approximately 7 days. The subcutaneous tissue left at the recipient site is vascular enough to nourish a split-thickness skin graft after an additional 5 days. The principal advantage of this procedure is to decrease the period of limb immobilization, such as would be involved with a cross-leg flap [220].

PEDICLED PERICRANIUM AS A BASE FOR SKIN GRAFTS. Saunders [286] has described the use of a flap of pericranium elevated from the skull through a small skin incision and moved to cover avascular defects of the frontal bone or medial canthal region. At the same operation, a full-thickness supraclavicular skin graft was applied to the vascular flap of pericranium.

Erol and Spira [98] experimentally used greater omentum with a split-thickness skin graft and converted it to a skin graft flap. In pigs, they mobilized the omentum on the right gastroepiploic vessels. The split-thickness skin graft was sutured to the omental flap, which converted an omental flap to a mobile pedicled skin graft flap. With the development of microvascular techniques, they successfully transferred the skin graft flap as a free flap.

## CHARACTERISTICS OF SKIN FLAPS POSTOPERATIVELY

### Color and Texture

The skin of a flap, even after transfer, maintains its original color and texture with little or no change, which is why skin flaps of head or neck origin are best for facial reconstruction. Skin flaps from such distant sites as the abdomen continue to maintain characteristics of abdominal skin following transfer to the face.

### Bulkiness

Pedicled tissue from the trunk, because it is too thick or has excess fat, may not compare favorably with the original tissue. This finding is especially true in the face, where the skin normally is thin enough to allow the underlying movements of facial muscles to register expression. It is also true in the hands, where the contours are complex, and on the fingers, where the clearance between parts may be small. The bulkiness in a flap may be further increased if the patient gains weight, as the flap continues to respond as though the tissue were still on the trunk.

Aggressive thinning of the flap at the time it is first developed to remove subcutaneous tissue, preserving only the subdermal plexus at the junction of dermis and subcutaneous tissue, prevents much of this bulkiness.

### Hair Growth and Sebaceous Secretion

Hair growth and sebaceous secretion continue to have the same characteristics in a skin flap as they did at their original site.

### Sensation and Sweating

Sensation and sweating, lost immediately after transfer of a flap, usually return some-time between 6 weeks and 3 years later [200]. These functions tend to acquire the characteristic pattern of the recipient site in much the same manner as occurs in a skin graft. Sensation returns by the ingrowth of nerve fibers from surrounding skin and from the recipient bed.

Sturman and Duran [320] have demonstrated on the tip of a reconstructed finger that the two-point discrimination of skin grafts, cross-finger flaps, and palmar flaps is close to that of the normal fingertip. Abdominal pedicled tissue transferred to the fingertip does not develop good two-point discrimination, presumably because of the excess fatty tissue.

When pedicled tissue is applied to a recipient area that has been the site of extensive tissue destruction, there rarely is good return of sensation and sweating. Scar tissue in the bed as well as along the junction between adjacent skin and the flap tends to block reinnervation.

Sweating, because of its dependence on the sympathetic nervous system, is usually restored at the same rate as pain, temperature, and touch sensation. McGregor [213] estimated that 70 to 80 percent of the sweat glands in a flap regain their function.

### Durability

A flap containing a good layer of fat usually provides bony prominences with a durable cover. The principal disadvantage is that for a long time following operation the flap is anesthetic, so prolonged pressure can result in painless ischemia of the tissues and a pressure sore. Occasionally, a neurovascular flap helps maintain some sensation at the point of pressure.

### Growth

A skin flap grows in proportion to body growth, a fact that has been demonstrated in growing rats observed over a 3-month period

[168]. Although initially the growth rate was reduced, this period was followed by growth that was faster than the growth of the total body surface.

MUSCLE FLAPS PLUS SKIN GRAFTS
Another type of arterialized flap is the muscle flap that is transferred with its intact neurovascular bundle into an adjacent recipient site and then covered with a split-thickness skin graft (see Fig. 1-17). These long muscle flaps have proved to be a valued addition to the tissues available for reconstruction in the lower extremity, trunk, and face.

Chapter 45 provides information on these flaps, including details on the anatomy of the musculocutaneous units and their sites of innervation and blood supply. Some of the commonly used muscle flaps in the lower extremity are derived from the gastrocnemius, soleus, flexor digitorum longus and brevis, abductor hallucis, and abductor digiti minimi muscles. Functional deficits caused by the loss of these muscles have been minor [340].

Ger and Levine [115], who pioneered the use of muscle flaps, had confidence in their application for the treatment of decubitus ulcers. The upper half of the gluteus maximus muscle can be rotated for coverage of a sacral ulcer, and the lower half can be rotated into the defect of an ischial ulcer. The rectus femoris or vastus lateralis muscles can be transposed into a trochanteric ulcer defect. Split-thickness skin grafts are then placed on the muscle at the initial procedure. The recurrence rate of these decubitus ulcers, as reported by Ger and Levine, was dramatically low. Additional information is included in Chapter 51.

The temporalis muscle flap has an important role in the reconstruction of operative defects of the upper face [17]. This broad, fan-shaped muscle receives its nerve and blood supply (from branches of the internal maxillary artery) on its deep surface near its coronoid insertion. Therefore all or part of the muscle can be detached from the side of the skull and rotated over the zygoma into the orbit or over exposed dura, after which a skin graft can be applied.

Pers and Medgyesi [261] have extended the use of muscle flaps: to repair the chest wall (serratus anterior muscle), to cover femoral vessels (sartorius and adductor longus muscles), for filling the retropubic cavity after surgical removal of the bladder (gracilis muscle), to control urinary or anal incontinence (gracilis muscle), for closure of vesicovaginal fistulas (gracilis muscle), and to restore the contour of the anterior axillary fold (latissimus dorsi muscle).

MYOCUTANEOUS FLAPS
Flaps of muscle and their attached overlying skin comprise another type of arterialized flap that can be used for reconstruction on the surface of the body (see Fig. 1-17). Hueston and McConchie [147] used such a flap of skin and pectoral muscle based on the shoulder to close a full-thickness defect of the upper anterior chest wall. If the muscle remains attached at its base and runs the full length of the flap, the blood supply through numerous musculocutaneous arteries augments the skin's blood supply, thereby providing a safe flap.

For decades now, muscle and myocutaneous flaps have become the most reliable tool for the reconstructive surgeon. The other flaps, previously mentioned, are now being used less and less often.

Myocutaneous flaps have been found useful for lower extremity reconstruction. Orticochea [253] used the gracilis muscle and its overlying skin as a cross-leg flap to cover a defect of the opposite ankle. Some of the myocutaneous flaps that have been used clinically involve the following muscles: gracilis, upper part of the trapezius, latissimus dorsi, lower portion of the sacrospinalis, upper rectus abdominis (island flap), lower rectus abdominis (island flap), thoracoepigastric, upper half of the sartorius, lower half of the sartorius, rectus femoris, and biceps femoris [210]. Vasconez and col-

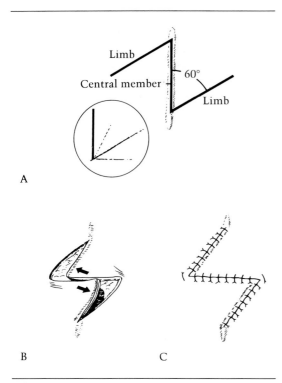

A

B                    C

**Figure 1-36** *Classic 60-degree angle Z-plasty. Inset shows method of finding the 60-degree angle by first drawing a 90-degree angle, then dividing it in thirds by sighting. The limbs of the Z must be equal in length to the central member.*

**Table 1-1** *Z-Plasty, angles, and theoretical gain in length*

| Angles of Z-plasty (degrees) | Theoretical gain in length (%) |
|---|---|
| 30–30 | 25 |
| 45–45 | 50 |
| 60–60 | 75 |
| 75–75 | 100 |
| 90–90 | 120 |

leagues detail their extensive experience with these lower extremity myocutaneous flaps in Chapter 45. Volumes by Mathis and Nahai as well as by McCraw provide excellent details on this subject [203, 204, 207].

## Z-Plasty

The Z-plasty is simply a technique by which two triangular flaps are interchanged, one for another.

GEOMETRIC PRINCIPLE

The Z-plasty geometrically consists of one central limb and two limbs positioned so they resemble a Z (Fig. 1-36). *The limbs of the Z must always be equal in length to the central member and must extend outward*

from it at an angle that varies between 30 and 90 degrees. For the classic Z-plasty this angle is 60 degrees. Clinical experience has repeatedly shown that 60 degrees is the largest angle that permits transposition of the triangular flaps while obtaining the maximal increased length in the direction of the central member. At the completion of the Z-plasty, the Z has been rotated 90 degrees and reversed (Fig. 1-36).

*Gain in Length*

The gain in length with the Z-plasty is in the direction of the central member, and it has been calculated mathematically. The gain depends on the angle and the length of the central member used in the design of the two triangles (Table 1-1).

A means by which the theoretical gain in length can be determined in any Z-plasty is illustrated in Figure 1-37. However, it must be emphasized that the theoretical gain in length is based on geometry and studies with paper models. In contrast, the biomechanical properties of skin that cause its tension to vary from loose and elastic to taut prevent surgery from being planned to such an exact science as geometry. The theoretical gain in length is determined as in Figure 1-37. Gibson and Kenedi [117] measured the theoretical and actual gain in length in four Z-plasties in humans. The actual gain in length was either less (14 and 16 percent less) or more (7 and 27 percent more) than calculated. Furnas and Fischer [110] have shown in experimental studies of Z-plasties on the skin of the trunk in dogs that the actual gain in length was always less than the theoretical gain. In a 60 degree angle Z-plasty, the actual gain in length was 28 percent less than that calculated for a Z-plasty with 8-cm limbs. As the limb length decreased, the gain in length decreased so that for a Z-plasty with 1-cm limbs it was 45 percent less than calculated.

To transpose the flaps of a Z-plasty, the skin in the base of these flaps must be loose or elastic enough to be pulled over into its new position. When the skin is contracted in a direction perpendicular to the central member of the planned Z, it may be impossible to do a Z-plasty. This situation occurs particularly after skin grafting a burned extremity, where the skin is often tight. One of the ideal factors when planning a Z-plasty is to be able to base the flaps in an area of loose skin [117].

*Variation of Angle Size and Length of the Central Member*

When planning a Z-plasty, the size of the angle created by the central member and each arm and the length of the central member are the only two factors that can be varied. It is important to remember that *the length of the limbs of the Z must remain equal to the length of the central member.*

ANGLE SIZE. A greater percentage gain in length is to be expected as the angle of each limb of the Z-plasty is increased (Fig. 1-38) [214]. The force required to transpose the Z-plasty flaps and pull them into their new position increases as the tip angle increases. On the trunk of the dog, the tension needed to close a 90 degree/90 degree angle and 8-cm-limb Z-plasty is approximately ten times that needed to close a 30 degree/30 degree angle 8-cm-limb Z-plasty [110].

The angle of the limbs from the central member can vary from 30 degrees to 90 degrees, and it is not necessary that the two angles be the same. Some examples of Z-plasties with varying angle sizes are illustrated in Figure 1-39.

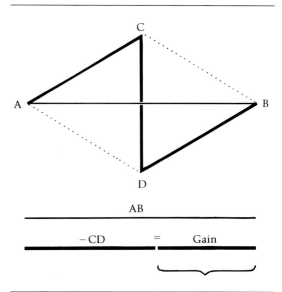

**Figure 1-37** *Calculating the theoretical gain in length of the Z-plasty. The theoretical gain in length is the difference in length between the long diagonal and the short diagonal. In actual practice the gain in length has varied from 45 percent less to 25 percent more than calculated geometrically owning to the biomechanical properties of the skin [232, 233].*

plasties with varying angle sizes are illustrated in Figure 1-39.

LENGTH OF CENTRAL MEMBER. The greater the length of the central member, the greater is the gain in length accomplished by the Z-plasty (Fig. 1-40). This result naturally follows because it has already been demonstrated that the length to be gained is a percentage of the length of the central member.

The scar resulting from a large Z-plasty is usually more noticeable than the one resulting from a series of small Z-plasties. Aesthetically, it is preferable on such areas as the face to keep the central member of the Z relatively short.

*Multiple Z-Plasties*

Any number of Z-plasties can be designed in series (see Figure 1-47A for an example of a

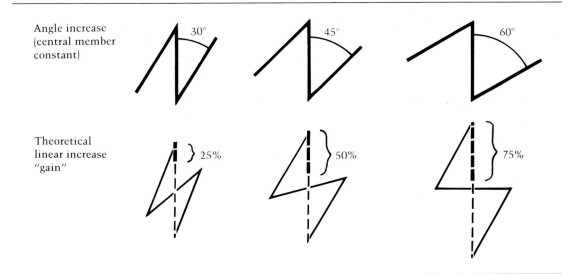

Angle increase (central member constant)

Theoretical linear increase "gain"

30°    } 25%

45°    } 50%

60°    } 75%

**Figure 1-38** *Theoretical gain in length of the Z-plasty calculated for angles of 30, 45, and 60 degrees. In actual practice the gain in length depends also on the varying degrees of rigidity or looseness of the skin being transposed to provide the increased length.*

multiple Z-plasty). However, it has been demonstrated in experiments in dogs that more length can be gained by making one Z-plasty with a long central member than by making multiple Z-plasties whose central member lengths collectively add up to the same total length. For example, a single 60

**Figure 1-39** *Examples of Z-plasties with varying angle sizes.*

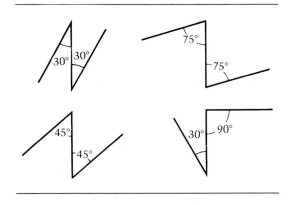

degree angle 8-cm-limb Z-plasty provided an actual gain in length almost twice that for a series of eight 60 degree angle 1-cm-limb Z-plasties [110]. Despite this fact, there is a place for the multiple Z-plasty when there is not sufficient tissue for a large Z and when the cosmetically superior appearance of a series of small Zs is a prime concern (i.e., the face).

*Four-Flap Z-Plasty*
In the four-flap Z-plasty variation, a 90 degree/90 degree angle Z-plasty is designed, and each flap is then subdivided into 45 degree angle flaps. This design permits a greater gain in length (124 percent) with less tension on the flaps (Fig. 1-41).

The four-flap Z-plasty is particularly effective for correcting web space contractures in the hand [353] (Fig. 1-42). Flaps with angles as large as 120 degrees/120 degrees have been subdivided into 60 degree angle flaps for the four-flap Z-plasty.

*Six-Flap Z-Plasty*
With the six-flap Z-plasty, an additional 45 degree angle flap is tacked on to each end of

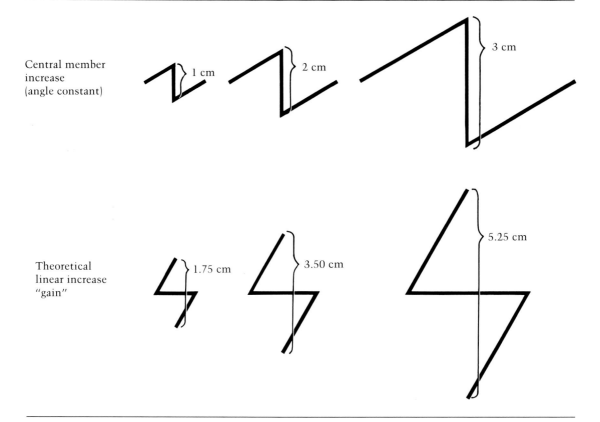

Central member
increase
(angle constant)

1 cm

2 cm

3 cm

Theoretical
linear increase
"gain"

1.75 cm

3.50 cm

5.25 cm

**Figure 1-40** *The greater the length of the central member, the greater is the gain in length accomplished by the Z-plasty.*

a 45/45/45/45 degree angle four-flap Z-plasty [230]. After the three 45 degree angle flaps have been incised at each end of the central member, all six flaps are transposed in the way that one interlocks one's fingers from the right and left hand. That is, one uses first a flap from one end of the central member, then a flap from the opposite end, and so on. The six-flap Z-plasty provides a theoretical gain in length in the direction of the central member of 180 percent.

Like the four-flap Z-plasty, the six-flap Z-plasty can be carried out in a stepwise fashion by first incising the 90 degree angle Z-flaps. If enough length is not gained by transposing these flaps and transverse tension is not too great, the 90 degree angle flaps can be divided into 45 degree angle flaps for a four-flap Z-plasty, which can be

temporarily sutured. If still more length is needed, 45 degree angle flaps can be added on to each end of the central member, creating a six-flap Z-plasty.

*Five-Flap* Y-V *Advancement
and* Z-*Plasty*
The combination of five-flap Y-V advancement and Z-plasty has been described as being effective for releasing transverse contractures of the dorsum of the interdigital web spaces and at other concave regions of the body (Fig. 1-43). The hypertrophic scar does not need to be excised but, rather, can be incised. Once the tension on the scar is released, it usually gradually involutes [282].

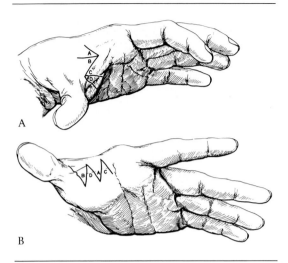

**Figure 1-41** *Four-flap Z-plasty. Each flap of a 90-degree/90-degree angled Z-plasty has been divided into two 45-degree angle flaps. (A and B, C and D). These four flaps are then easily transposed to provide greater lengthening of the central member than could be accomplished by a typical 60-degree/60-degree angled Z-plasty.*

*Method of Planning So the Completed Z-Plasty Is Properly Situated*

The central member of the completed Z-plasty must lie in the same direction as the skin lines whenever possible. For example, this central member finally lies in a direction parallel to the nasolabial fold whenever a Z-plasty is carried out in the region of this fold. In this manner, the direction of the final scar can be changed to correspond to the direction of the skin lines.

The length of the central member is first selected, and the central member is drawn so its midpoint lies on the skin line. A triangular flap is then constructed.

Although this technique effectively places the central member of the completed Z-plasty in the proper direction, it triples the length of the scar and adds two lines that are oblique to the direction of the skin lines. With the best results the eye visualizes the unconnected scars that form the limbs of the Z, with the central member of the Z being indiscernible.

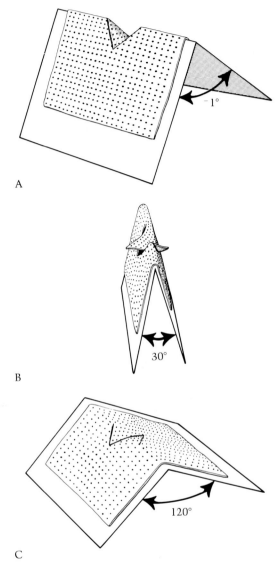

**Figure 1-42** *Z-plasty on webs. A. With a peak angle of 71 degrees, the flap of a 60-degree/60-degree angled Z-plasty lies easily in the cleft formed after transposition of the flaps. B. With a peak angle of 30 degrees, the tips of the 60-degree/60-degree angled Z-plasty flaps overhang redundantly and do not meet the deepest part of the cleft without tension. C. With a peak angle of 120 degrees, the Z-plasty flaps can be pulled into the cleft under tension.*

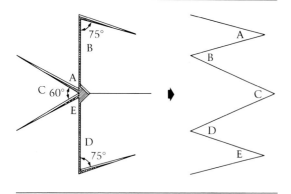

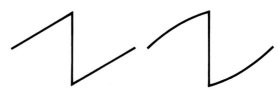

Figure 1-44 *Z-plasty flaps can be broadened by curving the limbs of the Z. This measure may decrease the likelihood of skin slough in burn-scarred tissue.*

Figure 1-43 *Five-flap Y-V advancement and Z-plasty. The central flap (C) is advanced in a Y-V fashion. The flaps of the two Z-plasties on each side of the central flap are transposed.*

USES OF Z-PLASTY

Z-Plasty has three major uses. It (1) increases the length of the skin in a desired direction; (2) changes the direction of a scar so it lies in the same direction as the skin lines; and (3) rotates the axis of the tissue included in the Z-plasty flaps.

*Increasing the Length of the Skin in a Desired Direction*

Most Z-plasties are used to increase the length of the skin in a desired direction.

LENGTHENING SCAR CONTRACTURES. Examples of scar contractures that can be lengthened by means of a Z-plasty are as follows.

**1.** Scars that cross flexion creases of the axilla, elbow, fingers, knee, or neck often contract and produce a bowstring type of scar that may limit extension. If the scar is a linear one and the adjacent skin is not burned or damaged, one or more Z-plasties can be performed to lengthen it. Clinical judgment is important for knowing when a contracture is too extensive for Z-plasty and must be released and skin grafted to obtain the maximal improvement.

**2.** With burn-scar contractures, the adjacent skin may have decreased vascularity because of the injury, making it a poor site

for a Z-plasty. There is always a risk that the tips of these densely scarred flaps will not survive [78]. To minimize this possibility, the width of the flaps near their tips can be maintained by curving the limbs of the Z-plasty incision (Fig. 1-44). Spina [313] has even advocated delaying the flaps of the Z-plasty in tissues with a poor blood supply. Wilkinson and Rybka [350] have demonstrated in the guinea pig that the incidence of necrosis of the tips of Z-plasty flaps was reduced from 20 percent to 0 percent by the use of skin tapes or wound adhesives rather than sutures. Another difficulty encountered when performing a Z-plasty in skin that has been burned is that the tightness and loss of elasticity make transposition of the flaps difficult. For these reasons, Z-plasties in skin scarred by burns must be approached with caution.

**3.** Scars or congenital skin webs that cross a concave surface invariably bridge the concavity. They can be lengthened and made to conform to the concave surface by placing a Z-plasty in the deepest part of the concavity. Examples of this type of problem are scars that lie transversely across the junction between the nose and the cheek or those that cross the slight hollow of the submandibular region. Pterygium colli is the classic example of a congenital skin web that can be corrected by a Z-plasty [85, 293].

**4.** U-Shaped scars are often elevated in the center because of the action of the contracting scar. Such scars in the face are unsightly. They can be improved by breaking the con-

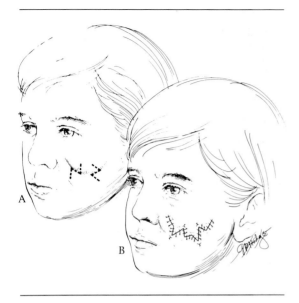

**Figure 1-45** *The fullness of the tissue encompassed by a U-shaped scar can best be improved by two Z-plasties near the bottom of the U.*

tracting line of the scar with one or two Z-plasties at or near the bottom of the U (Fig. 1-45). Attempts at correction of the U-shaped scar by simply trimming the excess tissue from underneath the elevated skin are usually unsatisfactory. The problem is one of contracture, not edema. Occasionally, small U-shaped scars can be removed by elliptical excision of the entire scar. It is un-

**Figure 1-46** *Siting the Z-plasty so the central member of the completed Z-plasty lies in the direction of the nasolabial fold. See text for the method of planning.*

wise to perform a Z-plasty in most cases as a primary procedure. The tissue that makes up the flaps of the Z-plasty has usually been traumatized at the time of injury, so the blood supply at this time may be precarious.

**5.** Circular scars of the extremities or body orifices can be released by a Z-plasty. Constricting scars of the arms or legs have traditionally been released in two stages, with a Z-plasty being carried out on about half the circumference of the scar in each stage [85, 319]. Congenital annular bands and grooves can be treated in a similar fashion. Circular contractures at orifices, such as the external auditory canal, urethra, colostomy openings, and vesicostomy openings, can be released (or prevented) by a series of Z-plasties around the opening. They can be performed in one operative procedure.

CLEFT LIP REPAIR. All of the techniques for repair of unilateral or bilateral cleft lip, with the exception of the straight line repair, make use of the Z-plasty. In this way the shortened lip at the cleft can be lengthened. Chapter 9 includes a complete discussion of cleft lip repair.

*Changing the Direction of the Scar*
Long scars on the face, except for those that lie in or adjacent to a skin line, are usually conspicuous. The line of scar can be changed by breaking it with a series of Z-plasties so situated that the central member of the Z lies in the same direction as the skin lines (Fig. 1-46). Thus the eye visualizes a series of

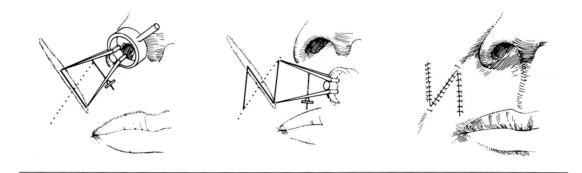

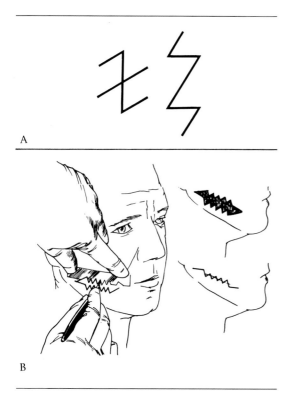

A

B

**Figure 1-47** *Methods of changing the direction of a scar. A. Multiple Z-plasties can be planned so that the central member of the completed Z-plasties lie in the direction of the skin lines. B. The W-plasty can also be used to break up a long scar that does not lie in the direction of the skin lines.*

unconnected short scars representing the limbs of the Z, with the central member of the Z being indiscernible; though longer than the original straight line scar, it is less noticeable. It is a rare long linear scar that does not cross a skin line at some point and that cannot be improved by breaking it up with one or more Z-plasties. The scar that makes up the central member of the Z-plasty can be excised in an elliptical fashion if it is not too wide. This method can be used whenever the smallest angle between the scar and the skin line is more than 30 degrees.

The W-plasty has been described by Borges [33–35] as another method of changing the direction of a linear scar. This method sim-

ply involves excising the scar in multiple small triangles that are so situated they interdigitate (Fig. 1-47B). A special metal instrument with the pattern of these triangles (or Ws) cut into it can be of assistance in making the triangles of equal size, but most often it is done free hand. Although the W-plasty changes the direction of the linear scar, it would only be by chance that one of the limbs of the W would lie in the same direction as the skin lines. However, usually one of the limbs is close to this direction. As a W-plasty does not lengthen a contracted scar line, it is best to use the Z-plasty for this purpose.

Both the Z-plasty and the W-plasty have the additional attribute of breaking up a linear scar into an accordion-like scar that has some degree of elasticity to it. This change permits the facial skin to be more mobile in its contribution to facial expressions. Each of these techniques has to its detriment the fact that it more than doubles the length of the scar. Thus these procedures are used only under appropriate circumstances for revising scars.

## References

1. Abbott, W. M., and Austen, W. G. Effectiveness and mechanism of collagen induced hemostasis. *Surgery* 78:723, 1975.
2. Acland, R. D. Discussion on experiences in monitoring the circulation in free-flap transfer. *Plast. Reconstr. Surg.* 68:554, 1981.
3. Allen, H. E., Edgerton, M. T., Rodeheaver, G. T., et al. Skin dressings in the treatment of contaminated wounds. *Am. J. Surg.* 126:45, 1973.
4. Anascombe, A. R., Hira, N., and Hunt, B. The use of a new absorbable suture material (polyglycolic acid) in general surgery. *Br. J. Surg.* 57:917, 1970.
5. Anderson, R. D. Expansion-assisted treatment of male pattern baldness. *Clin. Plast. Surg.* 14:469, 1987.
6. Angel, M. F., Narayanan, K., and Swartz, W. M. The etiologic role of free radicals in hematoma-induced flap necrosis. *Plast. Reconstr. Surg.* 77:795, 1986.

7. Angel, M. F., Ramastastry, S. S., Swartz, W. M., et al. Free radicals: Basic concepts concerning their chemistry, pathophysiology and relevance to plastic surgery. *Plast. Reconstr. Surg.* 79:990, 1987.

8. Antia, N. H., and Buch, V. I. Chondrocutaneous advancement flap for the marginal defect of the ear. *Plast. Reconstr. Surg.* 39:472, 1967.

9. Antonyshyn, O., Gruss, J. S., Zucker, R., et al. Tissue expansion in head and neck reconstruction. *Plast. Reconstr. Surg.* 82:58, 1988.

10. Arturson, G., and Khama, N. N. The effects of hyperbaric oxygen, dimethyl sulfoxide, and Complamin on the survival of experimental skin flaps. *Scand. J. Plast. Reconstr. Surg.* 4:8, 1970.

11. Ashley, F. L., Stone, R. S., Polak, R., et al. Further studies involving wound closure with a rapidly polymerizing adhesive. *Plast. Reconstr. Surg.* 31:333, 1963.

12. Astrup, P., Hellung-Laisen, P., Kjeldsen, K., et al. The effect of tobacco smoking on the dissociation curve of oxyhemoglobin. *Scand. J. Clin. Lab. Invest.* 18:450, 1966.

13. Aulenbacher, C. E., and Monafo, W. W. New spring wound dermatome for skin grafting under local anesthesia. *Am. J. Surg.* 118:131, 1969.

14. Austed, E. D., and Rose, G. L. A self-inflating tissue expander. *Plast. Reconstr. Surg.* 4:8, 1970.

15. Bagley, H. D., et al. Antibiotic concentration in human wound fluid after IV administration. *Ann. Surg.* 198:202, 1978.

16. Bakamjian, V. A technique for primary reconstruction of the palate after radical maxillectomy for cancer. *Plast. Reconstr. Surg.* 31:103, 1963.

17. Bakamjian, V. Y., and Souther, S. G. Use of temporal muscle flap for reconstruction after orbito-maxillary resections for cancer. *Plast. Reconstr. Surg.* 56:171, 1975.

18. Baker, G. C., and Watson, H. K. The mathematical principles in the use and design of serial Y-V advancements. Presented at the Plastic Surgery Senior Residents Conference, New Orleans, 1976.

19. Barnhill, R., and Ryan, T. S. Mechanical Considerations in New Vessel Growth. In M. Tsuchiya, et al. (eds.), *Basic Aspects of Microcirculation.* Amsterdam: Excerpta Medica, 1982.

20. Barron, J. N., Veall, N., and Arnott, D. G. The measurement of the local clearance of radioactive sodium in tubed skin pedicles. *Br. J. Plast. Surg.* 4:16, 1952.

21. Barton, F. E., Jr. Aesthetic aspects of partial nasal reconstruction. *Clin. Plast. Surg.* 8:177, 1981.

22. Barwick, W. J., Goodkind, D. J., and Serafin, D. The free scapular flap. *Plast. Reconstr. Surg.* 69:779, 1982.

23. Becker, H. Breast reconstruction using an inflatable breast implant with detachable reservoir. *Plast. Reconstr. Surg.* 73:678, 1984.

24. Berkowitz, R. L. Scalp: In search of the perfect donor site. *Ann. Plast. Surg.* 7:126, 1981.

25. Bertolami, C., and Donoff, R. B. The effect of full-thickness skin grafts on the actinomyosin content of contracting wounds. *J. Oral Surg.* 37:471, 1979.

26. Billingham, R. E., and Reynolds, J. Transplantation studies on sheets of pure epidermal epithelium and on epidermal cell suspensions. *Br. J. Plast. Surg.* 5:25, 1952.

27. Billingham, R. E., and Russell, P. S. Studies on wound healing, with special reference to the phenomenon of contracture in experimental rabbits' skin. *Ann. Surg.* 144:961, 1956.

28. Birch, J., and Branemark, P. I. The vascularization of a free full-thickness skin graft. I. A vital microscopic study. *Scand. J. Plast. Reconstr. Surg.* 3:1, 1969.

29. Birch, J., and Branemark, P. I. The vascularization of a free full-thickness skin graft. II. A microangiographic study. *Scand. J. Plast. Reconstr. Surg.* 3:11, 1969.

30. Birnstingl, M. A., Bringson, K., and Chakrabarti, R. The effect of short-term exposure to carbon monoxide on platelet stickiness. *Br. J. Surg.* 58:837, 1971.

31. Bloomenstein, R. B. Viability prediction in pedicle flaps by infrared thermometry. *Plast. Reconstr. Surg.* 42:252, 1968.

32. Bodenham, D. C., and Watson, R. The early ambulation of patients with lower limb grafts. *Br. J. Plast. Surg.* 24:20, 1971.

33. Borges, A. F. Improvement of antitension-lines scar by the "W-plasty" operation. *Br. J. Plast. Surg.* 12:29, 1959.

34. Borges, A. F. The W-plastic versus the Z-plastic scar revision. *Plast. Reconstr. Surg.* 44:58, 1969.

35. Borges, A. F. *Elective Incisions and Scar Re-*

*vision.* Boston: Little, Brown, 1973.

36. Borges, A. F. Unsatisfactory forehead scar following face lift. *Plast. Reconstr. Surg.* 78:526, 1986.

37. Brent, B. The acquired auricular deformity: A systematic approach to its analysis and reconstruction. *Plast. Reconstr. Surg.* 59:475, 1977.

38. Brent, B., and Bostwick, J., III. Nipple-areola reconstruction with auricular tissue. *Plast. Reconstr. Surg.* 60:353, 1977.

39. Brent, B., Upton, J., Aclard, R. D., et al. Experience with the temporoparietal fascial free flap. *Plast. Reconstr. Surg.* 76:177, 1985.

40. Brown, R. G., Vasconez, L. O., and Jurkiewicz, M. J. Transverse abdominal flaps and the deep epigastric arcade. *Plast. Reconstr. Surg.* 55:416, 1975.

41. Brunius, U. Wound healing impairment from sutures. *Acta Chir. Scand.* [Suppl.] 395:1, 1968.

42. Brunius, U., and Ahren, C. Healing during the cicatrization phase of skin incisions closed by non-suture technique. *Acta Chir. Scand.* 135:289, 1969.

43. Bucknall, T. E., and Ellis, H. *Wound Healing for Surgeons.* Philadelphia: Bailliere-Tindall, 1984.

44. Buhrer, D. P., Huang, T. T., Yee, H. W., et al. Treatment of burn alopecia with tissue expanders in children. *Plast. Reconstr. Surg.* 81:512, 1988.

45. Buncke, H. J., Furnas, D., Gordon, L., et al. Free osteocutaneous flap from a rib to the tibia. *Plast. Reconstr. Surg.* 59:799, 1977.

46. Bunnell, S. An essential in reconstructive surgery—"atraumatic" technique. *Calif. State J. Med.* 19:204, 1921.

47. Burget, G. C., and Merrick, F. J. Aesthetic restoration of one half of the upper lip. *Plast. Reconstr. Surg.* 78:583, 1986.

48. Burow, A. Zur Blepharoplastik. *Monatsschr. Med. Augenheilk. Cir.* 1:57, 1838.

49. Burton, A. C. Physiology of Cutaneous Circulation: Thermoregulatory Functions. In R. Rothman (ed.), *The Human Integument.* Washington, D.C.: American Association for the Advancement of Science, 1959.

50. Canepa, C. S., Miller, S. H., Buck, D. C., et al. Effects of phenylephrine on tissue gas tension, bleeding, infection and lidocaine absorption. *Plast. Reconstr. Surg.* 81:554, 1988.

51. Champion, W. M., McSherry, C. K., and Goulian, D. Effect of hyperbaric oxygen on the survival of pedicled skin flaps. *J. Surg. Res.* 7:583, 1967.

52. Cherry, G. W., Austad, E., Pasyk, K., et al. Increased survival and vascularity of random-pattern skin flaps elevated in controlled, expanded skin. *Plast. Reconstr. Surg.* 72:680, 1983.

53. Chin-Chun, Y., Tsi-Siang, S., and Wei-Shia, X. A Chinese concept of treatment of extensive third-degree burns. *Plast. Reconstr. Surg.* 70:238, 1982.

54. Chowdary, R. P., Berkower, A. S., Moll, M. L., et al. Fluorocarbons enhancement of skin flap survival in rats. *Plast. Reconstr. Surg.* 79:98, 1987.

55. Clemmesen, T. The early circulation in split skin grafts. *Acta Chir. Scand.* 124:11, 1962.

56. Clemmesen, T. The early circulation in split-skin grafts: Restoration of blood supply to split-skin autografts. *Acta Chir. Scand.* 127:1, 1964.

57. Clemmesen, T. Experimental studies on the healing of free skin autografts. *Dan. Med. Bull.* 14(suppl.)(2):1, 1967.

58. Coffman, J. D. Tobacco smoking and the peripheral circulation. *Heart Bull.* 19:89, 1970.

59. Cohen, I. K., and Turner, D. Immediate breast reconstruction with tissue expanders. *Clin. Plast. Surg.* 14:491, 1987.

60. Cohen, I. K., Ward, J. A., and Chandrasekkar, B. The pinwheel flap nipple and barrier areola graft reconstruction. *Plast. Reconstr. Surg.* 77:995, 1986.

61. Converse, J. M., and Ballantyne, D. L., Jr. Distribution of diphosphopyridine nucleotide diaphorase in rat skin autografts and homografts. *Plast. Reconstr. Surg.* 30:415, 1962.

62. Converse, J. M., and Robb-Smith, A. H. T. The healing of surface cutaneous wounds: Its analogy with the healing of superficial burns. *Am. Surg.* 120:873, 1944.

63. Converse, J. M., Ballantyne, D. L., Jr., Rogers, B. O., et al. "Plasmatic circulation" in skin grafts. *Transplant. Bull.* 4:154, 1957.

64. Converse, J. M., Uhlschmid, G. K., and Ballantyne, D. L., Jr. "Plasmatic circulation" in skin grafts—the phase of serum inhibition. *Plast. Reconstr. Surg.* 43:495, 1969.

65. Conway, H. Sweating function of transplanted skin. *Surg. Gynecol. Obstet.* 69:756, 1939.

66. Corps, B. V. M. The effect of graft thickness, donor site and graft bed on graft shrinkage in the hooded rat. *Br. J. Plast. Surg.* 22:125, 1969.

67. Corso, P. F. Variations of the arterial, venous and capillary circulation of the soft tissues of the head by decades as demonstrated by the methyl methacrylate injection technique, and their application to the construction of flaps and pedicles. *Plast. Reconstr. Surg.* 27:160, 1961.

68. Craig, S., and Rees, T. D. The effects of smoking on experimental skin flaps in hamsters. *Plast. Reconstr. Surg.* 75:842, 1985.

69. Crawford, B. S. An unusual skin donor site. *Br. J. Plast. Surg.* 17:311, 1964.

70. Crikelair, G. F. Skin suture marks. *Am. J. Surg.* 96:631, 1958.

71. Cronin, T. D. The use of a molded splint to prevent contracture after split skin grafting on the neck. *Plast. Reconstr. Surg.* 27:7, 1961.

72. Cuthbert, J. B. The "marsupial" skin flap. *Br. J. Plast. Surg.* 2:125, 1949.

73. Daniel, R. K., and Taylor, I. Distant transfer of an island flap by microvascular anastomoses. *Plast. Reconstr. Surg.* 52:111, 1973.

74. Daniel, R. K., Terzis, J., and Schwarz, G. Neurovascular free flaps. *Plast. Reconstr. Surg.* 56:13, 1975.

75. Daniel, R. K., and Williams, H. B. The free transfer of skin flaps by microvascular anastomoses. *Plast. Reconstr. Surg.* 52:16, 1973.

76. Das, S. K. The size of the human omentum and methods of lengthening it for transplantation. *Br. J. Plast. Surg.* 29:170, 1976.

77. Davis, J. C. *Hyperbaric Oxygen Therapy: A Committee Report.* Undersea Medical Society, 1983. Pp. 19–22.

78. Davis, J. S. Present evaluation of the merits of the Z-plasty operation. *Plast. Reconstr. Surg.* 1:26, 1946.

79. Davis, J. S., and Kitlowski, E. A. The immediate contraction of cutaneous grafts and its causes. *Arch. Surg.* 23:954, 1931.

80. Davis, T. S., Graham, W. P., and Miller, S. H. The circular excision. *Ann. Plast. Surg.* 4:21, 1980.

81. Dean, R. K., Kelleher, J. C., Sullivan, J. G., et al. Bilobed Flaps. In W. C. Grabb and M. B. Myers (eds.), *Skin Flaps.* Boston: Little, Brown, 1975.

82. DeHoll, D., Rodeheaver, G., Edgerton, M. T., et al. Potentiation of infection by suture closure of dead space. *Am. J. Surg.* 127:716, 1974.

83. Derganc, M., and Zdravic, F. Venous congestion of flaps treated by application of leeches. *Br. J. Plast. Surg.* 13:187, 1960.

84. Dinner, M. I., Peters, C. R., and Sherer, J. Use of a semipermeable polyurethane membrane as a dressing for split skin graft donor sites. *Plast. Reconstr. Surg.* 64:112, 1979.

85. Dingman, R. O. Some applications of the Z-plasty procedure. *Plast. Reconstr. Surg.* 16:246, 1955.

86. Dingman, R. O., and Walter, C. Use of composite ear grafts in correction of short nose. *Plast. Reconstr. Surg.* 43:117, 1969.

87. Donoff, R. B., and Grillo, H. C. The effects of skin grafting on healing open wounds in rabbits. *J. Surg. Res.* 19:163, 1975.

88. Dormandy, J. A. Influence of blood viscosity or blood flow and the effect of low molecular weight dextran. *Br. Med. J.* 4:716, 1971.

89. Douglas, B., and Bucholz, R. The blood circulation in pedicle flaps. *Ann. Surg.* 117:692, 1943.

90. Dupont, C., and Menard, Y. Transposition of the greater omentum for reconstruction of the chest wall. *Plast. Reconstr. Surg.* 49:263, 1972.

91. Edgerton, M. T., and Hansen, F. C. Matching facial color with split thickness skin grafts from adjacent areas. *Plast. Reconstr. Surg.* 25:455, 1960.

92. Edlich, R. F., Rodeheaver, G., Thacker, J. G., et al. Technical Factors in Wound Management. In T. K. Hunt (ed.), *Fundamentals of Wound Management.* New York: Appleton-Century-Crofts, 1979. Pp. 416–423.

93. Eklöf, B., Neglen, P., and Thompson, D. Temporary incomplete ischemia of the legs caused by aortic clamping in man. *Ann. Surg.* 193:99–104, 1981.

94. Eldh, J., Bartholdson, L., and Mobacken, H. Histological and histochemical studies on effects of some storage solutions on human split thickness skin grafts. *Scand. J. Plast. Reconstr. Surg.* 8:202, 1974.

95. Elek, S. D., and Conen, P. E. The virulence of Staphylococcus pyogenes for man: A study of the problems of wound infection. *Br. J. Exp. Pathol.* 38:573, 1957.

96. Ellenberg, A. H. Surgical tape wound closure: A disenchantment. *Plast. Reconstr. Surg.* 39:625, 1967.

97. Emmett, A. J. J., and Barron, J. N. Adhesive suture strip closure of wounds in plastic surgery. *Br. J. Plast. Surg.* 17:175, 1964.

98. Erol, O., and Spira, M. Omentum island skin graft flap. *Surg. Forum* 29:594, 1978.

99. Everett, W. G. Suture materials in general surgery. *Prog. Surg.* 8:14, 1970.

100. Feller, I. A., and DeWeese, M. S. The use of stored cutaneous autografts in wound treatment. *Surgery* 44:540, 1958.

101. Finseth, F., and Adelberg, M. Prevention of skin flap necrosis by vasodilator pharmacologic agents. *Plast. Reconstr. Surg.* 61:738, 1978.

102. Finseth, F., and Cutting, C. An experimental neurovascular island flap for the study of the delay phenomenon. *Plast. Reconstr. Surg.* 6:412, 1978.

103. Fischl, R. A. An adhesive for primary closure of skin incisions. *Plast. Reconstr. Surg.* 30:607, 1962.

104. Flinn, R. M. Knotting in medicine and surgery. *Practitioner* 183:322, 1959.

105. Forrester, J. C. Tape closed and sutured wounds. *Br. J. Surg.* 57:729, 1970.

106. Forrester, J. C. Suture material and use. *Br. J. Hosp. Med.* 8:578, 1972.

107. Forte, V., Middleton, W. G., and Briant, T. D. Expansion of myocutaneous flaps. *Arch. Otolaryngol.* 111:371, 1985.

108. Fujino, T., Harishina, T., and Aoyagi, F. Reconstruction for aplasia of the breast and pectoral region by microvascular transfer of a free flap from the buttock. *Plast. Reconstr. Surg.* 56:178, 1975.

109. Furnas, D. W. Freehand technique for cutting one-piece split-skin grafts from avulsed or excised skin and fat. *Plast. Reconstr. Surg.* 39:497, 1967.

110. Furnas, D. W., and Fischer, G. W. The Z-plasty: Biomechanics and mathematics. *Br. J. Plast. Surg.* 24:144, 1971.

111. Futrell, J. W., Johns, M. E., Edgerton, M. T., et al. Platysma myocutaneous flap for intraoral reconstruction. *Am. J. Surg.* 136:504, 1978.

112. Gallico, G. G., O'Connor, N. E., Compton, C. C., et al. Permanent coverage of large burn wounds with autologous cultured human epithelium. *N. Engl. J. Med.* 311:448, 1984.

113. Gatti, J. E., LaRossa, D., Brousseau, D. A., et al. Assessment of neurovascularization and timing of flap division. *Plast. Reconstr. Surg.* 73:396, 1984.

114. Gemberling, R. M., Miller, T. A., Caffee, H., et al. Dressing comparison in the healing of donor sites. *J. Trauma* 16:812, 1976.

115. Ger, R., and Levine, S. A. The management of decubitus ulcer by muscle transposition. *Plast. Reconstr. Surg.* 58:419, 1976.

116. Gibson, E. W., and Poate, W. J. The use of adhesive surgical tape in plastic surgery. *Br. J. Plast. Surg.* 17:265, 1964.

117. Gibson, T., and Kenedi, R. M. Biomechanical properties of skin. *Surg. Clin. North Am.* 47:279, 1967.

118. Gimbal, N. S., and Farris, W. Skin grafting. *Arch. Surg.* 92:554, 1966.

119. Gingrass, P. J., Grabb, W. C., and Gingrass, R. P. Rat skin autografts over Silastic implants: A study of the bridging phenomenon. *Plast. Reconstr. Surg.* 55:65, 1975.

120. Goetz, R. H. The diagnosis and treatment of vascular diseases. *Br. J. Surg.* 37:146, 1949.

121. Goetz, R. H. The rate and control of the blood flow through the skin of the upper extremities. *S. Afr. J. Med. Sci.* 8:65, 1963.

122. Goode, R. L., and Linehan, J. W. The fluorescein test in postirradiation surgery—a preliminary report. *Arch. Otolaryngol.* 91:526, 1970.

123. Goodman, G. *The Pharmacological Basis of Therapeutics* (5th ed.). New York: Macmillan, 1975. P. 950.

124. Gonzalez-Ulloa, M., Stevens, E., Alveres, F. G., et al. Espesor cutaneou; reporte de nuestro estudio microscopico. *Cir. Cir.* 24:455, 1956.

125. Goulian, D. A new economical dermatome. *Plast. Reconstr. Surg.* 42:85, 1968.

126. Grabb, W. C., and Oneal, R. The effect of low molecular weight dextran on the survival of experimental skin flaps. *Plast. Reconstr. Surg.* 30:649, 1966.

127. Grillo, H. C., and McKhann, C. F. The acceptance and evolution of dermal homografts freed of viable cells. *Transplantation* 2:48, 1964.

128. Haller, J. A., and Billingham, R. E. Studies of the vascularization in free skin grafts. *Ann. Surg.* 166:896, 1967.

129. Harii, K., Ohmori, K., and Ohmori, S. Successful clinical transfer of ten free flaps by microvascular anastomoses. *Plast. Reconstr. Surg.* 53:259, 1974.

130. Harii, K., Ohmori, K., and Sekiguchi, J. The free musculocutaneous flap. *Plast. Reconstr. Surg.* 57:294, 1976.

131. Harrison, D. H., Girling, M., and Mott, G. Experience in monitoring the circulation in free-flap transfers. *Plast. Reconstr. Surg.* 68:543, 1981.

132. Härting, F., Koorneff, H., and Peeters, H. J. F. Glue fixation of split thickness graft to the bony orbit following exenteration. *Plast. Reconstr. Surg.* 76:633, 1985.

133. Hartrampf, C. R., and Culbertson, J. H. A dermal-fat flap for nipple reconstruction. *Plast. Reconstr. Surg.* 73:983, 1984.

134. Hasson, H. M., Nicoloff, D., Ford, C. R., et al. New sutureless technique for skin closure. *Arch. Surg.* 111:83, 1976.

135. Hauser, W. H., Tauxe, W. N., Owen, C. A., Jr., et al. Determination of the vascular status of pedicle skin grafts by radioactive tracer studies. *Surg. Gynecol. Obstet.* 112:625, 1961.

136. Hayes, H. Cross-leg flaps after the age of fifty. *Plast. Reconstr. Surg.* 30:649, 1962.

137. Hayes, J. E., Robinson, D. W., Schloerb, P. R., et al. A simple method of testing the circulation of pedicle flaps. *Surg. Forum* 18:516, 1967.

138. Hermann, J. B. Changes in tensile strength and knot security of surgical sutures in vivo. *Arch. Surg.* 106:707, 1973.

139. Hermann, J. B., Kelly, R. J., and Higgins, G. A. Polyglycolic acid sutures. *Arch. Surg.* 100:486, 1970.

140. Hill, H. L., Brown, R. G., and Jurkiewicz, M. J. The transverse lumbosacral back flap. *Plast. Reconstr. Surg.* 62:177, 1978.

141. Hoffmeister, F. S. Studies on timing of tissue transfer in reconstructive surgery. *Plast. Reconstr. Surg.* 19:283, 1957.

142. Holden, I. A., Knoll, C. A., and Wesselman, J. Norfloxacin and silver-norfloxacin as topical antimicrobial agents: Results of in vitro susceptibility testing against bacteria and Candida sp. isolated from burn patients. *J. Burn Care Rx* 7:479, 1986.

143. Hong, C., Stark, G. B., and Futrell, J. W. Elongation of axial blood vessels with a tissue expander. *Clin. Plast. Surg.* 14:465, 1987.

144. Hooper, J. E. Pedicle Flaps: An Overview. In T. S. Krizek and J. E. Hooper (eds.), *Symposium on Basic Science in Plastic Surgery.* Vol. 15. St. Louis: Mosby, 1976.

145. Horton, C., Georgiade, N., Campbell, F., et al. The behavior of split thickness and dermal skin grafts in the peritoneal cavity. *Plast. Reconstr. Surg.* 12:269, 1953.

146. Howie, C. C. M. Refrigeration anesthesia for donor sites. *Br. J. Anaesth.* 43:616, 1971.

147. Hueston, J. T., and McConchie, I. H. A compound pectoral flap. *Aust. N.Z. J. Surg.* 38:61, 1968.

148. Hunt, T. K. (ed.). *Fundamentals of Wound Management.* New York: Appleton-Century-Crofts, 1979.

149. Hunt, T. K., Knighton, D. R., Thakrol, K. K., et al. Studies on inflammation and wound healing: Angiogenesis and collagen synthesis stimulated in vivo by resident and activated wound macrophages. *Surgery* 96:48, 1984.

150. Hutchison, J., Tough, J., and Wyburn, G. Regeneration of sensation in grafted skin. *Br. J. Plast. Surg.* 2:82, 1949.

151. Hynes, W. A simple method of estimating blood flow with special reference to the circulation in pedicled skin flaps and tubes. *Br. J. Plast. Surg.* 1:159, 1948.

152. Hynes, W. The "blue flap": A method of treatment. *Br. J. Plast. Surg.* 4:166, 1951.

153. Hynes, W. The treatment of scars by shaving and skin grafting. *Br. J. Plast. Surg.* 10:1, 1957.

154. Igel, H. J., Freeman, A. E., Broeckman, C. R., et al. A new method of covering large surface area wounds with autografts: Application of tissue culture expanded autograft. *Arch. Surg.* 108:724, 1974.

155. Jackson, D. M., Lowburn, E. J. L., and Topley, E. Chemotherapy of Streptococcus pyogenes infection of burns. *Lancet* 2:705, 1951.

156. Jenkins, H. P., Hrdina, L. S., Owens, F. M., et al. Absorption of surgical gut. III. Duration in the tissues after loss of tensile strength. *Arch. Surg.* 45:74, 1942.

157. Jervis, W., Salyer, K. E., Vargas Busquets, M., et al. Further application of the Limberg and Dufourmental flaps. *Plast. Reconstr. Surg.* 54:335, 1974.

158. Jesse, R. H., Jr., Anderson, B. C., and Healey, J. E., Jr. Fixation of split-thickness skin grafts with adhesive. *Plast. Reconstr. Surg.* 33:272, 1964.

159. Johnson, P. E., Kernahan, D. A., and Bauer, B. S. Dermal and epidermal response to soft tissue expansion in the pig. *Plast. Reconstr. Surg.* 81:390, 1988.

160. Jonsson, K., Hunt, T. K., Brennan, S. S., et al. Tissue oxygen measurements in delayed skin flaps: A reconsideration of the mechanisms of the delay phenomenon. *Plast. Reconstr. Surg.* 82:328, 1988.

161. Kazanceva, N. D. Growth characteristics of skin thickness in children and its significance in free skin grafts. *Acta Chir. Plast. (Praha)* 11:71, 1969.

162. Kazanjian, V. H., and Converse, J. M. *The Surgical Treatment of Facial Injuries* (2nd ed.). Baltimore: Williams & Wilkins, 1959.

163. Keenan, K. M., Rodeheaven, G. T., Kenney, J. G., et al. Surgical cautery revisited. *Am. J. Surg.* 147:818, 1984.

164. Kenigan, C. L. Skin flap failure: Pathophysiology. *Plast. Reconstr. Surg.* 72:766, 1983.

165. Kernanhan, D. A., and Littlewood, A. H. M. Experience in the use of arterial flaps about the face. *Plast. Reconstr. Surg.* 28:207, 1961.

166. Kernahan, D. A., Zingg, W., and Kay, C. W. The effect of hyperbaric oxygen on the survival of experimental skin flaps. *Plast. Reconstr. Surg.* 36:19, 1965.

167. Ketchum, L. D. Pharmacological alterations in the clotting mechanism: Use in microvascular surgery. *J. Hand Surg.* 3:407, 1978.

168. Kikuchi, I., and Omori, M. Demonstration of leaking vessels under skin grafts. *Plast. Reconstr. Surg.* 45:66, 1970.

169. Kirschbaum, J., and Rider, H. The surgical treatment of baldness. *Med. Times* 91:1037, 1963.

170. Kivisaari, J., and Niinikoski, J. Effects of HBO and prolonged hyperoxia on the healing of open wounds. *Acta Chir. Scand.* 141:14, 1975.

171. Klingenström, P., and Nylen, B. Timing of transfer of tubed pedicles and cross flaps. *Plast. Reconstr. Surg.* 37:1, 1966.

172. Knighton, D. R., Hunt, T. K., and Scheuenstuhl, H., et al. Oxygen tension regulated the expression of angiogenesis factor by macrophages. *Science* 221:1283, 1983.

173. Koehnlein, H. E., and Deitrich, E. E. Influence of different tension on growth of skin grafts. *Surg. Forum* 26:562, 1975.

174. Koehnlein, H. E., and Lemperle, G. Experimental studies on the effect of dimethyl sulfoxide on pedicle flaps. *Surgery* 67:672, 1970.

175. Kraissl, C. J. The selection of appropriate lines for elective surgical incisions. *Plast. Reconstr. Surg.* 8:1, 1951.

176. Krizek, T. J., and Robson, M. C. Evolution of quantitative bacteriology in wound management. *Am. J. Surg.* 130:579, 1975.

177. LaPiana, F. G., and Permer, R. Anaphylactoid reaction to intravenously administered fluorescein. *Arch. Ophthalmol.* 79:161, 1968.

178. LaTrenta, G. S., McCarthy, J. G., Epstein, M., et al. Bone graft survival in expanded skin. *Plast. Reconstr. Surg.* 81:406, 1988.

179. Lawrence, W. T., Murphy, R. C., Robson, M. C., et al. The detrimental effect of cigarette smoking on flap survival: An experimental study in the rat. *Br. J. Plast. Surg.* 37:216, 1984.

180. Leighton, W. D., Russell, R. C., Marcus, D. E., et al. Experimental pretransfer expansion of free flap donor sites. I. Flap inability and expansion characteristics. *Plast. Reconstr. Surg.* 82:69, 1988.

181. Leighton, W. D., Russell, R. C., Feller, A. M., et al. Experimental pretransfer expansion of free flap donor sites. II. Physiology, histology and clinical correlation. *Plast. Reconstr. Surg.* 82:76, 1988.

182. Lent, C. New medical and scientific uses of the leech. *Nature* 323:494, 1986.

183. Leonard, A. G., and Small, J. O. Tissue expansion in the treatment of alopecia. *Br. J. Plast. Surg.* 39:42, 1986.

184. Lie, K. K., Magargle, R. K., and Posch, J. L. Free full-thickness skin grafts from the palm to cover defects of the fingers. *J. Bone Joint Surg. [Am.]* 52:559, 1970.

185. Liedberg, N., Kuhn, L. R., Barnes, B. A., et al. Infection in burns. II. The pathogenicity of streptococci. *Surg. Gynecol. Obstet.* 98:693, 1954.

186. Limberg, A. A. *Planning of Local Plastic Operations on the Body's Surface: Theory and Practice.* Leningrad: Medgis, 1963.

187. Link, W. J., Incropera, F. P., and Glover, J. L. Plasma scalpel: Comparison of tissue damage and wound healing with electrosurgical and steel scalpels. *Arch. Surg.* 111:392, 1976.

188. Lister, G. D., and Gibson, T. Closure or rhomboid skin defects: The flaps of Limberg and Dufourmental. *Br. J. Surg.* 25:300, 1972.

189. Little, J. W., Fontana, D. J., and McCulloch, D. T. The upper-quadrant flap. *Plast. Reconstr. Surg.* 68:175, 1981.

190. Little, J. W., Munasafi, T., and McCulloch, D. T. One-stage reconstruction of a projecting nipple: The quadrapod flap. *Plast. Reconstr. Surg.* 71:126, 1983.

191. Littlewood, A. H. M. Seroma: An unrecognized cause of failure of split-thickness skin grafts. *Br. J. Plast. Surg.* 13:42, 1960.

192. Littlewood, M. Compound skin and sternomastoid flaps for repair in extensive carcinoma of the head and neck. *Br. J. Plast. Surg.* 20:403, 1967.

193. Lofgren, L. Recovery of nervous function in skin transplants with special reference to sympathetic functions. *Acta Chir. Scand.* 102:229, 1951.

194. Lopez-Mas, J., Ortiz-Monasterio, F., De-Gonzales, M. V., et al. Skin graft pigmentation: A new approach to prevention. *Plast. Reconstr. Surg.* 49:18, 1972.

195. Lucid, M. L. The interlocking slip knot. *Plast. Reconstr. Surg.* 34:200, 1964.

196. MacMillan, B. G. The use of mesh grafting in treating burns. *Surg. Clin. North Am.* 50:1347, 1970.

197. Manders, E. K., Au, U. K., and Wong, R. K. M. Scalp expansion for male pattern baldness. *Clin. Plast. Surg.* 14:469, 1987.

198. Manders, E. K., Saggers, G. C., Diaz-Alonso, P., et al. Elongation of peripheral nerve and viscera containing smooth muscle. *Clin. Plast. Surg.* 14:551, 1987.

199. Manson, P., Anthenelli, R. M., Im, M. J., et al. The role of oxygen-free radicals in ischemic tissue injury in island skin flaps. *Ann. Surg.* 198:87, 1983.

200. Maris, F., Jurkovic, I., Kobut, P., and Suchanek, A. Re-innervation of free and flap skin grafts. *Acta Chir. Plast. (Praha)* 5:57, 1963.

201. Marks, M. W., Argenta, L. C., and Thorton, J. W. Burn management: The role of tissue expansion. *Clin. Plast. Surg.* 14:543, 1987.

202. Masson, J. K. Exposure in free split-thickness skin grafts. *Arch. Surg.* 82:343, 1961.

203. Mathes, S., and Nahai, F. *Clinical Atlas of Muscle and Musculocutaneous Flaps.* St. Louis: Mosby, 1979.

204. Mathes, S. J., and Nahai, F. *Clinical Applications for Muscle and Musculocutaneous Flaps.* St. Louis: Mosby, 1982.

205. Mathes, S. J., Alpert, B. S., and Chang, N. Use of the muscle flap in chronic osteomyelitis: Experimental and clinical correlation. *Plast. Reconstr. Surg.* 69:815, 1982.

206. McCollum, M. S., and Grabb, W. C. Increasing the incidence and the size of successful experimental composite ear grafts by advance preparation of the recipient bed. *Plast. Reconstr. Surg.* 60:759, 1977.

207. McCraw, J. B., and Arnold, P. G. *Atlas of Muscle and Musculocutaneous Flaps.* Norfolk, VA: Hampton Press, 1986.

208. McCraw, J. B., and Dibbell, D. G. Experimental definition of independent myocutaneous vascular territories. *Plast. Reconstr. Surg.* 60:212, 1977.

209. McCraw, J. B., Dibbell, D. G., and Carraway, J. H. Clinical definition of independent myocutaneous vascular territories. *Plast. Reconstr. Surg.* 60:341, 1977.

210. McCraw, J. B., Dibbell, D. G., Horton, C. E., et al. Clinical definition of independent myocutaneous vascular territories. Presented at the Meeting of the American Association of Plastic Surgeons, Atlanta, 1976.

211. McDowell, A. J. Wound infections resulting from the use of hot wet sponges. *Plast. Reconstr. Surg.* 23:168, 1959.

212. McGrath, M. H., and Simon, R. H. Wound geometry and the kinetics of wound contraction. *Plast. Reconstr. Surg.* 72:66, 1983.

213. McGregor, I. A. The regeneration of sympathetic activity in grafted skin as evidenced by sweating. *Br. J. Plast. Surg.* 3:12, 1950.

214. McGregor, I. A. *Fundamental Techniques of Plastic Surgery* (2nd ed.). Edinburgh: Livingstone, 1962.

215. McGregor, I. A., and Jackson, I. T. The groin flap. *Br. J. Plast. Surg.* 25:3, 1972.

216. McIndoe, A. H. The treatment of hypospadias. *Am. J. Surg.* 38:176, 1937.

217. McKusick, V. (ed.). Ehrlos-Danlos Syndrome. In *Heritable Disorders of Connective Tissue.* St. Louis: Mosby, 1972.

218. McLean, D. H., and Buncke, H. J. Autotransplant of omentum to a large scalp defect, with microsurgical revascularization. *Plast. Reconstr. Surg.* 49:268, 1972.

219. Mercer, N. S., Beere, D. M., Bornemisza, A. J., et al. Medical leeches as sources of wound infection. *Br. Med. J.* 294:937, 1987.

220. Millard, D. R. The Crane principle for the transport of subcutaneous tissue. *Plast. Reconstr. Surg.* 43:451, 1969.

221. Millay, D. J., Cook, T. A., Brummett, R. E., et al. Wound healing and the Shaw scalpel. *Arch. Otolaryngol. Head Neck Surg.* 113:282, 1987.

222. Miller, J. M., Zoll, D. R., and Brown, E. O. Clinical observations on use of an extruded collagen suture. *Arch. Surg.* 88:167, 1964.

223. Miller, S. H., Buck, D. C., Woodward, W. R., et al. Alterations in local blood flow and tissue gas tension caused by epinephrine. *Plast. Reconstr. Surg.* 73:797, 1984.

224. Miller, T. A. The deleterious effect of split-skin homograft coverage on split-skin donor sites. *Plast. Reconstr. Surg.* 53:316, 1974.

225. Milton, S. H. The tubed pedicle flap. *Br. J. Plast. Surg.* 22:53, 1969.

226. Milton, S. H. Pedicled skin flaps: The fallacy of the length:width ratio. *Br. J. Surg.* 57:502, 1970.

227. Milton, S. H. Experimental studies on island flaps. I. The surviving length. *Plast. Reconstr. Surg.* 49:574, 1971.

228. Milton, S. H., and Corbett, J. L. Failure to increase the survival of experimental flaps by histamine and hypertension. *Plast. Reconstr. Surg.* 43:235, 1969.

229. Mir y Mir, L. The problem of pigmentation in the cutaneous graft. *Br. J. Plast. Surg.* 14:303, 1961.

230. Mir y Mir, L. The six-flap Z-plasty. *Plast. Reconstr. Surg.* 52:625, 1973.

231. Mladick, R. A., Pickrell, K. L., Thorne, F. L., et al. Ipsilateral thigh flap for total plantar resurfacing. *Plast. Reconstr. Surg.* 43:198, 1969.

232. Moncrief, J. A. Topical therapy for control of bacteria in the burn wound. *World J. Surg.* 2:151, 1978.

233. Morestin, H. La reduction graduelle des difformites tegumentaires. *Bull. Soc. Chir. Paris* 41:1233, 1915.

234. Moseley, L. H., Finseth, F., and Goody, M. Nicotine and its effect on wound healing. *Plast. Reconstr. Surg.* 61:570, 1978.

235. Mulliken, J. B., and Healey, N. A. Pathogenesis of skin flap necrosis from an underlying hematoma. *Plast. Reconstr. Surg.* 63:540, 1979.

236. Murray, J. F., Ord, J. V. R., and Gavelin, G. E. The neurovascular island pedicle flap. *J. Bone Joint Surg. [Am.]* 49:1285, 1967.

237. Myers, M. B. Wound tension and vascularity in the etiology and prevention of skin sloughs. *Surgery* 56:945, 1964.

238. Myers, M. B. Prediction and prevention of skin sloughs in radical cancer surgery. *Pacific Med. Surg.* 75:315, 1967.

239. Myers, M. B. Investigation of Skin Flap Necrosis. In W. C. Grabb and M. B. Myers (eds.), *Skin Flaps.* Boston: Little, Brown, 1975.

240. Myers, M. B., and Cherry, G. Enhancement of survival in devascularized pedicles by the use of phenoxybenzamine. *Plast. Reconstr. Surg.* 41:254, 1968.

241. Myers, M. B., and Cherry, G. Mechanism of the delay phenomenon. *Plast. Reconstr. Surg.* 44:52, 1969.

242. Myers, M. B., and Cherry, G. Functional and angiographic vasculature in healing wounds. *Ann. Surg.* 36:750, 1970.

243. Najarian, J. S., Crane, J. T., and McCorkle, H. J. An experimental study of the grafting of a suspension of skin particles. *Surgery* 42:218, 1957.

244. Neumann, C. The expansion of an area of skin by progressive distension of a subcutaneous balloon. *Plast. Reconstr. Surg.* 19:124, 1957.

245. Niinikoski, J. Viability of ischemic skin in hyperbaric oxygen. *Acta Chir. Scand.* 136:567, 1970.

246. Nordström, R. E. A., and Nordström, R. M. Absorbable versus nonabsorbable sutures to prevent postoperative stretching of wound area. *Plast. Reconstr. Surg.* 78:186, 1986.

247. O'Brien, B. A muscle-skin pedicle for total reconstruction of the lower lip. *Plast. Reconstr. Surg.* 45:395, 1970.

248. O'Brien, B., Morrison, W. A., Ishida, H., et al. Free flap transfers with microvascular anatomoses. *Br. J. Plast. Surg.* 27:220, 1974.

249. Oden, B. Microlymphangiographic studies of experimental skin autografts. *Acta Chir. Scand.* 121:219, 1961.

250. Omer, G., Day, D. J., Ratcliff, H., and Lambert, P. Neurovascular cutaneous island pedicles for deficient median nerve sensibility: New technique and results of serial functional tests. *J. Bone Joint Surg. [Am.]* 52: 1181, 1970.

251. Oneal, R. M., Knode, R. E., Grabb, W. C., et al. The effect of low molecular weight dextran on the survival of skin flaps in pigs vascularized either by a single artery and vein or by a subdermal plexus. *Plast. Reconstr. Surg.* 40:595, 1967.

252. Orentreich, N. Autografts in alopecias and

other selected dermatological conditions. *Ann. N.Y. Acad. Sci.* 83:463, 1959.

253. Orticochea, M. The musculo-cutaneous flap method: An immediate and theoric substitute for the method of delay. *Br. J. Plast. Surg.* 25:106, 1972.

254. Papaevangelou, E. J., and Edwards, S. W. Prevention of thrombosis after small artery endarterectomy with dextran and fibrinolytic agents. *J. Cardiovasc. Surg.* 16:554, 1975.

255. Pasyk, K. A., Argenta, L. C., and Hasset, C. Quantitative analysis of the thickness of human skin and subcutaneous tissue following controlled expansion with a silicone implant. *Plast. Reconstr. Surg.* 81:516, 1988.

256. Patterson, T. J. S., Berry, R. J., and Wiernik, G. The effect of x-radiation on the survival of skin flaps in the pig. *Br. J. Plast. Surg.* 25:17, 1972.

257. Patton, H. S. Split-skin grafts from hypothenar area for fingertip avulsions. *Plast. Reconstr. Surg.* 43:426, 1969.

258. Peacock, E. E., Jr. Reconstruction of the hand by the local transfer of composite tissue island flaps. *Plast. Reconstr. Surg.* 25:298, 1960.

259. Perrins, D. J. D. Influence of hyperbaric oxygen on the survival of split skin grafts. *Lancet* 1:868, 1967.

260. Perry, V. P. A review of skin preservation. *Cryobiology* 3:109, 1966.

261. Pers, M., and Medgyesi, S. Pedicle muscle flaps and their applications in the surgery of repair. *Br. J. Plast. Surg.* 26:313, 1973.

262. Polk, H. C., Jr. Adherence of thin skin grafts. *Surg. Forum* 17:487, 1966.

263. Ponten, B. Grafted skin—observations on innervation and other qualities. *Acta Chir. Scand.* [Suppl.]257:1, 1960.

264. Postlethwait, R. W. Long term comparative study of nonabsorbable sutures. *Ann. Surg.* 171:892, 1970.

265. Psillakis, J. M. Lymphatic vascularization of skin grafts. *Plast. Reconstr. Surg.* 43:287, 1969.

266. Radovan, D. Tissue expansion in soft-tissue reconstruction. *Plast. Reconstr. Surg.* 74:482, 1984.

267. Ragnell, A. The secondary contracting tendency of free skin grafts. *Br. J. Plast. Surg.* 5:6, 1952.

268. Randall, P. Problems in skin grafting. *Surg. Clin. North Am.* 40:1629, 1960.

269. Rees, T. D., Liverett, D. M., and Guy, C. L. The effect of cigarette smoking on skin flap survival in the face lift patient. *Plast. Reconstr. Surg.* 73:911, 1984.

270. Reinisch, J. F. Pathophysiology of skin flap circulation. *Plast. Reconstr. Surg.* 54:585, 1974.

271. Reinisch, J. F. The effect of local anesthesia with epinephrine on skin flap survival. *Plast. Reconstr. Surg.* 54:324, 1974.

272. Reinisch, J. F. The role of Arteriovenous Anastomoses in Skin Flaps. In W. C. Grabb and M. B. Myers (eds.), *Skin Flaps.* Boston: Little, Brown, 1975.

273. Reus, W. F., Robson, M. C., Zachary, L., et al. Acute effects of tobacco smoking on blood flow in the cutaneous microcirculation. *Br. J. Plast. Surg.* 37:213, 1984.

274. Rheinwald, J. G., and Green, H. Serial cultivation of strains of human epidermal keratinocytes: The formation of keratinizing colonies from single cells. *Cell* 6:331, 1975.

275. Rigbi, M., Levy, H., Eldon, A., et al. The saliva of the medicinal leech Hirudo medicinalis. *Comp. Biochem. Physiol.* 88:95, 1987.

276. Robinson, D. W. Blood loss from donor sites in skin grafting procedures. *Surgery* 25:105, 1949.

277. Robson, M. C., Krizek, T. J., and Heggars, J. P. Biology of Surgical Infections. In M. M. Ravitch (ed.), *Current Problems in Surgery.* Chicago: Year Book, 1973.

278. Rodeheaver, G. T., Rye, D. G., Rust, R., et al. Mechanism by which proteolytic enzymes prolong the golden period of antibiotic action. *Am. J. Surg.* 136:379, 1978.

279. Ross, D. S., and Gibson, T. A new dermatome for preparing large free skin grafts. *Med. Electron Biol. Eng.* 3:403, 1965.

280. Rudolph, R. Inhibition of myofibroblasts by skin grafts. *Plast. Reconstr. Surg.* 63:473, 1979.

281. Rudolph, R., and Klein, L. Healing processes in skin grafts. *Surg. Gynecol. Obstet.* 136:641, 1973.

282. Russo, M. Brulures dorsalis graves de la main. *Ann. Chir.* 29:1015, 1975.

283. Salisbury, R. E., Caines, R., and McCarthy, L. R. Comparison of the bacterial cleaning effects of different biologic dressings on granulating wounds following thermal injury. *Plast. Reconstr. Surg.* 66:596, 1980.

284. Salisbury, R. E., Wilmore, D. W., Silverstein,

P., et al. Biologic dressings for skin graft donor sites. *Arch. Surg.* 106:705, 1973.

285. Sasaki, G. H., and Pang, C. Y. Pathophysiology of skin flaps raised on expanded pig skin. *Plast. Reconstr. Surg.* 74:59, 1984.

286. Saunders, W. H. Pedicled pericranium as base for skin grafts. *Laryngoscope* 78:1088, 1968.

287. Sawhney, C. P., and Subbaraju, G. V. Healing of donor sites of split skin grafts—an experimental study in pigs. *Br. J. Plast. Surg.* 22:359, 1969.

288. Saxby, P. J. Survival of island flaps after tissue expansion: A pig model. *Plast. Reconstr. Surg.* 81:30, 1988.

289. Scothorne, R. J. Lymphatic repair and the genesis of homograft immunity. *Ann. N.Y. Acad. Sci.* 73:673, 1958.

290. Sekan, V., and Brozman, V. A survey of testing methods and techniques for free skin graft revascularization. *Acta Chir. Plast.* 28: 145, 1986.

291. Sellers, D. S., Miller, S. H., Demuth, R. J., et al. Repeated skin expansion to resurface a massive thigh wound. *Plast. Reconstr. Surg.* 77:654, 1986.

292. Serafin, D., Georgiade, N. G., and Smith, D. H. Microsurgical composite tissue transplantation for reconstruction of defects of the distal lower extremity: A comparison with older methods. *Plast. Reconstr. Surg.* 62:527, 1978.

293. Shearin, J. C., and DeFranzo, A. J. Butterfly correction of webbed-neck deformity in Turner's syndrome. *Plast. Reconstr. Surg.* 66:129, 1980.

294. Shepard, G. H. The storage of split-skin grafts on their donor sites. *Plast. Reconstr. Surg.* 49:115, 1972.

295. Shoul, M. I. Skin grafting under local anesthesia using a new safety razor dermatome. *Am. J. Surg.* 112:959, 1966.

296. Shuck, J. W., Pruitt, B. A., Jr., and Moncrief, J. A. Homograft skin for wound coverage. *Arch. Surg.* 98:472, 1969.

297. Siegel, R. J., Vistnes, L. M., and Iverson, R. E. Effective hemostasis with less epinephrine. *Plast. Reconstr. Surg.* 51:129, 1973.

298. Skoog, T. Porous tape in wound closure, skin grafting and wound dressing. *Acta Chir. Scand.* 126:383, 1963.

299. Smahel, J. The revascularization of free skin autograft. *Acta Chir. Plast. (Praha)* 9:76, 1967.

300. Smahel, J. Free skin transplantation on a prepared bed. *Br. J. Plast. Surg.* 24:129, 1971.

301. Smahel, J. The healing of skin grafts. *Clin. Plast. Surg.* 4:409, 1977.

302. Smahel, J., and Clodius, L. The blood vessel system of free human skin grafts. *Plast. Reconstr. Surg.* 47:61, 1971.

303. Smahel, J., and Ganzoni, N. Relay transplantation: A new method of expanding a free skin graft. *Plast. Reconstr. Surg.* 28:49, 1975.

304. Smith, F. *Plastic and Reconstructive Surgery, A Manual of Management.* Philadelphia: Saunders, 1950.

305. Smith, J. W. Clinical experiences with the vermilion bordered lip flat. *Plast. Reconstr. Surg.* 27:527, 1961.

306. Smith, J. W., Ringland, J., and Wilson, R. Vascularization of skin grafts. *Surg. Forum* 15: 473, 1964.

307. Smith, P. J., Foley, B., McGregor, I. A., et al. The anatomical basis of the groin flap. *Plast. Reconstr. Surg.* 49:41, 1972.

308. Snell, P. M. The pig as an experimental model for skin flap behavior: A reappraisal of previous studies. *Br. J. Plast. Surg.* 30:1, 1977.

309. Snow, J. W. Safety razor dermatome. *Plast. Reconstr. Surg.* 41:184, 1968.

310. Snyder, C. C., Bateman, J. M., Davis, C. W., et al. Mandibulofacial restoration with live osteocutaneous flaps. *Plast. Reconstr. Surg.* 45:14, 1970.

311. Southorn, P. A., and Powis, G. Free radicals in medicine. I. Chemical nature and biologic reactions. II. Involvement in human disease. *Mayo Clin. Proc.* 63:381, 1988.

312. Southwood, W. F. W. The thickness of the skin. *Plast. Reconstr. Surg.* 15:423, 1955.

313. Spina, V. "Z" plasty. *Rev. Paul. Med.* 36:347, 1950.

314. Stark, G. B., Hong, C., and Futrell, J. W. Rapid elongation of arteries and veins in rats with a tissue expander. *Plast. Reconstr. Surg.* 80:570, 1987.

315. Stark, R. B. *Plastic Surgery.* New York: Harper & Row, 1962.

316. Steffensen, W. H., and Worthen, E. F. Limitations of multiple excision. *Am. J. Surg.* 95:237, 1958.

317. Steiss, C. F. Utilization of the tube pedicle in

the reconstruction of facial defects. *Plast. Reconstr. Surg.* 4:545, 1949.

318. Stern, W. G., and Cohen, M. B. The intracutaneous salt solution wheat test. *J.A.M.A.* 87:1355, 1926.

319. Stevenson, T. W. Release of circular constricting scars by Z flaps. *Plast. Reconstr. Surg.* 1:39, 1946.

320. Sturman, M. J., and Duran, R. J. Late results of finger-tip injuries. *J. Bone Joint Surg. [Am.]* 45:289, 1963.

321. Sundell, B. Studies on the circulation of pedicle skin flaps. *Ann. Chir. Gynaecol. Fenn. [Suppl. 53]*133:1, 1963.

322. Sweeney, N. V. Composite grafts of skin and fat. *Br. J. Plast. Surg.* 26:72, 1973.

323. Szymonowski, J. von. *Handbuch der operativen Chirurgi.* Brunswick: Frederick Viewig, 1870.

324. Tagliacozzi, G. *De Curtorum Chirurgia per Insitionern.* Venetus: G. Bindonus, 1597.

325. Tauxe, W. N., Simons, J. N., Lipscomb, P. R., et al. Determination of vascular status of pedicled skin flaps by used radioactive pertechnetate ($^{99m}$Tc). *Surg. Gynecol. Obstet.* 130:87, 1970.

326. Tavis, M. J., Thornton, J. W., et al. Graft adherence to de-epithelialized surfaces: A comparison study. *Ann. Surg.* 184:594, 1976.

327. Tavis, M. J., Thornton, J. W., Harney, J. H., et al. Mechanism of skin graft adherence: Collagen, elastin and fibrin interactions. *Surg. Forum* 28:522, 1977.

328. Taylor, J. W. Scalp as a donor site. *Am. J. Surg.* 133:218, 1977.

329. Theogaraj, D. S. Personal communication.

330. Thompson, D. P., and Ashley, F. L. Use of stapler in skin closure. *Am. J. Surg.* 132:136, 1976.

331. Thompson, N. A clinical and histological investigation into the fate of epithelial elements buried following the grafting of "shaved" skin surfaces. *Br. J. Plast. Surg.* 13:219, 1960.

332. Thorne, F. L., Georgiade, N. G., and Mladick, R. The use of thermography in determining viability of pedicle flaps. *Arch. Surg.* 99:97, 1969.

333. Thorne, F. L., Georgiade, N. G., Wheller, W. F., et al. Photoplethysmography as an aid in determining the viability of skin flaps. *Plast. Reconstr. Surg.* 44:279, 1969.

334. Thorton, J. W., Marks, M. W., Izenberg, P. H., et al. Expanded myocutaneous flaps: Their clinical use. *Clin. Plast. Surg.* 14:529, 1987.

335. Thorvaldsson, S. E., and Grabb, W. C. The intravenous fluorescein test as a measure of skin flap viability. *Plast. Reconstr. Surg.* 53:576, 1974.

336. Trevaskis, A. E., Rempel, J., Okunski, W., et al. Sliding subcutaneous-pedicle flaps to close a circular defect. *Plast. Reconstr. Surg.* 46:155, 1970.

337. Turner, D. J., and Cohen, I. K. Personal communication.

338. Van Beek, A. L., and Adson, M. H. Tissue expansion in the upper extremity. *Clin. Plast. Surg.* 14:535, 1987.

339. Varma, S., Ferguson, H. L., Breen, H., et al. Comparison of seven suture materials in infected wounds—an experimental study. *J. Surg. Res.* 17:165, 1974.

340. Vasconez, L. O., Bostwick, J., and McCraw, J. Coverage of exposed bone by muscle transposition and skin grafting. *Plast. Reconstr. Surg.* 53:526, 1974.

341. Velander, E. Vascular changes in tubed pedicles: An animal experimental study. *Acta Chir. Scand. [Suppl.]*322:1, 1964.

342. Versaci, A. D., Balkovich, O. E., and Goldstein, S. A. Breast reconstruction by tissue expansion for congenital and burn deformities. *Ann. Plast. Surg.* 16:20, 1986.

343. Waris, T. Reinnervation of free skin autografts in the rat. *Scand. J. Plast. Reconstr. Surg.* 12:85, 1978.

344. Waris, T., Rechardt, L., Kyösola, K., et al. Reinnervation of human skin grafts: A histochemical study. *Plast. Reconstr. Surg.* 72:439, 1983.

345. Webster, J. P. Thoraco-epigastric tubed pedicles. *Surg. Clin. North Am.* 17:145, 1937.

346. Weisman, P. A. Microporous surgical tape in wound closure and skin grafting. *Br. J. Plast. Surg.* 16:379, 1963.

347. Westfall, T. C., and Watts, D. T. Catecholamine excretion in smokers and nonsmoker. *J. Appl. Physiol.* 19:40, 1964.

348. Wheeler, C. B., Rodeheaver, G. T., Thacker, J. G., et al. Side effects of high pressure irrigation. *Surg. Gynecol. Obstet.* 143:775, 1976.

349. White, W. L. Flap grafts to the upper extremity. *Surg. Clin. North Am.* 40:389, 1960.

350. Wilkinson, T. S., and Rybka, R. J. Experimental study of prevention of tip necrosis in ischemic Z-plasties. *Plast. Reconstr. Surg.* 47:37, 1971.

351. Willman, V. L., and Hanlon, C. R. The influence of temperature on surface bleeding: Favorable effects of local hypothermia. *Ann. Surg.* 143:660, 1956.

352. Winsten, J., Manalo, P., and Barsky, A. Studies on the circulation of tubed flaps. *Plast. Reconstr. Surg.* 28:619, 1961.

353. Woolf, R. M., and Broadbent, T. R. The four flap Z-plasty. *Plast. Reconstr. Surg.* 49:48, 1972.

354. Yannas, F. V., Burke, J. F., Orgill, D. P., et al. Wound tissue can utilize a polymeric template to synthesize a functional extension of skin. *Science* 215:174, 1982.

355. Zapata-Sirvent, R., Hansbrough, J. F., Carroll, W., et al. Comparison of biobrane and scarlet red dressings for treatment of donor site wounds. *Arch. Surg.* 120:743, 1985.

# 2

*Thomas J. Krizek*
*Albert E. Cram*

# Transplantation in Plastic Surgery

From its inception plastic and reconstructive surgery has been marked by transfer and transplantation of tissues. Most deformities, whether genetic or traumatic, involve a deficiency of tissue, and the history of the discipline has been punctuated by milestones in techniques of transplantation to fill this reconstructive need.

## History

History credits not necessarily the first to conceive of an idea but those who "give" it to the world. Susruta in his *Samhita* ("collection of writings") describes the first efforts to transfer tissue to repair ear lobes and parts of the nose [43]. The works of Saint Cosmos and Saint Damian are part lore, part fancy, and truly undocumented efforts to transplant a lower limb from one to another.

Many stories have been published of "replanting" of parts, and the milestone of Tagliocozzi's [64] nasal reconstruction from the tissue of the arm in the sixteenth century can more accurately be described as "transfer" rather than transplantation. The actual transplantation of tissue by techniques that involve a total separation from a blood supply for a period during the transfer is a relatively recent event. Baronio [7] explored the possibilities in what might be described as a "laboratory" setting (actually a stable) when he transferred "grafts" from the tail area of sheep to the back of the animal. Warren [69] performed a free graft of skin to the ala of the nose in 1830, but the significance of the event was not recognized. Some three decades later, J. L. Reverdin [57], a junior house officer in Paris, applied a thin, "epidermic" split graft to the granulating wound on the arm of his patient. A year later George David Pollock [56] employed the technique for the first time in a burned patient with success. Amazingly, he obtained some of his own skin and performed the first skin allograft. He watched the skin appear to grow and then dissolve as the allograft rejection phenomenon occurred. In the days marked by living donors (kidney: Boston, 1953; split livers: University of Chicago, 1989), Pollock set a remarkable standard whereby the surgeon served as the donor. Further advances in skin transplantation have been technical rather than conceptual, marked by the development of instruments to first make the grafts larger (dermatomes) and then smaller (mesher).

In the transplantation of composite tissue and internal organs, there was a flurry of activity at the University of Chicago when Alexis Carrel arrived in 1905 to work with Guthrie. Within a two-year period, before moving to New York, he developed much of the technology that was the foundation for the later experimental transfer of composite tissue [20]. This was performed later in animals by Krizek [41] in 1964 and O'Brien, Buncke, and many others in humans thereafter.

These exquisite developments in the technology of tissue transfer have been brought to clinical fruition in the transplantation of solid organs such as kidney, heart, liver, pancreas, and lung. For skin and composite tissues (as well as intestine), we have walked into the wall of our own limitations.

Between 1944 and 1948 Peter Medawar worked with Gibson at the Burn Center in Glasgow to understand the possibilities of skin allografts [45–47]. This experimental work and later work with Billingham and associates [10, 11] have been the cornerstone of our rapidly expanding study of transplantation biology.

Current methods of recipient immunosuppression are relatively nonspecific, and the side effects are such that allograft transplantation is limited primarily to life-threatening conditions. Future advances in the field of transplant immunology hold the promise of possible donor-specific immunosuppression and the vista of almost unlimited replacement of composite tissue defects by the plastic and reconstructive surgeon.

## Terminology

In this chapter we consider as transplants only those transfers of tissue in which the "graft" is completely separated from its bed and surrounding tissues. We use the terminology introduced by Snell [62] in 1964. An *isograft* (syngeneic graft) is a tissue transfer between genetically identical individuals such as identical twins or highly inbred strains of laboratory animals. An *autograft* is a graft transferred from one location to another on the same animal. An *allograft* (homograft) is a transfer of tissue between genetically disparate individuals of the same species. A *xenograft* (heterograft) is a graft between dif-

ferent species. Tissue transplanted to an anatomically similar site is referred to as an *orthotopic transplant;* tissue transplanted to a site anatomically or functionally different from its site of origin (e.g., vascularized omentum to an intracranial position) is referred to as a *heterotopic transplant.*

Current microsurgical techniques have allowed the heterotopic transplantation of composite autogenous tissues, such as myocutaneous flaps, with excellent maintenance of viability of the transplanted tissue. The more frequently performed free skin grafts depend on the acquisition of new vascular connections between the graft and the recipient bed by natural means. This requires that such transferred tissues remain viable during the 48 to 96 hours necessary for the establishment of circulation [74]. Some applications of tissue transplantation require only that the donated tissue remain physically present as a scaffold for the ingrowth of new host tissues, and in this case, the donor tissue need not be viable at the time of transplantation. Transplants can, therefore, be further subdivided into viable or nonviable donor tissues. Further complexity is added by the successful techniques of tissue banking and most recently by successful tissue cultures that allow either autogeneic or allogeneic transplantation from tissues preserved or grown in the laboratory. Finally, various tissue substitutes formed from biologic materials (primarily xenogeneic in origin) are gaining wide popularity in clinical applications, and these also represent tissue transplantation.

## Transplantation Immunology

The mechanism that allows us to recognize and tolerate "self" while rapidly identifying and rejecting "nonself" is an incredibly complex and precariously balanced miracle. Errors in this mechanism can be produced by trauma as in the severe immunosuppression seen in the massive burn injury, by various genetic errors, or by acquired disease most graphically illustrated by the acquired immunodeficiency syndrome (AIDS). The effects of these errors are well known (if poorly understood) even by the lay public. More subtle defects in the immune mechanism result in various autoimmune phenomena. The complexity of the subject is clearly indicated by the fact that more than 2000 articles on the subject of transplant immunology have appeared in the medical literature since 1978.

In the human, the recognition of self and nonself depends on the expression of both major and minor histocompatibility antigens. Each nucleated cell of the body carries the genetic code for the major histocompatibility antigens (HLA, -A, -B, -C) as well as an antigen complex identified in the human as DR and in the mouse as IA antigen. The genetic code is carried on the sixth chromosome in the human, and the A, B, and C components are expressed in the cell membrane of all nucleated cells. Although the code is present for the DR antigen in all nucleated cells, the expression of this antigen on cell membranes appears to be limited, under normal conditions, to cellular elements of the immune system—for example, lymphocytes and Langerhans cells. This genetic code is different for each individual, and the ability of the immune mechanism to recognize the minor variations in genetic protein sequences sets the stage for their ultimate rejection as nonself antigen.

The process of recognition begins with the initial contact between a foreign antigen and an antigen processing cell (APC). Although other cells can perform antigen processing functions, the macrophage migrating to the site of tissue injury and the Langerhans cell located within the epidermis are the two best described APCs. Contact with a foreign antigen results in activation of the macrophage or Langerhans cell, and at least one byproduct of this activity is the production of interleukin-1 (IL-1), a potent lymphokine, by the activated APC. In addition, the processed antigen is apparently modified to a form rec-

ognizable to specific subsets of the lymphocyte population responsible for humoral imunity (B lymphocytes) and cellular immune mechanisms (T lymphocytes). The IL-1 produced by the APC stimulates the proliferation and activity of a subset of T lymphocytes, designated *T helper cells.* T helper cells activated by IL-1 produce interleukin-2 (IL-2), and this potent lymphokine stimulates proliferation of both natural killer T lymphocytes and specific cytotoxic T lymphocytes. Interleukin-2–activated cytotoxic T cells produce gamma interferon and this in turn appears to activate natural killer cells of the T lymphocyte population. The end result of this activity is a growing population of cloned lymphocytes specifically cytotoxic to cells bearing the foreign antigen. This highly simplified concept describes the cellular arm of the immune mechanism, which appears to play the major role in transplant tissue rejection. Once stimulated by a specific foreign antigen, the system appears to have recall, and subsequent introductions of the same antigen will result in accelerated rejection reactions. Furthermore, this specific immunity can be transferred to a nonsensitized host by transfer of lymphocytes from a syngeneic sensitized animal.

The humoral (B lymphocyte) mediated arm of the immune mechanism is responsible for the production of a specific antibody. The recall phenomena are evident in this arm of the immune reaction also. Although circulating antibody to foreign protein can be detected after tissue transplantation, this appears to play a minor role in transplant rejection.

## Alteration of the Rejection Phenomena

The final barrier to the goal of ready transplantation of allogeneic tissue to replace significant tissue deficits has been breached in a number of "shotgun" nonspecific approaches. Methods currently in use depend on maintaining a delicate balance of relatively broad immunosuppression to prevent rejection while leaving the host with adequate immune mechanisms to deal with infection. It is apparent that in order to produce a donor-specific tolerance one must either render donor cells nonantigenic, or render the recipient incapable of responding to the specific donor major and minor histocompatibility antigens, either by impairing specific recognition or disabling the cytotoxic arm of the response to the specific donor antigen set. The only other alternative would be the production of syngeneic tissue via tissue culture techniques. Although progress has been made in some areas, such as skin and dermis, little evidence has been found that this technique will be successful in growing composite tissues commonly needed in reconstruction by any culture modalities currently available.

As major histocompatibility antigens were identified and tissue typing became possible, early efforts were aimed at finding closely matched combinations, usually with family members. This was perhaps most successfully carried out by Burke and associates [16] in grafting severely burned children with tissue from the closest tissue-matched related adult. Despite tissue matching and the known immunosuppression created by the massive burn injury, these patients required the best immunosuppressive measures available at the time to achieve clinically significant prolongation of allograft survival. It is obvious from the almost infinite combination of major and minor histocompatibility antigens possible that a "perfect match" can only occur in identical twins. Some reports have been published of improvements in allograft survival with close HLA matches, but for the most part these have been small increases in median allograft survival time and they are of minimal clinical significance to the patient [8]. Many of these early studies were performed using skin graft as the model and were carried out before the discovery of the DR antigen system. It is pos-

sible that more complete tissue typing, including DR matching, would produce further improvement in a median length of transplanted tissue survival, but even in animal systems with only one known minor mismatch, the prolongation of survival is measured in days rather than weeks.

Since tissue typing alone does not induce significant improvement in transplant survival, numerous agents and chemicals have been applied to transplant recipients in an attempt to produce immunosuppression. A significant dose of ionizing radiation applied to a recipient before foreign antigen exposure will result in marked inhibition of the rejection response. It has not been possible to define a level of radiation that prevents transplant rejection while leaving the host with adequate defense against generalized infection. Radiation, in addition to chemical immunosuppressive agents, has also been tried, but again, achieving the delicate balance between rejection and susceptibility to infection has proved a formidable barrier to general application of this technique. Nevertheless, radiation has been used along with closely matched allograft bone marrow to produce a "chimera" state. Graft-versus-host phenomena make this technique too risky for application in plastic and reconstructive surgical procedures.

A number of chemical agents have been used in an attempt to suppress allograft reaction. Cortisone was one of the earliest agents utilized and has been shown to delay rejection for a period of time. Its effects are primarily nonspecific impairment of the antigen recognition phase and probably some impairment of the production of lymphokines by APCs, as well as the response to lymphokines by the T helper cells. Steroids alone will not prevent rejection but have been used as an adjunct to other immunosuppressive agents.

A succession of alkylating agents (nitrogen mustards), antimetabolites (methotrexate, azathioprine, cyclophosphamide), and antibiotics (actinomycin C) have also been tried. All of these agents, in combination with steroids, have been shown to delay the rejection phenomena, but all render the patient susceptible to infection because they produce a severe generalized depression of the hemopoietic system.

As the cellular component became increasingly well defined, an attempt was made to alter recipient responses by developing antilymphocyte serum (ALS). This product, introduced in 1963, is produced by injecting lymphoid cells from the species in which it is to be used into another species [72]. Most of the ALS produced for human use consists of a globulin fraction isolated from horses injected with human lymphoid tissue. This agent has been refined by selection of thymus-derived lymphocytes, resulting in a serum that has a more specific activity against the effector arm of the rejection reaction. Both ALS and antithymocyte serum have been used experimentally and clinically to reverse rejection and in attempts to produce tolerance to transplant antigens. With development of the hybridoma techniques and improvements in our ability to identify and separate specific subsets of the T cell population, a number of monoclonal antibodies have been developed that are effective against specific subsets of this group. Work in our laboratory and others has shown that monoclonal antibody against Langerhans cells may eliminate the expression of DR antigen by the Langerhans cell. Monoclonal antibody is being used experimentally in renal transplantation and may well achieve clinical use in other transplant applications.

Attempts to alter donor antigenicity have been varied and largely unsuccessful. It has been shown that ultraviolet radiation of donor skin can result in prolongation of allograft survival [50]. It is hypothesized that this is due to the sensitivity of the Langerhans cell, which is the APC in the basal layer of the epidermis. Since this cell expresses the DR antigen, it is apparent that elimination of this antigen from skin can potentially prolong skin-graft survival, al-

though evidence shows that it does so only for a relatively short period of time. Others have noted that allograft skin stored at 4°C for a period of time exhibits prolonged survival, and again it is believed that this may be due to the loss of Langerhans cells, which seem to survive cold storage poorly.

Burke and associates [18] have attempted to alter donor tissue antigenicity in a xenogeneic substitute for human skin. They used a cross-link technique to disguise the bovine collagen in their "artificial skin," which has been tested successfully in burn patients. Although this material has been used with success in the clinical arena, it is likely that this nonviable transplant of xenogeneic tissue serves only as a scaffold for new host tissue. The efficacy of cross-linking tissue chemically to reduce immunogenicity is still under study, and this technique would not be applicable to transplantation in which viable tissue is needed. The treatment of donor tissue with specific monoclonal antibodies and complement to eliminate the expression of class 1 or 2 antigens, or both, remains in the very early investigative stage, and we can only speculate regarding its future use.

The induction of specific immunologic tolerance to an allotransplant antigen from a specific donor is possible experimentally using inbred animal strains. Creation of acquired tolerance during fetal development can be carried out before immunologic maturity. This has not found clinical application since the genetic barriers are much greater in an outbred population. Clinically and experimentally mild improvements have been made in transplantation survival when donor-specific lymphocytes have been transferred. Experiments have shown that this reaction may be dose dependent and again a fine balance is seen between the production of an accelerated rejection phenomenon and the production of a tolerant state. In addition, the possibility of producing a graft-versus-host reaction makes this technique unsuitable for application in reconstructive procedures at this time.

Cyclosporine A, a fungal metabolite described in 1976, has resulted in a significant advance in transplantation success at the clinical level [67]. This drug has increased kidney allograft survival by 25 percent over the more conventional forms of immunosuppression and has doubled the survival of liver allografts. Cyclosporine A acts primarily on the cellular arm of the immune reaction and is therefore much more specific than the antimetabolites used in the past. It appears to hamper the release of interleukin-1 and interleukin-2. Cyclosporine A does not have a suppressive effect on the hemopoietic system and has therefore been free of many of the problems previously inherent in other immunosuppressive methods. In addition, evidence has been found that cyclosporine A may allow emergence of recipient suppressor cells and thereby contribute to the tolerant state. Side effects of this drug in its usual dose of 15 mg per kilogram for induction, reduced to 5 to 10 mg per kilogram for maintenance, have been primarily those of mild nephrotoxicity, which seems to be reversible with dose reduction. It has been noted that the incidence of *Pneumocystis carinii* and cytomegalovirus infections is decreased.

## Transplantation in Current Use in Plastic Surgery

### SKIN

The transfer of split-thickness autograft is undoubtedly the most commonly practiced form of transplantation. These grafts are usually orthotopically placed to cover areas of skin or skin and soft-tissue loss. These grafts, taken with any of a variety of available dermatomes, can vary in thickness according to the recipient site needs and donor site skin thickness but generally are taken at approximately 12/1000 of an inch thickness. These grafts contain much or all of the epidermis and at least a portion of the dermis. Such grafts can be expected to "take" by obtaining a new blood supply from the recipient bed and will do so with great regularity, providing that certain conditions are met. Devitalized tissue in the recipient bed must be removed, the bed must have an adequate degree of vascularity, and the bacterial count must be fewer than $10^5$ microorganisms per gram of tissue [42]. The graft initially adheres via a fibrin "glue" and must be protected from inadvertent shearing motion while it is acquiring its vascular supply, which takes between 48 and 96 hours. Graft take can be destroyed by hematoma or seroma formation, so hemostatic techniques are critical to success. In the treatment of large surface area defects and massive burns, it is common to "expand" the skin by use of the mesher device, achieving skin expansions ranging from 1.5 to 1.0, up to 9 to 1. The larger expansions are difficult to work with, and closure of the interstices is extremely slow and requires protection with a biologic dressing to achieve a reasonable success rate.

Full-thickness skin grafts have the advantage of producing a final appearance that is close to the surrounding normal skin in texture and resilience. However, skin "take" is less certain than with partial-thickness skin, and great care must be taken to trim the underlying subcutaneous fat, so that early vascular connections can occur between the dermal vessels and the recipient bed. Donor sites for smaller full-thickness grafts can usually be closed primarily, but in very large full-thickness grafts, it may be necessary to create a second split-thickness donor site wound in order to close the open full-thickness donor site.

The transplantation of allogeneic, cultured epithelial cells is a relatively recent development, but Gallico and others [31] have shown that this technique can be useful in the management of patients with large burn injuries. A growing number of burn centers in the United States have developed the technical expertise to culture human epithelium, and full clarification of the indications and efficacy of this procedure should become clear in the next few years. It appears that the rate of growth of cells in culture depends somewhat on the age of the donor cells. The ultimate durability of such tissue culture transplants and the potential for senescent tumor formation remain a matter of speculation at this time.

### Skin Allograft

Skin is the largest and one of the most complex organs of the human body. It should therefore come as no surprise that skin is more antigenic than most tissues of the body. Because of its free accessibility and since rejection is easily observed, it was widely used in the earliest experiments of tissue transplantation. This was in some ways unfortunate, since the intense antigenicity may have led many early researchers to believe that histocompatibility barriers could not be overcome. Nevertheless, skin allotransplantation has become a common clinical procedure.

Allotransplantation of fresh or cold preserved human skin is practiced in many modern burn centers. The harvesting of cadaver skin up to 24 hours after clinical death provides large quantities of viable skin for transplantation. This can be used fresh or can be stored, either by a commonly used controlled-rate freezing technique or by storage at 4°C in a nutrient medium.

The freezing technique has the advantage of allowing storage for long periods of time but is technology intensive. The standard cooling technique has been shown to provide viable skin for up to 28 days after harvest, and in most burn centers the skin is used within that time period. In most centers, the skin is utilized as a "biologic dressing" and is regularly changed at intervals calculated to precede any evidence of active tissue rejection. As was noted earlier, however, the victims of massive thermal trauma exhibit a marked degree of immunosuppression secondary to the injury and may tolerate allogeneic skin grafts for prolonged periods of time. Burke and associates [17] and

others have used allogeneic split-thickness grafts and active immunosuppression to prolong the take of allogeneic cadaver or living related skin.

Cultured epithelial cells have been used by an increasing number of burn centers. They are of most functional value in structurally intact tissue such as partial-thickness wounds. Persistence of cultured epithelium from allogeneic sources has not been documented in humans.

### Xenogeneic Skin Grafts

Xenogeneic tissue has also been used in burn care as a temporary dressing. Commercially available pig skin has been utilized as a biologic dressing and must be changed every few days. This commercially available xenograft is nonviable, and a true graft take does not occur with this material.

The artificial skin developed by Burke and associates [18] consists of a "dermal" layer of enzymatically digested bovine collagen cross-linked with chondroitin-6 sulfate. This "dermal framework," covered by a thin adherent Silastic sheet, has been used successfully both clinically and experimentally as a skin substitute. This form of xenogeneic transplant is nonviable, and it appears likely that the bovine collagen framework is replaced by host collagen using the xenogeneic transplant as a scaffold or template. To achieve permanent closure of the wound, the Silastic layer must be removed after vascularization of the dermal component, and a thin (⁴⁄₁₀₀₀ of an inch) autograft of epithelium must be applied. This extremely thin autograft offers the practical advantage of more frequent harvesting of autologous donor sites, since the healing time for the donor site is related to the depth of the split-thickness graft taken. Burke and associates [16] and Heck and colleagues [36] have utilized a similar concept in applying cadaver allograft dermis, which is rendered nonviable by freezing. This dermal allograft is allowed to become vascularized and then autologous epithelium is obtained, using a blister formation technique and applied over the cadaver dermal allograft. Data are not adequate to state unequivocally that the nonviable cadaver dermal allograft is nonantigenic, but this form of transplant appears to be successful based on clinical observation. A report by Achauer and coworkers [1] regarding the use of split-thickness allograft skin and cyclosporine immunosuppression is encouraging but remains anecdotal in nature. The possibility that such allogeneic tissue can become a permanently tolerated transplant remains unproven to date. Such transplants may be very slowly rejected and concomitantly replaced by ingrowth of host tissue.

CARTILAGE

Cartilage has been a popular transplant material in plastic surgery in both autogenous and allogeneic forms since early in this century. Peer [55] reviewed the literature and stated that the works on cartilage transplantation since 1860 were too exhaustive to be summarized. John Sturge Davis [23] was studying the permanence of cartilage grafts in 1917. By the 1940s cartilage had received wide acceptance as an autologous graft and experiments have been carried out with xenograft cartilage [63].

Histologically, there are three varieties of cartilage: hyaline, elastic, and fibrocartilage. Clinically, the costal and nasal hyaline cartilage and the elastic cartilage of the ear are the most commonly used for autogenous transplants. The chondrocyte, which produces the matrix of the cartilage, is an extremely active cell from a metabolic standpoint. The oxygen consumption of cartilage is low, and it has been noted that the enzymes essential for anaerobic metabolism are present in articular cartilage.

The chondrocyte is a gel composed of approximately 75 percent water and 25 percent solids [65]. No blood vessels or lymphatics are contained in cartilage, and nourishment is derived by means of plasmatic diffusion. When injured, the cartilage possesses very little regenerative capacity. It is repaired primarily by scar formation in the form of connective tissue proliferation after injury. The perichondrium does not possess the regenerative capacity of the periosteum.

*Antigenicity*

Due to the lack of vascularization in cartilage and because the chondrocytes are protected from the environment by their surrounding matrix, the histocompatibility antigens of the chondrocytes are ordinarily not exposed to the antigen processing system of the recipient [27]. Dicing or crushing cartilage has been found to increase cartilage resorption, and this may be at least partly on the basis of exposure of allograft antigens to the host immune system.

Many clinicians have noted unpredictable distortion of fresh, autogenous cartilage graft. This warping of the graft generally occurs relatively early after operation and can often result in the need for secondary procedures to correct the deformity. Warping appears to be due to a difference in tension between the outermost and inner layers of the cartilage. Fry [30] has described the "interlocked stresses" found in cartilage. Gibson and Davis [32] carried out in vitro studies and described methods of carving costochondral grafts that prevented clinically significant warping. Others have attempted to overcome warping by various treatments, including irradiation of costal cartilage [34].

*Autograft Cartilage*

It appears that there is adequate evidence of long-term survival of autologous cartilage transplanted to either orthotopic or heterotopic sites. Cartilage can usually be obtained in sufficient quantities from the nasal septum, ears, or costochondral sources to meet most contouring needs. It is apparent that cartilage survives transplantation to heterotopic sites well since it retains its bulk without the need for functional stress factors that is required by some tissues such as bone. Autogenous cartilage appears to have lower absorption than bone when transplanted and is more easily carved and shaped.

Autogenous tissue can be stored, but there have not been sufficient studies to establish the optimum technique for maintaining chondrocyte viability. It has been shown that cartilage containing viable chondrocytes undergoes less resorption than that seen in nonviable transplants.

*Allogeneic Cartilage*
Available literature suggests that preserved homograft cartilage is subject to some degree of absorption in all cases [37]. The degree of absorption is variable and there appears to be calcification in grafts that are ultimately resistant to the resorptive phenomenon. Bardach [5] has reported fracturing of homograft, a problem apparently not seen with autologous cartilage. Despite these problems, preserved homologous cartilage has been used with good results in a number of reconstructive applications [51, 58, 59].

Absorption in these reports is usually cited at 20 percent. In general, it has been noted that larger cartilage grafts are more resistant than small grafts to the phenomenon of resorption.

*Xenograft Cartilage*
Despite the encouraging report by Ersek and associates [28], xenograft cartilage has generally proved inferior to either autograft cartilage or allogeneic transplants.

BONE
Bone is a complex combination of organic collagen and inorganic salts, with organic matter making up approximately 35 percent of the composite tissue and the minerals composing 65 percent. This proportion varies with age, location, and the function of bone, and the proportions are critical to creating a tissue that is rigid enough to bear significant stress loads but has enough elasticity to tolerate sudden stresses without breaking. The active cellular components are constantly reabsorbing and depositing collagen and minerals, and this allows bone to respond to external stresses during growth and with changes in function. The response of bone to stress was noted by Wolff [71] in 1892 when he stated, "All changes which may occur in the function of a bone are tended by definite alterations in its internal structures." This ability of bone to respond to changes in stress presents both a strength and a weakness from the standpoint of bone transplantation.

The role of the periosteum in bone regeneration remains a matter of some dispute. Some investigators have found that periosteal flaps without bone will not form new bone [21]. Skoog [61] found that a free tibial periosteum was capable of producing new bone in alveolar clefts. Thompson and Casson [66] found that grafts with retained periosteum performed better in transplantation than grafts from the same site without periosteum. Knize [40] reported that inlay bone grafts with retained periosteum gave the best result. All of these grafts do undergo resorption, however, and are ultimately replaced with fibrous connective tissue when they are placed in a heterotopic position. Zins and Whitaker [75] found consistently better survival in membranous versus endochondral bone grafts.

When transplanted as a free graft to a heterotopic position, bone gains a new blood supply from the surrounding tissues. Initially, the graft is surrounded by blood clot, and inflammatory cells are present during the first week after transplantation. During the second week there is invasion by fibrous granulation tissue and an increase in osteoblastic activity. It is clear that cancellous bone is revascularized much earlier than cortical graft. After vascularization new osteogeneic cells begin to appear and at least a few of the transplanted osteocytes probably contribute to this new cell population. Transplanted cortical bone repair takes place initially by osteoblastic resorption of bone, and ultimately osteoclasts appear and begin laying down new bone. In general, cancellous grafts tend to go on to complete repair whereas cortical grafts remain a mixture of viable and necrotic bone. When bone is placed in a weight-bearing location during transplantation, it has been found that fatigue fractures are frequent during the first 6 to 18 months after grafting; however, they decrease after this time [15].

There has been increasing use of autogenous vascularized autograft in the reconstruction of lower-extremity trauma as well as in some areas of facial reconstruction. The use of vascularized fibula in lower-extremity reconstruction or vascularized rib in conjunction with latissimus dorsi transplantation serves as an example of the former. Flaps of calvarial bone based on the temporalis blood supply are an example of the latter. This bone can be transferred on either periosteal or medullary endosteal blood supply.

Berggren and associates [9] have shown that bone can be stored at 5°C and will tolerate up to 25 hours of ischemia with survival of the cellular constituents. Moore [49] compared nonvascularized and vascularized autogenous bone grafts and showed that vascularized bone grafts were much stronger than the conventional, autogenous nonvascularized graft. It has also been demonstrated that vascularized bone grafts do well in an irradiated bed whereas nonvascularized autograft bone does poorly under such circumstances [54].

In summary, it appears that vascularized autograft provides bone of the greatest strength with the highest likelihood of bony union. Cancellous bone with associated muscle transfer appears to be the second choice for bone grafts, where needed, with cancellous bone showing better survival than cortical bone in all cases. Limited autogenous donor sites and donor site morbidity have resulted in increased interest and research efforts in bone allograft transplantation.

*Bone Allograft*
Bone allograft has enjoyed an increase in popularity in major orthopedic reconstructive procedures. Its primary use has been in large tissue defects secondary to surgical tu-mor ablation or in large defects secondary to trauma. In these cases, the donor site is inadequate for autogenous bone reconstruction. Current bone banking techniques primarily consist of preserving cadaver allograft bone in a frozen state. Although it may be possible in experimental settings to preserve living osteocytes in these grafts, the freezing of large bone segments undoubtedly leaves only the organic collagen matrix and associated inorganic salts. Thus, the graft can provide the objective of immediate rigidity and the lack of living cells undoubtedly results in a decrease in antigenicity of allografted bone. Large segment replacement requires long-term metal fixation techniques, and this allografted bone is replaced by creeping substitution over a prolonged time course. Since this bone is nonliving, it is unable to repair itself and stress fractures are therefore a significant problem with this technique. Nevertheless, many authors have reported good results using frozen osteochondral and intercalary allografts in clinical studies [19]. Allograft obtained from cadavers has also been used as a bone powder. Brown and associates [14] have shown that crushed bone is largely reabsorbed.

Urist and coworkers [68] have found that allogeneic, lyophilized decalcified transplants can induce the formation of new bone by host osteogeneic precursor cells. This bone induction factor appears to be an acid-insoluble protein and in some manner it stimulates new bone formation from cells migrating from the perivascular connective tissue to the interior of the implant. The specific protein involved appears to be a glycoprotein. This purified bone morphogenic protein induces the same response as autogenous bone matrix. Einhorn and colleagues [26] were able to show repair of surgically created bony defects in an animal model by 12 weeks using a demineralized bone matrix.

Both bone morphogenic protein and decalcified, freeze-dried, allogeneic, cortical bone grafts can be substituted for autogenous grafts, as they have minimal immunogenicity and both are capable of stimulating bone forma-tion [52]. These latter two products, how-ever, offer no immediate rigidity so that long-term internal and external skeletal sup-port is needed for weight-bearing applica-tions.

*Xenograft*

Fresh xenograft has been shown to elicit a strong immune response [33]. It is possible that freeze-dried xenograft preparations might produce a lesser immunogeneic response, but the current availability of human bone allo-graft renders this a moot point. In experi-mental studies of vascularized bone allograft transplanted across strong histocompatibil-ity barriers, evidence of rapid rejection was seen. Transplant rejection was directed at the donor vascular tissue. Against a weak histocompatibility barrier, the rejection was directed at the marrow. The clinical use of vascularized allograft remains highly exper-imental, but animal experiments with com-posite extremity grafts suggest that clinical success may be possible in the future.

NERVE

*Autograft*

The clinical use of autogenous nerves, such as the sural nerve to replace essential motor nerves in the forearm, has become a rela-tively common practice. The axons within the donor nerve sheath degenerate and, de-spite wallerian degeneration within the do-nor nerve sheath, the regenerating axons of the recipient nerve are able to use the sheath as a physical guide to the myoneural junc-tions. Although it is unlikely that all regen-erating axons complete the migration suc-cessfully, enough arrive at the myoneural junction to provide satisfactory functional recovery in many cases. It has been sug-gested, but is as yet unproved, that vascular-ized autogenous nerves allow quicker and more complete reenervation. The obvious disadvantage to autogenous nerve transplan-tation is the loss of function at the donor site. There are only limited donor nerves

(usually pure sensory nerves) whose func-tion can be spared. The search for a suitable substitute for autogenic nerve transplants to correct major motor nerve gaps has led some to suggest other autogenous tissue conduits. Chiu and associates [22] have suggested au-togenous vein to bridge nerve gaps and have shown successful reenervation in an animal model. Others have continued experimen-tation in the use of allogeneic nerve to serve as the conduit for axon reenervation.

*Allograft Nerve*

The first human nerve allograft was de-scribed in 1878 [4]. Despite a long history of attempted allograft use to overcome the problem of limited autogenous nerve suit-able for grafting, the consensus has been that nerve allografts are not useful in clinical practice. McKinnon and associates [44] stud-ied nerve allograft in animals with major histoincompatibility and animals with only minor histoincompatibility. They showed that in cases of major histoincompatibility in the rat, sensitization and the beginning of the rejection phenomenon could occur as early as the eighth day. In the case of a donor and recipient that were mismatched only at the minor histocompatibility, locus sensiti-zation and nerve rejection occurred as early as the tenth day. Administration of cyclo-sporine A was successful in delaying nerve allograft rejection for 80 days or longer. The authors suggest that nerve regeneration might take place through the allograft during this 80-day delay in sensitization so that reener-vation might be accomplished in cases in which only minor histoincompatibility exists.

Zalewski and Gulati [73] performed nerve allografts in recipients who were previously sensitized to the donor, using cyclosporine A immunosuppression. Control rats showed rapid rejection and host axons did not tra-verse the 4-cm-long nerve allografts. Sen-sitized rats treated with cyclosporine A (10 mg/kg/day) showed nerve allograft sur-vival, and numerous axons were seen to re-generate through the 4-cm length of nerve allograft. McKinnon and colleagues [44] have also assessed the use of immunosuppression in nerve allograft in the rat model. They showed that short-term, low-dose immunosuppression using hydrocortisone and azathioprine was as successful as a longer-term, higher-dose immunosuppressive regimen with these drugs. Nerve regeneration was significantly better than in an untreated nerve allograft control group. The authors also showed, however, that even immunosuppressed allograft transplants were inferior to autogenous nerve grafts. Aguayo and Bray [2] and Aguayo and associates [3] have suggested that in allogeneic grafts rejection will occur after cessation of immunosuppression. Despite the rejection of the allogeneic Schwann cells and connective tissue, the axons often continue to function, and the rejected nerve sheaths are replaced by host Schwann cells that have migrated down the rejecting nerve conduit [48]. McKinnon and coworkers [44] emphasize that neurotrophic factors from the distal end of the host nerve gap may be critical to the success of transplantation.

These studies suggest that short-term immunosuppression might be sufficient to allow axon regeneration and recovery of function, after which time the immunosuppression could be stopped and long-term function might well continue. The results from these recent studies are encouraging, and further research into allograft nerve and possibly even vein transplantation may lead to a solution for the nerve gap deficits that are often encountered in clinical practice.

## FASCIA, DERMIS, AND COLLAGEN

The transplantation of autogenous fascia and dermis in the repair of tissue deficits has been commonplace for many years. Survival of such tissue is almost assured since host fibroblast will either survive the transplantation or will repopulate the collagenous matrix and continue the balance between resorption of the collagen and the production of new collagenous ground substance. There may be some slight loss in overall bulk after transplantation so that mild overcorrection is often advised. The disadvantages of autogenous dermal graft include donor site scarring, occasional cyst formation, and calcification of any fat that may be transplanted with the dermis or fascia [53].

### Allogeneic Fascia, Dermis, and Collagen

There is evidence to suggest that cell-free dermal collagen does not excite an immune response in experimental allotransplantation [53]. In addition, treatment of collagen with glutaraldehyde may stabilize collagen against the action of collagenase, further decreasing the problem of graft resorption [6]. Griffiths and Shakespeare [35] studied allograft dermis treated with glutaraldehyde on implants to forearm and abdominal locations. They reported that over a three-year period no collagen resorption was observed, and they noted no immune or inflammatory response. They further reported that the implants were colonized by host fibroblasts although no specific tests were carried out to prove the origin of the fibroblasts within the grafts. Heck and colleagues [36] have used human allograft dermis for coverage of burn wounds in the clinical setting. They utilized frozen human cadaver skin on full-thickness injuries. Four days after transplantation, the donor epidermis was removed and vacuum blister prepared sheets of autologous epidermis were grafted over the exposed allograft dermal surface. The authors reported no graft loss and no significant wound contracture after this method of treatment.

Studies involving the development of living skin equivalents composed of allogeneic cultured fibroblasts and a collagen matrix with an overlying lattice of autogenous keratinocytes have shown that allograft fibroblasts do not provoke a rejection response even in presensitized animals [60]. The investigators suggest that cells such as fibroblasts that bear only class I antigen may be acceptable graft constituents if incorporated into a tissue equivalent that excludes cells expressing class I antigens. Bright and Green [13] have reported their experience in the use of freeze-dried fascia lata as an allograft material in orthopedic reconstruction. The results indicate that allograft fascia lata does survive and maintains its strength and anatomic integrity.

Webster and Werner [70] have looked at freeze-dried tendon allografts in an animal model. They found that these tendon grafts remained intact and were repopulated by host fibrocytes. Studies of mechanical strength showed the allografts to be similar in strength to implanted tendon autograft.

There has been a recent increase in the use of injectable collagen to correct small tissue deficits [24]. The commercial product currently in use is a xenograft consisting of bovine collagen. In Duts ring clinical trials of this material, the skin of approximately three percent of the subjects tested experienced local hypersensitivity reactions. It has also been stated that one percent of treated patients demonstrate symptoms of hypersensitivity at treatment sites. These injectable implants are composed of bovine type I collagen primarily, with a small percentage of bovine type III collagen. Clinical use has shown that treatment must often be repeated to maintain the contour improvement. The evidence available indicates that much of the fibrillar collagen injection is reabsorbed.

*Composite Tissue Allografts*

The dream of successful composite tissue transplantation was first satisfied in 348 A.D., when legend has it that Cosmos and Damian amputated a gangrenous leg and replaced it with a transplant from a recently deceased donor [38]. In the following centuries, no one has duplicated their result in humans. In numerous animal studies a number of immunosuppressive methods have been used, including azathioprine, steroids, 6-mercaptopurine, antilymphocyte serum, donor blood transfusions, and host antidonor serum, but these methods have met with little long-term success.

The introduction of cyclosporine has resulted in a marked resurgence in experimental composite tissue allografts and a notable increase in reported success using animal limb models. It is obvious from the research available that revascularized allograft muscle, bone, nerve, and blood vessels can survive and function for many months under continuous doses of cyclosporine immunosuppression. Skin appears to be the primary target of rejection. Fritz and colleagues [29] and Black and associates [12] have reported long-term composite graft survival even after cyclosporine withdrawal. However, this occurred in only a few animals in each series.

Kim and associates [39], using a specific rat model, could not show prolongation of limb survival after long-term cyclosporine immunosuppression. Egerszegi and colleagues [25] expanded the model for composite tissue transplantation to the primate. Using unrelated individuals in a baboon model, they achieved survival of neurovascular free flaps for 161 days with continuous application of cyclosporine. They also maintained hand transplants with anatomic viability at 150 days with continuous cyclosporine. Studies on the status of reenervation and function are in progress.

The prospect of lifelong immunosuppression for the maintenance of composite tissue allografts in young, otherwise healthy patients remains a formidable barrier to the current clinical use of such techniques. The present knowledge explosion in the field of transplant immunology, however, should encourage the plastic surgeon to follow this area of basic science closely. The development of donor-specific immune tolerance appears to offer the greatest hope for application of composite tissue grafts in the clinical situation.

## Summary

Autogenous tissue transplantation has become routine, and further refinements in technique will doubtless improve the success rate of major composite tissue autograft. Allotransplantation has become increasingly common in clinical practice and use of allograft materials will doubtless continue. Current concern regarding transfer of human immunodeficiency virus during cadaver tissue allotransplantation will certainly be of concern to all surgeons. Improvements in donor screening techniques are likely to develop, but these are also sure to increase the cost of allotransplantation. Until safe donor testing techniques have been developed, human allograft transplantation will and should remain confined to situations in which the transplantation of tissues will be life saving.

## References

1. Achauer, B. M., et al. Long-term skin allograft survival after short-term cyclosporin treatment in a patient with massive burns. *Lancet* 1:14–15, 1986.
2. Aguayo, A. J., and Bray, G. M. Experimental Nerve Grafts. In D. L. Jewett and H. R. McCarroll (eds.), *Nerve Repair and Regeneration.* St. Louis: Mosby, 1980.
3. Aguayo, A. J., et al. Myelination of mouse axons by Schwann cells transplanted from normal to abnormal human nerves. *Nature* 268:753, 1977.
4. Albert, E. Berichte, Des Naturwissenschaftligh-Medizinischen, in Innsbruck. *Innsbruck* 9:97, 1878.
5. Bardach, J. Problems of auricular reconstruction in microtia. *Acta Chir. Plast.* 6:264, 1964.
6. Barker, H., et al. Formaldehyde as a pretreatment for dermal collagen heterografts. *Biochim. Biophys. Acta* 632:589, 1980.
7. Baronio, G. *Degli Innesti Animali.* Milan: Stamperia e Fonderia del Genio, 1804.
8. Batchelor, J., and Haker, M. HLA-matching in treatment of burned patients with skin allografts. *Lancet* 2:581–583, 1970.
9. Berggren, A., Weiland, A. J., and Dorfman, H. The effect of prolonged ischemia time on osteocyte and osteoblast survival in composite bone grafts revascularized by microvascular anastomoses. *Plast. Reconstr. Surg.* 69:290, 1982.
10. Billingham, R. E., Brent, L., and Medawar, P. B. Quantitative studies on tissue transplantation immunity. III. Actively acquired toler-

ance. *Philos. Trans. R. Soc. Lond.* 239:375, 1956.
11. Billingham, R. E., et al. Quantitative studies in tissue transplantation immunity. I. The survival times of skin homografts exchanged between members of different inbred strains of mice. *Proc. Roy. Soc.* 143:43, 1954.
12. Black, K. S., et al. Composite tissue (limb) allografts in rats. *Transplantation* 39:365, 1985.
13. Bright, R. W., and Green, W. T. Freeze-dried fascia lata allografts: A review of 47 cases. *J. Pediatr. Orthop.* 1:13, 1981.
14. Brown, B. L., Kern, E. B., and Neel, H. B. Transplantation of fresh allografts (homografts) of crushed and uncrushed cartilage and bone, a one year analysis in rabbits. *Laryngoscope* 90:1521, 1980.
15. Burchardt, H. The biology of bone graft repair. *Clin. Orthop.* 174:28, 1983.
16. Burke, J. F., et al. Temporary skin transplantation and immunosuppression for extensive burns. *N. Engl. J. Med.* 290:269–271, 1974.
17. Burke, J. F., et al. Immunosuppression and temporary skin transplantation in the treatment of massive third degree burns. *Ann. Surg.* 182:183–195, 1975.
18. Burke, J. F., et al. Successful use of a physiologically acceptable artificial skin in the treatment of extensive burn injury. *Ann. Surg.* 194:413, 1981.
19. Burwell, R. B., Friedlaender, G. E., and Mankin, H. J. Current perspectives and future directions. The 1983 invitational conference on osteochondral allografts. *Clin. Orthop.* 197:141–157, 1985.
20. Carrel, A., and Guthrie, C. C. Anastomosis of blood vessels by the patching method and transplantation of the kidney. *J.A.M.A.* 47: 1648–1651, 1906.
21. Cestero, H. J., and Slayer, K. E. Regenerative potential of bone and periosteum. *Surg. Forum* 26:555, 1975.
22. Chiu, D. T. W., et al. Autogenous vein as a nerve conduit. *Surg. Forum* 31:550, 1980.
23. Davis, J. S. A comparison of the permanence of free transplants of bone and cartilage: An experimental study. *Ann. Surg.* 65:170, 1917.
24. DeLustro, F., et al. Reaction to injectable collagen: Results in animal models in clinical use. *Plast. Reconstr. Surg.* 79:581, 1987.
25. Egerszegi, E. P., Samulack, D. D., and Daniel, R. K. Experimental models in primates for re-

constructive surgery utilizing tissue transplants. *Ann. Plast. Surg.* 13:423, 1984.

26. Einhorn, T. A., et al. The healing of segmental bone defects induced by demineralized bone matrix. *J. Bone Joint Surg.* 66A:274, 1984.

27. Elves, N. W. Newer knowledge of the immunology of bone and cartilage. *Clin. Orthop.* 120:232, 1976.

28. Ersek, R. A., Rothenberg, P. B., and Denton, D. R. Clinical use of an improved process bovine cartilage for contour defects. *Ann. Plast. Surg.* 13:44, 1984.

29. Fritz, W. D., et al. Limb allografts in rats immunosuppressed with Cyclosporin A. *Ann. Surg.* 199:211, 1984.

30. Fry, H. J. H. Interlocked stresses in human nasal septal cartilage. *Br. J. Plast. Surg.* 19:276, 1966.

31. Gallico, G. G., et al. Permanent coverage of large burn wounds with autologous cultured human epithelium. *N. Engl. J. Med.* 381:448, 1984.

32. Gibson, T., and Davis, G. W. The restoration of autogenous cartilage grafts, its cause and prevention. *Br. J. Plast. Surg.* 10:257, 1957.

33. Gotfried, Y., et al. Histologic characteristics of acute rejection in vascularized allografts of bone. *J. Bone Joint Surg.* 69A(3):410, 1987.

34. Grabb, W. C. Costal cartilage homografts preserved by irradiation. *Plast. Reconstr. Surg.* 28:562, 1961.

35. Griffiths, R. W., and Shakespeare, P. G. Human dermal collagen allografts: A three year histological study. *Br. J. Plast. Surg.* 35:519, 1982.

36. Heck, E. L., Bergstresser, P. R., and Baxter, C. R. Composite skin graft: Frozen dermal allografts support the engraftment and expansion of autologous epidermis. *J. Trauma* 25:106, 1985.

37. Hoopes, J. E. Cartilage Grafts in Symposium. In T. J. Krizek and J. E. Hoopes (eds.), *Basic Sciences in Plastic Surgery.* St. Louis: Mosby, 1976.

38. Kahan, B. D. Cosmos and Damian revisited. *Transplant Proc.* 15:2211, 1983.

39. Kim, S. K., et al. Use of Cyclosporin A in allotransplantation of rat limbs. *Ann. Plast. Surg.* 12:249, 1984.

40. Knize, D. M. The influence of periosteum and calcitonin on inlayed bone graft survival. A roentgenographic study. *Plast. Reconstr. Surg.* 53:190, 1974.

41. Krizek, T. J., et al. Experimental transplantation of composite grafts by microsurgical vascular anastomoses. *Plast. Reconstr. Surg.* 36:538–546, 1965.

42. Krizek, T. J., et al. Biology of surgical infections. *Surg. Clin. North Am.* 55:1261, 1975.

43. Majno, G. *The Healing Hand.* Cambridge: Harvard University Press, 1975.

44. McKinnon, S. E., et al. The peripheral nerve allograft: An assessment of regeneration in the immunosuppressed host. *Plast. Surg. Forum,* ASPRS 79(3):436, 1987.

45. Medawar, P. B. Immunity to homologous grafted skin. I. The suppression of cell division in grafts transplanted to immunized animals. *Br. J. Exp. Pathol.* 27:9, 1946.

46. Medawar, P. B. Immunity to homologous grafted skin. II. The relationship between the antigens of blood and skin. *Br. J. Exp. Pathol.* 27:15, 1946.

47. Medawar, P. B. Immunity to homologous grafted skin. III. The fate of skin homografts transplanted to the brain, to subcutaneous tissue, and to the anterior chamber of the eye. *Br. J. Exp. Pathol.* 29:58, 1948.

48. Milward, T. M. Calcification in dermofat grafts. *Br. J. Plast. Surg.* 26:179, 1973.

49. Moore, J. B. A biomechanical comparison of vascularized and conventional autogenous bone grafts. *Plast. Reconstr. Surg.* 73:382, 1984.

50. Morrison, W. L., et al. The influence of PUVA and UVB radiation on skin-graft survival in rabbits. *J. Invest. Dermatol.* 75:331, 1980.

51. Muhlbauer, W. D., Schmidt-Tintemann, U., and Glaser, M. Long term behavior of preserved homologous rib cartilage and the correction of saddle nose deformity. *Br. J. Plast. Surg.* 24:325, 1975.

52. Oikarinen, J., and Korhonen, L. K. The bone inductive capacity of various bone transplanting materials used for treatment of experimental bone defects. *Clin. Orthop.* 140:208, 1979.

53. Oliver, R. F., et al. Incorporation of stored cell-free dermal collagen allografts into skin wounds, a short term study. *Br. J. Plast. Surg.* 30:88, 1977.

54. Ostrup, L. T., and Tam, C. H. Bone formation in a free living bone graft transferred by microvascular anastomosis. A quantitative microscopic study using fluorochrome markers. *Scand. Plast. Reconstr. Surg.* 9:101, 1975.

55. Peer, L. A. The fate of living and dead cartilage

transplanted in humans. *Surg. Gynecol. Obstet.* 68:603, 1939.

56. Pollock, G. D. Cases of skin grafting and skin transplantation. *Trans. Clin. Soc. Lond.* 4:37, 1871.

57. Reverdin, J. L. Greffes epiderminques: Expérience forte dans le service de M. le docteur Guyon, à l'Hôpital Necker, pendant 1869. *Bull. Soc. Imperiale Chir. Paris* 10(2), 1870.

58. Sailer, H. F. Experiences with the use of lyophilized bank cartilage for facial contour correction. *J. Maxillofac. Surg.* 4:149, 1976.

59. Schuller, D. E., Bardach, J., and Krause, C. J. Irradiated homologous costal cartilage for facial contour restoration. *Arch. Otolaryngol.* 103:12, 1977.

60. Sher, S. E., et al. Acceptance of allogeneic fibroblasts in skin equivalent transplants. *Transplantation* 36:552–557, 1983.

61. Skoog, T. The use of periosteum and Surgicel for bone restoration in congenital clefts of the maxilla. *Scand. J. Plast. Reconstr. Surg.* 1:113, 1967.

62. Snell, G. D. The terminology of tissue transplantation. *Transplantation* 2:655, 1964.

63. Stout, P. S. Bovine cartilage and correction of nasal deformities. *Laryngoscope* 43:976, 1933.

64. Taglicozzi, G. De curtorum chirurgia per Insitionem. Venice: Gaspare Bundoni, 1597.

65. Takapa, K. Enzyme histochemistry in bone tissue. *Acta Histochem.* 23:40, 1966.

66. Thompson, N., and Casson, J. A. Experimental inlay bone grafts to the jaws. A preliminary study in dogs. *Plast. Reconstr. Surg.* 46:341, 1970.

67. Towpik, E., Kupiec-Weglinski, J. W., and Tilney, N. L. The potential use of cyclosporine in reconstructive surgery. *Plast. Reconstr. Surg.* 76:312, 1980.

68. Urist, M. R., et al. The bone induction principle. *Clin. Orthop.* 53:243, 1967.

69. Warren, J. M. Rhinoplastic operations: With some remarks on the autoplastic methods usually adopted for the restoration of parts lost by accident or disease. Boston: Clapp, 1840.

70. Webster, D. A., and Werner, F. W. Freeze-dried flexor tendons in anterior cruiciate ligament reconstruction. *Clin. Orthop. Rel. Res.* 181:238, 1973.

71. Wolff, J. *Das Gesetz der Transformation der Knochen.* Berlin: A. Hirschwold, 1892.

72. Woodruff, M. F. A., and Anderson, N. Effect of lymphocyte depletion by thoracic duct fistula and administration of antilymphocyte serum on the survival of skin homograft in rats. *Nature.* 200:702, 1963.

73. Zalewski, A. A., and Gulati, A. K. Survival of nerve allografts in sensitized rats treated with Cyclosporin A. *J. Neurosurg.* 60:828–834, 1984.

74. Zarem, H. A., Sweifach, B. W., and McGehee, J. M. Development of microcirculation in full thickness autogenous skin grafts in mice. *Am. J. Physiol.* 212:1081, 1967.

75. Zins, J. E., and Whitaker, L. A. Membranous vs. endochondral bone: Implications for craniofacial reconstruction. *Plast. Reconstr. Surg.* 72:778, 1983.

# 3

*Darrick E. Antell*
*James W. Smith*

# Implantation Materials

As implied by the title, this chapter deals with materials that are inserted, embedded, or fixed firmly into living tissue. Materials are continually being developed in an effort to closely simulate the missing part and yet arouse a minimal reaction from the host. Among the more exciting materials are the injectable collagens and osseointegrated implants that were originally designed to replace teeth. Although initially buried, the osseointegrated implants are later exposed to allow attachment of a prosthesis, which is thus firmly anchored to the deep (bone) tissues of the body, bridging the internal and external environments.

The subject of implantation materials is one of the many areas in plastic surgery that merges the interests of dentistry and medicine. The addition of osseointegrated percutaneous implants to our armamentarium increases the selections available for reconstructive surgery.

With the exception of breast implants, most implant materials for plastic surgery are used in the face. However, advances in craniofacial surgery have increased the opportunities for recontouring the facial skeleton and in many cases have minimized or even eliminated the need for implants in situations where they were previously used. When developing the basic principles of cra-niofacial surgery, Tessier proposed the exclusive use of autogenous bone for graft onlays as well as for stabilizing the facial skeleton after it has been displaced. Particularly in the face, autogenous tissue has the advantage of healing even if part of it is exposed to the paranasal or paraorbital air sinuses. Autogenous tissue is incorporated into the body and becomes vascularized, but it also has the undesirable possibility of resorption.

Other concerns regarding the use of autogenous material (bone, cartilage, dermis, fat, fascia) are the following.

1. It requires additional surgery on the body for obtaining the graft.
2. It must be shaped at the time of the operation after it has been obtained, thereby prolonging the procedure.
3. The possibility of resorption remains.
4. Shift of the implant continues to be a problem.
5. A tight wad of scar tissue can result from a partially resorbed implant.
6. Only limited amounts of tissue are available.

These reasons as well as past training have contributed to the persistent use of alloplastic materials. In fact, there may be situations where alloplastic material is preferred to autogenous tissues. However, as a general concept, it is better to perform plastic surgery without the use of plastic, if possible.

The scope of this chapter does not include a discussion of autogenous graft materials. Rather, the focus is on tissue substitutes that are implanted into the body. Each clinical case must be decided separately with regard to the best material for substitu ing or replacing the missing tissues. As one considers the problem, the emphasis should be not only on the soft tissue defect but also perhaps on the underlying bony defect.

Moving along the reconstructive ladder when trying to solve a particular problem, one must assess both the quantity and the quality of the defect as well as address the problems of texture and color match. A history of radiotherapy or proposed irradiation of the area may also be significant. However, no matter what the defect, the basic issue that must be addressed is the quality of the "tissue envelope" that will hold this implant. If the implant is tight or if there is a marginal blood supply, as is often seen in irradiated tissues, the chance of implant extrusion is high. A tight soft tissue envelope also contributes to the possibility of bony resorption underneath the implant, as has been demonstrated in chin augmentation procedures. Once all of the available options have been explored, only then is one able to proceed with a choice of implant material.

## Tissue Substitutes

Scales, in 1953, described the ideal substitute qualities as the following [8].

1. Not physically modified by soft tissue
2. Not capable of inciting an inflammatory or foreign body reaction
3. Not capable of producing a state of allergy or hypersensitivity
4. Chemically inert
5. Noncarcinogenic
6. Capable of resisting strain

7. Capable of fabrication in the form desired
8. Capable of sterilization

During the implantation of foreign materials into the body most surgeons prefer to use antibiotics pre-, intra-, and postoperatively. Although it has never been studied specifically, one cannot fail to wonder if the patients who receive the implants should not continue to receive antibiotics in the future whenever they undergo a dental procedure or any other procedure causing a significant transient bacteremia. Patients with prosthetic heart valves or prosthetic hips always undergo dental work with prophylactic antibiotics. Perhaps, then, we should advise patients to have antibiotic coverage if they have other forms of implants as well, e.g., breast implants, chin implants, and cheek implants. It seems logical that these implants could also serve as a nidus for bacterial colonization. In addition to antibiotic prophylaxis, which should be maintained during the perioperative period, it is important for the surgeon to secure a complete description of the implant material as well a thorough understanding of its medical use and potential complications.

Certain materials tend to fall in and out of favor, such as the wide use of injectable silicone, which was popular during the early 1970s and has since fallen out of favor. However, the widespread use of injectable collagen and its success for correcting certain deformities has rekindled interest in injectable silicone, and the pendulum seems to be swinging at least a bit more toward injectable silicone. It is thus possible that this material may again gain popularity. It seems that with past usage, perhaps the lack of a mechanism for human control of its use, as well as poor quality control standards, allowed contaminated silicone samples to be injected and may have contributed to the complications that resulted from improper use of this product.

As a general concept, implant materials can be divided into two categories: soft and hard implants. *Soft implants* are the injectable implants, e.g., silicone or injectable collagen. *Hard implants* are composed of metals, textiles, and plastics. Safeguards for the use of these materials must be observed. With regard to hard implants, the following list of safeguards are recommended [8].

1. Shape the implant to avoid sharp corners and edges.
2. Bury the implant as deeply as possible under the skin and subcutaneous tissue.
3. Avoid tension in the adjacent tissues or tension against the overlying cutaneous coverage.
4. Place the incision line as far from the implant as possible.
5. Handle the implant with instruments to avoid soiling it with glove powder, lint, or fingerprints during and subsequent to the preparation period.
6. Utilize the proper stiffness of material; it should be as soft as is consistent with the application.
7. Do not use any hard material for soft tissue replacement.

Safeguards for "liquid" (injectable) implants include the following.

1. They should not be injected intravascularly.
2. One should always try to aspirate before injecting.
3. Care must be taken not to dissect new tissue planes during the injection process.
4. Extrusion through the needle tract hole must be prevented.

As a general concept, the hard implants can be removed should a problem occur. However, liquid injectable implants are more difficult to remove should it become necessary: They tend to track along their own planes and separate into small packets, whereas the hard implants tend to stay as a unit.

A conservative implant philosophy is basic to the successful use of any implant material.

Utilization of an inert foreign body material placed subcutaneously requires the following [8].

1. Comprehensive knowledge of the material, its properties, and its limitations
2. Intimate knowledge of the literature relating to any given implant material
3. Mastery of the particular surgical technique, with emphasis on minimal trauma to tissue during the implantation of foreign materials

## *Available Materials*

The literature is full of numerous reports of attempts at implantation of various materials, some of which include ivory, various organic rubbers, amber, silver, gold, platinum, paraffin, and zenogenic bone [8]. During maxillofacial surgery, Silastic, methylmethacrylate, Proplast, and tantalum are the most widely used materials [47]. Excluding breast implants (see Chap. 46), this chapter tends to focus on those types of implant that are most widely used in plastic surgery today. These materials fall under the following categories.

1. Metals (vitallium and pure titanium implants for osseointegration)
2. Textiles (Proplast)
3. Plastics (methylmethacrylate, polyurethane, polyethylene)
4. Fluids (injectable collagen, silicone)
5. Elastomers (rubbery materials)

METALS
Metal devices have been used in orthopedic surgery for the last several decades with great success. Adapting these techniques to craniomaxillofacial surgery has helped improve the rigid skeletal fixation and ultimate success of these procedures. Many techniques of skeletal fixation, including stainless steel wiring, K-wiring, threaded pins, and external fixation, have been employed.

However, introduction of the miniplate systems may decrease the relapse rate of elective LeFort osteotomy and provide increased stability to the mobilized segments, decreasing the length of time needed for intermaxillary fixation and sometimes eliminating the need for it. Although popular in Europe for many years, acceptance in North America was initially slow.

These plates had originally consisted of stainless steel, which when in contact with the electrolytes of the body could undergo corrosion after several years and on occasion require removal. The development of vitallium, a cobalt-chromium-molybdenum alloy, however, has maintained the characteristics of stainless steel in terms of strength yet added the ability to resist corrosion. As per the manufacturer (Homedica), vitallium consists of approximately 61 percent cobalt, 28 percent chromium, 4.5 percent molybdenum, and 1.5 percent nickel with less than 0.6 percent iron. It was initially developed as a casting material for dentistry in 1929; because of its continued success in that field, its applications have expanded, and it is now used for orthopedic and maxillofacial surgery. Compared with other techniques, miniplates provide stable fixation and can improve airway safety by minimizing the need for intermaxillary fixation in maxillofacial surgery. The complication rate is low, with infection rarely occurring. Like any alloplastic material, however, miniplates can also become exposed. Therefore meticulous technique when handling the plates is recommended [7]. Care should be taken also to provide adequate soft tissue coverage to prevent exposure of the plate.

Many metals have been used in dentistry with perhaps gold showing the least corrosion of the available materials. Gold does, however, lack the strength necessary for craniomaxillofacial applications. Nevertheless, it has been used in plastic and reconstructive surgery as a weight in the upper eyelid to allow closure of the eye in patients with seventh nerve palsy [24].

For bony fixation, metal miniplates have been developed in sets that can either provide or not provide compression. These two types of plate have different applications. Compression plates are designed for fracture repair and have an asymmetric hole on each side of the fracture site; placement and tightening of a screw into this hole allows compression of the bony segments along the fracture site, which in turn moves the fractured segments toward each other and allows compression of them. This type of movement, however, is not desirable in elective orthognathic surgery; therefore in nonfracture situations with elective osteotomies, the noncompression system is generally preferred to prevent movement of the segments once they have been positioned. The plates are provided in L,T, curved, and straight formats; the plate best suited to the particular situation is selected and then may require bending slightly for perfect adaptation to the bony segments. In addition, a double T-shaped plate is provided for genioplasty fixation. Although in this particular location the plates have not gained popularity, as they can occasionally be palpated underneath the skin. Other concerns about metal implants are potential allergic reactions, which may go unnoticed, as the plates are not visible at the completion of the case. Dermatologists are certainly aware of this type of reaction, as it is sometimes seen underneath inexpensive wrist watches or jewelry. In a review of the current literature on metallic implant biocompatibility, Smith [44] yielded the following conclusions.

1. Corrosion is a phenomenon common to all currently used implant alloys.
2. The process results in contamination of the local environment with metal constituents.
3. These corrosion products diffuse or are transported by mechanisms to sites not yet determined.
4. Potential exists for toxic effects at systemic sites of distribution or accumulation.

Remaining unanswered are questions of metallic implant biocompatibility over time as well as whether corrosion in the environment of the body is a cause for concern.

An additional application of metals in plastic and reconstructive surgery has been use of the osseointegrated percutaneous implant, which was originally developed as a dental implant system at the University of Gothenberg [8]. With the introduction of the osseointegrated implant, surgeons now have the ability to fix a prosthesis to the tissues with a permanent implant that is affixed to the bone but penetrating the skin or mucosa. These implants consist of 99.75 percent pure titanium with 0.05 percent iron, 0.10 percent oxygen, 0.03 percent nitrogen, 0.05 percent carbon, and 0.01 percent hydrogen [47]. A strict regimen for placement precludes touching the implant with any instruments manufactured with other materials, e.g., stainless steel.

Using gentle surgical technique, a small hole is drilled into the bone where the implant is to be placed, and the hole is then threaded with a pure titanium tap. Subsequently, the implant is gently screwed into this recipient site. The periosteum and overlying soft tissues are then sutured over the implant, and it is left buried for a minimum of 3 months to allow incorporation of the titanium implant into the bone, providing osseointegration [1]. At a second stage, the implant is uncovered and a permanent prosthesis can then be made for fixation to the implant.

A high degree of clinical success has been reported (95 to 100 percent) for all inserted implants [2]. The application of these implants allows restoration and reconstruction of many defects with prostheses that can be more securely anchored than was previously possible (Fig. 3-1).

TEXTILES
*Teflon*
Teflon is prepared by polymerization of tetrafluoroethylene gas at a high temperature and pressure [41]. Teflon is noncarcinogenic, can be sterilized, and is chemically inert with no known solvent. Teflon sheets (0.010 to 0.015 in. in thickness) are inexpensive, are contourable with gentle pressure, are easily sutured, and can easily be fitted into a specific defect. Most commonly, Teflon in this form is used to conform to the orbital floor and can be used as a prosthesis in this area as well as in a variety of facial fractures of both children and adults [5].

Alloplastic implants in the orbital region have become somewhat controversial owing to reports of complications related to the implant. Implant migration leading to ectropion, epiphora, diplopia, lacrimal obstruction, and late extrusion of the implant and infection have been reported [5]. Reports of orbital implant complication rates have been variable, from 0 to 14.6 percent. However, these studies included numerous types of implants with brief postoperative follow-up and without consistent surgical technique [5].

Aronowitz et al. [5] have shown the short-term complication rate with Teflon orbital implants to be as low as 3.9 percent and the long-term rate to be approximately 2.8 percent. Significantly, they noted that antral packing, when combined with a Teflon implant, led to a markedly higher risk of implant pocket infection. Recommendations were therefore made to not use alloplastic substances when antral packing was expected. Complication rates were further reduced with proper fixation, which included suturing, wiring, or a "tongue-like" flap; these measures prevented movement of the implant. The conclusion of that report was that the Teflon sheet is well tolerated in the orbital area. Using the above techniques, Aronowitz noted neither extrusion nor implant migration, although these problems did arise when no effort was made to fix the implant.

Use of Teflon for orbital floor reconstruction was also reported by Polley and Ringler [41], who noted a complication rate of 0.4

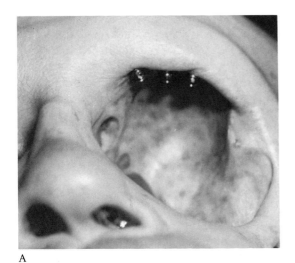

A

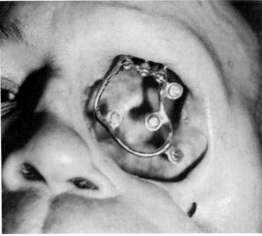

B

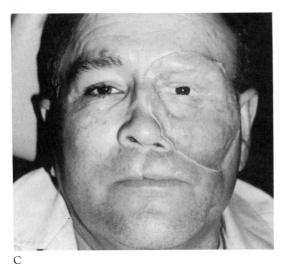

C

**Figure 3-1** *A. Osseointegrated percutaneous implants are seen protruding from the bone and are ready to receive the framework. B. The framework has been screwed into the implants, and magnets will affix the prosthesis to the framework. C. Prosthesis is in place. (Courtesy of Dr. Antell, New York, NY.)*

percent with only one infection requiring implant removal. That report covered a 20-year period, during which 230 Teflon implants were done for reconstruction of orbital floor defects. In addition, no extrusion or implant displacement was noted. Although the best method for reconstruction of the orbital floor in traumatic situations remains controversial, the use of Teflon implants in this area seems to be well established.

*Proplast*

Proplast, developed by Holmsey and reported in 1970, was the first of the synthetic biomaterials developed specifically for implantation in humans [21]. It was initially developed as a coating for the stabilization of skeletal implants; but the tissue ingrowth property that was observed led to applications in many surgical specialties. Today, block and sheet forms of Proplast may be easily shaped and contoured at the operating room table for the desired defect. In addition, preformed Proplast implants can be made for augmentation of the chin, zygoma, and periorbital rim area [28]. The initial Proplast material or Proplast 1, was made from a Teflon fluorocarbon polymer with black carbon fiber. The later addition of white aluminum oxide fiber provided Proplast 2, which found uses in more superficial areas and in lighter-skinned patients. For otologic reconstruction, ultrathin sheets have found wide application. In addition, the material has been formed into ossicle implants, which are now in general use [22]. Other uses of this material have been reported for reconstruction of the orbital rim, contour deformities of the maxilla and mandible, frontal bone defects, and nasal defects, as well as the correction of extensive pectus excavatum, rib cage deformities, and other hand and maxillofacial reconstructions. Size distribution of standard Proplast has been found to be optimal between 80 and 400 μm, at which point it has been found that rapid tissue ingrowth occurs maximally. Clinical advantages of Proplast include rapid stabilization of the implant by tissue ingrowth, ability to modify the implant and sculpt it, and an inherent firmness that maintains the prepared shape and contours while allowing flexibility for adaptation to the underlying bony contour. Studies on primates have demonstrated the ability for a high degree of tissue ingrowth as well as a rapid rate of tissue ingrowth. An additional advantage is the ability for vacuum impregnation of antibiotic solutions [27]. The overall infection rate with Proplast has been reported as minimal, with reports varying from less than 4 percent to as low as 2 percent [17].

Proplast has been found to be a good alternative to autogenous material and can often be prepared preoperatively. It is rapidly stabilized through fibrous tissue ingrowth, which provides dependable fixation and predictable results with less chance of extrusion. In addition, the porosity of the Proplast

allows added protection against infection because it can be impregnated with antibiotics preoperatively. Guidelines have been suggested by the manufacturer of Proplast (Vitek) that include the following.

1. Change to fresh, sterile gloves that have not touched the patient.
2. Rinse the gloves to remove the powder.
3. Do not overcompress the Proplast surface, as it may collapse the pores and inhibit tissue ingrowth.
4. Maintain the implant under antibiotic coverage by soaking it in a broad-spectrum antibiotic solution prior to implantation.

These techniques were well outlined by Sheen [42]. In Volume 1 of his book, an additional use of Proplast is demonstrated as a filler in the donor site of a cranial bone graft [42].

PLASTICS
*Methylmethacrylate*
Methylmethacrylate is a transparent resin with remarkable clarity. It has tensile strength in the range of 8500 lbs per square in., is stable, does not discolor in ultraviolet light, and has remarkable aging properties. It is chemically stable to heat and can be molded as a thermoplastic material at approximately 125°C [40]. As do all acrylic resins, it exhibits a tendency to take up water by a process of imbibition, which is why people who wear dentures are instructed to soak the dentures in a moist environment when they are not in the mouth. This material has been used with great success for denture construction. In plastic surgery it has been used to replace hard tissues, as in the chin area or the jaws, or as a replacement for missing cranial bone. Further application of self-curing acrylic has been in the external fixation devices for holding mandibular fragments together.

Methylmethacrylate may be either cold- or heat-cured. In either case, the density changes as the monomer is polymerized, causing shrinkage of the material. Consequently, when fitting acrylic into a defect, it must be constantly molded until it is fully set to ensure the fit of the final prosthesis. Additional advantages of the methylmethacrylate material are the following.

**1.** It is relatively inexpensive.
**2.** It can be hand-molded to fit a defect.
**3.** It can easily be trimmed during the setting phase.
**4.** Once it is set, it may still be trimmed using burrs and sanding instruments.
**5.** Using a moulage, it can be custom-fabricated preoperatively and later trimmed as needed.
**6.** As for denture construction, additional material may be added in selected locations even after the final set has been achieved.

Manson et al. reviewed the risk factors and choice of cranial vault reconstructive material [38]. They found that acrylic cranioplasties did not produce the complications expected (from previous reports in the literature). Although numerous materials have been tried for cranioplasty, at the present time acrylic appears to be the most widely used alloplastic material for this purpose.

Bone cranioplasty, although having the advantage of being the most tissue-compatible, has the disadvantage of potential contour deformities. Some have even advocated that an onlay of silicone or an acrylic material be placed over a bone cranioplasty to give a smoother, more satisfactory result [3, 9, 14, 19, 35]. An additional disadvantage of using autogenous bone as a cranioplasty material is its potential for variable resorption, leading to an irregular surface with possible soft areas developing postoperatively.

In a review of 42 frontal cranioplasties, Manson et al. [38] bone was generally preferred as the reconstructive material for extensive frontal orbital and nasal reconstructions. In all of the patients reviewed, the frontal sinus area was involved. Interestingly, in none of the acrylic cranioplasties

was infection noted. However, in 23 percent of the cranioplasties using bone, infection occurred that required bone or implant removal. These surprising results may be partially accounted for by the poor vascularity presumed in large bone defects, which might inhibit revascularization of the bone, thereby making it more susceptible to infection.

To draw the conclusion that acrylic is clearly preferred to autogenous material in cranial reconstruction is not accurate despite these statistics. However, it has been firmly established that acrylic as a cranial reconstructive material gives excellent results (Figs. 3-2 and 3-3). An additional recommendation for successful acrylic cranioplasty includes waiting at least 1 year in cases where a previous infection was present. At one time patients with infection, especially in the frontal area, were considered

*Figure 3-2* *A metal mesh reinforced methylmethacrylate cranioplasty had been performed on this 6-year-old abused patient. This radiograph was taken just before removal of the plate (because it had become infected).*

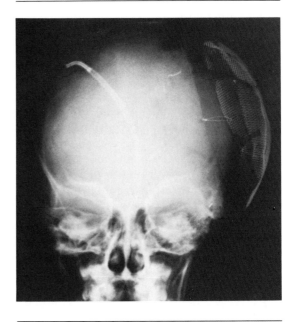

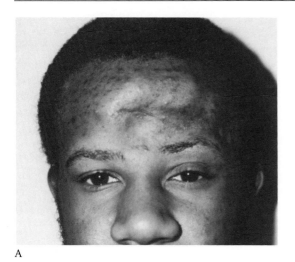

A

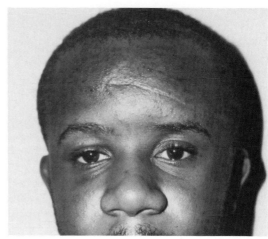

B

**Figure 3-3** *A. Frontal bone defect shown preoperatively. B. Postoperative result with methylmethacrylate cranioplasty. (Courtesy of Dr. Antell, New York, NY.)*

candidates only for bone reconstruction. However, more recent data suggest that the timing of the reconstruction may be more important than the choice of material [38].

Despite the success of acrylic cranioplasty, there remain those who believe that it represents a potential "time bomb" that, over time, will become infected, exposed, or extruded. Generally, craniofacial surgeons prefer to use autogenous material, and Wolfe reported a patient who demonstrated exposure of an acrylic cranioplasty 10 years after its insertion owing to breakdown of the overlying skin [46].

*Polyethylene*
Marlex is a popular surgical grade polyethylene that has been successfully used to reinforce hernia repairs as well as other abdominal and chest wall defects. Marlex has been used by the authors to reinforce large abdominal wall defects created after harvesting myocutaneous flaps in this area. No complications have been noted in our patients when Marlex was placed in a clean abdominal wound. We have, however, experienced exposure of the implant when it was used for chest wall reconstruction. This complication, most frequently related to infection, necessitated implant removal.

When rigid support is needed, Marlex is perhaps the most commonly used foreign body [18]. Marlex mesh on either side of a methylmethacrylate center has been used successfully for chest wall reconstruction [23] (Fig. 3-4). McCormack et al. [39] expanded the technique described by Hurwitz et al. [23] to incorporate steel mesh into the methylmethacrylate center, thereby strengthening the integrity of the implant and lessening the chances for fragmentation. However, we have observed that McCormack does not currently incorporate steel mesh within the methylmethacrylate as commonly as she once advocated. For reconstruction of chest wall defects, the to-and-fro motion of the chest can contribute to fragmentation of the implant; in selected cases where removal was necessary, the Marlex at least provided temporary support, allowing its removal without need for further skeletal reconstruction.

Infection is perhaps the biggest concern postoperatively when using Marlex mesh, and myocutaneous flaps have been em-

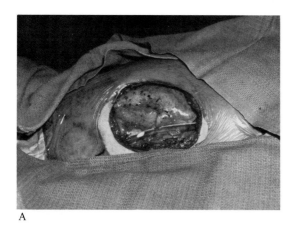

A

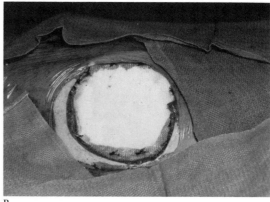

B

ployed as a form of closure over defects re-constructed with Marlex mesh. Such flaps often help ensure a good blood supply as well as providing a tension-free closure.

FLUIDS

The three structural proteins that support nearly all organic life on earth are chitin in the insect kingdom, cellulose in the plant kingdom, and collagen in the animal king-dom [4]. One might therefore presume that evolution has provided us with material of ideal qualities for application in the body to augment soft tissue defects.

*Collagen*

As the major connective tissue protein in animals, collagen accounts for 25 percent of the total body protein in vertebrates [4]. Col-lagen is a large protein composed of peptide chains arranged in a triple helix configura-tion.

The use of both human and bovine colla-gen in an injectable form for the correction of contour deformities in humans was first described by Knapp et al. in 1977 [33]. Bo-vine collagen has also been used for sutures and in hemostatic agents (Avitene, Gel-foam). Therefore a natural extension of its medical use was to augment soft tissues. Problems with other types of implant in-

*Figure 3-4* *For use in chest wall reconstruction, methylmethacrylate may be used sandwiched between Marlex mesh. A. Chest wall defect shown after resection, with lung exposed and chest tube in place. The patient's left arm is at the upper left of the picture. B. Sandwich of methylmethacrylate interposed between Marlex mesh is shown sutured in place. This defect was subsequently covered with a myocutaneous flap.*

clude capsule formation and migration. In-jectable collagen, however, is incorporated and biodegraded by the host tissue, though not encapsulated [32].

A highly purified form of injectable colla-gen was therefore derived from bovine col-lagen by the Collagen Corporation (Palo Alto, CA). The initial product, Zyderm I, has been in widespread use since 1981. Closely resembling human collagen, this material is administered via a fine-gauge needle by a se-ries of injections during multiple outpatient visits. Additional products—Zyderm II and Zyplast—have subsequently been developed for other indications. Reactions to the ma-terials have been temporary, of low inci-dence, and self-limiting. However, the im-munologic potential of this material, as it does represent a foreign body, has been a con-tinuing source of controversy and may be re-sponsible for attrition of the implant mate-rial over time.

In the proper setting, with patient selection being of the utmost importance and using proper technique, these materials have been demonstrated to provide benefit in the correction of small contour irregularities as well as small wrinkles. Like liquid silicone, injectable collagen can elevate depressions to the level of the surrounding skin.

Zyderm I and Zyderm II collagens are suspensions of sterilized fibrillar bovine collagen, with approximately 95 percent of the collagen being composed of type I collagen and the remainder type III. During the manufacturing process of injectable collagen, the telopeptide end regions are enzymatically digested for removal. These regions are thought to be the most antigenic sites on the molecule and are also the sites of greatest interspecies chemical variability. Their selective removal therefore renders the collagen hypoantigenic [45]. Zyplast implant, introduced in 1985, results from lightly cross-linking the collagen with glutaraldehyde. This relatively new form of injectable collagen is cross-linked for improved stability and longer survival than Zyderm I and Zyderm II. Zyplast has been shown to be more effective for treating deeper contour irregularities, though it has not shown a significantly longer persistence of correction when similar defects are treated.

These injectable collagens are suspended in saline and a 0.3% lidocaine solution. This method aids in administering the material through a fine-gauge needle, which must be used. The differences between Zyderm I and Zyderm II are concentration. Zyplast is the same concentration as Zyderm I, only it is treated with glutaraldehyde and cross-linked.

ZYDERM I. Zyderm I collagen remains the mainstay of the injectable collagens. It was the first to be introduced and has a collagen concentration of 35 mg per milliliter. As the least concentrated of the injectable collagens, it is useful for superficial dermal defects typically in thin skin. Such defects might include fine wrinkles, particularly in the periorbital and perioral area, as well as

superficial scars. The intended placement of this material is superficial within the dermis, and it is the Zyderm I collagen that is used for the initial skin test before later treatment with any of the available forms of injectable collagen.

ZYDERM II. Zyderm II collagen is distinguished by an increased concentration of collagen to 65 mg per milliliter. More collagen is therefore delivered per injection, and fewer treatments may be needed using Zyderm II, although it is more difficult to inject because it is a thicker material. Transient bumps or beads may result in the injection site, and so this material is usually reserved for thicker skin than at the sites where Zyderm I is most commonly used. Sites appropriate for the use of Zyderm II collagen include glabellar lines, nasolabial lines, transverse forehead lines, and acne scarring.

ZYPLAST. Zyplast collagen is the third commonly used form of injectable collagen, and it is a more rigid material than either Zyderm I or Zyderm II. It therefore does not distribute as easily within the superficial dermis and should be injected into the deep dermis to prevent a superficial bump.

During the preparation of Zyplast collagen, glutaraldehyde reacts with amino groups of lysine residues contained in these peptide chains to produce covalent bridges between the collagen molecules. Only about 10 percent of the available lysine residues are cross-linked in the reaction; however, it appears sufficient to stabilize the reaction and allows a longer period of correction of the skin defect. Although still a relatively new material, the Zyplast implant is thought to undergo little implant shrinkage compared to the Zyderm collagen implants, which shrink 30 to 40 percent of their implanted volume, as water is extruded from the implant [32]. Because of its thicker nature and better volume retention, it is recommended that Zyplast be used in glabellar folds, nasolabial folds, postrhinoplasty defects, and other areas where the material can be implanted into the deep dermis (in contrast to the superficial dermis).

INDICATIONS AND CONTRAINDICATIONS. When introduced properly, injectable collagen has been shown to provide effective correction of age-related wrinkles and scars induced by trauma or disease [25, 26]. The material can be used to touch up any fine lines that remain after a rhytidectomy, and it is particularly valuable for treatment of glabellar and nasolabial lines. Surgical depressions such as those that may occur after a rhinoplasty can also be treated with injectable collagen; and it may be used to correct contour deficiencies such as saucer-shaped acne scars as well as areas of steroid-induced atrophy. Perhaps one of the most common uses of this material is for treating crows' feet wrinkles in the perioribital area; however, extreme caution must be used when injecting this area, as there has been at least one reported case of partial loss of vision due to inadvertent injection into an artery in the extraorbital site that communicated with the central ophthalmic artery. This error is, however, a rare event; and it is estimated that at least 350,000 people have been treated with injectable bovine collagen in the United States with more than 3000 physicians having used the material [11].

Because of the different concentrations of Zyderm I and Zyderm II and the cross-linking of Zyplast, guidelines have been established, outlining the indications for their use (Table 3-1). These guidelines are meant to be only a suggestion, and of course clinical judgment must be used in each case to determine the best material for that particular situation.

In summary, the more superficial defects with soft, supple skin may be treated with Zyderm I and possibly Zyderm II. For deeper defects or where the tissues are thicker, Zyplast may be used. However, Zyplast must be injected into the deep dermis to prevent bumps, which may occur with superficial injections of this material.

Not all patients are suitable candidates for collagen injection. Prior to any treatment the patient must be adivsed about the need for skin testing, the length of the treatment, and the fact that multiple treatments are required as well as probable touch-up injections over time. The degree of correction that will be achieved should probably be understated, and the patient must clearly understand that the area has to be overcorrected initially to allow for absorption of the water carrier.

Contraindications to the use of collagen treatments include the following.

1. Tissue defects more amenable to treatment by other, established methods
2. Patients with a history of autoimmune disease
3. Viral pockmarks, deep acne scars (icepick-like), and indurated scars, which do not respond well to injectable collagen
4. Patients with a positive skin test or those who have had previous hypersensitivity reactions to injectable collagen
5. History of anaphylactoid reaction
6. Allergy to lidocaine

SKIN TESTING. Skin testing is performed to identify patients who may be sensitive to the injectable collagens. The skin test syringe is supplied with 0.1 ml of Zyderm I collagen. Zyderm I is always used for the skin test, regardless of whether the definitive treatment is to be with Zyderm I, Zyderm II, or Zyplast. All or as little as one-third of the test syringe contents may be injected into the superficial dermis of the volar forearm. Injection is done in a manner similar to that used for tuberculin testing [31]. The test site is examined within 3 days, as 70 percent of the test reactions occur during that time frame. The test site is then reexamined at 4 weeks and is considered positive if redness and swelling remain at the 1-month follow-up visit. Positive test reactions may resolve by the 4-week follow-up visit. Erythema, induration, tenderness, or swelling that persists for more than 6 hours

**Table 3-1** *Collagen implants in soft tissue defects*

| Zyderm I collagen | Zyderm II collagen | Zyplast implant |
|---|---|---|
| Perioral lines | Glabellar lines* | Acne scarring |
| Postorbital lines | Nasolabial lines | Glabellar furrows |
| Glabellar lines* | Transverse | Nasolabial furrows |
| Nasolabial lines |   forehead lines | Postimplant depressions |
| Transverse forehead lines | Acne scarring | Malar insufficiency |
| Acne scarring | Glabellar furrows | Subdermal atrophy |
| | Nasolabial furrows | Graft depressions |
| | | Rhinoplasty irregularities |

*Use with caution in this area.

or develops after 24 hours is considered positive, even if it has resolved by the 4-week follow-up. It is important to stress that the physician or a trained assistant must view the test site carefully, as the patient may ignore a positive test site reaction.

Patients who demonstrate a positive skin test reaction are excluded from further treatment. Hypersensitivity reactions to the localized intradermal test dose of Zyderm I collagen occur in approximately 3 percent of individuals tested. It generally manifests as an inflammatory response, indicating the patient's preexisting sensitivity to bovine collagen. The incidence of adverse reactions to the actual treatment is in the range of 1 to 5 percent at most [10, 13, 43]. The initial test injection yields the highest incidence of hypersensitivity reactions; and with each additional exposure, the incidence of reaction diminishes. Studies on a histologic level indicate that these hypersensitivity reactions represent localized granulomas with a lymphohistiocytic infiltrate surrounding the collagen implant [6]. Significantly, these immunologic responses appear to occur at the site of implantation and do not appear to significantly affect the host's surrounding connective tissues [15]. Although a small percentage of patients have been shown to develop hypersensitivity to injectable collagen, this response has not been shown to be cross-reactive with human collagen [12, 15, 16]. The incidence of adverse treatment reactions has been reported to be approximately 1.3 percent by the manufacturer. These responses involved typically localized erythema, swelling, induration, or pruritus. About 0.6 percent of these reactions developed subsequent to a negative skin test. All adverse responses, however, resolved over a period of months without sequelae and without therapeutic intervention.

TECHNIQUE. Having passed the stage of skin testing, the patient is then prepared for the initial treatment (Table 3-2). Three factors play a key role in maximizing the correction: (1) lesion selection; (2) amount of correction needed; and (3) tissue plane placement (superficial or deep dermis).

Substantial correction may be achieved in many soft tissue deformities so long as the material is injected properly. It must be placed in the superficial dermis with Zyderm I or Zyderm II and in the deep dermis with Zyplast to ensure good results. When using Zyplast, a greater angle (approximately 45 degrees) is used; with Zyderm, a more horizontal approach allows more superficial placement. A serial injection technique has been recommended by proponents who claim that this technique ensures proper placement and therefore gives consistently good results [30]. Once the site to be injected is identi-

**Table 3-2** Injectable collagen regimen (Zyderm I, Zyderm II, Zyplast)

| Visit | Time | Activity |
|-------|------|----------|
| 1 | 0 | Evaluate defects.<br>Secure patient history.<br>Administer collagen test dose (approx. 0.1 ml). |
| 2 | 3 days | Evaluate site at 3 days.<br>About 3% of patients have a sensitivity to the skin test; two-thirds of these reactions develop within 72 hours. |
| 3 | 4 weeks | Evaluate test site.<br>Administer first dermal injections. |
| 4 | 6–8 weeks | Evaluate result of first injection.<br>About 1.3% of patients have an adverse reaction (erythema, swelling, induration, pruritus).<br>Administer additional dermal injections PRN. |

fied, the area is cleaned and a 30-gauge needle is used to minimize patient discomfort and prevent extrusion of the material through the needle tract. Keeping the needle horizontal along the surface of the skin until it just penetrates the dermis helps ensure intradermal placement.

With proper positioning, only the bevel of the needle is inserted in the skin; it may be possible to see the needle tip through the skin. Once inserted, the needle tip is rolled toward the surface as the collagen is injected [32]. Proponents of the serial puncture technique recommend multiple deposits no more than 1/8 in. apart; with proper placement of the implant material, a wheal is subsequently apparent.

Using Zyderm I or Zyderm II collagen, overcorrection is essential when treating a lesion. This important point is critical as the saline carrier subsequently is absorbed, leaving only approximately 30 percent of the original injected volume. As a general guideline, the lesion should therefore be overcorrected 1.5 to 2.0 times the initial depth of the deficiency. A Zyplast implant, on the other hand, retains the volume that was implanted, and thus overcorrection is generally not advocated. The Zyplast implant, in contrast to the Zyderm implant, is placed in the deep dermis, not the superficial dermis. Overcorrection is also not recommended in thin skin areas, e.g., around the eyes or mouth; care is taken when using Zyderm II because of its high collagen content, which does not require as much overcorrection as with use of Zyderm I, which has roughly one-half the collagen concentration of Zyderm II.

Errors of injection technique include blood vessel occlusion or laceration, infection, and gross overcorrection. Reinjection for maintenance purposes is required within a 6- to 24-month period, although newer materials such as Zyplast may prove to have longer-lasting effects. In addition, depending on the patient's particular defect and skin type, up to 18 months of correction is achieved in some acne scars as well as other minor irregularities, e.g., those occurring after rhinoplasty [11]. In areas where mechanical stresses may be higher, e.g., areas of wrinkles, ongoing correction appears to be necessary, perhaps because of the activity of mechanical stresses in those areas, causing assimilation of the material.

According to the Collagen Corporation, the possibility of intravascular injection can be decreased by careful attention to details and using the following injection technique.

1. The needle is placed superficially in the papillary dermis, as recommended.
2. Loupe magnification of at least 2.5 times aids in visualizing correct needle placement.

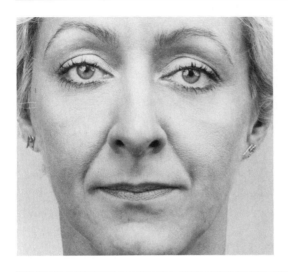 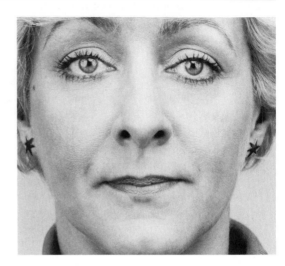

**Figure 3-5** *Before and after Zyplast collagen injection of nasolabial folds. (Courtesy of the Collagen Corporation, Palo Alto, CA.)*

**3.** If there is no blanching at the injection site, the needle is withdrawn immediately.
**4.** The serial puncture technique is used.

DISCUSSION. Injectable collagens have proved to be a useful adjunct to the armamentarium of the plastic surgeon. They give acceptable results in selected cases (Fig. 3-5). However, to achieve patient and physician satisfaction, it is important that the limitations be explained to and understood by the patient preoperatively. Early evidence suggests that injected Zyderm is replaced by host collagen [32]. This replacement collagen, by being not as highly cross-linked, may be more susceptible to the effects of forces causing wrinkles and may contribute to the recurrence of the deformity. The introduction of Zyplast may help alleviate this problem, at least in the deeper furrows, for which it is recommended. In addition, one must carefully select those patients in whom alternative procedures (e.g., facelifting, dermabrasion, chemical peel) are preferable. Injecting col-

lagen into postsurgical areas before they are fully healed may also contribute to resorption of the collagen. Generalized collagen turnover in a traumatized tissue would also contribute to turnover of the injectable collagens. This point is substantiated in the treatment of acne scars, where the longest-lasting and perhaps best results have been noted with injectable collagen. Minimal loss of correction has been noted in patients for as long as 2½ years postoperatively, suggesting that mature acne scars may not be as subject to dermal remodeling as areas of active inflammation [29].

The main concerns regarding the use of injectable collagens continue to focus on the need for repeated injections to maintain correction and the presence of circulating antibodies to the collagen. The concern of multiple injections has been previously addressed; although the issue has not been solved, the introduction of Zyplast may help maintain correction in certain clinical situations.

Hypersensitivity reactions are most frequently associated with the initial collagen injection. This reaction is a localized reaction focused at the site of injection, and the antibodies produced have not yet been shown to be cross-reactive with human collagen [15]. Future studies on the humoral immunity and biologic fate of injectable collagen will hopefully alleviate the present concerns about the efficacy and safety of these products. There must be continuing investigation regarding (1) preexisting immunity to animal collagens in patients who test positive with the skin test and (2) host responsiveness to collagen after repeated injections.

*Silicone*
The use of silicone in the practice of medicine has become widespread. Nearly all surgical specialties use silicone in some form: pacemakers, penile implants, joint replacement prostheses, myringotomy tubes, intraocular lenses, and ventricular peritoneal shunts, as well as for reconstructive and aesthetic surgery. In addition, silicone has found uses in the manufacture of intravenous catheters, intravenous tubing, and surgical drains. In its solid form silicone is thought to be a relatively inert substance, yet reports of failure with various silicone implants persist.

These failures are often associated with concomitant fibrosis, lymphadenopathy, silicone migration, hemorrhage, and fragmentation [34]. In an excellent, exhaustive article, Kossovsky et al. thoroughly reviewed the bioreactivity of silicone [34] and the plastic surgery experience with its implantation. The implantation of silicone in the breast is perhaps the most frequent use of this material. Complications are few, although local and distant reactions have been reported. Capsule formation with tight contraction is perhaps the most common complication after augmentation mammaplasty and may occur unilaterally in a patient with bilateral augmentation.

Examining capsules from patients who had had implants, Mandel and Gibbons identified silicone-containing compounds. They noted that the silicone polymer can be identified within the cells as well as in the intercellular matrix. These areas were associated with a macrophage and foreign body giant cell response [37]. Advocates of silicone implantation suggest that the granulomatous reaction and scar formation around these implants is a necessary consequence of the implantation of these materials.

Controversy remains, however, regarding the immunologic reaction to implantation of these materials. It has been suggested that once placed in the body silicone may act as a hapten-like incomplete antigen. It has been demonstrated that silicone is capable of eliciting a cellular immune response, as demonstrated by the migration inhibition technique [20]. Numerous types of breast implant have been developed with double and triple lumens to try to protect the body from exposure to the silicone material, but a penetrating injury to the patient that would expose the body to the silicone material is always possible.

As a liquid injectable material, silicone was once widely used for augmentation of soft tissue defects as well as for breast enlargement. Problems with migration of the material as well as infection and widespread abuse of this material caused it to be withdrawn from general use. Lemperle and Spitalny, discussing the use of liquid injectable silicones, stated that in their experience with approximately 50 cases of liquid facial injections the material tended to be affected by gravity, and the effect of the augmentation was gone after approximately 5 years [36]. In the same discussion, Jackson and Murray noted excellent results with the use of liquid injectable silicone for treating hemifacial atrophy, with a complication rate approaching zero. When complications did occur, however, they were difficult to treat [36]. At the present time, liquid injectable silicone is not available for widespread use.

ELASTOMERS
Silicone in a rubbery form is available as two major types. The heat-vulcanized type is

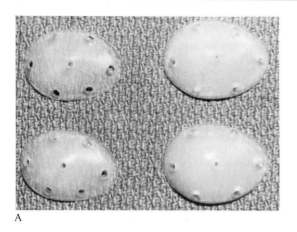
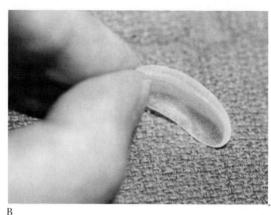

A                                        B

**Figure 3-6** *Preformed silicone implants.*
*A. Malar implants are shown in different sizes*
*with holes to aid in fixation of the implant.*
*B. Chin implant with concave surface designed*
*to fit over the pogonion. These implants come*
*in different sizes and may be trimmed for*
*additional contouring.*

supplied by the manufacturer in prepared
shapes: malar, nasal, and chin augmentation
prostheses (Fig. 3-6). Room temperature vulcanizing (RTV) silicone is also available and
can be used in areas where one wishes to
custom-fabricate an implant without causing a tissue reaction to the heat, as would be
required in the heat vulcanizing type of silicone. Supplied in a raw state, the RTV silicone rubbers can be mixed with a catalyst
and then cross-linked to form a rubbery
prosthesis in a few minutes at room temperature.

Silicone rubber implants can be obtained
prefabricated, or they can be custom-made for
specific defects. Once manufactured, they
tend to maintain their shape, although they do
have several disadvantages.

1. There is a lack of adaptation to the exact
   underlying contours during surgery.
2. Carving the silicone to the exact shape
   may leave rough, sharp edges, and the
   shaping is often difficult.

3. The material cannot be bent to conform
   to a defect owing to its inherent memory,
   which causes it to spring back to its original shape.
4. Stabilization of the implant often requires
   suturing it to adjacent tissues.
5. It may become displaced as capsule contracture occurs around the implant.

Despite persistent concerns, silicone implants have been widely used. Their success
has been repeatedly demonstrated for augmentation of contour deformities of the face
as well as their widespread use as implantation materials in virtually every surgical
specialty.

## References

1. Albrektsson, T., et al. The interference of
   some inorganic implants in vivo: Titanium
   implants in bone. *Ann. Biomed. Eng.* 11:1,
   1983.
2. Albrektsson, T., et al. Present clinical applications of osseointegrated percutaneous implants. *Plast. Reconstr. Surg.* 79:721, 1987.
3. Alexander, E., and Dillard, P. H. The use of
   pure polyethylene plate for cranioplasty. *J.
   Neurosurg.* 7:492, 1950.
4. Arem, A. Collagen modifications. *Clin. Plast.
   Surg.* 12:209, 1985.
5. Aronowitz, J. A., Freeman, B. S., and Spira, M.

Long term stability of Teflon orbital implants. *Plast. Reconstr. Surg.* 78:166, 1986.

6. Barr, R., et al. Necrobiotic granuloma associated with bovine collagen test site injections. *J. Am. Acad. Dermatol.* 6:867, 1982.

7. Beals, S. P., and Munro, I. R. The use of miniplates in craniomaxillofacial surgery. *Plast. Reconstr. Surg.* 79:33, 1987.

8. Blocksma, R., and Braley, S. Implantation Materials. In W. C. Grabb and J. W. Smith (eds.), *Plastic Surgery* (3rd ed.). Boston: Little, Brown, 1979.

9. Cabbage, E. B., Shively, R. E., and Malik, P. Cranioplasty for traumatic deformities of the frontoorbital area. *Ann. Plast. Surg.* 13:175, 1984.

10. Castro, F. F., and Krull, E. A. Injectable collagen implant—update. *J. Am. Acad. Dermatol.* 9:889, 1983.

11. Collagen Corporation. Personal communication, 1987.

12. Cooperman, L., and Michaeli, D. The immunogenicity of injectable collagen. II. A retrospective review of seventy-two tested and treated patients. *J. Am. Acad. Dermatol.* 10:647, 1984.

13. Cooperman, L. S., et al. Injectable collagen: A six year clinical investigation. *Aesthetic Plast. Surg.* 9:145, 1985.

14. Courtemanche, A. D., and Thompson, G. B. Silastic cranioplasty following cranio-facial injuries. *Plast. Reconstr. Surg.* 41:165, 1968.

15. DeLustro, F., et al. Reaction to injectable collagen: Results in animal models and clinical use. *Plast. Reconstr. Surg.* 79:581, 1987.

16. Ellingsworht, L. E., et al. The human immune response to reconstituted bovine collagen. *J. Immunol.* 136:877, 1986.

17. Freeman, B. S., and Wiener, D. R. Clinical uses of Proplast: Expectations and results. In L. R. Rubin (ed.), *Biomaterials in Reconstructive Surgery*. St. Louis: Mosby, 1983.

18. Graham, J., et al. Marlex as a prosthesis in repair of thoracic wall defects. *Ann. Surg.* 151:469, 1960.

19. Habal, M. B., and Chalian, V. A. Experience with prefabricated silicone implants for reconstruction in facially deformed patients. *J. Prosthet. Dent.* 32:292, 1974.

20. Heggers, J. P., et al. Biocompatibility of silicone implants. *Ann. Plast. Surg.* 11:38, 1983.

21. Holmsey, C. P. Bio-compatibility in selection of materials for implantation. *J. Biomed. Mater. Res.* 4:341, 1970.

22. Homsy, C. A. Proplast: Chemical and biological considerations. In L. R. Rubin (ed.), *Biomaterials in Reconstructive Surgery*. St. Louis: Mosby, 1983.

23. Hurwitz, D. J., Ravitch, M., and Wolmark, N. Laminated Marlex methylmethacrylate prosthesis for massive chest wall resection. *Ann. Plast. Surg.* 5:486, 1980.

24. Jobe, R. P. A technique for lid loading in the management of the lagophthalmos of facial palsy. *Plast. Reconstr. Surg.* 53:29, 1974.

25. Kamer, F. M., and Churukian, M. M. The clinical use of injectable collagen: A three year retrospective study. *Arch. Otolaryngol.* 110:93, 1984.

26. Kaplan, E. N., Falces, E., and Tolleth, H. Clinical utilization of injectable collagen. *Ann. Plast. Surg.* 10:437, 1983.

27. Kent, J. N., and Westfall, R. L. Presurgical infusion of Proplast: Primate facial augmentation. *J. Oral Surg.* 37:637, 1979.

28. Kent, J. N., Westfall, R. L., and Carlton, D. M. Chin and zygomaticomaxillary augmentation with Proplast: Long term follow-up. *J. Oral Surg.* 39:912, 1981.

29. Klein, A. W. Implantation technics for injectable collagen. *J. Am. Acad. Dermatol.* 9:224, 1983.

30. Klein, A. W. Implantation techniques for injectable collagen: Two and one-half years of personal clinical experience. *J. Am. Acad. Dermatol.* 9:224, 1983.

31. Klein, A. W., and Rish, D. C. Injectable collagen update. *J. Dermatol. Surg. Oncol.* 10:519, 1984.

32. Knapp, T. R., and Vistnes, L. M. The augmentation of soft tissue with injectable collagen. *Clin. Plast. Surg.* 12:221, 1985.

33. Knapp, T. R., Kaplan, E. N., and Daniels, J. R. Injectable collagen for soft tissue augmentation. *Plast. Reconstr. Surg.* 60:398, 1977.

34. Kossovsky, N., Heggers, J. P., and Robson, M. C. The bioreactivity of silicone. *CRC Crit. Rev. Biocompat.* 3:53, 1987.

35. Laub, D. R., et al. Accurate reconstruction of traumatic bony contour defects of periorbital area with prefabricated Silastic. *J. Trauma* 10:472, 1970.

36. Lemperle, G., and Spitalny, H. H. Long term experience with silicone implants in the face.

In E. P. Caronni (ed.), *Craniofacial Surgery.* Boston: Little, Brown, 1985.

37. Mandel, M. A., and Gibbons, D. F. The presence of silicone in breast capsules. *Aesthetic Plast. Surg.* 3:219, 1979.

38. Manson, P. N., Crawley, W. A., and Hoopes, J. E. Frontal cranioplasty: Risk factors and choice of cranial vault reconstructive material. *Plast. Reconstr. Surg.* 77:888, 1986.

39. McCormack, P., et al. New trends in skeletal reconstruction after resection of chest wall tumors. *Ann. Thorac. Surg.* 31:45, 1981.

40. Phillips, R. W. (ed.). *Skinner's Science of Dental Materials.* Philadelphia: Saunders, 1973.

41. Polley, J. W., and Ringler, S. L. The use of Teflon in orbital floor reconstruction following blunt facial trauma: A 20-year experience. *Plast. Reconstr. Surg.* 79:39, 1987.

42. Sheen, J. H. *Aesthetic Rhinoplasty* (2nd ed.). St. Louis: Mosby, 1987. P. 397.

43. Siegle, R. J., et al. Intradermal implantation of bovine collagen: Humoral immune responses associated with clinical reactions. *Arch. Dermatol.* 120:183, 1984.

44. Smith, G. K. Systemic aspects of metalic implant degradation. In L. R. Rubin (ed.), *Biomaterials in Reconstructive Surgery.* St. Louis: Mosby, 1983.

45. Timpl, R., et al. Characterization of conformation independent antigenic determinants in the triple-helical part of calf and rat collagen. *Immunology* 21:1017, 1971.

46. Wolfe, S. A. Discussion of "Frontal cranioplasty: Risk factors and choice of cranial vault reconstructive material." *Plast. Reconstr. Surg.* 77:901, 1986.

47. Wolfe, T. Autogenous bone grafts versus alloplastic material in maxillofacial surgery. *Clin. Plast. Surg.* 9:539, 1982.

*Julien Reich*

# 4

# *The Aesthetic Surgical Experience*

The surgical improvement in appearance for deviations that do not amount to an objective deformity can permanently relieve the patient of a preoccupation with his appearance. It does so by correcting the patient's inability to accept how he sees himself [2]. Obviously, then, the alteration in appearance is responsible for a change in mental attitude of a more fundamental nature than that produced by a superficial adornment. This fact is the raison d'etre of aesthetic surgery and is also the reason why "aesthetic" surgery is a more acceptable term than "cosmetic" surgery when referring to a surgical improvement in appearance.

In this context it is important to distinguish between the aesthetic surgical patient and the reconstructive surgical patient. The aesthetic surgical patient, because of his inability to accept how he sees himself, feels self-conscious about some aspect of his appearance, and it is this self-consciousness that affects his interpersonal relationships. In other words, he rejects himself and by inference feels rejected by others. The physically deformed person, on the other hand, is made to feel different either by unfavorable comments or ridicule, or by our often clumsy attempts not to direct attention to his disfigurement. In other words, he feels rejected by others and by inference may reject himself. It is thus clear that the practice of aesthetic surgery takes place against the background of an interpersonal triangle because it involves the patient, the patient's daily contacts, and the surgeon. Because their attitudes toward the justification and results of a surgical alteration in appearance may differ, we must examine these points separately before attempting to analyze the aesthetic surgical experience.

## *Aesthetic Surgery Patient*

The patient consults the surgeon because he is experiencing dissatisfaction with some aspect of his appearance. The trigger for the consultation is an urge for a change in appearance, which is linked to a desired change in the style or quality of his daily life.

PATIENT MOTIVATION

Most writings on the subject of motivation in aesthetic plastic surgery have distinguished between motivations at a conscious level and those at a subconscious level. Such a division may be useful if the subject is discussed from a purely psychological or psychiatric point of view. However, if we consider the everyday patient-surgeon relationship, motivation is best looked at in a different way.

Thus the force that initiates the request for aesthetic plastic surgery may be seen as an uneasiness in the mind of the patient associated with an urge for a change toward a more comfortable state of mind. In other words, we are dealing with an upset in the psychodynamic equilibrium of the patient that is experienced subjectively by the individual as dissatisfaction with his appearance, which may of course be focused on a particular feature. The upset in the psychodynamic equilibrium, or uneasiness of mind, is usually produced by an environmental stress. Thus it may be looked on as an insecurity in the life situation of the patient brought about by such factors as the realization of aging, employment problems, divorce, bereavement, or social isolation, whether self-inflicted or related to migration and associated ethnic problems.

The significant point of difference between the aesthetic surgery patient and the psychiatric patient is that with the former we are concerned with an individual who is actively trying to deal with his problem. Herein lies the justification of aesthetic plastic surgery: It enables the patient to accept how he sees himself and thus may lead to restoration of the patient's psychodynamic equilibrium.

The question we must ask ourselves in each case is this: What causes this particular individual to request a surgical procedure designed to effect an alteration in his appearance? In my practice there is considerable emphasis on allowing patients to express their feelings about their appearance and how they think it affects their lives. Although this approach takes valuable time, it is essential to understand the patient's point of view in order to ensure a successful result.

In a survey of more than 3000 patients, the predominant reasons for requesting aesthetic plastic surgery were as follows: In 60 percent of patients there was self-consciousness in in-terpersonal relationships. In another 25 percent, social isolation, including the problems of migrants, members of ethnic groups, and the elderly, played a part. In approximately 10 percent the employment situation appeared to be involved, and other adverse life situations were prominent in 5 percent.

Self-consciousness in interpersonal relationships in this context is associated with a feeling of dissatisfaction with one's mirror image, a growing preoccupation with a certain aspect of one's appearance, a constant and often frustrating effort to deal with this problem by some form of camouflage (e.g., makeup, changes in hairstyle, and clothing), or more drastically by attempts to change the body shape through dieting and exercise.

Social acceptance in our time relates less to social background than to one's ability to conform with current concepts of desirable social characteristics. These concepts, apart from a willingness to spend money, are centered on youthfulness, an acceptable appearance of the body, and at least the suggestion of physical fitness, even if it amounts only to the wearing of certain makes of tracksuit. The virtual explosion of outdoor activities and exposure of the body has led to an increasing demand for a surgical improvement in appearance.

Social acceptance is also related to one's ability to fit in with the predominant group in the country in which one lives. The tremendous migratory movements induced by the political and economic pressures of our time are responsible for many social problems. The older first-generation migrant usually alleviates these problems by congregating in ethnic groups and by intensifying his involvement with a traditional way of life, which makes his partly self-imposed social isolation more bearable. The younger first-generation migrant and those of succeeding generations, however, often actively try to assimilate and thus to become absorbed into the predominant group. Aesthetic plastic surgery can play an important part in helping to relieve those problems related to aspects of appearance that interfere with these aspirations.

In patients whose request for aesthetic plastic surgery is related to the availability of employment opportunities, preoccupation with appearance often commenced or was aggravated by remarks made during interviews for positions. Such remarks usually centered about the appearance of aging and its implied relation to efficiency. A much smaller proportion of patients were concerned with some particular aspect of appearance that affected employment in an appearance-sensitive field, e.g., photographic modeling or some areas of entertainment.

Coping with adverse life situations, such as bereavement or divorce, involves determined psychological rehabilitation after a period of stress. Some individuals appear to achieve this state best by undergoing a physical rehabilitation. The most familiar example is the woman who has experienced a minor stress but appears to feel better after application of lipstick or a visit to the hairdresser. In the same way, aesthetic plastic surgery is able to contribute to self-rehabilitation after major stresses. Symbolically here, the individual draws a line between an unhappy past and what is hoped to be a better future.

The aesthetic plastic surgeon is thus faced with an individual who is unable or unwilling to accept how he sees himself. The conscious aim of most patients who seek a surgical alteration in appearance is to be inconspicuous. They wish to lose the feeling of self-consciousness about an aspect of their appearance they believe draws unwelcome attention of others to them or that has had an unfavorable effect on some aspect of daily life.

SIGNIFICANCE OF PERSONALITY TYPE
Motivation of patients for aesthetic surgery can be discussed in general terms, but the patient's attitude to the motivating factor and indeed the period of patient-surgeon contact is often affected significantly by the patient's personality type. An understanding of these relationships is important to the aesthetic plastic surgeon.

Possibly the most important personality type from our point of view is the *obsessive personality*. These individuals are usually well organized and orderly, rigid or ritualistic individuals. They are often preoccupied with minute details of irregularities and asymmetries and are demanding in what they expect as a result of surgery. They demand guarantees and are prepared to go to any lengths to attain the desired improvement. They manage their feelings intellectually and become anxious when uncertain. These patients need to be supplied with precise details about the operation and the expected results. They require regular progress reports during the period in which they are under care. If anxiety develops in these patients, explanation is used rather than sedation. Even so, the likelihood of patient satisfaction is remote.

The *dependent personality* is one that constantly needs the support of others and expects their assistance. These persons are usually cooperative and grateful if they think that support is available. However, they may become manipulative or demanding of the surgeon or staff. They are prone to display helplessness, anxiety, depression, or anger if support is not available when they want it. On the other hand, they may display pseudoindependence, in which case they may not carry out specific orders given to them, or they may fail to keep postoperative appointments, even if it impairs the result. If problems arise, it is best to meet their demands to a reasonable extent or coax them into cooperation as one would a child. If handled correctly, they tend to be satisfied with reasonable results.

The third patient type to be considered is the *hysterical personality*. These individuals are warm and responsive and are able to express their feelings easily. They relate freely with others, even if somewhat superficially. Their thinking may be vague and unpredictable, and they are of interest because they are often preoccupied with attractiveness. Although they are definite in their desire for surgery, they nevertheless regard it as a threat that may generate anxiety. Once they have undergone the surgery, they become easily apprehensive about dressings, the removal of sutures, and indeed the outcome. These patients do best with frequent reassurance and the repetition of information, even if it is a tiresome task and the information has already been supplied to them on printed sheets. On the whole, however, they are pleasant patients to deal with and, if satisfied with the results of treatment, sing one's praises far and wide.

The recognition of psychotic illness characterized by a lack of contact with reality is essential in aesthetic surgery, as delusions related to physical appearance may be the only, or at least the predominant, manifestation of the illness. With this point in mind, we must consider two further personality types.

The *paranoid personality* type may be characterized as a sensitive individual who displays delusional thinking in relation to his actual or imagined deformity as well as suspicion, resentfulness, and even hostility. He takes offense easily, is distrustful, and tends to blame others for any problems. The latter applies especially to surgeons who have previously operated on them. These patients require great care and patience—if indeed they are accepted for surgery. A neutral attitude must be maintained in the face of complaints and accusations. It is important not to give these patients any guarantee nor to confront them or cause them to feel trapped. This type of patient poses a potential threat for the aesthetic surgeon. There have been several instances where a surgeon has been physically attacked and even killed by these patients. An excellent account of such a tragedy was given by Hinderer [1].

Finally, we must consider the *schizoid personality* type, which may be characterized as a shy individual who gives one the feeling of remoteness or perhaps eccentricity. It is not unusual for them to appear at successive consultations demanding entirely different procedures and appearing totally oblivious of previous requests and discussions. They display a passive attitude in relation to the requested operation and are found to be unappreciative, no matter how good the result of any operation carried out. Their remoteness makes it difficult to establish any close patient-surgeon relationship, and the nursing staff can expect little appreciation for their efforts.

Variations and combinations of the above personality characteristics are not unusual. From a practical point of view, however, a psychiatric label is not as significant to the aesthetic plastic surgeon as an understanding of how a patient feels, why he feels that way, and what we can do about it.

PATIENT'S AESTHETIC JUDGMENT

The patient is a human being who sees himself as an individual and a member of the society in which he lives. Although his appearance is basically the result of a genetically determined, proportionate relation of the structural features of his body, his image of it is not static but is subject to many influences, the direct result of being alive. It is thus clear that the individual cannot judge his appearance on aesthetic criteria applicable to works of art, such as sculptures.

Concern with his appearance centers around a particular social drive related to self-esteem and ego-identity—the need for an acceptable, well defined, consistent *body image*. Thus the individual must be able to accept how he sees himself. This image, formed in his mind as a result of the observed reactions of other people to him and reinforced by a comparison of himself with others around him, is subject to constant revision. Role-playing and the imagined requirements of the adopted role, so far as appearance is concerned, occasionally intrude on the individual's evaluation of his body image.

Several factors influence the individual's attitude toward his appearance: (1) prevailing concepts concerning a desirable appearance in the society in which he lives; (2) the attitudes of his daily contacts to his appearance; (3) the personality of the individual, particularly the existence of obsessive, dependent, or hysterical personality traits; (4) a tendency to seek overcorrection of a lack or excess of some portion of the body, which has been a source of preoccupation; (5) the symbolic significance to the individual of some aspect of his appearance (illustrated by the often observed fact that no matter how successful an abdominoplasty, it does not please the observer if the umbilicus has not been preserved); (6) transient influences, such as moods, interests, attitudes, and physical or mental condition; and (7) his aesthetic sense. The latter point possibly has a hereditary basis, but it is capable of being developed to varying degrees, e.g., by exposure to beautiful things and artistic activities. Current opinions as expressed in the media, especially advertising, further impose the profit-oriented dictates of fashion on the patient's own judgment.

DISSATISFACTION WITH APPEARANCE

Once an individual becomes dissatisfied with his appearance, certain psychological manifestations may develop that further influence his attitude about his appearance. He may display (1) anxiety, as a manifestation of a conflict between how he feels and what he sees in the mirror, such as feeling young and looking old, or feeling feminine and looking masculine; (2) focusing, as in the case of the rhinoplasty patient, who sees little else but his nose when he looks in the mirror; (3) rejection, or disgust with some aspect of appearance that is aesthetically unacceptable or cannot be reconciled with the way the individual sees himself (ranging from a purely physical problem such as dis-

comfort to a purely psychological phenomenon such as the subconscious rejection of femininity by a patient who requests virtual removal rather than reduction in size of her large breasts); (4) concealment or camouflage, in which the individual attempts to hide a feature that is a cause of preoccupation with his appearance (common examples are choosing hairstyles designed to balance a prominent nose, wearing dark glasses to cover baggy eyelids, using heavy makeup to hide a blemish, wearing high-necked garments to hide the neckline, and padding brassieres or wearing voluminous clothes to hide a figure defect. Apart from these attempts to deceive others, some individuals practice self-deception by extending their necks or making faces in front of a mirror in an attempt to influence their facial appearance by an aesthetically favorable alteration in posture or facial expression.); and (5) denial of the existence of some unfavorable aspect of appearance. Denial is often combined with focusing on some other aspect of appearance less obvious to an observer. The refusal of some patients to accept the preoperative photograph as a true record of their appearance is an example of the way denial is used as a psychologically self-protective mechanism. It is interesting to note that the tendency to denial is more marked among patients who are grossly unattractive than among those with slight irregularities.

It is thus clear that the patient's aesthetic judgment of his own appearance is influenced by a variety of factors and cannot be viewed merely on the basis of the classic concept of beauty established by the ancient Greeks.

## Aesthetic Plastic Surgeon

Many papers have been written on the psychological makeup of the aesthetic surgery patient, but few mention that of the surgeon. When one considers that the surgeon's personality may range from omnipotence and aggressive extroversion to the professional insecurity of a recently qualified plastic surgeon, it is obvious that plastic surgeons represent, by virtue of their personalities, a significant variable in interpersonal relationships. Although it may have been considered undesirable in the past to look at the surgeon in an analytic way, times have changed.

As members of the medical profession, we are open to scrutiny by the media and abuse by politicians. These influences have not been lost on the public, and the doctor of today faces attitudes and opinions about his or her motivation and actions that would have been unthinkable during the first half of this century.

It is thus essential that we look at ourselves and become aware of the factors that enter the patient-surgeon relationship and that exert powerful influences on the four desirable qualities of the plastic surgeon working in this field, i.e., professional judgment, aesthetic judgment, ethical behavior, and the degree of care he or she is prepared to give to any particular patient.

## MOTIVATIONAL AND RELATED FACTORS

Basically, of course, a surgeon wishes to *help* a patient, although if one reflects on this point considerable variations may be noted from surgeon to surgeon in the intensity of this desire to help. Another goal of the surgeon is *professional success*, as evidenced by the demands for one's services, appreciation by one's patients, and approval by one's peers. To this end, we join specialty societies, participate in their programs and symposia, seek office, try to have papers published or aspire to the editorship of multiple-authored books, and generally try to attract attention with the ostensible motive of "contributing" to our specialty.

We may choose to travel, establish contacts, and exchange hospitality with those who seem to matter in an attempt to appease our egos and to be regarded as a "some-body." Others, more concerned with mass approval than peer approval, resort to less desirable means of attracting attention.

How does all this activity affect our relationships with our patients? Basically, one might expect the intraprofessional activities to benefit the patients. The matter is not as simple as that, however, because in our time participation in these activities exposes the aesthetic surgeon to pressures that may prove detrimental to the patients.

Thus we are constantly being impelled to present something new. This need does not always lead to significant advances and usually interferes with long-term evaluation of previous ways of doing things. It is almost certainly responsible for a degree of dishonesty, which may mislead those who tend to accept things at face value. For instance, the supposed "breakthrough" is hailed by many, who rush off to try the untried. Soon variations, modifications, or other applications of the original material appear, compounding the situation. Indeed, it may be several years before reports of unsatisfactory results, disappointments, and denouncements provide further opportunities to get one's name into print. Any suggestion that this activity represents experimentation on humans would be rejected with indignant surprise. However, the increased litigation by dissatisfied patients in recent years is at least partly related to the risks inherent in current trends of professional practice.

One of the purposes of practicing a profession is to derive an income. As a motivational factor, *monetary reward* is sought not only to enable one to achieve a desirable life style but is increasingly important in our time because of economic uncertainties and the effects of inflation. The days have passed when only the well-to-do were able to attain an education, with the consequence that the professional endeavor is often the only source of income, especially for the younger surgeon. The need to consider the financial aspects of one's practice and to run it in a business-like manner may, however, lead to shortcuts in patient care.

Certain less clearly definable, *subsidiary motivational factors* related to the surgeon's personality makeup may enter the patient-surgeon relationship. Thus we may note moral judgment of the patient or of his motivation, hostility reactions to the patient's personality, erotic feelings toward attractive patients, and the existence of latent sadism, which may affect the degree of gentleness during the entire period of patient-surgeon contact.

Finally, we must consider the prevailing mood of the surgeon during the whole time of patient-surgeon contact. Both intrinsic and extrinsic factors influence this mood. Suffice it to say that intrafamilial problems with one's spouse or children, financial crises, ill health, and sundry irritations due to the ever-increasing growth of bureaucracy influence how the plastic surgeon feels on any one day and thus his or her attitude to any additional problems presented by the patient.

SURGEON'S AESTHETIC JUDGMENT

The term *aesthetic* relates to the perception of beauty. By inference, the aesthetic plastic surgeon is one who appreciates beauty so far as the human form is concerned.

Although purely aesthetic considerations are useful for the development and standardization of techniques, they are often not sufficient to ensure achievement of the desired result of aesthetic plastic surgery, i.e., to correct the patient's inability to accept how he sees himself. This goal is achieved only if the surgeon's aesthetic considerations correlate with the need of the patient and the attitudes of the latter's daily contacts [3].

We are thus faced with the question of whether a preoccupation with beauty is an adequate foundation on which to base our judgment of appearance. I do not consider it to be so, for the following reasons: (1) In Western society, human beauty is generally associated with women. Changes in popular standards of female beauty are occurring with ever-increasing frequency and are induced largely by the profit motivation of manufacturers of fashion and makeup items, supported by the media with a related interest. (2) Judgment of the human form may be based not only on purely aesthetic values but also on the strength of the sexual interest the form arouses in an observer. (3) The human form may be judged by association with certain memories, pleasant or unpleasant; that is, judgment is influenced by the emotional effect of reminding us of someone else in our past. (4) Finally, our judgment may be influenced by familiarity owing to repetitive exposure to a type of appearance common in our own environment or, conversely, by unusual or exotic features encountered on visits to other parts of the world.

Thus when we talk of a "sense of aesthetics" in relation to the human form, we are likely to mean a personal response to an appearance that is pleasant or attractive to the eye, rather than an appreciation of beauty in a philosophic sense, with its deeper quality of an appeal at an intellectual level.

SCULPTURE AND THE HUMAN BODY

For thousands of years, the artistic endeavors of Western culture have been rooted in the Greek and Roman worlds. According to Reich [3], the classic beauty ideal, as exemplified in ancient sculptures, is the beauty of a perfect but static form. Thus it differs from the live body, the appearance of which depends basically on a genetically determined proportionate relation of its various features. Added to this point is the dynamism of neuromuscular activity, which superimposes the effects of expression in the face and of posture and movement in the remainder of the body. Because the basic patterns of these dynamic features are modified by environment, education, health, and the need of the individual, the appearance of a face may be spoiled by certain, often habitual facial expressions and that of a body by poor posture and movement. This appearance can convey a sense of ugliness to an observer who might otherwise regard the component parts of the subject's body and their formal relation to each other as beautiful. Thus being beautiful requires not only a beautiful face and a meaningful expression but a body that conforms to acceptable proportions and moves with a natural ease and grace.

The aesthetic plastic surgeon can rarely, if ever, create beauty. He or she can help to reveal it when it is innately present but hidden by unattractiveness or ugliness of one of the features of the body or by imbalance in the arrangement of the various features. The surgical revelation of such innate beauty can be reinforced by education of the patient in the suitability of makeup, fashion, social behavior, facial expression, and body movement (deportment).

### SURGERY AS AN ART FORM

The surgical improvement in appearance could be regarded as a form of visual art, insofar as one of its aims is to arouse an acceptable aesthetic experience in an observer. Nevertheless, the aesthetic plastic surgeon differs from the creative artist in certain basic ways. Unlike that of the painter or sculptor, the surgeon's work cannot be essentially an expression of personal impulses or fantasies. Rather, it requires a technical approach based on an understanding of the medium, i.e., living tissues with their physiologic requirements and liability to pathologic change, coupled with the need to leave only minimal residual evidence of surgical interference. Furthermore, it requires a consideration of the needs of those for whom it is carried out, be they psychological, social, or economic.

It is thus clear from the above considerations that the surgeon represents a complex variable in the interpersonal aspects of the aesthetic surgical experience.

### Attitudes of the Patient's Contacts
#### PREOPERATIVE ATTITUDES

The attitudes of the patient's daily contacts are rarely based on purely aesthetic factors. Thus most patients who undergo aesthetic surgical operations report varying degrees of resistance from close members of their families. The most common reasons for this attitude are as follows: (1) fear for the patient's safety; (2) inability to see the need for the operation; (3) insensitivity to the patient's feeling about the deformity; (4) moral or religious reasons; (5) resentment on the part of a parent that a familial feature is regarded as objectionable by the patient; (6) fear of losing the affection or companionship of the marriage partner (because the improvement in appearance is expected to increase his or her appeal to others); and (7) economic factors.

In some families, however, the proposed improvement in appearance is regarded with favor and encouraged. The reasons for such favorable attitudes appear to be related to the following: (1) some members of the family are aware of the effects of the preoccupation on the life of the individual, having experienced a similar problem themselves; (2) having experienced the benefits of an aesthetic surgical procedure; (3) experiencing guilt feelings due to a sense of responsibility for the existence of the deformity; and (4) the hope that aesthetic surgery would increase the social or economic chances of an unattractive offspring.

In the case of close friends, the preoperative attitudes are often sharply divided between those who consider the operation unnecessary and those who encourage the operation. Those opposed may be expressing their ability to look beyond the deformity and base their friendship on deeper qualities. On the other hand, they may be subject to a possessive attitude, fearing loss of the friendship because of an expected increase in "popularity" of the patient after such an operation. In cases where close friends encourage the operation, they either display a high degree of empathy or are motivated by a desire to see an improvement in a feature they also find disturbing.

So far as casual daily contacts are concerned, the average person does not usually analyze the appearance of an individual in detail; he either likes it at first sight or he dislikes it. Basically, the judgment is an emotional one. As impressions based on appearance are often responsible for impulsive judgments, a situation arises that can have far-reaching psychological implications for the individual.

In some countries it is customary or mandatory for patients to see their general medical practitioners to obtain a referral to a plastic surgeon for a surgical improvement in appearance. The attitude of such general medical advisors may range from understanding and sympathy to doubt or even to a derogatory attitude and a refusal to be involved. The view that "cosmetic" surgery is frivolous and failure to appreciate the underlying motivation for such a request are not uncommon among general medical practitioners, who may attach greater importance to the quantity than to the quality of life. Because it often takes considerable courage for a patient to make this request for referral, an unsympathetic attitude or ridicule on the part of the doctor can produce considerable emotional stress. It must be noted, however, that many such patients do not abandon their desire for a surgical improvement in appearance and either seek the help of another, more sympathetic medical practitioner or approach a plastic surgeon directly, even if not until some months or years later.

Nursing staff in general hospitals and even in some plastic surgery units sometimes display unfavorable attitudes toward aesthetic surgery patients. It may represent an inter-personal incompatability, a resentment that someone else is able to undergo a surgical improvement in appearance, or the attitude that aesthetic surgery is unnecessary and not deserving of the use of hospital beds. Either way, guilt feelings are induced in the patient by virtue of the nurses' position. This source of problems must always be considered in patients who display undue anxiety during the period of treatment.

## AESTHETIC JUDGMENTS BY THE PATIENT'S CONTACTS

In the case of the patient's daily contacts, we deal with attitudes about appearance that may differ considerably from those of the patient or surgeon. These attitudes may or may not involve evaluation with or without preferences for certain types of appearance, and they are influenced by a number of factors: (1) the nature and closeness of their relationship, including such feelings as love, hate, empathy, antipathy, protectiveness, and guilt; (2) age, sex, education, and level of intelligence; (3) ethnic background; (4) socioeconomic background; (5) moral and religious attitudes; (6) personality traits; (7) previous personal experience with aesthetic plastic surgery, whether satisfactory or unsatisfactory; and (8) transient moods, interests, and attitudes, including their own physical and mental condition when the aesthetic judgment is made.

In any case, we are faced with two basic problems of criticism: (1) the ability of the patient's contacts to apply a rational interpretation and judgment of the results of surgery in relation to the preoperative appearance, and (2) their ability to choose appropriate words to express both their conscious and subconscious feelings on these matters. Be that as it may, the attitudes of a patient's contacts to questions of his appearance are important for revalidation of his body image after operation. The importance of influencing these attitudes for the benefit of the patient is discussed later in the chapter.

## Interaction Between Patient, Surgeon, and the Patient's Contacts

CONSULTATION IN AESTHETIC
SURGICAL PRACTICE

The patient consults the surgeon because of a strong urge to attain an alteration in appearance, yet strangely enough, he is often reluctant to discuss his preoccupation freely. Some surgeons tend to become impatient, and the patient, sensing it, experiences even greater difficulty communicating. A feeling of tension develops, and a satisfactory patient-surgeon relationship cannot eventuate.

What then is the purpose of the consultation? The patient thinks he has a problem. Despite his initial reluctance, he wishes to discuss the problem with someone he considers to have an understanding for such problems. Moreover, he would like something to be done to relieve him of this problem, and he expects the surgeon, by virtue of his specialization in plastic surgery, to be able to do it.

It is thus obvious that the primary object of the consultation is to establish mutual trust and then to ensure adequate communication. The establishment of mutual trust requires mutual perception. Observations allow categorization. The surgeon, then, must obtain an impression of age, appearance, personality type, social background, and financial status. Sometimes these items appear obvious, though in our time they have become less clear-cut.

The patient, on the other hand, wishes to assess the attitude, degree of involvement, and competence of the surgeon. Clearly, some individuals are able to obtain an early assessment, whereas others, lacking this skill, tend to become nervous and feel insecure. The sensitive surgeon is often able to help the patient by a relaxed attitude and appropriate facial expressions and gestures while gently inquiring about the purpose of the visit and displaying an understanding of the patient's problem when it is eventually revealed. The patient perceives this attitude as understanding on the part of the surgeon and experiences a satisfactory emotional reaction. Adequate communication now becomes possible.

Instinctive liking or disliking can occur between patient and surgeon. If feelings of disliking appear mutual, it is best to discontinue the association in a polite manner.

When adequate communication is possible between patient and surgeon, it is important to (1) establish what the patient desires, the realism of his expectations, and his ability to accept an imperfect result; and (2) inform the patient of the possible complications, the postoperative course, and the financial commitment.

A single consultation is often not sufficient patient-surgeon contact on which to base the decision to carry out elective aesthetic surgery with its far-reaching psychological implications. A second consultation is generally indicated to evaluate the medical and family history, social situation, and economic status and to check on the patient's understanding of the intended procedure and possible outcome. This visit also allows the patient to make the necessary social and financial arrangements for surgery. Occasionally, a patient returns for a third time to discuss some residual points of worry before making a decision on whether to undergo surgery.

If possible, the aid of a member of the family or a close friend is enlisted who is to be acquanted with the postoperative course and to whom the patient can turn when in doubt during that time. This point is particularly important for outpatient surgery, where many days often elapse before the patient is seen again after the operation.

WHEN *NOT* TO OPERATE

Dissatisfaction with the outcome of technically satisfactory aesthetic surgery can occur even in patients with realistic expectations and an apparently normal personality. Conversely, successful results can be obtained in patients assessed as psychotic. It appears that patient satisfaction with the result of aesthetic surgery is not definitely predictable by psychological, psychosocial, or psychiatric examination.

One, however, does avoid operation if the patient (1) is not certain which aspect of his appearance he would like to have changed; (2) is unable to contemplate a result that is "not perfect"; (3) has an obviously unstable personality or an unrealistic attitude; (4) is under emotional stress at the time of consultation or during the preoperative period; (5) complains of opposition by the family; or (6) requests operation at the insistence of others. When there is any doubt about the advisability of operating, the surgeon must avoid any suggestion that an aesthetic improvement is possible or, worse, agree to operate. Some method of delay can be adopted, as time sometimes solves these problems and permits operation with an uneventful postoperative course. Other patients occasionally change their own minds and thus their concern with appearance. Some return at intervals for further consultations without ever undergoing operation, which may well satisfy their needs. Finally, there are a few who can be induced to seek psychological, psychosocial, or psychiatric evaluation and help.

To simply reject the patient because the surgeon chooses not to be involved is not only unfair but potentially harmful to the patient. *Aesthetic plastic surgery involves patient care beyond the surgical improvement in appearance.*

PREOPERATIVE PHASE

Once the surgeon has indicated a willingness to operate, one of two types of psychological reaction may be observed in the patient. There may be a sudden relief in the feelings of anxiety that have existed in this patient. The obviously pleased patient then displays impatience. Any date proposed for operation seems too far ahead. This phase is a time for caution lest the patient rushes

into an operation with unrealistic expectations.

On the other hand, a surgeon may become aware of a state of anxiety at this stage. It appears that it is due to one or more of four factors: (1) a natural fear of the surgical experience; (2) apprehension about the change in appearance the patient is not able to approve of beforehand; (3) guilt feelings because of lack of approval or actual disapproval by close contacts; and (4) inability to afford the financial commitment.

The urge to undergo a surgical improvement in appearance is usually so great that the individual is capable of rationalizing his action and ignoring the above factors. There is no doubt that operating on the patient with unresolved anxieties is an important source of difficulties during the postoperative period. The solution of these problems is relatively easy to achieve. It involves free discussion with the patient and the contacts who matter most to the patient as well as a detailed explanation of the financial commitment. In countries where it is acceptable, charging a preoperative fee does much to remove the problems caused by an inability to afford the operation.

INFORMED CONSENT

The question of patient information and informed consent is approached in a positive manner. A consent form is used for each plastic surgical procedure; an operation is declined unless the patient has signed the relevant form, witnessed by an independent person who is not a member of the surgeon's staff. It is important to stress that from a purely legal point of view the consent form must contain a statement that the patient has read and understood the contents and that the contents have been explained to him.

In addition to the consent form, it is valuable to issue the patient with information sheets concerning the stay in hospital, the postoperative care, and the precautions and instructions to be observed during the pre- and postoperative phase. This point is especially important with patients treated in office surgical facilities. Patients often sign the forms without comprehending the contents. It is important therefore to adopt a policy of checking patient comprehension at a subsequent consultation or prior to operation. This practice not only prevents problems during the postoperative period but increases patient acceptance of the various stages of the healing phase.

In this context, the role of the paramedical staff in the surgeon's practice must be mentioned. The patients gain considerable reassurance about the surgical procedure and its outcome from members of the staff with whom they can discuss the matter during the preoperative period. They express their doubts and hopes to the staff often more freely than to the surgeon, especially if the latter has symbolic significance for the patient, who may thus find it difficult to express his apprehensions and fears.

Contact with the paramedical staff of the practice is infinitely more valuable and psychologically significant than placing a patient in front of a videotape or similar viewer to acquaint him with the planned procedure. The machine does not listen to the patient, nor does it answer personal questions as it unfolds its educational message on the viewing screen.

## THE OPERATION

The operative intervention represents a creative and technical challenge to the aesthetic plastic surgeon. Its significance to the patient, however, is that of a dual crisis. First, there is the physiologic trauma with its own attendant psychological effects, long since recognized in any surgical situation. Second, and more significant, is the invalidation of the patient's body image by the surgical procedure. The patient thus loses an important point of reference to a component of his self-concept. His reaction to this change may range from marked anxiety to a sense of depersonalization. Immediate and constant support must be available from those who attend the patient, especially the surgeon to whom he has entrusted himself. This support, in the form of firm confidence and frequent contact, must be available until the body image is revalidated.

It is particularly important that support by the surgeon be maintained even when the latter considers it desirable to request the aid of a psychiatrist to deal with any manifestations of anxiety or depression. To hand the patient over at this stage to someone who is, after all, a complete stranger may well aggravate the problem.

There is no doubt that with the widespread use of local anesthesia in aesthetic surgery, one needs to be cautious about conservations in the operating room. Premedication allows the patient to hear when he is unable to interpret. Amnesia, though usually complete, may be only partial, and the unintentional induction of emotional conflicts at this stage is a real possibility.

## EARLY POSTOPERATIVE PHASE

From a psychological point of view, the early postoperative period may be characterized in one of two ways. It may be uneventful and a pleasant experience for all concerned, or it may be marked by transient psychological disturbances—usually anxiety, though sometimes depression after 1 to 3 days. These moods are to a large extent related to the uncertainty of the outcome, the patient's personality structure, and the attitudes of those with whom the patient comes in contact during this period.

The attitudes of surgeon, nursing staff, and close family are important at this stage, as the patient searches for reassurance about the wisdom of his decision to undergo operation and the outcome. He must gain answers from the attitudes of others, as he can usually not reassure himself that all will be well by looking in the mirror. The site of operation is usually obscured by bandages, plaster splints, or swelling and bruising. A lack of available support, a failure to understand a patient's needs, or continuing reprimands by the family as a continuation of their original opposition to surgery are certain to allow the development of a marked emotional upset. These problems may be compounded through thoughtless remarks by members of the nursing staff or by their probing of the patient's motivations to satisfy their own curiosity.

It is important to ensure that all those who come into contact with the aesthetic surgical patient during the early postoperative period are familiar with the aims of such surgery, the usual conscious motivations, and the psychological mechanisms whereby anxiety may grow into an excessively demanding or critical attitude. Unless these factors are understood, interpersonal irritations and counterirritations can turn this period into a virtual nightmare for all concerned.

POSTOPERATIVE ATTITUDES
OF CONTACTS
The most common reaction of the immediate family to the result of operation is one of reserve. It applies not only to families who expressed their disapproval preoperatively but also to those who encouraged the patient to undergo operation. The reservation in expressing approval of the result of operation appears to be due to two main factors: First, there is an aesthetic factor that relates to the temporary postoperative distortion of the region; and second, there is a change in an appearance to which they had become accustomed. Usually, however, approval of the family is forthcoming in almost all cases after seeing the gradual resolution of tissue reaction and noting the change in the patient's attitude. It is particularly the case where the opportunity existed for a preoperative discussion with members of the family or friends about the expected postoperative course. The need for the approval of the family or close friends is significant. Such approval acts as a confirmation of the success

of the operation through the medium of a trusted opinion and is essential at a time when the unavoidable distortion due to the tissue reaction to operation and confusion due to invalidation of the previous body image makes it difficult for the patient to view his mirror image objectively. Such approval is also of importance to aid in the successful and speedy integration of a new body image, a process essential for achieving the desirable psychological results of surgery. There is no doubt that *unqualified approval by close contacts is the most important factor in ensuring patient acceptance of the result of aesthetic plastic surgery.*

In this context, it may be well to point out that some of the patient's contacts occasionally use this transitional period for their own aims and satisfy their aggressive tendencies, jealousies, resentments, or guilt feelings by consciously or subconsciously inducing conflicts in the patient by unfavorable comments. These responses may further undermine a patient's sense of security and produce an overwhelming state of anxiety. This state not only negates any potentially beneficial results of the operation but also produces tensions and conflicts that may become the basis of litigation.

LATE POSTOPERATIVE PHASE
The late postoperative phase includes that period after the tissue reaction to the operation has settled. The patient is able to assess the results in the mirror as well as the reaction of others to the change in his appearance. Psychologically, it is characterized by revalidation of the body image. The ideal situation obtains when a rapid revalidation of an acceptable body image occurs with a high degree of coincidence of body and mirror images and a favorable response on the part of the patient's contacts. The patient is pleased with the result of operation, feels comfortable, and is eager to get on with the task of living. Preoccupation with a particular aspect of appearance rapidly decreases and eventually disappears.

Less satisfactory is the slow revalidation of the body image with a vacillating attitude that may in fact result in an unacceptable body image. It may be due to slow resolution of the postoperative tissue reaction or failure to achieve aesthetic improvement especially if there is no likelihood of a successful revision.

More important as a cause of dissatisfaction with the result of aesthetic plastic surgery are the attitudes and responses of the patient's contacts. There is no doubt that patient dissatisfaction often develops only after his contacts had either failed to notice a change in his appearance, had made some disparaging remark, or had pointed out some residual asymmetries, irregularity, or a scar. Following such an encounter the patient notices increasing anxiety about the result, a compelling desire to check in the mirror frequently, and doubts about the adequacy of the operative procedure—even though the initial reaction to the result may have been satisfactory. A patient's dissatisfaction with the result of aesthetic plastic surgery is rarely accepted by him. It usually resolves in one of several directions: It may lead to the appearance of attention-seeking devices, accident-proneness in relation to the site of operation, the search for further aesthetic surgery elsewhere, or embarkation on a process of litigation. The psychotic individual may even entertain destructive action directed at the surgeon [1] or himself.

## Summary

The aim of aesthetic plastic surgery is to improve the quality of life of an individual who considers his appearance an unacceptable variant of the norm for the society in which he lives. It does so by eliminating self-consciousness, improving social acceptance and interpersonal relationships, and increasing the chances of obtaining employment, either in occupations where looks are important or in those where an appearance of youthfulness is considered desirable. Aesthetic surgery can also play a definite and useful role in achieving a change in outlook or in helping a patient start a new chapter of life after some personal crisis. In these cases the operation is symbolic of drawing a line between the old and the new chapters of life.

In the case of the individual with emotional instability or a disordered personality, aesthetic plastic surgery is not a substitute for psychotherapy when the latter is indicated. It can, however, help a patient resolve his psychological and social problems, especially if the reaction of others to the outcome of the operation is favorable. As such, it may achieve its purpose by itself or act as a valuable adjunct to psychotherapeutic management.

Interpersonal relationships are of considerable significance in determining the result of aesthetic plastic surgery. Speedy and successful revalidation of the body image requires that surgery be undertaken in an atmosphere of preoperative support and postoperative approval on the part of the patient's immediate contacts. This state requires adequate communication between surgeon, patient, and family or close friends who must be helped to appreciate the psychological, social, and personal factors in the patient's request for aesthetic plastic surgery and be acquainted with the postoperative course. Finally, the surgeon's constant interest and supervision are essential during the whole course of the aesthetic surgical experience to help the patient achieve the sole justifiable aim of such surgery, i.e., *to enable him to see himself in a way he can accept.*

## References

1. Hinderer, U. T. Dr. Vazquez Anon's last lesson. *Aesthetic Plast. Surg.* 2:375, 1978.
2. Reich, J. Factors influencing patient statisfaction with the results of esthetic plastic surgery. *Plast. Reconstr. Surg.* 55:5, 1975.
3. Reich, J. Aesthetic judgement in the surgery of appearance. *Aesthetic Plast. Surg.* 1:35, 1976.

# II
# Head and Neck

*Henry K. Kawamoto, Jr.*

# 5

# *Craniofacial Anomalies*

The craniofacial anomalies a plastic surgeon may experience are numerous, and, in fact, a separate book would be required to cover all the possible malformations. The constraints of space limit this chapter's focus to some of the more commonly encountered congenital deformities. Clefts of the lip and palate are discussed in Chaps. 9 and 10; the surgical management of some of the severe craniofacial malformations is discussed in Chap. 6.

In broad terms, craniofacial malformations can be grouped into those that involve a clefting phenomenon and those that are related to premature closure of the cranial sutures. Some of the anomalies have a characteristic concurrence of findings that facilitate their identification as a recognizable syndrome.

## *Facial Clefts*

Several classification schemes, such as those of the American Association of Cleft Palate Rehabilitation [20], Karfik [23], and Van der Meulen et al. [42], have been proposed. From a surgeon's point of view, the most effective classification integrates topographic clinical observations with the underlying skeletal disturbance. Because it correlates clinical appearance with surgical anatomy, the Tessier classification [25,41] has enjoyed popular acceptance.

In the Tessier classification, the orbit, nose, and mouth are key landmarks through which the craniofacial clefts follow constant axes. The clefts are numbered from 0 to 14, with the lower half of numbers representing the facial clefts and the higher numbers their cranial extensions (Fig. 5-1). Multiple and bilateral clefts can occur in the same patient. When a malformation traverses both hemispheres, a craniofacial cleft is produced that generally follows a set "time zone." Examples of these combinations include 0–14, 1–13, 2–12, 3–11, and 4–10 patterns. Although the craniofacial clefts tend to conform with these vertical precincts across the orbit, embryonic processes and vascular territories do not necessarily coincide with the "time zones." Thus it is difficult to explain the embryopathogenesis of some of the craniofacial clefts.

The concept of "time zones" is important, as it serves to heighten the awareness of the clinician. A conscious effort must be made to look up and down the tract in search of related deformities.

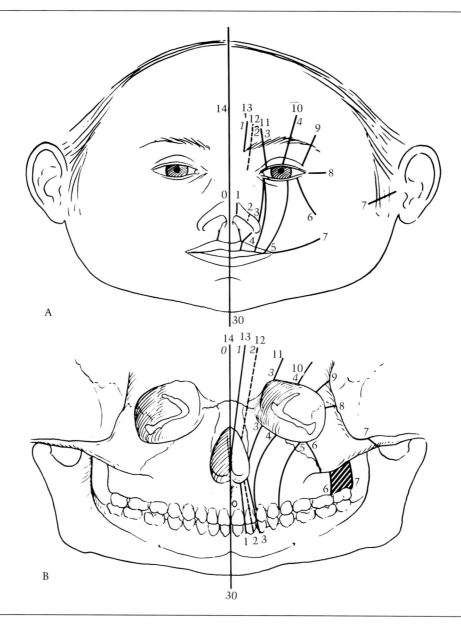

**Figure 5-1** *Tessier classification of clefts.
A. Path of various clefts on the face. B. Location
of the clefts on the facial skeleton. (Courtesy of
Dr. P. Tessier.)*

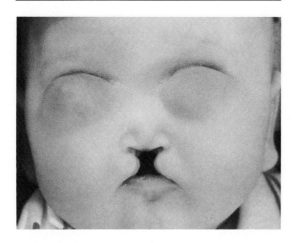

**Figure 5-2** *No. 0 cleft. Note absence of columella and prolabial segment of lip (false median left). Patient also has bilateral microphthalmos and rare infraorbital cysts, which transilluminate light.*

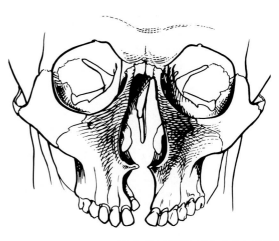

**Figure 5-3** *No. 0 cleft skeleton. Note the absence of the premaxillary segment and the hypoplastic neighboring structures of the mid-facial skeleton.*

**Figure 5-4** *No. 0 cleft. A. Patient with hypertelorbitism, bifid nose, a mild form of a true median cleft of the upper lip, and mild midline cleft of lower lip. B. Tongue of the patient is also bifid. (Courtesy of Dr. C. Raposo do Amaral.)*

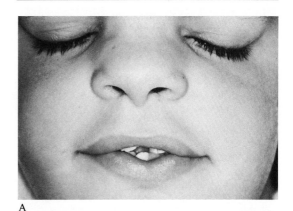

A

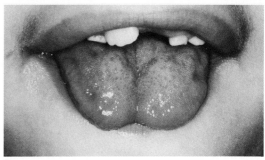

B

## NO. 0 CLEFT

Midline deformities of the upper lip and nose are included in the No. 0 cleft. When hypoplasia is the dominant theme, portions of these structures can be missing. Examples are a false median cleft lip and an absent columella (Fig. 5-2). The skeletal deficiencies are reflected by the absence of the premaxilla and nasal septum (Fig. 5-3). The holoprosencephaly malformation represents a craniofacial and hypoplastic combination of a No. 14 cleft.

At the other end of the spectrum, where there is a relative excess of tissue, a true median cleft lip can be seen as well as a bifid nose (Fig. 5-4). The labial frenulum can be duplicated, and a diastema is present between the central incisors. A midline cleft

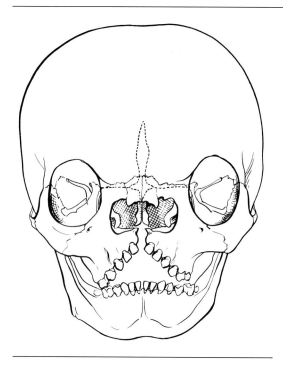

**Figure 5-5** *No. 0 cleft skeleton. Illustrated are the broadening of midline structures, cephalad cant of the midline of the maxilla, thickened nasal septum, and hypertelorbitism.*

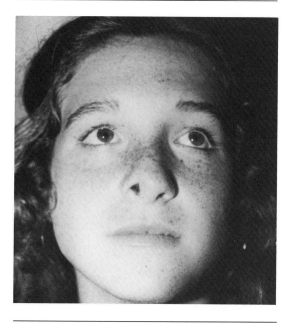

**Figure 5-6** *No. 1 cleft. Patient with a mild expression of the cleft as represented by the notch in the dome region of the nostril. (Courtesy of Dr. D. Cunningham.)*

with an upwardly titled premaxilla can exist with broadening of the nasal septum and the nasal bones (Fig. 5-5).

### NO. 1 CLEFT

The No. 1 cleft begins at Cupid's bow. The common cleft of the lip is an example of this malformation. The fault continues cephalad through the dome of the nostril (Fig. 5-6; see also Fig. 5-27).

The skeletal component cleft passes between the central and lateral incisors and through the alveolar process. The piriform aperture is violated lateral to the anterior nasal spine, but the nasal septum is spared.

### NO. 2 CLEFT

The soft tissue defect of the notably rare No. 2 cleft also begins in Cupid's bow, as

with a common cleft of the lip. The midportion of the nasal alar rim is hypoplastic and drawn upward (Fig. 5-7A).

On the maxilla, the cleft crosses the alveolus in the region of the lateral incisor. The piriform aperture is divided at its base. The nasal septum is intact but deviated by the surrounding distortion (Fig. 5-7B). A notch is frequently present near the junction of the nasal bone and the frontal process of the maxilla, which is widened.

### NO. 3 CLEFT

The No. 3 cleft is a well known entity that was described by Morian a century ago [30]. Although he called it an oblique facial cleft, it is commonly called an oro-naso-ocular cleft. As with the No. 1 and No. 2 clefts, it begins at Cupid's bow; hence any common cleft lip must be inspected closely for more telling structural faults. The cleft under-

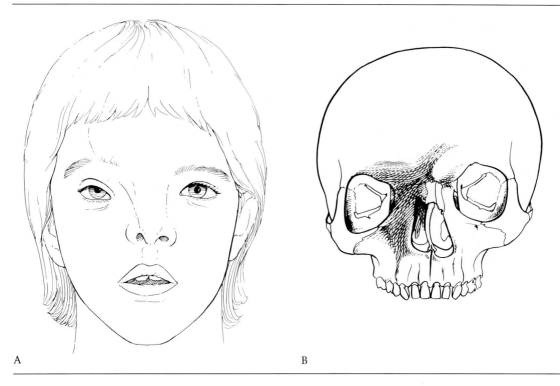

A                                                    B

**Figure 5-7** ▲ *No. 2 cleft. A. Line drawing showing hypoplasia of the midportion of the right alar and cephalad continuation as a No. 12 cleft, which spares the palpebral fissure and runs through the medial third of the eyebrow. B. Path of cleft through the broadened frontal process of the maxilla produces hypertelorbitism. (Courtesy of Dr. P. Tessier.)*

**Figure 5-8** ▶ *No. 3 cleft. Patient with a left form of the cleft. The cleft of the lip continues into the medial third of the lower eyelid, drawing the nasal ala toward the medial canthus. (Courtesy of Dr. J. Valero.)*

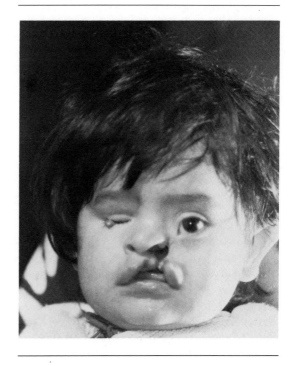

mines the nasal alar base and continues cephalad, just medial to the inferior punctum into the lower eyelid (Fig. 5-8). Its location coincides with the embryonic junction of the maxillary and frontonasal processes. Thus the nasolacrimal drainage system is disrupted and is prone to recurrent infections [19]. The lower canaliculus is malformed and beyond repair [40].

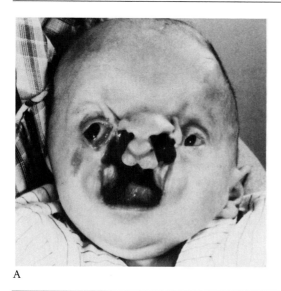

A

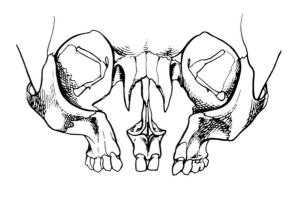

B

**Figure 5-9** *No. 3 cleft. A. Patient with a bilateral complete pattern and hypertelorbitism. B. Line drawing shows the confluence of the orbit, nose, maxillary sinus, and oral cavity as the fault enters the medial portion of the inferior orbital rim. (Courtesy of Dr. P. Tessier.)*

The skeletal disruption can be extensive, especially in its bilateral form (Fig. 5-9). The cleft passes between the lateral incisor and the canine to involve the neighboring alveolus and the secondary palate. The lateral portion of the piriform aperture is invaded, and the medial wall of the maxillary sinus is lacking. The frontal process of the maxilla is interrupted as the cleft terminates in the lacrimal groove. Thus a confluent cavity is formed between the mouth, nose, maxillary sinus, and orbit.

For treatment of the No. 3 cleft, the primary initial concern is preservation of a functional eye. Fortunately, the upper eyelid is usually not severely involved and functions sufficiently to provide the necessary protection. In the next step, the cleft of the lip can be repaired in the usual manner. The nasoocular component of the cleft can be managed at the same time. Almost without exception, local flaps can be used to close the defect and increase the vertical distance between the medial canthus and the nasal ala. The medial canthal tendon, being involved by the clefting phenomenon, cannot

be relied on for the canthopexy. Furthermore, it is difficult if not impossible to achieve proper placement of the medial canthus until the underlying medial orbital bony defect is corrected. The cleft of the palate is closed in the standard manner.

The osseous reconstruction can be postponed until a later date. The trough in the medial inferior orbital rim is obliterated with bone grafts. Additional bone grafts are required to construct the walls of the maxilla, and placement of the grafts along the orbital floor helps elevate the globe to a more normal position. A transnasal medial canthopexy, using the medial edge of the inferior tarsal plate, can now be performed (Fig. 5-10). Construction of the lacrimal drainage system and final eyelid repair are deferred until the osseous restoration is completed.

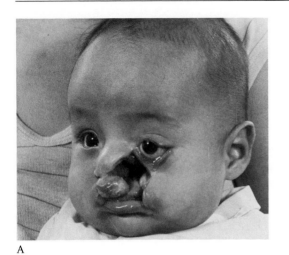

A

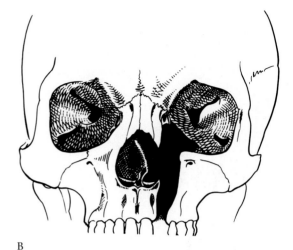

B

**Figure 5-10** *No. 3 cleft. A. Complete form of cleft with ala at the level of the medial canthus. B. Line drawing showing confluence of the orbit with maxillary sinus and nasal and oral cavities. (Courtesy of Dr. P. Tessier.) C. Postoperative appearance following initial protection of the globe by a medially based upper to lower eyelid banner flap followed by a V-Y advancement flap of nasal soft tissues to bring down the left ala and effect closure of the lip.*

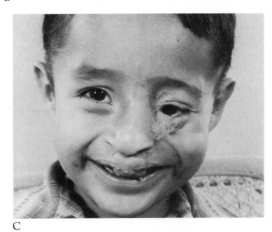

C

NO. 4 CLEFT

Boo-Chai [4] credited the first description of the No. 4 cleft to von Kulmus, who recorded the deformity in Latin in 1732. This oro-ocular cleft, unlike the first three clefts, begins lateral to Cupid's bow and shirts around the nose to end in the lower eyelid medial to the punctum (Fig. 5-11). The nose is basically intact but is distorted by the surrounding turmoil; its alar base is deflected upward.

**Figure 5-11** *No. 4 cleft. Patient with a bilateral form of the cleft, which starts lateral to Cupid's bow and passes to the medial third of the lower eyelid and spares the nose.*

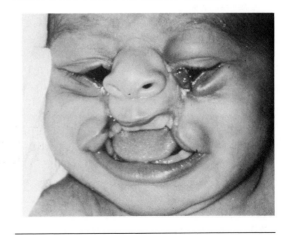

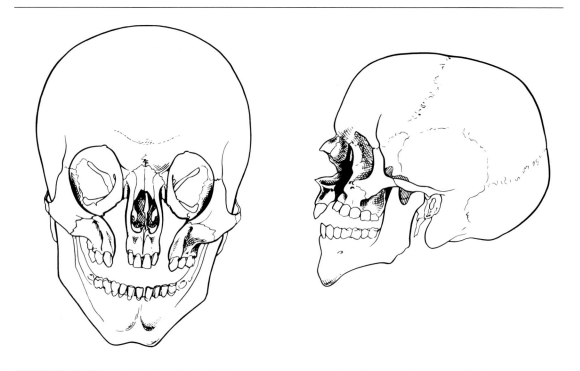

*Figure 5-12* No. 4 cleft skeleton. Bilateral form is depicted with communication of the orbit, maxillary sinus, and oral cavity. Piriform aperture retains its integrity. (Courtesy of Dr. P. Tessier.)

The osseous component starts between the lateral incisor and the cuspid. It spares the piriform aperture, nasolacrimal canal, and lacrimal sac as it courses into the medial portion of the inferior orbital rim (Fig. 5-12). A functional eye is usually present, but anophthalmia and intermediary grades of involvement can occur [34].

The basic steps and surgical principles involved in treating a No. 4 cleft generally follow those used for treatment of the No. 3 cleft with a few exceptions. Although it may sound like heresy, labial tissue between the ipsilateral philtral ridge and the cleft are removed (Fig. 5-13). Failure to do so results in an excessively wide, unnatural-appearing lip. The osseous defect is less extensive than the No. 3 cleft, as the piriform aperture and a nasal cavity remain intact.

NO. 5 CLEFT

The No. 5 cleft is a rare facial cleft that originates just medial to the oral commissure

(Fig. 5-14A). It traverses the cheek to enter the lower eyelid near its middle third. The upper lip and lower eyelid are drawn toward each other.

The path of the cleft on the facial skeleton is also distinct. It begins in the region of the premolars and travels lateral to the infraorbital foramen (Fig. 5-15). The orbit is penetrated in its lateral third. The orbital contents can prolapse into the maxillary sinus.

The soft tissue deficit of the No. 5 cleft must be corrected by increasing the distance between the mouth and the lower eyelid. Local transposition flaps can be used for this purpose with careful alignment of the vermilion–cutaneous border and the eyelid margin (Fig. 5-14B). The osseous restoration

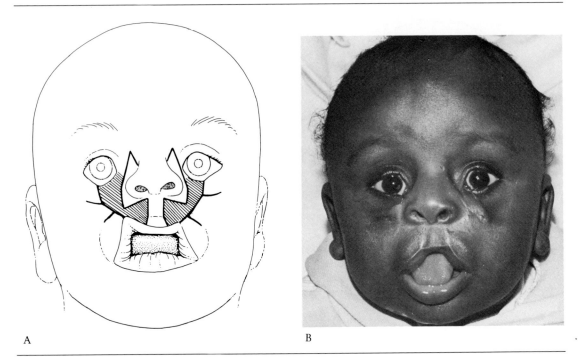

**Figure 5-13** *Treatment of No. 4 cleft. A. Design of flaps. Shaded area indicates tissue to be resected. Note that the prolabial segment lateral to the philtral ridge must be discarded to obtain normal labial contours. B. Postoperative view of the patient shown in Fig. 5-11. Further procedures are required to correct the position of the lower eyelids.*

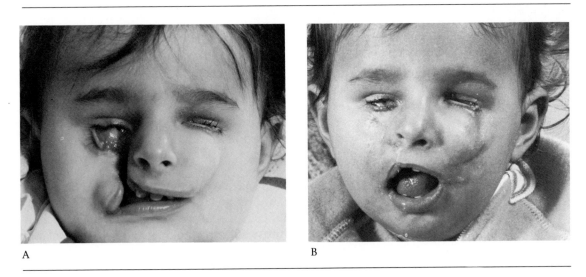

**Figure 5-14** *No. 5 cleft. A. Patient with a left No. 5 cleft that begins near the oral commissure and is directed into the medial third of the lower eyelid. On the right side is a No. 4 cleft. B. Postoperative view following soft tissue reconstruction with local flaps.*

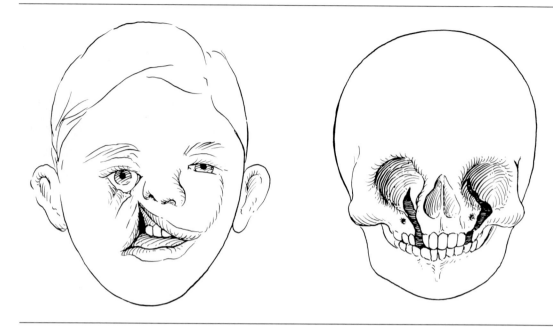

**Figure 5-15** *Nos. 4 and 5 clefts. The No. 4 cleft passes in the canine region and then medial to the infraorbital foramen. The No. 5 cleft begins closer to the oral commissure, crosses the premolar area, and trails lateral to the foramen. (From H. K. Kawamoto. The kaleidoscopic world of rare craniofacial clefts: Order out of chaos (Tessier classification). Clin. Plast. Surg. 3:529, 1976.*

consists mainly of building an orbital floor and an anterior wall of the maxilla, and filling the alveolar cleft with bone.

NO. 6 CLEFT

The No. 6 cleft represents an incomplete form of the Treacher Collins anomaly. Rogers believed that the original cases described by Treacher Collins were probably of this nature [35]. A mild coloboma of the lateral third of the eyelid marks the cephalic end of the cleft as it descends lateral to the oral aperture toward the angle of the mandible (Fig. 5-16). The palpebral fissures have an antimongoloid slant. The soft tissues over the zygomatic eminence are hypoplastic.

On the facial skeleton, the cleft passes through the zygomatico-maxillary suture and involves the lateral third of the inferior orbital rim (Fig. 5-17). The zygomatic arch remains intact.

Reconstruction for the No. 6 cleft includes correction of the lower eyelid coloboma and repositioning of the inferiorly placed lateral canthus. Establishing the os-

seous framework of the inferior orbital rim and the floor facilitates the soft tissue repair.

NO. 7 CLEFT

Various names have been assigned to the relatively common No. 7 facial cleft, the most popular of which are otomandibular dysostosis [16], hemifacial microsomia [5], first and second branchial arch syndrome [26], and craniofacial microsomia [11]. Closely related is the Goldenhar syndrome with its addition of an epibulbar ocular dermoid and vertebral abnormalities [17].

The incidence of the malformation is reported to be between 1:3000 [33] and 1:5642 [18] births. Males are more frequently affected than females [18], and bilateral forms

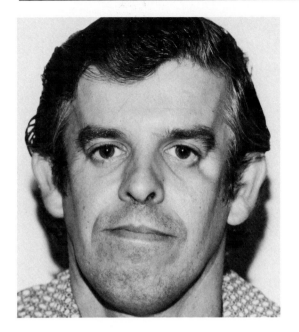
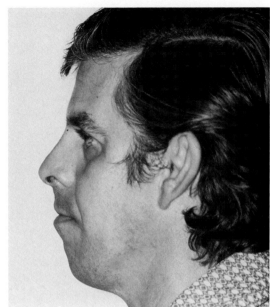

**Figure 5-16** *No. 6 cleft. Patient with an incomplete form of the Treacher Collins syndrome. The malar hypoplasia, lower eyelid colobomas, and antimongoloid slant of the palpebral fissures are mild.*

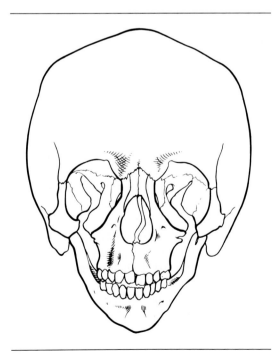

**Figure 5-17** *No. 6 cleft skeleton. The cleft separates the zygoma from the maxilla as it enters the lateral third of the orbit. The remaining zygomas are hypoplastic. (Courtesy of Dr. P. Tessier.)*

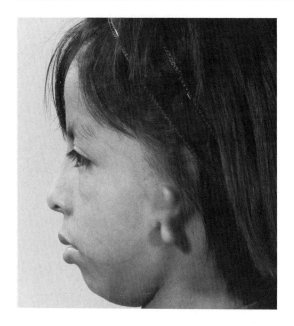

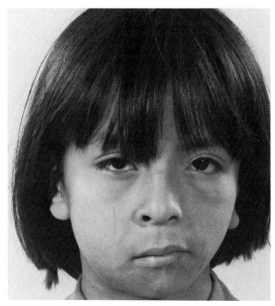

**Figure 5-18** *No. 7 cleft. Patient with craniofacial microsomia featuring macrostomia, microtia, and mandibular hypoplasia with the chin deviated to the affected side.*

occur. The inheritance pattern is sporadic. The malformation has been reproduced in animals by creating a localized hematoma in the embryonic otomandibular region [32].

The intensity of clinical expression of the cleft is variable. A preauricular skin tag may represent a microform of the malformation. In its complete form, the cleft begins as a macrostomia at the oral commissure and continues as a furrow across the cheek heading toward a microtic external ear (Fig. 5-18). The ipsilateral tongue, soft palate, and muscles of mastication can be underdeveloped. The parotid gland and duct can be absent. The seventh cranial nerve (CN VII) may be involved. When the external ear and middle ear ossicles are affected, conductive hearing loss is added to the list of defects.

The osseous manifestations also cover a wide range. The mandibular deficiency can be merely flattening of the condylar head or complete absence of the ramus with deviation of the mandible to the affected side (Fig. 5-19). The occlusal plane is canted cephalad, and there may be a maxillary alveolar cleft

in the region of the last molar and the tuberosity. The zygomatic arch may be missing with underdevelopment of the remainder of the zygoma and the temporal bone. The orbit is often depressed but elevated on lesser occasions.

Correction of the malformed parts of the No. 7 cleft is apt to be complex, as the facial soft deficits, the microtia, and the skeletal disarray require multiple integrated steps.

NO. 8 CLEFT
The No. 8 cleft extends from the lateral canthus to the temporal region (Fig. 5-20). It is seldom seen by itself, being more frequently associated with other clefts. A dermatocele often occupies the coloboma of the lateral commissure. The bony component is centered at the frontozygomatic suture.

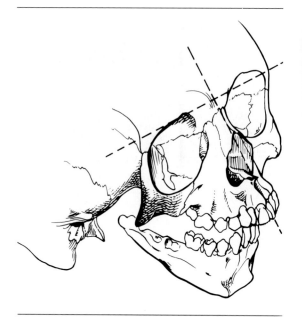

*Figure 5-19* No. 7 cleft skeleton. Absence of the condyle and portions of the ramus and zygomatic arch can be seen in the complete form.

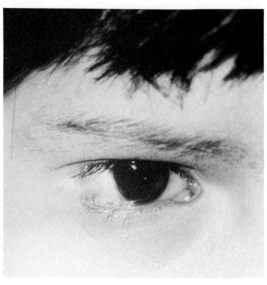

*Figure 5-20* No. 8 cleft. The lateral canthus is disrupted by the cleft with obliteration of the fornix. (Courtesy of Dr. B. Zide.)

*Figure 5-21* Nos. 6/7/8 cleft assembly. The osseous malformation is seen in the Treacher Collins syndrome and is hallmarked by the symmetric absence of the zygoma. The infraorbital foramen may be lacking, and the greater wing of the sphenoid bone now forms the lateral orbital rim.

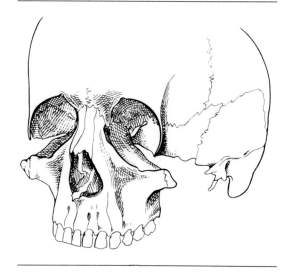

## NO. 6/7/8 CLEFT CONSORTIUM

Tessier thought that the combination of No. 6, 7, and 8 clefts was responsible for the Treacher Collins malformation. In 1889 Berry [2] first described the anomaly, but the syndrome is commonly referred to as that of Treacher Collins [9, 10]. Other popular names for the syndrome are mandibulofacial dysostosis and Franceschetti-Klein syndrome [15]. The inheritance pattern is autosomal dominant with variable expressivity. Rogers' analysis of 200 cases showed an equal distribution between the sexes [35]. Unlike craniofacial microsomia, Treacher Collins malformation is bilaterally expressed in a symmetric manner.

Absence of the zygoma characterizes the complete form of the malformation, with each cleft making a contribution (Fig. 5-21). The coloboma of the lateral third and the absence of eyelashes in the medial two-thirds of the lower eyelid are part of the No. 6 cleft,

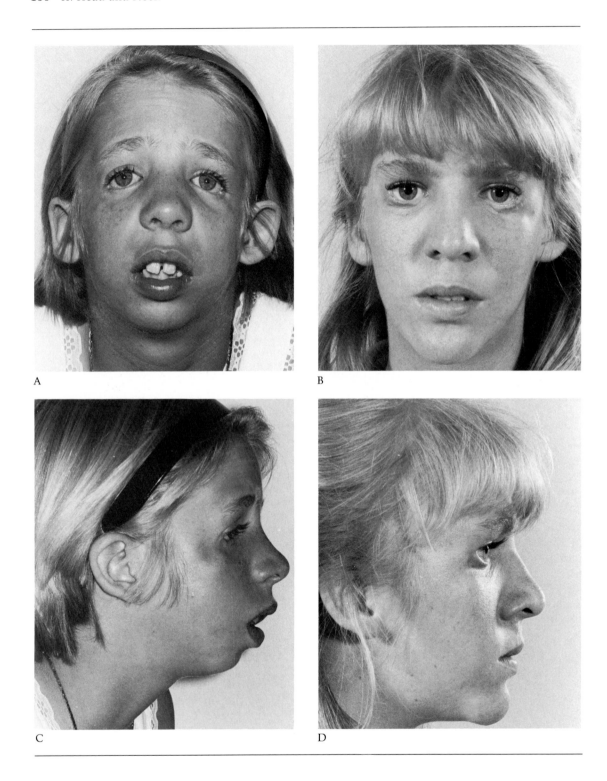

A

B

C

D

which is centered around the zygomatico-maxillary suture (Fig. 5-22). Because of the partial absence of the lateral portion of the inferior orbital rim and the infraorbital foramen, the infraorbital neurovascular bundle occasionally enters the soft tissues directly from the orbit.

The contributions of the No. 7 cleft, which involves the area of the zygomatico-temporal suture, are the microtia, mandibular deformity, and absence of the zygomatic arch. The external ear may have a normal appearance but is more likely to be a crumpled, hypoplastic mass. Conductive hearing loss is the rule. The ramus is short, and the antegonial notch is accentuated along a small mandibular body. An anterior open bite is present with a severely retruded chin. With the absence of the zygomatic arch, the temporalis is fused with the masseter, and the sideburns are anteriorly displace onto the cheeks. The No. 8 cleft undermines the frontozygomatic suture and is culpable for the absence of the lateral orbital rim. Additional findings may include macrostomia, cleft of the secondary palate, choanal atresia, and a nose that appears large because of the shallow nasofrontal angle and lack of malar prominences.

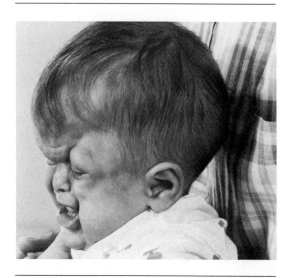

**Figure 5-23** *No. 9 cleft. A deep soft tissue groove through the lateral third of the eyebrow marks the path of the cleft. The underlying lateral superior orbital rim is absent, as is the neighboring roof.*

**Figure 5-22** *Nos. 6/7/8 clefts. A, C. Preoperative view of a patient with Treacher Collins syndrome. Symmetric malar flattening, antimongoloid slant of the palpebral fissures, lower eyelid colobomas with eyelashes only in the lateral third, anterior displacement of the preauricular hair, varying degree of microtia, and mandibular hypoplasia are notable features. B, D. Postoperative view following construction of zygomas with cranial bone grafts, laterally based upper to lower eyelid banner flaps, lateral canthopexies, and osseous genioplasty.*

### NO. 9 CLEFT
The No. 9 cleft is the rarest of the craniofacial clefts and with it begins involvement of the superior hemisphere of the orbit. The eyelid is divided in its lateral third, and the superior lateral angle of the orbital rim is involved (Fig. 5-23).

### NO. 10 CLEFT
The No. 10 cleft is located in the middle third of the eyebrow and eyelid (Fig. 5-24). It corresponds to the cranial extension of the No. 4 cleft. The soft tissue coloboma that disrupts the midportion of the upper eyelid covers the underlying defect of the central third of the superior orbital rim and roof. A frontoorbital encephalocele frequently fills the gap and displaces the entire orbit in an inferior and lateral direction to produce hypertelorbitism (Fig. 5-25).

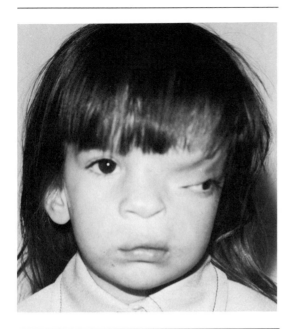

**Figure 5-24** *No. 10 cleft. Centered on the medial third of the superior orbital rim, the fault is usually occupied by a frontoorbital encephalocele. Asymmetric hypertelorbitism is produced. (From H. K. Kawamoto. The kaleidoscopic world of rare craniofacial clefts: Order out of chaos (Tessier classification).* Clin. Plast. Surg. *3:529, 1976.*

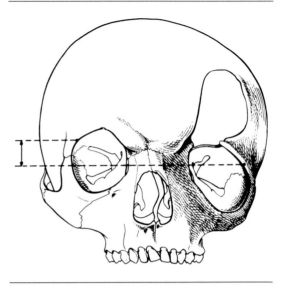

**Figure 5-25** *No. 10 skeleton. A frontoorbital encephalocele in the middle third of the superior orbital rim displaces the orbit in an inferolateral direction. (Courtesy of Dr. P. Tessier.)*

**Figure 5-26** *Intracranial path of a No. 12 cleft (bilateral). This drawing of the floor of the anterior cranium shows widening of the ethmoidal labryinth caused by the cleft. Arrows delineate the lateral divergence of the orbit. (Courtesy of Dr. P. Tessier.)*

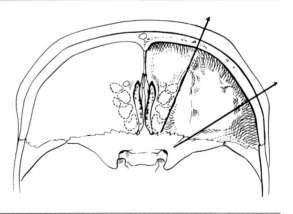

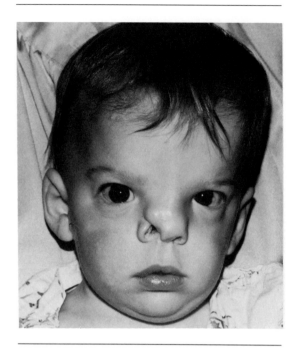

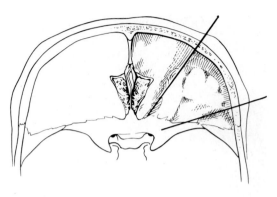

**Figure 5-28** *Intracranial path of a No. 13 cleft (bilateral). The cribriform plate and the olfactory grooves are widened, but the crista galli remains normal. The divergent lines represent the lateral displacement of the orbit. (Courtesy of Dr. P. Tessier.)*

**Figure 5-27** *No. 13 cleft. The patient has a No. 1 cleft that continues into the cranium as a No. 13 cleft and produces hypertelorbitism. An ipsilateral paramedian swirl of hair is seen at the frontal hair line.*

### NO. 11 CLEFT

The No. 11 cranial cleft occurs in combination with the No. 3 facial cleft. A small coloboma may be present in the medial third of the upper eyelid. The medial third of the eyebrow is also disturbed, as the fault extends into the frontal hairline.

The osseous path may pass lateral to the ethmoid bone (see Fig. 5-9) to create a cleft in the medial third of the superior orbital rim. An alternative trail is through the ethmoidal labyrinth, in which case hypertelorbitism is produced.

### NO. 12 CLEFT

The No. 2 facial cleft may be extended into the cranium as a No. 12 cleft. Topographically, the medial end of the eyebrow is involved. Hypertelorbitism is also present, as the skeletal split is directed through the frontal process of the maxilla or between this structure and the nasal bone (see Fig. 5-7). The cleft passes lateral to the olfactory groove and involves the ethmoidal labyrinth (Fig. 5-26).

### NO. 13 CLEFT

The No. 13 cleft is the cranial prolongation of the No. 1 cleft. In its paramedian location, it lies medial to the eyebrow; an omega-shaped distortion marks its entrance into the frontal hairline (Fig. 5-27). Hypertelorbitism is a constant feature with the cleft traversing the nasal bone (see Fig. 5-6), ethmoidal labyrinth, and olfactory groove. The cribriform plate is widened (Fig. 5-28).

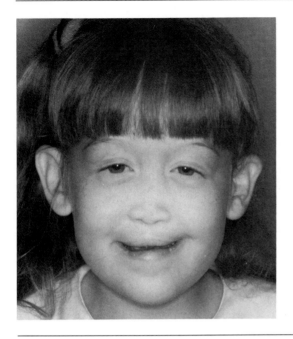
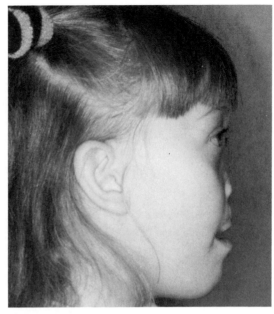

*Figure 5-29* *No. 14 cleft. Patient with hypotelorbitism due to a midline cleft with deficiency of tissue. The false median cleft of the upper lip has been repaired. Note hypoplasia of the nose, especially the columella.*

## NO. 14 CLEFT

A return to the midline is made with the No. 14 cleft. As with its partner, the No. 0 cleft, faults in reduction or excess of tissue are seen.

When hypoplasia is the dominant theme, all degrees of hypotelorbitism can be seen (Fig. 5-29). The holoprosencephalic malformations fall into this group. They range from cyclopia, ethmocephaly, and cebocephaly to a false median cleft lip. Embryologic division of the prosencephaly into two is faulty. The poorer the stage of forebrain differentiation, the greater is the facial malformation. The severely involved die shortly after birth. Those who do survive are generally seriously retarded.

In contrast, frontonasal dysplasia (medial cleft face syndrome) (Fig. 5-30) and frontonasal encephalocele (Fig. 5-31) are examples of midline malformations with excess material. The distance between the medial canthi is increased (telecanthus). Also exaggerated are the bony interorbital width (hypertelorbitism) and the breadth of the crista galli (Fig. 5-30). However, with frontonasal encephaloceles the splaying occurs more anteriorly, in the region of the nasal bones and the frontonasal processes of the maxilla; thus the span between the medial orbital walls can be normal. The intellect usually is normal except in those patients with an extreme degree of hypertelorbitism [14].

The surgical approach required to correct the malformation of Nos. 10 to 14 clefts depends a great deal on the magnitude of the interorbital separation and the presence or absence of vertical orbital asymmetries. In general, as the interorbital distance and the vertical discrepancy increase, so does the need for an intracranial approach. Details of surgical management are found in Chapter 6.

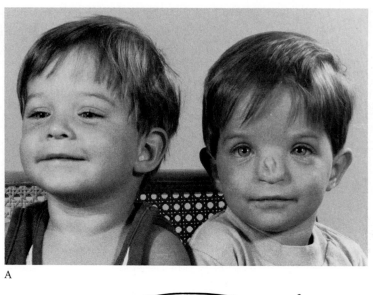

A

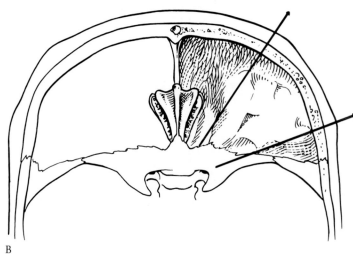

B

**Figure 5-30** *No. 14 cleft. A. Patient on right has frontonasal dysplasia with excess tissue along the midline, a corrugated bifid nose, and hypertelorbitism. Normal twin is on the left. B. Intracranial view with widening of the crista galli. Arrows indicate lateral displacement of the orbit. (Courtesy of Dr. P. Tessier.)*

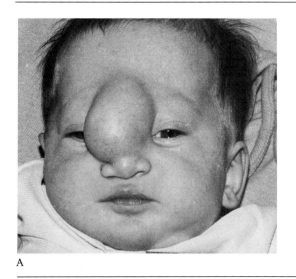
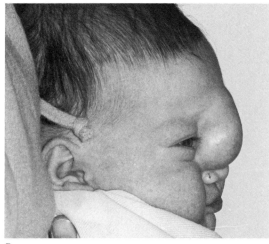

A

B

**Figure 5-31** *No. 14 cleft. A. Occupying the midline is a frontonasal encephalocele. Telecanthus is present. B. The nasal bones and medial canthi attachments are displaced by the defect caused by the frontonasal encephalocele; true hypertelorbitism is not produced, as the axis orbits are not displaced from the midline.*

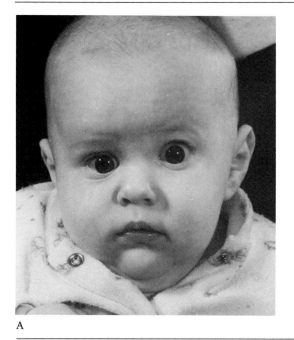
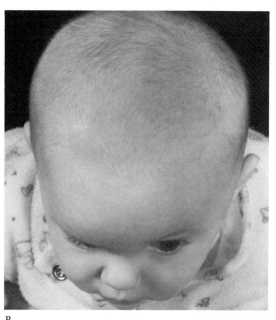

A

B

**Figure 5-32** *Unilateral coronal synostosis. A. Frontal view of patient showing increased vertical dimension and elevated orbit on the affected left side and deviation of the facial midline and chin to the contralateral side. B. Vertex view shows oblique orientation of the skull cap with ipsilateral flattening and compensatory bossing of the opposite forehead.*

## Craniosynostosis Malformations

When a cranial suture is prematurely closed, inhibition of growth at right angles to the involved suture and compensatory overexpansion at the open sutures occur to accommodate the normal growth of the brain (Virchow's law) [43]. The facial skeleton, by virtue of being attached to the undersurface of the anterior cranial base, can be secondarily deformed. A total of 57 syndromes with malformations of this type have been recorded [8]. In some, an associated inherent restriction of facial growth (faciosynostosis) compounds the distortion of the visage. When discussing the most common of these problems, it is convenient to organize the malformations in terms of the cranial suture that is prematurely fused.

### CORONAL SUTURE

Premature closure of the coronal suture can be unilateral or bilateral. Sometimes it is associated with well defined syndromes that can be inherited. Although overlapping features may fuel some confusion, it is important to establish a diagnosis as accurately as possible so that proper genetic counseling can be provided. A study of the clinical features provides the most information, as the chromosomes are usually unremarkable. Fortunately, intellectual potential is generally normal except for patients with Apert and Carpenter syndromes.

### Unilateral Coronal Synostosis

Premature closure in the form of unilateral coronal synostosis occurs in a sporadic fashion. On the side of fusion, the suture is represented as a palpable ridge, the forehead is tall and flattened, the vertical dimension of the face is decreased (see Fig. 5-32), and a "harlequin" appearance of the orbit is seen on a frontal skull radiogram. On the contralateral side, a variable degree of frontal bossing is present, and the eyebrow and orbit are lowered. The facial midline has a C-shaped curvature with deviation of the chin to the contralateral side. When the calvarium is viewed from above, it has an oblique orientation (plagiocephaly).

A similar clinical picture can be seen with muscular torticollis and cervical vertebral malformation, which restrict postural movements of the infant's head during sleep [24]. Unilateral premature closure of the lambdoidal suture also produces a plagiocephalic deformation. Because the treatment is radically different, these entities must be ruled out.

### Bilateral Coronal Synostosis

Several types of bilateral coronal synostosis can be easily distinguished. Discriminating features can be detected by augmenting the craniofacial examination with and inspection of the digits.

SIMPLE BILATERAL CORONAL SYNOSTOSIS. The malformation called simple bilateral coronal synostosis also occurs in a random manner. A ridge following the coronal suture can be palpated across the crown. The forehead is recessed, but the remainder of the face projects in a normal fashion (Fig. 5-33). The digits are also normal, as is the rest of the physical examination.

CROUZON SYNDROME (CRANIOFACIAL DYSOSTOSIS). Crouzon's malformation is named after the French neurosurgeon who described the syndrome in 1912 [13]. The mode of transmission is autosomal dominance. The calvarium is usually brachycephalic with a recessed forehead and a copper-beaten appearance of the inner table. Coupled with the faciosynostosis, exorbitism is present owing to the shallow orbits, and the midface is hypoplastic and retruded (Fig. 5-34). Divergent strabismus and a mild hypertelorbitism can be seen. The maxillary dentition is crowded on a constricted arch. An illusion of mandibular prognathism is evident, although the lower jaw is actually smaller than normal [12]. Upper respiratory flow is impeded by the crowded, confined oronasopharynx, and the dangers of obstructive sleep apnea are introduced. Ankylosis of the elbows and subluxation of the head of the

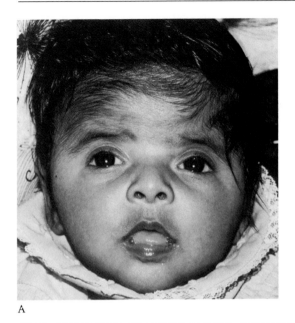

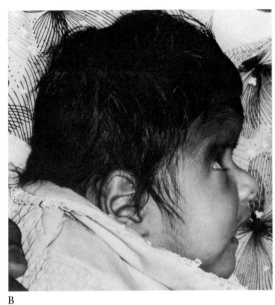

A                                                      B

radius may be seen, but the digits are normal [3].

APERT SYNDROME (ACROCEPHALOSYNDAC-TYLY). A Frenchman is credited for describing Apert's malformation, which bears his name [1]. Most cases occur in a sporadic manner, but an autosomal dominant transmission is suggested. Craniofacial features include a turribrachycephaly with a flattened high forehead, increased digital markings of the inner table of the calvarium, mild hypertelorbitism, exorbitism, and divergent strabismus (Fig. 5-35). The faciosynostosis augments the midfacial recession and the collapsed maxilla with its high, arched palate and Byzantine appearance. Pseudomandibular prognathism is present, even though the mandible is smaller than normal [3] and the bite is open in the anterior region. The upper airway can again be severely compromised.

A unique feature of the syndrome is the symmetric osseous and soft tissue syndactyly of the hands and feet (Fig. 5-36). The three central digits are often fused in a mass. Radial deviation of the distal phalanx of the

*Figure 5-33* Bilateral coronal synostosis. *A. Frontal view shows relative exorbitism because of the recessed superior orbital ridge and forehead. B. Brachycephaly with lack of projection of the forehead is seen on profile view. However, the mid-face is normally positioned.*

thumbs is also present. In addition, acne vulgaris of the face and forearms commonly appears during adolescence. Unlike the other synostosis problems, some degree of mental retardation may be observed.

PFEIFFER SYNDROME. Pfeiffer's malformation was described in 1964 and consists of turribrachycephaly and the hallmark of broadened thumbs and great toes [31]. The craniofacial characteristics are similar to those of Apert syndrome but are expressed to a milder degree. In addition, the intellectual potential is normal, acne vulgaris is not a feature, and the syndactyly of the hands and feet is mild and confined to the soft tissue webs. Genetic transmission is autosomal dominant.

CARPENTER SYNDROME (ACROCEPHALOPOLY-SYNDACTYLY). Originally described in 1901, polydactyly is a unique feature of Carpenter's

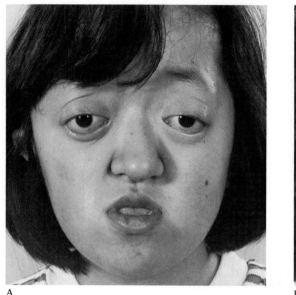
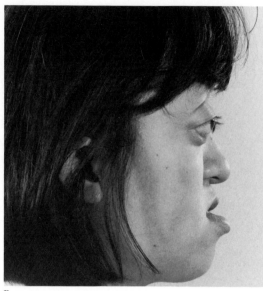

A                B

**Figure 5-34** *Crouzon syndrome. A. Frontal view. Exorbitism and exotropia are evident. B. Profile. Recession of the forehead and entire mid-face and relative mandibular prognathism with a retruded chin are characteristic.*

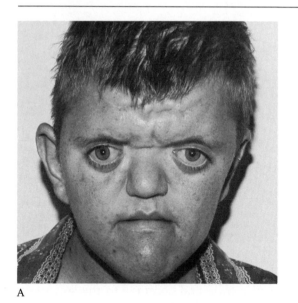
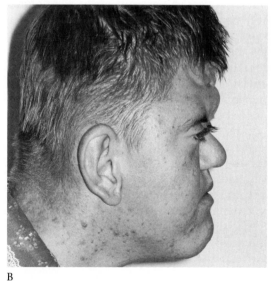

A                B

**Figure 5-35** *Apert syndrome. A. Frontal view. Mild hypertelorbitism, exorbitism, and exotropia are common ocular findings. B. Profile. Flattened forehead, parrot-beaked nose, hypoplastic retruded mid-face, and pseudomandibular prognathism are typical findings.*

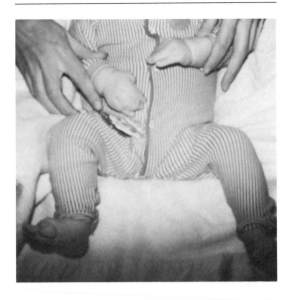

**Figure 5-36** *Hands and feet of Apert syndrome. Syndactyly of the hands and feet involving the bones are distinguishing features.*

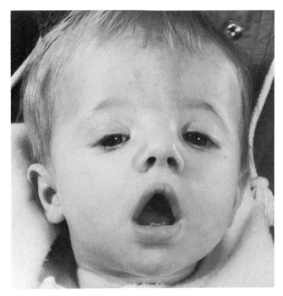

A

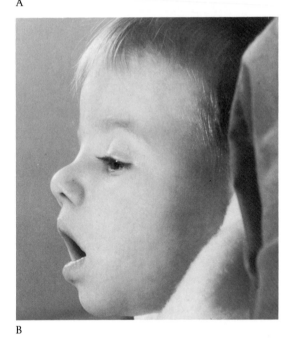

B

**Figure 5-37** *Saethre-Chotzen syndrome. A. Frontal view. Bilateral eyelid ptosis is a characteristic feature. B. Profile. A flattened forehead slopes backward, but the mid-face is normally developed.*

malformation [6]. In addition to the coronal sutures, other sutures can be prematurely fused. Mid-facial structures show a depressed nasal bridge and dystopia canthorum [39]. The inheritance pattern is autosomal recessive, and mental retardation usually accompanies the malformation. Soft tissue syndactyly is present on the hands and feet.

SAETHRE-CHOTZEN SYNDROME. Described separately by the individuals after whom this syndrome is named [7, 36], the major traits of Saethre-Chotzen syndrome are a low frontal hairline set on a backward sloping forehead and upper eyelid ptosis (Fig. 5-37). It is transmitted in an autosomal dominant manner. A mild soft tissue syndactyly is frequently seen between the second and third digits of the hands and feet. The mid-facial projection is normal, as is the intellect.

METOPIC SYNOSTOSIS
Premature closure of the midline suture separating the frontal bone results in a distinc-

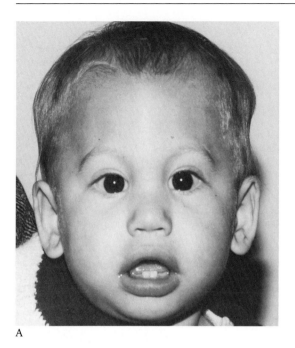
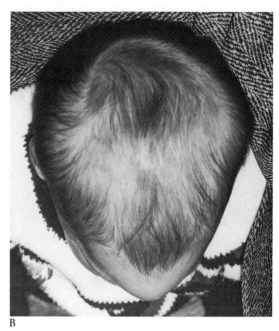

A                                         B

**Figure 5-38** *Trigonocephaly. A. Frontal view. Premature closure of the metopic sutures reduces the bifrontal width and the interorbital distance (hypotelorbitism). B. Vertex view. Prominent mid-forehead ridge with recession of the superolateral orbital rims highlights the triangular deformation of the calvarium.*

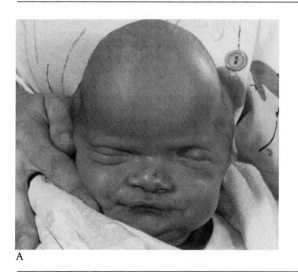
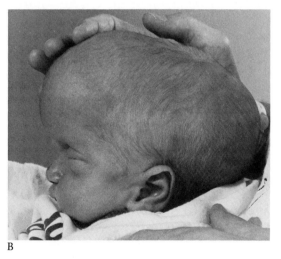

A                                         B

**Figure 5-39** *Scaphocephaly. A. Frontal view. The biparietal width is decreased, and the prematurely fused sagittal suture is palpable as a peaked ridge. B. Profile. Prominent bossing of the forehead and occiput with the elevated crown produces the upside-down boat appearance.*

tive trigonocephalic deformity called metopic synostosis. A palpable vertical ridge is centered on the forehead resulting in a V-shaped contour with recession of the lateral portions of the orbits (Fig. 5-38). A mild degree of hypotelorbitism is present. The occurrence is sporadic. Intellectual potential and the remainder of the physical examination are normal.

## SAGITTAL SYNOSTOSIS

Scaphocephalic deformation of the calvarium resulting from premature closure of the midline sagittal suture is one of the most common deformities. The upside-down boat shape deformation is easily recognized (Fig. 5-39). A palpable ridge is present along the site of the suture, and the forehead and occipital regions are prominent. The biparietal width is narrowed, and the vertex is tall. Occurrence is sporadic, and normal mental development is the rule.

## MULTIPLE SYNOSTOSIS

Although any combination of premature sutural fusion can be seen, the "cloverleaf" (kleeblatschädel) [22] anomalad is not easily forgotten (Fig. 5-40). The unmistakable trilobular deformation of the cranial vault is the result of premature closure of the coronal, lambdoidal, and temporoparietal sutures. The metopic suture can also be involved, with the brain bulging through an open sagittal suture. The anomalad can be found as an isolated entity or in patients with Apert, Crouzon, or Carpenter syndrome. Hydrocephalus is a frequent accompaniment.

## TREATMENT OF CRANIOSYNOSTOSIS

Although the surgical strategies depend on the individual malformation and patient, a few words on the general philosophy of treatment hold true for most of the craniosynostosis malformations. A major factor in the surgical management of premature closure of the cranial sutures is the growth of the brain. Accelerated enlargement of the

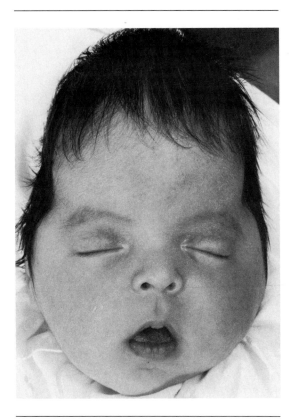

**Figure 5-40** *Kleeblatshädel (cloverleaf) skull. Premature closure of multiple sutures causes a trilobar deformation of the calvarium with protrusion of the brain through an enlarged open anterior fontanelle.*

brain takes place during the first year; it doubles in size and achieves half its adult size during this period [37, 44]. To take advantage of this phenomenon, it is desirable to intervene early, preferably during the first 6 months of life.

Furthermore, the deleterious aftermath of increased intracranial pressure on intellectual development and vision can be avoided by early intervention. Although the adverse effects of premature closure of multiple sutures is well known, Marchac and Renier have shown that 13 percent of patients with an isolated sutural involvement have increased intracranial pressure [28].

In the past, simple stripping of the involved sutures by the neurosurgeon has been the rule. However, better restoration of normal cranial form and aesthetic results are achieved when modern craniofacial surgical techniques are applied in consultation with a plastic surgeon. Infants tolerate these intracranial procedures surprisingly well. The details of treatment for each malformation are found in Chapter 6. Thus only general principles are described in this section.

The older methods of linear craniectomy with or without morcellation of the frontal bone successfully prevented subsequent cranial deformation in only approximately 60 percent of the cases [21, 38]. The accepted principle is to release the concerned suture and reposition the malposed calvarial structures to their normal position, not relying on catch-up growth [21, 27]. However, even with these methods, McCarthy et al. found that early operations did not prevent subsequent occlusal disharmony in those patients with a predilection for mid-facial inhibition of growth due to the underlying faciostenosis [29]. Consequently, measures to restore normalcy are required later in life (see Chapter 6).

## References

1. Apert, E. De l'acrocèphalosyndactylie. *Bull. Soc. Med. Paris* 23:1310, 1906.
2. Berry, G. A. Note on a congenital defect (? coloboma) of the lower lid. *R. Lond. Ophthalmol. Hosp. Rep.* 12:255, 1889.
3. Bertelsen, T. I. *The Premature Synostosis of the Cranial Sutures.* Copenhagen: Munksgaard, 1958.
4. Boo-Chai, K. The oblique facial cleft: A report of 2 cases and a review of 41 cases. *Br. J. Plast. Surg.* 23:352, 1970.
5. Braithwaite, F., and Watson, J. Three unusual clefts of the lip. *Br. J. Plast. Surg.* 2:38, 1949.
6. Carpenter, G. Two sisters showing malformations of the skull and other congenital abnormalities. *Rep. Soc. Study Dis. Child. (Lond.)* 1:110, 1901.
7. Chotzen, F. Eine eigenartige familare Entwicklungsstorung (Akrocephalosyndaktylie,

Dysostosis craniofacialis und Hypertelorismus). *Monatsschr. Kinderheilkd.* 55:97, 1932.
8. Cohen, M. M., Jr. Craniosynostosis and syndromes with craniosynostosis: incidence, genetics, penetrance, variability and new syndrome updating. *Birth Defects* 15:13, 1979.
9. Collins, E. T. 8. Case with symmetrical congenital notches in the outer part of each lower lid and defective development of the malar bones. *Trans. Ophthalmol. Soc. U.K.* 20:190, 1900.
10. Collins, E. T. 9. Case with symmetrical congenital notches in the outer part of each lower lid and defective development of the malar bone. *Trans. Ophthalmol. Soc. U.K.* 20:191, 1900.
11. Converse, J. M., et al. Craniofacial Microsomia. In J. M. Converse (ed.), *Reconstructive Plastic Surgery* (2nd ed.). Philadelphia: Saunders, 1977. P. 2359.
12. Costara-Volarich, M., and Pruzansky, S. Is the mandible intrinsically different in Apert and Crouzon syndromes? *Am. J. Orthop.* 85:475, 1984.
13. Crouzon, O. Dysostose cranio-faciale hérèditaire. *Bull. Soc. Med. Hop. Paris* 33:545, 1912.
14. DeMyer, W., Zeman, W., and Palmer, C. A. The face predicts the brain: Diagnostic significance of median facial anomalies for holoprosencephaly (arrhinencephaly). *Pediatrics* 34:256, 1964.
15. Franceschetti, A., and Klein, D. The mandibulofacial dysostosis: A new hereditary syndrome. *Acta Ophthalmol. (Copenh.)* 27:144, 1949.
16. Franceshetti, A., and Zwahlen, P. Un syndrome nouveau: La dysostose mandibulofaciale. *Bull. Schweiz. Akad. Med. Wiss.* 1:60, 1944.
17. Goldenhar, M. Association malformations de l'oeil et de l'oreille, en particular le syndrome dermoide épibulbaire-appendices auriculaires-fistula auris congenita et ses relations avec la dysostose mandibulo-faciale. *J. Genet. Hum.* 1:243, 1952.
18. Grabb, W. C. The first and second branchial arch syndrome. *Plast. Reconstr. Surg.* 36:485, 1965.
19. Gunter, G. S. Nasomaxilary cleft. *Plast. Reconstr. Surg.* 32:637, 1963.
20. Harkins, C. S., et al. A classification of cleft lip and cleft palate. *Plast. Reconstr. Surg.* 29:31, 1962.
21. Hoffman, H. J., and Mohr, G. P. Lateral can-

thal advancement of the supraorbital margin. *J. Neurosurg.* 45:376, 1976.

22. Holtermüller, K., and Wiedemann, H. R. Kleeblattschädel-Syndrom. *Med. Monatsschr.* 14:439, 1960.

23. Karfik, V. Oblique facial cleft. In: *Transactions International Society of Plastic Surgeons, Fourth Congress, 1967.* Amsterdam: Excerpta Medica, 1969. P. 105.

24. Kawamoto, H. K. Torticollis versus Plagiocephaly. In D. Marchac (ed.), *Craniofacial Surgery.* Berlin: Springer-Verlag, 1987. P. 105.

25. Kawamoto, H. K., Jr. The kaleidoscopic world of rare craniofacial clefts: Order out of chaos (Tessier classification). *Clin. Plast. Surg.* 3:529, 1976.

26. Longacre, J. J., DeStefano, A., and Holmstrand, K. The early versus the late reconstruction of congenital hypoplasia of the facial skeleton and skull. *Plast. Reconstr. Surg.* 27:489, 1961.

27. Marchac, D. Radical forehead remodeling for craniostenosis. *Plast. Reconstr. Surg.* 61:823, 1978.

28. Marchac, D., and Renier, D. *Craniofacial Surgery for Craniosynostosis.* Boston: Little, Brown, 1982. P. 12.

29. McCarthy, J. G., et al. Early surgery for craniofacial synostosis: An 8-year experience. *Plast. Reconstr. Surg.* 73:521, 1984.

30. Morian, R. Ueber die schrage Gesichtsspalte. *Arch. Klin. Chir.* 35:245, 1887.

31. Pfeiffer, R. A. Dominant erbliche Akrocephalosyndaktylie. *Z. Kinderheilkd.* 90:301, 1964.

32. Poswillo, D. The pathogenesis of the first and second branchial arch syndrome. *Oral Surg.* 35:302, 1973.

33. Poswillo, D. Orofacial malformations. *Proc. R. Soc. Med.* 67:13, 1974.

34. Rogalski, T. A contribution to the study of anophthalmia with description of a case. *Br. J. Ophthalmol.* 28:429, 1944.

35. Rogers, B. O. Rare Craniofacial Deformities. In J. M. Converse (ed.), *Reconstructive Plastic Surgery* (1st ed.). Philadelphia: Saunders, 1964. P. 1213.

36. Saethre, H. Ein Beitrag zum Turmschädelproblem (Pathogenese, Erblichkeit und Symptomatolgie). *Dtsch. Z. Nervenheilkd.* 117:533, 1931.

37. Sinclair, D. *Human Growth after Birth* (4th ed.). London: Oxford University Press, 1985. P. 85.

38. Shillito, J., Jr., and Matson, D. D. Craniostenosis: A review of 519 surgical patients. *Paediatrics* 41:829, 1968.

39. Temtamy, S. A. Carpenter's syndrome: Acrocephalopolysyndactyly: An autosomal recessive syndrome. *J. Pediatr.* 69:111, 1966.

40. Tessier, P. Colobomas: vertical and oblique complete facial clefts. *Panminerva Med.* 11:95, 1969.

41. Tessier, P. Anatomical classification of facial, craniofacial and latero-facial clefts. *J. Maxillofac. Surg.* 4:69, 1976.

42. Van der Meulen, J. C., et al. A morphogenetic classification of craniofacial malformations. *Plast. Reconstr. Surg.* 71:560, 1983.

43. Virchow, R. Uber den Cretinismus, namentlich in Franhen, und uber pathologische Schadelformen. *Verh. Phys. Med. Ges. Wurtzburg* 2:241, 1951.

44. White House Conference on Child Health and Protection. *Growth and Development of the Child. Part II. Anatomy and Physiology.* New York: Century Co., 1933. P. 232.

# 6

Joseph G. McCarthy
Gregory S. LaTrenta

# Craniofacial Surgery

The beginning of corrective surgery for maxillofacial deformities dates back to developments in military surgery during World War I, when severe bone and soft tissue facial injuries resulted from trench warfare. Maxillofacial surgery centers were established under the direction of Kazanjian, Gillies, and others. Gillies in 1920 proposed two principles of reconstructive surgery based on his experience in the treatment of war victims at the Queen's Hospital at Sidcup [25].

... as elsewhere, the aim is to estimate first the amount of loss; and secondly, the possibility of correcting displacement. It is often impossible to do so till one has undone some previous effort at repair. A moment's consideration will show that no estimation of the loss or distortion of soft tissues can be of use unless coupled with a knowledge of the *bony tissue.*

It was Gillies' concepts of knowing "the exact loss in terms of anatomical structure" and "replacing as early as possible [all normal tissue]" that initiated the immediate reduction of facial fractures and the correction of facial bone malunion with secondary surgery [25].

It is not surprising that 30 years later Gillies was the first to perform a modified Le Fort III advancement for the correction of a Crouzon deformity [26]. Despite the fact that the medial osteotomy was performed anterior to the lacrimal groove via a nasal infracture approach, the patient's exorbitism was improved. Seven and a half years later the patient underwent orbital expansion for persistent exorbitism. Gillies commented later that the procedure was too involved and should not be attempted again (J. M. Converse, personal communication). However, it was not until the work of Paul Tessier, in a collaboration between the plastic and neurosurgical teams at the Foch Hospital in Paris during the 1960s, that modern craniofacial surgery was born [75–78].

Tessier encountered his first patient with Crouzon's disease in 1957. He was familiar with the Gillies case and had studied Le Fort's experimental study of fractures of the upper jaw [41, 42, 68]. In this study Le Fort determined the three important lines of craniofacial skeletal weakness and fracture that bear his name. Tessier utilized this knowledge, first working on skulls and then practicing on cadavers before his first Crouzon patient. After the 25-mm mid-face Le Fort III advancement, "he was astonished by the size and the irregularity of the numerous bony defects which appeared ... instruments and the exposure were inadequate, the bone grafts did not fit the defects, the osteosyntheses were unsatisfactory, and the skeletal fixation was problematic" [68]. It was 3 years until Tessier saw another, similar case, but during the subsequent two decades he developed a repertoire of craniofacial procedures whose number was almost unlimited and that could be applied to both congenital and posttraumatic deformities.

Several fundamental principles can be distilled from his work.

1. The craniofacial skeleton should be adequately exposed through inconspicuous incisions.
2. Large segments of the craniofacial skeleton can be extensively devascularized, osteotomized, and translocated in multiple dimensions with retention of osseous viability.
3. The soft tissues, and especially the eyes, can be translocated with the bone segments without impairing vision [62].
4. Autogenous bone grafting is critical for filling residual defects, ensuring stability, and improving contour.
5. Rigid skeletal fixation must be attained by interosseous wiring or plating.
6. In general, skeletal reconstruction takes precedence over soft tissue repair.
7. The procedures must be undertaken only by an experienced, multidisciplinary craniofacial surgery team.

## Team Concept

Before initiating a craniofacial surgery program, the plastic surgeon must first organize a multidisciplinary team. The team consists of the craniofacial surgeon(s), anesthesiologist, audiologist, geneticist, neurologist, neuroradiologist, neurosurgeon, ophthalmologist, orthodontist, otolaryngologist, nurse specialist, pediatrician/internist, prosthodontist, psychiatrist, speech pathologist, and social worker. The team approach provides optimal care and aids in the collection of longitudinal data.

The patient is evaluated at a multidisci-

plinary conference attended by all members of the team. At this conference, the patient is available for examination and the data are presented, including medical photographs, cephalograms, panoramic radiographs, routine facial and skull radiographs, and computed tomography (CT) scans. The introduction of three-dimensional CT scans [47] has provided the craniofacial surgeon with realistic visualization of the craniofacial skeleton and allows for volume quantification [16] and more precise preoperative planning [14].

The geneticist helps to diagnose patients with congenital deformities and offers genetic counseling, supervising any chromosomal and genetic studies. A pedigree of the families of patients with congenital deformities is essential.

After the decision for surgery is reached, it is the surgeon who must warn the patient and the parents of the type of surgery being considered and its inherent risks.

The actual surgical procedure is designed by the surgeon, orthodontist, and neurosurgeon. The most valuable factor when planning is the clinical examination of the patient, aided by study of the photographs, radiographs, and CT scans. Cephalometric films provide multidimensional analysis of the osseous deformity and can be compared to normative controls by age and sex; they also permit longitudinal growth studies [94, 95].

The orthodontist takes dental cast impressions if jaw surgery is anticipated and provides interpretation of the cephalometric data. If intermaxillary fixation is required, the teeth are individually banded, preoperative orthodontic therapy is performed, and an interocclusal wafer is fabricated.

INTRAOPERATIVE MONITORING
Monitoring during the procedure is the joint responsibility of the craniofacial surgeon, neurosurgeon, and anesthesiologist. If an intracranial route is elected, the following are important: (1) Spinal drain. The catheter is inserted into the lumbar subarachnoid space

and connected to straight drainage (60 ml of cerebrospinal fluid is drained prior to temporary closure). (2) Central venous pressure line. The catheter is inserted via an antecubital vein and connected to a monitoring device. (3) Peripheral venous line. It is usually of large gauge for fluid administration. (4) Arterial pressure line. A 20 to 22-gauge line is inserted percutaneously or via cutdown into the radial artery at the wrist. (5) Foley catheter. (6) Rectal thermal probe. (7) Electrocardiographic leads. (8) Pulse oximeter. Intracranial pressure monitoring with a pressure screw that enters the posterior cranial subarachnoid space has also been recommended [19].

Transoral endotracheal anesthesia is administered unless intermaxillary fixation is planned, in which case transnasal intubation is performed with suture fixation to the membranous septum. The decision to perform a tracheostomy depends on the magnitude of the procedure and the status of the airway; if indicated, it is performed after induction of general anesthesia with an oral endotracheal tube. Hypotensive anesthesia technique is used for all craniofacial procedures to decrease blood transfusion requirements.

The combination of spinal drainage, hyperventilation technique (monitored by $PaCO_2$), and mannitol administration (1 gm/kg body weight) improves intracranial exposure. Postoperative spinal drainage assists the sealing of small dural lacerations. The drain is removed when the closed suction drains in the scalp wound are removed (between the third and fifth postoperative days).

Arterial blood gas analysis and hematocrit readings are recorded every 30 minutes intraoperatively. Serum electrolytes and coagulation profile, obtained preoperatively, are repeated intraoperatively if necessary. Continuous airway monitoring via a precordial stethoscope is important to detect accidental dislodgement of the airway.

For a major craniofacial surgical reconstruction, blood is crossmatched to a volume equal to 150 percent of the patient's blood volume. Packed red blood cells are administered via a blood warmer when the intraoperative hematocrit falls below 25 percent or when needed. Autogenous, parental, or sibling blood donation is encouraged if transfusion is required.

Intravenous antibiotics are administered preoperatively, intraoperatively, and postoperatively (7 days) according to pediatric and adult dosage guidelines.

POSTOPERATIVE PERIOD

After several hours in the recovery room, the anesthesiologist usually removes the patient's endotracheal airway. If jaw (maxillomandibular) surgery has been performed, the surgeon and anesthesiologist may elect to wait 24 to 48 hours for removal of the nasotracheal airway. At that time a small soft rubber nasopharyngeal airway is inserted and secured to guarantee patency of the nasal airway.

When cleared from the recovery room by the anesthesiologist, the patient is transferred to the intensive care unit. Neurosurgical vital signs are monitored for 24 to 48 hours, and the central venous line, arterial line, and light wraparound head dressing are discontinued upon transfer to the ward. Nasogastric suction is used for 24 hours postoperatively if intermaxillary fixation is established; otherwise, oral feeding is permitted on the first day postoperatively. The spinal drain and wound drains are discontinued between the third and fifth postoperative days, after which the peripheral intravenous line is discontinued and the patient is placed on oral antibiotics. Discharge follows the restoration of alimentation and the return of the patient's sense of well-being.

## Skeletal Anatomy
FRONTAL BONE

The two frontal bones, prominently situated and separated by the metopic suture during infancy, form the brow, forehead, and roof of

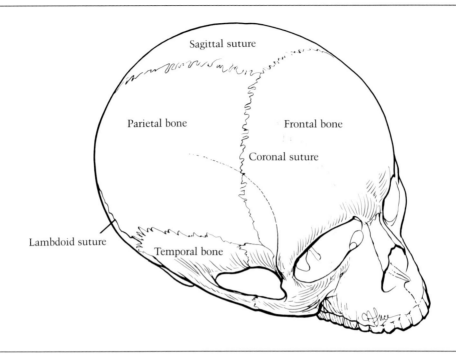

***Figure 6-1*** *Cranial bones and sutures.*

the orbit, nose, and ethmoid sinus (Fig. 6-1). The two orbital plates of the frontal bone, with the cribriform plate of the ethmoid and lesser wing of the sphenoid, form the support of the anterior cranial fossa [29]. Anterior to the ethmoid air cells within the orbital plate is the frontal sinus, which is responsible for the glabellar and supraorbital prominences. The frontal sinus communicates with the nasal cavity through the middle meatus via the frontonasal duct. On the internal surface of the squamous portion of the frontal bone is the sulcus for the superior sagittal sinus, the margins of which unite to form the frontal crest. This structure forms the attachments for the falx cerebri. The foramen cecum exists at the articulation of the frontal crest with the ethmoid bone. It can be the site for intranasal dermoid cysts and encephaloceles.

PARIETAL BONE

The parietal bone is the largest and thickest of the cranial bones (see Fig. 6-1). Crossing the external surface are the superior and in-ferior temporal lines, attachments for the deep temporal fascia and muscle, respectively. The parietal bone is quadrilateral in shape, articulating anteriorly with the frontal bone along the coronal suture, posteriorly with the occipital bone along the lambdoid suture, superiorly with the opposite parietal bone along the sagittal suture, and inferiorly with the greater wing of the sphenoid and the temporal bone along the squamosal suture. The *pterion* is the site near the sphenoidal angle where the parietal, sphenoid, temporal, and frontal bones approximate. The internal surface at this important external landmark is the middle cranial fossa. Occasionally, a deep groove is noted in the bone. It is caused by the frontal branch of the middle meningeal artery. The parietal bone is the preferred donor site for harvesting calvarial bone grafts.

TEMPORAL BONE

Along with the greater wing of the sphenoid, the temporal bone forms the base of the middle cranial fossa (see Fig. 6-1). The temporal bone develops from fusion of the three processes: the *squamous* process, which gives origin to the temporalis muscle; the *petromastoid* process, which encases the membranous labyrinth; and the small *tympanic* process interposed between the previous two. The squamous process articulates anteriorly with the zygoma. The glenoid fossa is bounded anteriorly by the articular tubercle of the zygomatic portion and posteriorly by the postglenoid and tympanic process of the temporal bone. The internal surface of the petromastoid process presents a deep, curved groove for the sigmoid sinus. Section of the mastoid process reveals mastoid cells, which communicate with the tympanic cavity. The styloid process takes origin from the inferior surface of the petrous process immediately in front of the stylomastoid foramen. It gives attachment to the stylohyoid and stylomandibular ligaments and to the styloglossus, stylohyoid, and stylopharyngeous muscles. Between the styloid process and the mastoid process lies the stylomastoid foramen, the exit for the facial nerve. The petrous portion is wedged between the sphenoid and occipital bones at the skull base. The anterior petrous surface contains the trigeminal ganglion, carotid canal, and hiatus of the facial canal for passage of the greater petrosal nerve. The posterior petrous surface forms the anterior part of the posterior cranial fossa and contains the internal acoustic meatus and canal, transmitting the facial and vestibulocochlear nerves as well as the facial canal. The tympanic process is wedged between the petrous and squamous processes.

## OCCIPITAL BONE

The occipital bone forms the most posterior aspect of the skull and cranial base. The large, quadrilateral segment anterior to the foramen magnum forming the posterior cranial base is the basilar process. On each side of the foramen are the lateral processes. The curved, expanded plates articulating with the parietal bones at the lambdoid suture are designated the squamous processes. The basilar process is joined to the sphenoid by a plate of cartilage, the sphenooccipital synchondrosis. The lateral processes articulate inferiorly with the atlas and superiorly with the petrous process of the temporal bone.

## SPHENOID BONE

The sphenoid bone (Figs. 6-2 and 6-3) is the vital link between the orbital, nasal, and cranial cavities and forms a major part of the temporal, infratemporal, and pterygopalatine fossae. The body of the sphenoid encompasses the sphenoid sinus and gives rise to the greater wings, lesser wings, and pterygoid plates. The anterior and inferior surfaces of the body articulate with the ethmoid bone and form part of the posterior wall of the nasal cavity. The rostrum of the inferior surface articulates with the vomer. The superior, or intracranial, surface contains the optic chiasmatic groove and canals, as well as the sella turcica, the petrosal process for articulation with the temporal bone, and the clivus for articulation with the occipital bone. The lesser wings of the sphenoid, which enclose the optic foramina, give rise to the anterior clinoid processes, which give attachment to the tentorium cerebelli. The upper surface of the lesser wings also forms part of the floor of the anterior cranial fossa, separating it from the middle cranial fossa. The greater wings are fairly complex, forming the floor of the middle cranial fossa and the lateral wall of the orbit, articulating with the frontal bone, parietal bone, temporal bone, and zygoma. Between the greater and lesser wings is the superior orbital fissure, which allows passage of the third, fourth, and sixth cranial nerves. The medial and lateral pterygoid plates are separated inferiorly by the pterygoid fissure, which encloses the pterygoid fossa and contains the medial pterygoid and tensor veli palatini muscles. The medial pterygoid plate ends at the pterygoid hamulus, around which the tendon of the tensor veli palatini glides.

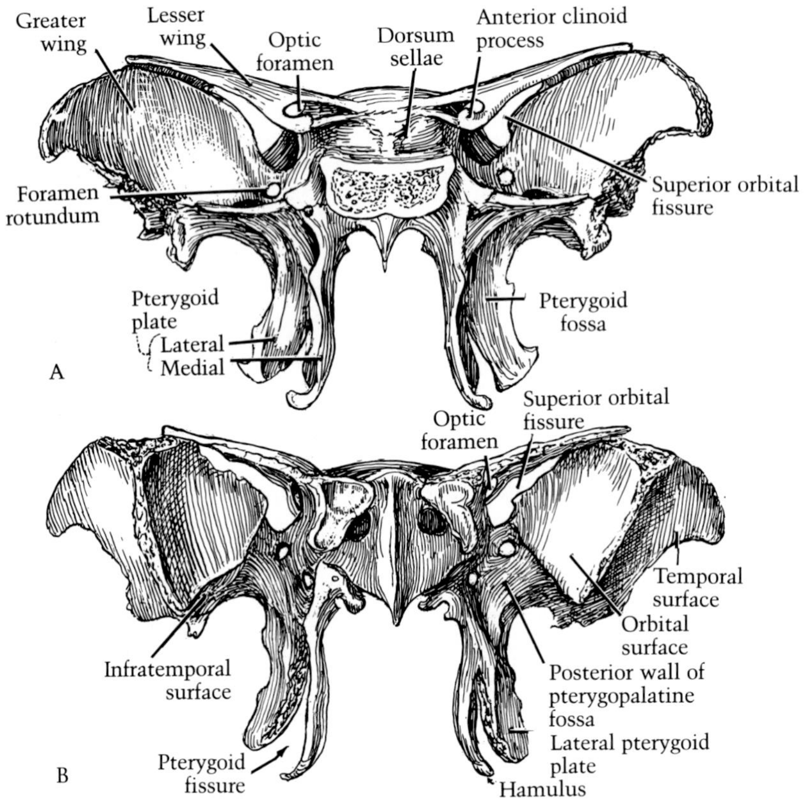

**Figure 6-2** *Sphenoid bone. A. Posterior view. B. Anterior view. (From J. M. Converse et al. Craniofacial surgery.* Clin. Plast. Surg. *1:499, 1974.)*

ORBIT

The orbits are the keystones of the face (Fig. 6-4). The bony orbit is somewhat pyramidal in shape with the sphenoid bone at its apex. The widest diameter, however, is located 1.5 cm within the orbital rim. The adult orbital height at the rim is approximately 35 mm with a width of 40 mm. The depth varies between 45 to 55 mm. The angle between the lateral walls of both orbits is 90 degrees, and the angle between the medial and lateral walls of each orbit is 45 degrees. The medial orbital walls are nearly parallel. The orbital axis varies from the visual axis by 23 degrees [92].

The *roof* of the orbit is composed anteriorly of the orbital plate of the frontal bone and posteriorly of the lesser wing of the sphenoid. The lacrimal fossa is located an-

terolaterally and the trochlear fossa anteromedially. The supraorbital extension of the frontal sinus abuts the anterior aspects of the roof.

The *lateral wall* of the orbit is stout, formed by the frontal process of the zygoma, the greater wing of the sphenoid, and the zygomatic process of the frontal bone. Whitnall's tubercle, which can be noted as a small bony promontory located within the rim, serves for attachment of the lateral canthal mechanism. The zygomaticofacial and zygomaticotemporal foramina provide exits for their respective complexes. The superior orbital fissure allows passage of CN III, CN

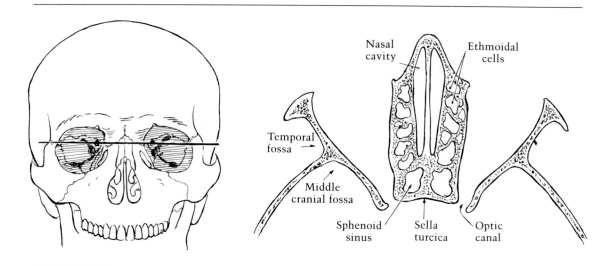

**Figure 6-3** *Transverse section showing the relation of the sphenoid bone and orbit to the temporal fossa and middle cranial fossa. (From J. M. Converse et al. Craniofacial surgery.* Clin. Plast. Surg. *1:499, 1974.)*

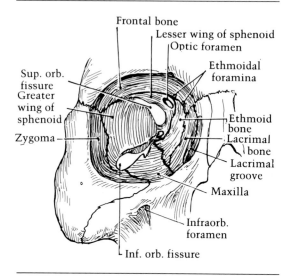

**Figure 6-4** *Frontal view of the right orbit. (From J. M. Converse (ed.).* Plastic Reconstructive Surgery. *Philadelphia: Saunders, 1977.)*

IV, and CN VI; it separates the roof from the lateral wall of the orbit and terminates between the greater and lesser wings of the sphenoid bone. The inferior orbital fissure, which contains the inferior orbital nerve, separates the greater wing of the sphenoid from the orbital floor and communicates with the infratemporal fossa. The posterior portion of the lateral wall of the orbit forms a border for the middle cranial fossa, which contains the temporal lobe of the brain.

The *medial wall* of the orbit is strongly reinforced anteriorly by the frontal process of the maxilla, but it is relatively fragile posteriorly. The posterior portion is composed of the lacrimal bone, lamina papyracea of the ethmoid bone, palatine bone, and the lesser wing of the sphenoid, the latter containing the optic foramen. The lacrimal groove, containing the nasolacrimal sac and duct, lies between the anterior lacrimal crest of the frontal process of the maxilla and the posterior lacrimal crest of the lacrimal bone. The fragile lamina papyracea is the largest component of the medial wall and is a frequent site of fracture. The anterior and posterior ethmoidal foramina lie between the roof of the orbit and the lamina papyracea. They communicate their respective vessels and nerves to the medial portion of the anterior cranial fossa.

The *floor* of the orbit, the most frequent site of fracture, is not sharply delineated from the medial wall. The floor is composed mainly of the orbital plate of the maxilla, containing the maxillary sinus, the zygomatic bone, and a small segment of palatine bone at its apex. The infraorbital groove extends across the floor, beginning near the midportion of the inferior orbital fissure.

The periosteum of the orbit communicates with the dura at the optic foramen, the superior orbital fissure, and the anterior and posterior ethmoid foramina. The optic canal is 4 to 10 mm in length and is contained between the lesser wing and body of the sphenoid bone, in close approximation to the sphenoid and ethmoid sinuses.

ETHMOID BONE

The ethmoid bone (Fig. 6-5), lying directly anterior to the body of the sphenoid, defines the interorbital space. Two lateral masses encompass the ethmoid air cells, which communicate with the sphenoid air cells via the sphenoethmoid recess. The lateral aspect of the ethmoid air cells forms the medial orbital walls (lamina papyracea) posterior to the posterior lacrimal crest. Both superior and middle nasal conchae are extensions derived from the lateral masses. The central perpendicular plate forms the posterosuperior bony portion of the nasal septum. The perpendicular plate articulates with the nasal and frontal bones anterosuperiorly, the quadrangular plate anteroinferiorly, the vomer posteroinferiorly, and the sphenoid body posterosuperiorly. In the roof of the nose the paired lateral masses converge to form the cribriform plate, separating the nose from the anterior cranial cavity. The cribriform plate lies between the orbital plate of the frontal bone and the crista galli, which is the intracranial projection of the perpendicular plate. Slender olfactory nerves penetrate the deeply grooved cribriform plate on either side of the crista galli

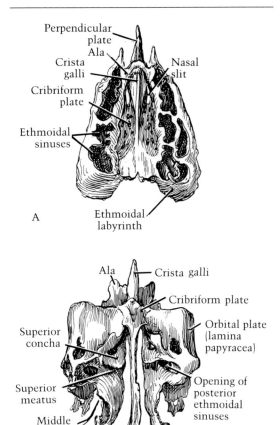

**Figure 6-5** *Ethmoid bone. A. View from above. B. Posterior view. (From J. M. Converse et al. Craniofacial surgery.* Clin. Plast. Surg. *1:499, 1974.)*

and supply the specialized olfactory mucosa of the superior nasal concha and adjacent septum. The olfactory bulb and tract lie underneath the frontal lobes in a paramedian position.

PALATINE BONE

The palatine bone is deeply situated between the posteromedial maxilla and the pterygoid plates of the sphenoid bone. The orbital process of the palatine bone gives a small contribution to the orbital floor.

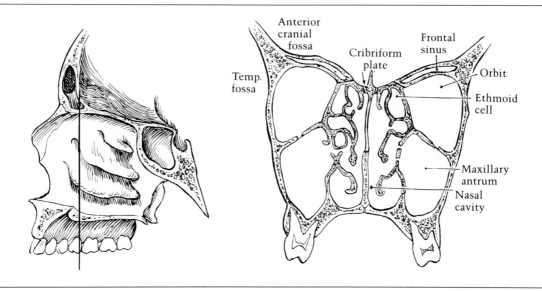

**Figure 6-6** *Frontal section showing the relation of the bony orbits and the interorbital space to the anterior cranial fossa, frontal sinus, temporal fossa, maxillary sinus, and ethmoidal sinus. (From J. M. Converse et al. Craniofacial surgery. Clin. Plast. Surg. 1:499, 1974.)*

The horizontal process of the palatine bone forms the posterior fourth of the hard palate and posterior nasal spine. The vertical process of the palatine bone, interpositioned between the maxilla and perpendicular plate, forms the superior, middle, and inferior meati. The sphenopalatine foramen, transmitting the sphenopalatine vessels and nerves, divides the superior from the middle meatus.

VOMER

The vomer articulates inferiorly with the midline maxillary and palatine crests, anterosuperiorly with the cartilaginous septum and the perpendicular plate of the ethmoid, and posterosuperiorly with the sphenoid body. The nasopalatine grooves, coursing downward and forward, are noted on each side for their respective vessels and nerves, exiting at the incisive foramen.

LACRIMAL BONE

The smallest and most fragile bone of the mid-face, the lacrimal bone, forms the posterior lacrimal crest, and together with the frontal process of the maxilla (anterior lacrimal crest), it also forms the lacrimal groove containing the lacrimal sac. The lacrimal bone articulates inferiorly with the inferior nasal concha and superiorly with the orbital plate of the frontal bone.

MAXILLA

The paired maxilla, or maxillae, are the largest bones of the mid-face (Fig. 6-6, 6-7). Each consists of a body and zygomatic, frontal, alveolar, and palatine processes. The *frontal process* extends upward to the medial orbital wall and nasal bones. The *zygomatic process* abuts the zygoma and, with the latter, forms the cheek prominence. The *palatine process* forms the anterior three-fourths of the hard palate. The *alveolar process* contains the teeth of the upper jaw.

The body of the maxilla, pyramidal in shape, contains the maxillary sinus. The anterior surface is sharply delimited by the infraorbital rims and piriform aperture. The posterior surface contains the alveolar canals for the posterosuperior alveolar vessels and nerves, as well as the maxillary tuberosities, which articulate medially with the pyramidal process of the palatine bone and laterally with the pterygoid plate of the sphenoid bone. The superior, or orbital, surface forms the greater part of the orbital floor medial to the inferior orbital fissure. Medially, it is bounded by the lacrimal groove. The medial or nasal surface forms both the lateral wall of the nasal cavity and the medial wall of the maxillary sinus. In addition, the perpendicular plate of the palatine bone, the uncinate process of the ethmoid, and the inferior nasal concha form part of the medial wall of the sinus. Anteriorly, the nasolacrimal duct passes via the nasolacrimal canal into the inferior meatus. The frontal, maxillary, and ethmoid sinuses drain into the middle meatus, and the sphenoid drains into the superior meatus. The greater palatine canal, formed by the posterior articulation of the maxillary tuberosity with the palatine bone, transmits the respective nerves and vessels to the hard and soft palate.

ZYGOMA

The zygomatic bone is quadrangular in shape and articulates laterally with the temporal bone via the arch, the maxilla anteroinferiorly, the sphenoid posteromedially, and the frontal bone superiorly (Fig. 6-7). The zygoma forms the cheek prominence, part of the lateral wall and floor of the orbit, and part of the bony wall of the temporal and infratemporal fossae.

NASAL BONES

The nasal bones are oblong and centered on the frontal process of the maxilla. They show great variability in size and form among individuals.

## Surgical Exposure

BICORONAL APPROACH

The eyes are protected prior to incision by eyelid closure with a 4-0 silk horizontal mattress suture. The preauricular incision

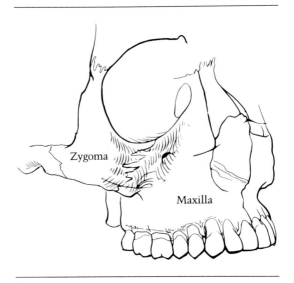

*Figure 6-7* *Zygoma and maxilla.*

(Fig. 6-8) begins at the tragus and extends across the scalp posterior to the coronal suture. The scalp is peeled toward the supraorbital rim with a periosteal elevator. The lateral dissection proceeds forward and remains superficial to the deep temporal fascia until the deep temporal fat pad is encountered. The dissection is then carried deep to the temporal fat pad until the zygomatic arch is encountered, a maneuver designed to avoid injury of the frontal branch of the facial nerve.

Orbital dissection begins in a subperiosteal plane. If the supraorbital vessels and nerves pass through a foramen rather than a fissure, a fine osteotome is used to remove the bony bridge while protecting the globe with a malleable retractor. Orbital dissection can safely proceed 25 to 30 mm posterior to the orbital rim for a full 360 degrees without disruption of the orbital apex (Fig. 6-9). Deep orbital dissection is safer along the superior and lateral walls. On the medial orbital wall, the anterior ethmoidal vessels are divided. The lacrimal sac is stripped from its fossa, care being taken to preserve the nasolacrimal duct as it passes through the canal. If access to the temporal and in-

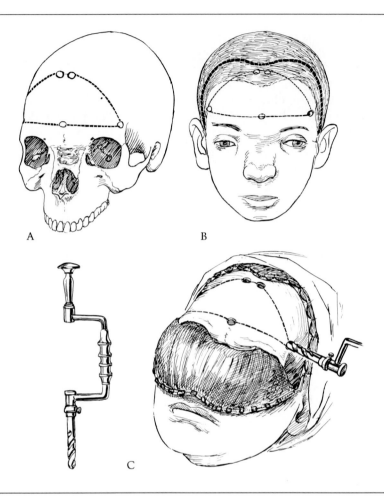

**Figure 6-8** Operative procedure for the correction of orbital hypertelorism. A. Site of burr holes preparatory to raising a frontal bone flap. B. Relation of the bicoronal scalp incision to the frontal bone flap. C. Drilling the frontal burr holes. (From J. M. Converse et al. Craniofacial surgery. Clin. Plast. Surg. 1:499, 1974.)

tratemporal fossae is necessary, the temporalis muscle can be mobilized off the parietal and temporal bones with a periosteal elevator. To prevent an hourglass deformity, this muscle must be reattached to the lateral orbital rim at the completion of the procedure. The lateral orbit, inferior orbital rim, zygoma, and anterior maxilla can be stripped of periosteum for full exposure without rim or eyelid incisions. Extension of the preauricular incision below the tragus may be necessary. *No traction or direct pressure* is placed on the periorbital envelope during this maneuver.

Complete nasofrontal subperiosteal dissection can then proceed to the level of the upper lateral cartilages, as well as to the medial orbital rim and adjacent maxilla. If a Le Fort III osteotomy is to be performed, subperiosteal stripping of the posterior maxilla and the pterygomaxillary fissure can be performed.

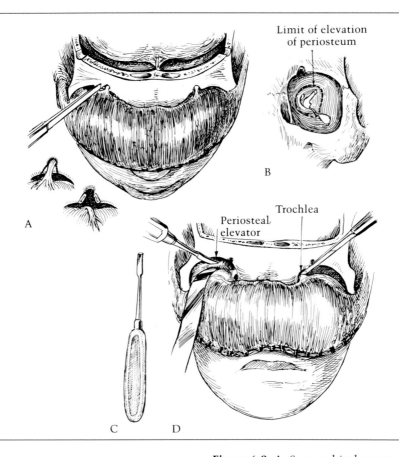

*Figure 6-9* A. Supraorbital nerves are liberated by resecting the inferior border of the supraorbital foramen. B. Dotted lines indicate the posterior limit of the periosteal elevation within the orbit. C. Elevator used for raising the periorbita. D. Trochlea is detached subperiosteally. (From J. M. Converse et al. Craniofacial surgery. Clin. Plast. Surg. 1:499, 1974.)

EYELID INCISIONS

If exposure of the inferior orbital rim, floor, and anterior maxilla is required and exposure is deemed inadequate with the bicoronal approach alone, either transconjunctival or subciliary eyelid incisions can be performed (Fig. 6-10).

*Transconjunctival Incision*

With corneal protectors in place, the lower eyelid is everted and the transconjunctival incision is performed through the conjunctiva below the tarsus with fine-needle-tipped Bovie cautery. The incision can be carried laterally to facilitate exposure. Dissection, in a plane anterior to the orbital septum, is carried down to the inferior orbital rim for full exposure. The periosteum is then incised.

*Subciliary Incision*

The subciliary incision is placed 2 to 3 mm below the lower lid margin. The skin is undermined to preserve the pretarsal orbicularis muscle, and a step incision is carried deep to the muscle. The skin–muscle flap is raised to the inferior orbital rim for full exposure. The periosteum is then incised as described above.

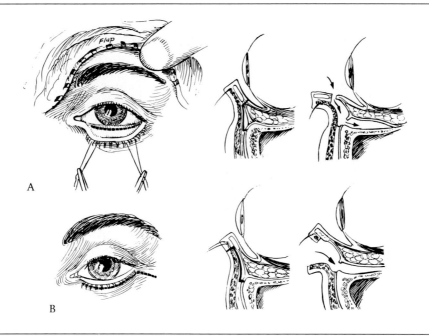

A

B

*Figure 6-10* A. Transconjunctival approach to the orbital floor. Note how the incision is made anterior to the septum orbitale. B. Subciliary approach to the orbital floor through an incision over the tarsus. (From J. M. Converse et al. Craniofacial surgery. Clin. Plast. Surg. 1:499, 1974.)

INTRAORAL INCISIONS

The upper buccal sulcus incision (Fig. 6-11) readily exposes the anterior and lateral maxilla as far superior as the inferior orbital rim. However, when bicoronal and eyelid incisions are used, intraoral incisions are rarely required. A buccal sulcus incision is used to perform osteotomies and introduce bone grafts and can be extended as far as the second premolar. Subperiosteal stripping can be extended posterolaterally as far as the pterygoid plates and superiorly as far as the inferior orbital rim, respecting the inferior orbital nerve. The nerve lies 7 mm inferior to the rim on a sagittal plane with the medial limbus of the eye. Dissection over and around the piriform aperture can be performed with an elevator if exposure of the

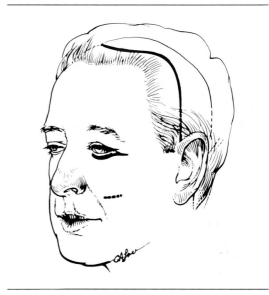

*Figure 6-11* Various craniofacial incisions: bicoronal, eyelid, and buccal sulcus. (From J. G. McCarthy (ed.). Plastic Surgery. Philadelphia: Saunders, 1990.)

nasal floor and walls is desired. The mucosa of the lateral wall and floor of the nose and mucoperichondrium of the septum can also be reflected with an elevator.

## Bone Grafts

### RIB

The rib graft is best used for correction of a contour deformity of the cranium, orbit, forehead, and zygoma. The incision for the harvesting of a rib graft is best made in the inframammary crease in females and along a line oblique and anterior to the posterior axillary line in males. The pectoralis, serratus, and rectus muscles are dissected bluntly off the chest wall. Through a relatively short incision, appropriately retracted, as many as four ribs can be removed: two sets of adjacent ribs with an intervening rib intact. Subperiosteal stripping of the entire rib from the costochondral junction to the posterior angle is facilitated by a periosteal elevator. If the parietal pleura is entered inadvertently, a red rubber catheter can be placed intrapleurally to evacuate the chest, the chest wounds closed in layers, and the catheter removed after several hyperinflations of the lungs by the anesthesiologist. Closed suction drainage facilitates wound closure.

The ribs are split with a straight osteotome to increase bone graft stock and increase cancellous exposure for greater graft survival.

### ILIUM

The ilium is the preferred donor site for grafting of the nasal dorsum and for harvesting large amounts of cancellous and cortical bone graft. The skin incision is placed well posterior to the crest to camouflage the resulting scar. The periosteum of the iliac crest is stripped over the inner and outer surfaces. To prevent a depressed hip deformity, the osteotomy begins on the inner surface below the crest. If inadvertent fracture of the crest occurs, it is repaired with wire prior to closure. Full-thickness or partial-thickness removal of bone can proceed, remaining posterior to the anterior iliac spine to avoid injury to the lateral femoral cutaneous nerve. Bone harvesting must not proceed too deeply, as the body of the ilium forms part of the acetabulum and greater sciatic notch. Repositioning of the periosteum over the crest is performed with closure. Closed suction drainage is advised.

The ilium can also be harvested and transferred as part of a flap based on the deep circumflex iliac vessels.

### CALVARIUM

The calvarium is the preferred donor site for reconstruction of calvarial, orbital, and zygomatic defects. If full-thickness calvarial bone has been harvested by the neurosurgeon, the inner and outer tables can be split with a sagittal saw and a sharp, curved osteotome. The preferred donor site for calvarial grafts is the parietal bone at a position posterior to the coronal suture and lateral to the midline. Split-thickness (in situ) harvesting can be facilitated by a high-speed burr. The outer table graft is outlined and scored to bleeding cancellous bone. Harvesting is performed with a large, curved osteotome. Bone wax facilitates hemostasis. No drains are necessary. Finally, a calvarial bone flap, based on the superficial temporal vessels, is especially indicated for onlay restoration of zygomatic defects where there is insufficient or irradiated overlying soft tissue.

## Canthopexies

### MEDIAL CANTHOPEXY

If the medial canthal tendon has been detached, transnasal medial canthopexy must be performed or telecanthus can result. After braided wire loops (transnasal) have isolated the medial canthal tendon, the loops can be wired tightly together through burr holes placed bilaterally at the posterosuperior aspect of the lacrimal groove [93] (Fig. 6-12). This maneuver provides nasoorbital sulcus depth and definition. Transnasal passage of the wires is performed with either a 16-gauge spinal needle or an awl.

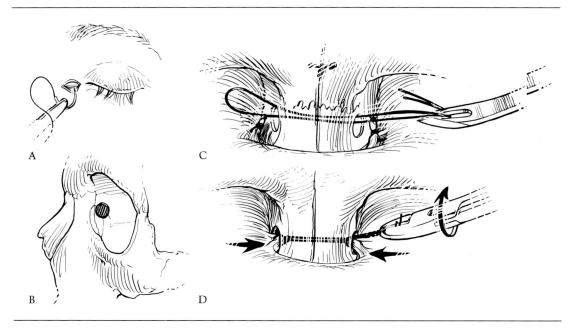

**Figure 6-12** *Medial canthopexy. A. Medial canthal tendon is identified by a small incision, and the tendon is labeled with a suture (Munro). B. Bony fenestration is made superior and well posterior to the lacrimal groove. C,D. Transnasal wire is sutured to both tendons and twisted under direct vision (on both sides). Note that the tendon is drawn into the bony fenestration. (From B. M. Zide and J. G. McCarthy. The medial canthus revisited—an anatomical basis for canthopexy.* Ann. Plast. Surg. *11:1, 1983.)*

## LATERAL CANTHOPEXY

Lateral canthopexy is often indicated to prevent lateral canthal drift and canthal dystopia. After subperiosteal identification and fixation of the lateral canthal mechanism with a braided wire suture, a small drill hole is placed in the lateral orbital wall at the level of Whitnall's tubercle, and the braided suture is fixed at the site (Fig. 6-13). The eyes are opened at this time, and the surgeon continually monitors the lower lid margin in relation to the inferior limbus for accurate and symmetric canthopexy. In the supine position it is best to achieve a lower eyelid (margin) height approximately 2 to 3 mm above the inferior limbus [43].

## Orbital Hypertelorism

Orbital hypertelorism is defined as an increased distance between the medial orbital walls. The distinction with telecanthus is fundamental, as telecanthus is an increased distance between the medial canthi (Fig. 6-14). The diagnosis is confirmed by an increased distance between the medial orbital walls on a posteroanterior cephalogram. Seventy percent of the adult interorbital distance (IOD) is attained by the age of 2 years [39]. The mean normal value ranges from 15 mm at birth to 23 mm at the age of 12 years [13]. The normal adult IOD is 23 to 28 mm (slightly less for women than for men).

Orbital hypertelorism is a physical finding (see Fig. 6-14), not a syndrome. It is usually secondary to a primary deformity, such as severe orbitofacial clefting, craniosynostosis, anterior encephaloceles and dermoids, or frontonasal dysplasia [82]. Tessier has classified hypertelorism into three types according to the IOD: type I, 30 to 34 mm; type II, 35 to 39 mm; type III, 40 mm or more [81]. In most cases there is a low-lying cribriform plate with a crista galli (duplicated or absent) and the optic canals are usually a normal

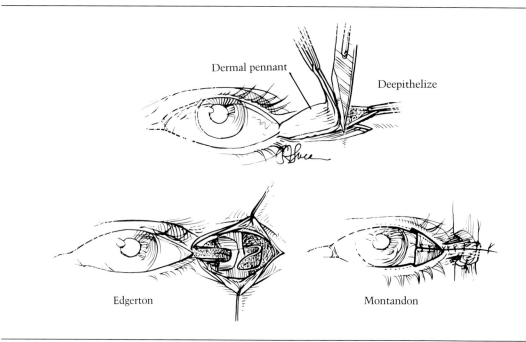

Dermal pennant

Deepithelize

Edgerton

Montandon

*Figure 6-13* *Lateral canthopexy. (From J. G. McCarthy (ed.).* Plastic Surgery. *Philadelphia: Saunders, 1990.)*

distance apart. The principal anatomic abnormality is horizontal widening of the ethmoid sinus, usually not affecting the posterior air cells or the sphenoid sinus [10]. The nasoorbital area is thickened and occasionally bifid. The medial orbital walls vary in configuration and shape, a property that influences the efficacy of the orbital translocation [63].

SURGERY
The major breakthrough in the surgical correction of orbital hypertelorism was made by Tessier and associates [86] when they recognized that a combined cranial and facial ("craniofacial") surgical approach was essential to ensure the safety and efficacy of the orbital translocation. They emphasized that the "functional orbital volume" (that portion of the orbit from the rims to a point posterior to the equator of the globe) must be mobilized to ensure secondary movement of the globes [86]. The original Tessier procedure was performed in two stages, but Converse and associates [10] developed a one-

stage procedure with osteotomies similar to those of Tessier, except that the cribriform plate and olfactory apparatus were preserved. Long-term studies demonstrated little change in gustatory or olfactory function following correction of orbital hypertelorism by the Converse technique [50].

EXTRACRANIAL APPROACH
When the cribriform plate is high and there is no associated frontal deformity, the infrabasal U osteotomy [85] is an effective technique for correcting orbital hypertelorism (Fig. 6-15). The procedure is somewhat similar to a Le Fort III osteotomy (mobilizing the medial orbital wall, floor, and lateral wall medially) and can be accomplished via a bicoronal or midline nasal approach.

INTRACRANIAL APPROACH
The intracranial approach is the most radical but is also the safest and most effective.

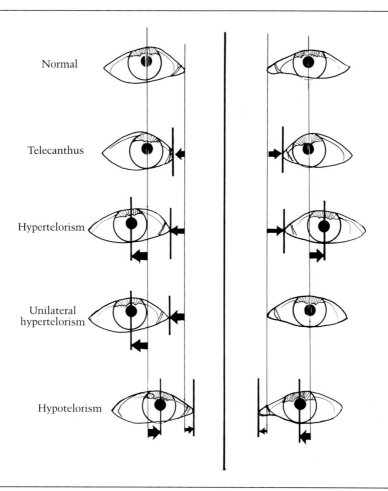

**Figure 6-14** *Comparison of normal and pathologic orbital anatomy. With telecanthus only the medial orbital walls are displaced laterally but the globes are in normal position. With orbital hypertelorism the entire (circumferential) orbits and globes are displaced laterally. The opposite is true for hypotelorism. The vertical lines designate the medial orbital walls (inner) and pupillary planes (outer). (Redrawn from M. H. Becker and J. G. McCarthy. Congenital Abnormalities. In C. Gonzalez, M. H. Becker, and J. Flanagan, (eds.),* Diagnostic Imaging in Ophthalmology. *New York: Springer-Verlag, 1984.)*

After exposure of the anterior cranial fossa by the neurosurgeon with preservation of a frontal bar, the plastic surgeon mobilizes the periorbita and the orbital contents in a subperiosteal plane (see Bicoronal Approach). The periorbita is freed in a circumferential fashion from the orbital roof, the medial and lateral walls, and the floor of the orbit as far posteriorly as the junction of the middle and posterior thirds. The medial canthal tendon is detached along the medial orbital wall, and the lacrimal sac is raised from the lacrimal groove, preserving nasolacrimal duct continuity. Subperiosteal dissection continues over the anterior maxilla, respecting the infraorbital nerves. Subciliary or transcon-

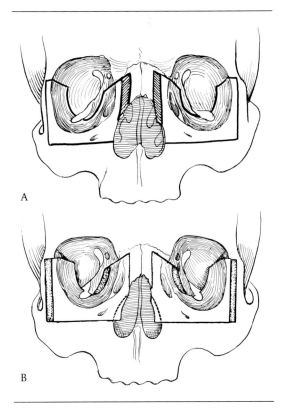

A

B

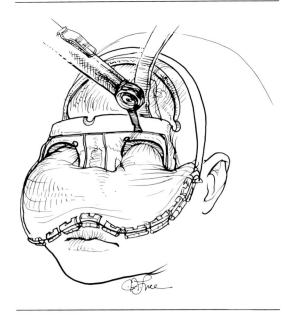

**Figure 6-16** *Supraorbital osteotomy is made inferior and parallel to the frontal bone flap osteotomy.*

**Figure 6-15** *Subcranial approach. A. Lines of osteotomy (U-shaped) and the paramedian bony resection. B. Mobilized orbits with bone grafts. (From J. M. Converse et al. Craniofacial surgery. Clin. Plast. Surg. 1:499, 1974.)*

junctival incisions can be used to facilitate anterior maxillary exposure for the transverse maxillary osteotomy. When there is excess nasal soft tissue or when exposure is required for correction of a bifid, foreshortened, or asymmetric nose, a midline incision along the dorsum to the nasal tip may be necessary.

The first osteotomy is in the supraorbital region along a line inferior and parallel to the neurosurgeon's craniotomy line. It is designed to preserve a frontal bar for stability and to allow horizontal orbital translocation (Fig. 6-16). The supraorbital osteotomy line, made with a mechanical saw approximately 1 cm above the roofs of the orbits, extends

above the lateral orbital wall; medially it joins the vertical osteotomies through the bone of the widened interorbital area. The latter osteotomies make possible resection of a measured section of bone either as a single median segment (Fig. 6-17) or as two paramedian segments. The latter technique also allows a solid recipient site for a nasal dorsal bone graft.

After medial ethmoidectomy (Fig. 6-18), which can be performed through either single midline (Tessier) [86] or paramedian (Converse) [10] osteotomies, and after vertical osteotomy of the lateral wall and malar bone, the orbital floor osteotomy and transmaxillary osteotomies are carried out. The transmaxillary osteotomy extends from the lateral aperture of the nose, below the infraorbital nerve, to join the lateral orbital osteotomy in the body of the zygoma (Fig. 6-19). For the most part, the lines of osteotomy are made with a mechanical saw, but the medial extension is usually completed with an osteotomy driven by a mallet.

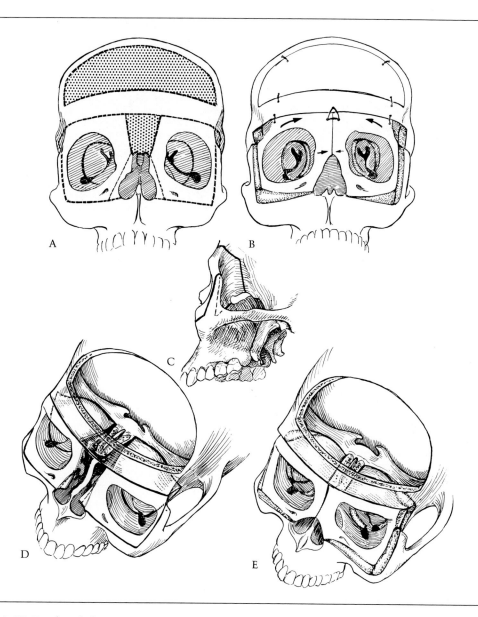

**Figure 6-17** *Total mobilization of the lateral orbital wall (after Tessier). A. Lines of osteotomy. Note the single median segment to be resected. B. After translocation of the orbits and bone grafting. C. Lateral orbital rim only (zygoma) has been osteotomized. The remainder of the lateral wall is mobilized after the indicated osteotomies have been performed. D. Technique of preservation of the cribriform plate. (From J. M. Converse (ed.).* Plastic Reconstructive Surgery. *Philadelphia: Saunders, 1977.) E. Bone grafting of the lateral orbital wall and anterior aspect of the maxilla.*

The predetermined measured segment(s) of bone can then be resected, exposing the interorbital space. The enlarged ethmoid air cells are exenterated on each side. If the septum is bifid, the skeletal framework is resected and the continuity of the mucosal lining with the cribriform plate is preserved to prevent interruption of olfaction.

A transverse line of osteotomy is extended across the roof of the orbit and through the

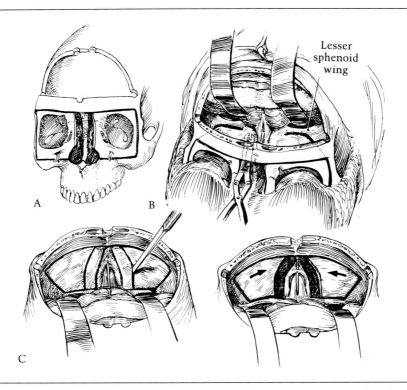

**Figure 6-18** *A. Resection of a median segment from the anterior wall of the interorbital space. The ethmoid cells and intranasal structures are exenterated. B. Osteotomies of the anterior cranial vault with preservation of the cribriform plate and bony resection along each side of the cribriform plate to permit orbital translocation without impinging on the olfactory nerves. C. The shape of the segments of bone resected from the anterior cranial fossa varies, depending on the type of translocation required to correct the deformity. (From J. M. Converse et al. Craniofacial surgery. Clin. Plast. Surg. 1:499, 1974.)*

medial wall of the orbit, remaining at least 10 mm anterior to the optic nerve (Fig. 6-20). It also passes across the floor of the orbit and joins the osteotomy through the lateral orbital wall. The orbital roof osteotomy stops at the cribriform plate. An area of bone forming the floor of the anterior cranial fossa, anterior and lateral to the cribriform plate, is outlined by the osteotomies and is resected. Osteotomies are facilitated with a fine, tapered osteotome and a right-angled oscillating saw.

At this point in the operation the completeness of the osteotomies is verified, and the sectioned orbit should be easily movable. If not, inadequate osteotomy of the thick frontal process of the maxilla or enlarged middle and inferior turbinates may be suspected. After translocation of the orbits, interosseous wiring (26-gauge stainless steel) is established between the mobilized orbits. The frontal bar ensures adequate stabilization. Interosseous wire or miniplate fixation is established at the junction of the frontal bar and medial walls of the mobilized segments. Bone grafts are wedged into the gap in the lateral orbital wall and the zygoma and are wired into place to maintain the medial position of the orbits. Bone grafts are placed along the anterior maxilla. The frontal bone flap is wired in place after the dura is checked for tears.

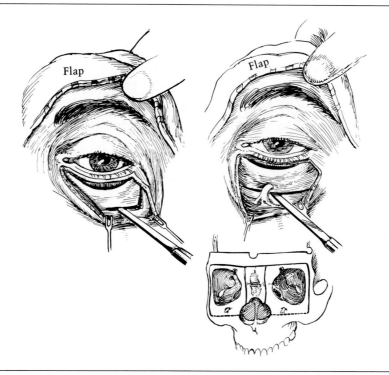

**Figure 6-19** *Infraorbital osteotomy through the anterior wall of the maxilla. (From J. M. Converse et al. Craniofacial surgery.* Clin. Plast. Surg. *1:499, 1974.)*

The canthal wires are placed in position through sufficiently wide drill holes placed high and posterior to the lacrimal groove on the medial orbital walls [93] (see Medial Canthopexy, above). The medial canthal tendons are inserted in the drill holes and secured by means of transnasal 28-gauge stainless steel wires.

Excess nasoglabellar soft tissue occasionally needs to be resected in a figure-of-eight fashion. In the bifid nose a bone graft is placed over the bony dorsum and its distal end secured under the reconstructed alar domes. The bone graft, which extends into the tip of the nose, is secured by transnasal wiring or miniplate or lag screw fixation. The nose can be lengthened by either a V-Y advancement or a Z-plasty performed in the region of the nasofrontal angle.

The lateral canthi may also be suspended by means of permanent sutures passed through each lateral canthal mechanism and anchored to holes drilled high on the lateral orbital rims (see Lateral Canthopexy, above).

The temporalis muscles are advanced and secured to the lateral orbital wall to prevent the hourglass deformity. Scalp closure is facilitated by a running nylon suture. The various cutaneous incisions are coapted. A dressing is applied with fluffed gauze under a meshed, light elastic dressing. The patient is awakened, and visual acuity is confirmed when the patient is awake.

COMPLICATIONS
*Anesthesia*
Anesthesia complications are basically related to inexperience with the procedure. Hypotensive anesthesia reduces fluid and blood replacement. Inability to shrink the

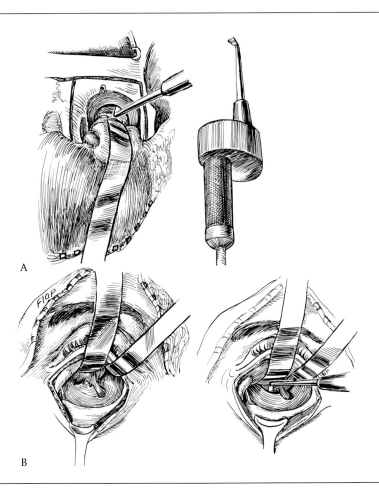

A

B

**Figure 6-20** *A. Osteotomy of the orbital roof and the posterior portion of the lateral wall. B. The orbital floor is sectioned on each side of the inferior orbital fissure with a right-angled oscillating saw. (From J. M. Converse et al. Craniofacial surgery.* Clin. Plast. Surg. *1:499, 1974.)*

brain completely to allow safe retraction of the frontal lobes is prevented by spinal drainage, hyperventilation, and administration of steroids.

*Neurosurgical Problems*
Intracranial anomalies are the rule. Care must be exercised when opening the cranial vault over the sagittal sinus. Failure to repair dural tears may cause a postoperative cerebrospinal fluid (CSF) leak (which is best treated by continuous external lumbar drainage until it stops spontaneously). Seizures, prolonged cerebral edema, and epidural hematoma have also been noted after intracranial hypertelorism correction [9].

*Reconstructive Problems*
Relapse was noted both clinically and radiographically in only 3 of 22 hypertelorism corrections in one longitudinal cephalometric study [53]. Two of the three patients were less than 5 years old. A remarkable degree of orbital stability was demonstrated despite moderate overcorrection (2–3 mm less than age-related IOD). Technical causes for relapse include inadequate exenteration of the

nasoethmoid complex (i.e., superior turbinates, ethmoid sinuses, or duplicated nasal septum) and failure to translocate the functional orbital volume [81]. Mulliken and associates have noted a high relapse rate in patients undergoing correction for second- and third-degree hypertelorism [60].

Tulasne surveyed eight growing patients 4 to 11 years of age operated on by Tessier and noted no adverse effect on maxillary growth despite hypertelorism correction [87]. In a similar study, McCarthy and associates failed to detect evidence of underdevelopment of the nasomaxillary complex after hypertelorism correction in the growing child unless there was an associated cleft palate or orbitofacial cleft [53].

Canthal drift is prevented by effective medial canthopexy [93]. It must not be confused with orbital (skeletal) relapse or relative soft tissue excess in the transverse axis of the nose resulting from resorption of the nasal bone graft [60]. Tessier has also reported hypertelorism correction without canthal tendon detachment [84].

### General Problems

A review of 793 patients, half of whom were under 4 years of age, who underwent craniofacial surgical procedures revealed 13 deaths (1.6 percent) [90]. Sepsis, airway mismanagement, neurosurgical complications, and inadequate blood replacement accounted for the deaths. The infection rate was 6.2 percent following intracranial procedures. Two patients reported decreased visual acuity, one permanent unilateral and one transient bilateral. CSF leakage occurred after 4.5 percent of intracranial procedures. Other complications included loss of bone grafts, ectropion, ptosis, nasolacrimal obstruction, and bone graft donor site morbidity (pneumothorax, contour irregularity, pain).

A review of 170 transcranial procedures revealed a comparable overall postoperative infection rate of 6.5 percent, with the infection rate in adults (23.5 percent) being much higher than in children (2.2 percent) [15].

Tracheostomy, residual frontal extradural deadspace, and lengthy operating time are factors contributing to the increased infection rate in adults.

In a series of 1092 patients, four cases of blindness (three temporary) were reported after craniofacial procedures [65].

## Orbital Hypotelorism

Orbital hypotelorism is defined as a decreased distance between the medial orbital wall (IOD) [8]. It is found in a variety of uncommon anomalies.

*1. Trigonocephaly:* a congenital cranial anomaly characterized by a small, pointed forehead. It has been attributed to premature closure of the metopic suture (see Fig. 6-29).

*2. Arhinencephaly:* a complex of faciocerebral malformations in which the olfactory nerves or other parts of the rhinencephalon ("nose-brain") are absent bilaterally (Fig. 6-21). It may be associated with midline or lateral clefts of the upper lip. Variants include (1) *cebocephaly*, in which there is a hypoplastic nose with a single nostril and without a septum or columella; (2) *ethmocephaly*, a more severe form with accompanying microcephaly and a penis-like proboscis; (3) *cyclopia*, the most extreme variant characterized by holoprosencephaly, a supraorbital proboscis, and a single or partly divided eye in a single orbit. Survival of any of these infants is rare [8].

*3. Binder's syndrome:* Binder described a syndrome of nasomaxillary dysostosis with orbital hypotelorism that is thought to be a variant of arhinencephaly [5]. The maxillary deformity consists of a deficient alveolar bone that slopes into a centrally excavated prenasal fossa. The anterior nasal spine is usually small and positioned on a lower, more posterior level. The maxillary hypoplasia extends radially from the anterior alveolar process to involve the frontal process and infraorbital margin [31]. Typical facial features include a dishface anomaly with a flat,

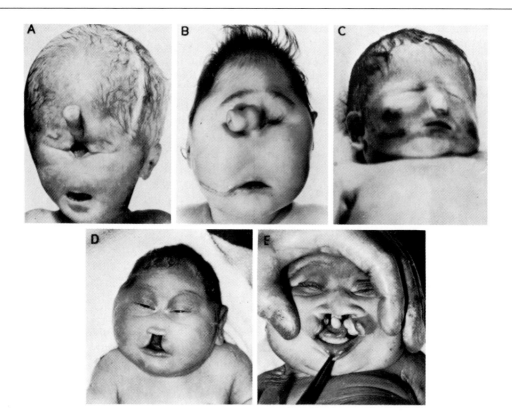

retruded nose (Fig. 6-22). Maxillary retrusion associated with a class III malocclusion occurs in one-half of the patients [31].

Treatment options depend on the severity of the syndrome and include septal advancement, a nasal L-shaped bone graft, onlay cartilage and bone grafts on the maxilla, and Le Fort I and II advancement osteotomies [32].

The correction of orbital hypotelorism follows the osteotomies used for hypertelorism, except bone is excised laterally, and the orbits are translocated laterally. The nasofrontal area is then filled with bone grafts [8].

### Orbital Dystopia

Vertical orbital dystopia can be defined as that condition in which one globe is located higher or lower than the other in the vertical

**Figure 6-21** *Spectrum of facies associated with holoprosencephaly-arhinencephaly. A. Cyclopia. B. Ethmocephaly. C. Cebocephaly. D. Orbital hypotelorism with medial cleft lip. E. Orbital hypotelorism with hypoplastic intermaxillary segment. (A is from E. L. Potter. Pathology of the Fetus and the Infant (2nd ed.). Chicago: Year Book, 1961; B–E are from W. DeMyer. Prenatal and Developmental Defects. In H. Barnett and A. Einhorn (eds.), Pediatrics (15th ed.). New York: Appleton-Century-Crofts, 1972.)*

plane. The skeletal pathology can vary from inferior displacement of the orbital floor and zygoma to a circumferential (360 degrees) lowering of the entire orbit (Fig. 6-23).

In a series of patients with vertical orbital dystopia, the etiology was as follows: 62 percent congenital (craniosynostosis, craniofacial microsomia, orbitofacial clefts, hypoplasia of the sphenoid); 26 percent posttraumatic (fractures and irradiation therapy in

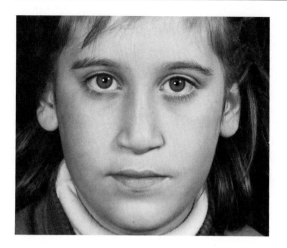
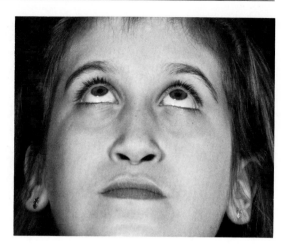

**Figure 6-22** Binder's syndrome. Note the retruded nose, hypoplastic mid-face, and acute nasolabial angle.

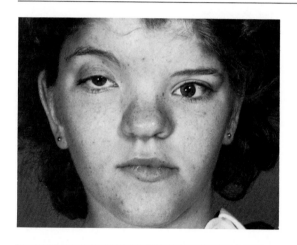
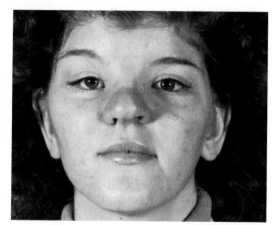

**Figure 6-23** Orbital dystopia of the congenital type (craniofacial clefting) corrected by lowering the right orbit. (From J. G. McCarthy (ed.). Plastic Surgery. Philadelphia: Saunders, 1989.)

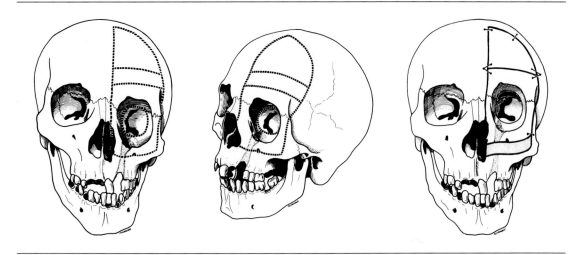

**Figure 6-24** *Correction of orbital dystopia.* Left. *Lines of osteotomy.* Center. *Note the osteotomy rectangle in the frontal bone.* Right. *After vertical mobilization of the orbit. The frontal bone segment has been placed in the maxillary defect. (Courtesy of Dr. P. Tessier.)*

children); 12 percent neoplastic (fibrous dysplasia, carcinoma of the maxillary antrum, intracranial lesions, neurofibromatoses); and miscellaneous (Romberg's disease) [18].

It must be emphasized that some patients can tolerate a severe degree of vertical dystopia and be free of diplopia, but the latter becomes apparent only after surgical transposition of the orbit. In general, surgical positioning of the globe in the *vertical* dimension produces visual disturbances much more commonly than in the *horizontal* dimension (e.g., correction of orbital hypertelorism).

## PREOPERATIVE EVALUATION

A complete ophthalmologic assessment is done that includes strabismus testing. Three-dimensional CT provides the best definition of the skeletal pathology. The scan is especially helpful for determining whether a *partial* or *subtotal* osteotomy/mobilization of the orbit is indicated.

## SURGICAL TREATMENT

A technique of *partial* osteotomy/mobilization of the zygoma-orbit was described for treatment of the malunited zygomaticoorbital complex and enophthalmos [36]. Mobilization of the osteotomized segment in

a superomedial direction also elevates the globe.

The *subtotal* osteotomy/mobilization of the orbit was described by Tessier [76] and involves movement of the circumferential orbit (360 degrees); the nasolacrimal apparatus, orbital apex, and optic stalk are spared. With this technique (Fig. 6-24) a limited anterior or frontal craniotomy provides exposure of the anterior cranial fossa to allow osteotomies of the orbital roof. A segment of bone (Fig. 6-24) is removed from the frontal bone, and the height (in millimeters) of this resection determines the amount of superior mobilization of the orbit. The remaining osteotomies are similar to those employed for correction of orbital hypertelorism: medial and lateral walls and floor of the orbit, zygoma, and anterior wall of the maxilla. The osteotomized orbital segment is translocated superiorly and the segment is placed in the resulting bony void in the anterior wall of the maxilla. The frontal bone flap is replaced, and all segments are secured

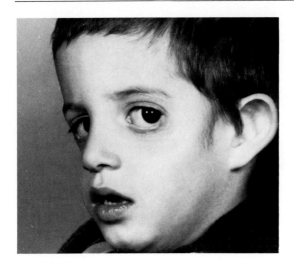 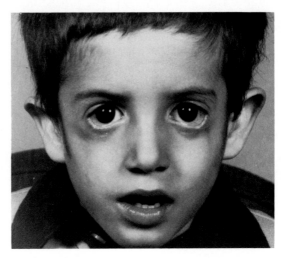

**Figure 6-25** *Treacher Collins syndrome. Note the colabomas, deficient zygomatic complexes, retruded chin, and abnormal sideburns.*

with miniplate fixation or interosseous wires. A medial canthopexy is usually indicated.

## Treacher Collins Syndrome

Mandibulofacial dysostosis, or Treacher Collins syndrome (Fig. 6-25), is an inherited condition characterized by hypoplasia and clefting of the orbitozygomatic complexes, antimongoloid slant of the palpebral fissures, eyelid colobomas, absence of the eyelashes in the medial third of the lower eyelids, malformations of the external ear, and tongue-shaped sideburns. Other malformations include macrostomia and a high, arched palate. Additional skeletal deformities include a short, acutely angled anterior cranial base, loss of the nasofrontal angle, and a short, obtusely angled mandible with an antegonial notch.

A review of three-dimensional CT scans in 14 Treacher Collins patients also revealed the following: partial to complete aplasia of the zygomatic process of the temporal bone, mild hypoplasia to aplasia of the frontal process of the zygoma, antimongoloid slant of the transverse orbital axis, and hypoplasia of the medial pterygoid plates and muscles. Asymmetry characterized all patients. The mandible was variably dysmorphic, ranging from normal to severe asymmetric dysplasia [49].

The treatment of mandibulofacial dysostosis is surgical, and the treatment design depends on the extent of the individual deformities. A series of reconstructive surgical procedures must usually be undertaken, some during childhood (e.g., augmentation of the malar region, eyelid reconstruction, and ear reconstruction), whereas others can be deferred to later in childhood or adolescence (corrective rhinoplasty, mandibular osteotomy, or genioplasty).

ZYGOMATICOMAXILLARY COMPLEX
Although many authors have recommended use of a variety of synthetic materials in the augmentation of the deficient zygomaticomaxillary complex, we prefer autogenous bone [44]. Our currently favored approach is a bicoronal scalp incision complemented by lower eyelid incisions. After the defect is defined, a vascularized calvarial bone flap is used to augment the deficient zygoma and

orbital rim (Fig. 6-26) [51]. The procedure is completed with a lateral canthopexy and a transposition flap of skin and orbicularis muscle from the upper to the lower eyelid.

MANDIBULAR HYPOPLASIA

Depending on the growth of the patient's mandible and the development of satisfactory dental occlusion, a horizontal advancement osteotomy of the mandible (genioplasty) (Fig. 6-27) with or without bone grafting is often required to achieve a satisfactory chin contour. It has been the author's experience that the majority of patients with mandibulofacial dystosis have an acceptable occlusion, and advancement osteotomy of the entire mandible is not indicated. If there is true retrognathia, the mandible can be advanced forward and rotated upward by a sagittal split osteotomy via the intraoral route (Fig. 6-28).

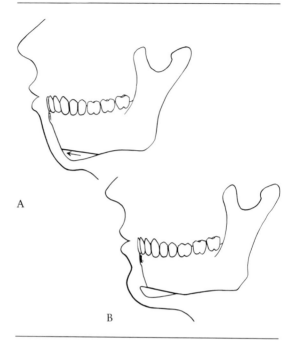

**Figure 6-27** *Horizontal osteotomy of the anteroinferior border of the mandible (genioplasty). A. Line of osteotomy. B. Following advancement.*

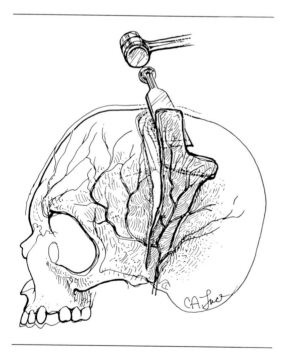

**Figure 6-26** *Vascularized calvarial bone flap for reconstruction of the deficient zygomatic complex. (From J. G. McCarthy and B. M. Zide. The spectrum of calvarial bone grafting: Introduction of the vascularized calvarial bone flap. Plast. Reconstr. Surg. 62:235, 1984.)*

**Figure 6-28** *Mandibular advancement (sagittal split or ramisection). A. An incision is made along the anterior border of the ramus following the oblique line. B. Subperiosteal elevation of both the medial and lateral surface is begun. C. The medial cortical osteotomy is placed above the level of the mandibular foramen and is continued anteriorly along the oblique line. D. Bone can be removed from the medial aspect of the anterior aspect of the ramus to permit a better view of the lingula and the mandibular foramen region. The Lindemann spiral burr or reciprocating saw cuts the medial cortex above the foramen. E. The medial section of the cortex is completed. F. A vertical cut through the lateral cortex in the region of the second molar tooth is made with a small round burr. G. The cortical line of section is indicated by the broken line over the medial aspect of the ramus and along the anterior border. The solid line represents the vertical cut through the lateral cortex of the body of the mandible. (From J. M. Converse (ed.). Reconstructive Plastic Surgery. Philadelphia: Saunders, 1977.)*

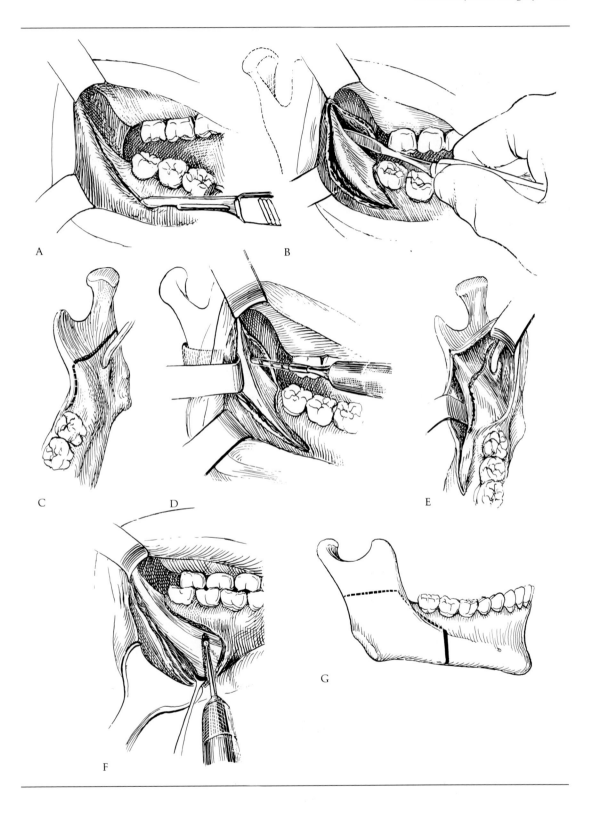

A

B

C

D

E

F

G

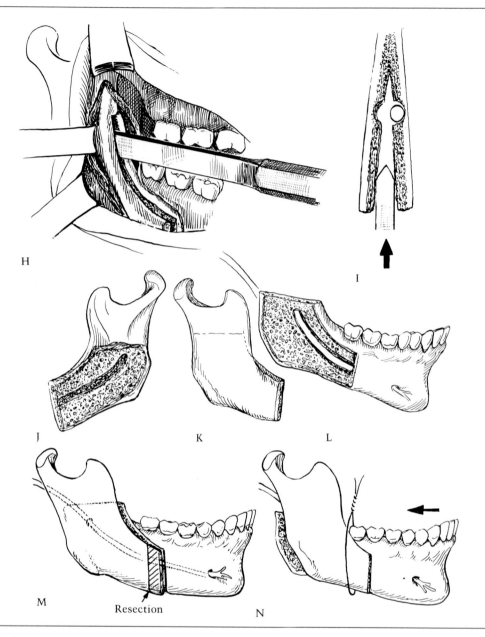

**Figure 6-28** *(continued)H. The sagittal splitting of the ramus is performed with a thick osteotome. I. The thick osteotome also acts as a wedge as it splits the ramus. J. View of the medial aspect of the lateral (condylar) fragment. K. The lateral aspect of the lateral (condylar) fragment. L. The medial (tooth-bearing) fragment. M. Excess bone (shaded area) must be resected from the anterior portion of the lateral fragment to allow for bony apposition after posterior displacement of the tooth-bearing fragment. N. Final position of the tooth-bearing portion of the mandible. A buried circumferential wire around the fragments or an interosseous wire is placed to approximate the fragments. Although not illustrated, the technique can be employed for mandibular advancement. (From R. Travner and H.L. Obwegeser. The surgical correction of manibular prognothism and retrognothism with consideration of genioplasty. I. Surgical procedures to correct mandibular prognothism and reshaping of the chin.* Oral Surg. *10:677, 1957.)*

NASAL DEFORMITIES

The nose of a patient with mandibulofacial dysostosis is frequently malformed, with a minimal or oblique nasofrontal angle, convexity of the nasal dorsum, and a depressed nasal tip. This combination gives the patient a fishlike profile when combined with other physical defects. The patients benefit from a rhinoplasty with or without a septoplasty.

EYELID DEFORMITIES

The lower eyelid deformity (coloboma) is characterized by shortage of skin, tarsus, and conjunctiva—therefore a full-thickness deformity. Correction of the deformity is usually best done at the same time as augmentation of the hypoplastic zygomaticomaxillary skeletal complex. A transposition flap of skin and orbicularis muscle from the upper to the lower lid is the preferred technique.

## Craniosynostosis

Craniosynostosis is a term that designates premature fusion of one or more sutures in either the cranial vault or the cranial base; the synostosis can occur either in an isolated fashion or as part of a syndrome [28]. Most cases of *isolated craniosynostosis* are sporadic, although there have been reported examples of autosomal dominant and autosomal recessive inheritance. In the familial cases the same suture or different sutures may be involved. The *craniofacial synostosis syndromes* share common features, such as suture synostoses, mid-face hypoplasia, abnormal facies, and limb abnormalities. Cohen has classified the craniosynostosis syndromes into types according to overall clinical similarity and genetic considerations [7]. The most common are Crouzon disease, Apert syndrome, Pfeiffer syndrome, Saethre-Chotzen syndrome, Carpenter syndrome, and kleeblattschädel anomaly. The mode of inheritance is usually autosomal dominant.

MORPHOLOGIC ASPECTS

*Isolated craniosynostosis*

There are several forms of isolated craniosynostosis (Fig. 6-29).

SCAPHOCEPHALY. Premature fusion of the sagittal suture is characterized by a narrow, elongated cranial vault and reduced bitemporal dimension. Scaphocephaly, the most common of the isolated suture synostoses, is usually nonfamilial and occurs predominantly in males [74].

TRIGONOCEPHALY. Premature fusion of the metopic suture (trigonocephaly) is characterized by a triangular forehead resembling a midline keel [48]. Orbital hypotelorism is usually associated.

BRACHYCEPHALY. Premature fusion of both coronal sutures (brachycephaly) is associated with a reduction of the anteroposterior dimension of the cranial vault and a compensatory increase in the bitemporal distance. A mild degree of exorbitism can be observed if the supraorbital rim is recessed. Underdevelopment of the mid-face is unusual.

PLAGIOCEPHALY. Premature fusion of one coronal suture (plagiocephaly) is associated with unilateral flattening of the forehead and recession and elevation of the brow. Frontal bossing, orbital dystopia, and occipital bulging occur on the opposite side. The nose and ear deviate to the affected side. There can be an associated lambdoid synostosis.

ACROCEPHALY (TURRICEPHALY). Multiple premature suture fusion (acrocephaly) in addition to bicoronal synostoses can result in an excess of skull height with vertical elongation of the forehead ("tower skull").

OXYCEPHALY. Multiple premature suture fusion (oxycephaly) is characterized by a retroverted forehead, tilted posteroinferiorly on a plane parallel with the nasal dorsum. The forehead, usually reduced in the horizontal dimension, is capped by an elevation in the region of the anterior fontanel.

KLEEBLATTSCHÄDEL ANOMALY. The kleeblattschädel anomaly is a three-lobed "clo-

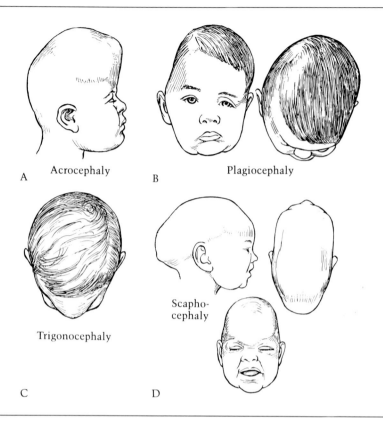

A   Acrocephaly

B   Plagiocephaly

Trigonocephaly

Scapho-cephaly

C

D

**Figure 6-29** *Skull deformities associated with craniosynostosis. A. Acrocephaly (turricephaly). B. Plagiocephaly. C. Trigonocephaly. D. Saphocephaly. (From J. M. Converse (ed.). *Reconstructive Plastic Surgery. *Philadelphia: Saunders, 1977.)*

verleaf" skull with bitemporal and vertex bulging. The spectrum of suture synostosis is wide, and newborns with the deformity may also show no evidence of sutural synostosis.

### Craniosynostosis Syndromes

CROUZON'S DISEASE. Described by a French neurologist in 1912, Crouzon's disease is characterized by craniosynostosis and a frog-like facies [12] (Fig. 6-30). In any large series of patients with Crouzon's disease, there is no regular pattern of the calvarial deformity; scaphocephaly, trigonocephaly, or oxycephaly may be present, depending on the site of the cranial suture synostosis [38]. The coronal, sagittal, and lambdoid sutures have all been found prematurely synostosed on radiographic study. The facial deformity consists of maxillary or mid-face hypoplasia and exorbitism as well as nystagmus, stra-

bismus, and hypertelorism. The pattern of inheritance is autosomal dominant with near-complete penetrance. Cranial vault and orbital anomalies, which reflect an elevated intracranial pressure, include a depressed sphenoid bone, a foreshortened anterior cranial fossa, and expanded and anteroinferiorly displaced middle cranial fossa, and a shallow orbit with marked reduction in the functional orbital volume. The maxillary hypoplasia is reflected in the shallowness of the orbital floor, the narrowness of the upper dental arch, bilateral crossbite, crowded dentition, a high and transversely compressed palate, compression of the zygomatic arch,

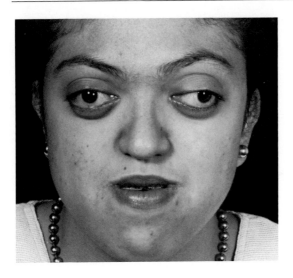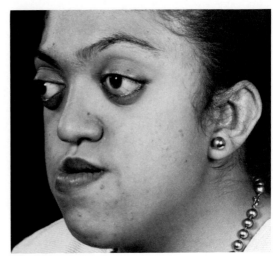

**Figure 6-30** *Crouzon's disease. Note the exorbitism, exotropian, and midface hypoplasia.*

and severe narrowing of the pterygomaxillary fossa. The chin is usually underdeveloped. Hypoplasia of the zygoma is variable.

APERT SYNDROME. The presence of syndactyly helps to distinguish Crouzon's disease from Apert syndrome (acrocephalosyndactyly) [4] (Fig. 6-31). It is autosomal dominant in inheritance. The Apert syndrome during childhood is characterized by craniosynostosis, exorbitism, mid-face hypoplasia, symmetric syndactyly of both hands and feet, and other axial skeletal deformities. In contrast to Crouzon's disease, the sutural synostosis in Apert syndrome is usually simple (coronal). There are also other findings more characteristic of the patient with Apert syndrome: acne, submucous clefts hidden in the arched palate, anterior open bite with crossbowing of the upper lip, oculomotor paralysis, asymmetry of the exorbitism, ptosis, overhanging of the upper frontal area with a transverse frontal skin furrow, and enlargement of the ear lobes [79, 80]. The usual hand deformity is a symmetric complex syndactyly consisting of bony fusion of the second, third, and fourth fingers with a single common nail.

PFEIFFER SYNDROME. Autosomal dominant in transmission, the pathognomonic findings in the craniosynostosis known as Pfeiffer syndrome are enlarged thumbs and great toes, in addition to exorbitism (variable) and mid-face hypoplasia [70]. The patients can have the same ocular and oral findings as previously described for the patient with Crouzon's disease or Apert syndrome.

SAETHRE-CHOTZEN SYNDROME. Described independently by Saethre and Chotzen, the syndrome that carries their names is transmitted in autosomal dominant fashion with full penetrance [6, 73]. Affected individuals show craniosynostosis, low hairline, ptosis, deviated nasal septum, and brachydactyly. Mild exorbitism is associated with retrusion of the brow or supraorbital rim. Maxillary hypoplasia is observed less commonly than with the other craniosynostosis syndromes.

CARPENTER SYNDROME. The Carpenter syndrome is characterized by craniosynostosis, polysyndactyly of the feet, and short hands with variable soft tissue syndactyly. The etiology is autosomal recessive.

FUNCTIONAL ASPECTS

*Increased Intracranial Pressure*

It has been assumed that increased intracra-

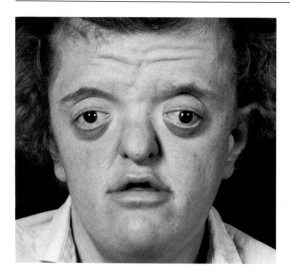
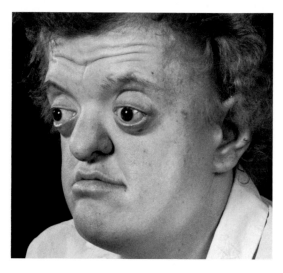

**Figure 6-31** *Apert syndrome. Note the mild frontal bossing, exorbitism, midface hypoplasia, and acne.*

nial pressure (ICP) is apparent in those cases of craniosynostosis in which there is the greatest disparity between intracranial volume and brain volume. In a series of 121 craniosynostosis patients, Marchac and Renier documented increased ICP in 42 percent of patients with multiple suture involvement and 13 percent of patients with single suture involvement [46]. Reduction of ICP was noted in those patients who underwent cranial vault remodeling. Longitudinal three-dimensional CT studies have documented significant increases in intracranial and ventricular volume after these techniques [17]. Papilledema is not an uncommon finding with increased ICP. It is more common in Crouzon's disease, Apert syndrome, acrocephaly, and oxycephaly; it is rarely seen in plagiocephaly and trigonocephaly [58].

*Hydrocephalus*
The true incidence of hydrocephalus in the various craniosynostosis syndromes is not known. Both communicating and noncommunicating types of hydrocephalus may be observed, but it is thought that the former is more common [21]. The incidence of hydrocephalus in scaphocephaly and in unilateral and bilateral coronal synostosis is lowest.

It is highest in multiple suture synostosis, especially the kleeblattschädel deformity where there is evidence of obstruction of cerebrospinal fluid flow at the level of the fourth ventricle [3]. As in the multiple suture synostoses, hydrocephalus is observed more frequently in patients with Crouzon's disease and Apert syndrome, but the true incidence is not known.

*Mental Retardation*
The incidence of mental retardation in the various craniosynostosis syndromes remains speculative. The incidence is certainly not as high as previously assumed, as the diagnosis of mental retardation had been made erroneously because of the facial appearance. In the past many patients had been relegated at an early age to institutional care with only minimal social-sensory stimulation. There is a paucity of objective psychometric data in the reported series. The risk of mental retardation is higher than in the general population, and the etiology of mental retardation associated with craniosynostosis has been attributed to several factors:

increased intracranial pressure (unrelieved) with cerebral atrophy, hydrocephalus, associated intracranial anomalies, meningitis, prematurity, or family history of mental retardation. The incidence of mental retardation is lowest in patients with involvement of a single suture, except in patients with metopic synostosis, where it is observed more frequently. The latter has been attributed to the associated forebrain anomalies observed in metopic synostosis (trigonocephaly). The highest incidence of mental retardation has been reported with the Apert syndrome and the kleeblattschädel deformity.

### Visual Disturbances

The incidence of optic atrophy has been reported to be common in brachycephaly, oxycephaly, Crouzon's disease and Apert syndrome [58]. It is a rare finding in trigonocephaly, plagiocephaly, and scaphocephaly [58]. Optic atrophy has been attributed to compression of the nerve by bony overgrowth of the walls of the optic canal [12], yet other investigators [46] have reported that the diameter of the canal is usually of normal caliber. Alternative theories proposed to explain the presence of optic atrophy include stretching of the nerve, compression by the carotid vessels, or a secondary effect of chronic papilledema and increased intracranial pressure.

In the presence of associated orbital hypertelorism, the patient may not develop binocular vision with resulting amblyopia. Approximately 50 percent of patients with Crouzon's disease or Apert syndrome show exotropia in the primary gaze position, and approximately two-thirds of these patients demonstrate a V pattern associated with overactivity of the inferior oblique muscle [54].

### TREATMENT

The trend in recent years has been toward early surgery for obvious psychological and functional benefit. Every effort is made to have the child look as good as possible at as early an age as possible to spare the psychological social trauma associated with craniofacial disfigurement.

Treatment can be divided into two stages: early (before 1 year of age) and late (after 1 year of age).

### Early Treatment (Before 1 Year of Age)

1. Shunt surgery for hydrocephalus
2. Strip craniectomies: limited and extended
3. Frontal bone advancement with or without strip craniectomies
4. Cranial vault remodeling
5. Monobloc or craniofacial advancement

### Late Treatment (After 1 Year of Age)

1. Frontal bone advancement
2. Subcranial Le Fort III advancement: (1) child; (2) adult
3. Intracranial Le Fort III
4. Monobloc or craniofacial advancement
5. Frontofacial bipartition
6. Le Fort III/Le Fort I advancement
7. Le Fort II advancement
8. Maxillary/mandibular osteotomies and ancillary procedures

### Early Surgery

The presence of hydrocephalus and ventricular enlargement can be assessed by CT scanning. It is preferable that *shunt surgery* is done prior to craniectomy and cranial vault remodeling.

Neurologic *strip craniectomies* have traditionally been advocated for infants before the age of 3 months. Although adequate cranial decompression is obtained, Shillito and Matson, after having reviewed 519 patients with craniosynostosis who had undergone strip craniectomies, noted that only 52 percent of the patients had satisfactory craniofacial form after surgery [74]. The best results were observed in infants with *isolated sagittal suture synostosis*. Coronal and sphenozygomatic suture stripping (to the inferior orbital fissure) is, however, a recommended surgical technique when there

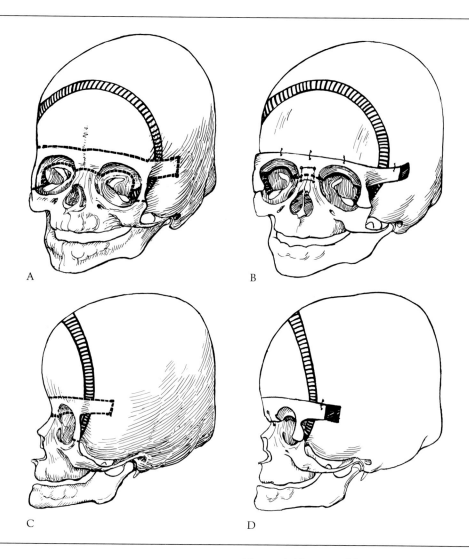

A

B

C

D

is mild bilateral coronal synostosis with brachycephaly, temporal bone bulging, and *minimal*, if any, exorbitism.

FRONTAL BONE ADVANCEMENT. *Brachycephaly/Oxycephaly.* Frontal bone advancement (Fig. 6-32) is indicated for infants with a craniosynostosis syndrome (e.g., Crouzon's and Apert disease) and for infants with isolated bilateral coronal synostosis with exorbitism and a foreshortened orbital roof. These findings suggest synostosis of the sphenoethmoidal, sphenozygomatic, frontoethmoidal, and frontosphenoidal sutures. The lateral lines of osteotomy encompass

**Figure 6-32** *Frontal bone advancement or frontoorbital remodeling. A,C. Lines of osteotomy-ostectomy. B,D. After advancement and recontouring. The forehead can also be reconstructed with a parietooccipital bone graft. (From J. G. McCarthy et al. Early skeletal release in the infant with craniofacial dysotosis: The role of the sphenozygomatic suture.* Plast. Reconstr. Surg. *62:235, 1978.)*

wide bony resection of the sphenozygomatic sutures as well. The procedure is performed with more facility in infants approximately 6 months of age [46, 52, 55].

After the frontal bone flap has been removed, the osteotomies are made across the

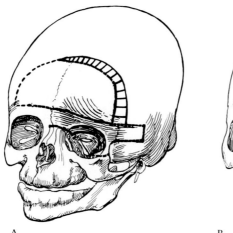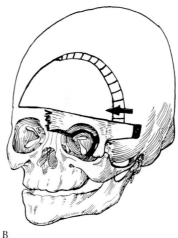

A                                    B

**Figure 6-33** *Frontal bone advancement or frontoorbital remodeling for plagiocephaly (left side). A. Lines of osteotomy-ostectomy. In many cases the deformity is treated with bilateral osteotomies. B. After advancement of the frontoorbital segment (arrow) and replacement of the forehead with a single-piece calvarial (parietooccipital) graft. (From J. G. McCarthy et al. Early surgery for craniofacial synostosis: An eight year experience.* Plast. Reconstr. Surg. 73:521, 1984.)

nasofrontal junction, across the roof of the orbit, and along the lateral orbital wall. Extensions are made into the temporal fossa to provide a tongue-in-groove arrangement, a maneuver that obviates the need for bone graft fixation. The frontal bone flap is wired to the advanced supraorbital bar, or the forehead is reconstructed by a parietooccipital bone graft. The frontal bone has been advanced as far as 20 mm with significant expansion of the orbital volume.

*Plagiocephaly.* For unilateral coronal synostosis, a unilateral (Fig. 6-33) or modified frontal bone advancement is indicated [30].

A supraorbital osteotomy is made approximately 1.5 cm above the roof of the orbit and carried into the temporal region; burr holes in the middle cranial fossa are usually required to prevent injury to the temporal lobe. A counter-osteotomy is made halfway up to medial orbital wall, across the roof,

and down the lateral wall in a full-thickness fashion. It is essential that the osteotomies be extended across the midline to the unaffected side, such that when the greenstick fracture is accomplished there is no resulting midline depression. The affected supraorbital arch is usually flat and lacks the desired convexity. Restoration of contour can be accomplished by bending the mobilized supraorbital segment after making posterior cuts or placing onlay bone grafts (removed from the frontal bone flap) on the anterior aspect of the supraorbital arch. The segment is then fixated in a slightly overcorrected position by placing stainless steel wires or a miniplate between the temporal extension and temporal bone. The resulting gap in the orbital roof does not require bone grafting. A calvarial bone graft obtained from a suitable portion of the parietooccipital region is used to restore forehead contour. It is important to remember that plagiocephaly, although caused by unilateral coronal synostosis, is often a bilateral deformity, and a bilateral frontal bone advancement is often indicated.

*Trigonocephaly.* Metopic synostosis is associated with a triangular forehead and a supraorbital rim that is usually recessed in the anteroposterior dimension. A supraorbital

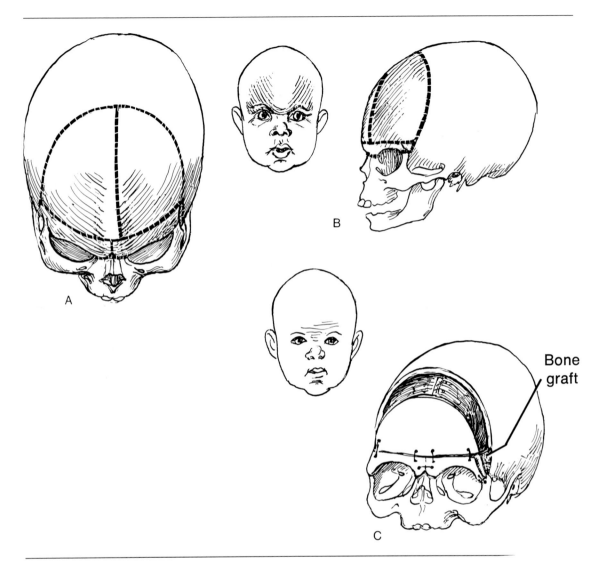

**Figure 6-34** *Surgical correction of trigonocephaly/metopic synostosis. A,B. Lines of osteotomy. C. After advancement of the frontal bone segment and replacement of the forehead with a single-piece calvarial bone graft. Bone grafts are also wedged in the lateral defect. (After D. Marchac. Radical forehead remodeling for craniostenosis. Plast. Reconstr. Surg. 61:823, 1978.)*

bar, according to the method of Marchac, is fractured in greenstick fashion at the midline and advanced as needed [45] (Fig. 6-34). A single piece calvarial graft from the lateral aspect of the frontal bone flap is selected for one-piece forehead reconstruction. Bone defects remaining at the conclusion of surgery in the newborn are usually replaced by new bone during the subsequent months [72].

*Cranial Vault Remodeling.* Munro described a radical calvariectomy or cranial vault remodeling for turricephaly correction

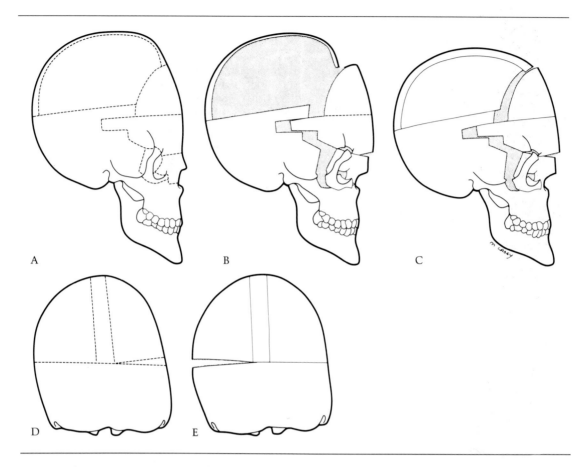

**Figure 6-35** *A. Cranial vault remodeling. Lines of osteotomy. B. The maxilla and the frontal bone have been advanced, and the lateral halves of the cranial vault are removed. C. The sagittal strip of bone is advanced inferiorly and forward to match the advanced frontal bone. The halves of the cranium are reshaped and replaced. D. To correct the plagiocephaly, a wedge of bone was removed from the left side of the cranium. E. The sagittal strip of bone was advanced to the right as well as forward, allowing closure of the wedge on the left and an opening on the right, which was filled with a bone graft. (After I. R. Munro. Reshaping the Cranial Vault. In J. M. Converse (ed.),* Reconstructive Plastic Surgery *(2nd ed.). Philadelphia: Saunders, 1977.)*

[61] (Fig. 6-35). The frontal bone is cut into three segments, the uppermost used at the end for a one-piece forehead. Above this point, a central piece of bone is preserved over the sagittal sinus. The midpiece of frontal bone is resected as required; the forehead is corrected with advancement and aligned with the sagittal segment. The parietal bones are removed, reversed, and replaced. Two-dimensional remodeling occurs: sagittal advancement with vertical reduction.

*Monobloc or Craniofacial Advancement.* With a severe craniofacial synostosis syndrome characterized by mid-face retrusion causing respiratory distress and exorbitism causing corneal ulceration, Muhlbauer and associates have recommended monobloc advancement [59]. This procedure involves simultaneous forehead, orbit, and mid-face advancement. Because of the danger of the procedure, it is reserved for infants with combined ocular and respiratory emergencies. If each is encountered alone, tracheostomy can relieve respiratory distress in the newborn, and a frontal bone advancement can successfully alleviate corneal exposure.

*Late Surgery*

FRONTAL BONE ADVANCEMENT. The frontal bone advancement technique as previously described is indicated in the older child or adult when there is retrusion of the supraorbital rims with a forehead deformity.

SUBCRANIAL LE FORT III ADVANCEMENT. As previously stated, Gillies and Harrison reported the first modified Le Fort III osteotomy for Crouzon's deformity [26].

The Tessier technique, reported in 1967, reproduced the classic Le Fort III fracture lines [86]. The osteotomy traversed the nasofrontal junction and then passed behind the lacrimal groove and across the floor of the orbit. The lateral wall of the orbit was split sagittally, the line of osteotomy extending downward through the body of the zygoma in a step-like fashion. The pterygomaxillary junction and nasal septum were severed. After the osteotomies were completed, the mid-face segment was advanced with disimpacting forceps.

Jabaley and Edgerton performed an osteotomy similar to that of Tessier [34]. The osteotomy in the zygomatic area differed, however, as the osteotomy was done through the zygomatic arch instead of the body of the zygoma. These investigators separated the hard palate from the pterygoid processes, cutting through the posterior wall of the maxillary sinus. Tessier subsequently published modifications of his original Le Fort III technique [80].

*Technique.* Exposure of the facial skeleton is obtained through three incisions: (1) scalp (bicoronal) incision; (2) conjunctival or subciliary cutaneous incision; and (3) buccal vestibular incision. The eyelid and buccal vestibular incisions can be avoided, but the operation is technically more difficult. The frontal scalp flap is raised in a subperiosteal plane to the roof and lateral wall of the orbit and to the root of the nose and the medial orbital wall. This area can communicate with that exposed through the conjunctival or eyelid incision. The latter incisions give access to the inferior orbital rims, orbital floors, and lower portion of the orbital walls. A buccal vestibular incision at the level of the bicuspids provides subperiosteal exposure of the pterygomaxillary fissure.

When mobilizing the periorbita from the orbit 360 degrees, care is taken to preserve the attachment of the medial canthal tendon and to elevate the lacrimal sac from the lacrimal groove.

The osteotomy begins at the nasofrontal junction with a mechanical saw. The line of section continues backward across the medial wall of the orbit on each side and downward (behind the lacrimal groove) to the floor of the orbit (Fig. 6-36). A narrow, tapered osteotome is the most suitable instrument for sectioning the delicate lamina papyracea of the ethmoïd, which forms the portion of the medial wall of the orbit posterior to the lacrimal bone. A transverse cut is made across the orbital floor with a fine osteotome as far as the inferior orbital fissure.

The lateral wall of the orbit is sectioned transversely in the region of the frontozygomatic suture line or above it. After retraction of the orbital contents medially and the temporalis muscle laterally, the lateral orbital wall is divided in a full-thickness fashion at its junction with the cranium. The osteotomy through the lateral orbital wall is continued inferiorly into the inferior orbital fissure.

The line of osteotomy through the lateral orbital wall is continued inferiorly and posteriorly across the maxilla to and through the pterygomaxillary fissure. Pterygomaxillary disjunction is best accomplished

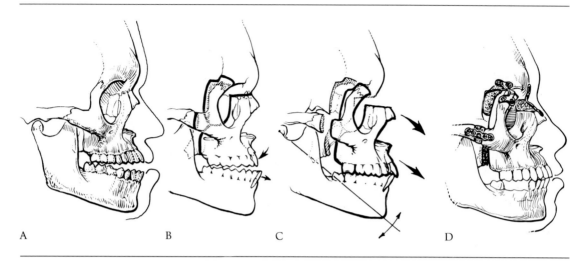

A              B              C              D

*Figure 6-36* *Subcranial Le Fort III advancement. A. Hypoplastic mid-face skeleton. B. Lines of osteotomy. The goals of preoperative orthodontic therapy are indicated by arrows. C. Anteroinferior translation of the osteotomized segment. D. Autogenous bone grafts are placed in the nasofrontal junction, lateral orbital wall, zygomatic arch, and pterygomaxillary fissure defects. Fixation is obtained by miniplates. (From J. G. McCarthy (ed.).* Plastic Surgery. *Philadelphia: Saunders, 1990.)*

through the mouth with a curved osteotome after the mucoperiosteum has been raised from the tuberosity of the maxilla. If a vestibular incision is not elected, a curved osteotome inserted into the pterygomaxillary fissure via the bicoronal incision can perform pterygomaxillary disjunction through the posterior wall of the maxilla. A combination of scissors and osteotome is employed to sever the posterior portion of the nasal septum. After all lines of osteotomy are verified, the mid-facial skeleton may be loosened and advanced with the Rowe-Kiley disimpaction forceps.

Autogenous bone grafts are placed in the defects of the nasofrontal junction, lateral orbital wall, and pterygomaxillary fissure. Intermaxillary fixation is established after appropriate anterior advancement. Additional fixation can be obtained with miniplate fixation across the nasofrontal, zygomaticotemporal, and zygomaticofrontal osteotomies. This technique stabilizes the advanced nasomaxillary segment, maintains the mandibular condyle in the glenoid fossa, and can obviate the need for intermaxillary fixation. A canthopexy is not required, as the medial canthal tendons were not detached from their skeletal attachments. The lateral canthal tendons can be secured to drill holes placed high in the lateral orbital wall.

INTRACRANIAL LE FORT III ADVANCEMENT. The combined intracranial approach is indicated when (1) the anteroposterior dimension of the roof of the orbit and brow must be increased ("frontal bone advancement"); (2) there is an associated correction of orbital hypertelorism with a low-lying cribriform plate; or (3) the middle cranial fossa is anteriorly situated and there is the risk of penetrating the temporal lobe when performing a subcranial procedure.

After the neurosurgeon has removed the frontal bone segment, the supraorbital osteotomy is extended horizontally to the region of the temporal fossa and continued in a stepwise fashion inferiorly toward the base of the skull; a posterior or temporal exten-

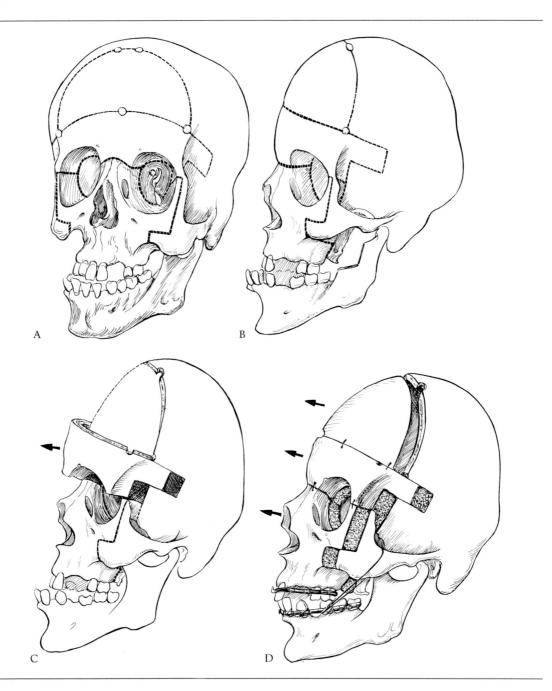

**Figure 6-37** *Combined Le Fort III–frontal bone advancement (after Tessier). A,B. Lines of osteotomy. C. Advancement of upper segment. D. Advancement of upper and lower segments.* *Rigid skeletal (miniplate) fixation is preferred (after Tessier). (From J. M. Converse (ed.).* Reconstructive Plastic Surgery. *Philadelphia: Saunders, 1977.)*

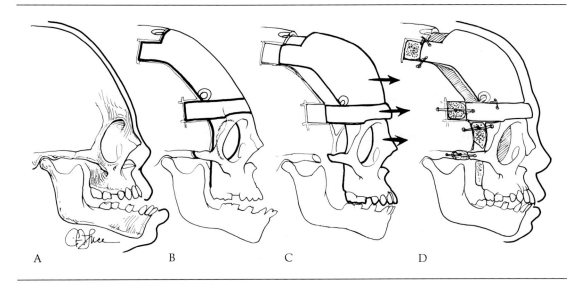

A    B    C    D

**Figure 6-38** *Monobloc advancement (after Ortiz-Monasterio and associates, 1978). A. Hypoplastic mid-face and orbitofrontal region. B. Lines of osteotomy. Note that the Le Fort III segment also incorporates the roof of the orbits. In addition, the frontal bone is remodeled in two segments. C. The three skeletal segments can be advanced to varying degrees. D. Final position with bone grafts. Rigid skeletal fixation can also be employed. (From J. G. McCarthy (ed.).* Plastic Surgery. *Philadelphia: Saunders, 1989.)*

sion is thus outlined that guides the skeletal advancement and maintains bony contact ("tongue-in-groove") (Fig. 6-37).

In a horizontal direction the osteotomy traverses the lateral orbital wall and follows a line across the orbital roof at approximately the midportion of the orbit. The procedure is then completed with the Le Fort III osteotomy.

Advancement proceeds as planned, and the carefully measured segments of bone graft are fixed in position. In this manner, a horizontal component approximately 2 cm in height is advanced, separate from the Le Fort III component. This segment contains the frontal bone, roof, and lateral wall of the orbit.

MONOBLOC ADVANCEMENT. Single skeletal segment advancement of the brow, orbits, and mid-face was popularized by Ortiz-Monasterio and associates [69]. The osteotomy lines are similar to those previously described for the combined Le Fort III–frontal bone advancement, except that the orbital, nasofrontal, and frontozygomatic regions are spared of osteotomies, and the frontal band and Le Fort III segment are advanced as a monobloc (Fig. 6-38).

The technique has the advantage of permitting concomitant hypertelorism correction but the disadvantages of an increased infection rate and limited orbital volume expansion [20]. The technique is best reserved for the craniosynostosis syndrome patient with mild exorbitism and class III malocclusion with a *well aligned* but retruded mid-face and brow.

FRONTOFACIAL BIPARTITION. A procedure (Fig. 6-39) developed by Tessier for correction of the Apert deformity [83], frontofacial bipartition was derived from the monobloc advancement of Ortiz-Monasterio et al. [69]. The orbital hypertelorism, mid-face retrusion (palatal constriction), and facial features of Apert syndrome are addressed in a single operation, which is usually performed in children 3 to 10 years of age. After the

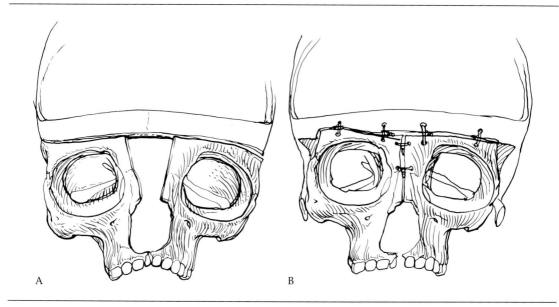

A                                              B

**Figure 6-39** *Frontofacial bipartition for correction of orbital hypertelorism and the deformity of the maxillary dental arch. A. The maxillary occlusion is arched and constricted, and the central nasoorbital segment has been excised. B. After medial translocation of the orbits and expansion and leveling of the maxillary arch with a palatal osteotomy. (From J. G. McCarthy.* Plastic Surgery. *Philadelphia: Saunders, 1990.)*

monobloc segments are mobilized, interorbital excision and palatal split are performed. The palate serves as a fulcrum on which the orbits and maxilla are advanced and torsioned together in opposing transverse directions. Replacement of the frontal bandeau, bending and narrowing of the frontoorbital region, and frontal bone transposition complete the cranial portion of the procedure. Fixation proceeds as with the monobloc advancement. Bone graft to the nasal dorsum and jumping bone flap genioplasty complete the skeletal reconstruction. Transnasal medial canthopexy, resection of the thick temporal fat pad, and alar cartilage reduction complete the soft tissue surgery.

LE FORT III/LE FORT I ADVANCEMENT. This procedure is best suited for patients with mid-face retrusion (exorbitism and maxillary hypoplasia) but an acceptable dental occlusion [66]. The Le Fort I osteotomy is performed first. The patient is placed in intermaxillary fixation; the Le Fort III osteotomy is then performed; and the upper midface segment is advanced as needed (Fig. 6-40). Miniplate fixation is achieved across the Le Fort I, nasofrontal, and zygomaticofrontal osteotomies.

The approach for the Le Fort I osteotomy is via the upper buccal sulcus incision (see Surgical Exposure). The osteotomy begins at the piriform aperture, taking a lateral course to the pterygomaxillary fissure. The line of osteotomy is superior to the apices of the teeth but well below the infraorbital nerves. Pterygomaxillary disjunction is performed with a curved osteotome, and the septum is severed. Intermaxillary fixation is established, and the upper Le Fort III segment is osteotomized and advanced into the desired position. Miniplate fixation and bone grafting proceed as described previously.

LE FORT II ADVANCEMENT. Although the least commonly performed of the Le Fort advancements, the Le Fort II advancement is indicated for the patient with mid-face hypoplasia and adequate zygomatic projection. The lines of osteotomy in the Le Fort II os-

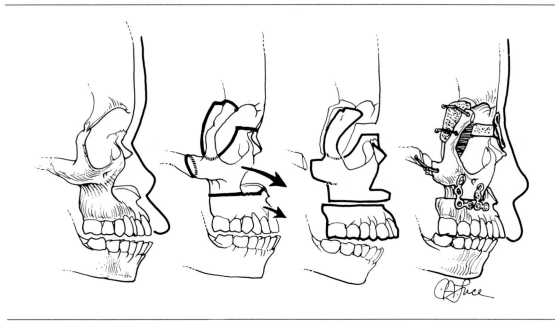

**Figure 6-40** *Combination Le Fort III and Le Fort I osteotomy offers differential advancement of the mid-face and maxillary segments. Autogenous bone grafts are placed in the defects, and fixation is established with a combination of wires and miniplates. (From J. G. McCarthy (ed.).* Plastic Surgery. *Philadelphia: Saunders, 1990.)*

teotomy (Fig. 6-41) commence at the nasofrontal junction, pass inferiorly on the medial orbital wall posterior to the lacrimal groove, and across the orbital floor to the infraorbital foramen bilaterally. The osteotomy is extended across the inferior orbital rim and maxilla to the pterygomaxillary fissure. Pterygomaxillary disjunction is performed. The Le Fort II segment is advanced and secured in position by the fixation techniques previously described.

ANCILLARY PROCEDURES. Jaw disharmonies (i.e., class III malocclusion and anterior crossbite) must be anticipated due to mandibular growth after Le Fort III advancement osteotomy in a growing child [56]. Various mandibular and maxillary osteotomies (see Chapter 7) may be required during adolescence.

In the patient with craniofacial synostosis who has undergone a mid-face advancement, there is often an obvious microgenia. Most of these patients require a genioplasty or advancement osteotomy of the anteroinferior border of the mandible. For patients in whom orbital and maxillary positions are satisfactory but zygomatic projection is lacking, isolated zygomatic advancement is indicated.

LONGITUDINAL STUDIES
Marchac, McCarthy, and their associates have reported their experience with frontoorbital remodeling for craniosynostosis [46, 55]. The authors were satisfied with long-term frontoorbital position, especially in the patients with bilateral and unilateral coronal synostosis. In the latter group there was also correction of the orbitonasal asymmetry with the passage of time. In those with the craniofacial synostoses syndrome (Crouzon's disease, Apert syndrome), however, the desired mid-face growth was not realized. Many patients in this group subsequently developed an anterior crossbite that required mid-face advancement. Mortality was less than 2 percent, and complications

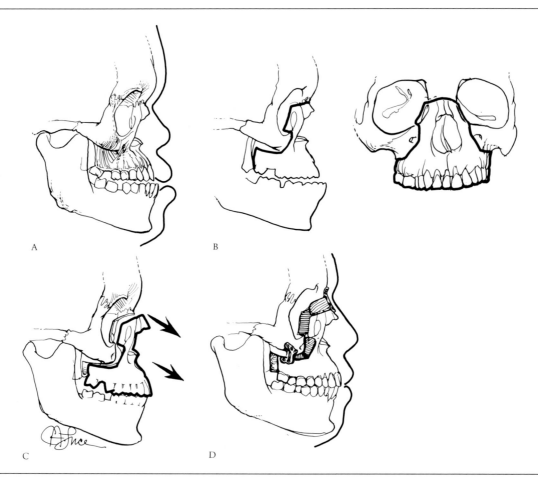

included infection, protruding wires, and contour irregularities or defects.

With the trend toward early mid-face advancement, critical questions have arisen as to the stability and growth of the advanced segment. Although preliminary longitudinal data after Le Fort III advancement in the growing child have demonstrated stability of the advanced skeletal segment, there has been little, if any, evidence of mid-face growth [23, 56].

## Craniofacial Microsomia

The first and second branchial arch syndrome (craniofacial microsomia) is usually unilateral but can be bilateral. The deformity is characterized by regional hypoplasia

of the temporomandibular and pterygomandibular complexes. The bilateral deformity must be distinguished from Treacher Collins syndrome, which is transmitted by autosomal dominant inheritance [22]. Distinguishing characteristics of craniofacial microsomia are malformations of the mandibular ramus and facial paralysis. Condylar hypo-

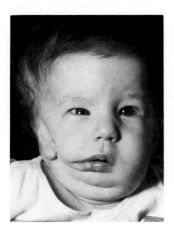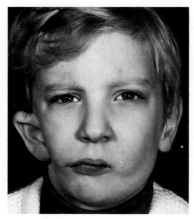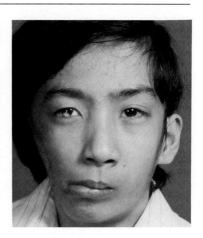

**Figure 6-42** *Variation in the clinical manifestation of craniofacial microsomia.*

plasia secondary to postnatal trauma or infection can also produce a similar mandibular deformity, often with associated temporomandibular ankylosis. Postnatal deformity is usually restricted to the mandible without causing the soft tissue, auricular, or temporal bone deformity associated with craniofacial microsomia. Similarly, severe orbitofacial clefts have an occlusal cant and a shortened mandibular ramus but without the pathognomonic condylar deformity of craniofacial microsomia.

Etiologic theories favor an intrauterine factor. The stapedial artery is the temporary vascular supply for the first and second branchial arch, and it is ultimately replaced by the external carotid system. Phenocopies of craniofacial microsomia have been produced by the administration of triazene to the mouse and thalidomide to the monkey [71]. Embryonic hematoma formation with spreading hemorrhage was noted prior to the formation of the stapedial artery. The extent and size of the hematoma correlated with the size of the anomalous defect. In the mouse experimental model the spectrum of defects was broad: a small aural hematoma producing a residual deformity of only the external ear and auditory ossicles and large hemorrhagic lesions affecting the condyle,

mandibular ramus, and zygoma. In addition, a decreased heat pattern was noted over the region of the external maxillary artery [91], possible evidence that a vascular event occurring during intrauterine life could produce the human syndrome [33]. Since that time there has been a report of a large number of newborns with first and second branchial arch anomalies following the widespread use of thalidomide (a hemorrhagic agent) during human pregnancy [37].

The major characteristic that defines craniofacial microsomia is the variation in the extent and degree of the deformity (Fig. 6-42). Because of this heterogeneous nature it is difficult to classify the individual deformity. In the severe form, all of the structures derived from the first and second branchial arches are hypoplastic, whereas in other types only auricular or jaw dysplasias may predominate. Radiographic studies have demonstrated that all cases of external auditory canal and auricular hypoplasia with middle ear deformity have some evidence of mandibular deformity on the affected side [11].

In cases of minor jaw deformities, careful clinical examination often shows a slight deviation of the mandible to the affected side. In other cases, the characteristic jaw deformity may be present without gross auricular or temporal bone maldevelopment. These

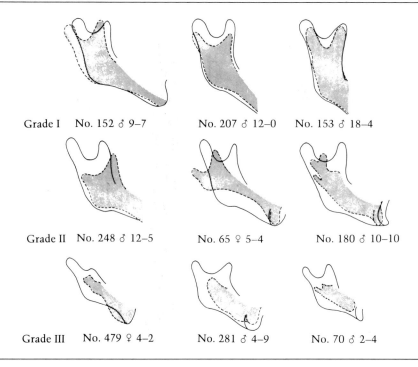

Grade I    No. 152 ♂ 9–7         No. 207 ♂ 12–0         No. 153 ♂ 18–4

Grade II   No. 248 ♂ 12–5        No. 65 ♀ 5–4           No. 180 ♂ 10–10

Grade III  No. 479 ♀ 4–2         No. 281 ♂ 4–9          No. 70 ♂ 2–4

**Figure 6-43** *Pruzansky classification of the mandibular deformity in unilateral craniofacial microsomia. The less affected ramus is traced in a solid outline. (From J. M. Converse (ed.).* Reconstructive Plastic Surgery. *Philaelphia: Saunders, 1977.)*

cases can be differentiated from postnasal deformity because they are present at birth. Formes frustes are also more frequent than acknowledged. They must be searched for in cases of slight facial asymmetry and auricular malformations without manifest jaw deformity. The most conspicuous deformity of unilateral craniofacial microsomia is hypoplasia of the mandible on the affected side (Fig. 6-43). The ramus and condyle are short or virtually absent. The condylar anomaly may represent the hallmark of the syndrome. The body of the mandible curves upward to join the short ramus. The chin is deviated to the affected side, and the body of the mandible on the "normal" side assumes a flattened contour with a straightened gonial angle. When there is hypoplasia of the temporal bone, the posterior wall in the glenoid fossa of the temporomandibular joint may be absent. Occasionally a distinct fossa cannot be identified. The hypoplastic ramus is often hinged on this flat surface

at a point anterior to the contralateral temporomandibular joint. As facial asymmetry increases during the formative years, the mandible deviates laterally and upwardly toward the affected side. The cant of the occlusal plane becomes higher on the affected side and lower on the unaffected side. The crowded dentition also tilts toward the affected side. The condyle and ramus shift medial to the growing temporal bone and glenoid fossa, with a resulting crossbite.

Craniofacial bones other than the mandible or maxilla can also be involved. The tympanic and mastoid portions of the temporal bone are affected, whereas the petrous portion is usually spared. The zygoma can be underdeveloped in all of its dimensions, with flattening of the malar eminence. Dis-

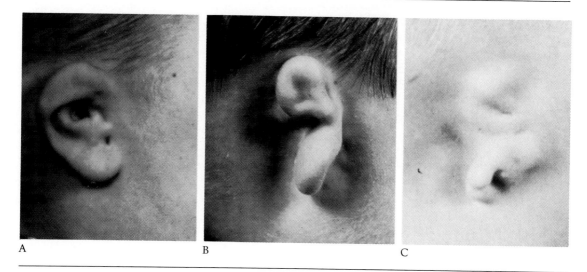

A          B          C

**Figure 6-44** *Meurmann classification of the auricular deformity. A. Grade I: the remnant is diminutive, but all elements are present. B. Grade II: a vertical remnant of cartilage and lobule. C. Grade III: only a vestigial remnant. (From J. G. McCarthy (ed.).* Plastic Surgery. *Philadelphia: Saunders, 1990.)*

parities in the vertical axis of the orbit (dystopia) with or without microphthalmos can be seen. Often in this situation there is flattening of the ipsilateral frontal bone, giving an appearance similar to plagiocephaly.

There is an associated muscular hypoplasia that involves the muscles of mastication: masseter, medial and lateral pterygoid, and temporalis. Muscle function, especially that of the lateral pterygoid, is impaired, resulting in severe limitation of mandibular protrusive and lateral movement. When the patient opens his mouth, deviation toward the affected side is produced not only by the skeletal asymmetry but by the minimal or absent contribution of the ipsilateral medial and lateral pterygoid muscles in countering the opposing actions of the muscles on the unaffected side. In many cases the coronoid process is absent, and there is reduction in the size of the temporalis muscle. The as-sociated masseter muscle is also grossly deficient.

Auricular malformations are a usual manifestation of the syndrome. Meurmann proposed a classification (Fig. 6-44) of the auricular anomalies: grade I, distinctly smaller malformed auricles with most of the characteristic components; grade II, vertical remnant of cartilage and skin with a small anterior hook and complete atresia of the canal; and grade III, auricle almost entirely absent except for only a small remnant, such as a deformed lobule [57]. In addition, the unaffected ear may manifest structural abnormalities. The type of hearing loss, although usually assumed to be conductive, can be determined only by audiometry.

A wide variety of cerebral anomalies exist with craniofacial microsomia, including ipsilateral cerebral hypoplasia [1], hypoplasia of the corpus callosum, hydrocephalus of the communicating and obstructive types, and unilateral hypoplasia of the brain stem and cerebellum [2]. Associated abnormalities include mental retardation and epilepsy [27]. The most common cranial nerve anomaly is facial paralysis secondary to agenesis of the facial muscles, an aberrant pathway of the facial nerve in the temporal bone, or hypoplasia of the intracranial portion of the facial nerve and facial nucleus in the brain stem. Congenital hearing loss may be due to a malformed inner ear or hypoplasia of the cochlear nerve and brain stem auditory nuclei. There can be hypoplasia and impaired function of CN IX through CN XII. Any cranial nerve, however, can be clinically involved in patients with craniofacial microsomia.

There is often a generalized soft tissue hypoplasia that involves the skin, subcutaneous tissue, and facial muscles. The musculature of the soft palate and tongue is occasionally less developed on the affected side. Occasionally, hypoplasia or aplasia of the parotid gland is noted, placing the branches of the facial nerve in a superficial and surgically vulnerable position. Transverse facial clefting, ranging from macrostomia to a full-thickness defect of the cheek, can be present.

### TREATMENT
#### Skeletal Restoration
Correction of the jaw asymmetry and crossbite by osteotomies and bone grafts has been practiced in children and adults, but the timing of the surgery has been the subject of considerable controversy. In general, the more severe the extent of the skeletal and soft tissue deficiency, the more extensive is the surgical procedure and the younger the age at which it is commenced.

In patients with an associated forehead or orbital deformity such as plagiocephaly, microphthalmos, or orbital dystopia, a combined intracranial approach is employed prior to 3 years of age to restore the skeletal anatomy. The plagiocephaly or forehead deformity and retruded brow can be repaired by the technique developed for the infant with unilateral coronal synostosis and plagiocephaly (see Fig. 6-33). In a similar manner the orbital dystopia (see Fig. 6-24) can be corrected prior to jaw reconstructive surgery.

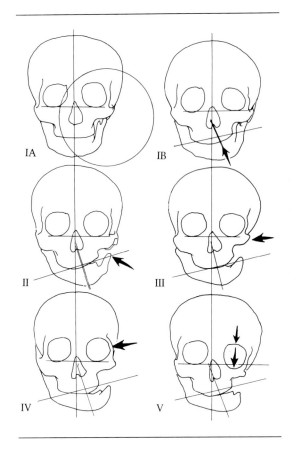

**Figure 6-45** *Munro and Lauritzen* [64] *classification of the skeletal deformity in craniofacial microsomia (see text for details). The occlusal and mid-sagittal planes are illustrated. (From J. G. McCarthy (ed.).* Plastic Surgery. *Philadelphia: Saunders, 1989.)*

Munro and Lauritzen proposed an anatomic/pathologic classification of craniofacial microsomia as an aid in designing the surgical procedure [64] (Fig. 6-45). Surgery is preferably performed at age 5 to 6 years for types II to V.

TYPE IA. The affected craniofacial skeleton is complete but hypoplastic. The occlusal plane (and labial fissure) is horizontal. Onlay bone grafts are added to the hypoplastic orbit, zygoma, maxilla, and mandible. The

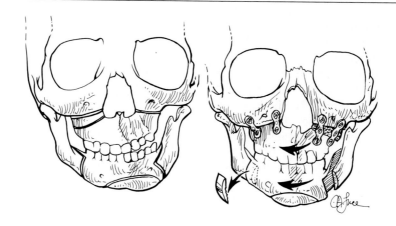

**Figure 6-46** *Treatment of the skeletal deformity with a combination of the Le Fort I osteotomy, bilateral sagittal split advancement of the mandible, and genioplasty (Obwegesser). (From J. G. McCarthy (ed.).* Plastic Surgery. *Philadelphia: Saunders, 1990.)*

procedure is usually delayed until age 8 when a sufficient amount of bone graft can be harvested.

TYPE IB. The facial skeleton is hypoplastic but complete. The occlusal plane, however, is tilted. The surgical treatment plan consists of a Le Fort I osteotomy with lowering and rotation of the affected maxilla, bilateral sagittal osteotomies of the mandibular rami, and genioplasty (Fig. 6-46).

TYPE II. There is absence of the mandibular condyle and part of the ascending ramus. A Le Fort I osteotomy, unilateral sagittal osteotomy of the remaining mandibular ramus, and genioplasty are employed as in the type IB patient. A costochondral rib graft is secured to the mandibular remnant on the affected side and directed laterally to the glenoid fossa to lengthen and reposition the mandible and to increase facial width.

TYPE III. In addition to the findings in type II, there is absence of the zygomatic arch and glenoid fossa. The latter are reconstructed with rib grafts, and the surgical reconstruction is otherwise as outlined for type II.

TYPE IV. The type IV deformity, which is uncommon, is characterized by hypoplasia of the zygoma and posterior and medial displacement of the lateral orbital wall. Correction can be achieved with a Le Fort III osteotomy of the affected side and Le Fort I osteotomy on the opposite side. Another approach is to insert rib grafts to reconstruct the zygomatic complex.

TYPE V. The most severe type (V) anomaly has either a microorbit or inferior displacement of the orbit. In the first surgical stage, performed through an intracranial route, the orbit is translocated as required. In the second stage, at least 6 months later, reconstruction is accomplished as previously described for types II and III.

COMMENT. Reconstructive jaw surgery may be indicated after age 12 for two reasons. The patient may not have sought surgical correction at an earlier age, or there is residual deficiency following skeletal surgery performed at an earlier age. The treatment program is designed according to the pathologic findings. Surgical correction ranges from simple autogenous onlay bone grafting to jaw osteotomies for mild deformities to extensive reconstruction of the zygomatic-orbital complex, maxilla, and mandible [67].

*Soft Tissue Restoration*

Soft tissue surgery (auricle and cheek soft tissue) is usually deferred until the underlying skeleton is reconstructed. Soft tissue hypoplasia is usually not as severe or as diffuse as in hemifacial atrophy (Romberg disease). It is most conspicuous in the parotid-masseteric and auriculomastoid areas. Improvement in the soft tissue deficiency has been obtained by insertion of a deepithelialized flap or a dermis-fat graft introduced subcutaneously to the preauricular area. In recent years deepithelialized microvascular free flaps of dermis and fat have been employed for correction of severe soft tissue atrophy [24, 89]. Soft tissue contour can also be restored by the microvascular transfer of omentum [88].

Auricular reconstruction is delayed until approximately age 6 or 7 years to allow development of adequate rib cartilage size and to permit reconstruction of the underlying craniofacial skeleton. Reconstructive techniques may also be required for correction of a deficit of the facial nerve.

## Fibrous Dysplasia

Orbital displacement and diplopia result from fibrous dysplasia. Involvement of the cranial bones, in general, is less frequent than involvement of the mandible or maxilla. However, when the cranial bones are involved, the order of occurrence is frontal, sphenoid, and ethmoid [40]. With orbital involvement the initial findings include proptosis, epiphora, and decreased vision.

Craniofacial surgical techniques permit globe repositioning after total or subtotal resection of the lesions with reconstruction of the orbit by bone grafts and orbital translocation.

## Neurofibromatosis

The orbital cavity is enlarged vertically and transversely in von Recklinghausen's disease, or neurofibromatosis. The basic defect involves hypoplasia or aplasia of the greater and lesser wings of the sphenoid and orbital plate of the frontal bone, as well as the malar bone.

With the craniofacial surgical approach, the orbital apex is opened widely into the anterior and middle cranial fossae. The intracranial approach allows repositioning of the globe and brain, division or separation of the cranial cavity and orbit, and reconstruction of the orbit with bone grafts [35].

## References

1. Aleksic, S., et al. Unilateral archinencephaly in Goldenhar-Gorlin syndrome. *Dev. Med. Child Neurol.* 17:498, 1975.
2. Aleksic, S., et al. Congenital trigeminal neuropathy in oculoauricular vertebral dysplasia-hemifacial microsomia (Goldenhar-Gorlin syndrome). *J. Neurol. Neurosurg. Psychiatry* 38:1033, 1975.
3. Angle, C. R., McIntire, M. S., and Moore, R. C. Cloverleaf skull: Kleeblattschädel deformity syndrome. *Am. J. Dis. Child.* 114:198, 1967.
4. Apert, E. De l'acricephalosyndactylie. *Bull. Soc. Med. Hop. Paris* 23:1310, 1906.
5. Binder, K. H. Dysostosis Maxillo-Nasalis, ein Arhinencephaler Missbildungskomplex. *Dtsch. Zahnaerztl. Z.* 17:438, 1962.
6. Chotzen, F. Unusual familial development disturbance of face (acrocephalosyndactylia, craniofacial dysostosis and hypertelorism). *Monatsschr. Kinderheilkd.* 55:97, 1932.
7. Cohen, M. M. An etiologic and nosologic overview of craniosynostosis syndromes. *Birth Defects* 11:137, 1975.
8. Converse, J. M., McCarthy, J. G., and Wood-Smith, D. Orbital hypotelorism: Pathogenesis, associated faciocerebral anomalies, surgical correction. *Plast. Reconstr. Surg.* 56:389, 1975.
9. Converse, J. M., Wood-Smith, D., and McCarthy, J. G. Report on a series of 50 craniofacial operations. *Plast. Reconstr. Surg.* 55:283, 1975.
10. Converse, J. M., et al. Ocular hypertelorism and pseudohypertelorism: Advances in surgical treatment. *Plast. Reconstr. Surg.* 45:1, 1970.

11. Converse, J. M., et al. Bilateral facial microsomia: Diagnosis, classification, treatment. *Plast. Reconstr. Surg.* 54:413, 1974.

12. Crouzon, O. Dysostose, cranio-faciale hereditaire. *Bull. Soc. Med. Hop. Paris* 33:545, 1912.

13. Currarino, G., and Silverman, F. N. Orbital hypertelorism, arhinencephaly and trigonocephaly. *Radiology* 74:206, 1960.

14. Cutting, C. B., et al. Three dimensional computer design of assisted craniofacial surgical procedures: Optimization and interaction with cephalometric and CT-based models. *Plast. Reconstr. Surg.* 77:877, 1986.

15. David, D. J., and Cooter, R. D. Craniofacial infection in 10 years of transcranial surgery. *Plast. Reconstr. Surg.* 80:213, 1987.

16. Dufresne, C. D., et al. Volumetric quantification of intracranial and ventricular volume following cranial vault remodeling: A preliminary report. *Plast. Reconstr. Surg.* 79:24, 1987.

17. Dufresne, C. R., et al. Volumetric quantification of intracranial and ventricular volume following cranial vault remodeling: A preliminary report. *Plast. Reconstr. Surg.* 79:24, 1987.

18. Edgerton, M. T., and Jane, J. A. Vertical orbital dystopia—surgical correction. *Plast. Reconstr. Surg.* 67:121, 1981.

19. Edgerton, M. T., et al. The feasibility of craniofacial osteotomies in infants and young children. *Scand. J. Plast. Reconstr. Surg.* 8:164, 1974.

20. Firmin, F., Coccaro, P. J., and Converse, J. M. Cephalometric analysis in diagnosis and treatment planning of craniofacial dysostoses. *Plast. Reconstr. Surg.* 54:300, 1974.

21. Fishman, M. A., Hogan, G. R., and Dodge, P. R. The concurrence of hydrocephalus and craniosynostosis. *J. Neurosurg.* 34:621, 1971.

22. Franceschetti, A., and Klein, D. The mandibulofacial dysostosis: A new hereditary syndrome. *Acta Ophthalmol. (Copenh.)* 27:144, 1949.

23. Freihofer, H. P. Results after midface osteotomies. *J. Maxillofac. Surg.* 1:30, 1973.

24. Fujino, T., Tanino, R., and Sugimoto, C. Microvascular transfer of free deltopectoral dermal-fat flap. *Plast. Reconstr. Surg.* 55:428, 1975.

25. Gillies, H. D. *Plastic Surgery of the Face.* London: Oxford, 1920. P. 5.

26. Gillies, H. D., and Harrison, S. H. Operative correction by osteotomy or recessed malar maxillary compound in a case of oxycephaly. *Br. Plast. Surg.* 3:123, 1950.

27. Gorlin, R. J., et al. Oculoauriculovertebral dysplasia. *J. Pediatr.* 63:991, 1963.

28. Gorlin, R. J., Pindborg, J. J., and Cohen, M. M. *Syndromes of the Head and Neck* (2nd ed.). New York: McGraw-Hill, 1976.

29. Gray, H. Osteology. In C. D. Clemente (ed.), *Gray's Anatomy of the Human Body* (30th ed.). Philadelphia: Lea & Febiger, 1985.

30. Hoffman, H. J., and Mohr, G. Lateral canthal advancement of the supraorbital margin. *J. Neurosurg.* 45:376, 1976.

31. Holmstrom, H. Clinical and pathologic features of maxillonasal dysplasia (Binder's syndrome): Significance of the prenasal fossa on etiology. *Plast. Reconstr. Surg.* 78:559, 1986.

32. Holmstrom, H. Surgical correction of the nose and midface in maxillonasal dysplasia (Binder's syndrome). *Plast. Reconstr. Surg.* 78:568, 1986.

33. Ide, C. H., Miller, G. W., and Wollschlaeger, P. B. Familial facial dysplasia. *Arch. Ophthalmol.* 84:427, 1970.

34. Jabaley, M. E., and Edgerton, M. T. Surgical correction of congenital midface retrusion in the presence of mandibular prognathism. *Plast. Reconstr. Surg.* 44:1, 1969.

35. Jackson, I. T., Laws, E. R., Jr., and Martin, R. D. The surgical management of orbital neurofibromatosis. *Plast. Reconstr. Surg.* 71:751, 1983.

36. Kawamoto, H. K. Late posttraumatic enophthalmos: A correctable deformity? *Plast. Reconstr. Surg.* 69:423, 1982.

37. Kleinsasser, O., and Schlothane, R. Dir Ohrm Bildungen in Rahmen de Thalidomide-embryopathie. *Z. Laryngol. Rhinol. Otol.* 43:344, 1964.

38. Kreiborg, S. Crouzon syndrome. *Scand. J. Plast. Reconstr. Surg.* [Suppl.] 18:1, 1981.

39. Laestadius, N. D., Aase, J. M., and Smith D. W. Normal inner canthal and outer orbital dimensions. *J. Pediatr.* 74:465, 1969.

40. Leeds, N., and Seaman, W. B. Fibrous dysplasia of the skull and its differential diagnosis: A clinical and roentgenographic study of 46 cases. *Radiology* 78:570, 1962.

41. Le Fort, R. The classic reprint: Experimental study of fractures of the upper jaw. I and II.

[Translated from French by Paul Tessier.] *Plast. Reconstr. Surg.* 50:497, 1972.

42. Le Fort, R. The classic reprint: Experimental study of fractures of the upper jaw. III. [Translated from French by Paul Tessier.] *Plast. Reconstr. Surg.* 50:600, 1972.

43. Lisman, R. D., et al. Experience with tarsal suspension as a factor in lower lid blepharoplasty. *Plast. Reconstr. Surg.* 79:897, 1987.

44. Longacre, J. J. *Craniofacial Anomalies: Pathogenesis and Repair.* Philadelphia: Lippincott, 1968.

45. Marchac, D. Radical forehead remodeling for craniostenosis. *Plast. Reconstr. Surg.* 61:823, 1978.

46. Marchac, D., and Renier, D. Craniofacial surgery for craniosynostosis improvers facial growth: A personal case review. *Ann. Plast. Surg.* 14:43, 1985.

47. Marsh, J. L., and Vannier, M. W. The "third" dimension in craniofacial surgery. *Plast. Reconstr. Surg.* 71:759, 1983.

48. Marsh, J. L., and Vannier, M. W. *Comprehensive Care for Craniofacial Deformities.* St. Louis: Mosby, 1985.

49. Marsh, J. L., et al. The skeletal anatomy of mandibulofacial dysostosis (Treacher Collins syndrome). *Plast. Reconstr. Surg.* 78:460, 1986.

50. McCarthy, J. G. A study of gustatory (taste) and olfactory function in craniofacial anomalies. *Plast. Reconstr. Surg.* 64:52, 1979.

51. McCarthy, J. G., and Zide, B. M. The spectrum of calvarial bone grafting: Introduction of the vascularized calvarial bone flap. *Plast. Reconstr. Surg.* 74:10, 1984.

52. McCarthy, J. G., et al. Early skeletal release in the infant with craniofacial dysostosis: The role of the sphenozygomatic suture. *Plast. Reconstr. Surg.* 62:235, 1978.

53. McCarthy, J. G., et al. Longitudinal Cephalometric Studies Following Surgical Correction of Orbital Hypertelorims: A Preliminary Report. In J. M. Converse, J. G. McCarthy, and D. Wood-Smith (eds.), *Symposium on Diagnosis and Treatment of Craniofacial Anomalies.* St. Louis: Mosby, 1979. P. 229.

54. McCarthy, J. G., et al. Extraocular muscle function following craniofacial surgery. In: *Transactions of the 6th International Congress of Plastic and Reconstructive Surgery.* Paris: Masson, 1976. P. 177.

55. McCarthy, J. G., et al. Early surgery for craniofacial synostosis: An eight year experience. *Plast. Reconstr. Surg.* 73:521, 1984.

56. McCarthy, J. G., et al. Le Fort III advancement osteotomy in the growing child. *Plast. Reconstr. Surg.* 74:343, 1984.

57. Meurmann, Y. Congenital microtia and meatal atresia. *Arch. Otolaryngol.* 66:443, 1957.

58. Montaut, J., and Stricker, M. *Dysmorphies Cranifaciales: Les Synostoses Prematuries (Craniostenoses et Faciostenoses).* Paris: Masson, 1977.

59. Muhlbauer, W., Anderl, H., and Marchac, D. Complete Frontofacial Advancement in Infants with Craniofacial Dysostosis. In B. Williams (ed.), *Transactions of the Eighth International Congress of Plastic Surgery,* Montreal, 1983.

60. Mulliken, J. B., et al. Facial skeletal changes following hypertelorbitism correction. *Plast. Reconstr. Surg.* 77:7, 1986.

61. Munro, I. R. Reshaping the Cranial Vault. In J. M. Converse (ed.), *Reconstructive Plastic Surgery* (2nd ed.). Philadelphia: Saunders, 1977.

62. Munro, I., Craniofacial Surgery. In W. C. Grabb and J. W. Smith (eds.), *Plastic Surgery,* Boston: Little, Brown, 1979. P. 131.

63. Munro, I. R. Improving results in orbital hypertelorism correction. *Ann. Plast. Surg.* 2:499, 1979.

64. Munro, I. R., and Lauritzen, C. G. Classification and Treatment of Hemifacial Microsomia. In E. P. Caronni (ed.), *Craniofacial Surgery.* Boston: Little, Brown, 1985. P. 391.

65. Munro, I., and Sabatier, R. D. An analysis of 12 years of craniomaxillofacial surgery in Toronto. *Plast. Reconstr. Surg.* 76:29, 1985.

66. Obwegeser, H. L. Surgical correction of small or retrodisplaced maxillae: The "dish-face" deformity. *Plast. Reconstr. Surg.* 43:351, 1969.

67. Obwegeser, H. L. Correction of the skeletal anomalies of otomandibular dysostosis. *J. Maxillofac. Surg.* 2:73, 1974.

68. Ortiz-Monasterio, F. Notes on the History of Craniofacial Surgery. In I. T. Jackson et al. (eds.), *An Atlas of Craniomaxillofacial Surgery.* St. Louis: Mosby, 1982. Pp. vii–xii.

69. Ortiz-Monasterio, F., Fuente del Campo, A., and Carrillo, A. Advancement of orbits and the midface in one piece, combined with frontal repositioning, for the correction of Crou-

zon's deformities. *Plast. Reconstr. Surg.* 61: 507, 1978.

70. Pfeiffer, R. A. Dominant erbliche Akrocephalosyndaktylie. *Z. Kinderheilkd.* 90:301, 1964.

71. Poswillo, D. E. The pathogenesis of the first and second branchial arch syndrome. *Oral Surg. Oral Med. Oral Pathol.* 35:302, 1973.

72. Reid, C. A., McCarthy, J. G., and Kolber, A. B. A study of regeneration in parietal bone defects in rabbits. *Plast. Reconstr. Surg.* 67:591, 1981.

73. Saethre, H. Oxycephaly (turmschadel), its neuro-psychiatric symptoms, pathogenesis and heredity. *Norsk. Mag. Laegevidensk.* 92:392, 1931.

74. Shillito, J., Jr., and Matson, D. D. Craniostenosis: A review of 519 surgical patients. *Pediatrics* 41:829, 1968.

75. Tessier, P. Osteotomies totales de la face: Syndrome de Crouzon, syndrome d'Apert, oxycephalies, scaphocephalies, turricephalies. *Ann. Chir. Plast.* 12:273, 1967.

76. Tessier, P. Traitement chirurgical des malformations orbito-faciales rares. *Comptes Rendus Premiere Congress International Neuro-Gen. et Neuro-Ophthalmology,* New York, 1968. Basel: Karger, 1968. Pp. 322–355.

77. Tessier, P. Dysostoses cranio-faciales: Osteotomies totales de la face. In: *Transactions of the Fourth International Congress of Plastic and Reconstructive Surgery.* Amsterdam: Excerpta Medica, 1969.

78. Tessier, P. Traitement des dysmorphies faciales propres aux dysostoses craniofaciales. *Chirurgie* 96:667, 1970.

79. Tessier, P. Relationship of craniostenosis to craniofacial dysostoses, and to faciostenoses: A study with therapeutic implications. *Plast. Reconstr. Surg.* 48:224, 1971.

80. Tessier, P. The definitive plastic surgical treatment of the severe facial deformities of craniofacial dysostosis, Crouzon's and Apert's disease. *Plast. Reconstr. Surg.* 48:419, 1971.

81. Tessier, P. Orbital hypertelorism. I. Successive surgical attempts: Materials and methods, causes and mechanisms. *Scand. J. Plast. Reconstr. Surg.* 6:135, 1972.

82. Tessier, P. Anatomical classification of facial, craniofacial, and lateral facial clefts. *J. Maxillofac. Surg.* 4:69, 1976.

83. Tessier, P. Facial Remodeling by Craniofacial Disjunctional Osteotomy: An Evolving Surgical Approach. In B. Brent (ed.), *The Artistry of Reconstructive Surgery.* St. Louis: Mosby, 1987. P. 607.

84. Tessier, P. The Surgical Correction of Hypertelorbitism. In B. Brent (ed.), *The Artistry of Reconstructive Surgery.* St. Louis: Mosby, 1987. P. 641.

85. Tessier, P., Guiot, G., and Derome, P. Orbital hypertelorism. II. Definitive treatment of orbital hypertelorism by craniofacial or by extracranial osteotomies. *Scand. J. Plast. Reconstr. Surg.* 7:39, 1973.

86. Tessier, P., et al. Osteotomies cranio-naso-orbitalies: Hypertelorisme. *Ann. Chir. Plast.* 12:103, 1967.

87. Tulasne, J. F. Maxillary Growth Following Total Septal Resection in Telorbitism. In E. P. Caronni (eds.), *Craniofacial Surgery.* Boston: Little, Brown, 1985. P. 176.

88. Upton, J., et al. Restoration of facial contour using free vascularized omental transfer. *Plast. Reconstr. Surg.* 66:560, 1980.

89. Wells, J. H., and Edgerton, M. T. Correction of severe hemifacial atrophy with a free dermis-fat flap from the lower abdomen. *Plast. Reconstr. Surg.* 59:223, 1977.

90. Whitaker, L. A., et al. Combined report of problems and complications in 793 craniofacial operations. *Plast. Reconstr. Surg.* 64:198, 1979.

91. Willie-Jorgensen, A. Dysostosis mandibulo-facialis (Franceschetti): Report of two atypical cases. *Acta Ophthalmol. (Copenh.)* 40:348, 1962.

92. Zide, B. M., and Jelks, G. W. *Surgical Anatomy of the Orbit.* New York: Raven, 1981. P. 1.

93. Zide, B. M., and McCarthy, J. G. The medial canthus revisited—an anatomical basis for canthopexy. *Ann. Plast. Surg.* 11:1, 1983.

94. Zide, B. M., Grayson, B. H., and McCarthy, J. G. Cephalometric analysis for upper and lower midface surgery. I. *Plast. Reconstr. Surg.* 68:816, 1981.

95. Zide, B. M., Grayson, B. H., and McCarthy, J. G. Cephalometric analysis. II. *Plast. Reconstr. Surg.* 68:961, 1981.

# 7
# Surgery of the Jaws

*S. Anthony Wolfe*

The function of the jaws is to chew. The surgeon who operates on the jaws should bear this statement in mind and perhaps should experience, if only in imagination, what it would be like if his teeth did not occlude properly and effortlessly, if his mouth opening were limited or painful, or if he bore a gross disfigurement of the lower third of the face. If a patient cannot chew properly after surgery, with either his own teeth or a denture, an operation cannot be considered a success from a functional point of view.

The jaws are the scaffolding for the teeth, and all surgical procedures on the jaws must start with a consideration of the teeth.

What is the state of dental repair and oral hygiene?

In what condition are the gums?

How do the teeth occlude?

Any surgeon who intends to operate on the jaws, regardless of whether he has dental training, must work in close collaboration with the various dental specialties of restorative dentistry, pediodontics, periodontics, endodontics, orthodontics, and prosthodontics. In emergency situations, he must be able to obtain dental models, fabricate splints, and recognize carious teeth that are beyond repair and should be extracted. He must have a knowledge of normal dental occlusion.

## Dental Terminology

**Mesial.** Toward the midline

**Distal.** Away from the midline

**Lingual.** Toward the tongue

**Buccal.** Toward the cheek

**Crossbite.** An abnormal buccolingual relation of the teeth (lingual crossbite of the upper incisors is called an anterior crossbite)

**Overbite.** Vertical overlap of the incisors, where the upper incisors are in a lower than normal position

**Overjet.** Horizontal overlap of the incisors, where the upper incisors are positioned anterior to their normal position

**Open bite.** Lack of contact between teeth in the mouth-shut position

The teeth may be referred to by their individual names, e.g., upper left cuspid (canine) or, in dental shorthand, as  3

| 87654321 | 12345678 |
|---|---|
| 87654321 | 12345678 |

227

***Tooth vitality.*** Sensate tooth with an intact pulpal nerve supply (A tooth may have adequate blood supply but is non-vital if a nerve supply is not present.)

***Curve of Spee.*** Curvature of the occlusal plane

***Centric occlusion.*** Position of the mandible where there is maximal intercuspation of the maxillary and mandibular teeth

***Centric relation.*** The most retruded position of the mandible, where the condyles are comfortably seated in the glenoid fossae

***Centric occlusion*** and ***centric relation.*** May be the same in a normal patient but may differ in cases of malocclusion (Centric relation can exist in the absence of teeth.)

***Ankylosis of a tooth.*** Solid fixation of a tooth resulting from fusion of the cementum and alveolar bone with obliteration of the periodontal ligament (The tooth is "locked" in bone and cannot be moved orthodontically.)

## Classification of Occlusion

As succinctly stated by physician and dentist Edward H. Angle in 1898, "The key to occlusion is the relative position of the first molars. In normal occlusion [Fig. 7-1] the mesiobuccal cusp of the upper first molar is received in the buccal groove of the lower first molar" [2]. This positioning is Angle's class I.

With class II malocclusion the lower first molar is located distal to this relation; with class III malocclusion the lower first molar is located mesial to this relation. The Angle classification of malocclusion describes the relation of the teeth but does not indicate the cause. Thus class III malocclusion may be caused by mandibular prognathia, maxillary retrognathia, or a combination of the two.

## Cephalometric Analysis

A cephalogram is a radiograph obtained from a standard distance (usually 60 in.) with the head held in a precise, reproducible position by a head holder. The lateral projection is particularly useful, with the teeth in their habitual occlusion or in the rest position. By taking tracings from S point (sella: the center of the sella turcica), Na point (nasion: the frontonasal suture), A point (subspinale),

*Figure 7-1 Normal dental occlusion. (From E. H. Angle. Treatment of Malocclusion of the Teeth and Fractures of the Maxillae: Angle's System. Philadelphia: S. S. White Dental Manufacturing Co., 1900. P. 6.)*

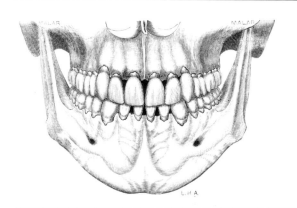
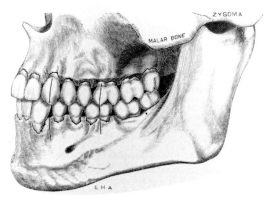

and B point (supramentale), angles such as SNA and SNB can be calculated and compared to various normative data [21]. Numerous other points and angles are used by cephalometricians, and the data obtained can be used for determining the anatomic basis of a malocclusion [39]. Experienced surgeons and orthodontists do not rely entirely on cephalometric analysis when planning corrective operations on the jaws: A careful examination of the patient's entire face and dental occlusion usually receive more weight. Cephalometric analysis in a patient who does not have an external auditory canal in which to position the head holder, or in a patient with an abnormality of the cranial base, must be evaluated accordingly. Unfortunately, the more complex the facial abnormality, the less help one can expect from cephalometry. Nevertheless, cephalometric records are still of great benefit when planning operations and are necessary to follow patterns of growth (or relapse) after surgical procedures.

## Other Radiologic Studies

*Occlusal* and *periapical films* provide information of the condition of individual teeth and supporting alveolar bone. An *orthopantomograph* is taken by rotating both the x-ray source and the film about the patient's head, so that all of the structures of the mandible from condyle to condyle are "opened up" and can be seen on the same film without overlap. The *Status-X* (Siemens) film is similar to the orthopantomograph, but the x-ray source is intraoral. Better detail of the mesial structures is provided, although the condyles are not seen. *Tomograms* of the temporomandibular joint in mouth-open and mouth-closed positions give the best detail of the condylar head and glenoid fossa. *Computed tomography* scans and *magnetic resonance imaging* may provide further information about the temporomandibular joint.

## Dental Models

The surgeon should be capable of making accurate stone casts of the maxillary and mandibular dentition, even though in most instances of elective surgery this task is performed by a dental technician. A wax bite impression is taken from the patient to establish the models in the patient's habitual occlusion, and the backs of the models are trimmed flat with the teeth in this relation. The casts can then be mounted on an articulator and model surgery performed to arrive at the desired postoperative occlusion. Even complicated articulators (Hanau, Dentatus, Obwegeser) with face bows do not exactly reproduce mandibular movements, and in most cases a simpler articulator can be used for model surgery. Acetate tracings of the cephalometric films can also be prepared and cut to simulate the surgical procedure, giving the surgeon a fairly precise idea of how much movement will be required in the various directions.

A *surgical splint*, when required, is made based on the dental models mounted on an articulator in the desired postoperative occlusion. The surgeon can do it by coating the teeth (of the model) lightly with Vaseline and making the splint from quick-curing acrylic, or it can be done in a dental laboratory. Splints are required when the postoperative occlusion does not "lock" into place, when overcorrection of a posterior bite is planned with the operation, or when segmental osteotomies are performed. Splints always introduce a source of error; if preoperative orthodontic treatment has independently prepared the two arches, they are not necessary. A surgical procedure can be done either before or after most of the orthodontic treatment; timing depends on the preference of the individual orthodontic/surgical team. Certainly an orthodontist should be involved in the treatment of every orthognathic surgical patient from beginning to end.

Many types of dental compensation occur in cases of malocclusion. In class III cases there can be a labial tilting of the maxillary incisors and a lingual inclination of the mandibular incisors. In class II cases the opposite situation may occur. If the skeletal structures are to be brought into a proper relation with one another, these dental compensations may need to be "decompensated" to allow proper skeletal correction. It may mean that as the teeth are brought into a proper axial inclination in the supporting basal bone, the malocclusion is made "worse." The class III problem may be more pronouncedly class III, and the class II problem may result in more of an incisal overjet. Orthodontists who are not accustomed to working with surgeons sometimes fall into the trap of thinking only about the occlusion and on occasion perform diligent orthodontic therapy in the wrong direction. Before the basic skeletal deformity can be surgically corrected, the orthodontic treatment must be done in the reverse (i.e., proper) direction. Fortunately, more and more orthodontists are becoming educated to the possibilities of surgery, and fewer and fewer think that surgery is a drastic step that should be avoided at all costs. Orthodontics can only tilt teeth and move them through alveolar bone; if the alveolar bone itself is out of position because

of malalignment of the jaws, surgery is usually required.

### Orthognathic Surgical Procedures

The mandible and the maxilla can be sectioned in myriad ways, either alone or together. Most of the surgical procedures commonly employed are not technically demanding given the proper instrumentation and training. It is again stressed that the most important portion of treatment lies in the preliminary planning: The wrong operation, no matter how brilliantly performed, gives a poor result. Preoperative and postoperative orthodontic treatment are of equal importance to the surgical procedure. An optimal result may require that the surgeon be able to carry out simultaneous or subsequent procedures on the soft tissues of the face.

The *genioplasty* was first proposed by Hofer [11] in 1942 and later popularized by Obwegeser [30] and Converse [6]. The intraoral approach is always used, and a hori-

***Figure 7-2*** *Chin deformities that can be associated with normal dental occlusion. (From S. A. Wolfe and S. Berkowitz.* Plastic Surgery of the Facial Skeleton. *Boston: Little, Brown, 1989.)*

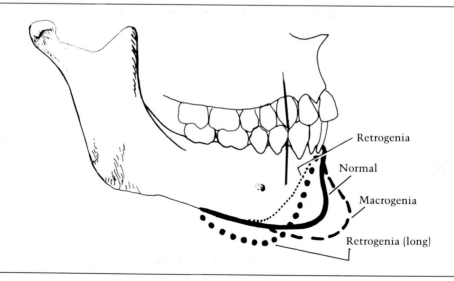

zontal osteotomy is performed below the roots of the teeth and the mental foramina (Figs. 7-2 and 7-3). (The procedure is obviously not used in children, who have dental roots below this level.) The geniohyoid and the genioglossus muscular attachments are maintained to the posterior border of the lower segment, so that it is a "myoosseous flap" with a good blood upply. The chin can be advanced, lengthened, or shortened, and lateral asymmetries can be corrected [35,37]. Although a genioplasty does not alter dental occlusion, it is frequently performed in concert with procedures that do (Fig. 7-4). Its main purpose is to alter the appearance of the chin, though in many cases a functional improvement is provided with better lip seal.

*Segmental osteotomies* (Fig. 7-5) do not require intermaxillary fixation in most cases, as stability can be provided by a splint attached to the remaining teeth. A segmental osteotomy of the anterior mandibular teeth, often referred to as a Köle procedure [13], was the first orthognathic surgical procedure of any type to be performed. Simon Hullihen, physician and dentist, performed the procedure in 1848 in Wheeling, Virginia (now West Virginia), on a patient with a mandibular deformity caused by a burn scar contraction [12]. The *Wassmund procedure* [33] is a premaxillary osteotomy done to correct a marked overjet/overbite relation. The *Schuchardt procedure* [23] is a posterior maxillary osteotomy with intrusion of the osteotomized segment into the maxillary sinus, usually done to correct an anterior open bite or extruded maxillary teeth because of the absence of their mandibular counterparts. If a tooth is extracted to allow performance of a segmental osteotomy, or if an adequate space of 4 to 5 mm can be created orthodontically, the vitality of the teeth on either side of the osteotomy generally remains good to carbon dioxide snow or electrical pulp testing. If an interdental osteotomy is performed between two teeth that lie a normal distance apart, the incidence of

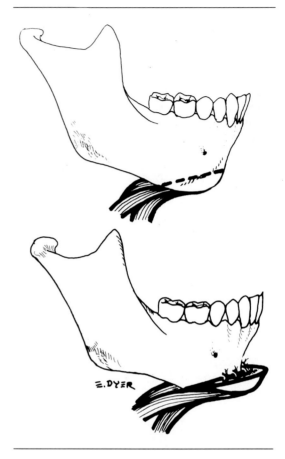

**Figure 7-3** *"Sliding" advancement genioplasty. (From P. Regnault and R. K. Daniel.* Aesthetic Plastic Surgery. *Boston: Little, Brown, 1984.)*

loss of tooth vitality requiring endodontic therapy increases [19].

*Mandibular body osteotomies* are rarely performed now because they require sacrifice of a tooth and a tedious unroofing of the inferior alveolar nerve. However, in cases where appropriate teeth are missing and there are major discrepancies in arch form, or in cases of extreme mandibular prognathism, they still may be the best operation available [7].

Of the *mandibular ramus osteotomies*, the sagittal splitting procedure (Fig. 7-6) is the most versatile because it can be used for both mandibular prognathia and retrogna-

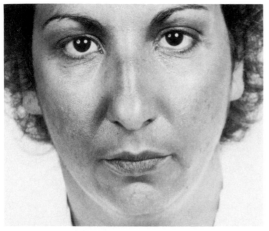

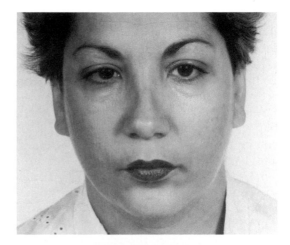

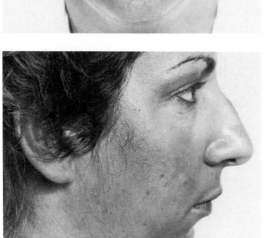

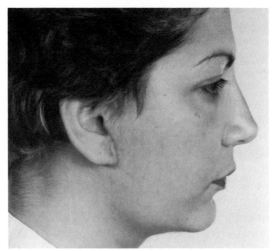

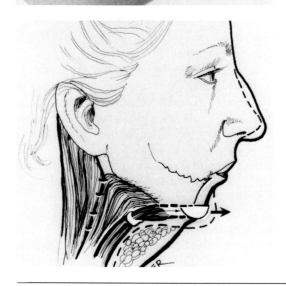

**Figure 7-4** *Before and after rhinoplasty, meloplasty, submental lipectomy, and sliding advancement genioplasty, performed in one stage. The improvement in the appearance of the neck is due to the removal of submental fat and the anterior pull on the geniohyoid muscle, which is provided by the genioplasty. (From S. A. Wolfe and S. Berkowitz.* Plastic Surgery of the Facial Skeleton. *Boston: Little, Brown, 1989.)*

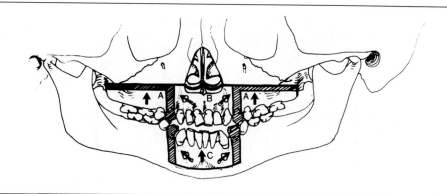

**Figure 7-5** *Segmental alveolar osteotomies commonly used to correct malocclusion. A. Schuchardt procedure. B. Wassmund procedure. C. Köle procedure.*

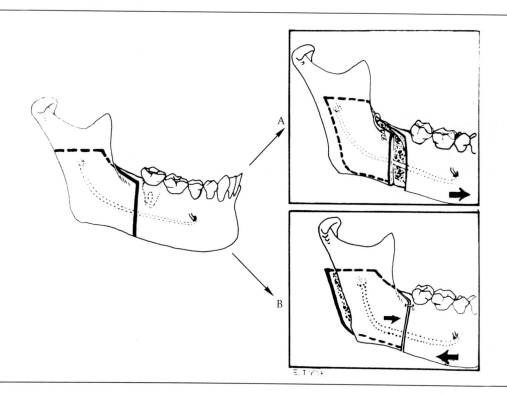

**Figure 7-6** *The sagittal splitting procedure is the most versatile ramus osteotomy, as it can be used for both mandibular advancement (A), or mandibular setback (B). The procedure is performed through an intraoral approach and requires special instrumentation to be performed with ease. Note that the osteosynthesis wire for mandibular advancement is placed in such a way that as it is tightened upward pressure is placed on the distal fragment, which tends to seat the condyle in the glenoid fossa. It is vital that the mandibular condyles be properly seated at the end of any mandibular osteotomy. If they are not, when intermaxillary fixation is removed they go back into the glenoid fossae with a resultant anterior open bite.*

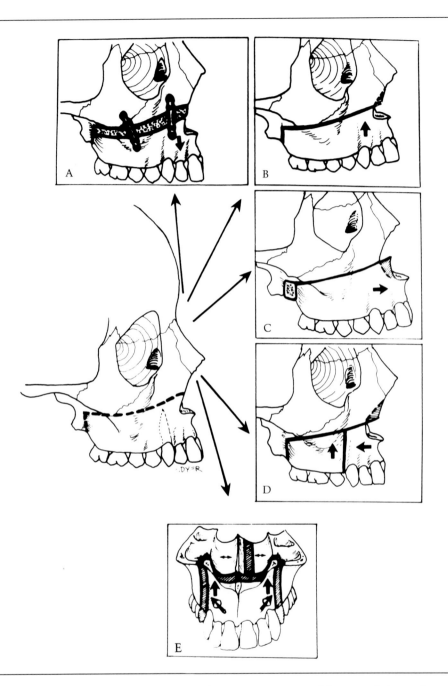

**Figure 7-7** *The Le Fort I osteotomy sections the maxilla transversely at a level between the roots of the teeth (note that the root of the cuspid may extend as high as the piriform rim) and the infraorbital foramen. After the lower portion of the maxilla is mobilized, movement in a number of directions is possible. A. Lengthening of the maxilla with an interpositional bone graft (note the use of miniplates for fixation). B. Shortening of the maxilla after resection of bone above the osteotomy line. C. Advancement of the maxilla, in this case with a retrotuberosity bone graft. D, E. Segmentalization of the maxilla after down-fracture and extraction of teeth.*

thia. The first sagittal splitting of the mandibular rami was reported in 1924 by Georg Perthes [20], who used an external approach; Trauner and Obwegeser [30] later popularized the intraoral approach. The intraoral vertical osteotomy is also commonly used for prognathia [9]. The inverted L osteotomy [32] is used for severe cases of retrognathia with anterior open bite and is performed through an external approach, usually with bone grafting.

The *Le Fort I* osteotomy (Fig. 7-7), the most commonly employed maxillary osteotomy, was first performed for correction of malocclusion by Wassmund [32], with further improvements by Axhausen [3], Schuchardt [22], and Obwegeser [18]. A Le Fort I osteotomy (note that it is *not* spelled Le Forte; the proper pronunciation is therefore "Le For") is performed at least 4 to 5 mm above the roots of the maxillary teeth (the canines are the highest). The osteotomy is carried across the anterior maxilla (below the level of the infraorbital foramen) and through the lateral and medial maxillary walls (below the nasolacrimal duct); the septum is then separated from the vomer. An osteotomy is performed between the maxillary tuberosity and the pterygoid plate of the sphenoid (through the palatine bone) with a thin, curved osteotome. At this point the maxilla can be down-fractured by digital pressure alone. The greater palatine vessels, in the posteromedial aspect of the sinus, are protected. The maxilla can be further mobilized with a blunt retrotuberosity lever or Rowe forceps. Movement of the maxilla in any direction is then possible, although upward or backward movement requires removal of bone, and downward movement necessitates an interpositional bone graft. In the down-fractured position, teeth can be moved and various segmental osteotomies performed. The palate can be split and the maxilla expanded. Virtually all patients with cleft lip and palate undergoing Le Fort I osteotomy receive autogenous bone grafts, which are placed across the anterior maxillary oste-

otomy line and in the pterygomaxillary space if the advancement is 7 to 8 mm or more. Bone grafts are used in cleft patients to provide greater stability and to improve the aesthetic result. Autogenous bone grafts routinely heal well even though they are exposed on one side to the maxillary sinus [17].

Velopharyngeal insufficiency may follow maxillary advancement. Usually, however, it occurs only in cleft patients who were borderline beforehand and who undergo substantial advancements [34].

## Particular Problems of Cleft Lip and Cleft Palate

Clefts of the lip often extend through the bony structures of the maxillary alveolus and hard palate. Teeth along the edges of the cleft are often absent or malformed, with the lateral incisor most often involved. Abnormalities of other teeth are not infrequent.

With skeletal rehabilitation, a cleft patient should achieve an intact maxillary alveolar arch before eruption of the permanent cuspid. Primary bone grafting of alveolar clefts has been generally abandoned because of subsequent interference with maxillary development, but late (5 to 10 years of age) bone grafting using iliac or cranial bone [38] provides a bony matrix through which permanent teeth can erupt with better eventual periodontal support and tooth longevity. If the alveolus is closed by periosteoplasty at the time of lip closure, good bone formation often occurs without the need for any bone grafting, but presurgical maxillary orthopedic care is generally necessary to bring the maxillary segments into close enough alignment to allow it to be done without extensive undermining. The long-term effects of this procedure on subsequent maxillary development are still unknown.

If a subsequent Le Fort I advancement is required in a cleft patient (and a certain number of patients require it no matter how they are treated primarily), management is easier if there is an intact maxillary alveolus instead of two or three maxillary segments.

*Combined maxillary and mandibular osteotomies* can be performed simultaneously (Fig. 7-8) or in stages (Fig. 7-9). In simultaneous bimaxillary procedures an intermediate split can be used to properly position the maxilla before completing the mandibular osteotomy. Combined procedures are indicated in patients with large anteroposterior discrepancies between the two jaws (15 to 20 mm or more), in situations where there are combined horizontal and anteroposterior discrepancies, and in cases where the occlusal plane is to be altered (hemifacial microsomia).

Almost all elective orthognathic surgical procedures can be done without a tracheostomy. As a rule, intraoperative steroids are not administered; but if more than a normal amount of postoperative swelling is anticipated, particularly in instances where both jaws are being operated on simultaneously, a short course of high-dose steroids may be indicated. It is prudent in certain cases to keep the patient intubated overnight, and careful surveillance of the patient's airway is maintained after extubation.

With fiberoptic equipment and an anesthesiologist skilled in its use, even patients with major mandibular deformities and limited mouth opening can usually be intubated. Having nasotracheal intubation in place of course precludes doing simultaneous correction of lip and nose deformities, but this procedure can be done much more precisely at a second operation.

The sequence of simultaneous Le Fort I osteotomy and sagittal split of the mandibular rami is as follows.

1. Perform the Le Fort I.
2. Perform the lateral and medial portions of the sagittal split.
3. Stabilize the maxilla in the desired position. An intermediate splint may be helpful, and miniplates provide the most stable fixation.

4. Finish the sagittal split and move the mandible into the final desired occlusal relation with the maxilla, with or without a splint.

The *Le Fort II osteotomy* was first performed for maxillary advancement in a nontrauma patient during the mid-1960s by Tessier [28], and it was later popularized by Henderson and Jackson [10]. This method, not the Le Fort I procedure, is a true "total maxillary osteotomy." It is indicated in cleft patients with severe maxillary hypoplasia involving the nose and infraorbital rims, in patients who may have markedly compromised palatal circulation, and in those with Crouzon's disease who do not show exorbitism [27]. Patients with exorbitism, even when it is mild, are best treated by a Le Fort III osteotomy [36].

### Fractures of the Jaw

*Fractures of the mandible,* if in good alignment and not prone to displacement by muscle pull (favorable fractures), can be treated by application of arch bars and intermaxillary fixation to the intact maxilla alone. If there has been displacement of the fractured segments and they cannot be accurately aligned by close reduction, open reduction and osteosynthesis are performed. In almost all instances the procedure can be done through an oral approach if the surgeon is familiar with intraoral orthognathic surgical

**Figure 7-8** *Patient with class III malocclusion due to mandibular prognathism, vertical maxillary excess, and macrogenia. In one stage, a Le Fort I osteotomy was performed with vertical impaction (shortening), along with a mandibular setback by sagittal splitting of the mandibular rami and a reduction genioplasty with advancement of the lower border fragment. The postoperative occlusal view shows that the absent right central incisor has been replaced by a pontic. (From S. A. Wolfe and S. Berkowitz.* Plastic Surgery of the Facial Skeleton. *Boston: Little, Brown, 1989.)*

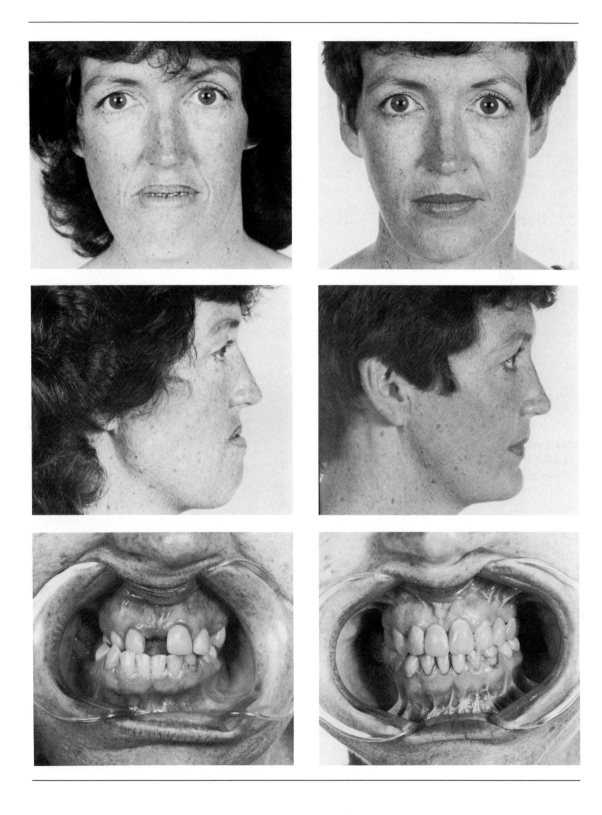

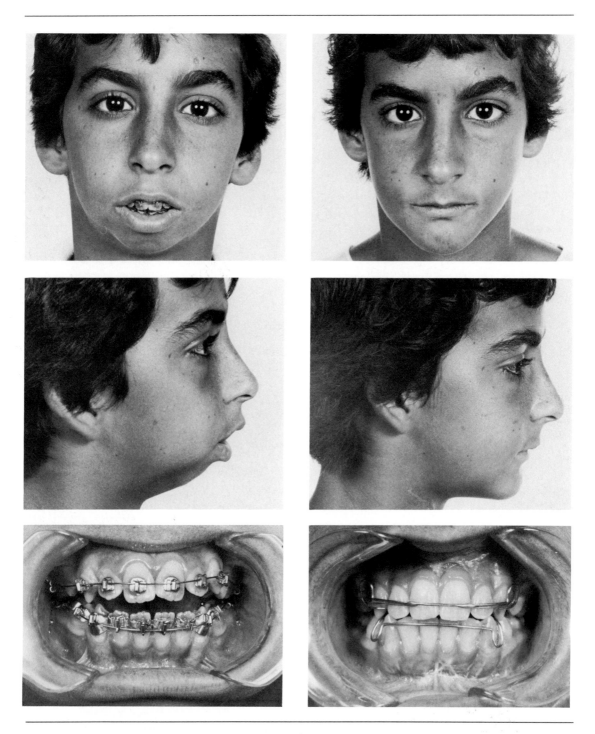

**Figure 7-9** *Patient with class II malocclusion due to mandibular retrognathia, premaxillary protrusion, anterior open bite, and microgenia. Correction was carried out in two stages.*

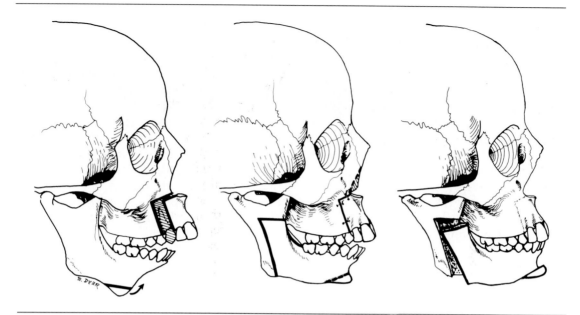

**Figure 7-9** (continued) First, a Wassmund procedure was performed along with extraction of two bicuspids and a jumping genioplasty. At a second stage, an inverted **L** osteotomy of the rami was performed with an interpositional iliac bone graft, and a second genioplasty (this time of the sliding variety) was performed through the previous genioplasty. (From S. A. Wolfe and S. Berkowitz. Plastic Surgery of the Facial Skeleton. Boston: Little, Brown, 1989.)

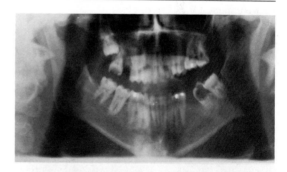

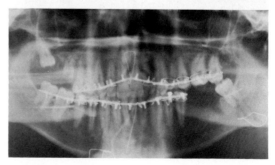

**Figure 7-10** Left ramus and right parasymphyseal fractures of the mandible due to a blow from a fist. The carious left lower first molar was extracted. The fracture passed distal to the roots of an otherwise healthy left lower second molar, which was not extracted. Upper and lower border wiring of the left ramus fracture and a lower border wire of the parasymphyseal fracture were performed through an intraoral approach. Arch bars were applied (note the piriform rim and circummandibular wires used for skeletal fixation), and the patient was maintained in intermaxillary fixation for 6 weeks. Healing proceeded uneventfully, and the patient was dispatched to his dentist for long-neglected dental restoration.

techniques and has the requisite instrumentation (Fig. 7-10). If a laceration over the fracture is present, the surgeon should by all means use this external approach; but if the skin is intact, Freihofer and Sailer [8] were right in stating that making an external incision should be looked on as a complication. Compression plating has been used extensively in Europe to provide more stable results with mandibular fractures, often without the need for intermaxillary fixation, and good results with a low infection rate have been reported [14].

*Fractures of the maxilla*, in the presence of an intact mandible and otherwise intact maxillary buttresses (nasomaxillary, zygomaticomaxillary), can be treated by reduction of the fracture and intermaxillary fixation if superior suspension to intact upper structures ("Adams suspension") [1] is performed to prevent development of a pseudoarthrosis at the fracture line. If these important facial buttresses have been shattered and comminuted, the best results are obtained if primary bone grafting is performed to restore the buttresses and maintain facial height.

## Reconstruction of the Mandible

With reconstruction of in-continuity defects of the mandible, a better than 90 percent success rate may be expected using autogenous bone grafts [4]. Excellent results have been obtained in nonirradiated patients by performing primary reconstruction if adequate soft tissue is present or can be provided [16]. If large intraoral or extraoral soft tissue defects are present, or if the soft tissues have been damaged by heavy irradiation, these problems must be dealt with before the mandible can be successfully reconstructed. It can be done in stages using various types of soft tissue flap from distant locations followed by a free bone graft, or in certain cases in one stage using composite skin–muscle–bone tissue transferred by microsurgical techniques [26]. The skull has been used as a donor site, transferred as a myoosseous flap pedicled on the temporal muscle [29]. In my experience, the best results have been obtained using only autogenous bone graft to replace missing segments of the mandible; large metallic trays or cadaver bone used as a crib serve only to complicate the issue and interfere with blood supply to the bone graft. Successful cases have been reported using these methods, but they are probably successful despite, rather than because of, the foreign bodies. Whatever the method of reconstruction employed, a mandibular reconstruction cannot be considered a complete success until the patient can be fitted for and comfortably wear a denture. It often requires vestibuloplasty [25], a procedure that cannot be performed over anything but an autogenous bone graft (Fig. 7-11).

*Figure 7-11* This patient had excision of a chondrosarcoma of the anterior mandible followed by two attempts at mandibular reconstruction using a metallic tray packed with cancellous bone. Both iliac regions were utilized for the previous reconstructive attempts. Reconstruction was accomplished according to basic principles. A. Deficient intraoral lining was replaced by an island flap of skin from the left supraclavicular region nourished by the platysma muscle and superficial cervical fascia (Barron-Tessier flap). B. Mandibular reconstruction was performed using autogenous bone only. Two ribs were harvested, split, and bent to the requisite shape, and additional cancellous bone was harvested from the tibia and packed into the "tray" made from the ribs. C. Vestibuloplasty has been performed over the bone graft using thick, split skin. D. The patient was fitted for a denture and can comfortably eat all types of food. The denture relies on fixation to the remaining mandibular molars, which are not in good condition, and it may be necessary in the future to contemplate an osseointegrated implant of the Branemark variety for stabilization of the denture.

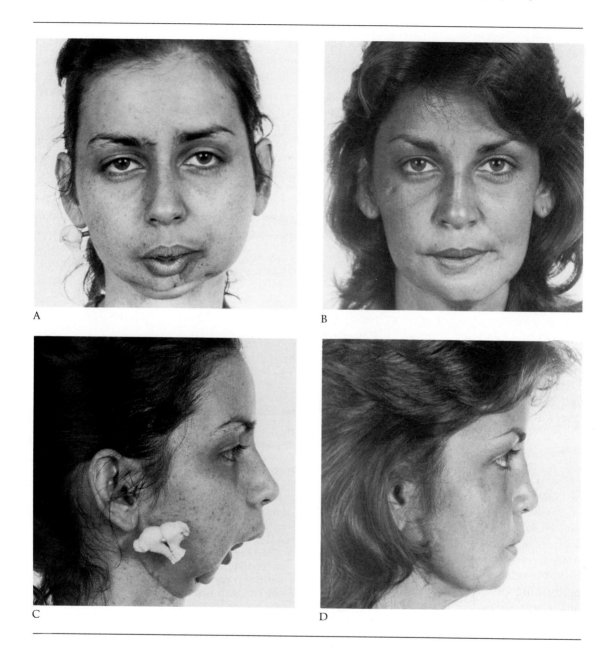

A

B

C

D

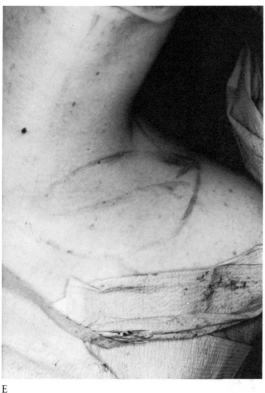

E

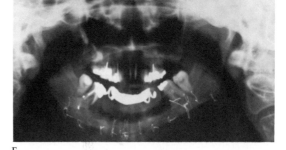

F

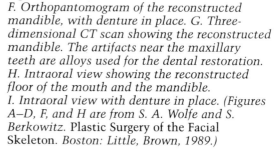

G

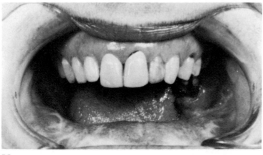

H

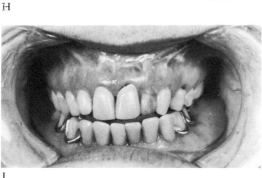

I

**Figure 7-11** (continued) E. Outline of the Barron-Tessier flap from the left supraclavicular region.
F. Orthopantomogram of the reconstructed mandible, with denture in place. G. Three-dimensional CT scan showing the reconstructed mandible. The artifacts near the maxillary teeth are alloys used for the dental restoration. H. Intraoral view showing the reconstructed floor of the mouth and the mandible.
I. Intraoral view with denture in place. (Figures A–D, F, and H are from S. A. Wolfe and S. Berkowitz. Plastic Surgery of the Facial Skeleton. Boston: Little, Brown, 1989.)

## What is New?

Miniplates used in maxillofacial surgery provide rigid enough fixation that in many cases intermaxillary fixation can be avoided altogether or used for a shorter period of time [5]. The Luhr system, which can provide compressive forces, has its best use in fractured mandibles. The Champy, Würzburg, and Medicon systems are smaller and have self-tapping screws. Guidelines for the use of miniplates remain to be established, and it is uncertain at present whether the plates must all be removed at a subsequent operation. Osseointegrated implants are finding increasing use in edentulous jaws, even after reconstruction.

Three-dimensional computed tomography scans provide valuable images of the facial skeleton [31], but metallic orthodontic appliances cause considerable scatter; and to date three-dimensional imaging has not been shown to be useful for planning orthognathic surgical procedures. Careful examination of the patient, the dental models, and cephalometric films remain the basis of treatment planning.

Hyperbaric oxygen treatment has improved the outlook for patients with osteoradionecrosis of the mandible [15] but has not been shown to improve the results of routine orthognathic surgery.

There is a perpetual search for bone substitutes, and waves of enthusiasm have come and gone for various substances. Bovine bone, human cadaver bone, demineralized bone, hydroxyapatite, and many other substances have been tried, but to date no material has been shown to consolidate as rapidly and resist infection as well as fresh autogenous bone graft containing primarily cancellous bone. Clinical trials of promising new bone substitutes will continue, but until the perfect material is found, plastic surgeons should learn how to harvest bone grafts quickly, with little blood letting and no permanent insult to the patient. The skull is increasingly popular as a donor source.

Good results are also obtained if one pays careful attention to technical fine detail when performing facial osteotomies: Primary bone healing occurs only when the bone segments are in tight abutment with less than 1 mm of separation [24]. There is much carpentry involved in this type of work, and the surgeon should not be surprised to find that much can be learned by watching a master cabinetmaker at work.

## References

1. Adams, W. M. Internal wiring fixation of facial fractures. *Surgery* 12:523, 1942.
2. Angle, E. H. *Treatment of Malocclusion of the Teeth and Fractures of the Maxillae: Angle's System.* Philadelphia: S. S. White Dental Manufacturing Co., 1900. P. 6.
3. Axhausen, G. Zur Behandlung veralteter disloziert geheilter Oberkieferbruche. *Dtsch. Zahn. Mund. Kieferheilk* 1:334, 1934.
4. Blocker, T. G., and Stout, R. A. Mandibular reconstruction in World War II. *Plast. Reconstr. Surg.* 4:153, 1949.
5. Champy, M., et al. Mandibular osteosynthesis by miniature screwed plates via a buccal approach. *J. Maxillofac. Surg.* 6:14, 1978.
6. Converse, J., and Wood-Smith, D. Horizontal osteotomy of the mandible. *Plast. Reconstr. Surg.* 34:464, 1964.
7. Dingman, R. Surgical correction of the mandibular prognathism. *Am. J. Orthodont.* 30:683, 1944.
8. Freihofer, H. P. M., Jr., and Sailer, H. F. Experience with intraoral transosseous wiring of mandibular fractures. *J. Maxillofac. Surg.* 1:248, 1973.
9. Hebert, J., Kent, J., and Hinds, E. Correction of prognathism by an intraoral vertical subcondylar osteotomy. *J. Oral Surg.* 33:384, 1970.
10. Henderson, D., and Jackson, I. T. Nasomaxillary hypoplasia—the Le Fort II osteotomy. *Br. J. Oral Surg.* 11:77, 1973.
11. Hofer, O. Die operative Behandlung der alveolären Retraktion des Unterkiefers und ihre Anwendungsmöglichkeit für Prognathie und Mikrogenie. *Dtsch. Kieferchir.* 9:(1), 1942. *Dtsch. Zahn. Mund. Kieferheilk.* 9:130, 1942.
12. Hullihen, S. Case of elongation of the under jaw and distortion of the face and neck caused

by a burn successfully treated. *Am. J. Dent. Sci.* 9:157, 1849.

13. Köle, H. Surgical operations on the alveolar ridge to correct occlusal abnormalities. *Oral Surg.* 12:227, 1950.

14. Luhr, H-G., et al. Comparative studies between the extraoral and intraoral approach in compression-osteosynthesis of mandibular fractures. In E. Hjorting-Hansen (ed.), *Proceedings from the 8th International Conference on Oral and Maxillofacial Surgery.* Chicago: Quintessence Publishing Co., 1985.

15. Marx, R. E., and Ames, J. R. The use of hyperbaric oxygen therapy in bony reconstruction of the irradiated and tissue-deficient patient. *J. Oral Surg.* 40:412, 1982.

16. Millard, D. R., Jr. Immediate reconstruction of the lower jaw. *Plast. Reconstr. Surg.* 35:60, 1965.

17. Obwegeser, H. Surgical correction of maxillary deformities. In W. C. Grabb, S. W. Rosenstein, and K. R. Bzoch (eds.), *Cleft Lip and Palate.* Boston: Little, Brown, 1971. Pp. 515–556.

18. Obwegeser, H. Surgical correction of small or retrodisplaced maxillae. *Plast. Reconstr. Surg.* 43:351, 1965.

19. Pepersack, W. Tooth vitality after alveolar segmental osteotomy. *J. Maxillofac. Surg.* 1:85, 1983.

20. Perthes, G. Der kieferöpfchens und ihre operative Behandlung. *Arch. Klin. Chir.* 1333:425, 1924.

21. Riolo, M. L., et al. *An Atlas of Craniofacial Growth: Cephalometric Standards from the University School Growth Study.* Ann Arbor: Center for Human Growth and Development, University of Michigan, 1979.

22. Schuchardt, K. Ein Beitrag zur chirurgischen Kieferorthopädie unter Berucksichtigung ihrer Bedeutung angeborener und erwoobener Kieferdeformationen bei Soldaten. *Dtsch. Zahn. Mund. Kieferheilk.* 2:73, 1942.

23. Schuchardt, K. Experience with the surgical treatment of some deformities of the jaws: Prognathia, microgenia and open bite. In A. B. Wallace (ed.), *Transactions of the International Society of Plastic Surgeons, Second Congress.* Baltimore: Williams & Wilkins, 1961. Pp. 73–78.

24. Shenk, R. K. Histologie der Primären Kno-

chenheilung. *Fortschr. Kiefer. Gesichtschir.* 19:8, 1975.

25. Steinhaüser, E. M. Vestibuloplasty—skin grafts. *J. Oral. Surg.* 29:777, 1971.

26. Taylor, G. I. The current status of free vascularized bone grafts. *Clin. Plast. Surg.* 10:185, 1983.

27. P. Tessier et al. (eds.), *Plastic Surgery of the Orbit and Eyelids.* Translated by S. A. Wolfe. New York: Masson, 1981. P. 213.

28. Tessier, P. Personal communication, 1975.

29. Tessier, P. Presented at the VIIth International Congress of Plastic Surgery, Montreal, 29 June 1983.

30. Trauner, R., and Obwegeser, H. Surgical correction of mandibular prognathism and retrogenia with consideration of genioplasty. *Oral Surg.* 10:677, 1957.

31. Vannier, M. W., Marsh, J. L., and Warren, J. O. Three-dimensional CT reconstruction images for craniofacial surgical planning and evaluation. *Radiology* 150:179, 1984.

32. Wassmund, M. Frakturen und Luxationen des Gesichtschadels unter Beruksichtigung des Komplikationen des Hirnschadels. In *Klinik und Therapie: Praktischen Lehrbuch* (Vol. 20). Berlin: Hermann Meusser, 1927.

33. Wassmund, M. *Lehrbuch der praktischen Chirurgie des Mundes und der Kiefer* (Vol. 1). Liepzig: Meusser, 1935.

34. Witzel, M. A., and Munro, I. R. Velopharyngeal insufficiency after maxillary advancement. *Cleft Palate J.* 14:176, 1977.

35. Wolfe, S. A. Aesthetic Procedures on the Chin. In P. Regnault and R. K. Daniel (eds.), *Aesthetic Plastic Surgery.* Boston: Little, Brown, 1984. Pp. 221–244.

36. Wolfe, S. A. A rationale for the surgical treatment of exophthalmos and exorbitism. *J. Maxillofac. Surg.* 5:249, 1977.

37. Wolfe, S. A. Chin advancement as an aid in correction of deformities of the mental and submental regions. *Plast. Reconstr. Surg.* 67:624, 1981.

38. Wolfe, S. A., and Berkowitz, S. The use of cranial bone grafts in the closure of alveolar and anterior palatal clefts. *Plast. Reconstr. Surg.* 7:629, 1983.

39. Zide, B., Grayson, B., and McCarthy, J. G. Cepahlometric analysis. Parts I, II, and III. *Plast. Reconstr. Surg.* 68:816,961, 1981; 69:155, 1982.

## Suggested Reading

Bell, W. H., Proffit, W. R., and White, R. P. *Surgical Correction of Dentofacial Deformities.* Philadelphia: Saunders, 1980.

Converse, J. M., et al. Deformities of the Jaws. In J. M. Converse (ed.), *Reconstructive Plastic Surgery* (Vol. 3). Philadelphia: Saunders, 1977.

Dingman, R. O., and Natvig, P. *Surgery of Facial Fractures.* Philadelphia: Saunders, 1964.

Epker, B. N., and Wolford, L. M. *Dentofacial Deformities.* St. Louis: Mosby, 1980.

Gabilisco, J. A. (ed.). *Stafne's Oral Radiographic Diagnosis.* Philadelphia: Saunders, 1985.

Gruss, J. S., et al. The role of primary bone grafting in complex craniomaxillofacial trauma. *Plast. Reconstr. Surg.* 75:17, 1985.

Harvold, E. P., Vargervik, K., and Chierici, G. (eds.). *Treatment of Hemifacial Microsomia.* New York: Liss, 1983.

Hinds, E. C., and Kent, J. N. *Surgical Treatment of Developmental Jaw Deformities.* St. Louis: Mosby, 1972.

Kawamoto, H. K., Jr., and Wolfe, S. A. Symposium on maxillofacial surgery. *Clin. Plast. Surg.* 9:1, 1982.

Manson, P. N., Hoopes, J. E., and Su, C. T. Structural pillars of the facial skeleton: An approach to the management of Le Fort fractures. *Plast. Reconstr. Surg.* 66:54, 1980.

McNamara, J. A., Jr. (ed.). *The Biology of Occlusal Development.* Monograph No. 7, Craniofacial Growth Series. Ann Arbor: Center for Human Growth and Development, University of Michigan, 1977.

Moyers, R. E. *Handbook of Orthodontics.* Chicago: Year Book, 1973.

Ramfjord, S. P., and Ash, M. M., Jr. *Occlusion.* Philadelphia: Saunders, 1971.

Van der Linden, F. P. G. M., and Duterloo, H. S. *Development of the Human Dentition.* New York: Harper & Row, 1976.

Whitaker, L. A., and Randall, P. (eds.). *Symposium on Reconstruction of Jaw Deformity.* St. Louis: Mosby, 1978.

*Jonathan S. Jacobs*
*Russell Bessette*

# 8

# *Temporomandibular Joint Deformities*

Surveys have estimated that between 4 and 28 percent of the adult population are affected by symptomatology of the temporomandibular joint (TMJ) [10, 34, 68], with a female/male ratio of 3:1 [25, 66]. Young to middle-aged women are most often affected. The common triad of symptoms include pain in the preauricular area, with popping and clicking of the TMJ, and limitation of mandibular movement. The mandible may deviate to the affected side, and the symptoms may be episodic. A strong psychological component has been implicated in many patients. It must be stated at the outset that most patients with these symptoms are best treated by nonsurgical therapy. However, each patient deserves an adequate evaluation to eliminate the possibility of organic disease. Conditions of neuralgia, paranasal sinusitis, dental pulpitis, central nervous system (CNS) neoplasms, and neuritis such as temporal arthritis can masquerade as TMJ syndrome. A complete head and neck physical examination remains the mainstay for evaluation of these patients. However, after a thorough examination, a significant number of patients complain of pain with no organic findings. This pain may be relieved by lidocaine infiltration of their joint. Special diagnostic testing is reserved for patients with suspected internal derangements of the TMJ, particularly if there is a history of trauma.

Most investigators consider malocclusion and long-term microtrauma to be of importance in the etiology. These problems may be secondary to either dental occlusal prematurity or overclosure of the mandible. Bruxism with microtrauma to the joint also has been implicated. These factors are thought to work alone or in conjunction with anxiety to produce masticatory muscle spasm. To denote the special role of muscle spasm, the term myofascial pain dysfunction (MPD) syndrome has been proposed [41]. Many investigators believe that the symptoms are secondary to dental malocclusion and subsequent muscle spasm. Their effort has been directed toward correcting occlusal function. Most notably, the vertical dimension of occlusion [17, 19] has been adjusted by either orthodontic or prosthetic means. If overclosure is thought to be a problem, it seems important to raise the height of the dentition, thereby opening the bite and increasing the vertical dimension. As part of the therapy, mandibular opening is limited to hinge movement only, as it eliminates the need for external pterygoid contraction. The construction of splints (Fig. 8-1) that disarticulate the occlusion has also been advocated. Splints function to change the position of the condyle in the fossa when the jaws are articulated. Therefore they help interrupt the pain–spasm cycle associated with bruxing [9]. They may be effective in "capturing" a subluxing disc by repositioning the condyle under the anteriorly positioned disc. Adjunctive treatments for muscle spasm are usually employed, including heat, ultrasonography, diathermy, exercises that decrease range of motion, and the use of muscle relaxants and antiinflammatory drugs.

## Normal Anatomy

The structure of the TMJ has been well described [11, 16, 24, 27], and its function has been confirmed on arthrograms [20, 34]. The meniscus is a dense, fibrous, connective tissue structure that encapsulates the condyle (Figs. 8-2 and 8-3). The joint space is in two compartments: an upper space and a lower space. Translatory movements of the joint take place in the upper space, whereas the lower space is reserved for rotatory movement (Fig. 8-4). This combination of joint movements allows the multiplicity of actions of the TMJ. The posterior attachment of the meniscus consists of fibrovascular

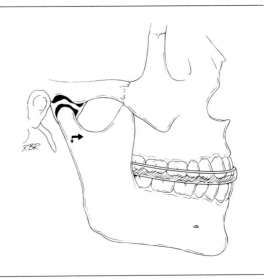

**Figure 8-1** A maxillary occlusal splint has been fabricated to disarticulate the mandible. The condyle is positioned anteriorly and downward in an attempt to capture a subluxed articular disc.

**Figure 8-2** TMJ with overlying vital structures. (a = superficial temporal artery; b = terminal fibers auriculotemporal nerve; c = internal maxillary artery; d = facial nerve; e = temporomandibular ligament (capsule); f = external pterygoid muscle.)

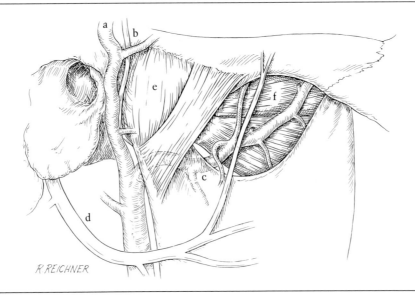

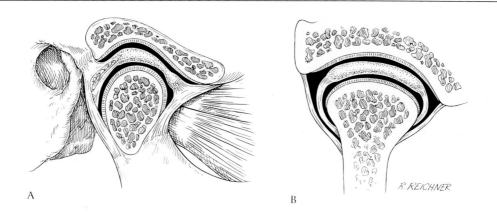

**Figure 8-3** *A. TMJ in sagittal section demonstrating the concave configuration of the articular disc, the bilaminar posterior attachment, and insertion of the external pterygoid on the disc and the condylar head. B. TMJ in coronal section demonstrating the position of the disc over the convexity of the condylar head and the separate attachments of the disc on the condyle in distinction from the capsule.*

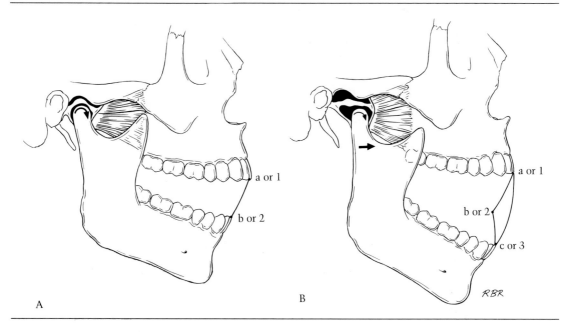

**Figure 8-4** *Normal range of motion. A. Lower joint space allows for rotation under the articular disc. B. Upper joint space adds translatory ability completing normal opening.*

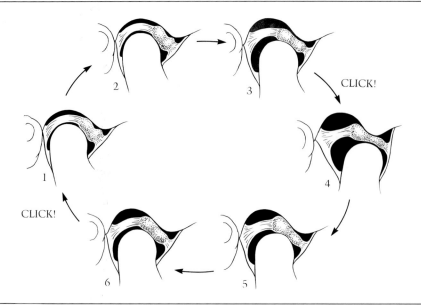

**Figure 8-5** *Mechanism of joint clicking: If the thickened posterior band of the articular disc is subluxed, opening produces a click as it is recaptured (between 3 and 4). A reciprocal click may be heard or palpated on closing if the disc again subluxes (between 6 and 1).*

connective tissue in two zones. The superior portion, consisting of predominantly elastic fibers, allows attachment of the posterior edge of the disc to the postglenoid tubercle area of the squamotympanic fissure. The inferior portion of this posterior attachment, which consists primarily of inelastic collagenous tissue, attaches the disc to the posterior aspect of the condylar neck (see Fig. 8-3A). Between these two attachments is a zone of high vascularity and the area through which the terminal fibers of the auriculotemporal nerve enter the joint space. It is thought that this so-called bilaminar zone is an important area in terms of the etiology of joint pain. Anteriorly, a portion of the superior head of the lateral pterygoid muscle attaches to the edge of the disc, with the remainder attaching to a depression on the anterior surface of the condylar head. The high elasticity of the superior aspect of the posterior attachment allows anterior movement of the disc with translation. The disc is thus a movable socket that advances with contraction of the external pterygoid and recoils passively with return of the condylar head posteriorly in the glenoid fossa (see Fig.

8-4). Maintenance of this function is integral to pain-free, noiseless joint function (Fig. 8-5).

## Neuromuscular Physiology

To maintain and operate the normal TMJ meniscal-condylar relation, it is necessary to have a harmoniously functioning neuromuscular system. The opening and closing muscles of the mandible are innervated by the motor nerves of the mandibular division of the trigeminal nerve. The complex activities of deglutition, mastication, and speech depend on a coordinated series of opening and closing muscle interactions. The positioning of the mandible is often guided by sensory input from the periodontal ligament receptors of the teeth and the TMJ capsule. Alterations in the dental occlusion or possibly the TMJ can lead to a deviated path of mandibular closing, which in turn produces masticatory muscle spasm. The muscle spasm may be seen in any or all of the muscles innervated by the fifth cranial nerve (CN V). Spasm is reported most frequently in the external pterygoid muscles. Of interest is that the tensor tympani muscles are innervated by the same motor divisions, and these muscles may go into spasm producing otalgia and possibly tinnitus [2, 12, 13, 22, 55].

As previously indicated, most TMJ problems are treated nonsurgically, and most investigators believe that the muscle spasm is the key etiologic factor in these cases. In an effort to eliminate aberrant proprioceptive input from the teeth and TMJ receptors, dentists have treated TMJ patients with various types of occlusal splint. The purpose of these splints has been to deprogram the CNS from the dental receptors and allow the mandible to open and close on a path dictated by a relaxed neuromuscular system. In addition, the splints impose forced relaxation of chewing and induce a period of TMJ and neuromuscular rest. The literature has reported varying degrees of success with these dental splints [23, 40–42, 54, 61, 64].

The decision to employ an occlusal splint is often based on empiric evidence. The clinician rarely depends on substantiating evidence of muscle spasm. It is for this reason that some investigators believe that splints may be inappropriately used. Many researchers have attempted to utilize electromyography (EMG) as a diagnostic tool, but the results have been difficult to interpret [21, 32, 33, 49, 52, 53, 57, 58].

We have reported on the use of measuring the duration of the masseteric silent period on EMG as an indicator of muscle spasm. Of particular interest is that this test may predict the response of nonsurgical patients to dental occlusal splint therapy [3–6].

It must be kept in mind that there are many patients who have normal diagnostic imaging of the joint and normal EMG studies yet show clinical signs of muscle incoordination. Many clinicians have advocated biofeedback therapy and transcutaneous nerve stimulation as alternative or adjunctive therapy to splints. These modalities are at present the object of numerous clinical investigations.

## Diagnostic Imaging of the TMJ
### RADIOGRAPHY

Radiographs of the TMJ represent one of the most valuable areas of demonstrative evidence and, simultaneously, one of the most fertile sources of misinterpretation. TMJ radiography poses a difficult, unique interpretive problem. The traditional radiographic views of the TMJ are transcranial films, tomography, and arthrography.

The transcranial view is frequently employed by dentists because of its adaptive use of standard dental x-ray equipment. Its disadvantage lies in the fact that it visualizes only the lateral, not the medial, pole of the mandibular condyle. Advocates of transcranial radiographs [19, 80] have shown that highly experienced practitioners can detect internal derangements of the TMJ through careful study of the joint spaces. However, these interpretations are subjective and require a clear understanding of skull anatomy and the dynamics of mandibular disorders.

Tomography provides the standard imagery for the TMJ. In an effort to overcome some of the criticisms of transcranial radiographs, tomographic cuts are made through the condyle at several points. It is important, however, that the radiographic planes section through the appropriate areas of condylar pathology. The average condyle is 15 mm in length from medial to lateral pole. Severe damage can exist on one portion of the condyle (usually the lateral third) but remains invisible if the plane of cut is through the middle or medial third. There also may be small osteophytes that are evident at surgery but are not seen in a specific cut through the joint.

It is important to recall that the bony surfaces of the TMJ may be completely normal, although the relation of the condyle to the fossa may be abnormal secondary to an internal derangement. This condition necessitates imaging the structure and function of the meniscus.

As radiographs of knees with injuries ranging from soft tissue contusion to ruptured ligaments and torn menisci may show no abnormality, so too may radiographs of the TMJ fail to demonstrate soft tissue pathology. It has been shown that up to 85 percent of patients with TMJ dysfunction demonstrate no abnormality on plain films [41, 69]. Therefore the diagnostic value of the conventional radiograph for detecting an internal derangement of the TMJ is questionable. In addition, it is well known that there is considerable variation in the position of the condyle within the fossa and in the condylar translation in asymptomatic individuals. As previously indicated, some clinicians consider the retruded condyle within the fossa as diagnostic of meniscus displacement. However, this controversial assertion has not been confirmed [7, 34]. Unilateral severe limitation of condylar translation is, however, suggestive of an acute meniscus displacement without reduction. Even in these cases, however, one may see normal condylar translation. To further cloud the diagnostic picture, it is clinically known that patients with tears or detachments of the bilaminar zone may show normal translation on the affected side.

Transcranial radiographs are not as sensitive to changes associated with degenerative arthritis as tomography. The earliest detectable osseous changes in patients with internal derangements appear to be erosions of the condylar surface. As the soft tissue damage progresses, the osseous abnormalities become more obvious, taking the form of deep erosions in the condylar surface. These changes are followed by progressive remodeling, which is associated with anterior and anterolateral osteophyte formation. Such changes may also be associated with areas of condylar sclerosis. As the disease progresses, there is increased osteophyte formation and flattening of the condyle. Long-standing internal derangements associated with meniscal tears or perforations may show flattening of the articular eminence. It is generally reported that only after severe and chronic disease is actual joint space narrowing apparent. All of the preceding changes can be seen in patients with internal derangements, but they are not limited to this group. They are also seen in patients with degenerative arthritis and arthritis associated with inflammatory joint disease, such as rheumatoid arthritis and psoriatic arthritis.

ARTHROGRAPHY

The TMJ arthrogram has emerged as the standard for imaging the structure and function of the meniscus [34] (Figs. 8-6 and 8-7). Patients are generally selected for arthrography based on clinical symptoms that suggest internal derangement, particularly if conservative treatment modalities have failed. The primary objective of the arthrogram is to assess the position of the meniscus, extent of meniscal movement, and meniscal integrity.

Contraindications to arthrography include a history of severe reaction to iodinated contrast media. Note that serious or life-threatening reactions to arthrography are rare. Bleeding disorders and anticoagulation medications are relative contraindications to arthrography. The procedure must not be performed in the presence of local skin infections because of the risk of introducing infection in the joint. An important practical consideration of TMJ arthrography are the technically demanding aspects of arthrography. Moreover, in some communities it is difficult for the surgeon to locate a radiologist comfortable with the procedure.

In preparation for arthrography, plain films or tomograms are obtained to stage the disease and assess joint space size. The patient is then placed on a fluoroscopic table in a lateral recumbent position with the head tilted on the table top. This positioning allows the joint to project over the skull above the facial bones. The side to be examined is

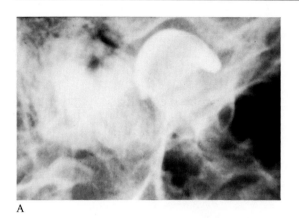

A

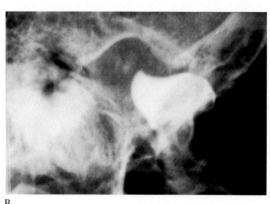

B

***Figure 8-6*** *Arthrogram of the TMJ. A. Lower joint space arthrogram demonstrating the normal meniscal position at the mandibular centric occlusion. B. Lower joint space arthrogram in the jaw-open position demonstrating the normal meniscal position. The contrast material is completely emptied from the anterior recess.*

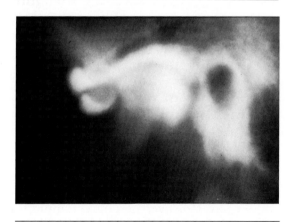

***Figure 8-7*** *Arthrogram demonstrating nonreducing meniscal displacement with perforation. Arrow denotes anteriorly displaced meniscus with contrast material in the lower joint space and anterior recess leaking into the superior joint space above the meniscus.*

uppermost, permitting skin preparation and draping. Instructing the patient to open and close the mouth several times under fluoroscopic observation allows rapid identification of the condyle of the affected joint.

Under fluoroscopic guidance, the posterosuperior aspect of the mandibular condyle is identified. Local anesthetic (1% lidocaine) is infiltrated locally. A 23-gauge scalp vein needle and attached tubing are filled with contrast material. The 23-gauge needle is introduced into the predetermined region of the condyle perpendicular to the skin. When the condyle is encountered, the patient is instructed to open the jaw slightly, and the needle is guided off the posterior slope of the condyle into the joint space. Correct positioning permits a test injection of contrast material to flow freely anterior to the condyle when the needle is properly placed in the lower joint space. The needle is then withdrawn, and fluoroscopic videotape images are recorded during opening and closing maneuvers of the jaw. Multidirectional tomograms are obtained for a more complete evaluation.

Abnormal arthrographic findings are as follows.

***1.*** *Meniscal displacement with reduction* (Fig. 8-8). Generally, though not exclusively, patients with clicking have this arthro-

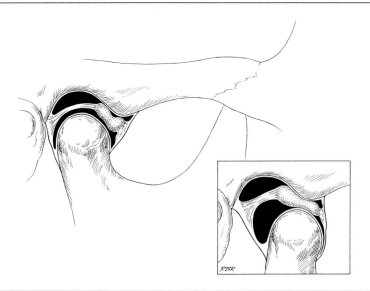

**Figure 8-8** *Anterior meniscal displacement with reduction. On opening, the disc is captured, and dye is squeezed from the anterior recess (inset). Prior to opening, the anterior recess has an abnormal peaked configuration.*

graphic finding. It represents a form of mechanical dysfunction caused by meniscocondylar incoordination during which the meniscus is in an anterior position relative to the oncoming condyle during jaw opening. As the condyle and meniscus "snap" into and out of correct anatomic position during a phase of jaw opening, the click is produced (Fig. 8-8). It occurs most often during the midopening position of the jaw. It is generally believed, though not proved, that such patients are best treated by mandibular repositioning splints; the rationale is to maintain the condyle underneath the meniscus and allow the attenuated bilaminar zone to heal. In some centers this jaw position can be recorded in quick-setting dental impression material, and a splint can be fabricated at the time of arthrography.

   2. *Meniscal displacement without reduction* (Fig. 8-9). This condition is the most significant mechanical dysfunction caused by anterior displacement of the meniscus and is often preceded clinically by painful clicking of the TMJ. It can be associated clinically with acute unilateral limitation of opening and deviation of the mandible to the affected side. The patient usually relates that clicking disappears once locking has occurred.

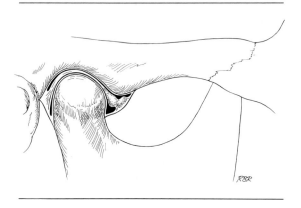

**Figure 8-9** *Anterior meniscal displacement without reduction. The anterior peaked configuration of dye is maintained, and jaw opening is limited by the displaced disc.*

The displaced meniscus may form a physical barrier to anterior translation. Incompetence of the posterior attachment (bilaminar zone) of the meniscus is probably the pathophysiologic mechanism, and it may be associated with damage to the fibroblasts and produce fibrosis. The force of the condyle on the well

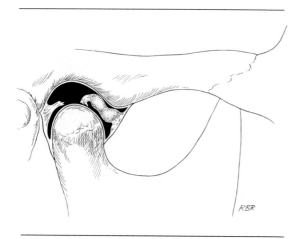

**Figure 8-10** *Anterior meniscal displacement with perforation. Dye injected in the lower joint space demonstrates an anterior peaked configuration. Dye is also seen in the superior joint space.*

innervated posterior meniscal attachment may be the major mechanism of pain. Because mandibular splint repositioning cannot recapture this meniscus, it is generally thought that surgical repositioning and meniscal repair comprise the best therapy for painful joints [17, 19] (Fig. 8-10).

**3.** *Meniscal displacement with perforation.* Almost all patients with perforations of the TMJ have anterior meniscus displacement. A high percentage of these patients shows osseous abnormalities that are compatible with a diagnosis of degenerative arthritis on tomographic evaluation. An interesting aspect of these cases is that condylar translation is nearly normal. However, these patients often relate a history of chronic limitation of opening that resolved slowly over time. Surgical findings in these patients often reveal that most perforations occur in the bilaminar zone. In some studies, a 15 percent incidence of false-positive perforations have been reported [45]. Generally, such a finding is due to straddling of the needle bevel between upper and lower joint spaces with simultaneous filling of compartments. However, note that virtually all perforations are associated with anterior menis-

cus displacement without reduction, which is the primary diagnosis.

**4.** *Early degenerative joint disease.* Arthrography is valuable for determining whether the arthritis is primary or secondary. We generally see a normal arthrogram with primary degenerative arthritis and a significant internal derangement related to meniscus dysfunction with the secondary form. Primary arthritis is treated symptomatically, whereas secondary arthritis requires correction of the internal derangement.

**5.** *Loose bodies ("joint mice").* Patients with internal derangement may or may not be calcified. Arthrography can ensure a correct diagnosis. The cause of this condition is generally unknown, but it is believed to be related to degenerative joint disease.

**6.** *Synovial chondromatosis.* This synovial disease is characterized by cartilagenous and osseous metaplasia. It is a rare disease of the TMJ and must be differentiated from loose bodies, with which there are generally only one or two filling defects.

COMPUTED TOMOGRAPHY
Computed tomography (CT), which has revolutionized the practice of radiology, has been used to evaluate the meniscus in TMJ patients. Conventional radiographs are obtained by recording the differences in attenuation of an x-ray beam passing through an object onto a film. This principle has several shortcomings when applied to the TMJ. First, subtle changes of the bone and soft tissue cannot be seen. To visualize the meniscus it must be coated with a contrast agent as for arthrography. Second, conventional radiographs record only the total attenuation of an x-ray beam passing through the object and indicate nothing of the object's homogeneity. Thus an object with high density peripherally and low density centrally may appear identical to an object of moderate density throughout. Computed tomography overcomes these disadvantages.

Essentially a CT scanner passes a thinly collimated x-ray beam through an object, and its attenuation is recorded by a detector.

The detector sends an electrical transmission to the computer based on the amount of attenuation and, along with the computer, records the exact position of the detector. After such a "pass," the x-ray tube and detector are shifted 1 degree, and the process is repeated. After 180 degrees of recordings are obtained, the computer reconstructs the attenuation data by assigning shades of gray to each attenuation value. This process produces a picture with cross-sectional anatomy depicted.

When evaluating fractures and tumors of the jaws, especially with soft tissue involvement, computed tomography has been shown to be superior to conventional tomography. It is also of great value for evaluating degenerative disease of the TMJ.

The distressing problems associated with using computed tomography occur when we attempt to visualize the meniscus without contrast instillation. The size of the meniscus is not the limiting factor (as modern CT scanners can resolve structures as small as 0.25 mm); rather, it is thought that the difference in density between the meniscus and surrounding muscle and fat might be too small to allow differentiation. Histologically, it is known that the meniscus is denser than muscle or fat. To emphasize this density attenuation, the scanner must be used in a "blink," or "identity," mode, which causes all the tissue of a particular density on a scan to be highlighted by blinking on and off. The density to be blinked can be manipulated so that different tissues (e.g., fat, bone, muscle) can be blinked separately. This procedure, however, requires some experience on the part of the radiologist, as false-positive results can be produced by improper blinking techniques (Fig. 8-11).

The advantages of computed tomography are a decreased radiation dose, its noninvasiveness, and the ability to examine both TMJs simultaneously. It has been estimated that more than 25 percent of patients with internal derangement have bilateral disease [35]. Its disadvantages lie in its high cost and

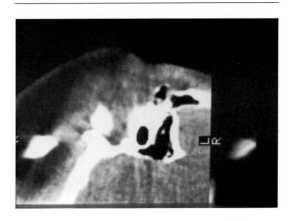

**Figure 8-11** *CT scan of the anteriorly displaced meniscus. Arrow denotes the meniscus, which is often enhanced on CT scan by use of "blink mode."*

the inability to assess the meniscus while it is functioning, as can be done with videotaped arthrography. In addition, considerable interpretive skill is required to distinguish (blink) the meniscus detail from surrounding soft tissue. It has been estimated that CT scanning is 85 percent reliable compared to arthrography [36].

MAGNETIC RESONANCE IMAGING

Even more dramatic than the revolutionary changes in diagnostic imaging provided by CT scanning is the outstanding soft tissue resolution provided by magnetic resonance imaging (MRI). This unique scanning method has the major advantages of not utilizing ionizing radiation and of being noninvasive. MRI is based on the manner in which certain nuclei behave in a magnetic field. Any nucleus with an odd number of protons or neutrons, or both, act as though it has a magnetic moment. Examples include hydrogen, phosphorus 31, sodium 23, and carbon 13. Of these substances, hydrogen is the most commonly used for magnetic imaging. When a tissue is placed in a magnetic field, the hydrogen atoms can be caused to align themselves in relation to the field. This align-

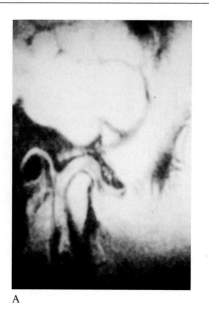

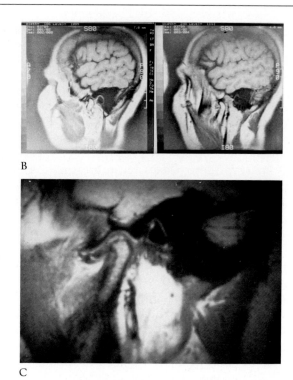

**Figure 8-12** *A. MRI scan of a normal TMJ in jaw-closed position. Arrow point rests on the superior junction of the meniscal posterior band and the retromeniscus. The blending of the anterior meniscal band and the tendon of the lateral pterygoid muscle can be visualized. The posterior band of the meniscus sets on the 12 to 1 o'clock position of the condyle. B. MRI scan of a normal TMJ in mouth-open position. Arrow point rests on the superior junction of the posterior band and the retromeniscus. The condyle can be visualized translating underneath the meniscus. C. MRI scan of the TMJ in jaw-closed position. Arrow denotes the posterior band of the meniscus. The meniscus lies anterior to the condyle and indicates meniscal displacement.*

ment can further be affected by pulsing the tissue with particular radiofrequencies. When the external radiopulse is turned off, the atoms tend to rearrange themselves into their equilibrium position and in so doing emit a radiofrequency of their own. This signal can be detected by the appropriate sensors and digitized for computer analysis to produce a reconstructed tissue image much like that seen on a CT scan.

Studies comparing MRI of the TMJ with arthrography and CT scanning demonstrate that MRI provided information about meniscal position, morphology, and histology that was not available with the other techniques. Because of these advantages MRI has become the preferred diagnostic technique for TMJ diagnosis (Fig. 8-12).

### Treatment
The patient with the condylar head that is positioned anteriorly in the glenoid fossa (stretching the posterior attachment) is subject to eventual development of TMJ dysfunction. If, on the other hand, the condylar head is being forced posteriorly, as with pos-

teriorly directed dental contacts, pressure may be exerted on the disc to dislocate [9]. Many clinicians advocate treatment of asymptomatic clicking or popping to avoid eventual symptomatology and secondary joint changes, which may be accomplished by splinting, orthodontic therapy, or dental realignment via prosthetic manipulation.

TREATMENT MODALITIES

Splints must be designed to recapture the subluxing disc while disarticulating the occlusion. The splint is constructed so the condylar head is brought under the posterior meniscal band, which eliminates the clicking and presumably allows the attenuated posterior attachment time to recall. Maintenance of splinting in this position for 3 to 6 months frequently eliminates further symptomatology. Some patients can become asymptomatic while "functioning" on the posterior band region or even completely off the disc. Because of stretching and pain about this band, however, external pterygoid muscle pain may occur. Use of adjunctive muscle relaxant therapy is sometimes helpful. Heat packs, ultrasonography, diathermy, antiinflammatory drugs, and limited range of motion with either soft diet or periods of liquid diet are advocated.

*Surgical treatment is indicated when conservative measures have failed to relieve pain and popping and to restore normal range of motion; moreover, correctable anatomic changes must have been documented.* This situation usually arises with internal derangements that are recalcitrant to conservative therapy, disc perforation, or in cases of advanced degenerative or rheumatoid arthritides. If degenerative joint disease is seen on plain films or tomograms, there may be no need for arthrography, CT scan, or MRI.

Surgical procedures have been designed to attack the problems as they present anatomically. When the articular disc is dislocated anteriorly, preventing opening, arthroplasty is carried out (Fig. 8-13). A preauricular in-

cision is used to expose the joint capsule. A flap of the lateral capsular elements is raised such that the closure after completion of the intraarticular procedure is possible. The articular disc is then repositioned by removing a wedge from the disc and its posterior attachment and then suturing the disc posteriorly. This maneuver tents the disc backward, repositioning it once again over the condylar head. It is important to remove the thickened portion of the posterior band with the resected specimen so that further difficulties with subluxation are obviated. In addition, it is thought that sectioning the posterior attachment helps to relieve pain. Some surgeons combine a high posteriorly angled condylar shave [29] with disc plication. We now advocate this step only if condylar head pathology warrants it. If disc pathology is severe, it may be appropriate to perform a total meniscectomy. This procedure had been the standard of care for many years [39].

If irreversible destruction of the condylar head is found, replacement is carried out (Figs. 8-14 and 8-15). It is important to reconstruct the height of the condylar head either directly or by glenoid fossa augmentation, thereby avoiding collapse of the ramus height. Multiple methods of joint reconstruction techniques have been advocated. We utilize the Proplast-coated metallic prosthesis [38], a Silastic sheet interpositional arthroplasty, or the ulnar head prosthesis [43, 71]. The type of prosthesis chosen depends on the clinical situation.

Surgical corrections of internal derangement of the joint have been intermittently popular [39, 56, 66, 77]. The most common procedures have been meniscectomy, condylar shave, or true condylectomy [29, 31, 39, 66]. All authors report satisfactory results. Some have questioned the appropriateness of meniscectomy [14, 31]. They reported failure to resolve pain, deviation of the meniscectomy to the side, and an inability to control symptoms when the disease has been long-standing. Indeed, even propo-

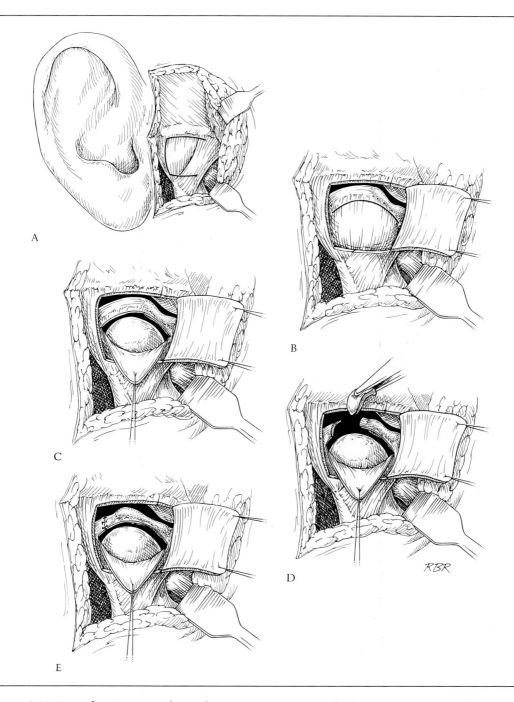

**Figure 8-13** *Disc plication procedure. The joint capsule is exposed under the body of the parotid gland through a preauricular incision. A. Anteriorly based flap of capsule is raised and access is gained to the upper joint space. B. Incision in the disc attachment then allows access to the lower space. C. A wedge is removed from the posterior attachment (D), which allows plication of the disc in a more posterior position (E) overriding the condylar head. The joint structures are then repaired in layers using nonresorbable suture.*

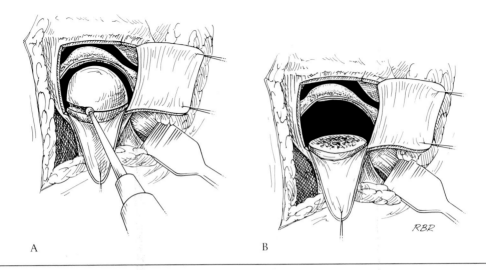

**Figure 8-14** High condylectomy. A. The condylar head is removed to the area of the neck through a preauricular approach. B. An attempt is made to leave the attachments of the external pterygoid on the neck intact.

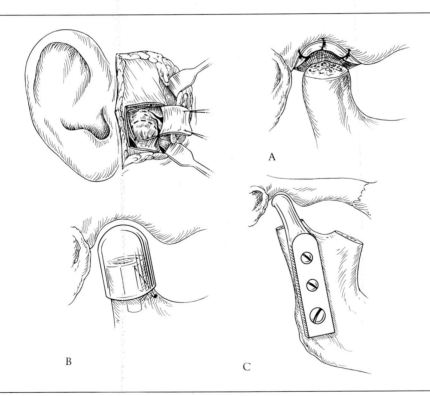

**Figure 8-15** Options for condylar head replacement after resection for ankylosis or severe degenerative disease. A. Silastic block arthroplasty secured to base of glenoid fossa. B. Condylar head replacement by Silastic ulnar head prosthesis. C. Proplast-vitallium ramus-condyle implant.

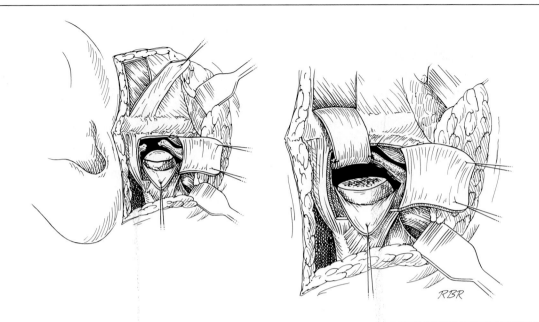

**Figure 8-16** *Repair of posterior attachment. When a large perforation is noted, it is possible to repair or replace the disc mechanism with a graft or flap of temporalis fascia (see text for details).*

nents of meniscectomy admit there is a small percentage of patients who go on to ankylosis following this procedure [66]. It seems logical to leave the meniscus as a cushion over the condylar head if it can be repaired such that normal joint function will return. A period of physical therapy is mandatory after any of these procedures to restore joint function. Proponents of condylectomy have had similar difficulties with deviation but most often with bite collapse and worsening symptoms. Condylar shaves have frequently not relieved symptoms. The use of the high posteriorly angled condylectomy in conjunction with disc plication [19] has been the most frequent procedure used in our experience. Shortening the posterior attachment and repositioning the disc are the anatomic corrections that we believe restore normal joint function in most cases,

thereby eliminating the painful symptomatology and joint noise. For this reason, we no longer perform a high posteriorly angled condylectomy on a routine basis. We see no advantage to removing normal condylar head cartilage and bone. If the condylar head is arthritic with bone spurs and osteophytes, conservative condylar shave is indicated.

Temporalis fascia as a flap has been used for repair of the posterior attachment [73]. This method has been combined with high condylectomy to restore function and leave an appropriate amount of joint space. This procedure has become the most frequently used for secondary repairs. Other repair materials have been advocated, but the use of viable fascia easily available through the same incision seems most appropriate [3] (Fig. 8-16). Silastic sheet interposition for the meniscus is sometimes well tolerated but has been found to fracture in some cases.

In patients requiring condylar replacement, a number of options are available (see Fig. 8-15). Silastic sheeting is most commonly used—not to restore the shape of the condylar head but to secure it to the undersurface of the glenoid fossa [20, 78]. The modified ulnar head prosthesis, readily available in most operating suites, provides an adequate condylar prosthesis [43, 71]. It restores the height of the ramus and can be secured by its "internal" suture to the area of the sigmoid notch so that it remains secure on the stump of the condylar head. The use of this prosthesis has been successful in most patients requiring replacement prosthesis (Fig. 8-16D).

Other techniques for condylar head replacement are also available, including replacement with autogenous material, metatarsal head, or costochondral grafts [44, 67, 79]. Other alloplastic materials have also been popular. The Proplast-coated metallic prosthesis has been advocated by Kent et al. [38]. It provides total replacement when no remnant of condylar head or neck is salvageable. It also has been well tolerated in most patients but requires an additional operative site (submandibular) for placement. It entails involved instrumentation and placement of a large foreign body.

## TMJ Ankylosis

Ankylosis of the TMJ is a different problem for both patient and reconstructive surgeon. The patient experiences difficulty with speech, mastication, oral hygiene, aesthetics, and often chronic pain. The surgeon is faced with a technically difficult problem that has inherent complications and requires the utmost patient cooperation. Instigation of surgical therapy requires careful detailed consideration. In 1938 Kazanjian classified ankylosis as true or false, *false ankylosis* being extraarticular and *true ankylosis* intraarticular [37]. True ankylosis is more common and is produced by any condition causing fibrous or bony adhesions between the condyle and fossa. False ankylosis can be caused by myogenic, neurogenic, and psychological factors, bony impingement, fi-

brous adhesions, and tumors. Major etiologies of end-stage ankylosis are trauma, intracapsular hematomas, birth deformities, and the arthritides—posttraumatic, postinfectious, and degenerative. Trauma was the responsible factor in 26 to 75 percent of cases. In another series [74] infection was responsible in 44 to 68 percent of cases [78].

Regardless of etiology, destruction of the meniscus and atrophy of the condyle and fossa cartilage are constant findings. Progressive destruction leads to narrowing of the joint space and formation of thick fibrous scar adhesions that blend with periarticular tissues (Fig. 8-17). Bony changes consist in severe erosions, lipping, osteophytes, and subcortical cysts with irregular condylar contour, flattening, and bony ankylosis.

Patients can masticate despite ankylosis. Rarely does it completely prevent opening. Thoma noted that elasticity of the mandibular bone and cranial sutures allows some opening [72]. Interincisal opening of 5 mm or less is indicative of complete bony ankylosis.

Facial deformity is often associated with ankylosis. Its severity is related to age at onset and degree of ankylosis. It consists in malocclusion with possible crossbite, incisor malalignment, class II relations with decreased ramus height, and anterior open bite. Protrusive function is absent in true ankylosis.

Radiographs are indispensable for the diagnosis of ankylosis. Anteroposterior and lateral tomograms or plain films usually provide adequate information. The Panorex, cephalometrogram, and submental vertex views are useful for determining the extent of ankylosis and associated dental-facial deformity. Enlargement of the coronoid process frequently accompanies ankylosis, and it must be diagnosed radiographically [1].

Prior to Esmarch's body ostectomy in 1851, ankylosis was thought to be incurable [18]. Humphrey performed the first condylectomy for ankylosis in 1854 [30]. Gap arthroplasty was advocated by Abbé in 1880

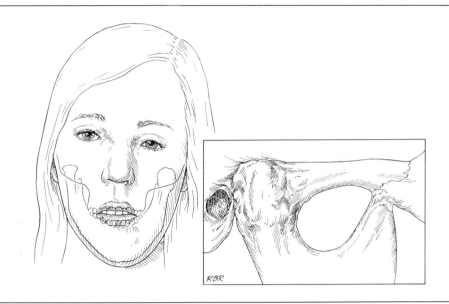

**Figure 8-17** *TMJ ankylosis. Long-standing ankylosis causes deviation of the mandible and subsequent malocclusion when it occurs during childhood years.*

and refined by Risdon in 1934 [59, 75]. Until Risdon's use of interpositional materials, ankylosis was fraught with recurrence. Topazian's review of gap arthroplasty without interposition found a recurrence rate of 53 percent [75]. Recurrence remains a problem in a small but significant number of patients despite interposition. Joint reconstruction with interpositional material returns the joint most closely to normal, provides the best mechanical results, and reduces the incidence of recurrence.

Dental-facial growth must be analyzed in the growing patient. These patients ideally have restoration of growth potential to the affected condyle. Currently, costochondral grafting is the most popular and the best available technique short of the use of vascularized bone [44]. However, growth of the graft is unreliable and unpredictable in terms of occurrence and degree. West re-

ported a patient in whom a costochondral graft outgrew the normal side and caused deviation toward the preexisting normal side [81]. Dingman and Grabb pioneered use of the fifth metatarsal and reported good results with minimum morbidity at the donor site [15]. Matucus, however, described an autogenous bicortical iliac crest bone graft with associated bilateral cartilagenous cap [46].

Condylectomy with gap arthroplasty by artificial or autogenous interpositional material is the basic technique for treating the nongrowing patient. Treatment of acquired dental-facial deformities may be necessary. If the ankylosis is not severe, a limited sculpting condylectomy of the condylar head may be adequate to produce joint motion. It minimally disturbs anatomy.

In condylectomy, excision is done as high as possible on the condyle to maintain the joint as close as possible to its normal position. This procedure maintains the class III level of the mandible and minimizes potential for posterior open bite. Interpositional material is used for any significant excision of the condyle. The most widely accepted material is Silastic rubber in block form; it usually performs well but has the usual problems associated with a foreign body. Condylectomy at the level of the condylar neck causes loss of ramus height and leaves only simple hinge motion. If this articulation is not balanced with the contralateral side by interposition materials, internal derangements and bony degeneration may occur on the contralateral side. Interpositional arthroplasty maintains posterior facial height and prevents formation of bony and fibrous adhesions but does not reduce normal anatomy and does not function as a glide and hinge joint.

Joint replacement more closely reproduces normal anatomy and function. Users of the condylar replacement made of Proplast-coated vitallium claim an 87 percent success rate in cases requiring functional TMJ rehabilitation [38]. Ninety percent of all successful prostheses used for ankylosis maintain or increase ramus height, incisal opening, and lateral excursions. Therefore the need for simultaneous correction of the dental-facial deformity and bony ankylosis may be an indication for a metallic condylar prosthesis in the nongrowing patient.

Silver and Carlotti advocated a condylar head prosthesis that uses an intramedullary stem secured by methylmethacrylate similar to a total hip replacement [65]. They claimed consistently acceptable long-term follow-up of up to 14 years. Complete evaluation of all patients is lacking. Use of the ulnar head prosthesis is another option. Alternatives must be constantly reevaluated.

Patients with active primary inflammatory arthritis and severe ankylosis present a special problem. They require condylar reconstruction with simultaneous correction of open bite and retrognathia. A costochondral graft may undergo resorption because of ongoing disease. A prosthesis may produce glenoid fossa erosion. Long-term follow-up of joint replacement is not available in these patients.

## Hypermobility and Dislocation of the Condyle

### ACUTE DISLOCATION

Acute dislocation of the condylar head occurs with its extension forward past the articular eminence. It occasionally luxates into the infratemporal fossa. Rapid spontaneous reduction usually occurs; however, the mandible can be repositioned manually with little difficulty.

Relocation is accomplished as follows. Facing the patient, the operator's thumbs are placed in the buccal sulcus adjacent to the mandibular bicuspids. The fingers of each hand are placed under the inferior border of the mandible body. Downward, anterior, and then posterior pressure is applied to the patient's mandible over several minutes to stretch the spastic elevator muscles and then relocate the condyle within the fossa. Intravenous sedation may be necessary prior to manipulation.

### RECURRENT DISLOCATION

Recurrent dislocation may cause recurrent TMJ pain and degenerative joint changes. Intraarticular injection of sclerosing agents to produce fibrosis of the capsular ligaments and thereby prevent dislocation has been advocated [47]. This indirect approach is rarely effective. If conservative therapy (i.e., training the patient to consistently avoid maximum opening) does not control the problem, several surgical procedures are available (Fig. 8-18). Tightening the capsule by excision of redundant tissue or plication is the simplest [48]. Mechanical interference in the condylar path may be increased by augmenting the articular eminence with Silastic or autogenous bone [63]. Removal of the articular tu-

*Figure 8-18 Options for treatment of chronic dislocation. A. Wedge bone graft to augment eminence. B. External pterygoid myotomy. C. Eminectomy. D. Fascial flap to limit translation. E. Capsulorrhaphy. F. Vitallium crib for eminence augmentation.*

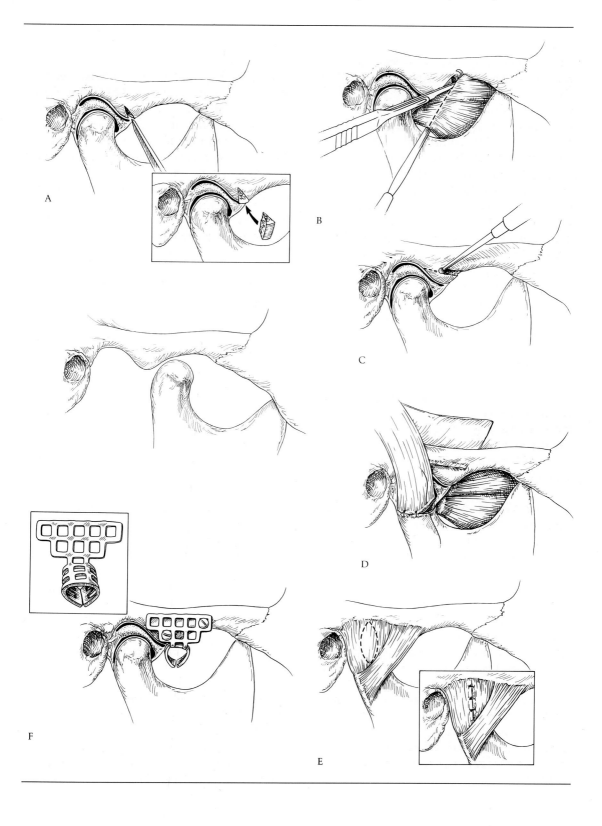

bercle prevents locking of the condylar head anterior to the articular eminence by its simple absence. It is effective, technically easy, and the current treatment of choice [26, 51].

## Coronoid Abnormalities Causing Limitation of Mandibular Movement

Abnormalities of the coronoid process may cause limited mandibular motion. Although rare, they must be considered when evaluating the TMJ [1, 60, 76]. The etiologies are bilateral or unilateral enlargement of the coronoid process, ossification of the temporalis tendon and muscle after trauma, and ankylosis of the coronoid process to adjacent body structures. All produce similar symptoms and differ only by the history of trauma associated with temporalis ossification. Plain films, tomograms, CT scans, or MRI scans are needed to make the diagnosis.

Satisfactory access can be obtained through intraoral incisions. This approach is less likely to injure vital nerves and vessels and maintains better cosmetic results. An incision can be made directly over the external oblique line and carried superiorly along the anterior edge of the ramus up the coronoid process. This incision can be extended downward and forward over bone to the distal buccal aspect of the second molar and then forward laterally in the gingival sulcus to the first premolar. The periosteum is reflected laterally, exposing the sigmoid notch, coronoid process, and tendon of the temporalis muscle. If ossified, a portion of the temporalis tendon or muscle is removed, the ankylosis is removed, or the coronoid process is excised. If the diagnosis was correct, the mandible opens widely with utilization of a mouth prop.

## Inflammatory Arthritis

After internal derangement, arthritis is the most common organic TMJ problem [25].

Osteoarthritis occurs most often, followed by rheumatoid arthritis. The TMJ is affected in as many as 50 to 60 percent of patients with rheumatoid arthritis. In one study, 68 percent of these patients had radiographic evidence of TMJ involvement. However, they rarely have severe handicapping temporomandibular symptoms. The most common symptoms are crepitus, limitation of motion (which may become progressive), and pain (usually mild).

In contrast, in juvenile rheumatoid arthritis, TMJ and facial growth involvement can be devastating. Progressive resorption of the condyle occurs. The adult condyle may be a mere remnant with shortened ramus height and resulting anterior open bite deformity. In the growing patient, this severely retarded mandibular growth can cause secondary growth deformities of the upper jaw. Treatment of these patients consists in surgical correction of the jaw and facial deformity to restore occlusion and facial form. When ankylosis is present or when significant TMJ damage is associated with debilitating pain, the surgical options are gap arthroplasty with interpositional alloplastic or autogenous material or total joint replacement [38].

Other diseases that occasionally cause arthritis of the TMJ include familial Mediterranean fever, collagen vascular syndromes (i.e., scleroderma, systemic lupus erythematosus), gout, Sjögren syndrome, infectious arthritis, and chronic psoriasis. Psoriasis occurs in 1.2 percent of the general population and TMJ psoriatic arthritis in 5.7 percent of the patients with chronic psoriasis [70]. Psoriatic arthritis is characterized by the triad (1) psoriasis, (2) erosive arthritis, and (3) negative results on a serologic test for rheumatoid factor. Involvement of the TMJ in patients with psoriatic arthritis is characterized by episodic, painful, unilateral inflammation, often with a sudden onset. Typically, spontaneous exacerbations and remissions occur. The painful episodes may last for months and are usually associated with the presence of skin lesions. Improvement of the arthritis usually follows improvement of the skin lesions. Radiographs of the TMJ may be normal, but necrosis and osteoporotic changes are often seen. Nonsteroidal antiinflammatory drugs may be helpful during exacerbation. To our knowledge, only one case of psoriatic arthritis of the TMJ leading to ankylosis has been reported in the English-language literature.

## Infectious Arthritis of the TMJ

The TMJ may become infected after an open operation or access procedure (arthrography, aspiration, or injection), by local spread of infection from adjacent regions (e.g., otitis media, mastoiditis, or parotitis), and rarely by hematogenous spread of a distant infection. Septic arthritis is rare but carries the potential for serious complications such as osteomyelitis and resulting ankylosis. Strict sterile techniques must be observed in all procedures. When infected, the joint requires incisions and drainage with sequestrectomy as indicated and appropriate antibiotics.

## Avascular Necrosis

Avascular necrosis of the mandibular condylar head is rare. It may develop several months after an untreated intracapsular fracture or inadvertent devascularization of the head during open reduction of a fracture. Clinical symptoms are pain in the TMJ on the affected side and limited opening of the mouth. Radiographically, the condylar head is characteristically eroded and irregular. Treatment consists in surgical removal of the necrotic condylar head and conservative débridement [62]. Eventual condylar replacement is indicated.

## Arthroscopy

It has become apparent that the upper joint space can be visualized by the needle arthroscope. Some workers have advocated arthroscopy and lysis of adhesions as bene-

ficial in the treatment of patients with disc subluxation and dislocation [8, 28, 50]. Scopes have been developed that range in diameter from 1.5 to 2.7 mm and have various angles of view. They can be inserted by percutaneous puncture, and allow simultaneous visualization with influent Ringer's lactate to lavage the joint, and require a separate puncture by a large-bore needle to remove joint effluent. To date, limited series have been developed, but complications have been infrequent. They include, however, hematoma, transient frontal branch of CN VII damage, and entrance into the middle ear. Microinstrumentation that allows manipulation of joint structure is under development.

It is fair to say that only limited application of this procedure, either diagnostically or for treatment, can be claimed. With improvement in instrumentation and technique, this situation may improve rapidly. There appears to be at least temporary relief of painful symptomatology associated with joint lavage. However, no claim at long-term relief of a true disc dislocation can be made. The argon laser has been additionally used to begin instrumentation of the internal joint as well as microshavers and bone rasps. We look forward to more information about the efficacy of these techniques.

## References

1. Allison, M. L., Wallace, W. R., and VonWyl, H. Coronoid abnormalities causing limitation of mandibular movement. *J. Oral Surg.* 27:229, 1969.
2. Bernstein, J. M., Mohl, N. D., and Spiller, H. Temporomandibular joint dysfunction masquerading as disease of the ear, nose, or throat. *Trans Am. Acad. Otolaryngol.* 73:1208, 1969.
3. Bessette, R., Bishop, B., and Mohl, N. Duration of masseteric silent period in patients with TMJ syndrome. *J. Appl. Physiol.* 30:864, 1971.
4. Bessette, R., Mohl, N., and Bishop, B. Contribution of periodontal receptors to the masseteric silent period. *J. Dent. Res.* 53:1196, 1974.
5. Bessette, R., Mohl, N., and DiCosima, C.

Comparison of results of electromyographic and radiographic examination in patients with myofascial pain dysfunction syndrome. *J. Am. Dent. Assoc.* 89: 1358, 1974.

6. Bessette, R., et al. Effect of biting force on the duration of the masseteric silent period. *J. Dent. Res.* 52:426, 1973.

7. Blaschke, D. D., and Blaschke, T. J. Normal TMJ bony relationships in centric occlusion. *J. Dent. Res.* 60:98, 1981.

8. Bronstein, S. Postsurgical TMJ arthrography. *J. Craniomandib. Pract.* 2:165, 1984.

9. Bronstein, S. L., Tomasetti, B. J., and Ryan, D. E. Internal derangements of the temporomandibular joint: Correlation of arthrography with surgical findings. *J. Oral Surg.* 39:572, 1981.

10. Bush, F. M., et al. Prevalence of Mandibular Dysfunction: Subjective Signs and Symptoms. In M. A. Littleton (ed.), *Occlusion: Diagnosis and Treatment. Plast. Reconstr. Surg.* 55:355, 1975.

11. Choukas, N. C., and Sicher, H. Structure of temporomandibular joint. *Oral Surg. Oral Med. Oral Pathol.* 13:1203, 1960.

12. Costen, J. B. Syndrome of ear and sinus symptoms dependent upon disturbed function of temporomandibular joint. *Ann. Otol. Rhinol. Laryngol.* 43:1, 1934.

13. Decker, J. C. Traumatic deafness as a result of retrusion of the condyles of the mandible. *Ann. Otol. Rhinol. Laryngol.* 34:519, 1925.

14. Dingman, R. O., Dingman, D. L., and Lawrence, R. A. Surgical correction of the temporomandibular joints. *Plast. Reconstr. Surg.* 55:355, 1975.

15. Dingman, Z., and Grabb, W. C. Reconstruction of both mandibular condyles with metatarsal bone grafts. *Plast. Reconstruct. Surg.* 34:2141, 1964.

16. Dixon, A. D. Structure and functional significance of the intra-articular disc of the human temporomandibular joint. *J. Oral Surg.* 15:48, 1962.

17. Dolwick, M. F., et al. Arthrotomographic evaluation of the temporomandibular joint. *J. Oral Surg.* 37:793, 1979.

18. Esmarch, F. Traitment du resserrement cicatriciel des machoires par la formation d'une fausse articulation dans la continuite de l'os maxillarie inferieur. *Arch. Gen. Med.* 5:44, 1860.

19. Farrar, W. B., and McCarty, W. L. The TMJ dilemma. *J. Ala. Dent. Assoc.* ;63:19, 1979.

20. Freedus, M. S., Ziter, W. D., and Doyle, P. K. Principles of treatment for temporomandibular joint ankylosis. *J. Oral Surg.* 33:757, 1975.

21. Garnick, J. An electromyographic and clinical investigation. *J. Prosthet. Dent.* 12:895, 1962.

22. Gelb, H. The role of the dentist and otolaryngologist in evaluating temporomandibular joint syndrome. *J. Prosthet. Dent.* 18:497, 1967.

23. Greene, C., and Laskin, D. Splint therapy for the myofascial pain dysfunction syndrome, a comparative study. *J. Am. Dent. Assoc.* 84: 624, 1972.

24. Griffin, C. J., and Sharpe, C. J. The structure of the adult human temporomandibular meniscus. *Aust. Dent. J.* 5:190, 1960.

25. Guralnick, W., Kaban, L. B., and Merril, R. G. Temporomandibular joint afflictions. *N. Engl. J. Med.* 229:123, 1978.

26. Hale, R. Treatment of recurrent dislocation of the mandible. *J. Oral Surg.* 30:527, 1972.

27. Harris, H. L. Anatomy of the temporomandibular articulation and adjacent structures. *J. Am. Dent. Assoc.* 19:584, 1932.

28. Hellsing, G., et al. Arthroscopy of the temporomandibular joint (examination of 2 patients with suspected disc derangement). *Int. J. Oral Surg.* 13:69, 1984.

29. Henny, F. A., and Baldridge, O. L. Condylectomy for the persistently painful temporomandibular joint. *J. Oral Surg.* 24:31, 1957.

30. Humphry, G. M. Excision of the condyle of the lower jaw. *Assoc. Med. J. (Lond.)* 160:61, 1856.

31. Ireland, V. E. The problem of "the clicking jaw." *Plast. Surg. Head Neck Med.* 44:363, 1951.

32. Jarabak, J. The adaptability of the temporal and masseter muscles; an electromyographical study. *Angle Orthod.* 24:193, 1954.

33. Jarabak, J. An electromyographic analysis of muscular and TMJ disturbances due to imbalances in occlusion. *Angle Orthod.* 26:170, 1956.

34. Katzberg, R. W., et al. Arthrotomography of the temporomandibular joint. *A.J.R.* 134:995, 1980.

35. Katzberg, R. W., et al. Normal and abnormal TMJ, MR imaging with surface coil. *Radiology* 158:183, 1986.

36. Katzberg, R., et al. Magnetic resonance imaging of the TMJ and meniscus. *Oral Surg. Oral Med. Oral Pathol.* 59:33a, 1985.
37. Kazanjian, V. H. Ankylosis of the TMJ. *Surg. Gynecol. Obstet.* 67:333, 1938.
38. Kent, J. N., et al. Temporomandibular joint condylar prosthesis: A ten-year report. *J. Oral Maxillofac. Surg.* 41:245, 1983.
39. Kiehn, C. L. Meniscectomy for internal derangement of temporomandibular joint. *Am. J. Surg.* 83:364, 1952.
40. Krough-Poulsen, W. G. Management of the Occlusion of the Teeth (part II). In L. L. Schwartz and C. M. Chayes (eds.), *Facial Pain and Mandibular Dysfunction.* Philadelphia: Saunders, 1968. P. 271.
41. Laskin, D. M. Etiology of the pain-dysfunction syndrome. *J. Am. Dent. Assoc.* 79:147, 1969.
42. Lerman, M. The hydrostatic appliance: A new approach to treatment of the TMJ pain-dysfunction syndrome. *J. Am. Dent. Assoc.* 89:1343, 1974.
43. Lewis, R. W., and Wright, J. A. Silastic ulnar head prosthesis for use in surgery of the temporomandibular joint. *J. Oral Surg.* 39:572, 1981.
44. Longacre, J. J., and Gilby, R. F. Use of autogenous cartilage graft in arthroplasty for true ankylosis of the temporomandibular joint. *Plast. Reconstr. Surg.* 7:271, 1951.
45. Manzione, J. V., et al. Computed tomography of the TM joint. *Radiology* 150:111, 1984.
46. Matucas, V. J. Management of ankylosis in the child using autogenous cartilagenous bone graft from the iliac crest. Presented at the 1979 Clinical Congress, S. E. Society of Oral Surgeons.
47. McKelvey, L. E. Sclerosing solution in the treatment of chronic subluxation of temporomandibular joint. *J. Oral Surg.* 8:225, 1950.
48. Morris, J. Chronic recurring temporomaxillary subluxation. *Surg. Gynecol. Obstet.* 50:483, 1930.
49. Moyers, R. An electromyographic analysis of certain muscles involved in TMJ movement. *Am. J. Orthod.* 36:481, 1950.
50. Murakami, K., and Kazumasa, H. Regional anatomical nomenclature and arthroscopic terminology in human temporomandibular joints. *Okajimas Folia Anat. Jpn.* 58:745, 1982.
51. Myrhaug, H. New method of operation for bilateral dislocation of mandible. *Acta Odontol. Scand.* 9:247, 1951.
52. Perry, H. Functional electromyography of the temporal and masseter muscles in class II, division I malocclusion and excellent occlusion. *Angle Orthod.* 25:49, 1955.
53. Perry, H. Muscular changes associated with TMJ dysfunction. *J. Am. Dent. Assoc.* 54:644, 1957.
54. Posselt, U. *Physiology of Occlusion and Rehabilitation.* (2nd ed.). Philadelphia: Davis, 1968. P. 99.
55. Prentiss, H. J. A preliminary report upon the temporomandibular articulation in the human type. *Dent. Cosmos* p. 505, 1918.
56. Pringle, J. H. Displacement of the mandibular meniscus and its treatment. *Br. J. Surg.* 6:385, 1918.
57. Ramfjord, S. Bruxism, a clinical and electromyographic study. *J. Am. Dent. Assoc.* 62:21, 1961.
58. Ramfjord, S. Dysfunctional temporomandibular joint and muscle pain. *J. Prosthet. Dent.* 11:353, 1961.
59. Risdon, F. Ankylosis of the temporomandibular joint. *J. Am. Dent. Assoc.* 21:1933, 1934.
60. Rowe, N. L. Bilateral developmental hyperplasia of the mandibular coronoid process: A report of two cases. *Br. J. Oral Surg.* 1:90, 1963.
61. Salzman, J. *Practice of Orthodontics.* Philadelphia: Lippincott, 1966. P. 572.
62. Sanders, B., McKelvy, B., and Adams, D. Aseptic osteomyelitis and necrosis of the mandibular condylar head after intracapsular fracture. *Oral Surg.* 43:5, 1977.
63. Schuchardt, K. *Fortschritte der Kiefer und Gesichts-Chirurgie.* Stuttgart: Georg Thieme Verlag, 1960.
64. Shore, N. A. *Occlusal Equilibration and Temporomandibular Joint Dysfunction.* Philadelphia: Lippincott, 1959. P. 131.
65. Silver, C., and Carlotti, A. Arthroplasty of the temporomandibular joint with use of a vitallium condyle prosthesis. *J. Oral Surg.* 35:909, 1977.
66. Silver, C. M., Simon, S. D., and Savestino, A. A. Meniscus injuries of the temporomandibular joint. *J. Bone Surg.* [Am.] 38:541, 1956.
67. Snyder, C. C., Levine, G. A., and Dingman, D. I. Trial of a sternoclavicular whole joint

graft as a substitute for the temporomandibular joint. *Plast. Reconstr. Surg.* 48:47, 1971.

68. Solberg, W. K., Woo, M. W., and Houston, J. B. Prevalence of mandibular dysfunction in young adults. *J. Am. Dent. Assoc.* 98:25, 1979.

69. Stanson, A. W., and Baker, H. L. Routine tomography of the temporomandibular joint. *Radiol. Clin. North Am.* 14:105, 1976.

70. Stimson, C. W., and Leban, S. G. Recurrent ankylosis of the temporomandibular joint in a patient with chronic psoriasis. *J. Oral Maxillofac. Surg.* 40:678, 1982.

71. Swanson, A. B. *Reconstructive Surgery of the Arthritic Hand and Foot.* Ciba Series Clinical Symposium 31, No. 6, 1979.

72. Thoma, K. H. Ankylosis of the mandibular joint. *Am. J. Orthol.* 32:259, 1946.

73. Toller, P. A. Temporomandibular capsular rearrangement. *Br. J. Oral Surg.* 11:207, 1974.

74. Topazian, R. G. Etiology of ankylosis of temporomandibular joint, analysis of 44 cases. *J. Oral Surg.* 22:227, 1964.

75. Topazian, R. G. Comparison of gap and interpositional arthroplasty in the treatment of temporomandibular joint ankylosis. *J. Oral Surg.* 24:405, 1966.

76. Van Zile, W. N., and Johnson, W. B. Bilateral coronoid process exostosis simulating partial ankylosis of the temporomandibular joint: report of case. *J. Oral Surg.* 15:72, 1957.

77. Wakely, C. The causation and treatment of displaced mandibular cartilage. *Lancet* 2:543, 1929.

78. Walker, R. V. Arthroplasty of the ankylosed temporomandibular joint. In: *Transactions of the Congress, International Association of Oral Surgeons* (Vol. 4), 1973. P. 279.

79. Ware, W. H. Growth centre transplantation in temporomandibular joint surgery. In: *Transactions, Third Congress, International Association of Oral Surgeons*, 1970. Pp. 148–157.

80. Weinberg, L. A. Role of condylar position in TMJ dysfunction syndrome. *J. Prosthet. Dent.* 41:636, 1979.

81. West, R. Surgical treatment of the growing patient. Presented at the ASOMS Annual Meeting, San Francisco, Spetember 1980.

# 9
# Cleft Lip

H. S. Byrd

## Historical Background

Numerous methods have been described for repair of the cleft lip deformity. Early techniques involved a straight line closure [3, 6], and these procedures still find applicability in the repair of microform (forme fruste) clefts [10].

Modern repairs have in common the use of a lateral lip flap to fill a medial deficit, a concept that can be accredited to Mirault [6]. The LeMesurier [3] repair involves a lateral, quadrilateral flap, whereas the Tennison [9] repair employs a lateral triangular flap. Both procedures introduce tissue in the lower part of the lip and share the advantage of producing a pouting tubercle (Fig. 9-1).

In 1955 Millard [4] described the concept of advancing a lateral flap into the upper portion of the lip combined with downward rotation of the medial segment. The technique preserves both the cupid's bow and the philtral dimple, and it has the additional advantage of placing the tension of closure under the alar base, thereby reducing flair and promoting better molding of the underlying alveolar processes.

Repairs involving a combined upper and lower lip flap were advocated by Skoog [8] and Trauner and Trauner [11]. However, emphasis has shifted away from skin flap design and has been placed on accurate and functional reconstruction of the orbicularis oris muscle [2, 7].

Surgical correction of the bilateral cleft lip deformity has yielded less satisfying results than correction of the unilateral deformity. Early procedures excised the prolabium or mistakingly assumed it to be a displaced columella [5], producing a lip that was grossly deficient horizontally. Later, the prolabium was used to form the upper central lip, its vertical height supplemented with excess tissue from the lateral lip; this technique resulted in a lip that was too long and too narrow [12]. These early repairs reflect the failure to recognize the potential of the prolabium to grow in width and height when attached to the dynamic lateral lip elements.

Modern techniques concentrate on using the prolabium for the entire central portion of the lip and are subdivided into straight line closures and closures involving the Z-plasty principle. The Z-plasties may be in the lower lip, the upper lip, or both (Fig. 9-2).

Whereas the trends in cleft repair may be accurately summarized, there is no agreement on the ideal timing and technique of repair. Advocates of differing methods may demonstrate results that are comparable, underscoring the fact that more than one treatment plan is acceptable. Total familiarity with the details and limitations of a tech-

STRAIGHT LINE

Rose-Thompson

LOWER LIP Z-PLASTIES

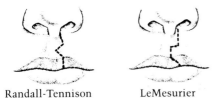

Randall-Tennison          LeMesurier

UPPER LIP Z-PLASTIES

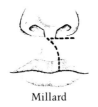

Millard

UPPER AND LOWER LIP Z-PLASTIES

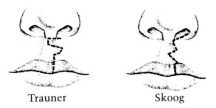

Trauner                   Skoog

*Figure 9-1*

nique is as important as the type of repair chosen. Accordingly, the remainder of this chapter focuses on a single, but coordinated, approach to cleft lip repair. The nuances that allow a predictable result are emphasized.

## Patient Evaluation and Classification

Initial evaluation ideally occurs during the newborn period. Unilateral clefts are placed in one of three categories for the purpose of treatment planning: microform cleft lip, incomplete cleft lip, or complete cleft lip. The associated nasal deformity is similarly categorized as mild, moderate, or severe. Mild nasal deformity is characterized by a wide alar base but normal alar contour and normal dome projection. Moderate nasal deformity has a wide alar base in association with either a depressed dome or alar crease. There is minimal hypoplasia of the alar cartilage. Severe nasal deformity has a wide alar base, a deep alar crease, and an underprojecting alar dome. Hypoplasia of the alar cartilage is present.

### MICROFORM CLEFTS
The microform cleft is characterized by a furrow or scar transgressing the vertical length of the lip, a vermilion notch, imperfections in the white roll, and varying degrees of vertical lip shortness [10]. Nasal deformity may be present and is sometimes more extensive than the associated lip problem. Surgery is generally indicated but must be approached cautiously to avoid a surgical deformity worse than the congenital defect.

### UNILATERAL INCOMPLETE CLEFTS
Unilateral incomplete clefts are characterized by varying degrees of vertical separation of the lip, but they all have in common an intact nasal sill, or Simonart's band. They are corrected with rotation advancement repairs. The associated nasal deformity is corrected at the time of lip repair, although the

degrees of alar mobilization and repositioning vary according to the magnitude of the deformity.

UNILATERAL COMPLETE CLEFTS
Unilateral complete clefts are characterized by separation of the lip, nostril sill, and alveolus (derivatives of the primary palate). Although the secondary palate may remain intact, complete clefts most commonly involve the entire palate. The critical factors for evaluating unilateral complete clefts are the position of the alveolar segments and the vertical height of the lateral lip element. The alveolar (maxillary) segments assume one of four positions: (1) narrow–no collapse; (2) narrow–collapse; (3) wide–no collapse; (4) wide–collapse. "Wide" is determined by an alveolus position lateral to the desired alar base position (i.e., with lip closure the alar base is sitting in the cleft). "Collapse" refers to a lingual position of the lateral maxillary segment as predicated by the arch configuration of the medial dental ridge (Fig. 9-3).

Clefts characterized as narrow–no collapse are prime candidates for rotation advancement lip repair with simultaneous correction of the nasal deformity. Clefts characterized as narrow–collapse are ideal candidates for presurgical palatal orthopedic expansion beginning at approximately 2 weeks of age and continuing to surgery, at which time definitive cheiloplasty is undertaken. Clefts characterized as wide–collapse benefit from presurgical palatal expansion to correct collapse followed by lip adhesion and a static "guiding" appliance to control the segments as the cleft narrows. Clefts characterized as wide–no collapse benefit from preliminary lip adhesion followed by a static "guiding" appliance to avoid collapse. With all wide clefts lip adhesion is advocated to improve alveolar segment relations and allow a more predictable nasal correction.

The short lateral lip segment may be identified when the vertical deficiency between

STRAIGHT LINE

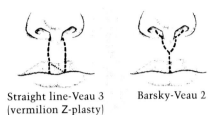

Straight line-Veau 3      Barsky-Veau 2
(vermilion Z-plasty)

LOWER LIP Z-PLASTIES

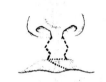

Tennison adaptation
(Cronin, Berkeley, Marcks)

UPPER LIP Z-PLASTIES

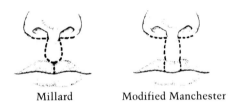

Millard         Modified Manchester

UPPER AND LOWER LIP Z-PLASTIES

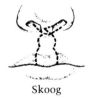

Skoog

*Figure 9-2*

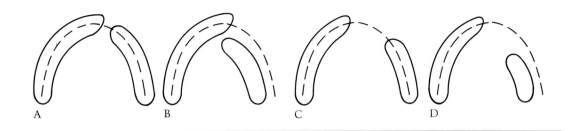

**Figure 9-3** *A. Narrow–no collapse. B. Narrow–collapse. C. Wide–no collapse. D. Wide–collapse.*

the alar base and cupid's bow peak on the cleft side forces one to borrow tissue beyond the acceptable anatomic limits of the lateral lip segment or alar base. The anatomic limit of the lateral lip segment is the point on the vermilion beyond which vermilion mismatch with the noncleft segment occurs. This limit should not be violated. The anatomic limit of the nose is the crease or groove joining the alar base and sill with the lip. This limit may be exceeded by several millimeters but requires special technical adjustment to avoid nasal deformity.

With all complete clefts, intravelar veloplasty is carried out at the time of initial lip repair or lip adhesion. The reconstruction of this posterior muscle sling is thought to balance the forces across the maxillary segments when the orbicularis oris is reconstructed. These muscle forces account for the improved arch relations that follow surgery. Active palatal expansion is terminated at the time of lip and velar closure. A stronger orbicularis oris muscle effectively transfers the lateral expansion forces posteriorly, placing the velar closure at risk for attenuation or dehiscence. Static appliances may be continued until the time of alveolar closure or until retention becomes a problem.

The primary benefit of a balanced noncollapsed arch configuration at the time of primary lip repair rests in the provision of a stable skeletal base on which the cleft nasal alar segment is positioned.

BILATERAL CLEFT LIP

Bilateral cleft lips may be incomplete, incomplete/complete, or complete. Evaluation of the bilateral cleft deformity focuses on the prolabium and the premaxilla. The quality of the prolabial white roll and the fullness of the prolabial vermilion must be assessed to determine if white roll vermilion flaps from the lateral lip segments are required to reconstruct the central tubercle. If a white roll is present and there is adequate vermilion fullness for a pouting tubercle, a modified Manchester repair is employed. If either the white roll or the vermilion is deficient, a Millard repair is used. Lip adhesion and staged repair of the two sides have not proved beneficial for bilateral clefts.

Assessment during the newborn period is essential if arch alignment of the maxillary segments is to be influenced. The vertically oriented or overly projecting premaxilla may be favorably influenced with elastic (headcap) traction. The lateral maxillary segments may be passively controlled with fixed palatal appliances, or they may be actively expanded if collapse is present. Retention of arch relations with a fixed appliance is frequently required following lip and velar closure. Closure of the premaxillary and maxillary alveolus with local mucoperiosteal flaps when the segments are 1 to 2 mm apart aids in stabilizing the arches. Surgical

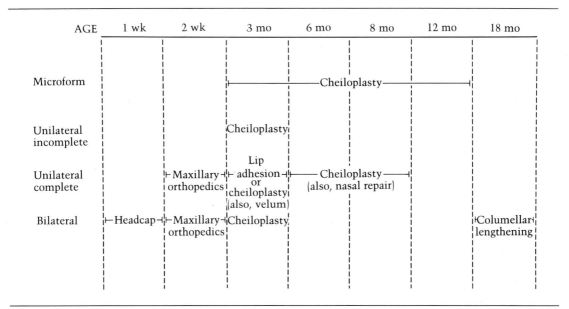

**Figure 9-4** *Management sequence.*

setback of the premaxilla at the time of primary repair is seldom if ever required.

## Timing and Treatment Planning

Elastic headcap traction for the overly projecting premaxilla in the bilateral cleft deformity must be initiated during the early newborn period if significant response is to be achieved. Treatment is initiated at age 1 week, with the maximal response occurring during the first 6 weeks. Expansion of the collapsed maxillary arches with dynamic palatal appliances is also initiated early. Treatment is initiated at age 1 to 2 weeks and continued until normal arch relations are achieved (usually before 3 months of age).

The initial lip procedure is deferred until 10 to 12 weeks of age, at which time simultaneous soft palate repair is undertaken. Lip adhesion is performed in those unilateral clefts with wide arch configuration, persistent collapse, or a short lateral segment. Definitive lip repair follows at 6 to 8 months of age. Primary definitive lip repair is per-

formed for all other clefts at the 10- to 12-week period (Fig. 9-4).

Closure of the residual hard palate cleft is accomplished at approximately 18 months of age. Alveolar closure is performed early with local mucoperiosteal flaps turned from the alveolar segments (not the vomer) when the segments are ideally aligned and approximately 2 mm apart. Bone grafts are not employed with only closure of the alveolus. If collapse is present or if the gap is too wide for closure with local turn-in flaps, closure is deferred until 7 to 8 years of age, when definitive two-layer closure and cancellous bone grafting is performed. The timing of this closure is mitigated by presurgical orthodontia to align the segments and with surgical closure and bone grafting prior to eruption of the permanent canines.

Correction of the nasal deformity in unilateral clefts is coupled with the rotation advancement repair. Septal repositioning and nasal osteotomies are deferred until late adolescence unless the deformity is severe, in which case they are coupled with alveolar cleft closure at 7 to 8 years of age. Correction of the nasal deformity in bilateral clefts is deferred until approximately 18 months of age, when the alar cartilages are mobilized, columellar lengthening is achieved, and hard palate closure is accomplished. Tip support with a columellar cartilage graft is generally added at the time of alveolar cleft closure. Definitive rhinoplasty is undertaken during late adolescence.

### Anesthesia
General endotracheal anesthesia is used for all stages of lip repair. With state-of-the-art pediatric anesthesia, risks are minimized and precise surgical detail is possible. After markings, 0.5% lidocaine with 1:200,000 epinephrine is injected in the velum. A volume of 2 to 3 ml is typically used. On completion of the veloplasty, the lip and nose are injected with a similar volume. A time interval of 1 hour generally elapses between injections. With these staggered doses of local anesthesia, high absorption peaks are avoided and toxic effects minimized even in small infants (weight approximating 10 kg).

### Operative Technique
MICROFORM CLEFT
The critical factor when evaluating the microform cleft is the vertical height of the lip. If the vertical height of the affected side approximates that of the normal side, imperfections in the vermilion along the skin furrow may be eliminated with an elliptical excision and a straight line repair (Fig. 9-5). Triangular flaps of the white roll and vermilion may be used to balance the closure.

When the vertical difference exceeds 1 to 2 mm, a rotation advancement repair is utilized (Fig. 9-6). The additional scar underneath the sill and columella is preferable to a loss of definition in the involved philtral column, which invariably results with straight line closure when the elliptical excision is extended to provide the desired lengthening.

The correction of a mild nasal deformity is deferred in the microform cleft requiring a

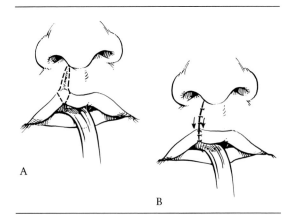

**Figure 9-5**  *Microform cleft: straight line repair.*

straight line repair, as the repair does not necessitate a perialar incision. If the deformity remains minimal, treatment is postponed until late adolescence, when a definitive rhinoplasty is done. If the deformity worsens with growth, alar mobilization and repositioning at age 7 to 8 years is accomplished. With a moderate nasal deformity and with mild deformities requiring a rotation advancement lip repair, correction of the nasal deformity is carried out with lip repair.

UNILATERAL INCOMPLETE CLEFT LIP
The markings for the rotation advancement repair are taken from Millard's description. Point 4 (in Fig. 9-6) is selected by matching anatomic features of the vermilion in lieu of measuring from the commissure. With this method two points are identified: one matching the vermilion with that of the cleft cupid's bow peak on the medial lip element, the other matching the vermilion with the noncleft cupid's bow peak, also on the medial lip element. Point 4 must lie on or between these points, its exact position being determined by the vertical lip requirements.

The vertical length of the noncleft side (alar base to cupid's bow peak) (see Fig. 9-6C–E) equals the length of the normal philtrum and is used to describe the length of the rotation flap (including back cut) and the advancement flap. As this length is transcribed from the nasal sill of the lateral lip element to the vermilion edge, point 4 is verified within its defined limits. If the dry vermilion mucosa at point 4 is thicker than that of the noncleft side, a triangular flap of the excess is interdigitated in a redline back cut of the noncleft side (see Fig. 9-6G). A smooth vermilion transition is thereby attained.

The rotation flap is marked as a gentle convexity following the cleft margin to the columellar base, where it extends transversely ending in a back cut prior to entering the normal philtrum. Its length equals the vertical lip length and the length of the advancement flap.

The cleft margins are cut on both the rotation and advancement flaps to preserve the orbicularis muscle and leave the mucosal parings based on the maxillary alveolus. The mucosal parings are frequently discarded to avoid tissue excess but may be used to supplement the labial sulcus.

Undermining on the medial rotation flap segment is less extensive than on the lateral side. A slight mucosal release on the sulcus is generally required, and the muscle is typically back cut slightly beyond the dermal incision. Adequate rotation of the medial lip element must be visually confirmed with leveling of the cupid's bow peak.

The advancement flap is cut free of the nostril sill and ala, leaving a full complement of muscle underneath the ala base. The advancement flap and lateral cheek musculature is dissected free of the maxilla in a plane superficial to the periosteum. Dissection extends to the level of the infraorbital nerve. The muscle underneath the ala base is also fully mobilized from fibrous connections between the piriform rim and lower lateral cartilage. These nasal attachments are densely adherent to the lining, but complete mobilization is necessary if correction of the nasal deformity is to be achieved.

The nostril sill and floor of the nose are elevated in continuity with the lateral alar musculature to the medial columellar and membranous septal area. The base of the medial crux is elevated in a C flap, and dissection between the medial crux is extended in the columella between the dome cartilages. Lateral dissection is superficial to the lateral crux in a subdermal plane and joins the medial dissection, thereby creating complete mobilization of the lower lateral cartilage. This dissection allows the C flap to lengthen the columella and the cartilage suspension sutures to hold the domes and lower lateral cartilages in their desired positions.

Prior to lip closure, the orbicularis oris muscle is dissected free of the skin and mucosa. On the medial segment, the skin and mucosal undermining is sufficient to allow accurate suture approximation in the muscle. On the lateral segment, undermining extends further laterally for a distance of 5 to 10 mm to allow complete unfurling of any bunched or gathered orbicularis fibers. Care is taken not to dissect the vermilion mucosa from the deep portion of the orbicularis oris, as fine balance of the vermilion is lost when the relation between muscle and mucosa is altered. The cut separating the ala base from the lateral lip segment also releases the aberrant attachments of the superficial orbicularis to the ala musculature.

Suturing begins with the placement of 5-0 clear nylon suture in the underside of the orbicularis muscle, above the back cut in the medial segment (see Fig. 9-6I). The suture is carried to the underside of the cephalic margin of the orbicularis, on the lateral segment several millimeters lateral to the tip of the orbicularis advancement flap. Securing this suture brings the lateral orbicularis in continuity with the medial segment, fixing it to the undissected portion underneath the nasal sill. This suture prevents overrotation or lengthening of the orbicularis and removes tension from the remaining muscle and skin repair. Chromic catgut sutures (4-0) are then used to complete the orbicularis repair. The second suture is placed deep in the orbicu-

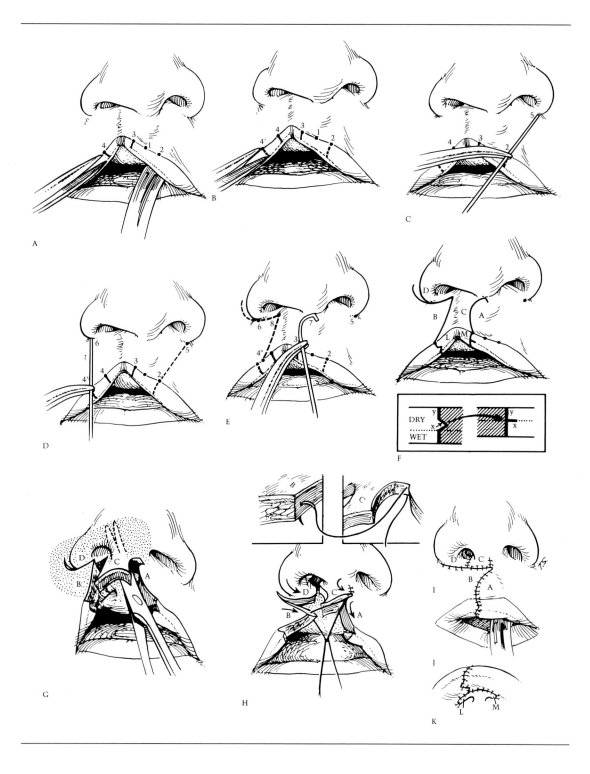

*Figure 9-6 Unilateral incomplete cleft: rotation advancement repair. A to E. 1 = tubercle; 2 and 3 = cupid's bow peak; 2–5 = vertical lip length; 4, 4' = possible peak locations, indicated by width of dry vermilion; 4 = cleft cupid's bow peak (matches vermilion at point 3); 4' = lateral limit for cupid's bow peak (matches vermilion at point 2); 4'' is between 4' and 4; 6–4 = 2–5; 4''–8 = 3–7 = 2–5. F. The advancement flap (B) equals the rotation flap (A). F (inset). x = excess dry vermilion on the lateral lip used to augment a medial deficiency. G. Nasal undermining. H to K. Sutures (see text).*

laris at the junction of the lip and vermilion musculature in the vicinity of the white roll. Remaining stitches between the medial and lateral muscles are placed to guarantee adequate rotation of the medial segment. A 5-0 chromic catgut suture is then placed in the vermilion musculature underneath the mucosa at the redline.

These sutures complete the muscle repair of the lip. The skin is generally closed with simple, interrupted 5-0 nylon sutures, although an occasional 5-0 chromic subdermal stitch is beneficial. The dry mucosa is similarly closed with a 5-0 nylon suture. The wet mucosa is closed with interrupted 4-0 chromic catgut. A Z-plasty is added to the underside of the lip to provide a step in the closure and to offset any fullness between the two sides of the repair (see Fig. 9-6K). This Z-plasty should be well removed from the visible portion of the lip vermilion. Several widely spaced chromic sutures are added to the labial sulcus to secure transposed mucosal flaps.

Suturing the nose begins with 5-0 clear nylon from the nasal spine to the retained muscle underneath the ala base. Placement of this suture in the alar musculature must be adjusted to allow the desired rotation and medial displacement of the ala base. Suspension sutures are added to the mobilized lower lateral cartilage, as needed. Skin closure about the nasal sill, c flap, and alar base is completed with interrupted 5-0 nylon sutures. Excess of sill tissue is mobilized me-

dially to create a fullness in the area of the base of the medial crux. Excision of nasal sill excess by completing the cleft is generally avoided, as it creates an unnatural break across an already deficient sill.

UNILATERAL COMPLETE CLEFT LIP

The cardinal markings of the repair of the unilateral complete cleft lip are made in the same manner as described for the incomplete cleft (Fig. 9-7). Mucosal parings are handled differently in that the lateral mucosal paring (L flap) is based on the lateral maxillary alveolus so that it can be used to augment the nasal lining (see Fig. 9-7B,C). The medial mucosal paring is based on the medial alveolar segment to augment sulcus closure. Dissection of the rotation flap and advancement flap proceeds as previously described. Mobilization of the ala base from its piriform fibrous attachments includes a full-thickness release of the lining along the piriform aperture and nasal bones. This release effectively separates the lower lateral cartilage and lateral portion of the upper lateral cartilage from its fibrous attachments. The defect created by this release is satisfied with an L flap. Dissection in the scroll arch between the upper lateral and lower lateral cartilages is avoided.

Suturing proceeds in the same manner as described for the incomplete cleft. The nasal floor is left unrepaired, although the sill is closed with the advancement of the ala base medially.

*Lip Adhesion*

Lip adhesion is of benefit for wide clefts and those with lateral maxillary collapse that do not respond to presurgical maxillary orthopedics. The adhesion improves maxillary arch alignment and enables a more predictable correction of the cleft nasal deformity. The improved nasal results are thought to be secondary to improved alar base arch support, which reduces the strain and relapse tendency for the mobilized lower lateral cartilage.

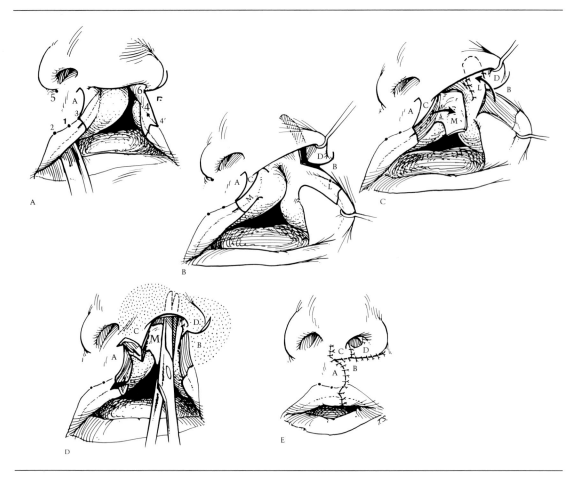

**Figure 9-7** *Unilateral complete cleft: rotation advancement. (M = medial mucosal flap; L = lateral mucosal flap).*

The adhesion is classified as a straight line muscle adhesion and begins with the complete marking of the rotation advancement cheiloplasty (Fig. 9-8). An L flap is elevated from the lateral segment beginning approximately 3 mm medial to point 4 (cupid's bow peak). This flap length provides adequate tissue for nasal release. The flap is turned 90 degrees into the nasal release along the lateral floor of the nose, which follows the piriform rim and the lateral portion of the nasal bones. A contiguous, maxillary sulcus incision is made through this nasal mucosal incision, and the lateral lip and cheek muscle mass is elevated in continuity from the maxilla and piriform aperture. The L flap is sutured into the nasal defect, and the lateral lip element is advanced medially for closure.

An M flap is also raised 3 mm from the cupid's bow peak to maintain symmetry of repair (see Fig. 9-8B). The mucosal flap is based on the maxillary alveolus and is turned into the alveolar cleft to augment closure. All dissection is maintained outside the margins for primary lip repair. No medial muscle dissection is done at this stage.

Closure is achieved with 4-0 chromic catgut sutures placed in the undissected orbicularis layer along the pared margin and is reinforced with a 4-0 chromic catgut mucosal closure between the M flap and the lateral lip mucosa. Skin is generally closed with interrupted 5-0 chromic catgut, with

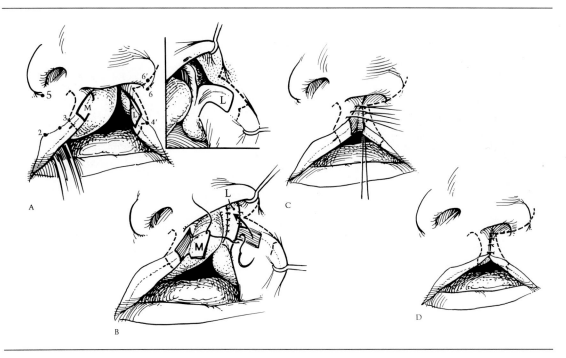

**Figure 9-8** *Straight line muscle adhesion. Lateral lip and ala are released from the maxilla and advanced medially. A. Markings for primary lip repair (dotted lines). Note adjustments for short lateral lip segment in 4', 6, and 6'. B. Medial (M) mucosal flap turned down to join lateral lining. L flap sutured intranasally along lateral side wall in area of release. C. Absorbable skin-muscle suture for closure. D. Adhesion designed so as not to violate primary repair. (L = lateral mucosal flap; M = medial mucosal flap.)*

sutures placed outside the markings for definitive cheiloplasty. The adhesion effectively closes the nasal sill and upper two-thirds of the lip. The forces for muscle closure have an immediate effect on the alveolar segments.

### Short Lateral Lip Segment

A short lateral lip segment is identified when the distance from the cleft side ala base to the lateral limit for point 4 is less than the vertical requirements for lip repair (distance from noncleft ala base to noncleft cupid's bow peak) (Fig. 9-9A–C). Moving point 4 farther laterally beyond its defined

limit ultimately results in vermilion mismatch and a horizontally tight upper lip (Fig. 9-9B). Accordingly, the needed tissue is obtained from the ala base and nostril sill (Fig. 9-9C). This step effectively raises the upper margin of the advancement flap marking into the sill and across the ala base. Other markings remain the same.

Dissection of the lateral advancement flap must be adjusted as the lateral segment is freed from the nose (Fig. 9-9D). The skin incision penetrates to the dermal level across the sill and ala base. Dissection is begun immediately underneath the dermis, preserving the fibromuscular structure of the ala base. The subdermal dissection extends down to the natural groove, separating the orbicularis from the nasal sill and ala base. With the dermal flap reflected, release of the orbicularis and the ala base is achieved, adhering to the same planes of muscle dissection as previously described.

At the time of lip closure, the perialar cheek skin is advanced over the denuded alar base and across the sill. Vertical lip

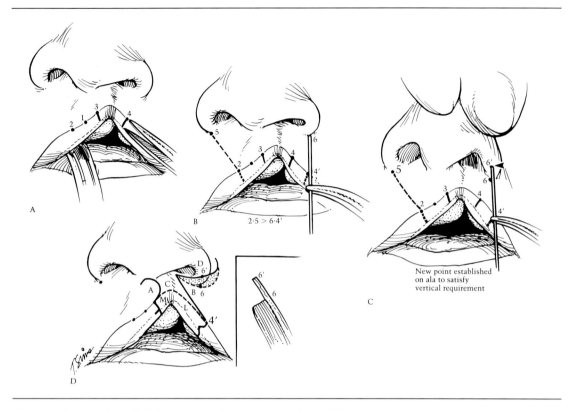

**Figure 9-9** *Complete cleft following adhesion: short lateral lip segment. (4′ = lateral limit for cupid's bow; 6–6′ = vertical deficiency skin flap from ala base.)*

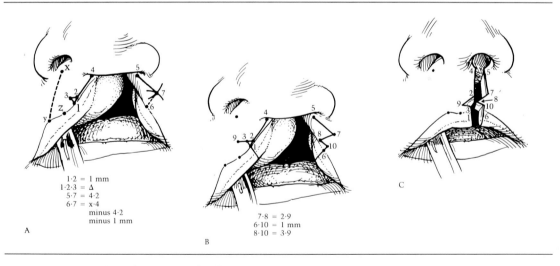

**Figure 9-10** *Complete cleft: triangular flap repair as modified by Brauer and Cronin.*

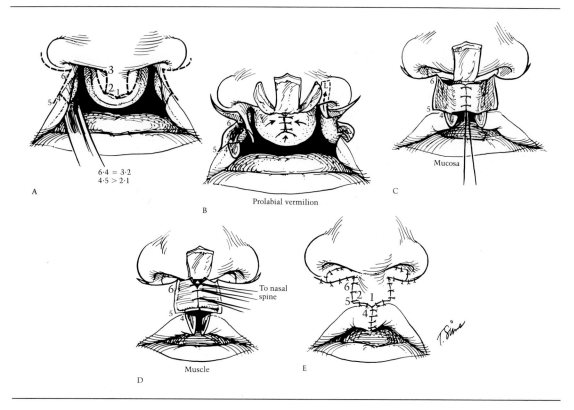

**Figure 9-11** *Bilateral cleft lip: Millard repair.*

length is maintained, and the definition of the ala base is preserved. A scar crossing the base is the result.

*Triangular Flap Repair*
Wide unilateral clefts, particularly those with a short lateral lip segment, present the greatest challenge to the rotation advancement repair. Although preliminary lip adhesion has been a useful adjunct, another alternative involves the lower triangular flap Tennison repair as modified by Brauer and Cronin [1]. The repair involves precise geometric planning (Fig. 9-10). The repaired side should be approximately 1 mm shorter than the noncleft side to avoid excess growth in vertical length. An offset in the incision immediately above the vermilion line avoids an oblique scar crossing the vermilion. Less

undermining is required, and simultaneous nasal correction can be achieved. The principal objection is the scar crossing the philtrum.

BILATERAL CLEFT LIP
*Millard Repair*
The Millard bilateral cleft repair augments the central prolabial vermilion, with white roll and vermilion flaps taken from the lateral lip elements (Fig. 9-11). Accordingly, it is the preferred repair when the prolabium is deficient of vermilion and has a poorly defined white roll.

The vertical length of the repair is determined by the natural prolabial length taken from columella base to cupid's bow peak (see Fig. 9-11A). The cupid's bow peaks are arbitrarily taken 2 to 3 mm from the central tubercle, and the line connecting tubercle to cupid's bow peak is slightly arched to accentuate the bow. The vertical line from cupid's bow peak to columella base is straight or slightly bowed because of the tendency of the philtrum to widen along the repair.

The point on the lateral lip segments where the white roll terminates and the vermilion becomes hypoplastic is the beginning of the white roll vermilion flap, which is used to augment the tubercle. A back cut is marked down the white roll 1 mm longer than the distance from cupid's bow peak to tubercle arc (see Fig. 9-11A). This lateral point coincides with the cupid's bow peak, and the vertical height of the lip is measured cephalad and along the cleft from this point. Excess lip length between nasal sill and the cephalad margin of the advancement is either excised or deepithelialized depending on the needs in the nasal sill.

Mucosal parings of the prolabium are turned in to line the premaxilla after the prolabium is elevated away from the premaxilla. Fork flaps are banked in the nasal sill with no medial advancement of the alar bases. Lateral cleft parings in incomplete clefts are used to augment the alveolar sulcus or are discarded, whereas in complete clefts they are used to augment the nasal lining along the lateral nasal floor. The lateral mucosa is advanced centrally and joined in the midline to complete the sulcus reconstruction (see Fig. 9-11C). Lateral orbicularis muscle flaps are sutured underneath the prolabium (see Fig. 9-11D). Wide undermining of the lateral lip and cheek is often required. The nasal deformity is not addressed at the initial stage of bilateral cheiloplasty.

*Modified Manchester Repair*

The modified Manchester repair is employed when the prolabium is characterized by a full vermilion with adequate white roll detail (Fig. 9-12). The philtral width is taken at approximately 4 mm between tubercle points. The full vertical length of the prolabium is used to establish the appropriate vertical lip length. Prolabial parings are banked as forked flaps, as previously described. Cupid's bow peak on the lateral

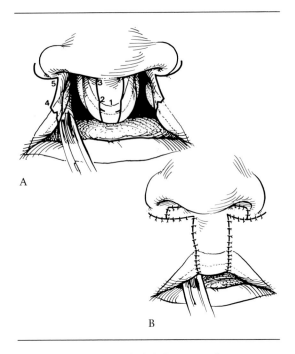

**Figure 9-12** *Bilateral cleft lip: Manchester repair.*

element is placed where the white roll terminates and the vermilion becomes hypoplastic. The vertical lip length is measured from this point using a distance equal to that determined by the prolabial length. A lateral release is made from this cephalad point across the sill and around the ala. Lateral prolabial parings are, again, used in complete clefts to augment nasal lining along the lateral floor. Lateral prolabial parings are also used to augment and close the prolabial sulcus; the vermilion and central prolabial skin is elevated to allow closure of the orbicularis across the premaxilla. The sulcus is closed with mucosa advanced from the lateral lip elements. The cupid's bow points from the lateral elements are sutured to the philtral points previously marked, and the lateral vermilion is closed with the prolabial segment in a similar manner. The repair differs from the Millard procedure in that the central prolabial vermilion is retained for tubercle, thereby limiting the amount of lateral lip tissue required in the closure.

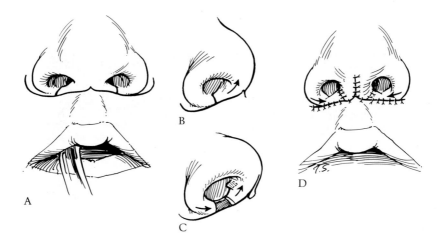

**Figure 9-13** *Columellar lengthening and second stage lip repair by combined forked flap and alar advancement.*

### Columellar Lengthening/Correction of Cleft Nasal Deformity

Columellar lengthening and correction of the cleft nasal deformity (Fig. 9-13) is undertaken at approximately 18 months of age. The procedure involves a combined Cronin advancement of the ala base, nostril floor, and sill with advancement of fork flaps into the columella. Closure of the nasal floor is completed with medial advancement of the lateral nasal tissues. Complete release of the ala from the piriform aperature and nasal bones is achieved. Wide undermining of the lower lateral cartilage from the skin is coupled with dissection between the medial crux and the columella. This mobilization allows for advancement of the medial and lateral crux toward the dome. Suspension sutures and sutures between the dome cartilages may be used to create central tip projection and definition. Although the procedure is adequate for positioning the ala bases, lasting tip support is generally not provided and secondary cartilage grafting to the columella is frequently required. The latter may be done for severe deformities at the time of alveolar bone grafting when the child is 7 to 8 years old, or it may be deferred until adolescence if the deformity is minimal.

## Postoperative Care

Feedings are administered with a catheter tip syringe fitted with a small red rubber catheter for the first 2 to 3 weeks postoperatively. Nipples are avoided to minimize strain on the muscle and skin sutures and to avoid trauma to the repaired velum. Diet is advanced to full-strength formula on the day of surgery to pacify the infant. Velcro arm restraints (No-No's) are used to protect the repair from flailing hands and fingers.

Suture line care consists in PRN cleansing with half-strength hydrogen peroxide followed with a liberal coating of polymyxin B–bacitracin ointment. Sutures are removed on the fifth postoperative day.

Routine diet and care are resumed about 3 weeks postoperatively. Parents are told to expect firmness in the lip scar and shortening across the repair that generally becomes maximum 4 to 6 weeks after surgery. Scars typically soften between 3 and 6 months postoperatively.

## Secondary Surgery

Scar revisions and touch-up adjustments are not part of the expected repair sequence. The best (least visible) lip scar is the product of the initial repair, as healing during the first year of life generally yields a scar superior to that produced during any other time period. When revisions are necessary, they are usually performed at preschool age.

## References

1. Brauer, R. O., and Cronin, T. D. The Tennison lip repair revisited. *Plast. Reconstr. Surg.* 71:633, 1983.
2. Kernahan, D. A., and Bauer, B. S. Functional cleft lip repair: A sequential, layered closure with orbicularis muscle realignment. *Plast. Reconstr. Surg.* 72:459, 1983.
3. LeMesurier, A. B. Method of cutting and suturing lip in complete unilateral cleft lip. *Plast. Reconstr. Surg.* 4:1, 1949.
4. Millard, D. R., Jr. A primary camouflage of the unilateral harlook. In T. Skoog (ed.). *Transactions of the First International Congress of Plastic Surgery, Stockholm, 1955.* Baltimore: Williams & Wilkins, 1957. Pp. 160–166.
5. Millard, D. R., Jr. *Cleft Craft—The Evolution of Its Surgery, Vol. II: The Bilateral and Rare Deformities.* Boston: Little, Brown, 1977.
6. Mirault, G. Deux lettres sur l'operation du bec-de-lievre considere dans ses devers etats de simplicite et de complication. *J. Chir. (Paris)* 2:257, 1844.
7. Nicolau, P. J. The orbicularis oris muscle: A functional approach to its repair in the cleft lip. *Br. J. Plast. Surg.* 36:141, 1983.
8. Skoog, T. A design for the repair of unilateral cleft lip. *Am. J. Surg.* 95:223, 1958.
9. Tennison, C. W. The repair of unilateral cleft lip by the stencil method. *Plast. Reconstr. Surg.* 9:115, 1952.
10. Thomson, H. G., and Delpero, W. Clinical evaluation of microform cleft lip surgery. *Plast. Reconstr. Surg.* 75:800, 1985.
11. Trauner, R., and Trauner, M. Results of cleft lip operations. *Plast. Reconstr. Surg.* 40:209, 1967.
12. Veau, V. Operative treatment of complete double harelip. *Ann. Surg. (Paris)* 76:143, 1922.

# 10

# Cleft Palate

*Peter Randall*
*Don LaRossa*

The *normal palate* (Fig. 10-1) is composed of the bony or hard palate anteriorly and the soft palate posteriorly. The alveolus borders the hard palate. Anteriorly and centrally the hard palate consists of the premaxilla, which gives rise to the incisor teeth; the premaxilla extends posteriorly to the incisive foramen. The major portion of the hard palate is made up of the paired maxillae. Posterior to the maxillae are the palatine bones.

The major *blood supply* comes from the greater palatine arteries via the major palatine foramina. A secondary blood supply comes through the lesser palatine foramina and incisive foramina.

The sensory *nerves* reach the palate through these foramina and from the nasal side of the soft palate by way of the posterior palatine nerve. These nerves are sphenopalatine branches of the maxillary nerve, the second division of the trigeminal nerve (cranial nerve V). The soft palate is densely attached to the posterior edge of the palatine bones by the palatal aponeurosis.

The major *musculature* consists of two sling-like muscles: (1) the levator palati muscles, which pull the palate upward and backward; and (2) the tensor palati muscles, which through a tendinous extension bend around the pterygoid hamulus, functioning as a pulley to allow these muscles to stretch the soft palate tightly. Other pairs of muscles contributing to speech and swallowing include the palatoglossus, the palatopharyngeus, the stylopharyngeus, and the superior pharyngeal constrictors. The innervation of the levator palati is by way of the pharyngeal plexus. The tensor palati and other swallowing muscles are innervated by way of the mandibular division of the trigeminal nerve [2, 3, 17].

## Anatomy of Prepalatal and Palatal Clefts

Clefts usually follow the lines of fusion so that anterior to the incisive foramen the cleft diverges between the maxilla and the premaxilla. It usually traverses the alveolus between the lateral incisor and the canine teeth. There may be some variation in the location of the cleft in the alveolus. In addition, rarely there is a midline cleft of these anterior structures [1].

The structures anterior to the incisive foramen (including the nasal tip cartilages, nasal floor, lip, and alveolus) are called the *prepalatal structures,* or the structures of the *primary palate.* Those posterior to the incisive foramen are called the *palatal structures,* or those of the *secondary palate.* These two areas are embryologically dis-

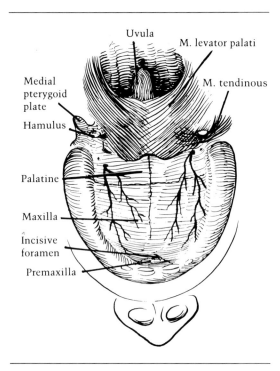

Uvula

M. levator palati

Medial
pterygoid
plate

M. tendinous

Hamulus

Palatine

Maxilla

Incisive
foramen

Premaxilla

***Figure 10-1*** *Normal palatal structures. The incisive foramen is the dividing point between clefts of the prepalatal structures and those of the palatal structures.*

tinct. These terms are interchangeable, but we prefer to use prepalatal and palatal rather than primary and secondary palate. It is awkward referring to the lip and nose as palatal structures, and the term *secondary* referring to the palate makes it sound less important than the *primary* palate, which probably is not true.

Clefts in the alveolus are usually associated with clefts in the lip. Without the restraining forces of the intact orbicularis oris muscle, the cleft alveolar segments are most often displaced outward from the normal position, causing anterior flaring of the premaxilla in a unilateral cleft and often marked protrusion in the bilateral cleft. The lateral maxillary segment is also usually laterally displaced prior to lip repair, but after lip repair it is compressed medially and often drifts to a lateral crossbite position. It

is usually lacking in vertical height as well. The teeth adjacent to the cleft are likely to be angled into the cleft, and their size and shape are frequently distorted. The lateral incisor tooth may be absent [19].

With unilateral clefts, the vomer is usually attached to the maxilla for its entire length on the noncleft side. With bilateral clefts of the prepalatal and palatal structures, the vomer is unattached laterally, which is also the case for palatal clefts involving only those structures posterior to the incisive foramen. Thus it seems that the clefting process in the midportion of the hard palate differs depending on whether the cleft occurs in conjunction with a unilateral cleft of the prepalate or is seen as an isolated palatal abnormality.

One of the most important anatomic distortions seen with cleft palate is in the *musculature of the soft palate.* Kraus [23] and Dickson and Dickson [9] have stressed again the findings of Veau [29] that in clefts of the soft palate the levator palati muscles, instead of being directed toward the midline as they should be, are oriented in a more longitudinal direction and are inserted not only along the posterior edge of the bony palate but often along the medial edge of the cleft as well.

Even in a submucosal cleft with most of the soft palate mucosa intact but with dehiscence of the underlying muscles in the midline, this abnormal orientation of the levator palati muscles usually can be seen as two longitudinal ridges in the soft palate on either side of the midline. Ideally, this abnormal attachment and orientation of the levator muscles must be corrected if the muscles are to function adequately [10].

The tensor palati muscles in patients with clefts are also abnormal, with little or no tissue found medial to the pterygoid hamulus. At times, fibers seem to bypass the hamulus altogether. Reconstruction of the tensor muscles does not seem to be important so far as speech is concerned. However, both the tensor and the levator palati muscles also insert along the eustachian tubes. This positioning seems to be of critical importance in children with clefts, as malfunctioning of the eustachian tube is usually a significant finding even in the newborn with a cleft palate. Persistent serous otitis media occurs in nearly 100 percent of children with palatal clefts [33, 34, 57, 61].

## Embryology and Etiology of Palatal Clefts

### PREPALATAL CLEFTS

In theory, prepalatal clefts in humans are caused by a lack of mesenchymal development. Stark [27] described three mesenchymal islands, one central and two lateral, that ordinarily develop and fuse. Lack of development of one or more of these three islands leaves an unstable condition, with ectoderm of the skin in contact with ectoderm of the oral mucosa; complete or incomplete breakdown occurs at this point.

This theory explains the various types of lateral cleft that are seen, depending on whether one or both lateral mesenchymal islands fail to develop. In addition, it explains the unusual midline cleft. The severe midline cleft defect, as seen in arhinocephaly, consisting of a midline loss of lip and columella, could be due to failure of all three islands to develop. This theory also explains the usual involvement of the nasal alar cartilages along with the lip and the associated defects of the alveolus in all prepalatal clefts. In addition, such a lack of mesenchymal development explains the hypoplasia seen in the adjacent maxillary structures [11].

### PALATAL CLEFTS

The palatal structures in a 7-week-old embryo are present as two shelves that lie in an almost vertical position, with their medial edges inferiorly placed alongside the tongue. Normally, the neck straightens from the flexed position, the tongue drops downward, and the shelves rotate upward to the horizontal position and fuse from anterior to posterior to form the intact palate by 12 weeks [27]. Whether the cleft condition is a result of the two halves never coming together or of an imperfect union and subsequent separation is open to some question [46]. Experimentally, it has been shown that in rodents the right palatal shelf reaches the horizontal position before the left one, leaving the left side vulnerable to interruption or interference in its normal development for a longer time than the right. This phenomenon may explain the more frequent occurrence of unilateral clefts on the left than on the right [13, 30].

Experimental clefts have been produced by a number of conditions, e.g., deficiencies of vitamin A, riboflavin, folic acid, panthothenic acid, and nicotinic acid. They have also been produced by an excess of vitamin A, fasting, hypoxia, nitrogen mustard, nucleic acid antagonists, corticosteroids, ACTH, irradiation, loss of amniotic fluid, and a number of other agents [7, 20, 24, 31–33]. The fetal alcohol syndrome also has been implicated and may indeed be significant over only a brief but critical period of embryologic development [5, 6].

Although the etiology in man is not known, heredity has been shown to play a significant part. The most frequent type of cleft in humans (left unilateral cleft of the palate and prepalate) is seen predominantly in male infants with a rather high hereditary background, whereas the second most frequent type of cleft (cleft palate alone) is predominantly seen in female infants with a fairly low hereditary background, suggesting entirely different causes. Because the defect is a frequent one, it is probably easily produced in humans and is likely to have a number of causes. A distinction should be made between those with a prepalatal cleft (with or without an accompanying palatal cleft) and those with only a palatal cleft [1, 14].

A number of monozygotic twins with discordant anomalies have been described by

Fogh-Andersen and others, which indicates that a slight environmental difference can alter the degree of manifestation or penetration of the anomaly [12, 53].

INCIDENCE

The incidence of various types of cleft was reported by Veau [29]. The overall incidence of clefts in the general population was reported by Fogh-Andersen [11, 12] as 1 in 665 and by Ivy [44] as 1 in 762 live births, placing it second only to club feet among congenital anomalies reported on birth certificates. Brogan and Murphy [2] reported a decrease in the incidence of clefts in western Australia, whereas Fogh-Andersen reported a slight increase in incidence in Scandinavia [12]. In general, there seems to be a greater incidence in Asians than in Caucasians and a decreased incidence in blacks. Fogh-Andersen found that the chances of cleft lip occurring in the child of parents, one of whom has a cleft, is about 2 percent. This figure increases to 14 percent if there is already a sibling with a cleft lip. If two normal parents have a child with a cleft lip, there is said to be a 4.5 percent chance that subsequent siblings will have the deformity. These figures hold true largely for clefts in the United States, Canada, and Western Europe. However, an interesting geographic distribution has been reported in the Scandinavian countries (Table 10-1). These figures raise intriguing questions as to etiology and inheritance [26].

## Classification of Clefts
PREPALATAL CLEFTS

The distinction between prepalatal clefts (clefts of the primary palate) and palatal clefts (clefts of the secondary palate) at the incisive foramen is made because embryologically these two types of cleft are different and because they can occur either separately or together. Prepalatal clefts involving the nasal tip cartilages, the floor of the nose, the lip, and the alveolus can occur unilaterally

**Table 10-1**  *Geographic distribution of isolated cleft palate*

| Country | % |
|---------|-----|
| Denmark | 25 |
| Finland | 57 |
| Iceland | 31 |
| Norway | 31 |
| Sweden | 31 |

Source: A. E. Rintala. Epidemiology of orofacial clefts in Finland: A review. *Ann. Plast. Surg.* 17:456, 1986.

or bilaterally and rarely in the midline. A further division is made depending on whether they are complete or incomplete (total or subtotal), which depends on whether the structures involved are completely or incompletely separated. Even more explicitly, the clefts can be described as being one-third, two-thirds, or three-thirds complete with added notes concerning rotation, protrusion, and measurements of the amount of separation between the involved parts [15].

PALATAL CLEFTS

Palatal clefts (posterior to the incisive foramen) are also classified as complete or incomplete (total or subtotal) depending on whether they extend all the way from the incisive foramen through the hard palate and soft palate or they involve only a part of this distance. Again, a more explicit classification describes the cleft involving one-third, two-thirds, or three-thirds of the soft palate or of the hard palate up to the incisive foramen. The most rudimentary form of cleft palate is the bifid uvula [21, 25, 28, 32] (Fig. 10-2).

Palatal clefts are considered to be midline clefts, but a note should be made in the records of those patients with a hard palate involvement describing any attachment of the vomer to either the right or left maxillary bone. Further notes should describe submucosal clefts when they are recognized. Certain combinations of clefts occur more frequently than others, the most frequent being a bifid uvula, as noted below. The next most frequent is a left unilateral complete cleft of the palate and prepalatal structures. The next most common is a midline cleft of three-thirds of the soft palate and part of the hard palate without a cleft in the prepalatal area. Bilateral clefts of the prepalatal area are usually accompanied by bilateral palatal clefts, and incomplete clefts in one area usually accompany incomplete clefts in the other. However, virtually any combination of clefts can occur. A hard palate cleft is almost never seen without a three-thirds cleft of the soft palate. We have seen only three such cases.

## BIFID UVULA

Meskin et al. reported an instance of bifid uvula in 2 percent of a large college population [50]. Most of the time, this abnormality is an incidental finding, and it is not associated with velopharyngeal incompetence or any other functional problem. However, it is a deformity that can be inherited as a palatal cleft and serves as a warning that, indeed, such a palate may be close to velopharyngeal incompetence so that adenoidectomy could render such a palate incompetent. When seen in a newborn, the bifid uvula raises immediate suspicion as to the possible presence of a submucosal cleft or a congenitally short palate with frank velopharyngeal incompetence.

## SUBMUCOSAL CLEFT

A bifid uvula may also be part of a complex known as a submucosal cleft with dehiscence of the levator muscles, disorientation of the levator muscle into a more longitudinal direction, a short anteroposterior dimension of the palate, and a submucosal cleft in the posterior third of the bony palate. Usually if these abnormalities are present, the midportion of the posterior third of the soft palate has a thin appearance on examination, called a zona pellucidum. It is easily demonstrated at operation if an elevator is placed behind the palate. On gagging, the

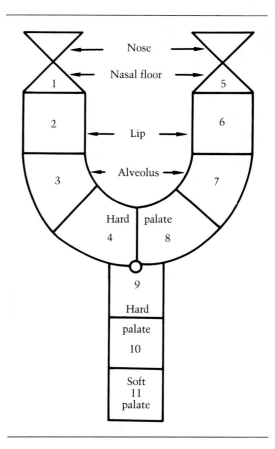

**Figure 10-2** *Classification: Millard's modification of Kernahan's diagrammatic Y. In Millard's description "to indicate a cleft, the area will be stippled; to indicate submucosal muscle and bony clefts, the area will be marked with horizontal lines; and to indicate the degree of nasal deformity, the top triangle will be lined horizontally in density, proportional to the severity of the distortion." (From D. R. Millard. Cleft Craft, Vol. 1. Boston: Little, Brown, 1976. P. 52.)*

displaced levator palati muscles stand out in their abnormal position. One should be able to palpate a notch in the posterior edge of the hard palate instead of the usual posterior nasal spine [8–10, 20, 93].

## ROBIN SEQUENCE

In clefts extending no further anteriorly than the incisive foramen, the mandible may be retropositioned or structurally small (or both). Under these conditions, the genio-glossus muscle, which normally holds the tongue in an anterior position (thus maintaining an adequate airway), has its bony attachment posteriorly displaced. A ball-valve type of inspiratory respiratory obstruction can occur owing to the glossoptosis. It is called the *Robin sequence* (or *Pierre Robin sequence*), which can vary widely in severity. Although usually associated with a cleft palate, the latter is not an essential part of the "sequence" (see Chapter 5) [18, 54].

## Soft Palate Movement and Speech

### SOFT PALATE MOVEMENT DURING SPEECH

The major action of the soft palate during speech (Fig. 10-3) consists in a rapid and voluntary, though subconscious, motion of the palate upward and backward, producing intimate contact with the posterior pharyngeal wall at the level of the adenoid pad. This movement is called *velopharyngeal closure.* The major muscles for achieving velopharyngeal closure are the paired levator palati muscles, which are efficient, contract rapidly and accurately, and fatigue slowly.

Velopharyngeal closure is also aided by the superior pharyngeal constrictor muscles, the palatopharyngeus muscles, and the musculus uvula. Skolnick et al. [89, 90] showed that there is considerable variation in the way velopharyngeal closure is achieved, even in the normal person. The motion appears to be truly sphincteric, with the greatest action being achieved by the levator palati. The terms velopharyngeal *competence* and velopharyngeal *incompetence* refer, respectively, to the presence or absence of velopharyngeal closure.

### PRODUCTION OF NORMAL SPEECH

Normal speech requires a competent speech mechanism plus adequate hearing, environment, and intelligence. So many factors go into speech production and there is so much variation under normal conditions that it is difficult to define "normal speech." Com-

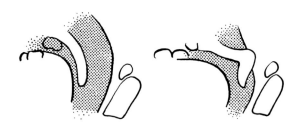

**Figure 10-3** *Outline of the posterior pharynx, soft palate, and tongue in sagittal cross section. At rest (left), the palate hangs free. Normal velopharyngeal closure (right) is achieved mostly by the levator palati muscles pulling the middle one-third of the palate upward and backward; firm contact is made at about the level of the adenoid pad.*

plete or nearly complete velopharyngeal closure is needed. All consonant sounds in the English language, with the exception of the "nasal consonants" (m, n) and the ng sound (as in "ring"), require the building up of intraoral air pressure. The sudden release of pressure produces an explosive sound, or a "stop plosive" consonant, such as p, t, and d. The production of sound by friction produces the consonants called continuants; when voiced, as v and z, they are called *fricatives,* whereas the more silent continuants are subclassified as *sibilants,* such as s and sh. The "nasal consonants" (m, n, ng) are pronounced with the oral port closed and the sound directed out through the nose, thus requiring an adequate nasal airway [62, 63].

### CLEFT PALATE TYPE SPEECH

Vowel sounds, when produced by patients with velopharyngeal incompetence, take on an excessively nasal quality that is called *hypernasality,* in contrast to the *hyponasality* heard with obstructed conditions such as choanal atresia, obstructing hypertrophied adenoids, or a simple "cold in the nose." Nasal resonance is due to vibrations in the nasal passages and paranasal sinuses. Thus one can describe normal nasal resonance, hypernasality, and hyponasality.

Because these structures are so small and the voice is high-pitched in the infant, even with velopharyngeal incompetence, hyper-nasality is difficult to hear. However, if present, it can be expected to get worse as the child grows and these passages enlarge and the voice deepens [71, 77].

Consonants, when enunciated by patients with velopharyngeal incompetence, are usually distorted by inadequate pressure, leading to *misarticulation* of the consonant sound. Another distortion is caused by the sound of air leaking into the nose as a sniffing or snuffing sound, referred to as *nasal escape*. Thus the speech of children with velopharyngeal incompetence can be distorted by hypernasality, misarticulation, and nasal escape. Each may be present to a greater or lesser degree, and all contribute to the *intelligibility*, or understandability, of the child's speech. The field of speech pathology has gone far in documenting and objectively assessing these abnormalities to provide good measures of speech evaluation.

Patients may *omit* consonant sounds that they are unable to produce or may *substitute* other sounds such as those produced by building up pressure behind the glottis, producing a plosive, called a *glottal stop*. For example, the word *daddy* becomes *ah-ee* with the consonants omitted or similar to *ga-gee* by substituting the glottal stop for the *d* sound.

Good speech requires not only a capable mechanism, adequate hearing, and intelligence but also a home and school environment where good speech is heard. A higher percentage of children with cleft palates develop normal speech if an adequate mechanism is provided before formal speech develops than if the child first learns incorrect speech owing to an incompetent palate, then has the palate repaired and tries to correct the errors. Even though a subsequent procedure provides an adequate speech mechanism, it is usually difficult for the patient who is accustomed to hearing his or her own incorrect speech to be comfortable with "normal speech," which sounds so different

to him or her. Some patients do, however, overcome this difficulty.

When testing speech it should be noted that a patient with borderline velopharyngeal incompetence can often put enough extra effort into his or her speech that no hypernasality or articulatory errors are made. Under these circumstances, poor speech is probably heard when the patient is more relaxed (as with conversational speech) or fatigued. The collaboration of a competent speech pathologist to help evaluate postoperative surgical results is helpful. Speech is the most important function to consider during cleft palate repair. Although few surgeons have had any training in speech pathology, they should be familiar with the essentials so as to understand the variations and to be able to do a rudimentary evaluation of their own patients [67–69, 72, 79, 91, 94, 95].

## General Care
### NEONATAL PERIOD
In addition to the cleft, there are four points to be emphasized regarding the treatment of young infants with clefts of the palate: (1) feeding; (2) maintenance of an airway; (3) middle ear disease; and (4) the possibility of other abnormalities.

### Feeding
Feeding a child with a cleft palate is difficult only because of the inability to develop suction, even though the infant may make sucking movements. Because swallowing is not normally affected, adequate nutrition is possible when milk or soft food is simply delivered to the posterior part of the oral cavity. Rarely, an abundance of breast milk can make breast feeding practical; otherwise, milk is given in such a way that suction is not needed. Artificial nipples can have the holes made larger so that the milk drips freely from an inverted bottle, or they can be deeply cross-cut so that suckling action

opens the tip sufficiently. The nipples can be attached to a Brecht-type feeder with a bulb syringe or simply to a plastic bottle that can be squeezed. It is helpful to hold the infant at about 45 degrees above the horizontal so that the milk flows to the back of the mouth, with minimal regurgitation into the nose. Note that more air than usual is swallowed, feeding takes longer than the average time, and the baby must be burped more frequently. With patience and understanding, feeding a child with a cleft is not difficult.

About the matter of feeding, it is important to urge the mother to take the most active part and to help regardless of how difficult the feedings might be. The mother can be expected to be timid at first, but she soon learns the tricks that are needed. In time, she should be more expert than anyone else in the feeding of her child. At this point, the baby is more dependent on the mother for survival than on any other person. Thus in a simple, subtle way, a strong, healthy mother–child bonding is begun. Advice from an experienced nursery nurse is helpful, but care must be taken that the nurse does not take over the complete feeding of the child, as many are likely to do. It is the mother's responsibility, and she must undertake it as soon as possible [43].

*Maintenance of an Airway*
Breathing can be a problem, particularly if the chin is retropositioned (short chin, micrognathic, retrognathic, undershot jaw), as in the Pierre Robin sequence. With retrognathia, the effectiveness of the genioglossus muscle is lost and the tongue falls backward, partly or completely blocking the airway on inspiration (Pierre Robin sequence; see Chapter 5).

*Middle Ear Disease*
The middle ear space, even during the neonatal period, is usually not properly aerated if the child has a cleft palate. Examination with an office otoscope is difficult because the infant usually squirms, the auditory canal is tiny, and the infant eardrum is oriented much more tangential to the long axis of the external auditory canal than that in older children. A pneumootoscope can be helpful for making this diagnosis.

A thorough examination with an operating microscope under a general anesthetic reveals abnormal fluid behind the eardrum in 90 to 100 percent of these infants. Usually, this fluid is thick but sterile; however, in older children evidence of prolonged infection is often encountered. Examination by an otolaryngologist is carried out using an operating microscope and is done virtually whenever a child with a cleft palate undergoes a general anesthetic. Malfunction of the eustachian tube appears to be the most likely cause of this problem. When a myringotomy is done, the incision is usually kept open with a small Silastic tube or grommet, which allows equalization of air pressure through the eardrum rather than by way of the eustachian tube. Otolaryngologic consultation and follow-up are obviously helpful. Bilateral myringotomy and ventilating tube insertion are usually done at the time of primary cleft palate repair or cleft lip repair. If the child has a cleft palate without a cleft lip, and the cleft palate is not to be repaired until after 12 months of age, some otolaryngologists elect to insert the ventilating tubes earlier.

Teen-aged children with cleft palate used to have about a 40 to 50 percent incidence of *permanent hearing loss* in the range of 30 to 40 decibels in one or both ears. With careful attention to ear problems, this incidence has virtually disappeared. Good hearing is important to the development of good speech, and so it is doubly important to guard it carefully [33, 34, 52, 61].

*Other Congenital Abnormalities*
Other congenital abnormalities occur more frequently in the cleft palate population than in the average infant. The incidence can be as high as 30 percent. A complete history and physical examination with the

usual laboratory studies are carried out. The history includes an inquiry about other clefts and deformities in the family and any known illness or problems that might have occurred during the early months of the pregnancy [6, 16, 19, 22, 31].

QUESTIONS FROM PARENTS

Most parents of children with cleft palate ask if there is a known cause and if the condition could have been prevented. They may ask about the chance of a cleft occurring in subsequent children. What can be done about the deformity? When can it be done? How much will it cost? Will the child be able to speak correctly? These queries should be answered simply, directly, and honestly but reassuringly. Even if they are not asked, they probably should be raised because if the answers are not supplied by a competent person they are likely to be volunteered by a less experienced person.

Parents are told that in most cases the exact cause of the cleft is not known, and that in some families it appears to be an inherited trait whereas in others it is not. In the absence of a significant family history, it has been helpful to describe the cleft as an "accident" in development. This description seems to convey a realistic appreciation of something that can be slight or severe and that can happen to anyone with or without known reason. In addition, it implies that some conditions can be corrected virtually completely whereas with others some stigmata of the "damage" may remain.

Parents are told that presently there is nothing known that can prevent the occurrence of clefts under most circumstances and that nothing could have been done during the pregnancy that was not done, nor was anything done that should not have been done. Despite this reassurance, a deep guilt complex frequently remains. Clefts have been diagnosed in utero by ultrasound, but only late in pregnancy.

In the absence of a strong family history of clefts, parents are told that, having had one child with a cleft, the likelihood of another being born with the same deformity is greater than in the general population. This increased likelihood, however, is probably so small that it should not interfere with plans to have more children, nor should it interfere with their child's plans to grow up, get married, and have a family, except that the child with a cleft should not marry another person with a cleft (if children are wanted). Consultation with a genetic counselor is offered.

The general time schedule of steps for correcting the defect is discussed. If appropriate, the cost of treatment, expected coverage from insurance, approximate duration of hospitalization, and availability of a cleft palate clinic or team facilities are explained. Articles written for lay consumption can be helpful and can be obtained from the American Cleft Palate Educational Foundation, 331 Salk Hall, Pittsburgh, PA 15261.

## *Age for Surgery*

In virtually every series where different ages for palate repair are compared, the best results, so far as speech is concerned, have been in the younger group. Most surgeons prefer to close the palate at 12 to 14 months of age. We believe that treatment at a much younger age could have definite advantages in that it would provide a functioning mechanism before the infant starts to learn to speak [39, 40, 55].

Piaget [81] believed that a 6-month-old infant can make *all* the necessary speech sounds, which the child then refines with development. The neurologic control necessary for this mechanical process must be complicated, and there is some evidence that if it is not put to work at the proper age it may indeed be bypassed in the process of development, never developing as it should.

Since 1965 we have been doing easy cleft palate repairs in selected cases at 3 to 6 months of age. At present, we prefer to repair virtually all clefts at 3 to 9 months of age, with some specific exceptions. One group is being studied at 3 to 6 months of age and another at 6 to 9 months of age; and as yet we do not know if there is a significant difference between these two groups or if 3 months of age is even young enough. The tangible evidence that early closure is better is at present confined to two series of patients. One study is by Dorf and Curtin [40], in which they showed a significantly increased incidence of persistent misarticulation in patients whose clefts were closed between 12 and 24 months of age (80 percent) compared with those closed in infants under 12 months of age (22 percent, $p < 0.0001$). The other study, by Randall et al., showed that among children whose soft palates were closed at 3 to 7 months of age fewer than one-third as many needed a subsequent posterior pharyngeal flap for velopharyngeal incompetence as those whose cleft palates were closed between 12 to 18 months of age ($p < 0.001$) [55]. A number of other studies have pointed out the *likely* advantages of early closure but with fewer hard data. For these reasons, we have preferred to close the soft palate at the early age of 3 to 9 months of age if the child is in good condition and *has not had any airway problems.* Patients with the Robin sequence, those with Treacher Collins syndrome, or those who have not been thriving are not operated at these early ages, and their repairs are postponed until they reach 12 to 14 months of age [54].

Often it is possible to close the soft palate at the time of the initial lip repair (3 to 4 months of age). If it is done, the hard palate cleft is left open to provide an additional airway, as swelling of the soft palate area can seriously impair the nasal airway and because we, like Davies [38], believe that closing the entire palate at one time when the child is this young constitutes considerably more surgery than doing just the lip and soft palate alone. In addition, when the lip and soft palate are repaired at the same time, one can expect to see marked narrowing of the hard palate cleft, so that closure of the hard palate as a secondary procedure 3 to 6 months later becomes much easier; in fact, if it is delayed too long, the cleft narrows so much that operation in such a confined area becomes difficult. In clefts of the palate only, the entire defect is closed at one stage.

With this approach, the speech mechanism is intact at an early age; moreover, the child has been described as eating better, speaking better, developing speech at an earlier age, being reunited into the family unit at a younger age, and having fewer middle ear problems. As previously noted, however, there are few hard data to confirm these reports.

Surgery at the younger ages is not particularly more difficult. The anesthesia must be superb. The tolerance for blood loss, prolonged surgery, borderline airway obstruction, and postoperative exhaustion is much less, so these patients must be handled carefully. Early soft palate closure is not an operation for the occasional or inexperienced surgeon without excellent anesthesia and postoperative support.

Malek et al. [49] suggested soft palate closure as the initial operation at 3 months of age followed within 2 to 3 months by primary lip and hard palate repair. The purpose is to bring the tongue forward as a restraining force behind the alveolar arches before achieving lip repair. This schedule is becoming popular in Europe, but we do not believe that a retro-placed tongue is often a problem; and if it is retro-placed, soft palate closure is indeed one way to bring it forward, although this technique is a risky way to manage the problem. In the long run, little difference will probably be proved between these two schedules.

DELAYED HARD PALATE CLOSURE
There has been renewed interest in the time schedule suggested by Schweckendeik and his father before him. Soft palate closure is carried out at the usual time, and hard palate closure is delayed until as late as 12 to 14

years of age. A dental obturator for the hard palate cleft is used. The purpose is to allow better growth of the bony tissue. Most surgeons following this schedule plan on hard palate closure at 6 to 7 years of age. However, careful studies have shown a high incidence of speech problems in these children. Even though Ross [122] and Olin and Spriesterbach [116] have shown slightly better facial bone growth in these children, the trade-off of poor speech hardly seems worthwhile [63, 70, 71, 73, 80, 99].

PRIMARY POSTERIOR
PHARYNGEAL FLAP

Stark and co-workers suggested during the 1960s that because at least 20 to 30 percent of cleft palate repairs are incompetent and need further surgery, why not do a posterior pharyngeal flap as part of the initial repair? They were pleased with the results of this "primary posterior pharyngeal flap," but hard data do not exist, to our knowledge, to confirm the benefits of this approach, though others have supported their aims [59, 60].

Should a primary palate repair be delayed for one reason or another until about 3 to 4 years of age, we usually expect a more difficult operation with a greater amount of blood loss than in infants, as well as a much poorer speech result. A primary posterior pharyngeal flap is usually used under these conditions. Now, with our preference of soft palate closure at a young age, the 12- to 18-month age group becomes "the older group" of children, and a primary posterior pharyngeal flap often is used with palate repair at this age. We were surprised that 48 percent of our patients in the 12- to 18-month age group eventually needed a posterior pharyngeal flap. One interpretation of this finding is that, in this group, nearly half of the children (closed at 12 to 18 months) would not obtain an adequate speech mechanism until the deficiency was recognized and treated. Often they were 3 to 5 years of age before a pharyngoplasty was done, and they would

then have good velopharyngeal competence. We already know that this great a delay leads to a high incidence of speech problems that are difficult to correct. For these reasons, we believe that the primary posterior pharyngeal flap should be considered in patients who are older than 12 months of age at the time of the palate repair, particularly if there is little soft palate tissue, little muscle, the cleft is particularly wide, or the anterior posterior dimension is short. A primary posterior pharyngeal flap is not considered if the patient has a Robin sequence, Treacher Collins syndrome, or failure to thrive.

We have carried out some of the primary posterior pharyngeal flap procedures at the early age of 3 to 6 months, but in two of six patients a severe amount of postoperative sleep apnea developed, and the flaps had to be taken down. Therefore we do not believe that a primary posterior pharyngeal flap should be considered with early soft palate closure [128].

There are two drawbacks to the primary pharyngeal flap. One is covered in the work of Subtelney and Nioto [145], who showed that with the attachment of a posterior pharyngeal flap there is some tendency to restriction of anterior growth of the maxilla. The other drawback was noted by Hamlen [131], who showed that the velopharyngeal closure achieved by patients with a posterior pharyngeal flap can be different from that achieved by the levator palati muscles without a flap.

Great variation is seen in the substance of the soft palate itself. Prior to surgery, some of these palates have a uvula that touches the posterior pharynx behind the adenoid pad; in others the uvula barely touches the posterior portion of the adenoids; in some it touches the anterior part of the adenoid pad; and in some it does not even reach the adenoid pad. We have arbitrarily called these uvulas types I, II, III, and IV, respectively, and note the length before and after surgery to see if a correlation with the eventual speech result can be determined. In some patients the cleft is narrow, whereas in others there is a huge horseshoe-shaped defect with little soft palate tissue. When dissecting out the levator muscles, as is described later, occasionally there is little muscle to be found on one or both sides. One would expect that the child who has a short palate with a wide defect in whom there is little levator muscle would have difficulty achieving good velopharyngeal closure with the usual cleft palate repair. Under these conditions, a primary posterior pharyngeal flap is considered.

Osada et al. [51] suggested another approach. They close the soft palate at 3 months of age, at the time of the lip repair, and leave the hard palate open for another 4 to 6 months. The infants are then examined nasendoscopically at monthly intervals. If the child is not able to achieve velopharyngeal closure by the time the hard palate is closed at age 7 to 9 months, a posterior pharyngeal flap is done at that time. We have used this approach in some patients (observing the soft palate directly at the time of hard palate repair rather than nasendoscopically), and indeed it may well be the best way to decide whether to construct an early posterior pharyngeal flap.

It should be noted that these primary posterior pharyngeal flaps do not need to be wide. About one-half to two-thirds of the posterior pharyngeal wall is used, and *under no circumstances is the "lateral port control" recommended at this young age* (discussed later). The danger of markedly obstructing the nasopharyngeal airway and producing serious sleep apnea and hyponasality or denasalized speech are too great to try to use a wide posterior pharyngeal flap with small lateral ports.

## Alveolar Arch Alignment

Much has been written about the advantages and disadvantages of moving the alveolar segments by dental plates before any surgery is started. This maneuver is referred to as or-
thopedics rather than orthodontics because at this age even the primary teeth may not have erupted and bony segments are moved. The steps can be done relatively easily and effectively and may help to provide a more even foundation on which to carry out the initial lip repair. If these segments are way out of line, as with the protruding premaxilla in the complete bilateral cleft, we prefer to do a lip adhesion or bilateral lip adhesion and to close the soft palate at the same time as the first step. The definitive lip repair and hard palate closure then is done 4 to 6 months later when the lip tissues have become soft. With a lip adhesion, good alignment of the alveolus is achieved in the most natural, gentle way; moreover, with a bilateral cleft the prolabium is stretched, providing ample tissue for a forked flap reconstruction of the columella if desired. Definitive closure of the lip then is done on what amounts to an incomplete cleft with minimal tension and good landmarks [107–110, 113].

Presurgical orthopedics has been claimed to be beneficial for a number of functions, such as feeding, facial growth, narrowing of the bony cleft, obturation of the cleft, and tongue position, as well as being satisfying to the parents. All but the last factor seem somewhat exaggerated. The "bottom line," however, is that in several series with good control the end results, so far as the *eventual occlusion in the permanent dentition* is concerned, show *no significant change or advantage*. For this reason, we seldom use this presurgical orthodontics or orthopedic control [112, 118]. There are still many proponents for manipulating these segments during early childhood. Hagerty has used a prosthesis that is held semipermanently in place with pins placed into the bone. Both Latham and Georgiade have more elaborate mechanisms for shifting alveolar bone. These steps may make the lip closure easier, but we believe that, if needed, the lip adhesion accomplishes the same purpose.

Furthermore, for severe bilateral clefts we

intentionally allow the lateral maxillary segments to slip medially behind the premaxilla, keeping the premaxilla forward and literally "locked out" of the upper dental arch. Others have preferred to expand the maxillary arches in bilateral clefts and to move the premaxilla back into the arch at an early age.

The biggest problem with growth and occlusion is seen in the older child. In older children with bilateral clefts, the premaxilla all too often is too far back instead of being anteriorly placed, as seen in the infant. The most frequently seen diminished growth in these children is in the anteroposterior direction, and often in later life one is constantly fighting a retruded premaxilla, a retruded middle third of the face, and a class III malocclusion. Many of these patients lack bony support to the nasal tip and even have hypoplastic malar bones. Follow-up evaluation of patients at 18 to 22 years of age who have had the premaxilla intentionally "locked out" of the upper dental arch in their early years have shown far better profiles, angles of convexity, and occlusion with less need for orthognathic surgical procedures than we have seen in the past. There can be difficult problems using this plan, however, such as an occasional anterior overjet. Also in a youngster age 5 or 6 the premaxilla may be excessively prominent, requiring some compromise in the overall plan [99, 114].

BONE GRAFTING
At present, we perform virtually no alevolar arch alignment in the infant or in the primary (deciduous) dentition. Orthodontia is begun with eruption of the permanent dentition, and the alveolar cleft is grafted with autogenous cancellous bone using gingival mucosal flaps for closure (at about 7 to 9 years of age). This approach has been worked out beautifully by the Norwegian teams and has produced the best reconstruction of the alveolar segment that we have seen. Without additional bone being placed in the alveolar cleft, the teeth adjacent to the cleft usually angle in toward the cleft instead of erupting in a vertical manner; there is poor bony coverage over the adjacent tooth roots, rendering them unstable so they are more likely to be lost; and there is no way that a displaced tooth can erupt into the empty space without a bone graft being placed there first. With bone replacement and gingival coverage, on the other hand, most of these unsatisfactory conditions are avoided. If a tooth needs to be replaced prosthetically, it can be bonded to the adjacent teeth using a "Maryland bridge." The prosthetic tooth rests on alveolar gingiva, which is much more natural in appearance and position than a cleft that is closed with buccal mucosa, and the bonded appliance is much less cumbersome than the usual denture. The adjacent teeth, however, must be stable [101–106, 115].

Bone grafting of these alveolar segments during infancy at the time of the initial lip repair did have a period of popularity, but because of evidence that this step restricted alveolar growth rather than helping it has led most surgeons to discard this approach [111, 117, 119, 120, 123–126]. However, two series of well studied patients—that of Nylen and Nordin at the Karolinska Institute in Stockholm and that of Rosenstein and Kernahan at the Children's Memorial Hospital in Chicago, stand out as achieving good results with excellent occlusion and alveolar ridge reconstruction when the surgery is done during infancy. The explanation may simply be the use of more careful techniques and follow-up [115, 121].

We are presently using some gingival flaps for alveolar reconstruction during infancy at the time of lip repair (but without bone grafts). It is done, however, only if it can be accomplished easily and in conjunction with mucosal closure of the nasal floor. These patients have not been followed long. Extensive surgery on the gingiva in infants risks damage to tooth buds located just below the anterior maxillary wall.

## *Preoperative Considerations*
### GENERAL CONDITION

Any elective surgical procedure is postponed if the child is not in good health and free from acute respiratory infection. With an open cleft palate, however, it is virtually impossible in some patients to be completely free from tenacious mucus or even mucopurulent material in the nasopharynx. Unless an acute inflammatory process is found, these conditions have not led to operative complications. As mentioned previously, pathologic changes in the middle ear are usual. Preoperative antibiotics may be indicated in the rare individual who continues to run a low grade fever despite repeated attempts to avoid infections [43].

A complete blood count, prothrombin time, partial thromboplastin time, and urinalysis are done routinely. Routine cultures of the nasopharynx are not carried out. In particularly difficult cases, older children, and adults, a crossmatch is done in preparation for a possible blood transfusion.

### ANESTHESIA

Excellent, well monitored oral endotracheal anesthesia is a joy to the surgeon. Monitoring includes electrocardiogram, pulse oximetry, expired carbon dioxide assay (capnography), blood pressure measurement, and airway dynamics. An oral Rae (preformed tracheal tube; NCC Division, Mallinckrodt, Argyle, NY) endotracheal tube is taped to the midline of the chin.

If an experienced anesthesiologist is not available, anesthesia can be administered by insufflation, with a heavy silk suture to hold the tongue forward and constant vigilance to keep the airway clear. The latter is a poor second choice but is preferable to inexpert handling of an endotracheal tube.

## *Operative Considerations*
### EQUIPMENT

The child is positioned at the end of the table with hyperextension of the neck. This extended position is aided by taking the foot mattress off the usual operating-room table and placing it under the trunk and shoulders.

Intravenous fluids are administered routinely during surgery with an attempt to supply about half of the daily feeding requirement while the patient is asleep. A proper mouth gag, such as the Dingman gag, is essential. It should provide a wide opening of the mouth, fixation of the endotracheal tube, and retraction of the corners of the mouth. Suction is essential but is used sparingly. An instrument table, placed several inches over the chest, allows ready access to a variety of instruments and permits the anesthesiologist to reach the anesthetic apparatus.

The surgical instruments include a variety of knife blades, such as the Bard-Parker No. 15 blade for making incisions, the No. 11 blade for excising cleft margins, and the No. 12 blade for reaching out-of-the-way places. The long knife handle is useful. Large and small scissors must be available. Forceps for handling tissues should have teeth, such as those found on the Adson forceps and on the Brown-Adson forceps, toothed arterial forceps, and the toothed bayonet forceps. Dural hooks are used for retraction. We use a Freer septal elevator, a Joseph nasal elevator, the flat palate elevator, the right-angle palate elevator, and the L-shaped palate elevator (Blair elevators).

A small dental "spoon" is helpful as a periosteal elevator in difficult-to-reach areas. Small chisels and a small bone drill are needed occasionally. A small right-angle knife (Cronin) [36, 37] and a septal knife are useful for obtaining mucosal flaps from the floor of the nostril; a small Webster needle holder is used, and a needle holder (Randall-Brown) with a hole in the jaws to allow end-on positioning of the needle is helpful for suturing in the posterior pharynx.

### PALATE CLOSURE

Soft palate closure used to be achieved by simple side-to-side suturing across the cleft with suitable relaxing incisions to relieve tension on the suture line. Accurate approximation of the muscular layer was considered important, and it implied complete release of the muscles from their attachment to the posterior edge of the bony palate [50]. Wide mucoperiosteal flaps were elevated off the hard palate, again with relaxing incisions.

Good results had been achieved with this von Langenbeck repair, but then steps were suggested which essentially used the flaps of mucoperiosteum from the hard palate to achieve an increase in the anteroposterior length of the hard and soft palates. Various V-Y advancements and transposition flaps known as the Veau flap, Kilner flap, and Wardill flap were added. Most of these flaps left significant denuded areas of membranous bone in the hard palate; although these surfaces can be expected to granulate and to epithelialize quickly, they do constitute areas of scar and usually cause some or considerable disturbance in bone growth and distortion in dental occlusion. In 1969 Kriens suggested an "intravelar veloplasty" operation to reorient and reconstruct the levator muscles. He preferred an end-on position of the redirected muscles; we prefer an overlap position for a tighter levator "sling" [47]. The addition of muscle reconstruction in our patients produced some improvement in function [35].

## FURLOW OPERATION

In 1978 Furlow [42] suggested an operation that achieved realignment of the misplaced levator muscles with reconstruction of a levator "sling" (Fig. 10-4). The operation uses two z-plasties: one from the oral mucosa and one oriented in the reverse direction from the nasal mucosa of the soft palate. The posteriorly based flap in each z-plasty also contains the levator muscle on that side. Lengthening is achieved within the soft palate, and realignment of the levator muscles is accomplished. Furthermore, this procedure has made it unnecessary to raise and shift large mucoperiosteal flaps from the

hard palate. Although it is a relatively new operation, it now is our procedure of choice and appears to achieve better results than we obtained before. To date, more than 165 cases have been completed with better speech and less need for subsequent pharyngoplasties than any other operation we have used [56].

The basic principle of the z-plasty is to achieve length at the expense of width. Note that when these flaps are oriented along the palatal cleft the posteriorly based limb of the z-plasty lies directly on top of the displaced levator muscle so that this muscle is included in the posteriorly based mucosal flap on one side. The anteriorly based flap from the opposite side contains just mucosa. When the limbs of the z-plasty are brought into position, the levator muscle is brought into a transverse orientation. A similar z-plasty is carried out on the nasal mucosa but in the reverse direction so that the posteriorly based flap is on the opposite side and includes the levator muscle from that side.

There are a number of fairly important details. The operation sacrifices width for length; however, in a wide cleft there may be little excess width. Ordinarily, the tendency is to use a larger z-plasty flap for a wider defect, but in this situation a smaller flap must be used or there is insufficient tissue. Furlow did not find this point to be a problem.

The levator muscle extends well beyond the limits of the mucosal flap and can be included in its entirety. The incision for the anteriorly based mucosal flap is not cut at the classic 60 degrees but closer to 80 degrees to bring the muscle flap into a more transverse position and to reduce the likelihood of the muscle becoming adherent to the posterior edge of the palatal bone on the opposite side. Although Furlow does not use lateral relaxing incisions, we do not hesitate to use them if the closure would otherwise be unduly tight. The area most likely to be short of tissue is the anteriorly based nasal mucosal flap. When raising this flap, its size can be augmented by including tissue along

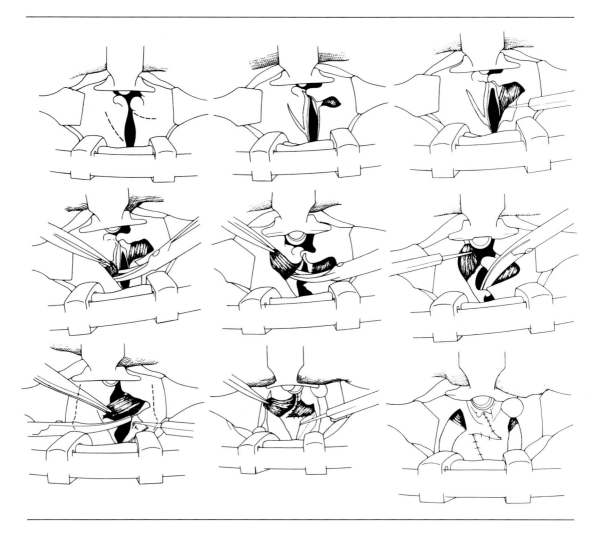

the edge of the cleft at the base of the uvula. This additional length to the anteriorly based flap can be obtained on the oral side as well. A primary posterior pharyngeal flap can be included, if desired, by raising turn-over flaps of nasal mucosa based along the posterior edge of the soft palate in the tissue between the edge of the palate and the muscular closure.

## HARD PALATE CLOSURE
Hard palate closure is achieved with a vomer flap (Fig. 10-5). Because the palatal shelves are usually directed more vertically than in

**Figure 10-4** *Furlow double-reversing Z-plasty. The levator muscle is included in the posteriorly based flap of the z-plasty. The z-plasty in the nasal mucosa is reversed so the posteriorly based flap is on the opposite side and includes the levator muscle from that side. The hard palate cleft is closed with a vomer flap that can be closed in one or two layers. Relaxing incisions can be made if needed. This maneuver achieves a lengthening step within the soft palate so large mucoperiosteal flaps do not need to be elevated from the hard palate. The muscles are reoriented in an overlapped position, which should enhance their function and add thickness to the soft palate. (From P. Randall, et al. Experience with the Furlow double reversing z-plasty for cleft palate repair. Plast. Reconstr. Surg. 77:569, 1986.)*

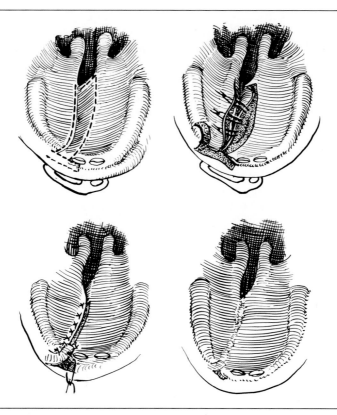

***Figure 10-5*** *Closure of the alveolar cleft and hard palate cleft by means of a flap of mucosa from the buccal sulcus and another from the vomer. These are interdigitated. The oral side of the vomer flap must granulate and epithelialize. This operation can be done at the time of lip closure or at the time of soft palate closure, or it can be delayed until the child is older, obturating the cleft with a dental "shell" or prosthesis.*

the uncleft palate, with minimal undermining at the cleft margins, a two-layer closure can usually be done. It may be performed either at the same time as the soft palate repair or at a second stage.

Among the advantages of this operation are repositioning and reorientation of the levator muscles with reconstruction of the levator sling placing the muscles in the overlapped position. This overlap adds thickness to the soft palate at the level of the levator eminence. A lengthening procedure within

the soft palate makes it unnecessary to raise large mucoperiosteal flaps from the hard palate. By keeping the levator muscles in continuity with one mucosal surface, less dissection is carried around these muscles, which will reduce fibrosis, it is hoped. The palate is repaired with a zigzag scar in the midline, rather than a straight-line scar, which has less tendency to contract and to shorten. The operation can be done in conjunction with a posterior pharyngeal flap, if desired, and lends itself well to muscle reconstruction in submucosal clefts. It can be done as a secondary procedure in soft palates where the original operation did not include reorientation of the levator muscles and where a lengthening procedure would be desirable.

The fistula rate (all of them small) among 160 patients has been 23 percent. A possible disadvantage is more scar if dehiscence occurs (which we have not seen). A secondary posterior pharyngeal flap for velopharyngeal incompetence would be disruptive if the soft palate has to be split. We usually can insert a superiorly based postpharyngeal flap into the nasal side of the soft palate with a turnover nasal mucosal flap by everting the posterior edge of the soft palate or by incising only the most posterior portion of the soft palate. The tightening of the levator sling with the overlapped position may increase the incidence of posterior dental crossbite, but it has not been a problem as yet.

OPERATIVE TECHNIQUE

After intubation and prior to preparing the skin with antiseptic solution, the anesthetist's laryngoscope is used and a 3- or 5-ml syringe with a 25-gauge spinal needle are employed to inject the operative area with 1% lidocaine and epinephrine 1:100,000. Small quantities are used to reduce the risk of inducing cardiac arrhythmias. In infants, epinephrine used in this way has had virtually no ill effects *so long as the $PCO_2$ is kept low.* Epinephrine has been safe even with halogenated anesthesia, though epinephrine 10 µg per kilogram or lidocaine 6 mg per kilogram is suggested as the maximum dose.

A note is made (as previously mentioned) about the position of the uvula in respect to the adenoid pad and posterior pharyngeal wall (type I, II, III, or IV). The same assessment is made at the end of surgery in an attempt to predict the functional outcome, though the bearing of these two assessments on the speech results has not yet been determined.

The edges of the cleft are incised followed by excision of the edges of the uvula to provide a broader surface for uvula reconstruction. Some surgeons prefer to excise all of the cleft margins, as they often seem to be cicatricial.

As noted by Furlow, a right-handed surgeon probably would want to place the posteriorly based oral mucomuscular flap on

the patient's left so the difficult dissection between this muscle and the nasal mucosa can be done more easily. The anteriorly based oral mucosal flap is fairly thick and is elevated first, dissecting down to the levator muscle and then continuing anteriorly at this level to the posterior edge of the palatine bone. Dissection is then continued forward between the mucoperiosteum of the hard palate and the underlying bone. A small dental "spoon" elevator helps in this dissection.

The same elevation is then continued between the mucoperiosteum and the maxilla on the left side; this dissection is then continued posteriorly to the insertion of the levator muscle into the posterior edge of the hard palate. The posteriorly based oral mucosal flap is incised down to muscle, and the small periosteal elevator is used to elevate the nasal mucosa off the maxilla on both sides. On the left side, by continuing this dissection of the nasal mucosa on posteriorly, past the posterior edge of the palatal bone, the insertion of the levator muscle to the palatal bone can be clearly identified, and it is cut across.

As noted above, the most difficult part of the dissection consists in developing a plane between the levator mucomuscular flap on the left side and the nasal mucosa. The flap is grasped gently by toothed bayonet forceps or arterial forceps, and the dissection is continued with either a No. 15 long-handled Bard-Parker scalpel or blunt scissors. Laterally, the muscle is separated from the adjacent tissue bluntly so as not to injure the innervation or blood supply. This dissection is carried well laterally along the muscle until it is conspicuously "free." The anteriorly based nasal mucosa flap is then developed using a back cut from the base of the uvula laterally to about the position of the eustachian tubes. The posteriorly based nasal mucomuscular flap on the right side then is dissected by detaching the attachment of the levator muscle to the palatine bone and cutting through the nasal mucosa, leaving an adequate rim of mucosa anteriorly for suturing. This cut also extends near the eustachian tubes.

At this point, an assessment is made as to whether lateral relaxing incisions are needed prior to closure. If so, they are made through the oral mucosa from just anterior to the anterior tonsillar pillar laterally to a point just lateral to the maxillary tubercle, then around the maxillary tubercle and forward on the hard palate for a short distance between the gingiva and the major palatine vessels. The pterygoid hamulus can be fractured medially with impunity if further relaxation is necessary [55]. The tissue deep to the relaxing incision is dissected bluntly. Dissection is carried around the major palatine vessels as they exit from the major palatine foramen using palatal elevators, and these vessels are gently stretched out of the foramen. If the hard palate is to be closed at the same time, a broad-based flap of mucosa is elevated from the vomer, with its base placed superiorly.

Closure is achieved using 4-0 chromic and 5-0 chromic catgut, though some surgeons prefer a more slowly absorbing suture. One point we believe to be important is that these sutures should not be tied tightly, as tightness leads to tissue necrosis and more scar. Several steps can be taken if the z-plasty flaps do not reach the apices of their intended incisions. The point of the flap can be left short of the intended position and the defect closed as a Y instead of a V. The lateral defect also simply can be left open and allowed to granulate and epithelialize, as there usually is good tissue covering the area. Additional adjacent mucosal flaps can be used if needed.

One or two sutures are placed between the two muscle flaps to obliterate any deadspace between them. The vomer flap is sutured well laterally on the nasal side of the opposite lateral mucoperiosteal flap, achieving an overlap with mattress sutures. Furlow has always been able to achieve a two-layer closure in the hard palate by dissecting the mu-coperiosteum off the maxilla for a short distance laterally. End-on mattress sutures are used to evert the edges. There is a potential deadspace between these two layers of closure, but it has not been a problem. We have not always been able to achieve a two-layer closure throughout the hard palate, but we believe the difference is not important so long as a good vomer flap is obtained. The most likely site of oronasal fistula is at the junction of the hard and soft palate closure, so great care must be used here to achieve accurate approximation.

BILATERAL CLEFTS

With bilateral clefts of the hard palate, we do not hesitate to use the mucosa from both sides of the vomer. As previously noted, closure in bilateral clefts at the level of the incisive foramen and further anteriorly in the alveolar cleft can be difficult. Often this area can be closed as part of the initial lip repair, gingival mucosal flaps being preferred in the alveolar cleft [41].

Jackson has noted that the oral mucosa is stretchable, so he does not hesitate to close the mucosa of the relaxing incisions a little at a time toward the end of the operation [45]. Some surgeons prefer to place packing in the relaxing incisions and on raw surfaces using *iodoform* gauze or *xeroform* gauze with either balsam of Peru or Whitehead's varnish. We usually do not use packing unless there is a persistent bleeding problem. Hemostasis at the end of the operation is critical; if necessary, all of the troublesome areas are reinjected with lidocaine and epinephrine. Suture ligatures, light electrocautery, or both also may be needed. A nasopharyngeal airway (18 to 22 French) is inserted, and a heavy (0 silk) tongue stitch may be placed deep in the tongue. This tongue suture is looped and taped loosely to the cheek so the tongue may be retracted manually if desired. The airway and tongue suture are usually removed in 24 hours but may be left in place longer if desired. Prophylactic use of antibiotics intraoperatively and for 48 hours postoperatively have reduced hospital stay and postoperative temperature elevation in our cases [48].

## Postoperative Care

Immediately postoperatively patients must be watched carefully for airway obstruction and bleeding. A semisitting position in bed is helpful; and parents are encouraged to hold their children, as they are frequently fussy and irritable. *Sedation must be used sparingly.* Codeine, 0.5 mg per kilogram, or meperidine hydrochloride, 0.75 mg per kilogram (Demerol; Winthrop Laboratories, New York, NY), is given infrequently on an individual dose basis as the need arises. Elbow splints are placed for restraint and are worn constantly for 3 weeks except when bathing. Sucking and blowing actions are avoided; and feedings are given by a cup, spoon, syringe with a pliable tube on the end, or plastic squeeze bottle with a Ross Nipple (Ross Laboratories, Columbus, OH).

Patients are usually returned to the surgical floor, though transfer to the surgical intensive care unit is indicated for some patients. A pulse oxygen saturation monitor has been an additional help. Postoperatively, clear liquid, milk, or formula is given by mouth in small amounts starting as soon as the child is responding well. After about 6 hours, any food that is liquid or mechanically soft (e.g., junket, custard, gelatin, ice cream, pureed food) is allowed. Intravenous fluids are continued as needed, and the patient usually is discharged from the hospital in 1 to 2 days postoperatively, when the temperature is within normal range and the oral intake is satisfactory.

The soft diet, elbow restraints, and avoidance of sucking and blowing actions are continued for 3 weeks after discharge. Food is offered by cup or syringe, though a spoon can be used if handled by an adult.

By 3 weeks after discharge the operative site is usually well healed, and most of the catgut sutures have disappeared so that the patient can be allowed to return to normal activity with no limitations on diet. At this point, it is stressed that the child should be brought up as normally as possible and that the parents must be particularly careful not to provide special restrictions or limitations unless they are necessary for other reasons.

Parents are urged to talk with their children and to begin speech stimulation. As the child grows, the use of picture books and magazines and the institution of gentle sucking and blowing exercises using whistles, mouth organs, soap bubble pipes, and drinking straws are carried out several times a day so long as they do not become tedious. *No attempt is made to correct speech errors* at this early age, but attention is directed toward developing a vocabulary and an outgoing, uninhibited personality, which can be a great help later if speech therapy is needed [59].

## Follow-Up Care

### RETURN VISITS

The patient is seen in 3 to 6 months and then at 6- to 12-month intervals unless more frequent visits are indicated. Careful attention is focused on the condition of the palate, appearance of the eardrums, hearing acuity, history of ear infections and leakage of liquids into the nose, condition and position of the teeth, and, most important, the development of speech. The coordinated efforts of a cleft palate team are particularly useful for following these patients while they grow.

### EAR PROBLEMS

Persistent middle ear effusions are frequent and can lead to hearing impairment, scarring, and permanent damage. The ears are examined, and audiometric testing is carried out regularly by the otolaryngologist. Examination with a pneumatic otoscope or tympanometry is helpful. The ear canals must be kept dry to avoid infection if ventilating tubes are in place. Children with chronic ear disease are checked frequently, particularly during the ages of increased respiratory tract infection. Audiometric examinations provide a further measure of middle ear disease. Conservative treatment is aimed at preventing permanent changes and requires close attention [33, 52, 61]. Removal of the tonsils and adenoids is advocated by some for repeated ear infection, yet the bulk of adenoid tissue can be important for adequate velopharyngeal competence, particularly if the soft palate is short and its excursion is limited by scar. For this reason, adenoidectomy is not done unless all other methods fail to prevent continued middle ear disease [57, 61, 92].

On the other hand, if the tonsils are huge, they can cause significant obstruction of the airway postoperatively. We do not hesitate to do a tonsillectomy (not an adenoidectomy) at the time of soft palate surgery or posterior pharyngeal flap under these conditions. Some prefer to do it as a separate procedure prior to the palatal or posterior pharyngeal flap surgery. Tonsillectomy does not alter velopharyngeal closure.

## Speech Problems
### VELOPHARYNGEAL INCOMPETENCE
Although the problems associated with cleft palate are many, the remaining remarks are concentrated on speech because, without question, it is the most important function to be considered. The surgeon interested in cleft palate surgery should develop a facility for handling children that encourages relaxed conversational speech at the time of their office follow-up visits. A gentle approach, a conversational tone with parents, the availability of children's picture books, or a school lunchbox filled with plastic toys can go a long way to bring out conversa-

tional speech in a young child. Unless the surgeon has this capability and can evaluate the results, the most important measure of his or her ability is missed as well as a considerable portion of the physician's own reward. The collaboration of a competent speech therapist or speech pathologist is needed for more detailed documentation of information and advice relative to therapy.

A high percentage of the patients develop "normal" speech without evidence of hypernasality, nasal emission, or articulation disorders due to the cleft palate. A hypernasal tone is usually one of the first indications of velopharyngeal incompetence. It is often accompanied by distortion of sibilant sounds in conversational speech and in simple test words and phrases [60, 62, 79, 91]. Direct observation reveals the length, flexibility, and excursion of the palate. If the patient can be induced to say *kah, kah,* a good view of the soft palate in motion can be obtained [74, 91]. The presence of scarring, dehiscence, or fistulas is noted, as is the excursion of the lateral pharyngeal wall and the presence or absence of Passavant's pad (a forward bulging of the posterior pharyngeal wall). Overactive use of the superior pharyngeal constrictor muscles usually indicates a soft palate that is not achieving full competence. Direct examinations, however, reveal little concerning the contour of the nasal side of the soft palate, the size of the adenoid tissue, and the ability of the levator palati muscles to approximate the two.

The simple use of fogging on a hand mirror held under the nose during speech, the blowing away of a piece of tissue placed under the nose, and the observation of "nasal grimacing" are of help when testing for nasal escape [60]. The ability to build up pressure and pronounce the letter *P* repeatedly with the use of a paper "paddle," as advocated by Bzoch, to demonstrate this ability or inability is helpful. Oral panendoscopy, pressure gauges, spirometer tests, sound spectrographic analyses, and instruments for measuring nasal airflow can also aid in the study of velopharyngeal closure, although children in the 2- to 4-year-old group usually cannot cooperate sufficiently for these tests. However, testing at this early age, in some way, is essential if velopharyngeal incompetence is to be diagnosed early [65, 66, 82, 83, 86, 88, 96, 97, 100].

Lateral static radiographs and cinefluorographic and video techniques do a far better job of demonstrating the presence or absence of velopharyngeal incompetence. These studies can show whether the patient is achieving velopharyngeal closure consistently, velopharyngeal closure occasionally, closure but only by virtue of an active superior pharyngeal constrictor muscle or by the help of a large volume of adenoid tissue, or no velopharyngeal closure at all [63, 64, 85, 98]. Skolnick described several anteroposterior views that are helpful for pointing out the level of the maximal lateral pharyngeal wall excursion [89]. We prefer the use of the Towne view, as it is more comfortable and yields reliable and reproducible results [76].

## NASENDOSCOPY

Nasendoscopy has provided a direct approach to visualizing the velopharyngeal port. It is difficult to do without cooperation; but with patience, gentleness, and topical anesthesia, it can be helpful. The instruments are small in caliber. Opinion varies as to the advantages of (1) the flexible tipped fiberoptic scope, which can literally be bent around so one can see down into the area of velopharyngeal closure, and (2) the fixed optic scope, which is inflexible and has a sharply angled objective and superior optical qualities [75, 82].

Sedation may be desired, though it is not usually necessary. Topical anesthesia is used, and the scope simply is slipped gently along the nostril floor. Observation during speech production demonstrates much in the way of excursion of the soft palate and pharyngeal wall, asymmetry, leakage, adequacy of closure, patterns of closure, or lack of closure.

## CLASSIFICATION OF VELOPHARYNGEAL COMPETENCE

It has been helpful to classify the palatal function after surgery into four broad categories.

I. *Velopharyngeal competence:* The soft palate is competent in every way.
II. *Partial or inconsistent competence:* The child may be able to achieve closure at some times but not at other times.
III. *Velopharyngeal incompetence:* Little or no evidence of velopharyngeal competence is present.
IV. *Indeterminate competence:* Speech samples and examination are insufficient for further classification.

The child with good velopharyngeal closure does not need to be examined as frequently or as extensively as the child with any degree of incompetence because this child rarely loses good function. Occasionally, with deepening of the nasopharynx and atrophy of the adenoid tissue, the child slips into velopharyngeal incompetence, but it does not happen often. At the other extreme, the child with severe incompetence, there is little reason to attempt even a trial period of speech therapy; and indeed extensive testing and verification are hardly justified if incompetence is clear-cut. A great deal can be gained in such a child by providing a competent palatal mechanism at the earliest possible age.

The good, crisp, accurate speech of a competent speech mechanism being well used is a joy to behold. On the other hand, the patient in whom velopharyngeal competence can be demonstrated but speech distortions are present that are due to incompetence should be given speech therapy to see if he or she can be taught to use the palate properly. If closure is borderline and speech is good to excellent, further surgery is difficult to justify; however, the patient is watched carefully, as deterioration can occur as the child grows.

As experience is gained with examination techniques, it becomes evident that two postoperative conditions are especially common: (1) Velopharyngeal closure can be achieved but barely so; this technique might be called "touch closure," with the soft palate barely touching the posterior pharyngeal wall. (2) Velopharyngeal closure can be achieved but only by excessive use of the superior pharyngeal constrictor muscles (seen on lateral radiographs as obliteration of the air shadow with the nasal side of the soft palate 2 to 3 mm from the posterior pharyngeal wall or by definite forward movement of the posterior pharyngeal wall). These children must be studied carefully to determine the best form of treatment. Fortunately, if speech is poor but some degree of velopharyngeal competence is achieved, such a patient usually is a good candidate for a secondary surgical procedure because little has to be done to this palate to render it competent. Furthermore, though intensive speech therapy may improve the quality of speech, it is unusual for speech therapy to overcome the incompetence completely, particularly if hypernasality is a major problem.

As mentioned previously, these conditions tend to get worse as the child grows; the paranasal sinuses and nasal chambers enlarge, and the nasopharynx deepens. We try to make the diagnosis of velopharyngeal incompetence at an early age if possible. Our preference for handling such a problem, at the present time, is a superiorly based posterior pharyngeal flap. A number of other surgical pharyngoplasties are preferred by others: Some clinics prefer to use a palatal lift prosthesis under these circumstances, and others fabricate a dental plate with an obturator to fit behind the soft palate. This obturator can be diminished gradually in size as function improves [58, 65, 78, 87]. Others prefer one of several varieties of biofeedback with or without electrical stimulation [86, 88]. The latter procedures require a fairly intelligent, mature patient for execution. With our stress on correction of in-

competence at an early age, these other approaches are not always usable. However, it is clear that a high percentage of success can be expected with a variety of pharyngoplasties and other methods of handling this problem of borderline incompetence; indeed it is difficult to determine if one method is significantly better than another.

Furthermore, it seems justified to be critical of the speech in these patients when studies demonstrate only borderline velopharyngeal closure. The reason is that, even though speech distortions are slight, a secondary surgical procedure usually has brought the level of speech well within the normal range in such cases. In addition, it has allowed these children to articulate with so much less effort that the patient frequently becomes appreciably more relaxed and happier as a result. As mentioned above, if not corrected these problems have a general tendency to become worse; or the patient may be able to speak well on testing and concentration but loses his or her "good speech" when speaking rapidly or when relaxed or fatigued. Some patients may even complain that the throat hurts after speaking for a period of time. Hoarseness and vocal cord nodules may occur under these conditions and may indicate a borderline or partial incompetence compensated for by straining at the laryngeal level [83].

Velopharyngeal incompetence is seen in a number of conditions in the absence of clefts of the palate. It may be the result of a congenitally short palate, deficiencies of neuromuscular control, a congenitally deep nasopharynx (often associated with cervical spine anomalies), and deficiencies due to ablative surgery and trauma [4, 84, 93]. Many of the tests for palatal incompetence and the techniques for correcting incompetence are applicable to these patients. In most patients, if marked incompetence is present, it can be demonstrated by the age of 2 to 5 years [85]. The handling of these problems may vary greatly. A short palate with good motion in it might simply have to be lengthened, or a surgical procedure might have to be carried out to bring the posterior pharyngeal wall forward (though these methods have met with limited success). If there is little motion in the soft palate, the superior pharyngeal constrictors must be used for valving, which can be improved with a wide posterior pharyngeal flap or with a dental plate and an obturating prosthesis. These patients also may be good candidates for initial prosthetic treatment by obturating the velopharynx, producing stimulation and activity in the lateral and posterior pharyngeal walls and then replacing the obturator with a posterior pharyngeal flap after stimulating the superior pharyngeal constrictor action. Velopharyngeal incompetence due to neuromuscular deficiencies can often be improved with a pharyngoplasty or a palatal lift prosthesis or obturator, but if there are problems in the speech mechanism in addition to the soft palate, complete correction of the speech problem is often impossible.

## *Secondary Palatal Procedures*
### PALATAL FISTULAS
Palatal fistulas are bothersome because they permit leakage of fluid into the nose, packing of food particles into crevices producing uncleanliness, and leakage of air into the nose causing articulation distortions, particularly with the sibilant sounds or even hypernasality. These speech distortions are usually not great. It has been shown that in the presence of a significant anterior oronasal fistula the soft palate does not have as much excursion as when the fistula is covered or obturated.

Closing a palatal fistula can be among the most difficult of all surgical techniques. Each failure and the scarring it produces makes additional attempts more difficult. In general, the tissue adjacent to a palatal fistula, particularly in the region of the hard palate, is not elastic. Closure must be achieved with complete excision of the epithelium of the fistula. Occasionally, this tissue is used as turnover flaps to aid in the closure. Complete relaxation of the adjacent

tissue is absolutely necessary, so that closure can be achieved without tension and preferably with the use of a fine surgical suture (e.g., 4-0 or 5-0 chromic catgut). In the region of the hard palate, it usually requires raising a surprisingly large adjacent pedicle flap and freeing it to the extent that it can literally fall or drop into place without tension. During the dissection, care must be taken to preserve the blood supply because it is usually limited at best. Sutures must not be tied tightly so as to avoid strangulation and necrosis of tissue. Occasionally in the soft palate area, relaxation incisions are needed. Closure in two layers is preferred if possible, but it is not always necessary or feasible. The closure of palatal fistulas is a good example of a big operation being needed for a small defect.

A two-layer closure in the area of the alveolus or anterior hard palate almost automatically means that, because of the presence of bone, there is a deadspace between these two layers of closure. This situation has led to a high degree of failure in these repairs and recurrence of the fistula. With the advent of alveolar reconstruction using gingival flaps and autogenous bone (see subsequent section), the incidence of failure in closing these fistulas has decreased markedly. Furthermore, a watertight closure over the bone grafts does not seem to be essential. Gingival flaps provide much more satisfactory closure in the alveolus, as is explained later. The use of bone and hydroxyapatite in the closure of fistulas in the hard palate has greatly improved the success of this operation. Hydroxyapatite may also be useful, but sufficient data have not accumulated to substantiate its being interchangeable with bone.

### TREATMENT OF VELOPHARYNGEAL INCOMPETENCE
In the United States and Canada today, the superiorly based posterior pharyngeal flap is probably the most widely used pharyngoplasty for the treatment of velopharyngeal incompetence. We have used this technique

extensively. It is a simple, direct, effective approach to this frequent problem, and it is described in detail here. This operation is not without failures or problems, however, and for that reason several other techniques also are mentioned. It has been almost impossible to compare these approaches, as they all seem to be associated with an appreciable measure of success and few failures [130, 139, 142].

The posterior pharyngeal flap probably improves palatal incompetence in several ways. As a static space-occupying tissue, it has an obturating effect and allows the medial movement of the lateral pharyngeal walls to be more effective. It tends to pull the soft palate posteriorly and adds bulk to the central part of the soft palate.

The superiorly based posterior pharyngeal flap can be raised with sufficient length to reach even the shortest soft palate; and with its base being located near the usual site of velopharyngeal closure, it has a natural tendency to shrink and to pull the soft palate in the direction of the adenoid pad. Initially, we reopened the soft palate to develop adequate turnover flaps from the nasal side of the soft palate for lining and to achieve a "high" insertion of the posterior pharyngeal flap onto the soft palate. This technique is sometimes necessary, but most of the time we simply evert the posterior edge of the soft palate forward into the mouth. Then, using a curved scalpel (No. 12 Bard-Parker), we elevate the turnover flaps from the nasal side of the soft palate, inserting the posterior pharyngeal flap into the posterior one-half to one-third of the palate. Lining on the bottom of the posterior pharyngeal flap is provided by the turnover flap of nasal mucosa.

*Superiorly Based Versus Inferiorly Based Posterior Pharyngeal Flap*

The superiorly based posterior pharyngeal flap is based fairly high in the posterior pharynx just below the adenoid tissue. At this level there may be less superior pharyngeal constrictor motion than more inferiorly in the pharynx. If the flap does not function adequately, one may want to make the lateral pharyngeal openings on either side of the posterior pharyngeal flap somewhat larger or smaller. It is more difficult to reach these openings in the superiorly based posterior pharyngeal flap than in the inferiorly based flap [142, 148, 149].

The inferiorly based posterior pharyngeal flap is constructed more easily than the superiorly based flap. It also has certain other advantages: (1) It acts somewhat as a sounding board to direct the airstream into the mouth; (2) it may well be located at a level where there is a greater amount of lateral pharyngeal wall motion; (3) its construction does not require reopening the soft palate; and (4) it lends itself well to secondary procedures that may be needed to make the lateral openings larger or smaller [58, 148].

Much attention has been directed toward reconstructing the posterior pharyngeal flap as a "tailor made" flap in terms of size [143] and location, depending on the findings in the particular patient. It is our belief that the surgeon does not have nearly so much control over the eventual size of the flap, the size of the lateral ports, the amount of shrinkage, or the level at which the base of the flap ends up as one would hope, despite what is planned. Usually the base of the superiorly based flap contracts inferiorly, and the inferiorly based flap tends to contract superiorly. As a result, each may end up at about the same location so that, except for the presence or absence of the uvula, it may be difficult to determine whether a given flap is superiorly based or inferiorly based [148]. Some inferiorly based flaps are indeed low and seem to have a marked tethering effect on the excursion of the soft palate. This situation can be improved simply by moving the base more superiorly. We, as surgeons, have little control over the healing forces that cause these changes.

Retrospective studies by Skoog [144] and Hamlen [131] and a prospective study by Whitaker and co-workers [148] have failed to show appreciable differences between the results obtained with the superiorly and inferiorly based flaps. Accordingly, we usually prefer the superiorly based flap; but if exposure is difficult, the patient is in poor condition, or the palate is so mobile that one is reluctant to make a through-and-through incision in the soft palate, we use the inferiorly based posterior pharyngeal flap. On the other hand, if the space to be bridged is great, a superiorly based flap must be used, or the palate would have to be lengthened at the same operation. If the radiographic examination described by Skolnick shows the maximal lateral pharyngeal wall motion to be "high" rather than "low," the superiorly based flap theoretically is better, and vice versa. If the amount of incompetence is slight but there is good palatal movement, in all likelihood *any method* of secondary palatal correction would produce a good result [142, 148, 149].

### Superiorly Based Posterior Pharyngeal Flap Operation

Because the superiorly based posterior pharyngeal flap operation is the pharyngoplasty that we and most surgeons prefer, it is described here in detail. The technique for the posterior pharyngeal flap requires endotracheal anesthesia, a good mouth gag, and a local infiltration with 1% lidocaine with epinephrine 1:100,000. If a wide flap is desired, an incision is made longitudinally through the mucosa and muscle on each side of the posterior pharyngeal wall at its junction with the lateral pharyngeal wall, elevating the entire width of the posterior pharynx (Fig. 10-6). If little is needed to overcome the velopharyngeal incompetence, a smaller flap can be used, consisting of only one-half to three-fourths of the posterior pharyngeal flap wall. When the flap is used as a primary posterior pharyngeal flap in conjunction with primary closure of the cleft palate, the narrower flap is used. Each incision is carried down through the pharyngeal constrictor muscle to the prevertebral fascia by sharp and blunt scissor dissection. Dissection is then carried medially along the prev-

ertebral fascia, by either curved scissors or a palate elevator, until the dissection from the opposite side is reached, thus raising a flap of mucosa and the superior pharyngeal constrictor muscle. If the flap is to be based superiorly, it is cut across transversely inferiorly. If it is to be based inferiorly, the palate is retracted and the flap cut across just below the adenoid pad. Note that the internal carotid artery lies just lateral to this incision; rarely a sizable aberrant artery or tortuous carotid artery is located between the superior constrictor muscle and the prevertebral fascia. This unusual finding can be seen as an abnormal pulsation in the posterior pharyngeal wall. If seen, the posterior pharyngeal flap procedure probably should not be done.

Disposable suction cautery is useful for obtaining good hemostasis in this area. The lateral margins of the donor area are approximated with interrupted 3-0 chromic catgut; if this approximation tends to pull the edges away from the prevertebral fascia, the sutures can include prevertebral fascia to obliterate this deadspace. A needle holder with a hole in the jaws to allow an "end-on position of the needle" (Randall-Brown needle holder; Storz Instrument Company, St. Louis, MO) can be helpful. Some surgeons prefer to leave the donor site open.

As previously noted, the soft palate usually is relaxed enough that it can be everted sufficiently to allow elevation of turnover lining flaps from the nasal mucosa without reopening the midline repair. Sometimes the midline incision of the soft palate must be reopened and nasal mucosal flaps elevated on either side to line the underside of the posterior pharyngeal flap. Closure is achieved using a through-and-through 3-0 chromic catgut suture at each corner and a third suture through the center of the pharyngeal flap. The edges of the flap are sutured to the edges of the recipient site with simple 3-0 chromic catgut. The turnover lining flaps of the nasal mucosa are held in place with 4-0 chromic catgut. If the midline palate incision had to be reopened, it

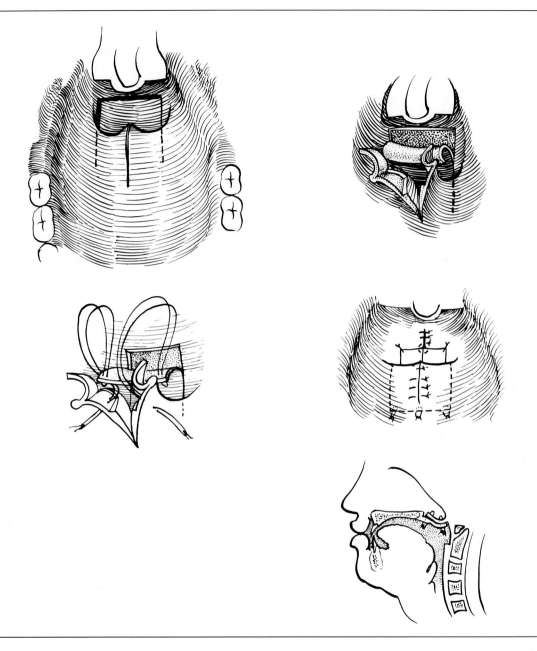

**Figure 10-6** *A superiorly based posterior pharyngeal flap. The lateral incisions in the posterior pharyngeal wall are at the junction of the posterior and lateral walls (unless a narrower flap is needed, as in a primary posterior pharyngeal flap done at the time of initial palate repair). They are carried down to the prevertebral fascia, and the flap is elevated to include the superior pharyngeal constrictor muscle. The soft palate may have to be reopened with a longitudinal incision to develop a lining flap from the nasal side of the soft palate with its base at the free edge of the palate.*

is closed in layers with 4-0 or 5-0 chromic catgut. This posterior pharyngeal flap can survive even when sutured under a slight amount of tension. Most authors seem to favor placing the superiorly based flap in the "high" position close to the posterior edge of the hard palate, which we believe is not necessary; we prefer to suture it into the muscular part of the soft palate rather than at the free edge of the palate, as others suggest.

### Lateral Port Control

Hogan [132] popularized the "lateral port control" operation where he put a 16 French catheter on either side of the superiorly based posterior pharyngeal flap. He sutured the closure down around this catheter to "control" the size of the lateral ports. The purpose is to provide a cross-sectional airspace, which is still compatible with velopharyngeal competence. (Warren and Dalston had noted that, even with as much as a 10 mm$^2$ persistent opening, effective velopharyngeal valving was achieved [147].) We believe that this criterion is misleading and, to some degree, risky. The importance of the 10 mm$^2$ noted by Warren and Dalston [147] does not refer to the measurement in an anesthetized patient with the sutures tightening the mucosa around the catheter; rather, it refers to the maximum amount of closure in an awake patient who is trying to achieve active velopharyngeal closure—a different situation entirely. Furthermore, we do not believe that suturing the mucosa around a rubber catheter in any way ensures what the size of this opening will be after healing has taken place. More important, it is our thought that lateral port control is likely to overobturate the nasopharynx, producing an excessive amount of obstruction, hyponasality, and an inadequate nasal airway. Postoperatively, sleep apnea has been reported by Levine et al. [138] in every patient on whom they carried out this procedure. The 16-gauge catheters are insufficient for an adequate nasopharyngeal airway, and a dangerous amount of airway obstruction can result.

Occasionally, in the older patient who is severely incompetent, one indeed must create a posterior pharyngeal flap that is wide with small lateral ports, literally aiming to *overcorrect* the problem. Even so, it may be necessary to come back later and make the lateral ports larger. In our experience, the latter has been the exceptional, rather than the usual, case.

### Trauner Operation

In patients with severely scarred posterior pharyngeal walls and those whose palates are long, the Trauner procedure has been helpful. Here, the soft palate is displaced posteriorly until it touches the posterior pharyngeal wall. At this point, a transverse incision is made in both opposing surfaces, and the soft palate is fixed to the posterior pharyngeal wall with through-and-through sutures [146].

### Other Operations for Velopharyngeal Incompetence

PALATAL LENGTHENING. Various lengthening operations, when used alone, have been disappointing for overcoming velopharyngeal incompetence. A lengthening procedure combined with repositioning and reconstruction of the levator muscles has gained popularity in the United States and may be worthwhile if these steps were not taken at the time of the initial palate repair and if only a small amount of improved function is needed. A lengthening operation combined with a posterior pharyngeal flap is a good alternative.

POSTERIOR PHARYNGEAL AUGMENTATION. Insertion of retropharyngeal implants using various kinds of material to build the posterior pharyngeal wall forward is another approach to the problem of velopharyngeal incompetence. This technique is particularly valuable when the incompetence is small (2 to 3 mm gap on lateral radiographs) and the excursion of the soft palate is good. Shredded

Teflon [57] in glycerine seems to be the most reliable material so far as extrusion of the implant is concerned, but these patients must be selected carefully and this material loses about 50 percent of its initial volume after absorption of the glycerin. *It is no longer approved for use in the United States.* Autogenous tissues, such as cartilage and muscle flaps, have been suggested but with little follow-up. The implant of a Silastic pillow or cushion as suggested by Brauer [129] may hold some promise, but none of these techniques has provided a panacea. Good palatal motion and a small amount of deficiency remain key criteria for these approaches.

LATERAL PHARYNGEAL FLAPS. Laterally based posterior pharyngeal flaps, as described by Kapetansky [137], appear to preserve more of the superior pharyngeal constrictor muscle in the flaps than other designs, but his technique requires separation of the levator muscles at the site of inset of the flaps into the soft palate, and that step appears to be detrimental to soft palate motion. Approximation of the posterior tonsillar pillars apparently provides significant speech improvement but does not seem to improve function at the level of the levator muscle.

ORTICOCHEA PHARYNGOPLASTY. Orticochea has popularized a technique using the palatopharyngeus muscle located within the posterior tonsillar pillars. Fortunately, the blood and nerve supplies allow these structures to be based medially, so the lateral inferior portions of the flaps can be brought around to the posterior pharyngeal wall and sutured either into a posterior pharyngeal flap or as a shelf all the way around the pharyngeal wall, somewhat similar to the old Hynes pharyngoplasty. This method has achieved considerable popularity because of the ability of this tissue to contract and literally provide another "sphincter." However, it appears that only about one-third of these flaps ever do contract, and a high percentage of Ortichochea's patients have had persistent hypernasality postoperatively [133–136, 140, 141].

*Postoperative Care After Operation for Velopharyngeal Incompetence*
Postoperatively, these patients are handled in much the same way as those who had had primary cleft palate repair. Antibiotics have reduced postoperative fever and hospital stay [48]. If healing progresses rapidly, the time schedule is accelerated. A nasopharyngeal airway (18 to 24 French), a tongue stitch, or both are particularly useful in these patients, especially if the patient is young. These patients must be handled just as carefully in terms of postoperative airway obstruction and bleeding as those with primary palate repair. Similarly, sedation must be carefully administered.

Three steps are suggested to ensure an adequate airway postoperatively. If a child is small, the mandible is short, or bleeding has been a problem, it is particularly important to use a nasopharyngeal airway, either at the time the posterior pharyngeal flap is sutured into place or at the end of the operation. If difficulty is encountered passing such a tube, a small tube may be passed first and used as a guide. It can even be placed in a retrograde manner if need be. Second, a tongue suture of heavy (0 or 1) silk can be placed. A deep bite is taken far back in the tongue, a big loop tied, and the ends taped loosely to the cheek. If it is necessary to retract the tongue, it must be held by hand. Taping it in the retracted position is not a reliable method. Finally, if the tonsils are huge, we do not hesitate removing them at the beginning of the operation because otherwise the nasopharyngeal space will be severely compromised and a dangerous amount of airway obstruction can occur. Some prefer to do the tonsillectomy as a separate operation before the posterior pharyngeal flap surgery. As previously noted, the adenoids are not removed.

BLEEDING. Bleeding after the primary or the secondary palatal repair can be a major problem, and possible bleeding idiosyncrasies must be ruled out preoperatively. If bleeding is noted at the end of the operation, the area is reinjected with lidocaine and epinephrine; alternatively, suture ligatures are used. Pressure is held on the area for 4 to 5 minutes (by the clock) and then the area watched for 3 to 4 minutes to be sure the bleeding does not begin again. Unfortunately, it is difficult to determine postoperatively how much blood the child is losing because it is generally swallowed. If there is much bleeding, the child usually vomits clotted blood. These children are not routinely crossmatched for blood transfusions at the time of surgery, but if bleeding is found to be a problem postoperatively, crossmatching is done without delay.

Under direct vision, an area of bleeding often can be seen with a good headlight, tongue blade, and suction. During the early postoperative period, it usually can be handled simply by reinjecting the area with lidocaine and epinephrine. A 25-gauge spinal needle is helpful for this maneuver; the tongue suture and occasionally a laryngoscope also can help achieve exposure. If these measures fail, suture or cauterization under local anesthesia is occasionally done; otherwise, the child is taken back to the operating room, general anesthesia administered, and complete hemostasis obtained.

SPEECH AFTER SECONDARY PHARYNGOPLASTY. Some patients achieve immediate and lasting "normal" speech, whereas a few show only slight improvement. Hypernasality is almost always diminished or obliterated. Some patients have shown initial improvement, apparently due to postoperative swelling and blood clot formation, which is then followed by degeneration almost to the preoperative level. These patients may continue to have poor speech until the operative area becomes comfortable and the tissues soft and pliable. When the patient becomes aware of how to use this newly constructed mechanism, gradual and steady improvement in speech may be expected. Speech therapy can be helpful with these patients and is begun 6 to 12 weeks postoperatively to help the child adjust to the new mechanism as it heals, softens, and matures.

Many older patients, however, have been so accustomed to hearing their voices with hypernasal characteristics and articulatory distortions that speech produced in a non-nasal manner, with good, crisp articulation, sounds distinctly abnormal to them. Under these conditions, it is difficult to teach the patient to speak normally even though he or she may possess the mechanisms to do so. The "overcorrection" of the problem with a wide posterior pharyngeal flap and small lateral ports, described by Hogan as "lateral port control," can be useful under these conditions even if the openings must be made larger at a later date. A tape recorder to allow the patient to hear his or her own voice as others hear it can be helpful.

Occasionally these posterior pharyngeal flaps produce hyponasal speech because the lateral openings are too small. This problem is usually due to edema and is transient. If it should persist, the lateral openings can be made larger by z-plasties. Rarely the openings are too large and have to be made smaller, in which case reverse z-plasties can be used. At times the flap base on the posterior pharyngeal wall scars in such a way that it shifts inferiorly and actually tethers palatal movement upward and backward. If it is a problem, the flap can be detached from the posterior pharyngeal wall and reinserted just below the adenoid pad. Flap revisions are usually helpful in the hypernasal patient, especially if an anatomically correctable problem is identified. Flap revision in the patient with postoperative hyponasality has been less successful [128].

## Alveolar Reconstruction

As previously noted, alveolar reconstruction is carried out at about 7 to 10 years of age, at a time when the adjacent permanent teeth are erupting into the area of the cleft. Initial orthodontic alignment of the alveolar segments is carried out. At surgery, the area is opened widely by elevating gingival flaps, and considerable autogenous bone is packed into the defect. We have preferred iliac cancellous or cranial membranous bone [106, 127]. Minced bone from the rib also can be used. If a plate of bone is needed to stabilize a floating premaxilla, the bone can be obtained from rib, ilium, or outer table of the skull and is wired into place. One advantage to using rib bone is that it also allows procurement of costal cartilage for nasal tip support. Closure with nasal mucosa superiorly and gingival flaps orally has achieved good coverage for the bone grafts and usually closes any oronasal fistulas in this area. Indeed, alveolar oronasal fistulas are difficult to close without bone grafts.

By bone grafting the alveolar defects, the adjacent tooth roots gain considerable stability, displaced unerupted teeth have a bony matrix through which they can erupt, and the alveolar ridge is reconstructed as well. If a prosthetic tooth is needed, it can be bonded to the adjacent teeth (Maryland bridge) and rest on an acceptable looking gingiva, with improved stability of the teeth adjacent to the cleft. Even with incomplete alveolar clefts an appreciable bony defect may be present. The stability that bone grafts provide the adjacent tooth roots appears to be well worthwhile in these cases too.

Definitive orthodontia is done after bone grafting. Tooth replacement using a "Maryland bridge" bonded to the adjacent teeth has worked well. Teeth are much more secure, eruption has taken place through these bone grafts, and good reconstruction of the gingiva has been achieved. In older patients in whom teeth do not have to be moved, hydroxyapatite has been used in place of autogenous bone. This substance can be used in the same way as bone grafts, but after healing it has no flexibility. Furthermore, its interchangeability with bone for closure of alveolar clefts has not yet been proved.

Surgery of the cleft palate is an ever-changing art, requiring careful coordination with the fields of dentistry and speech pathology. Long-term follow-up for facial growth and fully developed speech patterns are needed for the evaluation of treatment schedules.

## References

ANATOMY, EMBRYOLOGY, ETIOLOGY, AND CLASSIFICATION

1. Brescia, N. J. Anatomy of the Lip and Palate. In W. C. Grabb, S. W. Rosenstein, and K. R. Bzoch (eds.), *Cleft Lip and Palate.* Boston: Little, Brown, 1971.
2. Brogan, W. F., and Murphy, B. P. The incidence of cleft lip and palate in Western Australia. Presented at the 3rd International Symposium on Early Treatment of Cleft Lip and Palate. Zurich, September 1984.
3. Broomhead, I. W. The nerve supply of the muscles of the soft palate. *Br. J. Plast. Surg.* 4:1, 1951.
4. Calnan, J. S. Congenital large pharynx. *Br. J. Plast. Surg.* 24:263, 1971.
5. Clarren, S. K. Recognition of fetal alcohol syndrome. *J.A.M.A.* 245:2436, 1981.
6. Cohen, M. M., Jr. Syndromes with cleft lip and cleft palate. *Cleft Palate J.* 15:306, 1978.
7. Cohlan, S. Q. Excessive intake of vitamin A as a cause of congenital anomalies in the rat. *Science* 117:535, 1953.
8. Croft, C. B., et al. The occult submucous cleft and the musculus uvulae. *Cleft Palate J.* 15:150, 1978.
9. Dickson, D. R., and Dickson, W. M. Velopharyngeal anatomy. *J. Speech Hear. Res.* 15:372, 1972.
10. Fara, M., and Dvorak, J. Abnormal anatomy of the muscles of the palatopharyngeal closure in cleft palate. *Plast. Reconstr. Surg.* 46:488, 1970.
11. Fogh-Anderson, P. *Inheritance of Harelip and Cleft Palate.* NYT Nordisk Forlag. Copenhagen: A. Busck, 1942.
12. Fogh-Anderson, P. Incidences and Etiology. In M. Edwards and A. C. H. Watson (eds.), *Advances in the Management of Cleft Palate.* Edinburgh: Churchill Livingstone, 1980.
13. Fraser, F. C. Etiology of cleft lip and palate. *Am. J. Hum. Genet.* 22:125, 1970.
14. Fraser, F. C. The Genetics of Cleft Lip and Palate: Yet Another Look. In R. Prat and R. L. Christiansin (eds.), *Current Research*

*Trends in Prenatal Craniofacial Development.* Amsterdam: Elsevier North Holland, 1980.

15. Fritzell, B. The velopharyngeal muscles in speech. *Acta Otolaryngol. [Suppl.] (Stockh.)* 250:1, 1969.

16. Gorlin, R. J., Pindborg, J. J., and Cohen, M. M., Jr. *Syndromes of the Head and Neck.* New York: McGraw-Hill, 1976.

17. Gray, H. The Peripheral Nervous System. In C. M. Goss (ed.), *Anatomy of the Human Body* (28th ed.). Philadelphia: Lea & Febiger, 1966.

18. Hanson, J. W., and Smith, D. W. U-shaped palatal defect in the Pierre Robin anomalad: Developmental and clinical relevance. *J. Pediatr.* 87:30, 1975.

19. Jordan, R. E., Kraus, B. S., and Neptune, C. M. Dental abnormalities associated with cleft lip and/or palate. *Cleft Palate J.* 3:22, 1966.

20. Kaplan, E. N. The occult submucous cleft palate. *Cleft Palate J.* 12:356, 1975.

21. Kernahan, D. H., and Stark, R. B. A new classification for cleft lip and clefts palate. *Plast. Reconstr. Surg.* 22:435, 1958.

22. Kitamura, H., and Kraus, B. S. Visceral variations and defects associated with cleft lip and palate in human fetuses: A macroscopic description. *Cleft Palate J.* 1:99, 1964.

23. Kraus, O. Anatomy of the velopharyngeal area in cleft palate. *Clin. Plast. Surg.* 2:261, 1975.

24. Ortiz-Monasterio, F., et al. A study of untreated adult cleft palate patients. *Plast. Reconstr. Surg.* 38:36, 1966.

25. Pashyan, H. M. Nomenclature of facial clefts. *J. Clin. Dysmorphol.* 2:20, 1984.

26. Rintala, A. E. Epidemiology of orofacial clefts in Finland: A review. *Ann. Plast. Surg.* 17:456, 1986.

27. Stark, R. B. The pathogenesis of hare lip and cleft palate. *Plast. Reconstr. Surg.* 13:20, 1954.

28. Tessier, P. Anatomical classification of facial, craniofacial, and lateral facial clefts. *J. Maxillofac. Surg.* 4:69, 1976.

29. Veau, V. *Division Palatine.* Paris: Masson, 1931.

30. Walker, B. E. The association of mucopolysaccharides with morphogenesis of the palate and other structures in mouse embryos. *J. Embryol. Exp. Morphol.* 9:22, 1961.

31. Warkany, J., Roth, C. B., and Wilson, J. G. Multiple congenital malformations: A consideration of etiologic factors. *Pediatrics* 1:462, 1948.

32. Watson, A. C. H. Classification of Cleft Palate. In M. Edwards and A. C. H. Watson (eds.), *Advances in the Management of Cleft Palate.* Edinburgh: Churchill Livingstone, 1980.

GENERAL PATIENT CARE AND PRIMARY
PALATAL PROCEDURES

33. Bluestone, C. D. Eustachian tube obstruction in the infant with cleft palate. *Otol. Rhinol. Laryngol.* 29(suppl. 2):1, 1971.

34. Bluestone, C. D., Wittel, R. A., and Paradise, J. L. Roentgenographic evaluation of eustachian tube function in infants with cleft and normal palates. *Cleft Palate J.* 9:93, 1972.

35. Brown, A. S., Cohen, M., and Randall, P. Levator muscle reconstruction: Does it make a difference? *Plast. Reconstr. Surg.* 72:1, 1983.

36. Cronin, T. D. Method of preventing raw area on nasal surface of soft palate in push-back surgery. *Plast. Reconstr. Surg.* 20:474, 1957.

37. Cronin, T. D. Pushback Palatorrhaphy with Nasal Mucosal Flaps. In W. C. Grabb, S. W. Rosenstein, and K. R. Bzoch (eds.), *Cleft Lip and Palate.* Boston: Little, Brown, 1971.

38. Davies, D. The one-stage repair of unilateral cleft lip and palate. *Plast. Reconstr. Surg.* 38:129, 1966.

39. Desai, S. N. Early cleft palate repair completed before the age of 16 weeks: Observations on a personal series of 100 children. *Br. J. Plast. Surg.* 36:300, 1983.

40. Dorf, D. S., and Curtin, J. W. Early cleft palate repair and speech outcome. *Plast. Reconstr. Surg.* 70:74, 1982.

41. Dunn, F. S. Results of the vomer flap technique used in surgery of the cleft palate during the past eleven years. *Am. J. Surg.* 92:825, 1956.

42. Furlow, L. T. Double Reversing Z-plasty for Cleft Palate. In D. R. Millard (ed.), *Cleft Craft, Vol. 3: Alveolar and Palatal Deformities.* Boston: Little, Brown, 1980.

43. Grabb, W. C. General Aspects of Cleft Palate Surgery. In W. C. Grabb, S. W. Rosenstein, and K. R. Bzoch (eds.), *Cleft Lip and Palate.* Boston: Little, Brown, 1971.

44. Ivy, R. H. Modern concept of cleft lip and

cleft palate management. *Plast. Reconstr. Surg.* 9:121, 1952.

45. Jackson, I. Personal communication.

46. Kaplan, E. N. Cleft palate repair at 3 months? *Ann. Plast. Surg.* 7:179, 1981.

47. Kriens, O. B. Fundamental anatomic findings for an intravelar veloplasty. *Cleft Palate J.* 7:27, 1970.

48. LaRossa, D., Vaniver, K., and Randall, P. The effect of perioperative antibiotics on postoperative morbidity in patients with cleft lip and palate: A retrospective study. Presented at the American Cleft Palate Association meeting, New York, 1986.

49. Malek, R., Psaume, J., and Genton, N. New timing and new sequence for operative interventions in CLP patients. Presented at the 5th International Congress on Cleft Palate and Related Craniofacial Anomalies, Monte Carlo, 1985.

50. Meskin, L. H., Gorlin, R. J., and Isaacson, R. J. Abnormal morphology of the soft palate: In the prevalence of cleft uvula. *Cleft Palate J.* 1:342, 1964.

51. Osada, M., et al. The studies on the nasopharyngeal closure in small children aged 1–3 years old. Presented at the 5th International Congress on Cleft Palate and Related Craniofacial Anomalies, Monte Carlo, 1985.

52. Paradise, J. L., and Bluestone, C. D. On the universality of otitis media in fifty infants with cleft palate. *Pediatrics* 44:35, 1969.

53. Randall, P. A triangular flap operation for the primary repair of unilateral clefts of the lip. *Plast. Reconstr. Surg.* 23:331, 1959.

54. Randall, P. Micrognathia and glossoptosis with airway obstruction in the Pierre Robin syndrome. In J. M. Converse (ed.), *Reconstructive Plastic Surgery.* Philadelphia: Saunders, 1964.

55. Randall, P., et al. Cleft palate closure at 3 to 7 months: A preliminary report. *Plast. Reconstr. Surg.* 71:624, 1983.

56. Randall, P., et al. Experience with the Furlow double reversing z-plasty for cleft palate repair. *Plast. Reconstr. Surg.* 77:569, 1986.

57. Spriesterbach, D. C., et al. Hearing loss in children with cleft palates. *Plast. Reconstr. Surg.* 30:366, 1962.

58. Stark, D. B. Nasal lining in partial cleft palate repair. *Plast. Reconstr. Surg.* 32:75, 1963.

59. Stark, R. B., and DeHaan, C. R. The addition of a pharyngeal flap to primary palatoplasty. *Plast. Reconstr. Surg.* 26:378, 1960.

60. Stark, R. B., and Frileck, S. Primary Pharyngeal Flap and Palatorrhaphy. In W. C. Grabb, S. W. Rosenstein, and K. R. Bzoch (eds.), *Cleft Lip and Palate.* Boston: Little, Brown, 1971.

61. Stool, S., and Randall, P. Unexpected ear disease in cleft palate patients. *Cleft Palate J.* 4:99, 1967.

## SOFT PALATE MOVEMENT AND SPEECH

62. Adisman, I. K. Cleft Palate Prosthetics. In W. C. Grabb, S. W. Rosenstein, and K. R. Bzoch (eds.), *Cleft Lip and Palate.* Boston: Little, Brown, 1971.

63. Bardach, J., Morris, H. L., and Olin, W. H. Late results of primary veloplasty: The Marburg project. *Plast. Reconstr. Surg.* 73:207, 1984.

64. Blackfield, H. N., et al. Cinefluorographic analysis of the surgical treatment of cleft palate speech. *Plast. Reconstr. Surg.* 31:542, 1963.

65. Blakely, R. W. The rationale for a temporary speech prosthesis in palatal insufficiency. *Br. J. Disord. Commun.* 4:134, 1969.

66. Blocksma, R. Correction of velopharyngeal insufficiency by Silastic pharyngeal implant. *Plast. Reconstr. Surg.* 31:268, 1963.

67. Brookshire, B. L., Lynch, J. I., and Fox, D. R. *A Parent–Child Cleft Palate Curriculum: Developing Speech and Language.* Tigard, OR: C. C. Publications, 1980.

68. Bzoch, K. R. Articulation proficiency and error patterns in pre-school cleft palate and normal children. *Cleft Palate J.* 2:340, 1965.

69. Bzoch, K. R. Etiological Factors Related to Cleft Palate Speech. In W. C. Grabb, S. W. Rosenstein, and K. R. Bzoch (eds.), *Cleft Lip and Palate.* Boston: Little, Brown, 1971.

70. Cosman, B., and Falk, A. S. Delayed hard palate repair and speech deficiencies: A cautionary report. *Cleft Palate J.* 17:27, 1980.

71. Fara, M., and Brousilova, M. Experiences with early closure of hard palate. *Plast. Reconstr. Surg.* 44:131, 1969.

72. Fletcher, S. C. *Diagnosing Speech Disorders from Cleft Palate.* Orlando, FL: Grune & Stratton, 1978.

73. Hotz, M. M., et al. Early maxillary orthopedics in CLP cases: Guidelines for surgery. *Cleft Palate J.* 14:405, 1978.

74. Hynes, W. The examination of imperfect speech following cleft palate operations. *Br. J. Plast. Surg.* 10:114, 1958.

75. Ibuki, K., Karnell, M. P., and Morris, H. L. Reliability of the nasopharyngeal fiberscope (NPF) for assessing velopharyngeal function. *Cleft Palate J.* 20:97, 1983.

76. LaRossa, D., et al. Video-radiography of the velopharyngeal portal using the Towne's view. *J. Maxillofac. Surg.* 8:203, 1980.

77. Mason, R. M., and Warren, D. W. Adenoid involution and developing hypernasality in cleft palate. *J. Speech Hear. Disord.* 45:469, 1980.

78. Mazaheri, M. Indications and contraindications for prosthetic speech appliances in cleft palate. *Plast. Reconstr. Surg.* 30:663, 1962.

79. McWilliams, B. J., Morris, H. L., and Shelton, R. L. *Cleft Palate Speech.* St. Louis: Mosby, 1987.

80. Perko, M. A. Two-stage closure of cleft palate. *J. Maxillofac. Surg.* 7:76, 1979.

81. Piaget, J. *Play, Dreams and Imitations in Childhood, Part I.* Translated by C. Gettegno and F. M. Hodgson. New York: Norton, 1962.

82. Pigot, R. W. The nasendoscopic appearance of the normal palatopharyngeal valve. *Plast. Reconstr. Surg.* 43:19, 1969.

83. Randall, P. Surgery and speech. *Surgery* 56:810, 1964.

84. Randall, P., Bakes, F. P., and Kennedy, C. Cleft palate-type speech in the absence of cleft palate. *Plast. Reconstr. Surg.* 25:484, 1960.

85. Randall, P., O'Hara, A. E., and Bakes, F. P. A simplified x-ray technique for the study of soft palate function in patients with poor speech. *Plast. Reconstr. Surg.* 21:345, 1958.

86. Shelton, R., et al. Videoendoscopic feedback in training velopharyngeal closure. *Cleft Palate J.* 15:6, 1978.

87. Shelton, R. L., Lindquist, A. F., and Chisum, L. Effect of prosthetic speech bulb reduction on articulation. *Cleft Palate J.* 5:195, 1968.

88. Shelton, R. L., et al. Panendoscopic feedback in the study of voluntary velopharyngeal movements. *J. Speech Hear. Disord.* 40:232, 1975.

89. Skolnick, M. L. Videofluoroscopic examination of the velopharyngeal portal during phonation in lateral and base projections: A new technique for studying the mechanism of closure. *Cleft Palate J.* 7:803, 1970.

90. Skolnick, M. L., et al. Patterns of velopharyngeal closure in subjects with repaired cleft palate and normal speech: A multiview videofluoroscopic analysis. *Cleft Palate J.* 12:369, 1975.

91. Spriesterbach, D. C., and Sherman, D. (eds.) *Cleft Palate and Communication.* New York: Academic Press, 1968.

92. Subtelny, J. D., and Baker, H. K. The significance of adenoid tissue in velopharyngeal function. *Plast. Reconstr. Surg.* 17:235, 1956.

93. Trier, W. C. Velopharyngeal incompetency in the absence of overt cleft palate: Anatomic and surgical considerations. *Cleft Palate J.* 20:209, 1983.

94. Trost, J. E. Articulatory additions to the classical description of the speech of persons with cleft palate. *Cleft Palate J.* 18:193, 1981.

95. VanDemark, D. R., Morris, H. L., and Vande-Harr, C. Patterns of articulation abilities in speakers with cleft palate. *Cleft Palate J.* 16:230, 1979.

96. Warren, D. W. PERCI: A method for rating palate efficiency. *Cleft Palate J.* 16:279, 1979.

97. Warren, D. W., and DuBois, A. B. A pressure-flow technique for measuring velopharyngeal orifice area during continuous speech. *Cleft Palate J.* 1:52, 1964.

98. Williams, W. N., and Eisenbach, C. R. Assessing V. P. function: The lateral still technique cinefluorography. *Cleft Palate J.* 18:45, 1981.

99. Witzel, M. A., Salyer, K., and Ross, R. Delayed hard palate closure: The philosophy revisited. *Cleft Palate J.* 21:263, 1984.

100. Zwitman, D. H. Velopharyngeal physiology after pharyngeal flap surgery as assessed by oral endoscopy. *Cleft Palate J.* 19:36, 1982.

## BONE GRAFTING AND MAXILLARY ORTHOPEDICS

101. Abyholm, F., et al. Secondary bone grafting of alveolar clefts. *Scand. J. Plast. Reconstr. Surg.* 15:127, 1981.

102. Backdahl, M., and Nordin, K. E. Bone defect

in cleft palate. *Acta Chir. Scand.* 122:131, 1961.

103. Backdahl, M., et al. Bone grafts to the maxillary defect in cleft lip and palate by the method of Backdahl and Nordin. In *Transactions of 3rd International Congress of Plastic Surgery.* Amsterdam: Excerpta Medica, 1964. P. 193.

104. Bergland, O., Semb, G., and Abyholm, F. E. Elimination of the residual alveolar cleft by secondary bone grafting and subsequent orthodontic treatment. *Cleft Palate J.* 23:175, 1986.

105. Bergland, O., et al. Secondary bone grafting and orthodontic treatment in patients with bilateral complete clefts of the lip and palate. *Ann. Plast. Surg.* 17:460, 1986.

106. Boyne, J. P., and Sands, N. R. Secondary bone grafting of residual alveolar and palate clefts. *J. Oral Surg.* 30:87, 1972.

107. Burston, W. R. The pre-surgical orthopaedic correction of the maxillary deformity in clefts of both primary and secondary palate. In *Transactions of the International Society of Plastic Surgeons.* Edinburgh: Livingstone, 1960.

108. Burston, W. R. The early orthodontic treatment of alveolar clefts. *Proc. R. Soc. Med.* 58:767, 1965.

109. Georgiade, N. C. The management of premaxillary and maxillary segments in the newborn cleft palate patient. *Cleft Palate J.* 7:411, 1970.

110. Jacobson, B. N., and Rosenstein, S. W. Early maxillary orthopedics: A combination appliance. *Cleft Palate J.* 2:369, 1965.

111. Johansen, B., and Ohlsson, A. Bone grafting and dental orthopaedics in primary and secondary cases of cleft lip and palate. *Acta Chir. Scand.* 122:112, 1961.

112. Mazaheri, M., Harding, R. L., and Nanda, S. The effects of surgery on maxillary growth and cleft width. *Plast. Reconstr. Surg.* 40:22, 1967.

113. McNeil, C. K. *Oral and Facial Deformity.* London: Pitman, 1954.

114. Monroe, C. W., Griffith, B. H., and McKinney, P. Surgical recession of the premaxilla and its effect on maxillary growth in patients with bilateral clefts. *Cleft Palate J.* 7:784, 1970.

115. Nordin, K. E. Bone grafting to the alveolar process clefts following orthodontic treatment of secondary cleft palate deformity. In *Transactions of the International Society of Plastic Surgeons.* Baltimore: Williams & Wilkins, 1957. P. 228.

116. Olin, W. H., and Spriesterbach, D. C. *Cleft Lip and Palate Rehabilitation.* Springfield, IL: Thomas, 1960.

117. Pruzansky, S. Pre-surgical orthopedics and bone grafting for infants with cleft lip and palate: A dissent. *Cleft Palate J.* 1:164, 1964.

118. Pruzansky, S., and Aduss, H. Arch form and the deciduous occlusion in complete unilateral clefts. *Cleft Palate J.* 1:411, 1964.

119. Rehrmann, A. H., Koberg, W. R., and Koch, H. Long-term postoperative results of primary and secondary bone grafting in complete cleft of the lip and palate. *Cleft Palate J.* 7:207, 1970.

120. Robinson, F., and Wood, B. Primary bone grafting in the treatment of cleft lip and palate with special reference to alveolar collapse. *Br. J. Plast. Surg.* 22:336, 1969.

121. Rosenstein, S. W., et al. A case for early bone grafting in cleft lip and cleft palate. *Plast. Reconstr. Surg.* 70:297, 1982.

122. Ross, R. B. Prediction of facial growth in patients with cleft lip and palate. Presented at the V International Congress on Cleft Palate and Related Craniofacial Anomalies, Monte Carlo, 1985.

123. Schmid, E. Die aufbanende Kieferkamplastik. *Os. Z. Stomatol.* 51:582, 1954.

124. Schmid, E. Die osteoplastick bei Lippen-Kiefer-Gaumenspalten. *Langenbecks Arch. Klin. Chir.* 295:868, 1960.

125. Schuchardt, K., and Pfeifer, G. Primary and secondary operations for cleft palate. *J. Int. Coll. Surg.* 38:237, 1962.

126. Stellmach, R. Primare Knochenplastic bei Lippen-Kiefer-Gaumenspalten am Sauglingunter-besunderer Berucksichtigung der Transplantatdeckung. *Langenbecks Arch. Klin. Chir.* 292:865, 1959.

127. Tessier, P. Autogenous bone grafts taken from the calvarium for facial and cranial applications. *Clin. Plast. Surg.* 9:531, 1982.

## FOLLOW-UP CARE AND SECONDARY PALATAL PROCEDURES

128. Barot, L. R., Cohen, M. A., and LaRossa, D. Surgical indications and techniques for pos-

terior pharyngeal flap revisions. *Ann. Plast. Surg.* 16:527, 1986.

129. Brauer, R. O. Retropharyngeal implantation of silicone pillows for velopharyngeal incompetence. *Plast. Reconstr. Surg.* 51:254, 1973.

130. Dingman, R. O., Grabb, W. C., and Bloomer, H. Posterior pharyngeal flap. In *Transactions 3rd International Congress of Plastic Surgery.* Amsterdam: Excerpta Medica, 1964. p. 220.

131. Hamlen, M. Speech results after pharyngeal flap surgery. *Plast. Reconstr. Surg.* 46:437, 1970.

132. Hogan, V. M. A clarification of the surgical goals in cleft palate speech and the introduction of the lateral port control (L.P.C.) pharyngeal flap. *Cleft Palate J.* 10:331, 1973.

133. Hynes, W. The results of pharyngoplasty by muscle transplantation in "failed cleft palate" cases, with special reference to the influence of the pharynx on voice production. *Ann. R. Coll. Surg. Eng.* 13:17, 1953.

134. Hynes, W. Pharyngoplasty by muscle transplantation. *Br. J. Plast. Surg.* 3:128, 1956.

135. Jackson, I. T. Discussion: A review of 236 cleft palate patients treated with dynamic muscle sphincter. *Plast. Reconstr. Surg.* 71:187, 1983.

136. Jackson, I. T., and Silverton, J. S. Sphincter pharyngoplasty as a secondary procedure in cleft palates. *Plast. Reconstr. Surg.* 59:578, 1977.

137. Kapetansky, D. I. Bilateral transverse pharyngeal flaps for repair of cleft palate. *Plast. Reconstr. Surg.* 52:52, 1973.

138. Levine, N. S., Buchanan, R. T., and Orr, W. The effect of cleft palate repair and pharyngeal flap surgery on upper airway sleep patterns. Presented at the V International Congress on Cleft Palate and Related Craniofacial Anomalies, Monte Carlo, 1985.

139. Morris, H. L., and Spriesterbach, D. C. The pharyngeal flaps as a speech mechanism. *Plast. Reconstr. Surg.* 39:84, 1967.

140. Orticochea, M. Construction of a dynamic muscle sphincter in cleft palates. *Plast. Reconstr. Surg.* 41:323, 1968.

141. Orticochea, M. A review of 236 cleft palate patients treated with dynamic muscle sphincter. *Plast. Reconstr. Surg.* 71:180, 1983.

142. Owsley, J. Q., Jr., et al. Experiences with the high attached pharyngeal flap. *Plast. Reconstr. Surg.* 38:232, 1966.

143. Shprintzen, R. J., et al. A comprehensive study of pharyngeal flap surgery: Tailormade flaps. *Cleft Palate J.* 16:46, 1979.

144. Skoog, T. The pharyngeal flap operation in cleft palate. *Br. J. Plast. Surg.* 18:265, 1965.

145. Subtelney, J. D., and Nioto, R. P. A longitudinal study of maxillary growth following pharyngeal flap surgery. *Cleft Palate J.* 15:118, 1978.

146. Trauner, R., and Doubek, F. I. A new procedure in velopharyngeal surgery for secondary operations on too short soft palates. II. The speech results compared with other surgical or prosthetic methods. *Br. J. Plast. Surg.* 8:291, 1956.

147. Warren, D. W., and Dalston, R. M. The diagnosis of velopharyngeal inadequacy. *Clin. Plast. Surg.* 12:685, 1985.

148. Whitaker, L. A., et al. A prospective and randomized series comparing superiorly and inferiorly based posterior pharyngeal flaps. *Cleft Palate J.* 9:304, 1972.

149. Williams, H. B., and Woolhouse, F. M. Comparison of speech improvement in cases of cleft palate after two methods of pharyngoplasty. *Plast. Reconstr. Surg.* 30:36, 1962.

## Selected Readings

Bardach, J., and Salyer, K. *Suggested Techniques in Cleft Lip and Palate.* Chicago: Year Book, 1987.

Bixler, D. Genetics and clefting. *Cleft Palate J.* 18:10, 1981.

Blocksma, R. Correction of velopharyngeal insufficiency by Silastic pharyngeal implant. *Plast. Reconstr. Surg.* 31:268, 1963.

Bluestone, C. D., and Stool, S. E. (eds.). *Otolaryngology* (Vol. 2). Philadelphia: Saunders, 1983.

Bluestone, C. D., et al. Teflon injection pharyngoplasty. *Cleft Palate J.* 5:19, 1968.

Braithwaite, F. Cleft Palate Repair. In T. Gibson (ed.), *Modern Trends in Plastic Surgery.* London: Butterworth, 1964.

Bzoch, K. R. Clinical studies of the efficiency of speech appliances compared to pharyngeal flap surgery. *Cleft Palate J.* 1:275, 1964.

Calnan, J. S. V-Y Pushback Palatorrhaphy. In W. C. Grabb, S. W. Rosenstein, and K. R. Bzoch (eds.), *Cleft Lip and Palate.* Boston: Little, Brown, 1971.

Calnan, J. S. Diagnosis, prognosis and treatment of "palatopharyngeal incompetence" with special reference to radiographic investigations. *Br. J. Plast. Surg.* 8:265, 1956.

Calnan, J. The error of Gustav Passavant. *Plast. Reconstr. Surg.* 13:275, 1954.

Calnan, J. S. Movement of the soft palate. *Br. J. Plast. Surg.* 5:286, 1953.

Converse, J. M. (eds.). *Reconstructive Plastic Surgery* (Vol. 4, 2nd ed.). Philadelphia: Saunders, 1977.

Conway, H. Effect of supplemental vitamin therapy on the limitation of incidence of cleft lip and cleft palate in humans. *Plast. Reconstr. Surg.* 22:450, 1958.

Conway, H., and Stark, R. B. Inferiorly based pharyngeal flap in speech rehabilitation of complicated cleft palate cases. In *Transactions of the International Society of Plastic Surgeons.* Baltimore: Williams & Wilkins, 1957.

Croft, C. B., Shprintzen, R. J., and Rakoff, S. J. Patterns of velopharyngeal valving in normal and cleft palate subjects: A multiview videofluoroscopic and nasendoscopic study. *Laryngoscope* 91:265, 1984.

Dalston, R. M. Photodetector assessment of velopharyngeal activity. *Cleft Palate J.* 19:1, 1982.

Dingman, R. O., and Grabb, W. C. A rational program for surgical management of bilateral cleft lip and cleft palate. *Plast. Reconstr. Surg.* 47:239, 1971.

Dorrance, G. M. *Operative Story of Cleft Palate.* Philadelphia: Saunders, 1933.

Dreyer, T. M., and Trier, W. C. A comparison of palatoplasty techniques. *Cleft Palate J.* 21:251, 1984.

Grabb, W. C., Rosenstein, S. W., and Bzoch, K. R. *Cleft Lip and Palate.* Boston: Little, Brown, 1971.

Holdsworth, W. G. *Cleft Lip and Palate* (3rd ed.). London: Heineman, 1963.

Hotz, M., et al. (eds.). *Early Treatment of Cleft Lip and Palate.* Bern: Hans Huber, 1986.

Kalter, H., and Warkany, J. Experimental production of congenital malformations in strains of inbred mice by maternal treatment with hypervitaminosis A. *Am. J. Pathol.* 38:1, 1961.

Kernahan, D. A., and Berner, B. S. Cleft Palate. In N. C. Georgiade et al. (eds.), *Cleft Palate Essentials of Plastic Maxillofacial and Reconstructive Surgery.* Baltimore: Williams & Wilkins, 1987.

Kraus, B. S. Some aspects of the anatomy of normal and cleft palate development in man. Presented at an American Cleft Palate Association meeting. Los Angeles. April 1964.

Kremanak, C. R., Jr., Huffman, W. C., and Olin, W. H. Maxillary growth inhibition by mucoperiosteal denudation of the palatal shelf bone in non-cleft beagles. *Cleft Palate J.* 7:817, 1970.

Krogman, W. M. The problem of cleft palate fade. *Plast. Reconstr. Surg.* 14:370, 1954.

Latham, R. A., Long, R. E., and Latham, E. A. Cleft palate velopharyngeal musculature in a five-month old infant: A three-dimensional histological reconstruction. *Cleft Palate J.* 17:1, 1980.

McWilliams, B. J., Morris, H. L., and Shelton, R. L. (eds.), *Cleft Palate Speech.* Philadelphia: B. C. Decker, 1984.

Musgrave, R. H., and Brenner, J. C. Complications of cleft palate surgery. *Plast. Reconstr. Surg.* 26:180, 1960.

Noone, R. B., et al. The effect on middle ear disease of fracture of the pterygoid hamulus during palatoplasty. *Cleft Palate J.* 10:23, 1973.

Melnick, M., Bixler, D., and Shields, E. D. *Etiology of Cleft Lip and Cleft Palate.* New York: Liss, 1980.

Millard, D. R. *Cleft Craft* (Vols. 1, 2, 3). Boston: Little, Brown, 1976, 1977, 1980.

Randall, P. Report on a foundation trip in Europe in 1959. *Plast. Reconstr. Surg.* 26:69, 1960.

Riski, J. E., and DeLong, E. Articulation development in children with cleft lip/palate. *Cleft Palate J.* 21:57, 1984.

Schuchardt, K., Pfeifer, G., and Kriens, O. Primary osteoplasty in patients with cleft lip alveolus and palate. In *Transactions IV International Congress on Plastic and Reconstructive Surgery, 1967.* Amsterdam: Excerpta Medica, 1969.

Schultz, R. D. A survey of European and Scandinavian bone grafting procedures for cleft palate deformities. *Cleft Palate J.* 1:188, 1964.

Schweckendiek, H. Zur zweiphasigen Gaumenspalten-operation bei primarem Velumverschluss. *Fortschri. Kiefer. Gesichtschir.* 1:73, 1955.

Schweckendiek, W. Primary veloplasty: Long-term results without maxillary deformity—a twenty-five year report. *Cleft Palate J.* 15:268, 1978.

Shelton, R. L. Oral Sensory Function in Speech Production. In W. C. Grabb, S. W. Rosenstein, and K. R. Bzoch (eds.), *Cleft Lip and Palate.* Boston: Little, Brown, 1971.

Slaughter, W. B., and Pruzansky, S. The rationale for velar closure as a primary procedure in the repair of cleft palate defects. *Plast. Reconstr. Surg.* 13:341, 1954.

Song, I. C., and Bromberg, B. E. Pharyngopalatoplasty with free transplantation of palmaris longus. *Br. J. Plast. Surg.* 27:337, 1974.

Trier, W. C. Velopharyngeal incompetency in the absence of overt cleft palate anatomic and surgical conditions. *Cleft Plate J.* 20:209, 1983.

VanDemark, D. R. Predictability of velopharyngeal competencey. *Cleft Palate J.* 16:429, 1979.

Walker, B. E., and Crain, B., Jr. Effects of hypervitaminosis A on palate development in two strains of mice. *Am. J. Anat.* 107:49, 1960.

Warren, D. W. Nasal emission of air and velopharyngeal function. *Cleft Palate J.* 4:148, 1967.

Watson, A. C. H. Secondary Surgery. In M. Edwards and A. C. H. Watson (eds.), *Primary Surgery in Cleft Palate.* Edinburgh: Churchill Livingstone, 1980.

*Richard C. Schultz*

# 11

# *Soft Tissue Injuries of the Face*

Facial injuries deserve special attention because of their enormous functional and aesthetic significance. Although facial injuries can logically be divided into soft tissue injuries and facial bone fractures, each form of injury interrelates and bears on the approach to management of the other. (Facial bone fractures are discussed in Chapter 12.)

## *Initial Care of the Patient*

*Triage,* the sorting of patients according to the seriousness of their injuries for priorities of treatment, also applies to the individual patient with multiple injuries. Victims of multiple injury must always be viewed with the following priorities [29]: First, a clear airway is ensured; then hemorrhage is controlled, shock is treated, and associated injuries are evaluated. Only then are facial injuries diagnosed and treated.

### CLEAR AIRWAY
Blood, dentures, or vomitus can fully or partially obstruct the upper airway, resulting in an agitated or nearly lifeless patient. These obstructions can usually be cleared quickly by sweeping a finger deeply into the mouth and oral pharynx [31]. Aspiration and tracheostomy are never as prompt, effective, or informative as use of a finger in these circumstances. Partially aspirated foreign bodies or occluding edema from a fractured larynx or trachea requires prompt surgical attention, but only after the mouth and oral pharynx have been cleared [35]. The condition of a patient with an airway problem stemming from uncontrolled facial hemorrhage or grossly displaced facial tissue can often be dramatically improved simply by sitting the patient upright [29]. When patients with facial injuries make violent efforts to sit up or to thrust the head forward, they should be allowed to do so, as they almost invariably are exhibiting a protective reflex to maintain the upper airway. Strapping or forcibly holding prone a patient with extensive facial injuries could result in death [31].

### CONTROL HEMORRHAGE
Although hemorrhage from facial wounds can appear alarming, it is seldom of such magnitude as to be the sole cause of systemic shock, except in the case of close-range shotgun wounds [12,13] Extensive arterial hemorrhage from facial wounds usually results from injury to the external maxillary artery, the superficial temporal artery, or the angular artery [30]. Hemorrhage from these arteries can almost always be controlled at least temporarily by direct pressure to the wound. The vessel can then be ligated directly through the wound. The most dangerous aspect of facial hemorrhage

**325**

is the possibility that it might obstruct the upper airway [29]. Also, if the patient swallows large amounts of blood, gastric irritation and vomiting may result, further complicating the management of the patient [22].

TREAT SHOCK

Shock is only occasionally caused by facial injury alone. Penetrating or avulsing ocular injuries may initiate the shock syndrome through pain and apprehension. Extensive facial injuries, even including facial bone fractures, seldom cause great pain. When a patient with facial injury is found in shock, associated injuries should be suspected and evaluated as the cause [26].

EVALUATE ASSOCIATED INJURIES

Once a clear airway is ensured and hemorrhage and shock have been controlled, consideration is given to associated injuries before undertaking treatment of the facial injuries themselves [32]. Patients do not die from facial injuries, but patients with facial injuries die from associated injuries [27].

## Diagnosis of Facial Injuries

A comprehensive diagnosis and classification of facial injuries are made before initiating definitive treatment [31]. Observation of a facial injury logically begins with the surface for indications of soft tissue injuries. Eyelids are always opened to look for associated ocular injury [8, 9].

Soft tissue injuries include contusion with or without hematoma, abrasion, accidental tattoo (numerous small particles embedded in the dermis), retained foreign bodies, puncture, laceration (subdivided into simple, beveled, tearing, and burst or stellate type), avulsion flap (undermined laceration), and avulsion injury (loss of tissue) [31].

After life-threatening problems have been resolved, soft tissue injuries amenable to repair under local anesthesia are usually treated first. One exception is the close-

range shotgun wound of the face [31]. Such a complex facial injury with tissue loss and extensive fractures can seldom be treated immediately, as these patients are usually poor candidates for a general anesthetic.

When definitive care must be postponed, the simplest type of accurate tissue approximation helps promote a better end result. If necessary, soft tissue injuries can wait without repair up to 24 hours without compromising the final result, provided that bleeding has been controlled and the wounds have been properly cleaned and dressed [35]. Systemic antibiotics are advisable when significant delay in soft tissue repair is anticipated.

Proper records of facial injuries include diagnosis of type, anatomic location, and, in the case of soft tissue injury, measurements. In addition, a photograph of every extensive facial injury should be taken before definitive treatment begins [35]. Such a record of injury can subsequently prove invaluable for understanding and explaining secondary problems and the nature of final healing (as well as be useful in the event of medicolegal problems) [31].

## Preparation for Treatment of Soft Tissue Injuries

Attempting to repair extensive soft tissue injuries of the face in a corner of the emergency room with inadequate light and without assistance invites frustration and second-rate results. Such injuries should be repaired in the operating theater with the help of at least a scrub nurse and a circulating nurse.

When a penetrating injury extends through the scalp, beard, or moustache, the hair is shaved around the wound to facilitate suturing—but the eyebrow is *never* shaved [35]. The shape and periphery of the eyebrow provide a valuable landmark for accurate repair. Once an eyebrow has healed with misalignment of its edge, it becomes exceedingly difficult to correct.

## Anesthesia

With a reasonably cooperative patient, local anesthesia is unquestionably preferable for repair of most soft tissue injuries [23] from the standpoint of safety and ultimate patient comfort, as victims of acute trauma often arrive in the emergency room with their stomachs filled with food, alcohol, or blood. In addition, local anesthesia allows the surgeon far greater access to the face. When possible, the patient's comfort can be significantly enhanced under local anesthesia by supplemental oral, intramuscular, or intravenous sedation with promethazine (Phenergan), diazepam (Valium), or meperidine (Demerol).

For most extensive soft tissue facial injuries, my choice of agent is 1% lidocaine (Xylocaine) with epinephrine (1:100,000). When only small quantities of solution are injected, such as into the eyelids, a 2% solution is preferred. The discomfort of the injection can be minimized by introducing it through the cut edge of the wound rather than through the adjacent intact skin [4].

The sensory nerve distribution to the face lends itself fairly well to local nerve block anesthesia. In common practice, there are five areas on the face that are amenable to local block anesthesia: (1) supraorbital, (2) nasal, (3) infraorbital, (4) maxillary (second division of the trigeminal nerve), and (5) mandibular (the third division of the trigeminal nerve) areas. Maxillary and mandibular blocks require the most technical skill and are the most difficult to achieve. Cocaine (5% solution) is still the best topical anesthetic agent available for nasal mucous membranes. It is introduced into the nose on cotton pledgets, cotton dental rolls, or cotton-tipped applicators.

When soft tissue injuries are being repaired in small children and local anesthesia is used, authoritative assurance can often make the patient cooperative. If not contraindicated by associated injuries, a combination of narcotic and tranquilizing drugs given by injection (varying the dosage according to weight and age [31] helps achieve a cooperative patient in about 15 minutes. The sedative mixture may be composed of meperidine 50 mg (1 ml), promethazine 12.5 mg (0.5 ml), and chlorpromazine (Thorazine) 12.5 mg (0.5 ml); the dosage is 1.5 ml for an 18-kg child and 2 ml for a 27- to 45-kg child.

When the child continues to be agitated, comfortable physical restraint is appropriate. It can be provided by a skillful assistant if the repair can be done quickly. When more time is needed, the patient's trunk and extremities can be "mummied" with an ordinary sheet. When it is necessary to restrain all extremities, the head, and the torso, an infant restraining board with Velcro straps is more suitable [31].

When general anesthesia becomes necessary (e.g., when the repair involves multiple injuries), a brief preinduction discussion with the anesthetist is appropriate. This step facilitates selection of compatible anesthetic agents (if the surgeon intends to inject a solution containing epinephrine for purposes of hemostasis) and positioning of the anesthetic equipment.

## Treatment of Soft Tissue Injuries
### CONTUSION (WITH OR WITHOUT HEMATOMA)

Contusion is a bruising injury caused by blunt trauma. It seldom results in serious injury to the skin, and cleaning and observation are usually sufficient treatment. However, such injury can be associated with an underlying hematoma.

Small hematomas of the face often spontaneously resorb; those that become encapsulated, however, usually require surgical treatment. Left untreated, such hematomas form permanent subcutaneous scar deformities. Proteolytic enzyme preparations given systemically have not proved helpful for reducing hematomas in my experience.

When still in the "currant jelly" stage, a hematoma is best evacuated by incision [20]. As further liquefaction takes place, aspiration with a large-bore needle (18 gauge or larger) may be possible.

## ABRASION

Abrasion injuries are best treated by cleaning with mild, nonirritating soap. It is usually best to leave abrasions uncovered, but when the pain is significant, the abrasion may be protected from the air by a thin layer of antibiotic ointment, such as bacitracin (Neosporin). The injury may also be covered with a light, serum-absorbent dressing, such as cellulose acetate gauze, which is then covered with ordinary cotton dressing gauze. Such dressings are removed after 1 to 2 days. Healing is usually prompt, leaving no apparent residual scar unless the abrasion approaches third-degree depth or becomes infected.

## ACCIDENTAL TATTOO

Small dermis-embedded particles must be removed promptly from an abrasion before they become tissue-fixed, which usually occurs within 12 hours. If the area involved does not lend itself well to treatment under local anesthesia, general anesthesia must be used. Scrubbing with a stiff, sterile scrub brush and mild soapsuds, if done early, is adequate to remove most tattooing foreign bodies. When grease or oil is present in or about the wound, it can usually be dissolved and removed by small amounts of ether, acetone, or xylol.

Once foreign particles have become fixed in the tissues, a formal surgical abrasion is necessary [11]. If the area is extensive, the procedure is planned under general anesthesia. It is best done with power equipment, either electric or air-driven.

With all methods of abrasion, including scrubbing, care must be taken not to penetrate the deep dermal layers, lest permanent scarring results. Occasionally, when isolated foreign bodies are deeply embedded, a scalpel blade can be used as a spud to tease out or excise these particles individually.

The dressing applied over a surgical abrasion should be absorptive but nonadherent. Cellulose acetate gauze is ideal for this purpose.

When left untreated, accidental tattoos result in permanent, unattractive discoloration in the skin. Additional material on this subject is included in Chapter 31.

## RETAINED FOREIGN BODIES

Retained foreign bodies are larger than the particles that cause accidental tattoos and should routinely be removed from the face, with the exception of metal fragments from missiles. (Bullets or missile fragments usually are sterile when they enter the face and commonly penetrate deeply [12]. If there is minimal reaction, more harm is often done by attempting to remove them than by leaving them in place.) Glass, ornamental metal, wood splinters, and dental fragments require removal.

Failure to remove foreign bodies originating in the mouth can lead to severe cellulitis and subsequent abscess formation [24].

## PUNCTURE

Puncture wounds of the face are uncommon; such small wounds must alert one to the possibility of injury to deeper structures. Swelling about puncture wounds is most often due to hematoma. However, an arteriovenous fistula may form after puncture wounds, particularly in the parotid and preauricular regions.

Graphite fragments from lead pencils, paint chips, rust particles, and wood splinters are the most common foreign bodies implanted by puncture. They must be removed to prevent infection, scar formation, and pigmentation. The puncture wound itself must sometimes be excised to achieve the best healing.

The possibility of pathogenic inoculation requires prophylactic treatment for tetanus and early follow-up examination [34].

## SIMPLE LACERATION

Laceration is the most common form of facial injury [31]. Repair is undertaken only after underlying structures have been put in order. The time lapse between injury and repair is important in terms of the possibility of infection and the choice of repair techniques. After observing the effects of varying time intervals between injury and repair, I have concluded that, with the exception of shotgun wounds, animal bites, and accidental tattoos, most soft tissue wounds of the face, properly cleaned and dressed, can await primary repair for up to 24 hours without serious risk of infection and without jeopardizing the final aesthetic result [26].

Wound toilet consists in cleaning, irrigation, and débridement. Tissue that is devitalized must be cut away, regardless of its location or its former importance [25]. Although débridement should be conservative, it must be adequate. Ragged, tangential, severely contused wound edges are conservatively excised to provide perpendicular skin edges that will heal primarily with a minimum of scar [28]. Closely parallel lacerations can be converted to a single wound by excising the intervening skin bridge, thus facilitating repair and reducing scar formation.

Displaced tissue is returned to its original position. Only occasionally is there an indication for immediately changing the direction of a wound by Z-plasty or for making tissue allowance for scar contracture at the time of primary wound repair.

*Suturing*
Muscular and subcutaneous tissue is best closed with plain catgut suture to minimize dead space and the accumulation of blood and serum [35]. In the event of infection, the more rapid resorption of plain catgut suture proves to be an advantage. Similarly, interrupted sutures of 5-0 or 6-0 nylon are ideal for skin closure; if hematoma or pocketing of serum or pus occurs, one or two sutures can be removed to permit drainage leaving the remainder of the repair intact. Running over-and-over sutures accurately placed can also provide an excellent repair and can also save time in cases of multiple extensive lacerations.

*Removal of Sutures*
Facial wounds have the advantage of a rich vascular supply, which contributes to early healing. Where the skin is thin, as in the eyelids, sutures are removed in 3 to 4 days; elsewhere on the face they are left 4 to 6 days. Sutures in the ears are often left in place 10 to 14 days with definite advantage when there has been injury to underlying cartilage, as scars over divided ear cartilage tend to thicken and spread when sutures are removed too early. Suture scars on the ears are not usually noticeable.

AVULSION FLAP
The avulsion flap is an undermined laceration that can be one of the most disfiguring of all soft tissue injuries (Fig. 11-1). Broad, tangentially located scar tissue in the dermis and subcutaneous tissue interferes with free circulation of venous blood and lymph to adjacent skin. The resulting venous engorgement and lymphedema swell the flap and partially contribute to the spreading and subsequent depression of the peripheral scar. Furthermore, as the scar contracts, the avulsion flap tissue bordered by it assumes a heaped-up appearance [31].

It is important therefore to minimize the thin, beveled portion of these flaps (Fig. 11-2). If the flap is small and the location fortunate, it can be totally excised, which solves the problem [28]. When avulsion flaps are larger or involve features, a more conservative approach to repair must be taken. The thinnest peripheral portions of the flap are cut away to create perpendicular edges for skin closure. After this débridement, closure is performed in essentially the same manner as for simple laceration.

Small avulsion flaps and gouges, as seen in injuries sustained on current automobile windshields [10] (Fig. 11-3), are best managed by complete excision following normal skin lines whenever possible. Left untreated or managed solely by a pressure dressing, these tiny avulsion flaps and full-thickness gouges heal with a pebbly skin surface that

of blood clots from the globe can be hazardous because iris tissue may be bound to the clot or confused with it [8]. A wound that penetrates deeply into the orbit through the upper eyelid or globe must be considered a potential intracranial injury, as the superior orbital plate is thin and fragile.

Eyelid infection is rare because the blood supply is abundant; nevertheless, eyelid lacerations are cleaned by irrigation with saline. Avulsed eyelid tissue is gently cleaned in saline and replaced as an autograft whenever possible [1, 35].

Eyelid lacerations can be divided into two groups: superficial and deep. Superficial lacerations can be further divided into those that parallel the lid margin and those that are perpendicular to it. Superficial lacerations that run parallel require only simple closure of the skin, and smaller ones may not require sutures. Those that are perpendicular to the lid margin cross normal skin lines and tend to gape; they require absorbable sutures in the underlying muscle and subcutaneous tissue prior to skin closure. Many small conjunctival lacerations heal well without suture repair, but when suturing is necessary, 6-0 catgut on a swaged ophthalmologic needle is used.

Deep lacerations are anesthetized and retracted to search for injury to underlying structures. Division of the levator palpebrae or superior rectus muscles is repaired [7]. Lacerations extending through the lid margin are repaired promptly. Wound gaping and notching of the lid margin result from contracture of the orbicularis muscle fibers that encircle the palpebral fissure. If repair is delayed for 7 to 10 days, these muscle fibers fibrose, the tarsal plate thickens and retracts, and the wound edges can no longer be approximated [31].

Surgeons inexperienced in repairing eyelid lacerations often feel compelled to perform complicated procedures, such as staggered or Z-plasty repairs, in an effort to prevent contracting deformities. The simplest type of anatomically accurate approximation with sutures is generally the best. Greatest care should be taken to approximate the tarsus and ciliary margin accurately. Once these structures have been sutured, the remainder of the eyelid falls into place.

Care must also be taken to preserve the integrity of the lacrimal apparatus and the canthal ligaments. A divided and grossly displaced lacrimal system may require cannulation with a fine polyethylene catheter and repair with overlying fine suture. (A 3-0 nylon suture acts as an excellent probe or splint for the lacrimal duct.) However, in instances of incomplete division, the lacrimal system may simply be approximated with expectation of good functional return, often without direct suture. Injury to the upper canaliculus alone rarely results in epiphora.

DACRYOCYSTORHINOSTOMY

Despite the apparent logic of performing dacryocystorhinostomy early, it is most often a secondary reconstructive operation performed months after healing of the original nasoorbital injury [31]. It is indicated to relieve epiphora and secondary obstructive dacryocystitis. These symptoms of obstruction in tear flow are caused by a missed or inadequately repaired lacrimal canaliculus, sac or duct injury, secondary scarring and stenosis, or obstruction in the lacrimal collecting system as a result of injury to adjacent bone or medial palbebral ligament [3].

Though many surgical techniques for dacryocystorhinostomy have been described, their shared underlying principle is the reestablishment of unobstructed tear drainage from the conjunctival sac into the nose [19]. When reestablishing the lacrimal collecting system, the medial canthal ligament must frequently be relocated and reattached to adjacent bone of the medial orbital wall. Also, because of bone resorption in the healing of comminuted, telescoped fractures of the nose or ethmoids, secondary bone reconstruction, often with bone grafts, is indicated. Therefore medial canthoplasty and reconstruction of the nasal pyramid are fre-

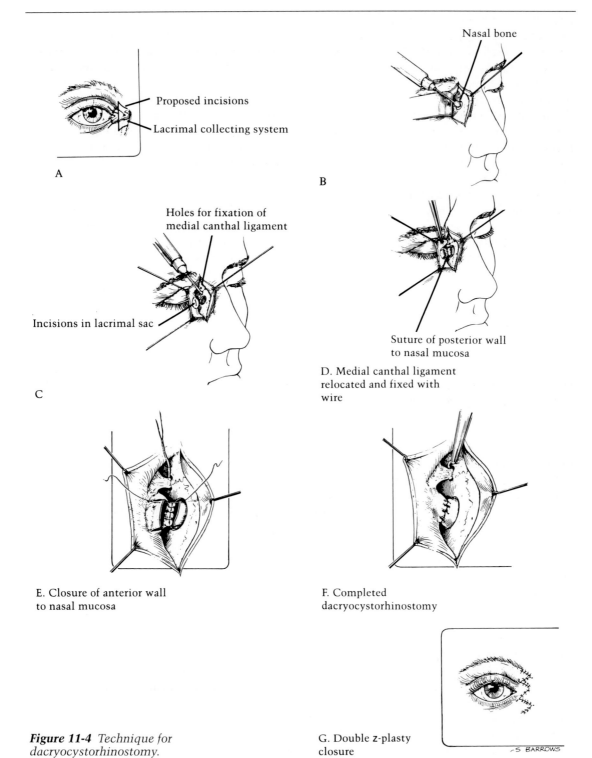

A

Proposed incisions

Lacrimal collecting system

B

Nasal bone

C

Holes for fixation of
medial canthal ligament

Incisions in lacrimal sac

Suture of posterior wall
to nasal mucosa

D. Medial canthal ligament
relocated and fixed with
wire

E. Closure of anterior wall
to nasal mucosa

F. Completed
dacryocystorhinostomy

G. Double z-plasty
closure

-S BARROWS

***Figure 11-4*** *Technique for
dacryocystorhinostomy.*

quently performed in conjunction with a dacryocystorhinostomy. If these procedures are done independently, the later operations become increasingly difficult owing to scar formation that results from the previous dissections.

The essence of one operation to reestablish unobstructed lacrimal flow is shown in Figure 11-4. A polyethylene catheter, small red rubber catheter, or Pyrex Jones tube keeps the newly formed drainage system open for 3 to 4 weeks until epithelialization of the constructed lacrimal tract has occurred.

The number of surgical techniques to correct this problem is an indication of the persistent problems seen with all of them. There are numerous instances in which the most logically planned procedure and the most refined surgical technique have had a disappointing outcome. It is likely that the best way to achieve a high rate of success with this procedure is to perform it within 1 to 2 days following injury [31].

When lower eyelid skin is avulsed or when it is resected because of nonviability, replacement is ideally accomplished either by transposition of skin from the adjacent upper eyelid (Fig. 11-5B) or by a full-thickness skin graft from the opposite upper eyelid or postauricular area. Thin split-thickness skin grafts fail to provide adequate elasticity, and eyelid contractures result. Similarly, stretching adjacent eyelid skin to cover any but the smallest defect is apt to result in eyelid distortion, especially in the lower lids.

EARS

Primary ear reconstruction is important, as secondary repair is not only considerably more difficult but the outcome is usually much less satisfactory [17].

Tissues making up the external ear are unique, and there is no good donor area for their substitution. Reconstruction becomes tedious and requires special skills. Therefore surgical débridement should be conserva-tive, and every effort is made to return tissue to its position of origin. Cutaneous blood supply is abundant, so that narrow, pedicled avulsion flaps and even avulsed or amputated composite tissue segments often survive if relocated anatomically. If the perichondrial-cutaneous sutures provide sufficient support, sutures in the cartilage may be unnecessary, especially in the conchal region. When sutures are required, nonabsorbable 5-0 monofilament nylon is a good choice, if it is not tied so tightly as to cut through the cartilage. Absorption of the suture material deep to the perichondrium is slow, making the use of catgut sutures in this area somewhat risky.

Information on treatment of amputated portions of the ear and hematoma of the ear is included in Chapter 13.

NOSE

With the exception of avulsion or amputation, soft tissue injuries to the nose are generally uncomplicated. Good healing can usually be obtained simply by accurate tissue approximation and refined suture technique. Soft tissues of the nose consist essentially of skin, cartilage, and mucous membrane. The superficial muscle fibers of the nose are sparse and, for the most part, adherent to the skin. Once the bony framework is put right, soft tissues need only be approximated with anatomic accuracy, taking special pains to align the nostril borders accurately.

Septal hematoma can be diagnosed with a nasal speculum. It is evacuated immediately through a small mucosal incision. An untreated septal hematoma typically results in chondromalacia, resulting in loss of septal cartilage, especially if infected, leaving a "saddle nose" deformity [6].

For injuries penetrating all soft tissue layers of the nose, it is easiest to repair the mucous membrane lining first, using 4-0 plain catgut suture. Torn septal, upper lateral, alar, and columellar cartilages can usually be reapproximated under direct vision through the wound and held in good position simply

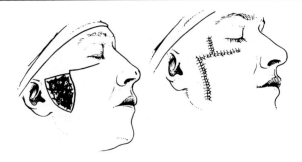

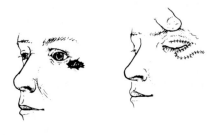

A. Rotation-advancement flap

B. Transposition flap

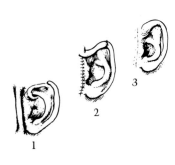

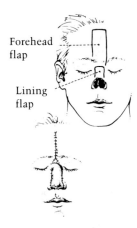

C. Tube pedicle flap

D. Direct distant pedicle flap

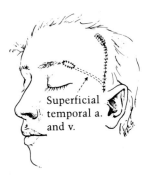

E. Subcutaneous island
pedicle flap

**Figure 11-5** *Five types of regional flap for repair and reconstruction of avulsion defects of the face.*

by accurate repair of the underlying mucous membrane and the overlying skin. Subcutaneous sutures are usually unnecessary if deep bites are taken through the skin and the sutures tied to achieve a slight eversion of skin edges. Interrupted sutures of 5-0 monofilament nylon are ideal.

Packing the nose with petrolatum-impregnated gauze is sometimes done to maintain the position of cartilaginous or bony fragments. However, if the supporting structures of the nose are accurately repositioned, packing is usually unnecessary and should be avoided when possible [31]. Not only do such packs interfere with the natural drainage of the nose and the beneficial effects of circulating air, but they are uncomfortable; moreover, removal of nasal packs may cause additional bleeding and separation of the repaired mucous membrane.

Skin grafts of the nose are ideally done with full-thickness postauricular grafts, which give the best possible match of color and texture. Thick split-thickness skin grafts can be used, however, and they are best obtained from exposed body areas, such as neck or arm, for good color match.

CHEEKS AND CHIN
Laceration of the cheek is the most commonly encountered facial injury. The superficial aspects of this repair are relatively simple, and the outcome is ordinarily satisfactory. However, important structures lying within the cheek deserve special mention: (1) branches of the facial nerve; (2) parotid gland and Stensen's duct; and (3) muscles of mastication and expression.

*Branches of the Facial Nerve*
Soft tissue injuries are of greatest concern when located in the posterior and inferior aspect of the cheek. Within this vital area lie the branches of the facial nerve, the parotid gland and duct, and the masseter muscle.

Major branches of the facial nerve are deep in the cheek, well protected by overlying soft tissue, and are seldom injured by accidental trauma. Exploration is not necessary to determine injury of this nerve; if division has occurred, unmistakable signs of lost muscle function will be present.

The most severe functional deficit of the face from division of a single nerve branch is that of the temporal branch, as it causes paralysis of the eyelid and subsequent exposure of the cornea. The marginal branch of the facial nerve is sometimes injured with lacerations about the lower jaw. This branch is always deep to the platysma muscle when posterior to the facial artery; it then courses near the lower border of the mandible, sometimes 1 cm below it.

Division of nerve branches anterior to the region of the parotid duct (midpupillary line) does not result in permanent loss of muscle function because the superficial facial muscles are innervated in their posterior portions and cross over from the contralateral side. Repair of these anterior branchings is therefore unnecessary. When there has been a clean division of the posterior portion of the facial nerve branches, as with a razor, the nerve sheaths are carefully approximated in fascicular units with fine soft suture. When there is greater damage, such as that caused by a blunt, penetrating object, the nerve ends require exploration and débridement prior to repair. This dissection is facilitated by use of a magnifying loupe or operating microscope. If portions of the nerve adjacent to the division have been damaged, the severed ends are sharply excised prior to anastomosis [2, 14]. A significant amount of nerve regeneration may occur following such a repair, but complete return of function is rare. In general, use of free nerve grafts or crossed anastomosis with other nerves is imprudent at the time of initial care [5].

*Parotid Gland and Stensen's Duct*
The parotid gland and duct are more superficial than the branches of the facial nerve and therefore are more exposed to injury. In-

jury is suspected when clear fluid is seen leaking from a wound of the posterior cheek. Drooping of half of the upper lip may also be associated with such an injury. The buccal branch of the facial nerve runs parallel to, and sometimes obliquely across, the parotid duct, and they are therefore often divided simultaneously.

The gland itself need not be sutured, but patency of the duct should be determined before the wound is closed. The parotid duct courses along a line from the tragus of the ear to the midportion of the upper lip. A parotid gland fistula usually closes spontaneously within a few days and almost always within 3 to 4 weeks [2]. If the fistula persists for several months, the severed duct can be sutured over a soft tubular splint.

A fine polyethylene catheter, such as an Intracath, may be used to cannulate Stensen's duct. When it is obvious that the duct has been divided and the external wound overlies the point of division, cannulation is most easily done in a retrograde fashion from the point of division. When the point of division is not easily accessible through the external wound, or if division of the duct is uncertain, intubation is through the ostium opposite the crown of the upper second molar tooth.

Catheterization through the ostium is made easier by retracting the cheek outward, thereby straightening the angulated portion of the cut. The portions of the duct that overlie the masseter muscle are more easily repaired, as the duct is fixed and thicker there. Once catheterized, the divided ends are approximated with fine, soft suture material, such as 6-0 silk, on an atraumatic cutting needle. If the duct has been only partially divided and there is relatively little associated injury in the area, the catheter may be safely removed following repair. If the duct has been completely divided or if there is other local injury, it is best to leave this catheter in place 5 to 7 days, or until most of the edema has resorbed. The catheter is best kept in place by looping it out of the mouth and taping the end low on the cheek or chin to encourage gravitational flow of parotid secretion.

When there is extensive damage to the duct or loss of duct tissue without laceration of the gland, the proximal cut end of the duct can be sutured to a new ostium in the oral mucosa as an alternate procedure to maintain parotid function. The proximal portion of the duct also may be ligated, following which the parotid gland atrophies and ceases to function.

Fascia, subcutaneous tissue, and skin are closed over a lacerated parotid gland. If the duct is patent, a subsequent parotid fistula eventually closes spontaneously.

*Muscles of Mastication and Expression*
Divided muscles of mastication and facial expression are repaired routinely. Tissue is returned to its original location whenever possible. Healing and return of function almost always occur even when these muscles are not repaired, but depression and broad overlying scars can then be anticipated.

Relatively superficial lacerations of the posterior chin may damage the marginal mandibular branch of the facial nerve, which may account for drooping of half of the lip by the loss of innervation of both levator and depressor muscles (mentalis and quadratus labii inferioris) of the lip. Therefore every effort is made to discover and repair such a division.

A unique injury can occur at the chin: The soft tissues are avulsed up from the anterior mandible, and the oral cavity is penetrated at the base of the lower lip [28]. The wound is tangential and enters the mouth at the level of the lower labial sulcus. It is important that this perforation into the mouth be recognized and repaired, as delayed healing and oral cutaneous fistula may result. The intraoral repair requires delicate tissue handling aided by the use of small atraumatic needles, as the gingival portion of the lower buccal sulcus is vital to proper closure but is easily torn if treated roughly.

## LIPS

Lip repair is always performed with respect to the vermilion border. "Step-off" or puckering in this area is not only unsightly but often difficult to correct later [16, 18].

Lip musculature is closed first, using 3-0 or 4-0 catgut. Blood is then completely cleaned from the vermilion border to make an accurate approximation.

The mucous membrane is closed next to avoid strain and "seesawing" of sutured skin. The mucous membrane is closed effectively with 3-0 or 4-0 vicryl sutures. As intraoral mucous membrane is highly elastic, this closure is done with concern for the vermilion border to avoid an excess of tissue on one or the other side.

## INTRAORAL INJURIES

Intraoral soft tissue wounds deserve special emphasis, as many reputable medical educators still teach that they may be left to heal spontaneously. This philosophy may have its origin in the observation that intraoral wounds and defects close rapidly by epithelialization [21]. Unfortunately, such uncontrolled and imprecise healing results in uncontrolled scarring and imprecise function, just as it does elsewhere in the body.

Intraoral war wounds are managed under different circumstances, and therefore delayed treatment and secondary reconstruction are often necessary [12]. Similar to war wounds are injuries from animal bites and neglected wounds; in general, these wounds are surgically débrided and approximated loosely. This treatment allows drainage and prevents abscess formation while minimizing scarring. A culture for bacteria and sensitivity studies are essential to the management of such injuries. Specific antibiotic therapy and attention to hygiene, such as rinsing with half-strength hydrogen peroxide, promote uncomplicated early healing.

In the mouth, as in the skin, nonabsorbable sutures cause less tissue reaction. On the other hand, absorbable sutures (e.g., catgut or synthetics) are easy to work with in the mouth and do not require removal. This convenience is especially appreciated in work with children, in whom suture removal is difficult and trying for both patient and physician.

## ANIMAL BITES

Facial injuries due to dog bites are the most common in the category of animal bites; they are usually sustained by young children. The injuries are invariably soft tissue wounds of a tearing nature and tend to follow a rather typical pattern: a crescent-shaped, deep laceration of the cheek, often extending to the oral commissure [34]. There are frequently parallel wounds on the cheek and occasionally a laceration or avulsion defect of the nasal tip. Such wounds of the cheek tend to gape and, at first glance, give the mistaken appearance that tissue is missing [16]. Human bites, though not as severe in appearance, have routinely proved to be more virulent from the standpoint of infection.

Animal bite wounds are heavily contaminated with microorganisms from the mouth of the animal; for this reason they are more apt to become infected than are other injuries (with the exception of the human bite wound). Because of this special concern, these wounds are best treated by prompt excision. If the patient is seen more than 6 hours after the injury, a more conservative surgical approach is followed, anticipating infection. Antibiotics are indicated, but frequently their use does not prevent infection [36].

Knowledge of the health of the animal is important. When the species and whereabouts of the animal are unknown, the physician is faced with the decision of whether to begin rabies vaccination. Persons bitten by rabid dogs are infected in only 10 to 20 percent of instances, the risk varying with wound site and the character of the bite. Bites about the face and neck are the most dangerous. The dog is infectious several days before symptoms appear. The virus is pres-

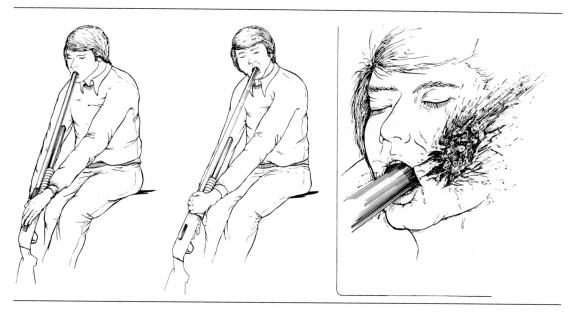

**Figure 11-6** *Attempting suicide with a shotgun placed in the mouth or underneath the chin is sometimes unsuccessful, creating instead extensive avulsion wounds of the cheek and facial bones. (From R. C. Schultz. Gunshot Wounds of the Face. In* Facial Injuries *[3rd ed.]. Chicago: Year Book, 1988. P. 496.)*

ent in the dog's saliva, and even an abrasion bathed in saliva may result in rabies infection. In humans the incubation period varies between 2 and 8 weeks, whereas in dogs the incubation period is thought to be shorter. This time differential is the basis for the observation of the confined animal before initiating antirabies treatment of the person who was bitten.

In suburban areas, where most dogs are known and commonly immunized for rabies, the risk of rabies is minimal. The ideal situation for all concerned is to have the animal confined under observation of a veterinarian. In this way, if the animal shows signs of rabies within 10 days, the patient can be treated by rabies vaccination within the incubation period. If the animal is killed, however, it is absolutely essential to have a microscopic examination of the brain for Negri bodies or the fluorescein antibody test to de-

termine if the animal was rabid [31]. When results are positive, rabies vaccination of the patient must begin at once.

## Gunshot Wounds of the Face

Gunshot wounds of the face can appear trivial or be among the worst injuries imaginable, depending on the range, velocity, and caliber of the shot [31]. The small-caliber wound of entrance may appear inconsequential, but damage created along its course may be extensive. Conversely, point-blank shotgun wounds inflict such severe damage to both soft tissue and bone that patient survival may appear doubtful. However, unless death is immediate, the latter injuries are usually survivable, despite the grotesque destruction of facial features. Surprisingly, those who attempt suicide by placing shotguns underneath the chin or in the mouth often survive because the length of the barrel is such that to pull the trigger the gun must be angled away from the central nervous system, thereby injuring only the face (Fig. 11-6). If the patient survives transportation to the hospital, he or she must be considered salvageable.

Missiles of smaller caliber with low velocity create much less damage, and the shot is often found harmlessly embedded in the face and, unless symptomatic, can often be left undisturbed. Shotgun wounds are ordinarily serious only when the gun has been fired at close range, especially at less than 10 feet. Nonsymptomatic, deeply embedded metallic missiles are best left alone when exploration is apt to cause further damage.

The primary objective of immediate care is maintenance of the upper airway. During transportation, sitting the patient upright may be all that is required; certainly, forceably strapping the patient supine is contraindicated. When surgery is imminent, an awake orotracheal intubation with a cuffed endotracheal tube of the largest appropriate size is ideal. An emergency tracheostomy may be necessary but can be difficult when there is massive bleeding and the patient is thrashing about in the semirecumbent position. Tracheostomy is best done over an endotracheal tube at the end of the initial operative procedure. Simultaneously, massive hemorrhage must be controlled accurately, as frenzied clamping of raw tissue can seriously damage functional structures. Hypovolemic shock is treated by lactated Ringer's solution and plasma until whole blood can be typed and crossmatched.

Débridement of all nonmetallic foreign bodies and nonviable tissue is performed at this stage along with stabilization of the bony framework of the face. Definitive rigid fixation of the facial fractures with and without bone grafts is ideally done at the onset, provided the patient can tolerate prolonged surgical time and adequate soft tissue coverage can be found. When such definitive care is not possible immediately, intermediate surgical procedures become necessary once the patient has stabilized. Interosseous rigid fragment fixation is accomplished by wiring, plates and screws, bone grafts, and even K wires. All fragments of viable soft tissue are preserved and replaced anatomically whenever possible, but definitive soft tissue

reconstruction is commonly a multistaged surgical undertaking stretched out over several years, depending on infection and the rapidity of scar maturation.

## Postoperative Care
### PSYCHOLOGICAL ASPECTS
All patients with extensive soft tissue facial injuries are fearful of disfigurement, especially women. They may even become hysterical in their fear. Firm reassurance by the surgeon, rather than sympathy, is the most effective remedy. However, in this effort to allay fear and reduce anxiety, one must be careful not to promise too much [33]. Implying to the patient that there will be no disfigurement or scars may lead to legal action later. If the patient needs unusual amounts of reassurance, one gives as much comfort as needed, but some responsible member of the family should be realistically informed [31].

The surgeon is commonly asked, "Will I have scars on my face?" Any penetration of the dermis results in scarring, and the patient should not be misinformed in this regard. With the techniques described, scars can often be kept minimal; and when the scars are mature, some become unnoticeable.

### INFECTION, ANTIBIOTICS, AND IMMUNIZATIONS
Infections in facial wounds are uncommon because of the rich vascular supply in this area, but they become far more common following massive bacterial inoculation, as with animal or human bites. It is for this reason that highly contaminated wounds are often excised prior to closure.

Infection of a facial injury is a serious detriment to healing and subsequently to function and appearance. Moreover, the infection is particularly dangerous because of ready communication of the organisms through the venous system to the cavernous sinuses. For these reasons, infections of the face deserve prompt attention. Bed rest, warm compresses locally, and specific systemic antibiotics are ordinarily all that is required. When buried foreign material is contributing to the infection, it must be removed.

As with any other wound, the danger of tetanus infection must be considered with facial injuries, especially puncture wounds. Because tetanus toxoid immunization has become widespread, there is now rarely an indication to use the tetanus antitoxin. When a booster dose of alum-precipitated tetanus toxoid seems insufficient to protect against tetanus, human tetanus immune globulin (Hyper-Tet) is much safer to use for the prevention of tetanus infection.

## Scars and Revisional Procedures

The *nature of facial scars* is often determined more by the character and location of the wound than by the technique of repair. A flat "hairline" scar without distortion of features is the aim of the surgeon.

Scars may heal with bumpy irregularity. This situation is seen when one side is higher or partially overlaps the other as well as after the healing of small avulsion flaps. Such scars can often be improved by surgical excision or abrasion.

Circular or U-shaped scars or those crossing natural skin folds usually benefit from some form of revision involving change in direction, lengthening, or staggering. Revision can be accomplished by Z-plasty, W-plasty, or V-Y techniques [31]. Skin grafting is occasionally necessary when skin has been avulsed or excised, leaving broad areas of contracting scar. However, grafting is avoided whenever other methods are applicable, as matching facial skin color and texture with a graft is difficult and the results may prove aesthetically disappointing.

### SCAR REVISION

Once scars have matured sufficiently, they may be revised. Red, raised, indurated, ugly scars are the most tempting to revise for the novice. However, these scars are the ones that are not ready for revision. The best results are obtained with revision after these scars have softened, faded, and flattened. These signs of maturation indicate control of inflammation and the establishment of capillary and lymphatic flow. The error lies not in waiting too long but in beginning too soon.

Most scar revisions of a limited area can be performed under local anesthesia and on an outpatient basis. As is the case for all elective facial operations, these patients are prepared with a scalp shampoo and oral hygiene; male patients are clean-shaven. The patient comes to the operating room with all cosmetics removed. If the patient has dentures, they are worn, as the appearance and apparent location of scars about the lower face may be changed considerably by the dentures.

First, the scar is outlined with methylene blue or a skin marking pen. This step is especially helpful when the periphery is irregular. It is much easier to correct mistakes made with the marker than those made with a scalpel.

After the scar is outlined, local anesthetic solution containing epinephrine is slowly injected about its periphery. A relatively bloodless field is available if the surgeon waits 7 minutes until the epinephrine takes effect.

Scars are excised as outlined through the full thickness of the skin into the subcutaneous tissue. Most of the subcutaneous portions of the scar are excised, but compulsive removal of all visible scar tissue is unnecessary and contributes to damage to adjacent structures or subsequent depression.

When scar excision extends deeply into the subcutaneous tissue or involves fascia and muscle, these deeper layers are best approximated with 4-0 plain catgut suture. For closure of the more superficial layers, a nonabsorbable soft suture, such as Vicryl or Mersilene (4-0 or 5-0), can be used. This suture should substantially incorporate the dermis in the closure, with the knot buried underneath the dermis. These sutures not only bring the skin surface into apposition and decrease dependence on the skin sutures but also help prevent subsequent spreading of revised scars. Depending on the location, length, and configuration of the scar, the skin may be approximated with intracuticular, interrupted, or continuous running monofilament nylon suture.

ALTERING SCAR POLARITY

Linear scars crossing normal skin folds contract and become hypertrophied. Lengthening and altering the polarity of such a scar by staggering relieves the contracture and greatly improves its appearance.

*Staggering*

Simple staggering can be accomplished by putting a deliberate angled limb in the scar, directly in or parallel to the skinfold at the site where the scar crosses it. Such a procedure may suffice, but the classic and more definite correction of linear scar contracture is the Z-plasty.

*Z-Plasty*

Z-plasty not only staggers a linear scar but lengthens it by interposing flaps of adjacent tissue. The principle of this simple procedure must be well understood so that it can be modified when necessary to adapt to a particular location on the face.

It is advisable to begin by marking the proposed incisions with a skin marker, as angles and flap lengths may be altered several times before obtaining the pattern desired. Although the classic Z-plasty is described as having equal triangular flaps drawn 60 degrees from the line of contracture, both size and angle may be varied considerably to accommodate a particular feature or facial area. Ideally, Z-plasty flaps comprise the full length of the contracted scar, but often it is not possible because of adjacent features. In these instances, either the flaps are made somewhat dissimilar for accommodation or multiple smaller Z's are used.

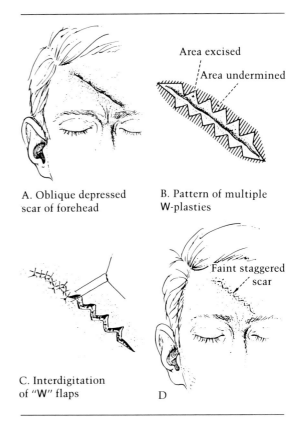

A. Oblique depressed scar of forehead

B. Pattern of multiple W-plasties

C. Interdigitation of "W" flaps

D

*Figure 11-7* Technique for W-plasty.

In a well planned Z-plasty, the flaps, once cut and undermined, often transpose themselves if relocation of tissue in the area is vital. Z-plasties should seldom be tiny, even when in series, as the total area of resulting scar then retains a linear orientation. Polarity is thus reestablished and contracture reappears.

*W-Plasty*

Another procedure designed principally for staggering linear scars is the W-plasty. Because this technique requires excision of multiple small triangles of normal skin to facilitate closure by interdigitation, little is gained in scar lengthening (Fig. 11-7).

Prior skin marking is important to ensure proper interpositioning of these small triangular flaps. This procedure is probably best

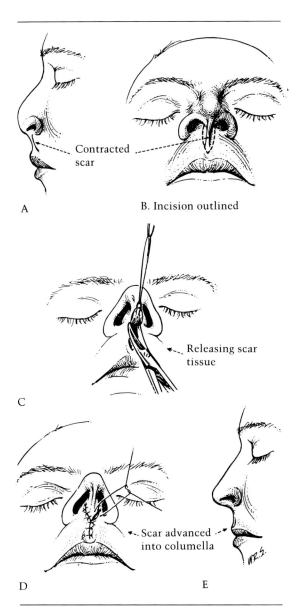

A

B. Incision outlined

Contracted scar

C

Releasing scar tissue

D                    E

Scar advanced into columella

**Figure 11-8** *Operative technique for V-Y-plasty at nasolabial angle.*

for long, depressed linear scars running obliquely across the forehead, cheeks, or chin.

Because of the multiplicity of flaps, angles, and adjacent surfaces, this type of closure sometimes heals with a pebbly surface. If it does, surgical abrasion using a motor-ized rotary abrader may offer additional improvement once the revised scar has matured.

### V-Y-*Plasty*

Just as the W-plasty is principally used to stagger linear scars, so the V-Y plasty is used principally to lengthen. In practice, converting a V to a Y scar has a minimal lengthening effect unless the scar is lengthened where redundancies form; however, the change in configuration is often beneficial to the surface contour on which the scar lies.

A broad V-shaped scar may become particularly disfiguring owing to contracture and edema of the central flap. If the scar is excised, a V-shaped defect results. By closing the bottom of the V in a linear manner, a Y-shaped scar is formed. It also facilitates closure of the long sides to the short sides of the surgical defect. Removal of these "dog ears" further lengthens the scar.

The procedure is especially useful for revising scars bridging the nasolabial angle at the columella (Fig. 11-8), as well as V-shaped scars at the oral commissures and palpebral canthi.

### AVULSION FLAPS AND U-SHAPED SCARS

Among the most disfiguring scars are those resulting from superiorly based avulsion flaps, particularly from windshield injuries. These crescent or U-shaped scars usually are depressed when they heal, thereby contributing to edema of the flap. Extensive undermining of the flap and tearing of its borders serve to interpose a broad scar between the flap and its bed. Use of continuous pressure immediately after repair not only diminishes deadspace and resulting fibrosis but also improves pressure gradients for venous and lymphatic return from the flap, thus reducing edema.

Softening and maturation of these scars sometimes takes more than a year. Even after several years the appearance is usually disappointing. When avulsion flaps are relatively small and their location is appropriate, they may be excised with their surrounding scar; if primary closure can be accomplished, the problem is immediately solved. When it is not possible, revision of the peripheral scar with staggering or Z-plasty procedures is indicated. The Z-plasties are placed at the curved portions of the scars where they cross normal skin lines. In addition to interrupting the constricting nature of the scar in this area, flaps of adjacent tissue interpolated with flaps cut from the avulsion flap bring in undamaged venous and lymphatic channels for improving drainage. Defatting the edematous flap is not corrective and produces still more fibrosis under the flap.

# References

1. Argenta, L. C., et al. The versatility of pericranial flaps. *Plast. Reconstr. Surg.* 76:695, 1985.
2. Barton, N. W., Miller, S. H., and Graham, W. P., III. Managing lacerations of the parotid gland, duct, and facial nerve. *Am. Fam. Physician* 13:130, 1976.
3. Becker, F. F. Reconstructive surgery of the medial canthal region. *Ann. Plast. Surg.* 7:259, 1981.
4. Bromberg, B. B. Soft-Tissue Injuries of the Face. In W. C. Grabb and J. W. Smith (eds.), *Plastic Surgery*. Boston: Little, Brown, 1975.
5. Bunkis, J., et al. The evolution of techniques for reconstruction of full thickness cheek defects. *Plast. Reconstr. Surg.* 70:319, 1982.
6. Clark, G. M. Trauma to the cartilaginous skeleton of the nose. *Eye Ear Nose Throat Monthly* 49:284, 1970.
7. Crawford, J. S. Ptosis as a result of trauma. *Can. J. Ophthalmol.* 9:244, 1974.
8. Ellingham, T. R. The immediate care of eye injuries. *Anesthesia* 31:433, 1976.
9. Goldberg, M. F., and Tessler, H. H. Occult intraocular perforations from brow and lid lacerations. *Arch. Ophthalmol.* 86:145, 1971.
10. Huelke, D. F., Grabb, W. C., and Dingman, R. O. Facial injuries due to windshield impacts in automobile accidents. *Plast. Reconstr. Surg.* 37:324, 1966.
11. Iverson, P. C. Surgical removal of traumatic tattoos of the face. *Plast. Reconstr. Surg.* 2:427, 1947.
12. Kathak, F. F., and Dubrul, E. L. The immediate repair of war wounds of the face. *Plast. Reconstr. Surg.* 2:110, 1947.
13. Kerster, T. E., and McQuarrie, D. G. Surgical management of shotgun injuries of the face. *Surg. Gynecol. Obstet.* 140:517, 1975.
14. McCabe, B. F. Facial nerve grafting. *Plast. Reconstr. Surg.* 45:70, 1970.
15. Mladick, R. A., and Carraway, J. H. Ear reattachment by the modified pocket principle. *Plast. Reconstr. Surg.* 51:584, 1973.
16. Musgrave, R. H., and Garrett, W. S. Dog bite avulsions of the lip. *Plast. Reconstr. Surg.* 49:294, 1972.
17. Ohlsen, L., Skoog, T., and Shon, S. A. The pathogenesis of cauliflower ear. *Scand. J. Plast. Reconstr. Surg.* 9:34, 1975.
18. Pitts, W., Pickrell, F., and Quinn, G. Electrical burns of lips and mouth in infants and children. *Plast. Reconstr. Surg.* 44:471, 1969.
19. Putterman, A. M., and Eipstein, G. Combined Jones tube canalicular intubation and conjunctival dacryocystorhinostomy. *Am. J. Ophthalmol.* 91:513, 1981.
20. Schultz, R. C. Organized hematoma. *J.A.M.A.* 189:215, 1964.
21. Schultz, R. C. Intraoral sutures. *J.A.M.A.* 195:400, 1966.
22. Schultz, R. C. Facial injuries from automobile accidents: A study of 400 consecutive cases. *Plast. Reconstr. Surg.* 40:415, 1967.
23. Schultz, R. C. Facial injuries from automobile accidents. *Surg. Gynecol. Obstet.* 127:151, 1968.
24. Schultz, R. C. 760 Consecutive cases of facial injury. *Dent. Abstr.* 13:29, 1968.
25. Schultz, R. C. The changing pattern and management of soft tissue windshield injuries. In D. Huelke (ed.), *Proceedings of the 1970 Meeting of the American Association for Automotive Medicine*. Ann Arbor: University of Michigan Press, 1970.
26. Schultz, R. C. One thousand cases of major facial injury. *Rev. Surg.* 37:394, 1970.
27. Schultz, R. C. One thousand major facial injuries from auto accidents. In *Proceedings of the International Association for Accident and Traffic Medicine*. Ann Arbor, MI: Highway Safety Research Institute, 1971.

28. Schultz, R. C. The changing character and management of soft tissue windshield injuries. *J. Trauma* 12:1, 1972.
29. Schultz, R. C. The nature of facial injury emergencies. *Surg. Clin. North Am.* 52:1, 1972.
30. Schultz, R. C. Facial Injuries. In R. E. Condon and L. M. Nyhus (eds.), *Manual of Surgical Therapeutics* (3rd ed.). Boston: Little, Brown, 1975.
31. Schultz, R. C. *Facial Injuries* (2nd ed.). Chicago: Year Book, 1977.
32. Schultz, R. C., and Baker, S. P. Recurrent problems in emergency room management of maxillofacial injuries. *Clin. Plast. Surg.* 2:65, 1975.
33. Schultz, R. C., and deCamara, D. L. Athletic facial injuries. *J.A.M.A.* 252:3395, 1984.
34. Schultz, R. C., and McMaster, W. C. The treatment of dog bite injuries, especially those of the face. *Plast. Reconstr. Surg.* 49:494, 1972.
35. Schultz, R. C., and Oldham, R. J. An overview of facial injuries. *Surg. Clin. North Am.* 57:987, 1977.
36. Shannon, G. M. Treatment of dog bite injuries of eyelids and adnexa. *Ophthalmic Surg.* 6:41, 1975.

# 12

# Facial Fractures

*Paul Manson*

The treatment of facial fractures has undergone significant change in the last ten years. The advent of computed tomographic scanning [46, 48, 140, 141] has allowed visualization of both soft tissue and bone with unexcelled clarity, and regional trauma centers provide improved diagnostic capabilities and supportive care for the multiply injured patient. Prompt definitive evaluation of all injuries allows the plastic surgeon to operatively approach facial injuries at an early time. Finally, the application of craniofacial techniques [80, 171], extended open reduction [106], immediate bone grafting [56], and the use of plate-and-screw fixation [146] have improved the quality as well as the functional and aesthetic results of facial fracture treatment.

The etiology of facial injuries in the United States is frequently a motor vehicle or motorcycle accident. Victims often present with multiple injuries [59, 102, 116, 150] that require the simultaneous coordinated effort of a multiple specialty team. The use of seatbelts [21], observance of the speed limit, and avoidance of driving while intoxicated have fortunately lowered the incidence of such fractures. Other common

causes of facial injuries are physical altercations, athletic injuries, and home accidents. Early definitive treatment of maxillofacial injuries need not compromise the survival of a multiply injured patient. Prompt treatment maximizes functional and aesthetic results and yields grateful patients who are more fully able to return to productive roles in society.

## Priorities of Care in Maxillofacial Injury Treatment

Care for the patient with maxillofacial injuries may be organized according to three priorities: (1) emergency care; (2) early care; and (3) nonemergent definitive treatment.

### EMERGENCY TREATMENT
The emergency care of facial injuries identifies conditions that require immediate treatment for the prevention of life-threatening complications. Such conditions include (1) maintenance of the airway; (2) prevention of hemorrhage; (3) identification and prevention of aspiration; and (4) identification of other injuries, e.g., cervical spine, intracranial, thoracic, and abdominal injuries.

### Maintenance of the Airway
Maintenance of the airway and the provision of adequate ventilation is of supreme impor-

This chapter uses material from P. Natvig and R. K. Dortzbach. Facial Bone Fractures. In W. C. Grabb and J. W. Smith (eds.), *Plastic Surgery* (3rd ed.). Boston: Little, Brown, 1979.

347

tance for patients with fractures of the facial bones. Facial fractures may impair ventilation in several ways. Facial bone fragments may be displaced with airway obstruction. An example is the comminuted mandibular fracture with posterior displacement, in which the unsupported tongue falls against the posterior wall of the pharynx and obstructs ventilation. Blood may interfere with respiration or may be aspirated into the trachea. The hemorrhage accompanying facial fractures produces swelling, edema, and hematoma, which may narrow the airway. Any of these conditions may compromise the airway. Fractured or avulsed teeth, blood clots, broken dentures or bridgework, and foreign materials (e.g., glass, metal fragments, clothing) may be forced into areas where the airway is impaired. The examiner must remove these items. In those patients who demonstrate compromise of the airway or respiratory embarrassment, endotracheal intubation or tracheostomy is completed. Airway obstruction is usually a prolonged threat in patients with burns, concomitant fractures of the upper and lower jaws, concomitant fractures of the nose and maxilla, fractures of the larynx, and injuries that result in significant swelling of the neck, floor of the mouth, pharynx, or soft palate. Symptoms that indicate impending respiratory obstruction include noisy respirations, stridor, hoarseness, retraction, drooling, and inability to swallow or handle secretions. Cyanosis is an extreme condition signifying complete inability to breathe and impending demise. The alert examiner anticipates the respiratory emergency and performs tracheal intubation or tracheotomy before complete respiratory obstruction demands a chaotic "emergency" tracheotomy or a "crash" intubation.

TRACHEOTOMY. A tracheotomy is performed to relieve obstruction at or above the larynx. It consists in making an artificial opening into the trachea. Patients with multiple fractures of the facial bones are often best managed with a tracheotomy in preference to prolonged endotracheal intubation if

intermaxillary fixation is necessary. Simultaneous requirements for nasal packing and interdental fixation compromise the airway; in these cases a tracheotomy is often preferable to prolonged nasal intubation. Skilled anesthesiologists may change the location of the endotracheal tube from the nose to the mouth during an operative procedure to facilitate fracture reduction. Operative procedures are often more easily accomplished and the provision for precise occlusal relations and intraoral surgery more certain if a tracheotomy is performed. The danger of accidental extubation during the postoperative period rests in the inability to reintubate a patient in intermaxillary fixation with significant facial and neck swelling.

Tracheotomy is considered for the following fractures: (1) panfacial fractures (combined maxillary, nasal, and mandibular fractures); (2) the multiply fractured mandible with significant swelling of the neck and floor of the mouth; (3) patients who require intermaxillary fixation who also have significant head or chest injuries (the patient is unlikely to be able to manage his airway within 1 week); and (4) the patient with significant soft tissue swelling (burns). Tracheostomy may be avoided if a stable (plate-and-screw) fixation system is utilized for facial fracture treatment, which makes postoperative intermaxillary fixation unnecessary.

A tracheotomy is usually performed through a transverse incision located two fingerbreadths above the suprasternal notch (Fig. 12-1). A roll placed under the shoulders allows extension of the neck (if not contraindicated by cervical spine injury), which facilitates exposure. The skin is incised and the subcutaneous tissue divided down to the strap muscles. A vertical fascial incision in the midline is used to separate the strap muscles. The thyroid isthmus, if it intervenes, is divided and the trachea identified. A hook is used to elevate the trachea, and a vertical incision is made in the third and fourth tracheal rings. No segment of trachea should be excised, nor should cruciate inci-

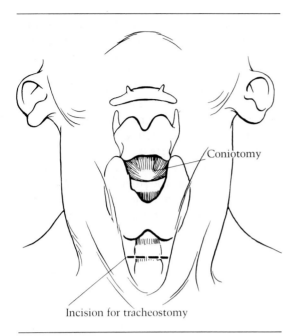

Coniotomy

Incision for tracheostomy

***Figure 12-1*** *The skin incision for tracheostomy is indicated between the third and fourth tracheal rings. The trachea is opened with a single vertical incision. The site for an emergency coniotomy (above) is located between the thyroid and cricoid cartilages. A coniotomy is converted to a tracheostomy as soon as possible.*

sions be made. An appropriately sized tube is placed in the trachea, and the flanges are both sutured to the skin; a tie is then placed about the neck to prevent the tube from becoming dislodged. Complications of tracheostomy include innominate vein erosion, tracheal stenosis, pneumothorax, and accidental decannulation [19, 115].

In an extreme emergency, a coniotomy (cricothyroidotomy) (see Fig. 12-1) can be performed, as this procedure is more easily accomplished than a formal tracheostomy, with less dissection and chance of hemorrhage. This "superior tracheotomy" is performed through the cricothyroid (conic) ligament, which connects the thyroid and cricoid cartilages. A horizontal incision is made between the thyroid and cricoid cartilages, and the subcutaneous tissue and the

conic ligament are divided. A tube is inserted into the trachea. A standard tracheotomy is then done and the coniotomy closed as soon as the situation permits. The coniotomy is not allowed to remain for an extended period, as laryngeal or tracheal stricture and fibrosis are possible.

It is emphasized that a tracheotomy or intubation is performed if there is reasonable suspicion that airway obstruction is possible. Death from upper respiratory obstruction is almost always a preventable complication, and intubation "in the field" in appropriate instances is a life-saving maneuver.

*Profuse Hemorrhage*
Major hemorrhage accompanying maxillofacial injuries may occur from open wounds and lacerations or may accompany closed facial fractures. The bleeding that accompanies facial lacerations may result in significant hemorrhage, particularly if a large artery has been partially divided by the injury. External bleeding is controlled with digital pressure until precise identification of *only* the bleeding vessel is accomplished. Blind probing with clamps in the area of important cranial nerves, such as the facial nerve, must be avoided, as permanent damage may be produced by crushing clamps.

Bleeding in closed facial fractures usually results from lacerations of arteries and veins adjacent to the walls of fractured sinuses. Significant hemorrhage may result and presents from the nose and mouth. Bleeding from the nose may occur in association with any of the following: nasal, zygomatic, orbital, frontal sinus, nasoethmoidal, maxillary, or anterior cranial fossa fractures. It is not specific for a nasal injury alone. The most significant nasopharyngeal bleeding accompanies Le Fort maxillary fractures. Several steps allow control of such hemorrhage from closed injuries.

***1.*** *Reduction of fractures.* Gross malalignment of facial bone fractures contributes to hemorrhage; frequently manual repositioning of the fracture segments reduces bleeding. Maxillary fractures, for instance, display less hemorrhage when the patient is placed in intermaxillary fixation.

*2. Anteroposterior nasal packing.* Anteroposterior packing of the nose is the most efficient method for controlling profuse nasopharyngeal bleeding. A posterior pack serves as an obturator in the nasopharynx and may be either an inflated Foley catheter balloon or a gauze pack. The nasal cavity may then be tightly packed with antibiotic-impregnated gauze against this posterior pack or Foley balloon. If the hemorrhage persists through the packing, the anterior packing is removed and the cavity repacked, as it is likely that the packing has not been properly placed for tamponade of the bleeding. The packing is generally removed in 24 to 48 hours. Caution is exercised not to exert excessive prolonged pressure on the columella or septum, which would produce necrosis. Early removal of the packing is considered if a cerebrospinal fluid leak is present. It is possible to enter the orbit or cranial cavity with packing material if significant orbital or cranial base fractures are present.

*3. Soft wraparound facial compression dressing.* This measure may provide additional pressure over a short period to decrease hemorrhage accompanying facial fractures. Excessive pressure on soft tissue over bony prominences may produce tissue necrosis.

*4. External carotid ligation.* When profuse hemorrhage from closed fractures has not responded to the above maneuvers, arterial ligation may be considered, though it is rarely necessary. If employed, the bilateral external carotid and superficial temporal arteries are ligated. The external carotid is approached through a transverse incision in the upper neck, and the superficial temporal artery is approached through an incision in the hair above the ear. The combination of these arterial ligations most effectively reduces blood flow in the internal maxillary artery, which is the usual cause of profuse uncontrolled hemorrhage. Selective arterial liga-

tions, such as the internal maxillary or ethmoidal artery, may be performed, but in the presence of acute profuse hemorrhage, these procedures may be difficult and the results disappointing.

*5. Blood replacement.* In patients with profuse hemorrhage, coagulation factors may be depleted. Bleeding abnormalities are noted early in patients with cerebral injuries. The hourly assessment of coagulation with a prothrombin time and a partial thromboplastin time is an important assessment of patients with continuing hemorrhage. Patients with brain injuries often have a diffuse coagulopathy in the absence of hemorrhage.

### Aspiration
Aspiration of blood, saliva, and gastric contents frequently accompanies maxillofacial injuries. It is an underappreciated mechanism of respiratory insufficiency and occurs commonly, especially in patients with cerebral injuries. Endotracheal intubation or tracheostomy limits aspiration if the tube cuff is inflated. During the operative treatment of facial fractures, the use of a throat pack prevents irrigation fluids and blood from entering the larynx and protects against pulmonary injury. The surgeon must remember to remove this pack at the end of the procedure.

### Accompanying Regional Injuries
CERVICAL SPINE INJURIES. Patients with facial fractures are frequently the victims of cervical fractures or head injuries [6, 16, 100]. The examiner must be alert to confirm that these injuries are not present. There is an association between mandibular fractures and upper cervical spine fractures [100], and the presence of a mandibular fracture prompts careful evaluation of the cervical spine. Cervical spine fractures most likely to be overlooked are those occurring at either the upper or the lower end of the spine [100]. If the entire cervical spine is not visualized radiographically and the absence

of symptoms confirmed, the patient must be managed as if a cervical fracture were present, protecting him by proper immobilization. Standard approaches to facial fractures may require modification if the cervical fracture does not permit rotation or extension of the neck [100].

INTRACRANIAL INJURIES. Intracranial injuries often accompany facial fractures [10, 57], especially those of the upper face [110, 118]. If significant intracranial injury exists, a craniofacial evaluation with computed tomography is mandatory. If a patient with a significant intracranial injury requires a general anesthetic, monitoring the intracranial pressure during the procedure is considered so that any deterioration in intracranial condition can be immediately identified. The use of intracranial pressure monitoring has allowed safe anesthesia for those patients who demonstrate brain injury and facial fractures [99]. Pressures in excess of 25 torr usually contraindicate the safe operative treatment of facial injuries. Evaluation with the Glascow Coma Scale [163] (Table 12-1) facilitates classification of head injuries when combined with analysis of the computed tomography (CT) scan.

REMOTE INJURIES

Patients with dramatic facial injuries are often rapidly assigned to subspecialty services with an incomplete multisystem evaluation. Every patient with the possibility of multiple injuries [59, 102, 116, 150] must have an evaluation of the chest with an upright radiograph to identify conditions such as pneumothorax, pulmonary contusion, aspiration, or a widened mediastinum (indicating possible aortic vascular injury). Abdominal paracentesis and lavage disclose the possibility of significant injury to an abdominal viscus. A film of the pelvis discloses fractures that can result in silent retroperitoneal hemorrhage. The identification of these ancillary injuries allows accurate assessment of the total patient and permits

*Table 12-1* *Glascow coma scale*

| Criteria | Points |
| --- | --- |
| Eyes open | 5 |
| Spontaneously | 4 |
| To speech | 3 |
| To pain | 2 |
| None | 1 |
| Best verbal response | |
| Oriented | 5 |
| Confused | 4 |
| Inappropriate | 3 |
| Incomprehensible | 2 |
| None | 1 |
| Best motor response | |
| Obey commands | 5 |
| Localize pain | 4 |
| Flexion to pain | 3 |
| Extension to pain | 2 |
| None | 1 |

safe early treatment of facial injuries. It is important that subspecialists *confirm* that this multisystem evaluation has been properly performed to avoid complications under general anesthesia.

In the past, it was desirable to defer operations on facial fractures to allow the progress of occult intracranial, intrathoracic, or intraabdominal injuries to be assessed over days to weeks. In the absence of the more invasive diagnostic maneuvers described, it was a prudent course. Nowadays, however, delayed treatment is neither necessary nor desirable. Many patients with facial injuries benefit from definitive early treatment, which is allowed by the multisystem evaluation.

EARLY MAXILLOFACIAL INJURY CARE

The early care of patients with maxillofacial injuries consists of a history and physical examination, appropriate radiographic examinations, closure of soft tissue lacerations, application of arch bars and intermaxillary fixation devices, preparation of models and fabrication of splints, and early fracture reduction.

*History*

The events of the injury are ascertained and a complete history of the accident or injury documented in the chart. The patient's medical history is also obtained, as medical diseases may influence the type or timing of treatment to be rendered.

*Physical Examination*

A thorough physical examination is performed, concentrating on the areas of injury. Consultations from other specialists, such as an ophthalmologist and a neurosurgeon, are obtained when appropriate.

FACIAL LACERATIONS. The location, length, and apparent depth of facial lacerations are documented. Lacerations, contusions, and bruises imply damage to deeper structures, and, if present, a complete functional examination of the region is performed. It is assumed that there is a fracture under each bruise or laceration until an appropriate clinical examination with appropriate radiographs has shown otherwise.

SYMPTOMS OF FACIAL FRACTURES. Facial structures are examined in an orderly fashion, proceeding from the upper to the lower face or vice versa. The symptoms produced by facial injuries may include the abovementioned soft tissue injuries, tenderness or pain, crepitation from underlying bony movement, numbness in the distribution of a sensory nerve, paralysis in the distribution of a motor nerve, malocclusion of the teeth, visual disturbance (diplopia or diminution of vision), facial asymmetry, deformity, obstructed respiration, air in soft tissues, intraoral lacerations, and nasopharyngeal bleeding.

An accurate clinical examination begins with an evaluation of the symmetry of facial structures. Comparison of the sides of the face is important, and reference can be made to old photographs often contained in the patient's identification. Such photographs document preexisting asymmetry. After a thorough visual inspection and comparison, all bony surfaces are palpated, running the fingers over the orbital rims, nose, brows, zygomatic arches, malar eminences, and borders of the mandible.

Gloves are worn for the intraoral examination, which involves palpation of the maxillary and mandibular dentition, carefully noting any avulsed or loose teeth or intraoral lacerations. The dental arches are assessed for movement laterally and anteroposteriorly. Localized tenderness and abnormal movement indicate underlying fracture.

Facial sensation is noted, examining the supraorbital, infraorbital, and mental branches of divisions of the trigeminal nerve. Absent or diminished sensation in the distribution of a sensory nerve indicates that a fracture may be present somewhere along the course of a nerve.

Facial expression is noted and its symmetry compared between frontal, orbital, buccal, and marginal mandibular branches. Extraocular movements and pupillary response are noted, again evaluating symmetry. Pupillary size, eyelid excursion, and the presence of palpebral or subconjunctival hematoma are noted.

An intranasal examination allows identification of lacerations, hematoma, or areas of obstruction inside the nose. The excursion of the jaws is noted, and any pain present on movement is identified. Deviation of the jaws on movement or the presence of an abnormal relation of the dentition is confirmed by careful examination of the patient in occlusion. Often the patient's subjective sensation of malocclusion is an important guide to a mandibular or maxillary fracture. The presence of fractured or missing teeth indicates the possibility of maxillary or mandibular fracture. Dentures and nonfixed bridgework are removed to permit accurate evaluation.

The presence of a significant periorbital hematoma should not prevent examination of the globe and assessment of vision and intraocular pressure. Indeed, one should suspect an intraocular injury when there is a hematoma in the periorbital area. Clear fluid draining from the nose indicates cerebrospinal fluid rhinorrhea and signifies a fracture of the anterior cranial fossa. Usually these fractures involve the cribriform plate of the skull.

CLASSIFICATION OF FACIAL FRACTURES. Facial fractures are classified as closed or open injuries as well as by the anatomic region involved. The latter serves as the major basis for classification. The anatomic areas in the upper face are the frontal bone, frontal sinus, and supraorbital areas. The orbit is divided into the rim and the internal orbit. Rim fractures are classified in three sections and the internal orbit in four sections. The upper portion of the orbital rim is the supraorbital region; the medial portion of the orbital rim is the nasoethmoidal region; and the inferior and lateral orbital rim constitutes the zygomatic region. The internal orbit consists of the medial (ethmoidal) orbit, the inferior orbit (orbital "floor"), the lateral orbit, and the superior (roof) portions. Maxillary fractures are classified according to the general scheme of Le Fort. The nose and mandible complete the anatomic regional areas of the face.

The biomechanical basis for facial injuries involves an impact [126, 159, 160] with inbending of bone at the area of impact. Fractures also may occur distant to the impact [49, 78, 96, 159, 160], at areas of reciprocal "outbending;" usually the "outbending" occurs in areas of weak bone.

### Radiographic Examination

Radiographic examination provides important evidence to confirm the findings of the physical examination [5]. The appropriate radiologic examination of the patient usually includes plain radiographs, a CT scan, and special radiographs, such as a Panorex or apical views of specific teeth.

Plain radiographs consist in the following views, which may be reversed if the patient cannot be turned.

1. Water's view of the skull. This view is the single most valuable radiograph and identifies the lateral and inferior orbital rim, the lateral walls of the maxillary sinuses, and the nose. The zygoma, nasal bones, nasal septum, and mandible can also be visualized.
2. Towne's view of the skull. This view is helpful for evaluating condylar and subcondylar fractures in the mandible.
3. Posteroanterior (Caldwell) skull view. The frontal bone, zygomaticofrontal suture, frontal sinus, medial orbital rim, and ethmoidal areas are visualized. The ramus of the mandible and angle region are also shown.
4. Lateral skull film. The frontal sinus is visualized, as are the roofs of the orbit and the facial bones in lateral projection.
5. Posteroanterior and lateral oblique films of the mandible. These specialized films show the mandibular symphysis and parasymphysis areas; and the lateral oblique films demonstrate the mandibular body, ramus, condylar, and coronoid areas.
6. Panorex examination. This examination utilizes a rotating x-ray tube and may not be possible if the patient cannot stand and cooperate. It shows the entire mandible and lower maxilla on one radiograph and is the most valuable film for evaluation of the mandibular fracture.

A CT scan is essential for evaluation of mid and upper facial fractures [46, 88, 140, 141]. Its use is routine for fractures involving the frontal bone, frontal sinus, orbit, nasoethmoidal, zygomatic, and maxillary areas; it is helpful in the evaluation of condylar fractures and dislocations. Its use has virtually replaced plain films for the mid and upper face.

### Dental Impression and Models

For fractures involving the dentition, it is often helpful to obtain an alginate impression of the maxillary and mandibular dental

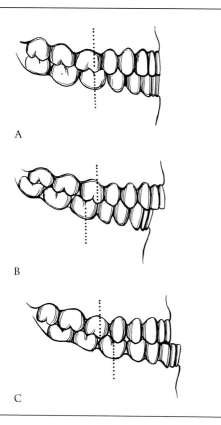

A

B

C

**Figure 12-2** *Angle classification of occlusion. A. Class I, normal occlusion. B. Class II, retroocclusion or mandibular deficiency. C. Class III, prognathic occlusion (maxillary deficiency or mandibular excess).*

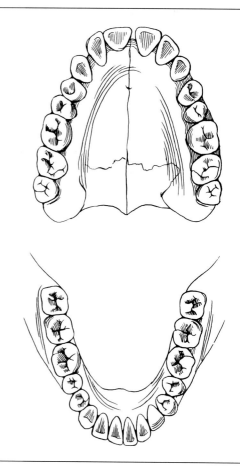

**Figure 12-3** *Normal adult dental arches contain 32 teeth, 16 in each arch. There are three molars, two bicuspids, a cuspid, and two incisors on each half of both maxillary and mandibular dental arches.*

arches. These impressions are utilized for the preparation of stone models, which serve as a patient record and allow leisurely study of the occlusion between the fracture fragments [72]. The ideal dental relation can be identified after the stone model is sectioned at the sites of fracture. The sections are then replastered and used to construct acrylic splints to assist fracture reduction and immobilization. The dental impressions are best obtained at the time of the initial evaluation and prior to placement of intermaxillary fixation devices.

OCCLUSION AND DENTAL RELATIONS. Occlusion is the relation of the upper and lower teeth as they fit together. The determination of occlusal relations and the reduction of fractures often demands knowledge of precise occlusal relations. Although a wide variety of dental relations is possible, occlusal relations are defined in terms of the Angle classification system [5] (Fig. 12-2). Identified in this system are relations between the first molar, cuspid (or canine), and incisor teeth. The incisor relation and prominence of the jaws is noted. The permanent or secondary dentition is composed of 32 teeth (Fig. 12-3): two central incisors, two lateral incisors, four premolars, and three molars in

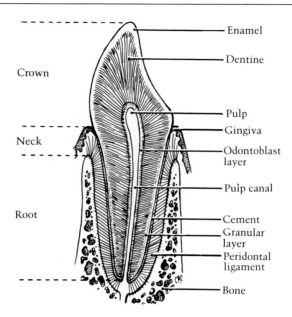

Crown

Neck

Root

Enamel

Dentine

Pulp

Gingiva

Odontoblast
layer

Pulp canal

Cement

Granular
layer

Peridontal
ligament

Bone

**Figure 12-4** *Structure of the normal tooth. The anatomic areas of a normal tooth are identified. The crown is the projecting portion. The periodontal ligament secures the tooth to the bone. Note the location of the pulp canal for the neurovascular vessels with the entrance of the vessels and nerve at the apex of the tooth. Fractures through the apex of the tooth devitalize the pulp and predispose to abscess formation.*

each of the upper and lower dental arches. The anterior teeth consist of the incisors and canines. The posterior teeth consist of the premolars and molars.

TERMS SIGNIFYING DIRECTION IN DENTAL ANATOMY. The surfaces of the teeth that face an imaginary line drawn between the central incisors in the midsagittal plane are known as the *mesial surfaces*. The surfaces that face away from this line are identified as *distal surfaces*. The term *mesial* thus identifies a direction toward the midline, and the term *distal* identifies a direction away from the midline. For the lower teeth, *labial* and *buccal surfaces* indicate those areas that face either the cheek or the lip. *Lingual surfaces* face the tongue. The *occlusal surfaces* of the

teeth face the adjacent upper or lower dental arch. The *interproximal space* is the potential space between the teeth. For the upper jaw, the *palatal surface* of the teeth faces the palate, and the buccal and labial surfaces face the cheek and the lip, respectively.

The anterior teeth have knife-like incisal edges that allow the tearing of food. The occluding surfaces of the premolar and molar dentition are suited for grinding functions. The incisors and canines have a single root. The premolars have one or two roots, and the molars have two or three roots. The third molars may be fully or partially erupted or impacted (submerged) within alveolar bone.

The teeth are located in a projecting bony process of the mandible and maxilla called the *alveolar process*. Each tooth has its own socket, or alveolus. The portion of a tooth projecting above the gum line is termed the *crown* and that below it the *root* (Fig. 12-4). The crown is covered by glistening enamel and the root by cementum. The inner structure of the tooth consists of dentin and a root canal or pulp chamber containing the nerve and blood supply to the tooth. Each

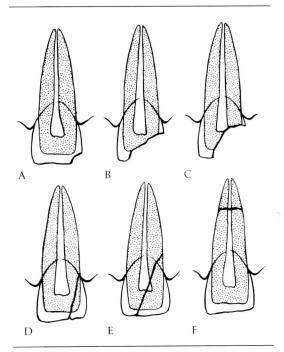

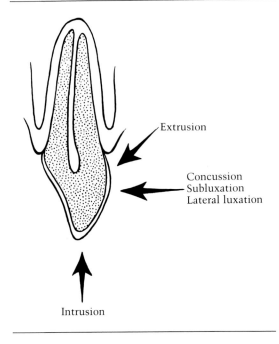

**Figure 12-5** *Dental injuries. A. Enamel fracture. B. Fracture extending into dentin. C. Fracture extending into the pulp (requires emergent treatment). D. Fracture of the crown. E. Fracture of the crown extending into the root structure and involving the pulp. F. Fracture of the root. (If the apex of the tooth is involved, necrosis of the pulp is likely.)*

**Figure 12-6** *Dislocations involving teeth. Extrusion tends to force the tooth out of the socket. The tooth is replaced and stabilized. Concussion, subluxation, and lateral luxation tend to force the tooth posteriorly, sideways, or anteriorly in the socket. Replacement and stabilization are indicated. Intrusion forces the tooth into the alveolus. The tooth is allowed to reerupt.*

tooth is anchored in its socket by a strong periodontal ligament, which attaches the tooth to alveolar bone.

Prior to eruption of the permanent dentition, primary or deciduous teeth are present. The deciduous teeth consist of 20 teeth divided between the two arches. There are two central and two lateral incisors, two canines, and four molars in each dental arch. The permanent 6-year molar erupts behind the second deciduous molar.

TEETH IN THE LINE OF FRACTURE. Fracture lines in the mandible or maxilla often travel through or around a tooth socket. The tooth may be fractured (Fig. 12-5) or loosened in its socket (Fig. 12-6). With the advent of antibiotics and more accurate fixation devices,

many teeth can be salvaged [82, 127, 149], and it is not necessary to extract every tooth adjacent to or involved in a fracture. Loose or carious teeth are removed, and generally third molars in a fracture site are removed unless the removal would create fracture displacement and necessitate open reduction of a fracture that otherwise would be amenable to closed reduction.

INTERMAXILLARY FIXATION. The standard immobilization technique for fractures involving the upper and lower jaws consists of ligating arch bars to the teeth of each jaw (Fig. 12-7). These arch bars can then be connected with intermaxillary wires, which hold the teeth of the upper and lower jaws in a specific dental relation. Arch bars are

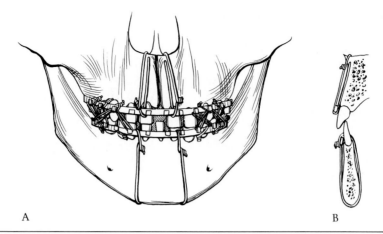

A                                                    B

*Figure 12-7* A. Placement of arch bars involves ligating metal bars with lugs to the molar, premolar, and cuspid teeth. The maxillary and mandibular bars may then be connected with wires or elastics to accomplish intermaxillary fixation. These bars, especially in the partially dentulous patient or the patient with mixed dentition, are stabilized with circummandibular and piriform aperture wires as indicated. B. Lateral view of the relation of the piriform aperture and circummandibular wires to the arch bars and the maxillary and mandibular alveolar processes and basal bone of the maxilla and mandible.

generally ligated to the molar, premolar, and cuspid teeth under local or general anesthesia. The arch bars are connected by wires or elastics and generally remain in place for 4 to 8 weeks. The intermaxillary wires may be omitted until the danger of vomiting or respiratory obstruction has passed in those patients recovering from a general anesthesia. If control of fracture fragments makes immediate intermaxillary fixation mandatory, appropriate consideration is given to prolonged nasotracheal intubation or tracheostomy, so that the patient's airway is protected.

A number of dental arch bars are available. The usual bar employed is the Erich arch bar, which has small metal hooks for intermaxillary fixation (see Fig. 12-7). The bar is malleable and is conformed and cut to the length of the maxillary and mandibular den-

tal arches. The hooks are oriented superiorly for the maxillary and inferiorly for the mandibular arch. No. 24 wire is used to ligate the bar to the necks of the molar, premolar, and cuspid teeth. Wire ligatures placed around the incisors may extrude them, and these teeth are generally omitted from ligature. In cases where additional fixation is necessary, circummandibular or piriform aperture wires are used, as shown in Figures 12-7 and 12-8. The maxillary and mandibular arch bars may be connected either with wires around the hooks or by elastic bands. The patient is instructed to cleanse the mouth frequently and to brush the teeth to promote oral hygiene. Intermaxillary fixation remains in place for 3 to 4 weeks for subcondylar mandibular fractures, 4 to 6 weeks for most fractures of the mandible, and 6 to 8 weeks for Le Fort maxillary fractures. When the intermaxillary fixation is released, the stability of the maxilla or mandible is determined by palpating movements and by persistent observation of the occlusion. The patient is observed over a 1- to 2-week period for any deviation in occlusal relation while functioning. If no deviation is seen, the intermaxillary fixation devices are removed. In those patients who demonstrate incomplete union of fractures, a short additional period of intermaxillary fixation usually results in healing. Radiographs often demonstrate persistent lucency at fracture sites in the facial bones and are not helpful for determining the adequacy of bone healing. The clinical examination with appropriate stress on the site of fracture is the most accurate means to identify those fractures demonstrating incomplete union.

On release of intermaxillary fixation, the patient cannot open the mouth more than a centimeter or so. Several weeks of gradual exercise allows the jaw to regain its normal range of motion, which in the adult exceeds 30 mm and is usually 45 to 55 mm of incisal opening. The range of motion may continue to improve for more than a year after injury. The most important determinant of the final result is the vigorous pursuit of physical therapy by the patient.

When a rigid fixation system is utilized for facial fracture reduction, the patient may be released from intermaxillary fixation at the end of the operative procedure. The arch bars are left in place and the occlusion observed at intervals to confirm proper fracture alignment. A soft diet is prescribed for the patient for the period of fracture healing. Early motion facilitates good function, decreases weight loss, and permits better hygiene.

### External Fixation and the Use of Headframes

Headframes and external fixation [47] are utilized in patients with bone loss or those who demonstrate severe comminution of maxillary or mandibular fractures where stabilization is difficult to achieve with the usual techniques of interfragment wiring. Plate-and-screw fixation has eliminated the need for external fixation in most cases. Patients with combined soft tissue and bone loss require external fixation to preserve bony relations while soft tissue reconstruction is accomplished. Bone reconstruction is begun once soft tissue reconstruction is complete.

One of the previous indications for the use of a headframe was to preserve the position

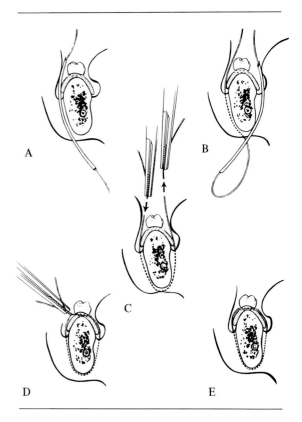

**Figure 12-8** *Circumferential wiring of the patient's artificial denture to the mandible. A. A curved passing needle armed with the wire punctures the skin at the inferior border of the mandible and passes upward on the lateral surface of the bone into the buccal vestibule. The passing needle is then pulled through the mouth and is slipped off the wire. B. Another passing needle, similarly armed with a wire, is inserted through the same puncture wound in the skin and is directed on the medial surface of the mandible into the lingual sulcus. The passing needle is then slipped off the wire and is removed from the mouth. C. A seesaw motion is applied to the wire to cut through any small fibers of tissue that are trapped in the wire loops; this action ensures contact of wire with the inferior border of the bone. D. The wire from the lingual side is passed through a burr hole and the artificial denture and is then twisted securely with the wire from the buccal side. E. The twisted double wire is cut, and its end is pressed firmly against the dentures so that the end does not irritate the buccal mucosa. Plate-and-screw fixation may obviate the need for splints or dentures.*

of the mandible relative to the cranial base with concomitant bilateral subcondylar and Le Fort fractures. The use of a headframe in this situation allowed the mandible to be positioned correctly in relation to the cranial base; midface height and projection are thus preserved (see Fig. 12-29). Headframes were generally employed for 6 to 8 weeks. Subcondylar open reduction and rigid fixation have replaced headframe use. Although some headframe devices provide only simple traction (e.g., the Georgiade device), others (University of Tennessee) provide rigid spatial fixation of fracture fragments. The headframe may be connected to the mandible by means of Joe Hall Morris pins, or it may be connected to a Morris biphasic appliance, which provides mandibular external fixation. The mandibular biphasic external fixation appliance involves the use of bone screws connected by an acrylic connector. Two bone screws are placed in each fragment of a mandibular fracture, and the fragments are temporarily aligned with an assemblage of rods and clamps prior to application of the acrylic connector. The clamp assembly is removed after the acrylic connector is applied. The facial nerve may be injured if there is inappropriate placement of incisions for pin bolt fixation.

## Facial Bone Fractures
### SOFT TISSUE INJURIES
Soft tissue injuries may be classified as blunt (contusion) injuries, lacerations, and avulsions, where pieces of tissue are missing. Whereas the latter two categories demand immediate attention—débridement [61, 101, 143] and repair—the blunt injury has not commanded the same degree of attention as the open wound. Contused tissue, filled with hematoma, undergoes a reorganization process with the development of an internal network of scarring. The tissue becomes thick and rigid, and it assumes the architecture of the underlying bony structural support. If the bone is not in its anatomic position when this reorganization occurs, the soft tissue reorganization becomes fixed in the position of the bony deformity and requires correction at a later date. It is thus important for this soft tissue healing to occur over an anatomically aligned bony skeleton.

### FRACTURES OF THE NOSE
The nose consists of the nasal bones, the frontal processes of the maxilla, nasal cartilages, and nasal septum. The nasal septum consists of the quadrilateral cartilage, the perpendicular plate of the ethmoid, and the vomer. Fractures of the nose may involve only the cartilaginous nasal septum or the nasal bones as well. A specific classification of fractures of the nose is difficult to organize. Two such classifications are illustrated.

Figure 12-9 shows a classification of nasal fractures according to Dingman, Natvig and Dortzback. Figure 12-10 illustrates the classification of nasal fractures according to Stranc and Robertson [158]. Stranc's classification is especially useful because it analyzes posttraumatic nasal dislocation into lateral and anteroposterior displacements. Figure 12-10 indicates the types of "frontal impact" fractures. Fractures with anteroposterior displacement are divided into "degrees of severity," with the first representing minimal injury and the third a severe (nasoethmoidal orbital, or midface, crush) injury.

The patient with a nasal fracture generally presents with swelling over the external surface of the nose, and frequently a small laceration is present. Symptoms associated with fractures of the nose include pain, swelling, and respiratory obstruction. In the absence of epistaxis, the diagnosis must be questioned. The physical signs of a nasal fracture are swelling, the presence of a laceration, lateral or anteroposterior displacement of the nasal bones, symptoms of crepitation or movement on palpation, and epistaxis. Intranasal examination may disclose a septal hematoma (which is drained) or obstruction from turbinate swelling or displacement of the septum. Mucosal lacer-

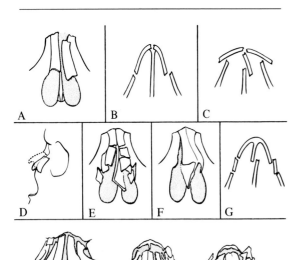

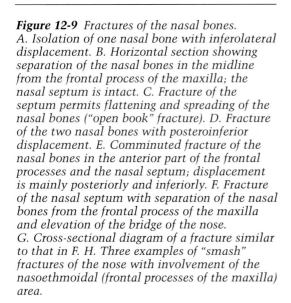

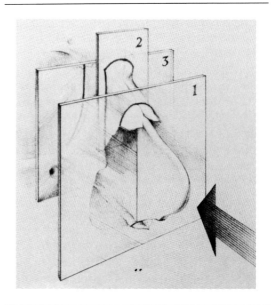

**Figure 12-9** *Fractures of the nasal bones.*
*A. Isolation of one nasal bone with inferolateral displacement. B. Horizontal section showing separation of the nasal bones in the midline from the frontal process of the maxilla; the nasal septum is intact. C. Fracture of the septum permits flattening and spreading of the nasal bones ("open book" fracture). D. Fracture of the two nasal bones with posteroinferior displacement. E. Comminuted fracture of the nasal bones in the anterior part of the frontal processes and the nasal septum; displacement is mainly posteriorly and inferiorly. F. Fracture of the nasal septum with separation of the nasal bones from the frontal process of the maxilla and elevation of the bridge of the nose. G. Cross-sectional diagram of a fracture similar to that in F. H. Three examples of "smash" fractures of the nose with involvement of the nasoethmoidal (frontal processes of the maxilla) area.*

**Figure 12-10** *Nasal fractures are analyzed according to displacement laterally and anteroposteriorly. "Lateral" and "frontal impact" forces and fracture displacement are thus classified. Frontal impact nasal fractures occur in varying degrees of severity and are illustrated here. According to Stranc, type I frontal impact nasal injuries involve the anterior portion of the nasal pyramid and the septum (1). Type II injuries result in more comminution of the nasal pyramid and more dislocation of the septum (2). Type III frontal impact nasal fractures involve the frontal processes of the maxilla and are, in reality, nasoethmoidal orbital fractures (3). (From M. F. Stranc and G. A. Robertson. A classification of injuries to the nasal skeleton.* Ann. Plast. Surg. *2:468, 1978.)*

ations may be present inside the nose and may be repaired or the mucosa approximated with packing.

*Radiographic Evaluation*
Radiographic evaluation of the nose consists of views of the nasal bones, a lateral view of the nose, and a Water's view. Nasal frac-

tures are accurately demonstrated on a CT scan, and one should be obtained if there is the possibility of a nasoethmoidal orbital (Stranc type III frontal impact) nasal fracture. Nasal films do not assist the surgeon in treatment of the nasal fracture. They do, however, provide documentation of the injury and may disclose fractures in adjacent bones, such as the maxilla, orbit, and zygoma.

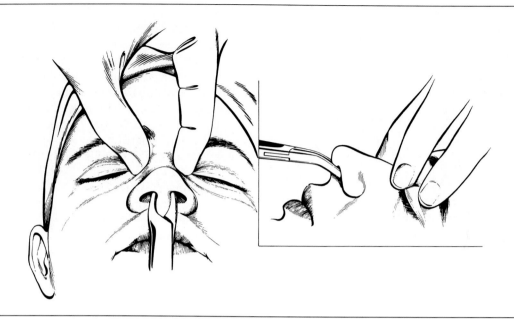

**Figure 12-11** *Asch forceps applied intranasally for reduction of a fracture of the nose. Remolding reforms the nasal pyramid.*

*Treatment*

Treatment of nasal fractures involves reduction of both the nasal pyramid and the nasal septum under local or general anesthesia. The septum is reduced by manipulation with an Asch forceps, completing the fracture. Simple septal fractures are often U-shaped, with the open end of the U projecting anteriorly. More complex fractures show complicated patterns.

To reduce the nasal pyramid, the nasal bones are first "out"-fractured, completing any incomplete components of the fracture. This manipulation of the nasal pyramid is accomplished with a Walsham or Asch forceps (Fig. 12-11), Rubershod elevator, or knife blade handle. The nasal bones are then pressed into position by digital manipulation (Fig. 12-11). Proper reduction is assessed by palpation and visual inspection; fractures older than several hours may have too much

edema and swelling to permit analysis of the accuracy of reduction. A period of 5 to 7 days is then needed before accurate operative inspection is possible. After the nasal pyramid reduction has been completed, the septum is reduced, and terramycin-soaked Adaptic packing is placed in each nostril to retard bleeding and centralize the septum. A nasal splint is applied to the nose and maintained for 7 days.

Nasal fractures frequently display some deformity after healing. They may benefit from a formal rhinoplasty after at least 6 months have elapsed to improve breathing or correct residual nasal deformity.

FRACTURES OF THE ZYGOMA

The zygoma forms the lateral structure of the midfacial skeleton and comprises the lateral and inferior orbital rim and malar eminence. Its projections articulate with the sphenoid bone in the lateral orbit, with the frontal bone superiorly, the maxilla medially, and the maxillary alveolus inferiorly. Like the nose, the prominent position of the zygoma make it susceptible to traumatic injury, and its prominence accounts for its

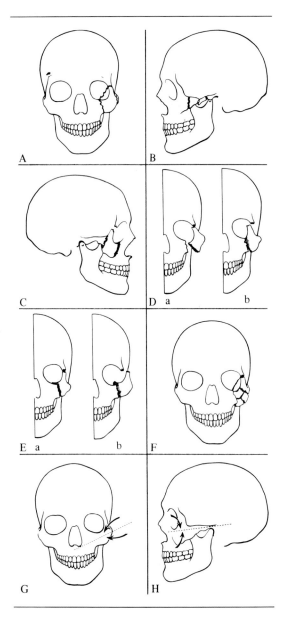

**Figure 12-12** *Fractures of the zygoma. A. Group I: no significant displacement. B. Group II: zygomatic arch fractures. C. Group III: unrotated body fractures. D. Group IV: medially rotated body fractures; outward displacement at zygomatic prominence (a) and inward at zygomatic frontal suture (b). E. Group V: laterally rotated body fractures; upward at infraorbital margin (a) and outward at zygomaticofrontal suture (b). F. Complex fractures. G and H. Directions of force and rotation.*

fracture frequency. Zygomatic fractures, with the exception of zygomatic arch fractures, always include a component in the orbital floor; such injuries may be linear or a more severe (orbital blow-out) fracture [162]. The common types of fracture displacement include medial, lateral, inferior, and posterior dislocation (Fig. 12-12) [36, 48, 50, 83, 86, 89, 94, 172]. The fracture may be an isolated zygomatic arch fracture (Fig. 12-12B) or a significant comminution (Fig. 12-12F).

The strongest articulation of the zygoma is that at the zygomaticofrontal suture. The articulations with the maxilla at the inferior orbital rim and with the maxillary alveolus at the zygomaticomaxillary buttress usually fracture first, with the more incomplete fracture generally occurring through the zygomaticofrontal junction. The presence of this incomplete fracture is the basis for the success of closed reduction techniques by manipulation [94]. Fractures demonstrating little displacement of the zygomaticofrontal suture are those that have been treated with reasonable success by closed reduction. Fractures with displacement at the zygomaticofrontal suture require open reduction [172]. Fractures of the zygomatic arch with inward displacement may impinge on the coronoid process of the mandible and limit excursion.

The symptoms of zygomatic fractures almost always include the combination of a periorbital and subconjunctival hematoma and numbness in the infraorbital nerve distribution. The absence of these two symptoms makes the diagnosis questionable. As fractures of the zygoma injure the lining of the maxillary sinus, ipsilateral epistaxis is present. Inferior displacement of the zygoma alters the position of the lateral canthus, producing an inferior cant to the palpebral fissure. The numbness in the infraorbital nerve distribution involves the ipsilateral upper lip, side of the nose, and upper anterior teeth. Occlusion or range of motion of the mandible is disturbed if there is significant swelling around the arch or displacement of the arch, impairing the movement of the coronoid process of the mandible. A hematoma may be observed intraorally in the upper buccal sulcus. Loss of prominence of the malar eminence may be perceptible if there is not a significant component of cheek swelling. The physical signs of fracture of the zygoma include the periorbital and subconjunctival hematoma, loss of prominence of the malar eminence, numbness in the distribution of the infraorbital nerve, depression (by palpation) of the infraorbital margin, a slight occlusal disturbance or impairment of motion of the jaw, and a hematoma in the buccal sulcus. Inferior displacement of the palpebral fissure may be perceptible. If there is a significant component of an orbital fracture, impairment of extraocular muscle motion may be noted, or the position of the globe may drop downward and backward with loss of orbital floor support. "Step" deformities of the orbital rim may be palpated, and tenderness occurs at the sites of fracture.

*Radiographic Evaluation*
Zygomatic fractures may be visualized on plain facial radiographs or by computed tomography. The computed tomogram more accurately assesses the internal orbit and periorbital soft tissue injury, and thus, for all practical purposes, it has replaced the plain radiograph. A "Caldwell" radiograph is most appropriate for assessing displacement at the zygomaticofrontal suture. The Water's radiograph demonstrates displacement at the inferior orbital rim and zygomaticomaxillary buttress areas. The submental vertex view is necessary to assess the zygomatic arch fracture and also displays posterior displacement of the malar eminence.

*Treatment*
Treatment of fractures of the zygoma involves reduction and immobilization. Classically, immobilization has been obtained by passing wire ligatures through holes drilled adjacent to the ends of the fracture frag-

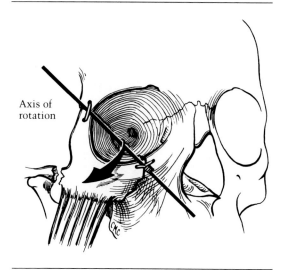

**Figure 12-13** *Classic treatment of zygoma fractures has involved reduction and interfragment wiring at the zygomaticofrontal suture and infraorbital rim. Small drill holes were placed adjacent to the fracture site, and No. 26 or No. 28 wire was used to link the fragments together. This wiring, which does not fully stabilize a comminuted zygoma fracture, creates an axis of rotation about which the zygoma can rotate. The masseter muscle acts as the force for this displacement. The malar eminence rotates inferiorly and posteriorly, and the orbit may become enlarged, contributing to enophthalmos and orbital dystopia.*

ments at the zygomaticofrontal suture and infraorbital rim (Fig. 12-13). K-wires [14, 15] were used as supplemental fixation. Today additional points of fixation have been included, such as the zygomaticomaxillary buttress adjacent to the maxillary alveolus; and, for more extensive injuries, where there is lateral dislocation of the zygomatic arch, coronal incision is employed. Rigid internal fixation may be performed throughout the zygomatic arch (Fig. 12-14). Access to the fracture sites is through incisions in the upper lateral eyebrow, lateral limb of an upper eyelid blepharoplasty, or incisions in the infraorbital region. The zygomaticomaxillary buttress is approached through a gingival-buccal sulcus incision. Bone grafts replace

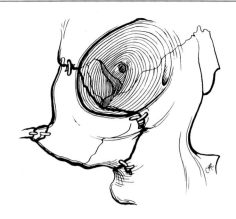

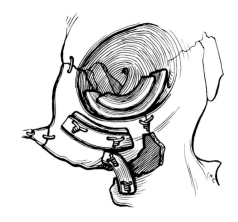

**Figure 12-14** *Wiring at the zygomaticofrontal suture, infraorbital margin, and zygomaticomaxillary buttress contributes to additional stability. The zygomaticomaxillary buttress can be approached intraorally through a gingival-buccal sulcus incision. With more complicated fractures such as a LeFort fracture, the zygomatic arch can also be wired, contributing to the anterior projection of the zygoma. A coronal incision is utilized for the arch reduction and repair of adjacent fractures (e.g., supraorbital and frontal bone fractures). Plate-and-screw fixation is the most stable form of fixation and has largely replaced classic interfragment wiring.*

**Figure 12-15** *Zygomatic fractures may require intraorbital bone grafts, depending on the extent of the fracture. Bone grafts can also be used for malar augmentation or for replacement of comminuted bone such as that at the zygomaticomaxillary buttress area. This technique demonstrates the stabilizing effect of "buttressing" bone grafts. Rigid fixation is now preferred instead of interfragment wires.*

unusable bone support (Fig. 12-15). The zygomatic arch if medially displaced, may be reduced with an elevator through the Gillies temporal approach. In those circumstances (lateral dislocation) where an open reduction of the arch is to be accomplished, a coronal incision is appropriate. The displaced zygoma may be elevated by direct repositioning or by passing an elevator behind the malar eminence either through the Gillies temporal approach, the brow (Dingman) approach, or intraorally through the maxillary sinus.

For isolated zygomatic arch fractures the Gillies (temporal) approach, an incision in the temporal hair-bearing scalp, is carried through skin, subcutaneous tissue, and fascia until the temporal muscle is exposed. An elevator is then slipped between the fascia and the muscle to gain access to the under-

surface of the zygomatic arch or malar eminence. Care is exercised that no excess pressure is applied to the temporal skull, which is thin and may fracture. A less desirable alternative is to place a towel clip about the zygomatic arch and effect reduction by lateral traction.

Plate-and-screw fixation of zygomatic fractures has been used routinely. The use of plate-and-screw fixation (Figs. 12-16 and 12-17) minimizes postreduction displacement, which has been observed with interfragment wiring alone. Plates should be utilized at the zygomatic frontal suture and the inferior orbital rim. For more comminuted injuries, the zygomaticomaxillary buttress and the zygomatic arch should also be stabilized with open reduction and rigid fixation. In complex injuries, multiple points of alignment and fixation need to be utilized to attain proper position.

Ankylosis of the zygoma to the coronoid process is occasionally seen with severe injuries. It may be managed by intraoral resection of the coronoid process.

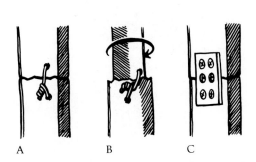

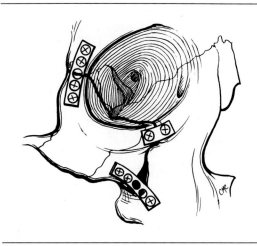

**Figure 12-16** *A. Interfragment wire creates a one-directional force of apposition. B. This wire does not prevent fracture segment tipping or rotation. C. Angulation and rotation are controlled by plate-and-screw fixation. Two screws per fragment are necessary for stabilization, and the plate-and-screw fixation is more stable if the screws are bicortical.*

**Figure 12-17** *Use of plate-and-screw fixation for treatment of a zygomatic fracture with open reduction of the zygomaticofrontal suture, the infraorbital rim, and the zygomaticomaxillary buttress. Such fixation is stable.*

FRACTURES OF THE INTERNAL ORBIT

Fractures of the internal orbit may involve the medial wall, floor, lateral wall, and orbital roof. The most frequent internal orbital fracture observed is the *blow-out fracture* [8, 91, 133], which is usually confined to the floor (Fig. 12-18A) and lower medial wall (Fig. 12-18B) of the orbit. Depressed fractures of this portion of the orbit allow orbital soft tissue to be displaced into the maxillary and ethmoid sinuses [8, 27, 152, 162]. Fractures of the internal orbit may be isolated or associated with orbital rim fractures.

**Figure 12-18** *Orbital blow-out fractures. A. A small orbital blow-out fracture is confined to the orbital floor and located medial to the groove or canal for the infraorbital nerve. The fracture involves the "bulging" section of the orbital floor and usually extends posteriorly adjacent to the inferoorbital fissure. B. A larger blow-out fracture extends to involve the medial orbit as well. The lamina papyracea of the ethmoidal cells is involved. Larger defects may extend far posteriorly.*

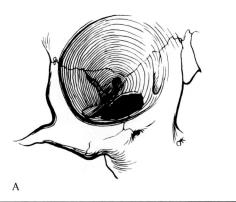

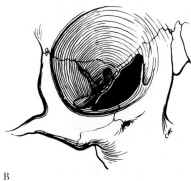

A

B

*Anatomy of the Orbit*

The orbital space may be conceptualized as a modified cone or pyramid. The orbital rim consists of thick bone, and thinner bone comprises the inner walls of the orbit. Posterior to the globe, the orbital walls converge and the dimensions of the orbit constrict, contributing to globe support. In the posterior portion and floor of the orbit are located fissures for blood vessels and cranial nerves to enter the orbit. The optic foramen is specifically for the optic nerve. A blow-out fracture most commonly involves the orbital floor medial to the groove for the infraorbital nerve. This portion of the floor is thin, and, with the adjacent lamina papyracea of the ethmoid, it represents the weakest portion of the orbit. Frequently, a "blow-out fracture" extends from the orbital floor up into the medial ethmoidal area. In the posterior orbital floor the infraorbital nerve lies in a groove. This groove becomes a canal in the anterior portion of the orbital floor, and the infraorbital nerve then passes through the rim to exit into the tissue of the cheek 1 cm below the rim. It sends small branches to the upper anterior teeth in the anterior wall of the maxillary sinus. These nerves are often damaged in orbital fractures, resulting in hypesthesia. Small fractures in the orbital floor may incarcerate orbital soft tissue contents. Frequently, this soft tissue is fat adjacent to the inferior rectus muscle, which can tether the action of this muscle by restricting movement [87] (Fig. 12-19). It is rare for the muscle itself to be physically entrapped in the fracture. Ischemia of the muscle [153] has also been suggested as a mechanism of diplopia. The inferior oblique muscle, located more anteriorly, is usually not as involved as the inferior rectus muscle in the restriction caused by inferior orbital fat entrapment. A branch of the oculomotor nerve, however, travels adjacent to the inferior rectus muscle along the floor of the orbit and is frequently contused during the fracture process. Care should be taken, when exploring the orbital floor, to avoid this nerve and the inferior rectus muscle, which travel close to

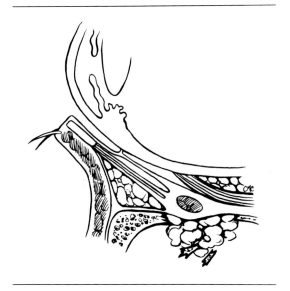

**Figure 12-19** *Orbital blowout fracture involving the thin portion of the orbital floor. Fat and interconnecting fascia are trapped within the blow-out fracture segments and limit the excursion of the inferior oblique and inferior rectus muscles. Diplopia is produced in up or down gaze.*

the floor of the orbit posterior to the equator of the globe.

*Mechanism of Blow-Out Fractures*

Blow-out fractures were long thought to result from transmission of intraorbital pressure to the floor of the orbit [49, 78]. The application of a force to the globe and the incompressibility of orbital soft tissue results in transmission of this force to the walls of the orbit [8] and fracture in the thinnest portion of bone. This weak area "blows out," forcing orbital soft tissue into the fracture site [43, 78] (Fig. 12-19). When the force is released, the soft tissue might remain incarcerated in the fracture site. This incarceration (or contusion) accounts for the restriction of extraocular muscle motion.

It has been demonstrated in experiments that other mechanisms may produce blow-out fractures as well. Indeed a force applied to the orbital rim [44] that is not sufficient to fracture the rim is transmitted to the thin

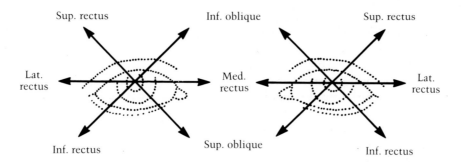

Sup. rectus    Inf. oblique    Sup. rectus

Lat. rectus    Med. rectus    Lat. rectus

Inf. rectus    Sup. oblique    Inf. rectus

**Figure 12-20** *Analysis of diplopia consists in identification of the field in which diplopia is produced. The muscle usually responsible for the diplopia is indicated. If the injury is bilateral, placing a "red glass" over one eye causes the most peripheral object images to be that of the affected eye. The affected eye "underrotates" as a rule, projecting the object image onto a more peripheral portion of the retina. (Adapted from Richards, R. D.* Ophthalmic Disorders. *Flushing, N. Y. Medical Examination, 1973.)*

portion of the orbit, resulting in a fracture that first occurs distant to the point of application of the force. Thus it seems that several mechanisms may be responsible for the usual blow-out fracture injury. The rim and thin (central) portion of the orbit fracture first and act to protect the posterior portion of the orbit (with its important nerves and vessels in the superior orbital fissure and optic foramen) from injury. The thin portions of the orbit serve additionally to protect the globe from rupture. If the orbit consisted entirely of thick bone, globe rupture would occur more frequently than is currently observed.

*Physical Signs of an Orbital Fracture*
The patient usually provides a history of blunt injury to the periorbital area. There may or may not be complaints of double vision that is exaggerated when looking to the upward or downward extremities of gaze. The extraocular range of motion may be limited on either upward or downward gaze or medial to lateral gaze depending on whether there is inferior (floor) or medial wall in-

volvement. The patient with an orbital floor fracture invariably has a periorbital and subconjunctival hematoma. Numbness in the inferior orbital nerve distribution is almost always present with orbital floor fractures. It is imperative that the globe be examined for visual acuity and the possibility of globe rupture, hyphema, retinal detachment, and similar injuries.

Orbital fractures have a significant (10 to 25 percent) incidence of associated ocular injury [65, 73, 119, 128, 132, 168]. Although many of these injuries are minor, a significant number are not; therefore any periorbital injury demands precise evaluation of the integrity of the globe and visual system. The visual examination includes assessment of visual acuity and confrontation fields, determination of intraocular pressure, and a forced duction test. A funduscopic examination is performed. The visual acuity can be assessed by having the patient read a visual examination card, checking each eye individually. Confrontation fields are evaluated by having the patient look directly at the examiner's nose and signal when he or she sees a finger entering the peripheral field of gaze. The range of extraocular motion is then assessed by having the patient look laterally, assessing globe motion and double vision. Double vision may be attributed to contusion of nerve and muscle or to entrapment and physical restriction of motion (Fig. 12-20).

The *forced duction test* is used to document incarceration of orbital soft tissue in a fracture site. This test is performed by instilling a drop of anesthetic in the conjunctival sac. A delicate forceps is then used to grasp the insertion of the inferior rectus muscle through the conjunctiva. The globe is then gently rotated upward and downward, assessing any restrictive component.

The traction test is useful for distinguishing physical entrapment from muscular or nerve contusion. Force generation may be perceived by noting the force through the forceps as the patient tries to move the globe. Entrapment of soft tissue occurs more frequently with small than with large fractures. The large fracture, however, is responsible for displacement of the globe, enophthalmos [24], and ocular dystopia.

*Enophthalmos*
Several mechanisms for enophthalmos have been postulated [8, 107, 108, 134]. Large fractures of the orbital floor allow orbital fat and soft tissue behind the globe to escape into the maxillary sinus, resulting in reduced globe support. Tissue (e.g., muscle and fat behind the globe) may be caught in the fracture site and hold the globe in a posteriorly displaced position. The fracture causes enlargement of the orbital cavity relative to its soft tissue contents. When sufficient damage occurs to the ligament support system of the globe and periorbital soft tissues, the orbital soft tissue may be permitted to sink backward and downward into the enlarged orbital cavity (Fig. 12-21). Finally, injury to the orbital soft tissue may result in atrophy of orbital fat, which contributes to loss of soft tissue volume and globe support.

Periorbital injuries are usually accompanied by significant hemorrhage and edema. Proptosis or exothphalmos is frequently observed during the first several days, and usually the perception of the possibility of enophthalmos is thus not possible. Enophthalmos develops once the hemorrhage and edema have subsided. Globe position may be measured relative to the lateral or inferior orbital rim and the measurement is accurate if they are not displaced. However, if the or-

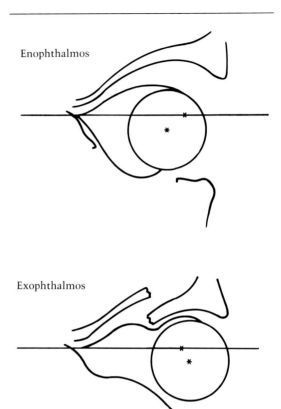

**Figure 12-21** *Enophthalmos (top) is produced by a defect in the floor and medial wall of the orbit. The globe sinks downward, backward, and medially; the shape of the orbital soft tissue, formerly a modified pyramid or cone, becomes more spherical. Normally the orbital floor bulges upward behind the globe. In enophthalmos cases, the orbital floor bulges inferiorly into the maxillary sinus. Bottom. The deformity of exophthalmos may be produced by a fracture of the superior orbital rim and superior orbital roof. These segments are usually dislocated inferiorly and posteriorly and give rise to a "downward" and "forward" position of the globe. The size of the orbit is reduced.*

bital margin is displaced, the measurement of globe position relative to the rim is no longer accurate and must be assessed by a measurement on a CT scan of the optic foramen. Globe position is best evaluated clinically by assessing the patient from an inferior (worm's eye) view. Enophthalmos of less than 2 to 3 mm is usually not cosmetically deforming. Usually enophthalmos or posterior displacement of the globe is accompanied by some inferior displacement (dystopia) of the globe as well (see Fig. 12-21). A supratarsal hollow and ptosis of the upper eyelid are usually present. The deformity of enophthalmos may be improved by immediate or late bone reconstruction to replace the soft tissue into its usual position.

### Radiographic Evaluation

Orbital floor fractures may be visible in plain (anteroposterior or Water's view) radiographs. These films do not document the orbital soft tissue injury or display the deformity in thin bone as well as the CT scan, which must be obtained in both axial and coronal projections. The exact position and the areas of fracture may be clearly demonstrated; incarceration of muscle or fat in fracture fragments may be precisely observed. The use of the computed tomogram has replaced both tomographic evaluation and plain films.

### Treatment

In many cases the symptoms of a blow-out fracture are mild and substantially resolve within a short period of observation. Surgery is therefore often not indicated [37, 41, 134]. Frequently double vision is transient or present at the extremities of gaze but not in a "functional" field of vision. Surgery would therefore not be indicated. There are two major indications for surgery: (1) muscle entrapment, confirmed by forced duction or CT scan, that is severe or does not respond to a short (less than 7 day) period of observation. Entrapment can be implied with the traction test or CT scans; it may be assessed

additionally with saccatic velocities, which involve determination of the range of acceleration of movement in a particular muscle's field of action [2]. Significant orbital fractures (more than 2 cm$^2$) begin to permit the possibility of globe displacement (enophthalmos and globe dystopia). Generally, the size of the fracture can be accurately estimated on CT scans; the potential for enophthalmos is then discussed with the patient and a correction pursued on the basis of the concern about aesthetic results.

The operation may be performed at any time during the first 7 to 10 days following injury; however, early treatment is preferred for surgical candidates. The surgical approach is generally through a lower eyelid incision (Fig. 12-22), either a subciliary incision with skin muscle flap or a conjunctival incision with lateral canthotomy. With the former, a skin muscle flap is developed to the level of the inferior orbital rim. A periosteal incision is made on the anterior surface of the rim, the periosteum is reflected, and the zygoma and inferior orbit are exposed. The entire orbital floor is then explored, identifying all the edges of the fracture. The defect may then be covered with an alloplastic implant, which must be thick enough to provide rigid support (similar to the bone previously present); alternately, a bone graft from rib, calvarium, or the iliac areas may be contoured to recreate the normal bony architecture and size of the orbital cavity (Fig. 12-23). Any incarcerated orbital tissue is gently and delicately removed from the fracture site. The branch of the oculomotor nerve to the inferior oblique or to the inferior rectus muscle may be inadvertently damaged with careless dissection. In cases where visualization of the incarcerated tissue is difficult, the fracture may be enlarged through an intact portion of bone, allowing easy visualization of the inferior margin of the entrapped tissue and gentle retrieval of the tissue to the normal confines of the orbit. If alloplastic material is utilized for orbital floor reconstruction, we generally pre-

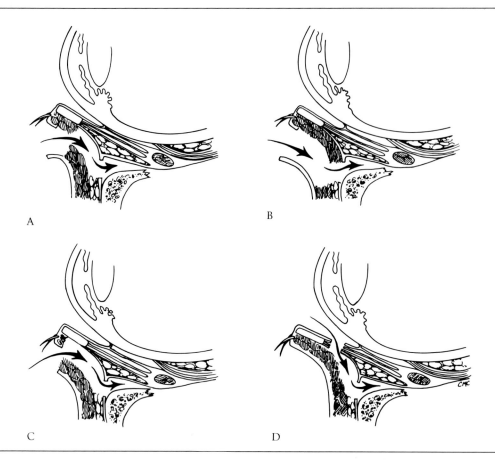

A

B

C

D

*Figure 12-22* *Eyelid incisions for zygoma and orbital floor fracture reduction. A. Converse muscle-splitting incision. B. Skin-only flap (this incision is not recommended, as a high incidence of ectropion results). C. Skin–muscle flap. This approach is preferred for zygoma or orbital fracture reduction. The lateral canthal ligament can be detached, allowing exposure of the zygomaticofrontal suture through this single lower eyelid incision. D. Conjunctival incision. The lower eyelid retractors are divided inferior to the tarsal plate, allowing exposure of the zygoma and orbital floor if a lateral canthotomy is utilized. The canthal ligament can be released, allowing exposure of the zygomaticofrontal suture. The approaches in C and D produce the least noticeable scars.*

fer Medpor. The thickness should be at least 1 mm to provide proper floor support. Alloplastic implants have a 2 percent long-term risk of infection, but this complication has not been a major problem in our experience. Autogenous bone grafts [25, 174] are more physiologic but are more difficult to obtain and involve potential donor site morbidity, which varies with the site chosen. The bone graft is patterned to be slightly larger than the defect and appropriately curved to the configuration of the orbit in that location. Once the implant or bone graft is in proper position, it may be wired to the orbital rim or screwed to intact bone to prevent migration. Before closure of the incision, a traction test is performed to confirm that the implant is not restricting extraocular mus-

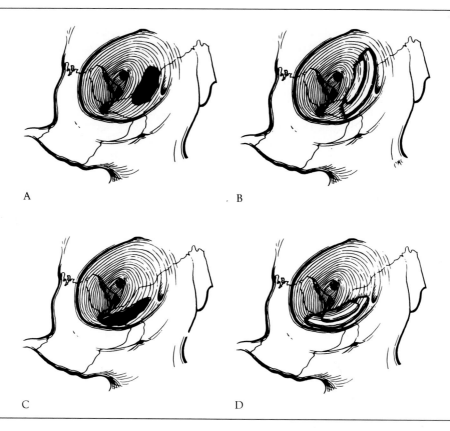

A

B

C

D

**Figure 12-23** *A. Medial blow-out fracture.*
*B. Bone graft for repair of medial blow-out*
*fracture. C. Inferomedial blow-out fracture.*
*D. Bone graft for repair of inferomedial blow-*
*out fracture.*

cle motion. No periosteal closure is performed anteriorly, as shortening of the orbital septum is a frequent accompaniment of this suturing. The skin is closed with a subcuticular 6-0 nylon suture and a frost stitch placed in the lower eyelid margin and taped to the brow to encourage redraping of eyelid tissue in the anatomic position. A protective eye dressing is applied and remains in place for 48 to 72 hours. Antibiotics may be utilized at the discretion of the surgeon.

CALDWELL-LUC APPROACH. Although the Caldwell-Luc approach has been described for orbital fracture treatment, there is no indication for its use as an isolated approach. Visualization of the floor of the orbit is im-

portant when releasing incarcerated soft tissue or reconstructing the orbital floor. The literature contains the records of injury from blind reduction or pressure of bone fragments displaced into orbital structures, such as the optic nerve.

*Complications of Surgery*
Diplopia may be worsened by muscle damage at the time of surgery [104, 113]. It is not unusual for diplopia to take 6 months to improve or stabilize. No eye muscle surgery is contemplated until this recovery is complete. In many instances, diplopia improves sufficiently that the patient is not bothered in straightforward (functional) gaze, although diplopia may be detected in the peripheral fields of gaze. This double vision at the extremes of gaze is of more academic than functional interest and is not usually functionally limiting. Often diplopia in the

inferior field of gaze is more handicapping than that in the superior field of gaze.

Hematoma may occur either within the orbit or within the lid. A hematoma in the orbit can contribute to pressure on the optic nerve through the mechanism of retrobulbar hemorrhage. It is essential that hemostasis be established prior to closing the incision. It is also essential for surgeons performing orbital surgery to have a precise knowledge of the landmarks of the orbit so that damage to the structures in the superior orbital fissure and optic foramen is avoided. A hematoma within the lid, if localized, is evacuated, which can often be accomplished with local anesthesia. Hematomas contribute to ectropion and increased scleral show, two complications of surgical approaches through the lid. These complications are more frequent with upper incisions than rim incisions in the lower eyelid. Aesthetically, the subciliary incision yields the best results but has an increased propensity for complications. Incisions through the inferior portion of the lower eyelid are made in "eyelid" skin rather than "cheek" skin and are "stepped" through skin, muscle, and periosteum to avoid adherence of skin to the orbital rim. In patients who desire relief of double vision without eye muscle surgery, the use of prisms can be considered.

UNDERCORRECTION AND OVERCORRECTION OF ENOPHTHALMOS. The conditions leading to enophthalmos (i.e., absence of bone in the posterior portion of the orbit and displacement of orbital soft tissue) are frequently undercorrected at the time of the initial surgery. As the swelling subsides, residual enophthalmos is apparent. Too much emphasis has been placed on eye position obtained at the time of surgical correction. Because of the presence of edema and swelling, the eye position may not be a correct indication of the amount, placement, and volume of bone graft material to be placed within the orbit. The surgeon tries to reconstruct the bony orbit to its preinjury dimensions rather than place the emphasis on eye position obtained

at the time of surgery. Correction of enophthalmos can be pursued secondarily by: (1) total release of the orbital soft tissue from bone to a pedicle consisting of the optic nerve and structures in the superior orbital fissure; and (2) bone grafting the orbit to its preinjury dimensions. Usually, improved eye position results. Frequently enophthalmos is accompanied by inferior dystopia (lowered position) of the ocular globe. Many patients need correction of the position of the inferior and lateral orbital rim as well, which are accomplished by marginal (rim) osteotomy with interpositional bone grafting. Although alloplastics are not subject to absorption, as is bone, the use of alloplastics for enophthalmos correction is usually not recommended initially because of the large open communications with the sinus cavities. The use of cartilage grafts can be considered for acute and late orbital fracture treatment, but they are more difficult to work with than bone. Overcorrection of eye position, both vertically and anteroposteriorly, is usually present immediately after fracture repair or late surgical correction of enophthalmos and orbital floor fractures. Several months must elapse for swelling and edema to go down before the eye position can be criticized.

INCREASED SCLERAL SHOW AND ECTROPION. An increased amount of sclera visible underneath the inferior limbus of the cornea on the involved side is a temporary, frequent sequela to lower lid surgery. Usually it improves with time, but it may be permanent as a result of scarring within the lower eyelid. Surgical treatment involves release of all adhesions to the orbital septum and usually release of the lower eyelid from the inferior orbital rim and anterior portion of the orbital floor. The deformity frequently recurs.

Ectropion may follow lower lid incisions and, if present, usually improves greatly with time, massage, and orbicularis muscle exercises. Protection of any corneal irritation or tendency to drying is important, as is patient reassurance. Persistent ectropion requires surgical correction, which usually involves release of any adhesions present and perhaps a full-thickness skin graft when lid skin is deficient.

INFECTION. Infection is an uncommon complication of orbital surgery. An obstructed maxillary antrum or an obstructed ethmoid sinus is frequently the cause. Adequate drainage of these structures is confirmed at the time of surgical exploration. Many prefer to leave a drain within the maxillary sinus for several days using a Caldwell-Luc approach.

IMPLANT DISLODGEMENT OR EXTRUSION. Alloplastic implants, if not fixed, may dislodge and present as a palpable mass or an extrusion through the lower lid structures. Their removal is not usually accompanied by any significant change in globe position because scar tissue that forms around the implant provides globe support. Implants may, if inappropriately placed, produce pressure on the optic nerve or structures in the superior orbital fissure. Again, it is important to know the location of these structures so that implants may be properly designed.

CHRONIC EDEMA. Chronic edema follows vertical lacerations or dissections through the lateral portion of the lower eyelid. The lymphatic vessels draining this area are compromised by lacerations or inferior orbital rim incisions that are carried too far laterally. Usually edema of the lower eyelid improves slowly over the course of several months. Occasionally, excision of lymphadematous tissues or lower orbital fat improves the appearance.

LACRIMAL SYSTEM OBSTRUCTION. The surgeon must be aware of the position of the inferior oblique insertion, lacrimal system, and nasolacrimal duct to avoid damaging these structures during orbital explorations. The inferior oblique muscle attaches just lateral to the nasolacrimal canal and must also be protected during surgical exploration. Epiphora, or tearing, may be due to nasolacrimal obstruction, ectropion, damage to the orbicularis oculi muscle, or medial canthal malposition.

INFRAORBITAL NERVE DAMAGE. Hypesthesia or anesthesia in the distribution of the infraorbital nerve is frequently detected as a permanent sequela to orbital floor or zygomatic fractures. Usually, enough return of sensation occurs that the patient is not disabled by the symptoms. Trigeminal neuralgia in this nerve distribution may follow the injury. During exploration of the orbit or zygomatic fracture repair, medially displaced bone fragments impinging on or compressing the nerve are removed or restored to their proper position, as permanent anesthesia in the infraorbital nerve distribution is disabling.

LE FORT MAXILLARY FRACTURES

Fractures of the maxilla in reality involve not only the maxilla but the bones and structures of the midfacial region [31, 104, 106, 117, 118, 123, 154]. A classification developed by Le Fort [96] (Fig. 12-24) is commonly applied. In low level (Le Fort I, transverse, or Guerin) fractures, the maxillary alveolus is separated from upper midface structures at the level of the piriform aperture. Upper Le Fort fractures consist of Le Fort II and III types. In the Le Fort II type, a pyramidally shaped central fragment containing the maxillary dentition is separated from the upper craniofacial skeleton through the inferior orbital rims and nasofrontal junction. These fractures are called pyramidal fractures because of the shape of the central fragment. In the craniofacial dysjunction, or Le Fort III fracture, the upper level of the fracture lines travel through the zygomaticofrontal junction, across the orbit, through the lateral wall, floor, and medial wall, across the nasofrontal junction, and through the other orbit. Le Fort fractures are usually more comminuted on one side than the other [104, 106], and thus it is common to see a Le Fort III fracture on one side coexist with a Le Fort II level fracture on the other. The fracture would thus consist of a zygomatic fracture plus a Le Fort II fracture. In 10 percent of Le Fort fractures, the palate is split in a sagittal direction [105], which increases instability and makes preservation

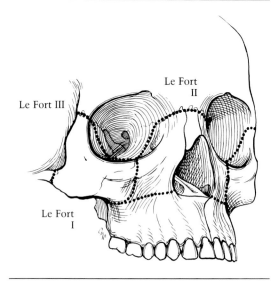

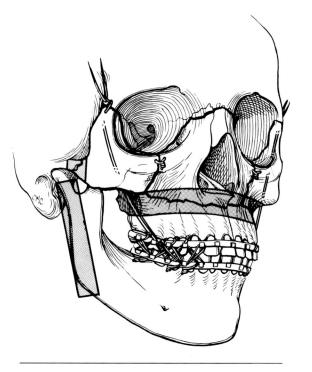

**Figure 12-24** Le Fort fractures. Le Fort I, a horizontal or transverse fracture, separates the maxillary alveolus at the lower margin at the piriform aperture and extends through the maxillary sinus. Le Fort II fracture separates a pyramid-shaped segment from the upper craniofacial structures. The fracture lines extend from the Le Fort I level upward through the inferior orbital rims and across the bridge of the nose in either a high or a low fashion. Le Fort III fracture separates the cranial from the facial bones. It is a "craniofacial disjunction" with fracture lines separating the frontal bone from the zygoma and orbits. The fracture lines extend across the floor of the orbit and up through the nasofrontal area. If this area is comminuted, a nasoethmoidal orbital fracture may be produced.

**Figure 12-25** Formerly, the "Adams fixation" of Le Fort fractures utilized wiring at the fracture sites around the orbital rim. The patient was placed in intermaxillary fixation utilizing arch bars. The Le Fort I level, nasoethmoidal area, and vertical height of the mandibular ramus, if involved by fracture, were not addressed in the usual pattern of Adams fixation. Suspension wires extended from above the highest level of fracture on each side to either the maxillary or the mandibular arch bar to assist stabilization. Midface shortening and retrusion occur with comminuted fractures.

of the normal occlusal relation a challenge. This fracture is often accompanied by the presence of a palatal laceration oriented sagittally and the presence of lateral mobility within the upper dental arch.

Maxillary fractures are encountered less commonly than other types of facial injury. They may be isolated to the midface or accompanied by injuries to the frontal bone, nasoethmoidal region, or mandible [104, 106].

The symptoms of maxillary fractures include periorbital hematomas, profuse naso-

pharyngeal bleeding, pain, malocclusion, and intraoral lacerations. The symptoms of zygomatic, orbital, or nasoethmoidal fractures depend on the level of the maxillary injury. The most important physical sign of a maxillary fracture is mobility of the maxillary dental arch. The level at which this mobility occurs indicates the level of the Le Fort fracture. Occasionally, Le Fort fractures are not mobile and are either impacted or incomplete. The patient would therefore have a malocclusion without maxillary mobility.

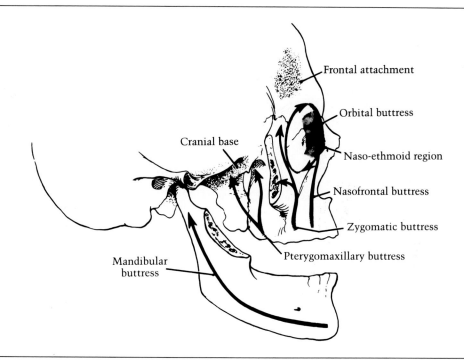

Frontal attachment

Orbital buttress

Naso-ethmoid region

Nasofrontal buttress

Zygomatic buttress

Pterygomaxillary buttress

Cranial base

Mandibular buttress

**Figure 12-26** *Buttresses of the maxilla and mandible. The maxilla consists of thick and thin portions of bone. The thicker portions form buttresses that extend from the maxillary alveolus to the frontal cranium. There are three vertical buttresses on each side: a nasofrontal buttress extending along the piriform aperture and medial orbital rim, a zygomatic buttress extending from the maxilla up through the zygoma to the zygomaticofrontal area, and a pterygomaxillary buttress extending to the cranial base from the posterior portion of the maxilla. Horizontal buttresses include the frontal bar at the frontal cranium (superior orbital rim), orbital buttress, and palate. The mandible has vertical and horizontal segments that must be stabilized in proper relation with the cranial base.*

Le Fort fractures are frequently accompanied by profuse nasopharyngeal bleeding with moderate or massive swelling in the midface and periorbital area. Facial elongation and midface retrusion occur if the patient is not placed in intermaxillary fixation shortly after the injury. The midface elongation occurs both through the orbits and at the Le Fort I level. The maxilla is retruded and tilts with premature contact with the mandible in the molar occlusion. An open bite is present anteriorly. Cerebrospinal fluid rhinorrhea and pneumocephalus [74] may accompany Le Fort II and III fractures and, if carefully sought, are found in at least 25 percent of these injuries.

*Treatment*
The most important concept in the treatment of maxillary fractures is stabilization of the occlusal relations with the mandible [104, 138]. Stabilization is generally accomplished by placing the patient in intermaxillary fixation (Fig. 12-25) after application of arch bars. Adams suspension wires were formerly utilized and led to a point above the highest level of fracture on each side. With more modern techniques, the maxilla may be held in position with plate-and-screw fixation, which can decrease or eliminate the period of intermaxillary fixation in selected patients.

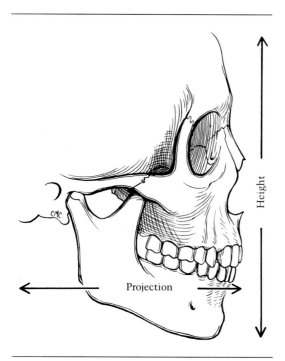

Height

Projection

CMC

**Figure 12-27** *For treatment of a pan-facial fracture, restoration of the proper facial aesthetics requires preservation of midface height and projection. This goal is accomplished with stabilization of both midface and mandible by restoration of mandibular and anterior midfacial buttresses. The occlusal relation is intraoperatively stabilized with intermaxillary fixation and possibly the use of splints. Intermaxillary fixation is the key to the initial alignment of the dentition.*

LE FORT I FRACTURES. Frequently, the Le Fort I fracture can be treated by placing the patient in intermaxillary fixation alone. Alternately, the gingivobuccal sulcus incision at the Le Fort I level exposes the fracture site and facial buttresses (Figs. 12-26 and 12-27), allowing either interfragment wiring or plate-and-screw fixation. Although some have used suspension wires [1, 2] (Fig. 12-25) (wires passed from the mandibular or maxillary arch bar to a point above the highest level of fracture on each side), we have not utilized this method of fixation over the past few years. Suspension wires are cumber-

some and aggravate the tendency toward midface shortening, which occurs with most Le Fort injuries. They do not precisely control lower midface position and thus are less useful than other types of open reduction and fixation of the anterior and middle maxillary buttresses.

LE FORT II FRACTURES. The patient is placed in intermaxillary fixation. Fractures at the orbital rims, nasofrontal junction, and the Le Fort I level in the zygomaticomaxillary buttresses are opened and fixation secured either with interfragment wiring or plate-and-screw fixation (Fig. 12-28). Le Fort II fractures may be accompanied by a nasoethmoidal injury that requires an open reduction in this area. Significant defects or enlargement of the orbit are treated by immediate bone grafting. Intermaxillary fixation (in the absence of plate-and-screw fixation) is usually maintained for 4 to 8 weeks depending on the stability of the reduction and the method of fixation. If rigid fixation techniques are utilized, the arch bars are left in place and the patient may have the intermaxillary fixation released postoperatively. A soft diet is prescribed. The occlusion must be carefully observed so that any displacement is identified early. Accompanying mandibular fractures are openly reduced to provide a stable base for intermaxillary fixation, especially if a subcondylar fracture is present. In the presence of bilateral subcondylar fractures, the maxilla and mandible together retrude and displace superiorly (Fig. 12-29).

LE FORT III FRACTURES. Generally, a Le Fort III fracture does not consist of a single bone fragment but exists as comminuted segments of other types of Le Fort fracture (Fig. 12-28). The segment carrying the maxillary alveolus is usually a Le Fort I or Le Fort II segment, which is then accompanied by a zygomatic injury, a nasoethmoidal injury, or both. With severe fractures, supraorbital fractures are also present. Reduction of these fractures by region is accomplished in the same manner as for zygomatic and orbital

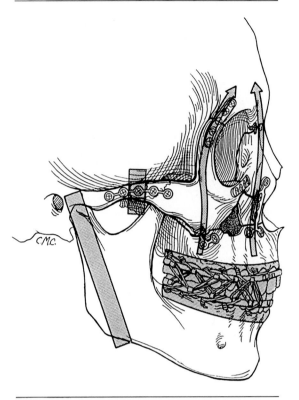

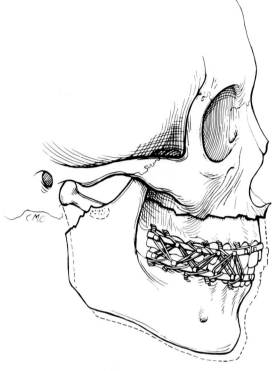

**Figure 12-28** *Treatment of a Le Fort midface fracture. Interfragment wiring is indicated to link the fragments; plate-and-screw fixation then secures the reduction. Maxillary and mandibular dental arches are united by intermaxillary fixation. Nasomaxillary and zygomatic buttresses are stabilized with interfragment wiring or plate-and-screw fixation. The pterygoid buttress (indicated by the midface bar) is not approached surgically. If there are concomitant mandibular subcondylar fractures, the vertical height of the mandibular ramus must be stabilized by open reduction and plate-and-screw fixation as well. This stabilization is indicated by the bar in the mandibular ramus.*

**Figure 12-29** *When concominant bilateral subcondylar fractures exist with a Le Fort fracture, the maxilla and mandible placed in intermaxillary fixation can drift posteriorly and superiorly. Such displacement can be opposed by open reduction in the maxilla but is more effectively prevented by the addition of open reduction of the subcondylar fracture. The relation of the low maxilla and mandible to the cranial base is thus preserved [64].*

floor fractures. Nasoethmoidal orbital fractures must have an open reduction. The fractures at the Le Fort I level are then exposed through a gingivobuccal sulcus incision, and fixation is secured with interfragment wiring or plate and screw fixation.

SAGITTAL FRACTURES OF THE MAXILLA
Sagittal fractures of the maxilla [105] are subject to lateral displacement (Fig. 12-30) and require a palatal splint or open reduction (Figs. 12-31 and 12-32) to preserve the transverse width of the upper dental arch and prevent palatal rotation of the maxillary teeth. This palatal rotation is aggravated by the use of intermaxillary fixation, which tends to tip the maxillary segments toward the palate (see Fig. 12-30). The palatal splint is made

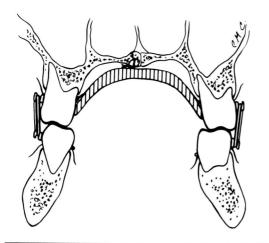

**Figure 12-30** *Sagittal fracture of the palate accompanies 10 percent of Le Fort fractures. It divides the halves of the maxillary alveolus. The force of intermaxillary fixation tends to tip the palatal segments medially, preventing proper occlusal relations with the use of intermaxillary fixation alone (arrows).*

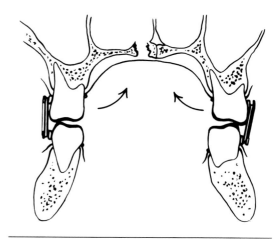

**Figure 12-31** *A palatal splint fashioned from acrylic can be utilized to prevent this palatal rotation of the maxillary segments accompanying a palatal fracture. A wire may be placed in a posterior portion of the palatal bone to ensure approximation of bone segments. The acrylic splint is made from a dental model after it has been sectioned at the site of the fracture and repositioned appropriately.*

from a dental model that has been sectioned at the sites of fracture and restored to its correct relation with the mandible prior to molding the splint. When rigid fixation is used in the palatal vault, the splint may be omitted intraoperatively and postoperatively.

With severe maxillary fractures, treatment is organized according to the various regions as described.

FRONTOBASILAR FRACTURES

Fractures of the frontal skull, frontal sinus, supraorbital areas, and nasoethmoidal orbital regions are encountered less commonly than other types of facial fracture. Their severity warrants precise diagnosis and treatment according to neurosurgical and craniofacial principles. These fractures are frequently accompanied by frontal brain injury and dural fistula, such as cerebrospinal fluid rhinorrhea or pneumocephalus. A combined neurosurgical-plastic surgery evaluation and approach to treatment is important for reducing complications and improving aesthetic results.

**Figure 12-32** *The palatal splint may be either ligated to the maxillary teeth with circumdental wires or secured with a circumpalatal wire. This wire extends from the anterior portion of the palatal splint up over the surface of the piriform aperture, across the floor of the nose, and down through the soft palate adjacent to the posterior portion of the palatal bone to secure the posterior portion of the acrylic splint. This technique provides stable fixation.*

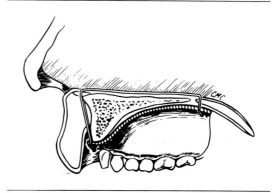

## SUPRAORBITAL FRACTURES

Supraorbital fractures involve the frontal bone and the lateral two-thirds of the superior orbital rim [29, 56, 120, 139, 151, 157]. They may be of limited extent (rim) producing few symptoms or may involve the entire lateral portion of the frontal bone, the "lateral frontalorbital" fracture (Fig. 12-33). More extensive injuries are always accompanied by dural and cerebral injuries [114, 118] and produce dramatic displacement of the globe (see Fig. 12-21). The signs of a supraorbital fracture include lacerations, periorbital hematoma, and deformity. The symptoms include the above with a downward and forward displacement of the ocular globe. Ptosis due to contusion or damage to the levator muscle may be present, as may superior rectus palsy; and anesthesia may occur in the distribution of the supraorbital nerve. Fractures extending to the superior orbital fissure or optic canal produce either the superior orbital fissure syndrome or blindness if they result in excessive pressure on nervous or vascular structures.

## SUPERIOR ORBITAL FISSURE SYNDROME

Fractures involving the superior orbital fissure produce a combination of cranial nerve palsies known as the superior orbital fissure syndrome [90] (Fig. 12-34). This syndrome consists in ptosis of the eyelid, proptosis of the globe, paralysis of cranial nerves III, IV, and VI, and anesthesia in the distribution of the first division of the trigeminal nerve. The occurrence of superior orbital fissure syndrome accompanied by blindness indicates involvement of the optic foramen [58, 85, 103] as well, and the fractures involve the entire posterior portion or "apex" of the orbit. A CT scan demonstrates the fractures involved. If blindness occurs at the onset of the injury, optic nerve decompression [45] is generally not thought to be of benefit. If blindness occurs suddenly and late (after a period of intact vision), optic nerve decompression is considered; however, the value of surgical maneuvers is open to considerable question. CT scans demonstrating displaced bone fragments may confirm optic

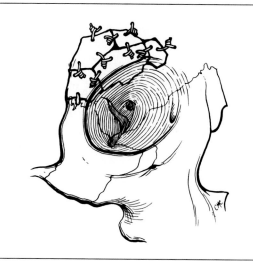

**Figure 12-33** *Supraorbital fractures may be small, consisting in segments of the rim, or may extend up into the frontal bone. After débridement and repair of any brain or dural injury, the segments are replaced and connected with interfragment wires. A bone graft may be utilized to reconstruct the orbital roof if necessary. Plate-and-screw fixation may stabilize the supraorbital bar if wire fixation is unstable.*

nerve impingement. The release of this pressure by removing bone fragments seems to be indicated; however, the results of these surgical procedures leave the ultimate value of this difficult surgery open to considerable question.

Although supraorbital fractures may be visualized on plain (Caldwell) posteroanterior radiographs, they require a thorough craniofacial CT scan for precise evaluation.

Displaced supraorbital fractures require open reduction with repair of dural lacerations and evacuation of epidural hematoma. Usually, continuity of the frontal skull is reconstructed by interfragment wiring with plate-and-screw fixation of the frontal bar replacing missing bony fragments with split calvarial grafts (see Fig. 12-33). Approximately 5 percent of open reductions demonstrate infection. Fractures involving the orbital roof may be bone-grafted if the defect is significant. A bone graft may be placed un-

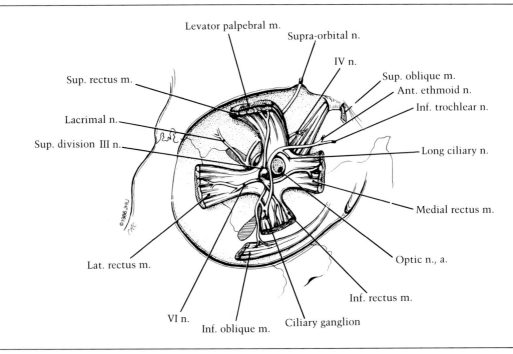

Levator palpebral m.
Supra-orbital n.
IV n.
Sup. oblique m.
Ant. ethmoid n.
Inf. trochlear n.
Sup. rectus m.
Lacrimal n.
Sup. division III n.
Long ciliary n.
Medial rectus m.
Lat. rectus m.
Optic n., a.
Inf. rectus m.
VI n.
Inf. oblique m.
Ciliary ganglion

***Figure 12-34*** *The contents of the superior orbital fissure are indicated; they consist in cranial nerves III, IV, and VI and sensory divisions of V. The branches of the ophthalmic division of the trigeminal nerve are indicated. Fractures compromising the superior orbital fissure produce anesthesia in the first (ophthalmic) division of the trigeminal nerve and paralysis of the extraocular muscles and the levator palpebrae superioris.*

der the edges of a small roof defect within the orbit, with the pressure of the orbital soft tissue holding the bone graft in position. Large grafts require fixation. The failure to bone-graft the roof of the orbit can result in position abnormalities of the globe or the transmission of cerebral pulsations to orbital soft tissues, producing the condition "pulsating exophthalmos."

CAROTID CAVERNOUS SINUS FISTULA
Severe fractures of the basal skull may result in a fistula between the carotid artery and the cavernous sinus [17]. The symptom of a pulsating globe is usually accompanied by the superior orbital fissure syndrome or blindness. The globe pulsations are visible, and a thrill can be auscultated when placing a stethoscope on the globe. Demonstration of the fistula requires an angiogram. Treatment is usually balloon occlusion or embolization, which may be accomplished with invasive radiologic procedures.

FRONTAL LOBE INJURIES
Frontal lobe injuries commonly accompany fractures of the bones of the frontobasilar skeleton. Because of the "silent" nature of frontal lobe function, there may be minimal evidence of underlying brain injury. The patient may demonstrate slight confusion or no symptoms despite evidence of significant contusion on CT scan. Patients with frontobasilar fractures are subjected to CT scanning in all cases and most certainly prior to any operative intervention.

CEREBROSPINAL FLUID LEAKS
Cerebrospinal fluid fistulas may accompany fractures of the anterior or middle cranial

fossae [12, 30, 39, 63, 71, 76, 84, 95, 98, 121, 125, 135, 161, 167]. Treatment is operative closure if the injury is accompanied by depressed or open skull fractures. Antibiotics have not proved to be helpful when used on a prolonged basis but may be useful during the immediate operative period [12, 30, 39, 63, 71, 76, 84, 95, 98, 121, 125, 161, 167]. Cerebrospinal fluid fistulas from isolated basal skull fractures or from nasoethmoidal orbital fractures usually close spontaneously within several days. Rarely, persistent or late leaks require localization by metrizamide [145] contrast instillation and operative repair. Late leaks occasionally occur and should be treated operatively, as the incidence of meningitis is high [148].

NASOETHMOIDALORBITAL FRACTURES
Nasoethmoidal orbital fractures consist of injury to one or both frontal processes of the maxilla (medial orbital rims) and the nose [26, 54, 109, 111, 156]. The medial orbital rim is dislocated, allowing displacement of this structure with its associated medial canthal ligament. By virtue of their extensions, these fractures often involve the orbital roof, frontal sinus, and frontal bone. They result from direct blows to the nasofrontal and glabellar area and frequently accompany Le Fort or frontal cranial fractures.

They are injuries of significance and are surprisingly easily missed in the presence of swelling. One should suspect the presence of a nasoethmoidal orbital injury in nasal fractures with posterior displacement and when lacerations of the frontal and nasal area and bilateral periorbital hematomas (spectacle hematomas) are present. The spectacle hematoma, for instance, signals the possible presence of a fracture of the anterior cranial fossa.

One-third of nasoethmoidal fractures are unilateral, occurring either as an isolated medial orbital rim injury or with other fractures through the inferior or superior portion of the orbit. Bone fragments may penetrate the dura, which is tightly adherent to the bone in the frontal region and anterior cranial fossa. The dural fistula present may manifest either as leakage of cerebrospinal fluid (CSF) into the nose (CSF rhinorrhea) or as entry of air in the subdural space (pneumocephalus). The presence of bloody nasal drainage often obscures the perception of a CSF leak during the first several days after the injury. Thus the presence of a CSF leak is suspected in patients with fractures adjacent to the frontal cranium or anterior cranial fossa. Nasoethmoidal orbital fractures invariably injure the nasolacrimal duct in its passage through the maxilla, which can (in 5 percent of patients) result in late lacrimal system obstruction with epiphora. Many patients with obstruction are not symptomatic. The early proper operative reduction of these fractures limits the symptomatic problem of epiphora.

The diagnosis of a nasoethmoidal fracture is suggested by the presence of nasal bleeding, a depressed, comminuted nasal fracture, pain and tenderness over the frontal process of the maxilla, or medial canthal ligament bone crepitation in this area and bilateral eyelid hematomas.

*Radiographic Evaluation*
Fractures in the nasoethmoidal area are best visualized by computed tomography. Plain radiograms do not display this area as precisely as a CT scan, which must demonstrate fractures surrounding the medial orbital rim as the sine qua non of the nasoethmoidal injury. The CT scan may demonstrate fractures extending into adjacent bones, such as the orbital roof, frontal sinus, frontal bone, zygoma, and orbital floor. The most reliable clinical sign of a nasoethmoid fracture is movement on direct pressure of the frontal process of the maxilla immediately under the medial canthal ligament. This movement may be appreciated by a bimanual examination, placing a clamp in the nose in subtle injuries. Movement signals instability of the lower two-thirds of the medial orbital rim and predicts the ne-

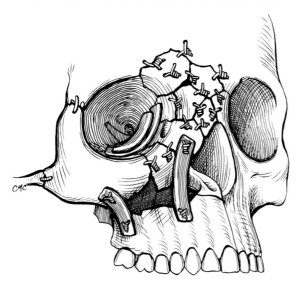

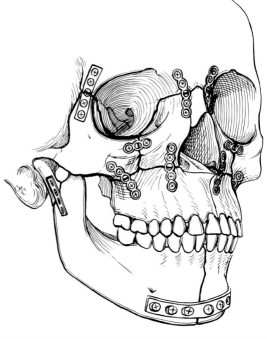

**Figure 12-35** *Scheme for open reduction and internal fixation of the nasoethmoidal orbital fracture. The fracture fragments are wired to each other, and any missing fragments are replaced with bone grafts through the buttress area. The medial and inferior internal orbit is bone-grafted. The most important principle in the reduction of a nasoethmoidal fracture is the passage of a wire through the frontal processes of the maxilla adjacent to the posterior lacrimal crest. This wire is placed transnasally behind the canthal ligament; it represents transnasal reduction of the medial orbital rims. The wire is covered by the medial orbital bone graft in this photograph.*

**Figure 12-36** *Plate-and-screw fixation can be adapted to the treatment of a nasoethmoidal orbital fracture coexisting with Le Fort and subcondylar fractures, as indicated. If sufficient fixation is obtained, intermaxillary fixation may not be necessary.*

### Treatment

Nasoethmoidal orbital fractures require a definitive open reduction with interfragment wiring (Fig. 12-35) or plate-and-screw fixation (Fig. 12-36) linking all fragments. It can be accomplished either through a coronal incision (preferred in all patients, especially those who do not have suitable lacerations) or with local incisions of the vertical midline or Converse "open sky" type. The vertical midline nasal incision is perhaps appropriate in those with glabellar wrinkles and may be preferable to a coronal incision in a bald Caucasian patient for a localized fracture alone. The H-type incision is not indicated; a transverse incision in a crease over the bridge of the nose may provide ad-

cessity for open reduction. Traumatic telecanthus (increase in the distance between the medial orbital rims) may be observed immediately in severe injuries. In less severe injuries, fractures may demonstrate lesser degrees of mobility, canthal deformity, and malposition during the early postinjury period. Additional deformity cannot be perceived until the swelling has resolved. With fractures that are grossly unstable, the canthus is seen to move if traction is applied to the lower eyelid (eyelid traction test).

equate exposure. Both of these local incisions have limited application.

It is important to perform a transnasal open reduction of the medial orbital rims to prevent telecanthus and to preserve the interorbital distance (see Fig. 12-35). This situation is not ensured by simple fragment-to-fragment wiring alone, and the performance of transnasal reduction of the medial orbital rims [109] is the most important step in treatment of a nasoethmoidal orbital fracture. Such transnasal reduction is performed posterior and superior to the attachment of the medial canthal ligament on the frontal process of the maxilla. The canthal ligament is not detached during reduction of a nasoethmoidal orbital fracture. The frontal process of the maxilla may be subperiosteally stripped, except for the area of canthal attachment, through a combined coronal [80, 171] and subciliary approach without detaching the medial canthal ligament or the structures in the nasolacrimal fossa. The medial orbital rim may thus be united to the contralateral orbital rim with two transnasal wires. The canthal ligament need not be involved in this reduction. Bone grafts [54, 56] are usually required to reconstruct medial and inferior (internal) orbital wall fractures and to preserve the contour and dorsal height of the nose. These bone grafts may be taken from the calvarium, iliac crest, or rib areas. The CSF leak accompanying isolated nasoethmoidal orbital fractures may not need definitive dural closure. Neurosurgical exploration is reserved for those displaying the usual criteria of depressed or open frontal skull or frontal sinus fractures and conditions such as intracerebral or epidural hematoma requiring neurosurgical intervention. The frontal sinus is invariably injured in the floor area in nasoethmoidal orbital fractures. Frontal sinus treatment is not necessary unless there are displaced fractures of the anterior and posterior walls of the frontal sinus. It is important that nasoethmoidal orbital fractures be treated within the first few days after the injury, as the soft tissue begins to undergo thickening and fibrosis, which makes proper reduction more difficult.

LACRIMAL SYSTEM

The lacrimal system is frequently injured in lacerations involving the medial portions of the eyelids. It may also be damaged in fractures involving the bones surrounding the nasolacrimal duct [54, 55]. Usually a nasoethmoidal orbital fracture is present in these injuries. Evaluation of the lacrimal system after trauma [79] may include irrigation of the system with fluorescein dye or saline, which may be detected either in the wound after lacrimal transection or in the nose when an intact lacrimal system is present. Transections of the canalicular lacrimal system are repaired with fine sutures under magnification. The lacrimal system is usually intubated with fine tubes (0.025 inch) of silicone [18] intubating the upper and lower puncta. These tubes are then brought through the nasolacrimal canal into the nose where they remain for several weeks to "stent" the repair. The absence of tearing indicates a functioning, patent lacrimal system.

FRONTAL SINUS FRACTURES

The frontal sinus occupies the central portion of the frontal bone and consists of two paired but unequal cavities that drain through the floor of the frontal sinus via the nasofrontal ducts. Each sinus cavity has its own duct that extends down through the ethmoidal cells to empty into the middle portion of the nose. The frontal sinus begins to develop between 5 and 10 years of age and forms a significant pneumatized cavity in the lower frontal bone during the late teenage years. The bone is thus weak in this area when compared to the lateral or supraorbital segments of the frontal bone.

The extent of the frontal sinus is variable in addition to being asymmetric. In unusual cases, it involves virtually the entire frontal bone and supraorbital region, whereas its usual extent is confined to the central one-third of the frontal area. The two sinus cavities are separated by an intrasinus septum.

Frontal sinus fractures cause few acute symptoms and are suspected when contusions, bruises, or lacerations occur in the central portion of the forehead. Frequently the deformity due to a depressed fracture of the anterior wall is not perceived until the swelling has resolved. Associated fractures in the supraorbital, nasoethmoid, or anterior cranial fossa area are commonly present. The frontal sinus may be accurately assessed only by computed tomography demonstrating integrity of the bony structures or fractures involving the posterior wall, anterior wall, or nasofrontal duct area. Cerebrospinal fluid leaks and pneumocephalus frequently accompany frontal fractures, as the posterior wall of the frontal sinus forms the boundary between the cranial and sinus cavities. Epistaxis may accompany these injuries.

### Radiographic Evaluation

Plain films such as Caldwell and Water's radiographs may show linear or comminuted fractures with depression and frontal sinus opacification or an air-fluid level. An accurate evaluation of the injury always requires a CT scan, including thin cuts showing the anterior and posterior walls of the frontal sinus, floor of the frontal sinus, roof of the orbits, and nasofrontal duct area. Posterior table fractures are significant because of the possibility of injury to the underlying dura.

### Treatment

Treatment of frontal sinus fractures includes a variety of procedures [3, 33, 34, 69, 70, 92, 131, 144, 169]. Treatment depends on the anatomic area involved by the fracture. For fractures involving only the floor of the frontal sinus, such as the isolated nasoethmoid orbital fracture, no frontal sinus treatment is specifically necessary unless persistent obstruction is demonstrated. The patient is observed periodically for evidence of sinus opacification or obstruction, which should be treated by frontal sinus obliteration.

For isolated anterior wall fractures displaying displacement [169], a surgical approach via a local or coronal incision is recommended. A local incision is rarely appropriate for a significant fracture and is aesthetically more conspicuous than a well healed coronal incision. Depressed anterior wall fragments are exposed and ragged mucosa débrided [144]. The patency of the nasofrontal duct is ensured, and the anterior wall fragments can be fixed in position with interfragment wires. Late frontal sinus obstruction may occur in these patients, or a mucocele (mucous cyst) may develop within the sinus that requires late surgical intervention. Patients with a history of frontal sinus fracture are kept under periodic observation. In fractures where significant dislocation of the anterior and posterior walls of the frontal sinus have occurred, or in fractures where the nasofrontal duct is obstructed, the mucosa is removed and the walls of the sinus lightly burred with an abrasive bit [69, 70, 92]. This step eliminates small mucosal invaginations into the bone and prevents regeneration of frontal sinus mucosa. The nasofrontal duct orifice is plugged with a properly designed bone graft; the cavity may be filled with cancellous bone (preferred) or fat, or it may be left open to obliterate with a combination of scar tissue and bone. The latter process is termed *osteoneogenesis.* The anterior wall of the frontal sinus is then reconstructed with interfragment wires or rigid fixation using existing fragments or bone graft materials. Alternately, the sinus may be "exenterated," which involves thorough removal of the mucous membrane and débridement of bone fragments. The skin is allowed to collapse against the posterior wall of the frontal sinus or the dura. This procedure eliminates the potential space created by the reconstruction of the anterior wall of the frontal sinus, and it is the safest procedure in terms of the subsequent

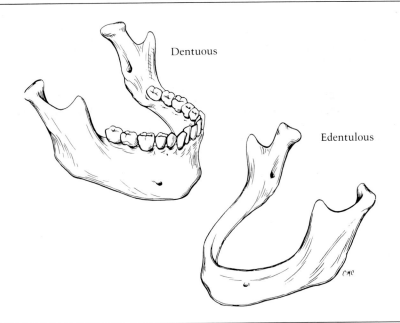

*Figure 12-37 Comparison of the dentulous and edentulous mandible. The loss of the alveolar process and the teeth weakens the mandible in the region of the angle. The angle is thus the most common area to fracture in an edentulous mandible and the second most common area for fracture in the subcondylar area. In the dentulous mandible the most common fracture is observed in the subcondylar area with the angle and the parasymphysis symphysis area being frequently involved. The third molar and long root of the cuspid teeth weaken these areas. Many fractures of the mandible are multiple, and a second fracture should be sought if one fracture is identified.*

incidence of infection. It is not routinely utilized, however, as it is cosmetically deforming and requires cranioplasty with alloplastic or autogenous material. It is utilized only in the presence of established infection following primary reconstruction [124]. Patients demonstrating infection after immediate reconstruction must undergo débridement of devitalized bone fragments. A 6- to 12-month period then elapses before the patient undergoes frontal cranioplasty. Remnants of the frontal sinus and any communication with the nose must be eliminated

and any residual ethmoidal disease eradicated before a cranioplasty is undertaken.

MANDIBULAR FRACTURES
The mandibular fracture is a common facial injury, especially in the multiply injured patient. The prominent position of the mandible renders it susceptible to trauma. Frequently mandibular fractures are multiple, and a second mandibular fracture is suspected if one fracture is identified. Mandibular fractures may be classified according to the state of the dentition (Fig. 12-37) and the region of the mandible in which the fracture occurs [60] (Fig. 12-38). Finally, they are classified as closed or open depending on whether they have a communication with a skin laceration or with an intraoral laceration. Mandibular fractures frequently coexist with cervical spine injuries, other facial fractures, and head injuries. The sites and frequency of mandibular fractures vary with the age of the patient and the state of the dentition [60] (see Figs. 12-37 and 12-38).

Generally, mandibular fractures occur in structurally weak areas, such as the subcondylar area, the angle region of the mandible that is weakened by the presence of a third molar tooth, or the cuspid region where the long root of the cuspid tooth weakens the bone structure. In the edentulous mandible, the most common area to be fractured is between the body and the angle, an area that is weak owing to the loss of alveolar bone. The subcondylar fracture is frequently observed in both dentulous and edentulous mandible fractures. Treatment of mandibular fractures involves establishing a proper occlusal relation with the upper jaw.

The mandible conceptually may be considered to have horizontal and vertical segments. The vertical segment consists of the condyle, the condylar neck, and the ramus with the coronoid process. At the angle, the horizontal segment joins the vertical segment. The horizontal segment of the mandible consists of the body, parasymphysis, and symphysis areas. Fractures are additionally classified in terms of their direction, such as oblique, transverse, comminuted, or greenstick. Fractures that have teeth adjacent to both sides of the fracture are class I fractures. With class II fractures, there are teeth present on only one side of the fracture, and open reduction is usually required. With class III fractures, there are no teeth on either side of the fracture, and open reduction is usually required if significant displacement has occurred.

*Diagnosis*

The diagnosis of mandibular fractures is suggested by the presence of pain, swelling, tenderness, and malocclusion. Fractured teeth, gaps or level discrepancy in the dentition, asymmetry of the dental arch, the presence of intraoral lacerations, loose teeth, and crepitus indicate the possibility of a mandibular fracture. Frequently the patient volunteers that the teeth do not feel like they are "coming together properly." Numbness in the distribution of the mental nerve may accompany fractures of the body, angle, or ramus areas. Bleeding may be observed from

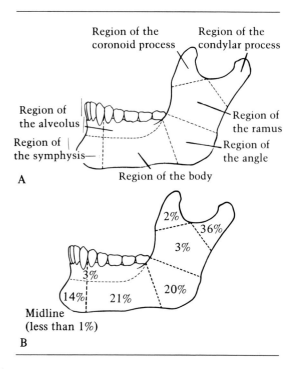

**Figure 12-38** *A. Anatomic regions of the mandible. B. Frequency of fractures in those regions.*

lacerations or from a tooth socket. Fractured, missing, or dislocated teeth are frequently present. Trismus (pain on moving the jaw) is noted. An open bite occurs if there is inability to fully occlude the teeth anteriorly, laterally, or bilaterally. The jaw may deviate toward one side on opening. The patient may not be able to bring the teeth into full intercuspation. Condylar fractures or dislocations frequently lacerate the ear canal and produce bleeding from this area. The presence of an alveolar fracture of the mandible is indicated by instability of a section of the mandibular dentition relative to the basal bone of the mandible. An alveolar fracture indicates that there has been separation of alveolar bone from the basal bone of the mandible.

The mandible has strong muscular attachments that result in displacement following injury (Fig. 12-39). The function of the mus-

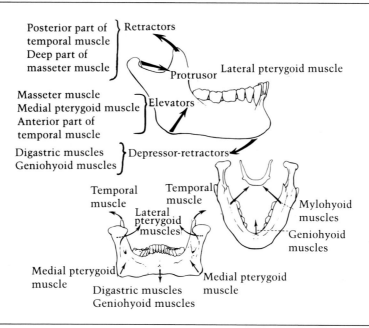

**Figure 12-39** *Main directions of the composite forces of the mandibular muscles.*

cular groups attaching to the mandible may be divided according to the displacement produced. Muscles that elevate the mandible include the masseter, medial pterygoid, and temporalis. The protrusor muscles include the lateral pterygoids. The depressor-retractor group of muscles include the geniohyoid and digastric muscles. The mylohyoid muscle may result in lingual rotation of the mandible.

The direction of a fracture line may oppose fracture displacement. Analysis of the vertical and transverse directions of the fracture may be utilized to predict fracture stability following closed reduction techniques in that the direction of the fracture line should oppose the forces of displacement caused by the muscles attached to the mandible (Fig. 12-40).

*Radiographic Evaluation*
Radiographic evaluation consists in a Panorex examination, lateral oblique films of the mandible, posteroanterior views of the mandible, and a Towne's skull view. Lateral oblique views of the mandible visualize the body, angle, and ramus area. The posteroanterior view demonstrates the mandibular symphysis, angles, and lower ramus. The Towne's view demonstrates the condyle and subcondylar area. The Panorex examination is the single best examination of the mandible but requires patient cooperation and usually travel to a dental facility. Specialized dental films, such as occlusal, palatal, or apical views of the teeth, may be indicated but again involve travel to a dental facility.

*Treatment*
Intraoral and extraoral lacerations are closed; bone fragments are débrided; and fractured or grossly loose teeth are removed. The principal treatment for mandibular fractures is the application of intermaxillary fixation devices to hold the teeth in occlusion with the maxilla. Alternately, plate-and-screw fixation techniques [23, 146, 147, 155, 166] may be employed to permit early motion without intermaxillary fixation postoperatively.

Isolated subcondylar fractures are usually treated by intermaxillary fixation alone [20] or with functional therapy [165]. Rarely, open reduction [174] is necessary. Fractures in the region of the angle, body, or symphysis may be treated by either open or closed reduction techniques [11, 22, 35, 75, 93, 164] depending on the displacement and the "favorable" or "unfavorable" direction of the fracture line. The use of a lingual splint [72] is necessary for some fractures, such as the parasymphysis fracture occurring with bilateral subcondylar neck fractures. The application of a lingual splint prevents rotation of the mandibular body segments and the increase in the transverse width of the mandible through the angles. Splints may be discontinued postoperatively when rigid fixation is employed. Fractures of the coronoid process [42, 136] are uncommon and usually require no treatment or perhaps a short period of intermaxillary fixation. Fractures in edentulous mandibles may be treated with a soft diet if minimal displacement has occurred [97, 173]. Alternately, they may require open reduction with plate-and-screw fixation (Figs. 12-41 and 12-42), which is preferable to interfragment wiring supplemented by the use of a denture modified to provide intermaxillary fixation. Edentulous atrophic mandibles may require bone grafting at the time of fracture reduction. Studies have shown that the height on the bone in the edentulous mandible is a predictor of complications such as nonunion. When the height exceeded 2 cm, union was universal; 20 percent of the nonunions were observed in the group in whom the height ranged from 1 to 2 cm. Eighty percent of the complications were observed when the height was less than 1 cm—thus the recommendation for immediate bone grafting when this fracture requires open reduction [97, 173].

CLOSED REDUCTION AND INTERMAXILLARY FIXATION. The fracture is manipulated into the proper position with closed reduction and arch bars applied to the teeth and connected to the maxilla with intermaxillary wires. Intermaxillary fixation is maintained for 3 to 4 weeks for condylar fractures and

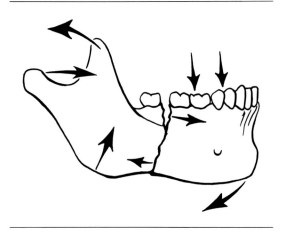

**Figure 12-40** *Displacement of mandibular segments in a proximal body fracture produced by the composite actions of the muscle forces described in Fig. 12-39.*

for 4 to 6 weeks for fractures in other areas of the mandible. It is important to maintain oral hygiene during the period of intermaxillary fixation and to provide a sufficient nutritional liquid diet for patients unable to chew.

OPEN REDUCTION. Open reductions may be performed intraorally [22, 165, 166, 170] or extraorally. In the region of the angle of the mandible, intraoral reduction may be performed by placing an interfragment wire or plate along the upper or lower border (or both borders) of the mandible across the fracture site. In the symphysis and parasymphysis areas, the use of a gingivobuccal sulcus incision allows exposure of the entire parasymphysis–symphysis area and unexcelled exposure of this region. For fractures of the body, intraoral reduction may be more difficult: An external incision is made along the inferior border of the mandible, with care taken to preserve the marginal mandibular branch of the facial nerve [32]. The fracture site is exposed, the fracture is reduced, and small drill holes are made on both sides of the fracture. Stainless steel wire (No. 24) is threaded through the holes and twisted to maintain fracture alignment. The use of a

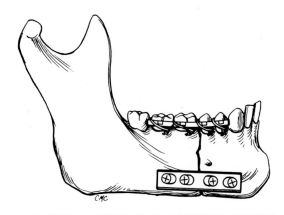

**Figure 12-41** *Treatment of a mandibular fracture by application of an arch bar and compression plating at the inferior border. The arch bar acts as a "tension band" uniting the superior alveolus. Intermaxillary fixation is not necessary.*

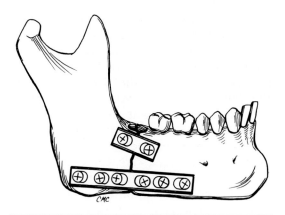

**Figure 12-42** *Treatment of an angle fracture with compression plating. The third molar has been removed in the course of the open reduction. A compression plate is applied at the inferior border and a tension band plate at the superior border. Such fixation is stable and permits immediate function without intermaxillary fixation. The screws are bicortical and precisely measured to the thickness of the mandible. The plates must be carefully bent to exactly conform to the bone contour desired.*

plate and screws [146, 147, 155] or lag screws [129] for fragment fixation allows increased stability and in practice has replaced inter-fragment wiring techniques for fractures requiring open reduction. The period of inter-maxillary fixation is reduced and may be eliminated if a stable (A-O plate) fixation is utilized.

Complications include nonunion, delayed union, and infection [49]. Delayed union usually responds to a brief period of increased intermaxillary fixation and is usually not perceived when intermaxillary fixation is utilized. Nonunion indicates failure of union at 3 months, at which point débridement, bone grafting, and rigid fixation are required. Infection requires débridement of devitalized bone, removal of involved teeth (apical films are helpful), stabilization with internal or external fixation, and possible bone grafting.

## Gunshot and Shotgun Wounds

The treatment of ballistic injuries to the facial region depends on the amount of bony and soft tissue injury and loss [13, 38, 52, 66, 68, 112]. These conditions relate directly to the mass and velocity of the projectile. With low velocity (civilian) gunshot injuries [122] there is minimal soft tissue injury and the bone injury is of limited extent. These injuries are managed as simple fractures with overlying lacerations, and the techniques described under the regional treatment of fractures are appropriate. In higher velocity gunshot or close-range shotgun injuries, significant soft tissue loss occurs, and primary closure of the soft tissue may not be possible. Initial skin-to-muscosa closure is followed by serial (every 48 hours) débridement until all devitalized soft tissue has been removed. During this period, fracture fragments may be held in position with either plate-and-screw fixation or external fixation devices. Soft tissue reconstruction may then proceed with completion of fixation and bone grafting.

Close-range shotgun injuries involve areas

of bone and soft tissue injury and areas of bone and soft tissue loss. The areas of loss determine the treatment required. In general, bone fixation is achieved in the anatomic position with the use of rigid internal or external fixation compensating for areas of bone loss. Soft tissue reconstruction is then accomplished, and areas of bone loss are replaced with bone grafts. It is important to achieve anatomic reduction of existing bone during the first stages of injury treatment and to maintain this position until soft tissue reconstruction and bone reconstruction have been completed. Facial deformity is thus minimized. In general, the fracture treatment for each region is the same as that described above, emphasizing the use of rigid internal fixation techniques. Reconstruction of these devastating injuries has been worthwhile despite the fact that the injuries frequently represent suicide attempts [51, 57].

## Facial Fractures in Children

Facial fractures in children account for about 5 percent of all facial fractures [7, 40, 53, 62, 67, 81, 130, 137, 142]. Most of these fractures occur in children over 5 years of age. Children's bones are cancellous and soft, and they frequently displace without fracture as they are subject to lesser injury forces. After a fracture, bone healing progresses rapidly. Sinuses are small. Some adjustment occurs with growth, such that minor occlusal deformity after a fracture may be eliminated by the adaptive potential of alveolar bone and the development of secondary dentition.

Treatment of children's fractures in the upper face follows the same principles described for adults, with the emphasis on early or immediate treatment, as healing occurs rapidly. (It may be difficult to reduce a Le Fort fracture properly after even 1 week.) It may also be difficult to apply intermaxillary fixation devices to children with mixed dentition, and the added use of a piriform aperture, circumandibular wires, or suspension wires is recommended when intermaxillary fixation is necessary to stabilize the arch bars. Children have shallowly rooted teeth, especially during the period of mixed dentition, and the shape of the crowns may make application of arch bars difficult. An acrylic splint may improve alignment of mandibular fractures for closed reduction techniques and prevent an open reduction. Intermaxillary fixation, when utilized, must be present only for a 3-week period for treatment of mandibular and maxillary fractures in children. Any malocclusion is undesirable; however, children are able to compensate for small degrees of malocclusion with developing growth and the eruption of the secondary dentition.

A frequent injury in children is subcondylar fracture of the mandible. If the child can bring the mandible into a proper occlusal relation with the maxilla, only a soft diet is necessary. Alternately, a short period of intermaxillary fixation is recommended to preserve occlusal relations. If open reduction of a mandibular fracture is performed, one must be careful to avoid the tooth roots and tooth buds, as they extend close to the inferior border of the mandible.

## Temporomandibular Joint Injuries

Temporomandibular joint injuries consist in dislocations and injuries to the intraarticular structures. A common acute dislocation of the mandible without fracture involves dislocation of the condyle anterior to the articular eminence [77]. This dislocation usually occurs bilaterally, and the patient is unable to close the mouth. Reduction is achieved by placing the thumbs of both hands on the occlusal side of the molar teeth (or the alveolar ridge, if edentulous). The mandible is displaced downward and backward. Usually reduction can be achieved with this maneuver. A local anesthetic may be injected into the joint to relieve pain and muscle spasm, permitting reduction of the dislocation. In some instances, general anesthesia must be used.

Injuries to the internal joint mechanism and meniscus can produce clicking or locking with pain. These situations require selective evaluation by arthrographic techniques and reconstructive surgery for intrajoint structures.

## References

1. Adams, W. M. Internal wiring fixation of facial fractures. *Surgery* 12:523, 1942.
2. Adams, W. M., and Adam, L. H. Internal wire fixation of facial fractures: A 15 year follow-up report. *Am. J. Surg.* 92:12, 1956.
3. Adkins, W. Y., Cassone, R. D., and Putney, F. J. Solitary frontal sinus fractures. *Laryngoscope* 89:1099, 1979.
4. Angle, E. H. Classification of malocclusion. *Dent. Cosmos* 41:248, 1899.
5. Ayella, R. J. The Face. In *Radiologic Management of the Massively Traumatized Patient*. Baltimore: Williams & Wilkins, 1978. P. 33.
6. Babcock, J. L. Cervical spine injuries: Diagnosis and classification. *Arch. Surg.* 111:646, 1976.
7. Bales, C. R., Randall, P., and Lehr, H. B. Fractures of the facial bones in children. *J. Trauma* 12:56, 1972.
8. Barkowski, S. B., and Krzystkowa, K. M. Blow out fracture of the orbit: Diagnostic and therapeutic considerations, results in 90 patients, *J. Maxillofac. Surg.* 10:155, 1982.
9. Barton, F. E., and Berry, W. L. Evaluation of the acutely injured orbit. In S. J. Aston et al. (eds.), *Third International Symposium of Plastic and Reconstructive Surgery of the Eye and Adnexae*. Baltimore: Williams & Wilkins, 1982.
10. Becker, D. P., et al. The outcome from severe head injury with early diagnosis and intensive management. *J. Neurosurg.* 47:491, 1977.
11. Bochlogyros, P. N. A retrospective study of 1,521 mandibular fractures. *J. Oral Maxillofac. Surg.* 43:547, 1985.
12. Brawley, B. W., and Kelly, W. A. Treatment of basal skull fractures with and without cerebrospinal fluid fistulae. *J. Neurosurg.* 26:57, 1967.
13. Broadbent, T. R., and Woolf, R. M. Gunshot wounds of the face; Initial care. *J. Trauma* 12:229, 1972.
14. Brown, J. B., and McDonnell, F. Internal wire pin fixation for fractures of upper jaw, orbit, zygoma and severe facial crushes. *Plast. Reconstr. Surg.* 9:276, 1952.
15. Brown, J. D., Fryer, M. P., and McDonnell, F. Internal wire-pin immobilization of jaw fractures. *Plast. Reconstr. Surg.* 4:30, 1979.
16. Bucholz, R. W., et al. Occult cervical spine injuries in fatal traffic accidents. *J. Trauma* 19:768, 1979.
17. Cahill, D. W., Rao, K. C., and Ducker, T. B. Delayed carotid cavernous sinus fistula and multiple cranial neuropathy following basal skull fracture. *Surg. Neurol.* 16:17, 1981.
18. Callahan, M. A. Silicone intubation for lacrimal canaliculi repair. *Ann. Plast. Surg.* 2:355, 1979.
19. Cambell, D. A. Discussion. In W. W. Glas, O. J. King, Jr., and A. Andlui. Complications of tracheostomy. *Arch. Surg.* 85:62, 1962.
20. Chalmers, J. Lyons Club Lecture: Fractures involving the mandibular condyle: Post treatment survey of 120 cases. *J. Oral Surg.* 5:45, 1947.
21. Christian, M. S. Non-fatal injuries sustained by seatbelt wearers: A comparative study. *Br. Med. J.* 2:1310, 1976.
22. Chuong, R., and Donoff, R. B. Intraoral open reduction of mandibular fractures. *Int. J. Oral Surg.* 14:22, 1985.
23. Chuong, R., Donoff, R. B., and Goralnick, W. C. A retrospective analysis of 327 mandibular fractures. *J. Oral Maxillofac. Surg.* 41:305, 1983.
24. Converse, J. M., and Smith, B. Enophthalmos and diplopia in fracture of the orbital floor. *Br. J. Plast. Surg.* 9:265, 1957.
25. Converse, J. M., and Smith, B. Reconstruction of the floor of the orbit by bone grafts. *Am. J. Ophthalmol.* 44:1, 1950.
26. Converse, J. M., and Smith, B. Naso orbital fractures and traumatic deformities of the medial canthus. *Plast. Reconstr. Surg.* 38:147, 1966.
27. Converse, J. M., et al. Orbital blow-out fractures: A ten year study. *Plast. Reconstr. Surg.* 39:20, 1967.
28. Cramer, L. M., Tooze, F. M., and Lerman, S. Blow-out fractures of the orbit. *Br. J. Plast. Surg.* 18:171, 1965.
29. Curtin, H. D., Wolfe, P., and Schramm, V. Orbital roof blow-out fractures. *A.J.R.* 139:969, 1981.

30. Dagi, T. F., Meyer, F. B., and Poletti, C. A. The incidence and prevention of meningitis after basilar skull fractures. *Am. J. Emerg. Med.* 1:295, 1983.

31. Dawson, R. L., and Fordyce, G. L. Complex fractures of the middle third of the face and this early treatment. *Br. J. Surg.* 41:25, 1953.

32. Dingman, R. O., and Grabb, W. C. Surgical anatomy of the mandibular ramus of the facial nerve based on the dissection of 100 facial halves. *Plast. Reconstr. Surg.* 29:266, 1962.

33. Donald, P. J. Frontal sinus ablation by cranialization. *Arch. Otolaryngol.* 108:142, 1982.

34. Donald, P. J., and Bernstein, L. Compound frontal sinus injuries with intracranial penetration. *Laryngoscope* 88:225, 1978.

35. Eid, K., Lynch, O. J., and Whitaker, L. A. Mandibular fractures: The problem patient. *J. Trauma* 16:658, 1976.

36. Ellis, E., el Attar, A., and Moos, K. An analysis of 2067 cases of zygomatic-orbital fracture. *J. Oral Maxillofac. Surg.* 43:417, 1985.

37. Emery, J. M., von Noorden, G. K., and Schlernitzauer, D. A. Orbital floor fractures: Long-term follow-up of cases with and without surgical repair. *Trans. Am. Acad. Ophthalmol. Otolaryngol.* 75:802, 1971.

38. Finch, D. R., and Dibbell, D. G. Immediate reconstruction of gunshot injuries to the face. *J. Trauma* 19:965, 1979.

39. Finney, L. A., Reynolds, D. H., and Yates, B. M. Comminuted subfrontal fractures. *J. Trauma* 4:711, 1964.

40. Fortunato, M., Fielding, A. F., and Guernsey, C. H. Facial bone fractures in children. *Oral Surg. Oral Med. Oral Pathol.* 53:225, 1982.

41. Fradkin, A. H. Orbital floor fractures and ocular complications. *Am. J. Ophthalmol.* 72:699, 1971.

42. Frim, S. P. Fracture of the coronoid process. *Oral Surg. Oral Med. Oral Pathol.* 45:978, 1978.

43. Fueger, G. F., Bright, J., and Milauskas, A. The Roentgenological Anatomy of the Floor and of the Orbit. In G. M. Bleeker and T. K. Lyle (eds.), *Fractures of the Orbit.* Baltimore: Williams & Wilkins, 1970.

44. Fujino, T., and Makino, K. Entrapment mechanisms and ocular injury in orbital blow-out fracture. *Plast. Reconstr. Surg.* 65:571, 1980.

45. Fukado, Y. Results in 400 cases of surgical decompression of the optic nerve. *Mod. Probl. Ophthalmol.* 14:474, 1975.

46. Gentry, L. R., et al. High resolution analysis of struts in facial trauma. 1. Normal anatomy. 2. Osseous and soft tissue complications. *A.J.R.* 140:523, 1983.

47. Georgiade, N., and Nash, T. An external cranial fixation apparatus for severe maxillofacial injuries. *Plast. Reconstr. Surg.* 38:142, 1966.

48. Gillies, H. D., Kilner T. P., and Stone, D. Fractures of the malar-zygomatic compound with a description of a new x-ray position. *Br. J. Surg.* 14:651, 1927.

49. Giordano, A. M., et al. Chronic osteomyelitis following mandibular fractures and its treatment. *Arch. Otolaryngol.* 108:30, 1982.

50. Godoy, J., and Mathog, R. H. Malar fractures associated with exophthalmos. *Arch. Otolaryngol.* 111:174, 1985.

51. Goodman, J. M., and Kalsbeck, J. Outcome of self-inflicted gunshot wounds of the head. *J. Trauma* 5:636, 1965.

52. Goodstein, W. A., Stryker, A., and Weiner, L. J. Primary treatment of shotgun injuries to the face. *J. Trauma* 19:961, 1979.

53. Graham, G. G., and Peltier, R. J. Management of mandibular fractures in children. *J. Oral Surg.* 18:416, 1960.

54. Gruss, J. S. Naso-ethmoid-orbital fractures: Classification and role of primary bone grafting. *Plast. Reconstr. Surg.* 75:303, 1985.

55. Gruss, J. S., et al. The pattern and incidence of nasolacrimal injury in naso-ethmoidal orbital fractures: The role of delayed assessment and dacryocystorhinostomy. *Br. J. Plast. Surg.* 38:116, 1985.

56. Gruss, J. S., et al. The role of primary bone grafting in complex craniomaxillofacial trauma. *Plast. Reconstr. Surg.* 75:17, 1985.

57. Gurdjian, E., and Webster, J. Mechanism of head injury. In *Head Injury.* Boston: Little, Brown, 1958. P. 58.

58. Guyon, J. J., Brant-Zawadzki, M., and Seiff, S. R. C.T. demonstration of optic canal fractures. *A.J.R.* 143:1031, 1984.

59. Gwyn, P. P., et al. Facial fractures—associated injuries and complications. *Plast. Reconstr. Surg.* 47:225, 1971.

60. Hagan, E. H., and Huelke, D. F. An analysis of 319 case reports of mandibular fractures. *J. Oral Surg.* 19:93, 1961.

# 13

James M. Stuzin
Barry M. Zide

# Scalp, Calvarium, and Forehead Reconstruction

The coalescence of several bones around the brain forms a protective covering known as the calvarium (or calvaria). This bony armor serves to absorb the shock of blunt and sharp injuries and is itself protected by the overlying soft tissue of the scalp. Loss of this protective covering often leads to desiccation of the calvarium and the development of infection and sequestration.

Numerous reports, beginning with the Egyptians in 3000 BC and extending to efforts during the Industrial Revolution, attest to the difficulty of these injuries and the lethality associated with lack of prompt soft tissue coverage of exposed calvarium. A review of the early literature indicates that many of these unfortunate patients were doomed to die because of prolonged infection and intracranial complications. Those who survived had chronic wounds, with denuded bone, sequestrations, and dense scar. These chronic ulcers often terminated in scar carcinomas [14].

The basic principle when approaching defects of scalp, calvarium, and forehead is early soft tissue coverage of exposed bone. Bony reconstruction to restore contour and skull integrity remains secondary to adequate wound closure. Conversely, soft tissue coverage alone over a bony defect does not provide adequate protective covering of in-

tracranial contents and is often lacking in proper contour. Reconstructive efforts in this region must thus look at scalp, forehead, and calvarium as a single reconstructive unit.

## Anatomy

The scalp and forehead are part of the same structural anatomic unit. This region is generally described as being comprised of five distinct anatomic layers: skin, subcutaneous tissue, galea, loose areolar tissue, and pericranium [16]. The main differences between scalp and forehead are the lack of hair-bearing tissue present in the forehead skin and the presence of the frontalis muscle anteriorly (Fig. 13-1). The skin is thickest in the occiput and decreases in thickness as one moves anteriorly and temporally.

The subcutaneous layer, formed of dense connective tissue and fat, binds the skin to the underlying galea. The subcutaneous layer contains the principal arteries and veins of the scalp, as well as the sensory nerves and lymphatics.

The galea aponeurotica is the tough fibrous layer of the scalp. It is extensive in its attachments and is, in reality, a part of the subcutaneous musculoaponeurotic system (SMAS) of the face [31, 46]. It connects the

397

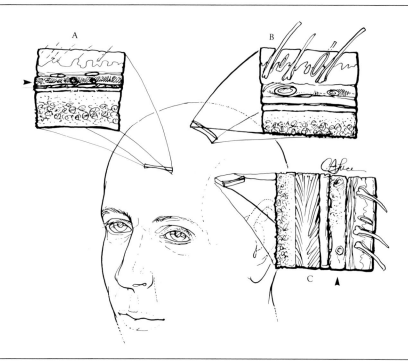

**Figure 13-1** *A. Forehead layers: skin, subcutaneous tissue, galea (dart)/frontalis, subaponeurotic cellular layer (Merker's gap), periosteum, bone. B. SCALP layers (using the mnemonic):* S*kin,* C*onnective tissue (tight)/ subcutaneous tissue with hair follicles,* A*poneurosis (and blood vessels),* L*oose connective tissue,* P*eriosteum, (bone).* *C. Temporal layers: skin, superficial temporal fascia, innominate fascia (dart), temporalis fascia, temporalis muscle, (no real periosteal layer), bone.*

occipitalis muscle posteriorly with the frontalis muscle anteriorly. It is similarly continuous with the auricularis muscles posterolaterally and the SMAS of the face below. Laterally, overlying the temporalis muscle, it becomes continuous with a thin, highly vascular layer of moderately dense connective tissue, which has been termed the temporoparietal fascia, or superficial temporal fascia. Although the galea and the temporoparietal fascia are continuous, their junction is indistinct. The temporoparietal fascia becomes more firmly attached to the scalp and its subdermal layer as it approaches the vertex, and it is usually indistinct from galea beginning at a point 12 cm above the ear [8].

The loose areolar space underneath the galea is composed of thin, avascular connective tissue and has been termed the subaponeurotic layer [11]. It may easily be dissected sharply or bluntly, and most avulsion injuries occur in this plane. A number of fine perforating vessels cross this space from the galea to the pericranium and extend to the underlying calvarium [15]. The laxity present within the subaponeurotic layer provides the mobility of the scalp.

The innermost layer of the scalp, the pericranium, is densely adherent to the outer table of the skull. The pericranium contains an ample vascular network that allows it to serve as a recipient bed for skin grafts as well as be fashioned as random flaps to cover exposed areas of calvarium [72]. When mobilizing the scalp, dissection should stay superficial to the pericranium, leaving this layer intact.

## Basic Principles of Scalp Reconstruction

Lacerations, contusions, and small avulsion injuries of the scalp are common, most often due to blunt trauma. The scalp is endowed with a rich blood supply, and if properly managed primary healing can be expected. Bleeding may be underestimated and extensive, especially with partially lacerated vessels. It is managed by pressure or precise suture ligation, as well as replacement when necessary.

Scalp lacerations require proper local care prior to closure, with thorough irrigation and débridement of devitalized tissue or foreign material. Hemostasis is crucial, as subgaleal hematoma is a common predecessor to subgaleal abscess formation, facial and periorbital cellulitis, and, in its most extreme form, intracranial infection extending via the diploic vessels. After adequate wound preparation, scalp lacerations may be closed in a single layer, preferably with interrupted nonabsorbable sutures (2-0, 3-0, or 4-0), including the galea in the closure. This method secures the supragaleal vessels, preventing hematoma formation. Alternatively, a two-layer closure, securing the galea and subcutaneous tissue with buried suture followed by a permanent suture material to close the skin, provides adequate wound closure. Large scalp lacerations may be drained by suction catheter or Penrose drains, again to prevent subgaleal collections.

After debridement or substantial tissue loss, the scalp may require extensive undermining in the loose areolar level underneath the galea prior to closure. The galea may require scoring to provide laxity. For lacerations of the posterior and peripheral areas of the scalp, it is always best to take advantage of the relative looseness of the skin in the nape of the neck by extensive undermining in this region. This step can greatly aid in wound closure, although attention must be given to prevent noticeable distortion of the hairline.

The scalp has a particularly rich blood supply arising from four principal arteries and lesser contributing vessels (Fig. 13-2). The occipital and superficial temporal arteries on each side are the key vascular input channels. The posterior auricular and the small branches of the external carotid artery extensively contribute to the scalp, as do the supraorbital and supratrochlear vessels, which are terminal branches of the internal carotid system. These vessels travel in the layer above the galea and form abundant communications, such that the whole scalp can survive on one major vessel, as demonstrated by successful replantation efforts [10, 26, 45].

The lateral territory of the scalp is supplied primarily by the superficial temporal artery. This artery is the largest and longest vessel of the scalp and supplies the greatest area. This terminal branch of the external carotid artery becomes superficial just in front of the tragus of the ear as it emerges from the parenchyma of the parotid gland. The superficial temporal artery then travels within the temporoparietal fascia after it crosses the zygomatic arch and provides extensive vascularity to this layer. About 2 cm above the zygomatic arch the artery bifurcates, sending a frontal branch anteriorly and a parietal branch posteriorly. The main continuation of the artery is its posterior branch, which courses in a gentle arc through the parietal region of the scalp [65].

The posterior auricular artery supplies the posterolateral territory. It divides into small tributaries that are short in length and adherent to the mastoid process. Flaps based on this vessel provide a short pedicle.

Posteriorly, the occipital artery is the dominant vessel. The occipital vessels pass deep to the muscles of the cranial base and enter the scalp at the supranuchal line where they divide into two medial and lateral branches. The main vessel may be found about 2 cm lateral to the midline at the supranuchal line.

Anteriorly, the supratrochlear and supraorbital vessels enter the scalp vertically from the

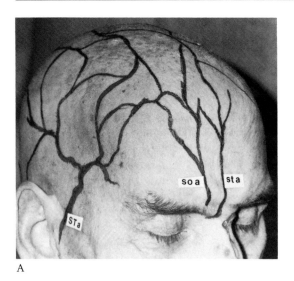

A

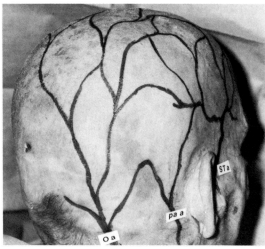

B

*Figure 13-2* *Arteries of the scalp; dominant vessels are in italics. A. soa = supraorbital; sta = supratrochlear; STa = superficial temporal. B. STa = superficial temporal; paa = posterior auricular; Oa = occipital.*

supraorbital rims. They are easily seen and preserved in this region when caudally undermining below the frontalis muscle and above the pericranium. These vessels traverse the frontalis muscle at the brow to travel along the superficial surface of the muscle. They anastomose to form a rich vascular network in the frontoparietal region of the scalp with the other scalp vasculature.

In general, this vascular network sends multiple perforators to the pericranium and through it to the outer cortex of the calvarium. It is the understanding of this principle that has allowed the development of pedicled flaps of vascularized calvarial bone based on axial galeal flaps and its extension laterally as superficial temporal fascia. Bone flaps pedicled on deep temporal fascia [11] and temporal muscle have also been described [71].

The scalp has multiple sensory nerves. The anterior portion of the scalp and forehead is supplied by the supraorbital and supratrochlear nerves, terminal branches of the fifth cranial nerve (CN V). A branch of the second or third cervical nerve (CN II or CN III), the lesser occipital, supplies the posterior scalp, and the great auricular nerve

provides sensation to the posterior auricular region, earlobe, and angle of the jaw. The temporal region receives sensory input from the auriculotemporal nerve, a branch derived from the trigeminal, mandibular root. This nerve may be found accompanying the superficial artery and vein just above the zygomatic arch.

## Avulsion Injuries
PARTIAL-THICKNESS LOSSES
Avulsion injuries commonly produce partial-thickness losses in the subgaleal layer. Small avulsion injuries can be managed by primary closure in a fashion similar to that for simple scalp lacerations (i.e., after undermining and galeal scoring). Large avulsion losses with intact pericranium provide the plastic surgeon with several options for obtaining initial wound closure, which can be followed by secondary reconstruction at a later date.

Lu, in 1969, successfully treated a large scalp avulsion in a child by replacing the avulsed segment as a free composite graft [37]. Although successful in isolated cases, this technique has proved to be an unreliable form of management, as the volume of tissue replanted as a free graft is too great to be nourished by the underlying pericranial bed. Others have successfully defatted the avulsed segment and replaced it as a full-thickness skin graft [55]. However, it is generally agreed that skin grafting of the exposed pericranium is the proper initial management of these injuries. The graft can be taken from a minimally injured or avulsed part or, preferably, from a distant site, such as buttocks or thigh. Secondary scalp reconstruction can then proceed after initial wound healing. Of course, if the graft is taken from the avulsed scalp, it is not expected to grow hair, and the patient must be so informed.

FULL-THICKNESS DEFECTS
Full-thickness defects, involving loss of all layers, including pericranium, are more difficult problems. Skin grafting does not "take" on exposed outer table devoid of pericranium. Furthermore, exposed calvarium deprived of its periosteal blood supply is prone to necrose and sequestrate unless it is kept from drying out. These wounds thus mandate a more aggressive approach to primary wound closure. The technique used may vary with the cause and size of the defect and the quality of the surrounding local tissue. The basic methods used to cover exposed bone are the following.

1. Outer table removal with direct or delayed grafting
2. Pericranial flap and skin graft
3. Local scalp flap(s) with galeal scoring
4. Distant or microvascular flap transfer
5. Expansion

The outer table can be removed by drill and chisel down to bleeding diploë and a skin graft immediately applied [21]. Such grafts are knobby and prone to ulcerate, but they are expeditious. The graft rarely takes 100 percent, but local ointments usually produce slow secondary healing. Another, similar technique involves using small drill holes placed close together down to the diploic spaces, which in time produce granulation tissue. This development occurs slowly over 3 to 5 weeks. When the bed is ready, a skin graft can then be applied.

The senior author (B.Z.) prefers to remove the outer table by first scoring with a drill and then chiseling off the squares of the outer table. The wound is dressed postoperatively to avoid drying. Two layers of Adaptic, followed by gauze and head wrap, are placed. An irrigating catheter (i.e., 16-gauge Intracath) is incorporated in the dressing. The nurses are instructed to add 10 to 30 ml bacitracin solution each shift—enough to keep the dressing slightly moist. The first dressing is changed at 48 hours, then once a day thereafter. Two thicknesses of Adaptic are used as the contact layer each time. Within 12 to 18 days a perfect granulating bed has developed. Excellent, stable graft take is the rule. For basal or squamous cell tumors, this method provides excellent coverage and ease of follow-up (Fig. 13-3).

As alternatives to removal of the outer table, full-thickness losses can be reconstructed using pericranial flaps with overlying skin grafts or local flaps, which also bring hair-bearing tissue into the area of the deficit. Scalp expansion, followed by closure with a local flap, is also an acceptable method of closure, though temporary coverage of exposed bone should be obtained prior to undergoing expansion. Finally, distant flaps may be transferred using microvascular techniques.

FULL-THICKNESS DEFECTS USUALLY
LESS THAN 6 CM
The basic principles of wound preparation, wide undermining, galeal scoring, and primary closure may apply to the treatment of small full-thickness defects. More commonly, the use of local flaps is the best

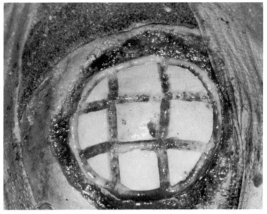

A

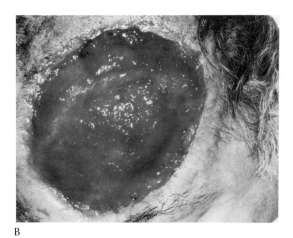

B

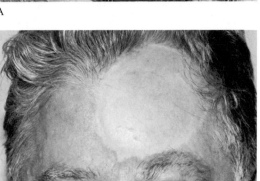

C

**Figure 13-3** *A, B. Basal cell cancer approached the periosteum. The outer table required removal. After burring to diploë, a chisel was used to remove the outer table in sections. Meticulous dressings were then carried out to prepare the bed for grafting. C. Grafted result. The patient is a candidate for expansion at a later date.*

method to close these wounds. These flaps are raised above the pericranium and are based peripherally to include a major nutrient vessel, which can be localized by Doppler imaging or by simple palpation examination. The nonstretchable scalp can be made to cover a larger area by making multiple incisions through the galea according to the techniques of Kazanjian and Converse [5, 14, 53, 54]. This step is performed by placing the surrounding scalp under tension after undermining and making a number of incisions through the galea, approximately 1 cm apart and perpendicular to the direction of tension. Great care must be used to not injure the vessels in the supragaleal plane

when performing galeal scoring; magnifying loupes may be helpful. If the flap must also be widened, the galea may be cross-hatched to relieve tension and permit closure without vascular compromise of the flap. Almost all scalp flaps require galeal scoring to provide successful closure.

*Rotation Flaps*
Quarter scalp rotation flaps are particularly suited for closure of defects up to 6 cm in diameter (smaller in children) (Fig. 13-4). These flaps are designed to take advantage of neck laxity when possible. Some donor defects can be closed primarily, but others require grafting on the pericranium, depending

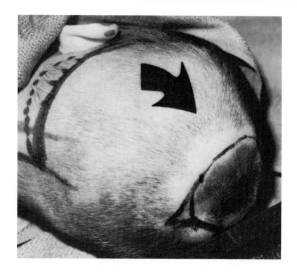 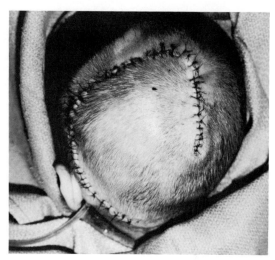

**Figure 13-4** *Partial scalp rotation flaps may be used if the defect is 3 to 6 cm in diameter. Considerable undermining and scoring are required for closure.*

on back cut and advancement. Double opposing flaps, based peripherally, are particularly well suited to closure of defects involving the vertex of the scalp. They can then be revised at a later date, following tissue expansion. Mobilization of scalp adjacent to the donor defect, with galeal scoring, may aid in donor site reduction.

*Advancement Flaps*

Advancement flaps [35] can be used to close full-thickness defects. Large areas of posterior scalp may be closed by advancement, taking advantage of loose neck skin and head extension. When advancement is chosen for other areas, maintenance of a major vessel and heavy galeal scoring are important (Fig. 13-5). The main problem with this type of flap design is its limited ability to move. In addition, advancement of anterior scalp to cover any defect might raise the brows to an objectional height.

*Pericranial Flaps*

The pericranium is the contacting layer of connective tissue overlying the calvarium and below the galea and subaponeurotic layer. It is similar to the periosteum of long bones except that it is thicker, especially in young patients [25]. Endowed with a rich vascular network, it may be utilized as a pedicled flap that provides coverage of denuded bone and acts as a bed for skin grafting [23, 72, 74]. It can also be used as a vascular covering over areas of bone grafting for calvarial reconstruction to enhance bone graft survival.

Pericranial flaps are designed fairly large compared to the defect to be closed and are broad-based. Intact scalp is first raised in the subgaleal plane overlying the pericranium to be used in the flap. Then the pericranium itself is raised using a blunt elevator, with care to not lacerate the pericranium.

The great advantage of pericranial flaps is their minimal donor site morbidity and their dependability as a bed for skin grafting (if properly designed). When resurfacing large areas, pericranial flaps can be used to cover the more central area of the defect, and local scalp flaps can be used to provide the periph-

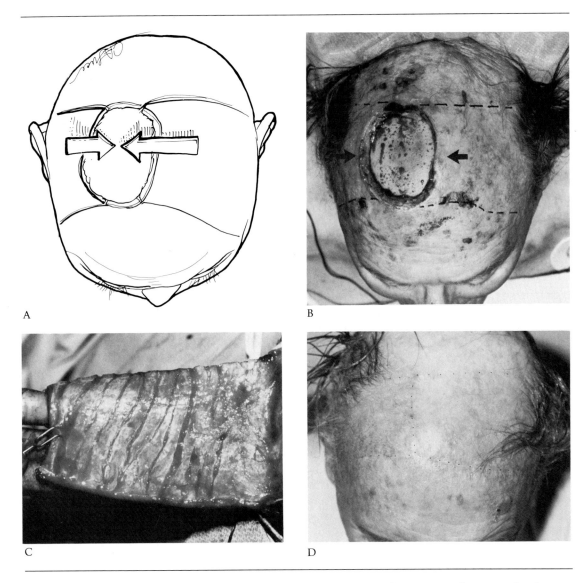

A

B

C

D

*Figure 13-5* *Advancement flaps may be done by scoring the galea or after expansion. A, B. The defect will be closed with scored axial flaps advanced medially. C. Galeal scoring. D. Final result.*

eral wound closure. The small central area is then covered with a skin graft, which can be easily revised at a later date or camouflaged by proper hairstyling.

## MEDIUM-SIZED DEFECTS, USUALLY MORE THAN 6 CM

When dealing with larger defects, the reconstructive options are more complex, although the principles of closure remain the same. If the pericranium is intact, skin grafting allows primary wound closure followed by secondary reconstruction. This method is especially useful in the severely injured patient with associated injuries. For full-thickness defects, large broad-based pericranial flaps, often of the rotation-type design, provide a vascular bed for grafting and a simpler means of closure in the severely injured patient. Large transposition flaps with split-thickness skin grafting of the donor sites offer another initial solution. Replantation of the avulsed segment is a final option in appropriate circumstances, as is tissue expansion.

*Multiple Flaps/Single Subtotal Flap*

As initial management in properly selected patients, as well as for secondary reconstruction of moderately sized defects, the use of multiple axial flaps has been useful. This concept, popularized by Orticochea [53], was initially described as a four-flap technique, utilizing the entire remaining scalp to close the defect. In 1971 this technique was modified to a three-flap technique in which two smaller flaps adjacent to the defect are used to provide primary wound closure and a third larger flap, consisting of the entire remaining scalp, is used to close the donor defect following rotation of the two smaller flaps [53, 54].

This multiple flap technique can generally be used to close defects up to one-third of the scalp surface area. These flaps must be based on known vascular territories, and each flap has its own vascular pedicle included in its base, which can be identified by Doppler examination (Fig. 13-6).

Flaps used to reconstruct anterior scalp and forehead must include the superficial temporal artery and vein. Posteriorly based flaps and flaps used for occipital reconstruction must carry the occipital and hopefully the posterior auricular vessels as well. The width of the two smaller flaps should be at least one-half the width of the primary defect so that when mobilized and juxtaposed they automatically cover the raw surface. The large flap (flap No. 3) essentially includes the rest of the scalp. The pedicle of this flap can be designed on either side when closing midline wounds. If the area to be reconstructed is lateral to the midline, it is

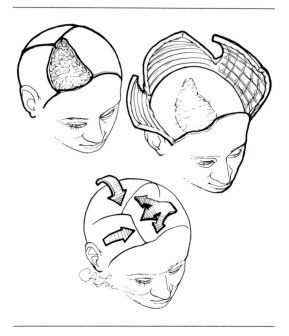

**Figure 13-6** *Orticochea method for large defects. Each flap must have at least one main vessel. The posterior flap may be back cut, sacrificing one occipital vessel if necessary. This method still leaves another to nourish the flap.*

preferable to base the pedicle of the large scalp flap on the contralateral side of the defect.

The three flaps are elevated in the subgaleal plane above the pericranium. Extensive undermining is performed into the remaining scalp, forehead, and nape of the neck; great care is required peripherally in the area where the vascular pedicles enter the scalp to avoid injury to these nutrient vessels. Galeal scoring is required prior to insetting the flaps, and if a great degree of expansion is required, the scoring can be done both perpendicularly and parallel to the axis of the flaps. The circulation of these flaps can be checked with fluorescein after suturing has begun [5] unless epinephrine has been injected. If necessary, the secondary defects can be partially skin-grafted and then revised by excision and lateral expansion at a later date.

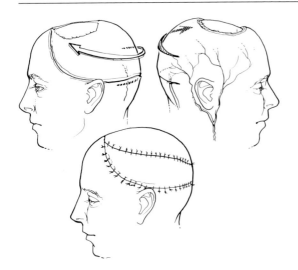

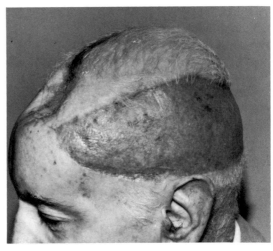

**Figure 13-7** *Single subtotal flap. The entire scalp can survive on any one dominant vessel. In this case, a 9-cm deeply invasive tumor was removed including bone. A single scalp flap based on contralateral superficial temporal and posterior auricular vessels was rotated, leaving a large donor site, which was grafted.*

The advantages of the Orticochea concept of multiple rotation/transposition flaps are that large flaps can be reliably designed based on axial blood supply, the defects can be primarily closed, and closure is obtained with hair-bearing scalp tissue, which provides an excellent aesthetic result. Great care in planning is required to use this technique successfully for single subtotal reconstruction.

When the defect is large (8 to 10 cm) and anterior but more to one side, a single subtotal scalp flap may be raised. Based on the superficial temporal and posterior auricular branches, the remaining scalp may be transposed with a large donor deficit that must be grafted. The patient is appraised preoperatively regarding the size of the graft. The back cut in the occipital region may require special attention (e.g., padding), as it may break down if the patient lies on it (Fig. 13-7).

*Expanders*
Because no other tissue in the human body adequately replaces scalp tissue, expansion is uniquely qualified for reconstruction in this area [3, 4, 35, 40]. Expanders are useful for the initial treatment of large scalp nevi and are valuable after another type of wound

closure has been achieved to avoid infectious complications from the expander prosthesis. For secondary reconstruction, such as to cover an area of previous skin grafting, the prosthesis is placed in the subgaleal space through what will become the advancing edge of the flap. Expansion is then performed over several weeks, the expanders removed, and the flaps advanced. Hair growth has been found to proceed normally during expansion and following transfer of these flaps [3] (Fig. 13-8). A composite (Fig. 13-9) is presented to outline the variations for large defects.

LARGE DEFECTS (MORE THAN
ONE-THIRD OF SCALP) AND TOTAL
SCALP AVULSION
Large defects and total scalp avulsion injuries mandate immediate coverage of exposed calvarium. The best form of reconstruction is replantation of the avulsed tissue [1]. If the avulsed tissue is so badly injured it is

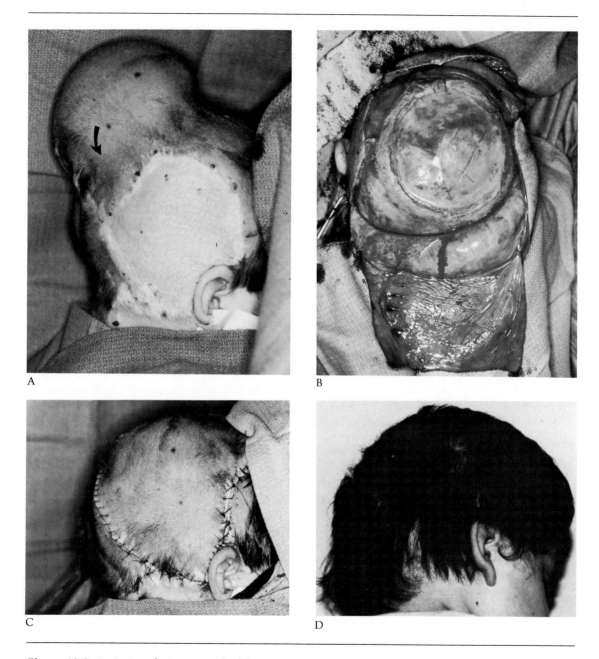

**Figure 13-8** *A. A giant hairy nevus had been excised and the wound partially closed by Ortichochea flaps and a large skin graft. The skin-grafted area is not closed by the scalp flap behind the left ear. Expander is in place. Skin for rotation is indicated by the arrow. B. Note the circular capsule on the skull. The expanded flap is reflected. C. Flap inset. D. One year after hair growth.*

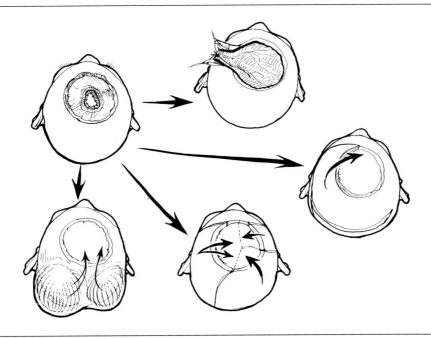

**Figure 13-9** *Overview of methods for closure of large defects. Pericranium may be rotated for grafting (top right). A subtotal scalp flap or smaller axial flaps (Orticochea) are possible. Adjacent tissue may be expanded for later advancement or rotation.*

not replantable, coverage with free tissue transfer is performed if skin grafting is not applicable.

*Replantation*
Replantation is the treatment of choice for the totally avulsed scalp if there are no other injuries and the patient is in a stable enough condition to tolerate a long anesthesia. Miller and colleagues [45] performed the first successful scalp replantation, and since then multiple successful scalp replantations have been performed [7, 9, 49, 64, 70]. Extended periods of ischemia can be tolerated with scalp avulsions because of the lack of muscle in this tissue, particularly if the part has been cooled. Anastomosis must be done to uninjured vessels away from the zone of injury. This move often requires the use of vein grafts, especially for the arterial inflow. The superficial temporal vessels are most commonly used, although in most series multiple arterial and venous anastomoses have been performed to ensure viabil-

ity. Nonetheless, as demonstrated by Nahai et al. [49], the entire scalp can survive on a single microvascular anastomosis of one artery and one vein, showing that the midline of the scalp is not an absolute barrier for segmental blood supply. After successful replantation, regrowth of hair can be expected, producing the best results obtainable in these difficult injuries.

*Free Tissue Transfer*
When faced with acute large scalp defects, whether of traumatic, infectious, or ablative etiology, and when skin grafting is not appropriate, coverage via a free tissue transfer may be the preferred treatment. McClean and Buncke [44] were the first to use the free vascularized omental transfer for scalp cov-

erage. The gastroepiploic vessels were the donor vessels for this flap. The omentum was molded to the scalp defect and then covered with a split-thickness skin graft. The necessity for laparotomy and the availability of other, less morbid flaps, however, has limited the usefulness of this transfer.

The groin flap, based on the superficial circumflex iliac vessels, has similarly been used to cover scalp defects [28]. A short vascular pedicle, variable anatomy, and lack of reliability has made it a difficult flap to use, and in most centers other forms of free tissue transfer are used today.

The latissimus dorsi muscle, which can be transferred as a myocutaneous unit or as free muscle only and covered with a split-thickness skin graft, was first used by Maxwell et al. in 1978 to cover a scalp defect [42]. The muscle itself is large enough to cover the entire scalp and is reliable in its anatomy. The vascular pedicle to the flap is the thoracodorsal artery and vein. These vessels provide a long pedicle that aids in the usefulness of this flap. The muscle can be easily molded into the scalp defect and is also useful for providing coverage in areas of bony defect. The main disadvantage with the use of the latissimus dorsi muscle is that it provides excessive bulk, which may be difficult to revise at a later date.

The parascapular flap, based on the terminal branch of the circumflex scapular artery, has been used to close scalp defects [12]. This flap is less bulky than the latissimus myocutaneous flap, its vessels are large and reliable, and no functional muscle is sacrificed. Its main disadvantage is that it does not cover the entire scalp as does the latissimus unit.

The disadvantage of free tissue coverage includes both the long anesthesia involved in free tissue transfer and the morbidity of the donor site. In general, these flaps are also poor from an aesthetic point of view and do not restore hair-bearing tissue to the scalp. They accomplish primary wound closure but then must be followed by hairline recon-

struction or coverage with the use of wigs, scarves, and hats.

*Hairline Reconstruction*
Considerable progress has been made in terms of hairline reconstruction [32, 51]. Most of these techniques have been developed for the treatment of male pattern baldness and can similarly be applied for treating other forms of alopecia. Most efforts are directed at first reconstructing the anterior hairline and then reducing areas of alopecia by a combination of techniques including scalp reduction, hair grafting, the use of local flaps, and the use of tissue expanders.

The punch graft involves the transfer of free plugs of hair-bearing tissue taken from an uninjured donor site and transferred to the frontal region to reconstruct the anterior hairline. The patient must have an acceptable donor area and a healthy recipient site of reasonable thickness to provide a successful bed for grafting.

In a similar fashion, scalp can be taken as a strip graft [69] or as a square scalp graft [13] to reconstruct the anterior hairline. According to its proponents, in selected patients these methods produce a more natural hairline than when free punch grafts are used.

Temporo-parieto-occipital flaps, as popularized by Juri [32], involve the use of long, thin flaps of scalp delayed and pedicled on the parietal branch of the superficial temporal artery. The flap is centered at 2 cm on either side of this vessel, extending to the posterior occiput and transposed to the anterior hairline after two surgical delays (Fig. 13-10). The donor site is closed primarily after wide undermining. A similar flap from the contralateral side can furnish a second row of hair-bearing tissue following reconstruction of the anterior hairline.

The lateral scalp flap, as described by Elliot [20], involves the use of a similarly based flap taken from the temporal scalp and transposed anteriorly. As this flap is short, it does not require a delay but only recon-

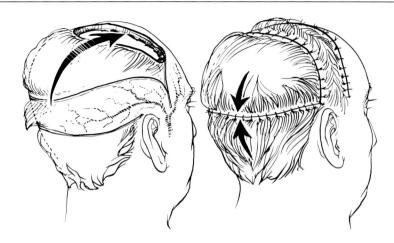

structs the anterior hairline up to the midline of the forehead.

Similar temporooccipital flaps have been transferred as free flaps by microvascular anastomoses, as described by Ohmori [52]. These flaps can be harvested based on the superficial temporal or occipital vessels and are usually anastomosed to the contralateral superficial temporal artery and vein anteriorly. The advantage of this technique is that a relatively large flap can be transferred in a single stage; moreover, when properly performed, it is reliable in producing hair growth after transfer. It also provides a freedom in design so that the donor area can be properly oriented to provide hair growth in the proper direction after transfer.

Tissue expansion techniques similar to those used for treatment of male-pattern baldness can also be useful for restoring hair-bearing tissue to the scalp. Bilateral expansion of normal scalp followed by scalp reduction with elimination of large areas of alopecia, damaged scalp, or previously placed skin grafts can be accomplished with this method [2, 39].

Sideburn reconstruction is approached in a similar fashion, though hairstyling can often camouflage this area. If the posterior auricular scalp remains intact, it can be transposed as a random transposition flap in a reliable fashion, producing good aesthetic results [22].

## Calvarial Reconstruction

As emphasized previously, the establishment of soft tissue coverage is essential prior to undertaking bony reconstruction. Exposed, desiccated calvarium usually starts the sequence of sequestration, osteomyelitis, and chronic ulceration. Although skin grafts over pericranium or over the decorticated outer table provide soft tissue coverage, they do not provide suitable resurfacing for secondary reconstructive cranioplasties, which must be delayed until thicker, definitive coverage is obtained.

Calvarial reconstruction is undertaken to provide adequate protective coverage of intracranial contents and restore calvarial contour to improve aesthetic deformity. The location and size of the defect often dictate the method of treatment and the surgical approach. Defects in the frontal region warrant cranioplasty for both cosmetic and protective reasons. Obviously, injuries to the frontal sinus must be properly dealt with, and reconstruction with autogenous material may be preferable, though this subject is controversial. Wolfe [75] related no incidence of infection among 73 cranioplasties using autogenous bone grafts. Conversely, Manson et al. [41] reported no statistical difference of infection in the use of autogenous bone versus mesh-acrylic in reconstructions involving the frontal region. Defects in the parietal and occipital areas may represent less of a problem from a cosmetic point of view but may still require a cranioplasty for protective purposes [59]. Defects in the temporal region are less obvious, being somewhat protected by the overlying temporalis muscle, and thus less frequently require cranioplasty. In general, defects larger than 10 cm$^2$ are reconstructed [59].

The timing of reconstruction depends on many factors, including the condition of the patient, associated injuries, and the size and nature of the underlying defect. Numerous alloplastic materials have been used to restore bony skull defects. Metals were originally used, including vitallium, tantalum, and stainless steel. In general, ideal wound conditions must exist to use alloplastic materials successfully, the main disadvantage being the development of infection and extrusion. Nonetheless, numerous studies show that, in properly selected patients, these synthetic materials, the most common being acrylic, can be successfully used in cranioplasty, providing ease of reconstruction and no donor site morbidity [41].

For most plastic surgeons autogenous bone remains the material of choice for reconstructing calvarial defects [6, 33, 43, 48]. The advantages of reconstructing with like tissue are many, although, most important, the use of autogenous bone grafting is associated with a low incidence of infection and graft loss. It is noteworthy that exposure and infection in a wound containing alloplastic material usually means removal of the implant and loss of the cranioplasty. An autogenous bone graft involved in a wound infection may undergo resorption or may develop a local area of osteitis, but sepsis in these wounds can often be managed without complete graft loss. When dealing with the acute reconstruction of posttraumatic deformity, the use of autogenous material is clear. Another advantage of bone grafting is that the graft heals with a strength that simulates calvarium and, in children, grows with the patient. Its primary disadvantage relates to donor site morbidity.

The successful use of bone grafting requires broad bone-to-bone contact, complete immobilization of the graft, and good soft tissue coverage to provide a bed for uncomplicated revascularization of the graft.

ALLOPLASTIC MATERIAL

The most commonly used alloplastic material for cranioplasty today is methylmethacrylate. It has many advantages, including durability, poor conduction of heat, economy, and the ease with which it is used. As previously stated, infectious complications remain its main disadvantage. Rish et al. [59], in a series of patients, showed an overall 3.7 percent incidence of infectious complications with the use of acrylic. In patients with a history of infection near the calvarial defect, the incidence of infection following cranioplasty rose to 32 percent. Other criticisms with the use of methylmethacrylate relate to problems with traumatic fracture of the acrylic plate or its dislocation following a blow to the area of cranioplasty. However, as noted by Manson et al. [41], the incorporation of mesh stabilizes the acrylic greatly.

If acrylic is to be used, it is recommended that cranioplasty be delayed a minimum of 1 year after the initial débridement surgery. If previous infection has been noted during the preoperative period, it is thought by some authors [27, 59] that surgery should be delayed for a second year. The use of acrylic reconstruction during the immediate postinjury period is thus discouraged.

Stainless steel mesh has similarly been

used for cranioplasty. It is easily contoured to the bony defect and can be securely fixated, providing relatively good protective covering. As noted, acrylic and mesh work well together [41].

AUTOGENOUS MATERIAL
*Rib*
Split rib grafts remain an excellent technique for reconstructing large calvarial defects. Longacre and De Stefano [36] showed that split rib grafts can be used to fill in enormous defects of the cranium. They reported a 0 percent incidence of infection with the use of this technique. Similar success has been reported by others [33, 48].

The ribs are usually harvested through a short anterolateral thoracotomy incision over the seventh rib. Only alternate ribs are removed to minimize respiratory and aesthetic deformity, and usually only three ribs are removed on each side. Ribs are harvested subperiosteally; if necessary, the total length of rib can be removed.

An osteotome is used to split the rib, which doubles the amount of available bone for reconstruction and increases revascularization by exposing inner cancellous bone. The ribs are bent to fit the defect using a bone bender and then are wedged within the bony defect of the calvarium. They are securely wired to calvarium as well as to each other in a "chain-link fence" configuration to ensure bone-to-bone contact and bony stability [48]. Small gaps between ribs that are not in direct contact are filled with bony chips or bone paste.

The rapid revascularization of rib grafts is the main reason for its high rate of take and low incidence of infection. Its main disadvantage is donor site morbidity, which can be minimized by careful technique during the harvesting and wound closure. In addition, the final contour tends to resemble a washboard, which may require subsequent acrylic overlay (Fig. 13-11). In general, we commonly use rib in cranioplasties performed

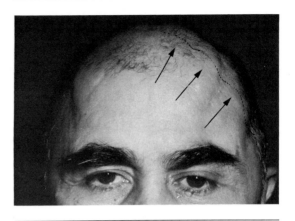

**Figure 13-11** *Rib graft skull reconstruction leaves the patient with a solid calvaria with a "washboard" configuration (arrows).*

behind the hairline, where this washboard configuration would not be noticeable; we rarely use rib to reconstruct the forehead. Donor rib regenerates in almost 100 percent of patients if the ribs are harvested subperiosteally.

*Iliac Bone*
Iliac bone grafting is excellent for reconstruction of moderately sized defects. The donor site is acceptable, particularly in adults, and the bone itself is useful for repair in the frontal region because the bone plate can be shaped to obtain an excellent contour match for frontal bone.

Iliac bone can be harvested in many ways. Preferably, the iliac crest is left in situ, and either a full-thickness or partial-thickness plate of bone is harvested by medial dissection from the region below the crest. Also, cancellous bone can be harvested from between the inner and outer tables to provide bone chips in areas of bony gap.

A unicortical graft is preferable from a revascularization point of view, and full-thickness grafts are split prior to insertion into calvarial defects. Contouring of the graft and secure wiring to the surrounding skull, with

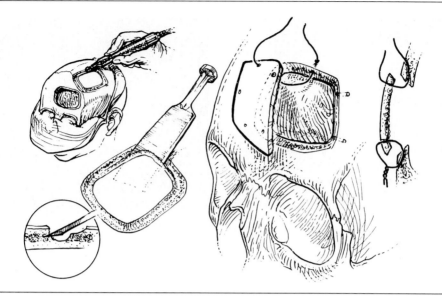

**Figure 13-12** *Calvarial bone graft. A template is made of the defect after the edges are stepped or burred to maximize bone contact. Bone is taken preferably from the parietal area (more posteriorly than drawn). A burr is used to go around the donor area. The trough is cut to allow an osteotome to pass into the diploë. Multiple osteotomies are used to lift the graft. The graft is wired into position, and bone contact is maximized.*

adequate bone-to-bone contact, are important technical points to ensure a successful reconstruction.

*Calvarial Bone*

For most defects, calvarial bone grafts have several advantages [43, 68]. First, these bone grafts, harvested from intact calvarium, are in the same operative field and do not require a distant donor site. Second, there is a good deal of evidence [76] to suggest that calvarial (membranous) bone is revascularized earlier and undergoes less resorption than endochondrial bone, forming a more durable material for reconstruction. Finally, calvarium is easily contoured to resurface calvarial defects. The main disadvantage of using calvarium is the possibility of violating the in-

ner table, the dura, or both when harvesting the graft.

The preferred area from which to harvest these grafts is the posterior parietal area, where the skull is thickest [56] (Fig. 13-12). The grafts are usually harvested with an osteotome at the level of the diploic spaces between the inner and outer tables. Alternatively, a full-thickness graft can be obtained, then split away from the operative field, with the inner surface used to reconstruct the donor site and the outer table used to reconstruct the calvarial defect (Fig. 13-13).

*Bone Paste*

Bone dust, harvested from the cranium at the time of an ablative procedure [6] or from the ilium [26], has been used alone or combined with elastomer-coated mesh to reconstruct calvarium [63]. The bone dust is spread over the exposed dura and then is covered with oxycellulose or mesh to protect it from disruption and provide a matrix for bony growth. According to Habal et al. [26], the newly formed bone follows the contour of the undersurface of the mesh, which acts purely as a template for bony growth.

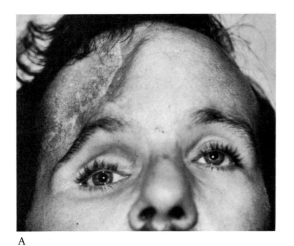
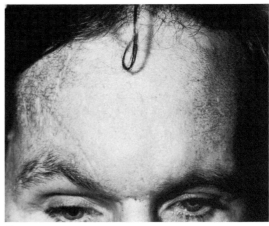

A

B

*Figure 13-13* *A. Preoperative defect of the right forehead. B. After calvarial bone graft.*

## Forehead Reconstruction

Although usually considered a part of the general facial anatomy, the forehead is, in reality, an anterior extension of the scalp and calvarium. Reconstruction in this region, then, must similarly be considered in terms of soft tissue deformity and bony reconstruction. The frontal sinus requires special consideration and, if not properly managed, can lead to serious problems, often after extended periods. Although forehead skin does not bear hair, attention must be given to anterior hairline reconstruction as well as to minimizing eyebrow deformity. Also, blunt frontal trauma can produce direct or indirect globe and optic nerve injury, and careful ophthalmologic evaluation is of the utmost importance for evaluating patients with severe injuries to the frontal region [66].

### FRONTAL SINUS FRACTURE

Located prominently above the roof of the nose, the frontal sinus is prone to injury, usually by blunt trauma. Injuries to this area can present in one of three ways: fracture of the anterior wall with contour depression; obstruction of the nasofrontal duct with a subsequent sinusitis or mucocele; and fracture of the posterior wall, dura, or both with subsequent cerebrospinal fluid (CSF) leak and possible contamination and meningitis.

A high index of suspicion followed by facial radiographs often confirms the diagnosis of frontal sinus fracture, showing bony deformity or opacification of the sinus. Polytomography and CT radiographs provide better delineation of bony pathology, although controversy exists regarding the accuracy of these modalities for predicting patency of a nasofrontal duct [73].

The size of the frontal sinus may vary considerably from one side to the other. The median septum always starts inferiorly in the midline, as seen on radiographs, but it may then veer off based on the growth of the frontal sinus on each side. Frontal sinus fractures are rare in children, as pneumatization begins at 8 years of age and continues past puberty.

The treatment of frontal sinus fractures remains controversial. Some recommend surgical exploration of most frontal sinus fractures, whereas others use surgery selectively [34, 38, 47]. Although therapy must be individualized, guidelines to the acute management of these fractures are based on the anatomic location of the injury. Superb radiographs are critical, as therapy depends on adequate evaluation. Prophylactic antibiotics are usually recommended for management of these fractures.

ANTERIOR TABLE FRACTURES

Fractures of the anterior table present problems primarily from an aesthetic point of view and must be explored if contour irregularities are noted. The main difficulty with these fractures is the possibility of an associated nasofrontal duct injury or obstruction, which if not diagnosed leads to sinusitis or mucocele, pyocele, and orbital cellulitis [73].

Minimally displaced fractures may be treated conservatively and the patient followed closely to ensure re-aeration of the frontal sinus. A significantly displaced anterior table fracture must be explored, as must those fractures associated with a persistent frontal sinus air-fluid level. These fractures are best approached via a bicoronal incision, although an overlying laceration at times provides useful exposure. At the time of exploration, bony fragments are elevated and, if unstable, wired into place. The nasofrontal duct must be inspected and irrigated to determine patency. The median septum is best removed to allow drainage via the other duct if a question exists regarding patency. The patient is not released from follow-up until the sinus cavity is completely aerated and the forehead contour is satisfactory [50].

NASOFRONTAL DUCT INJURY

Approximately one-third of frontal sinus fractures involve the nasofrontal duct [50]. If the injury to the floor of the frontal sinus is such that the mucosal orifice of the nasofrontal duct is obstructed, exploration of the frontal sinus is advisable. It is best performed via a bicoronal scalp incision. The frontal sinus is exposed through an inferiorly based osteoplastic* flap through the anterior table.

In general, attempts at ductal reconstruction are prone to stenosis and the development of sinusitis. If the ductal injury is unilateral, sinus drainage may be restored by removing the intersinus septum and establishing drainage through the contralateral duct. If both ducts are occluded, consideration is given to sinus obliteration. It is performed by meticulous removal of all mucosa lining the frontal sinus, usually with the use of cutting and polishing power burrs [17]. The nasofrontal duct mucosa is then inverted into the duct, and the duct is occluded with the use of autologous tissue (e.g., temporalis fascia, muscle, or cancellous bone) to plug the duct. The space of the frontal sinus is then obliterated, and both free fat grafts as well as cancellous bone grafts have been used for this purpose.

Luce [38] advocates primary reconstruction of the nasofrontal ducts following ductal injury. Small indwelling catheters, left in place for 2 weeks and traveling through the duct into the nose, are thought to be an alternative treatment to sinus obliteration.

POSTERIOR TABLE FRACTURES

Posterior table fractures may be complicated by laceration of the frontal dura or underlying frontal lobes, or the development of a subdural hematoma. A fracture of the posterior wall of the frontal sinus is, by definition, a compound fracture involving the cranial vault, and it connects the intracranial cavity with the sinus cavity and nasal airways. Displaced posterior table fractures that lacerate the dura can be complicated by CSF rhinorrhea. The development of meningitis or cerebral abscess formation can similarly result from posterior table fractures.

Nondisplaced fractures of the posterior table are not explored unless the nasofrontal duct is occluded or CSF rhinorrhea persists longer than 3 weeks [30]. In general, rhinor-

---

*Osteoplastic: The anterior bone plate is left attached to the overlying soft tissue. The surgeon measures the sinuses on a radiograph, cuts a template, and thus knows where to enter the superior sinus area.

rhea is unusual following nondisplaced posterior table fractures [61].

Displaced fractures of the posterior table are explored and the dura is examined and repaired as soon as the patient's general condition permits. The repair requires an intracranial approach via a bicoronal incision in conjunction with neurosurgery. Any posterior table fragments present are elevated and removed, and the dura is repaired directly with autogenous fascia or pericranial grafts.

The keystone to treatment of these injuries is obliteration of the sinus cavity and sealing of the connection between the brain and the nasal airways [62]. If a good dural seal is obtained and comminution is not too severe, the sinus should be obliterated. As a last resort, in the case of poor dural seal and severe bony comminution, the anterior table and orbital rims can be removed to collapse the wound and close the dura with forehead tissue [58]. This maneuver, unfortunately, creates a severe contour defect that must be secondarily reconstructed and provides poor protection for intracranial contents.

As an alternative, Donald and Bernstein [17–19] proposed "cranialization" for severe injuries involving the posterior table of the frontal sinus. It is performed by removing all of the posterior table, meticulous burr excision of all frontal sinus lining, obliteration and inversion of the nasofrontal duct mucosa, and allowing the frontal lobes to expand to fill and obliterate the prior frontal region. The anterior table is thoroughly débrided, cleansed of its mucosal lining, and wired into place to restore contour and provide protection for the frontal lobes. Replacement by calvarial grafts may be required. The key to successful cranialization is meticulous excision of frontal sinus mucosa. The dangers of recurrent mucocele and pyocele in close proximity to frontal lobes demand technical excellence to obtain good results with this procedure.

SECONDARY RECONSTRUCTION

The final surgical challenge of severe frontal bone fractures is frequently contour restoration. Although somewhat controversial, it is our belief that autogenous material must be used for all reconstruction following frontal sinus injuries because of the risk of a secondary infection. Calvarial grafts are most commonly used, optimizing bone-to-bone contact in reconstruction (see Fig. 13-13).

In general, a bicoronal incision is used when dealing with secondary frontal bone reconstruction, with the incision distant from the implant site. All communications between nasal passages and graft sites are sealed to prevent contamination, and soft tissue coverage is equivalent to the normal soft tissue present within the forehead.

*Forehead Skin*

The amount of glabrous forehead varies from person to person but also depends on hairstyling or the presence of male-pattern baldness. To perform an adequate reconstruction of this region, the surgeon must have an appreciation for forehead skin contour and color, the frontalis muscles and associated nerves, and the fixed aesthetic structures such as eyebrows and the anterior and lateral hairlines.

*Anatomy*

Like the scalp, the forehead consists of several layers including skin, subcutaneous tissue, frontalis muscle (which, on its deep surface, is covered by a thickened fascial layer that is continuous with the galea), a loose areolar plane, and pericranium overlying the frontal bone. The skin of the forehead is paler than that of the lower face and is usually smoother and somewhat thicker in texture. The lines of relaxed skin tension run horizontally, except in the glabellar region, where they are vertical.

The musculature of the forehead includes the frontalis, procerus, and corrugator muscles. These muscles provide symmetric forehead movement and are innervated by the frontal branch of the facial nerve.

The frontal branch of the facial nerve lies on a line between the lobule of the ear and a point 1.5 cm from the lateral eyebrow [57].

Though numerous branching patterns of this nerve exist, the frontal branch always travels in a constant anatomic plane as it traverses the temporal region toward the frontalis muscle. After crossing the zygomatic arch, the frontal branch travels along the undersurface of the temporoparietal fascia until it enters the frontalis muscle superficially approximately 1.5 cm above the eyebrow. The subaponeurotic plane, where

**Figure 13-14** *Cross section of the temporal region showing fascial relations to the zygomatic arch. The superficial layer of deep temporal fascia inserts along the superficial surface of the arch. The deep layer of the deep temporal fascia inserts along the deep surface of the arch. The superficial temporal fat pad adjoins the superior surface of the arch. The recommended path of dissection to the arch is within the subaponeurotic plane until approximately 2 cm above the arch. The dissection then deepens to penetrate the superficial layer of deep temporal fascia, dissecting within the fat pad inferiorly to the arch periosteum. (From J. M. Stuzin et al. Anatomy of the frontal branch of the facial nerve: The significance of the temporal fat pad. Plast. Reconstr. Surg. 83:265, 1989.)*

dissection is commonly carried when operating in the scalp and forehead, lies immediately deep to the frontal branch in this region and offers little protection to the nerve as one dissects inferiorly toward the zygomatic arch. In those situations when surgical dissection must proceed within the temporal region or subperiosteal exposure of the zygomatic arch is required, we recommend carrying the dissection deep to the superficial layer of the deep temporal fascia, which offers greater anatomic protection against injury to the frontal branch [67] (Fig. 13-14).

Sensory innervation to the forehead occurs primarily from the supraorbital and supratrochlear nerves, branches of the ophthalmic division of the trigeminal nerve. They exit from the supraorbital grooves or foramina at the junction of the medial and middle one-third of the orbital rim. The supratrochlear branches exit the orbit at the superomedial corner. The supraorbital, supratrochlear, and anterior branch of the superficial temporal artery provide a generous blood supply to the forehead, allowing the development of dependable axial and random flaps in this region.

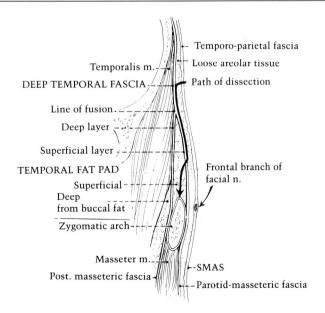

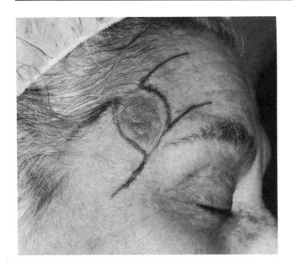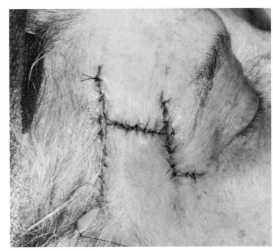

**Figure 13-15** *Advancement flaps place incisions in a good direction. Triangles are removed in crow's feet and the scalp. Wider undermining may have been done, and only the inferior flap could have been used if so desired.*

### General Principles

Excision flaps or scar revisions are optimally located to align the final scar along relaxed skin tension lines (Fig. 13-15). Surprisingly, scars oriented perpendicular to relaxed skin tension lines often produce acceptable results with careful suturing. Scars running diagonally on the forehead produce the least satisfactory appearance and often require revision. In general, simple excisions are horizontally oriented in the forehead and vertically oriented in the glabellar region. The surgeon must take into consideration the effect of excisions on the eyebrow. The eyebrow should not be moved excessively. Grafts placed on the forehead tend to look like a patch and are avoided unless a high suspicion of tumor recurrence is likely.

Because hairline and eyebrows form rigid boundaries, the skin used to close forehead defects ideally comes from within these boundaries, and hair-bearing scalp tissue is not brought into the area of reconstruction. Flaps should be the same thickness as that of the skin excised, and to avoid asymmetry, if possible, the frontalis muscle and the frontal branch of the facial nerve are not injured.

In many instances, it is possible to assess forehead mobility by placing the skin between two fingers and moving it in all directions. This practice enables one to estimate how the scalp will redistribute to aid in wound closure. The forehead does not contain a great deal of excess skin, and some degree of tension is usually present following the development and closure of forehead flaps. Galeal scoring, with care to not injure the innervation of the frontalis muscle, can aid in closure in a similar fashion to its use for scalp defects. At the center of the forehead, up to 4 cm may be closed primarily after wide undermining and scoring of the medial frontalis muscles and galea. Immediate tissue expansion is another useful modality for obtaining additional skin recruitment (1.0 to 2.5 cm) at the time of closure of large frontal soft tissue defects [60].

Rotation flaps are dependable and aesthetically acceptable, but they may leave the an-

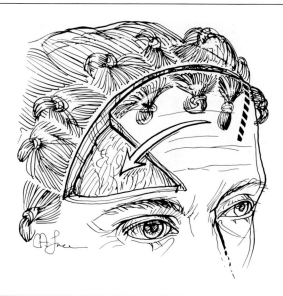

**Figure 13-16** *The forehead and anterior hairline may be rotated around for lateral defects. The nerve to the frontalis muscle enters in the first 2 cm above the lateral brow.*

terior scalp insensitive. Galeal scoring and back cuts can provide additional flap length if required. A large defect can be resurfaced by a large rotation flap that rotates the whole remaining forehead into the defect (Fig. 13-16). The incision for this repair lies just within the hairline and extends down into the temporal region. The galea is scored, and the forehead skin is then rotated, producing a horizontal scar above the brow and slight lowering of the hairline. Although large supraorbital lesions can be excised as a triangle and closed with a unilaterally based rotation flap, median forehead flaps also work well. Large lesions in the midaspect of the forehead can similarly be closed by triangular excision followed by the use of bilateral rotation flaps, the bases of which follow a horizontally oriented skin line.

*Transposition Limberg Type Flaps*
Small, randomly based transposition flaps are not generally useful for forehead reconstruction, whereas a median flap is an excel-

lent choice for reconstructing small defects. Laterally based defects are often more amenable to using local transposition flaps and, similarly, advancement flaps (Fig. 13-17).

The rhomboid principle can be adapted to forehead reconstruction. Hexagon excision and closure [29] using a triple rhomboid flap has been proposed as useful for upper forehead excision, especially in bald men when distortion of the frontal hairline is not a consideration. The multiple scars produced from this technique are a disadvantage, as is the precise planning necessary for its success. Nonetheless, this technique can provide acceptable results in properly selected patients.

*Large Forehead Defects*
Defects greater than one-third of the forehead are too large to be closed only with the use of forehead skin unless greatly expanded. In these situations, the use of scalp flaps, bringing scalp hair-bearing tissue onto the forehead, can provide wound closure, although they are aesthetically troublesome.

If pericranium remains, a split-thickness skin graft can be used to close the defect, which can be secondarily revised. If pericra-

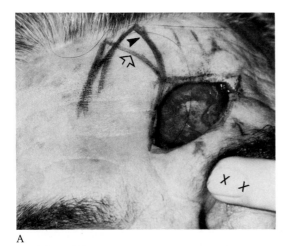

A

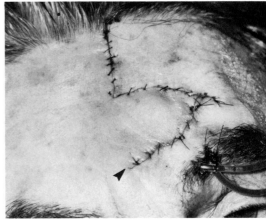

B

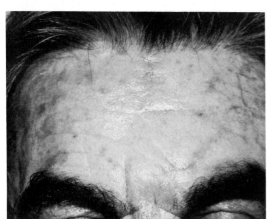

C

*Figure 13-17* *A. When defects occur over the brow, the eyebrow should not be lifted by the closure (xx). The open arrow depicts the Limberg flap, and the arrowhead shows the bullet-shaped transposition flap that was used. B. Flap transposed. A small dog-ear (arrowhead) will be removed with vertical excision later. Butterfly drains are placed through eyebrow. C. Result prior to dog-ear excision.*

nium is not present, the outer table of the frontal bone can be burred down to bleeding tissue and a split-thickness skin graft applied to this surface in a fashion similar to that used for skin grafting on calvarium. Great care must be used to not enter the frontal sinus. Skin grafting is also useful following tumor excision in situations where recurrence may be high. This area can then be more definitively reconstructed at a later date, after a period of observation.

Skin expansion can also be useful for secondary reconstruction of large defects. The expander is placed in a subgaleal position in the remaining forehead skin, expanded over a period of time, and then rotated as a unit when adequate tissue is available.

## *References*

1. Alpert, B., Buncke, H., and Mathes, S. Surgical treatment of the totally avulsed scalp. *Clin. Plast. Surg.* 9:145, 1982.
2. Anderson, R. D. Expansion-assisted treatment of male pattern baldness. *Clin. Plast. Surg.* 14:477, 1987.
3. Argenta, L., Marks, M., and Pasyd, K. Advances in tissue expansion. *Clin. Plast. Surg.* 12:159, 1985.
4. Argenta, L., Watanabe, M., and Grabb, W. The use of tissue expansion in head and neck reconstruction. *Ann. Plast. Surg.* 11:31, 1983.
5. Arnold, P., and Rangarathnam, C. Multiple flap scalp reconstruction: Orticochea revisited. *Plast. Reconstr. Surg.* 69:605, 1982.
6. Bakamjian, V., and Leonard, A. Bone dust cranioplasty. *Plast. Reconstr. Surg.* 60:784, 1977.
7. Biemer, E., et al. Successful replantation of a totally avulsed scalp. *Br. J. Plast. Surg.* 32:19, 1979.
8. Brent, B., et al. Experience with the temporoparietal fascial free flap. *Plast. Reconstr. Surg.* 76:177, 1985.
9. Buncke, H., et al. Successful replantation of two avulsed scalps by microvascular anastomosis. *Plast. Reconstr. Surg.* 61:666, 1978.
10. Buncke, H., et al. Microvascular transplant of two free scalp flaps between identical twins. *Plast. Reconstr. Surg.* 70:605, 1982.
11. Casanova, R., et al. Anatomic basis for vascularized outer-table calvarial bone flaps. *Plast. Reconstr. Surg.* 78:300, 1986.
12. Chiu, D., Sherman, J., and Edgerton, B. Coverage of the calvarium with a free parascapular flap. *Ann. Plast. Surg.* 12:60, 1984.
13. Coiffman, F. Use of square scalp grafts for male pattern baldness. *Plast. Reconstr. Surg.* 60:228, 1977.
14. Converse, J. M. *Reconstructive Plastic Surgery* (2nd ed.). Vol. 2. Philadelphia: Saunders, 1977. P. 822.
15. Cutting, C., McCarthy, J., and Berenstein, A. Blood supply of the upper craniofacial skeleton: The search for composite calvarial bone flaps. *Plast. Reconstr. Surg.* 74:603, 1984.
16. Dingman, R., and Argenta, L. The surgical repair of traumatic defects of the scalp. *Clin. Plast. Surg.* 9:131, 1982.
17. Donald, P. The tenacity of the frontal sinus mucosa. *Otolaryngol. Head Neck Surg.* 87:557, 1979.
18. Donald, P. Frontal sinus ablation by cranialization. *Arch. Otolaryngol.* 108:142, 1982.
19. Donald, P., and Bernstein, L. Compound frontal sinus injuries with intracranial penetration. *Laryngoscope* 88:225, 1978.
20. Elliot, R. Lateral scalp flaps for instant results in male pattern baldness. *Plast. Reconstr. Surg.* 60:699, 1977.
21. Feierabend, T., and Bindra, R. Injuries causing major loss of scalp. *Plast. Reconstr. Surg.* 76:189, 1985.
22. Fodor, P., and Liverett, D. Sideburn reconstruction for post rhytidectomy deformity. *Plast. Reconstr. Surg.* 74:430, 1984.
23. Fonseca, J. Use of pericranial flap in scalp wounds with exposed bone. *Plast. Reconstr. Surg.* 72:186, 1983.
24. Gatti, J., and LaRossa, D. Scalp avulsions and review of successful replantation. *Ann. Plast. Surg.* 6:177, 1980.
25. Habal, M., and Maniscalco, J. Observations on the ultrastructure of the pericranium. *Ann. Plast. Surg.* 6:103, 1981.
26. Habal, M., et al. Repair of major cranio-orbital defects with an elastomer-coated mesh and autogenous bone paste. *Plast. Reconstr. Surg.* 61:394, 1978.
27. Hammon, W., and Kempe, L. Methyl methacrylate cranioplasty: Thirteen years experience with 417 patients. *Acta Neurochir. (Wien)* 25:69, 1971.
28. Harii, K., Ohmori, K., and Ohmori, S. Successful clinical transfer of tear free flaps by microvascular anastomoses. *Plast. Reconstr. Surg.* 53:259, 1974.
29. Jackson, I. *Local Flaps in Head and Neck Surgery.* St. Louis: Mosby, 1985. P. 43.
30. Jacobs, J. *Maxillofacial Trauma: Cerebrospinal Fistula.* Baltimore: Williams & Wilkins, 1984. P. 297.
31. Jost, G., and Levet, Y. Parotid fascia and face lifting: A critical evaluation of the SMAS concept. *Plast. Reconstr. Surg.* 74:42, 1984.
32. Juri, J. Use of parieto-occipital flaps in the surgical treatment of baldness. *Plast. Reconstr. Surg.* 55:456, 1975.
33. Korlof, B., Nylen, B., and Rietz, K. Bone grafts of skull defects. *Plast. Reconstr. Surg.* 52:378, 1973.

34. Larrabee, W., Travis, L., and Tabb, H. Frontal sinus fractures—their suppurative complications and surgical management. *Laryngoscope* 90:1810, 1980.

35. Leonard, P., and Small, J. Tissue expansion in the treatment of alopecia. *Br. J. Plast. Surg.* 39:42, 1986.

36. Longacre, J., and De Stefano, G. Further observations of the behavior of autogenous split-rib grafts in reconstruction of extensive defects of the cranium and face. *Plast. Reconstr. Surg.* 20:281, 1957.

37. Lu, M. Successful replacement of avulsed scalp. *Plast. Reconstr. Surg.* 43:231, 1969.

38. Luce, E. A. Frontal sinus fractures: Guideline to management. *Plast. Reconstr. Surg.* 80:500, 1987.

39. Manders, E. K., Au, V. K., and Wong, R. K. M. Scalp expansion for male pattern baldness. *Clin. Plast. Surg.* 14:469, 1987.

40. Manders, E., et al. Soft tissue expansion: Concepts and complications. *Plast. Reconstr. Surg.* 74:493, 1984.

41. Manson, P. M., Crawley, W. A., and Hoopes, J. E. Frontal cranioplasty: Risk factors and choice of cranial vault reconstructive material. *Plast. Reconstr. Surg.* 77:888, 1986.

42. Maxwell, P., Steuber, K., and Hoopes, J. A free latissimus dorsi myocutaneous flap. *Plast. Reconstr. Surg.* 62:462, 1978.

43. McCarthy, J., and Zide, B. The spectrum of calvarial bone grafting: Introduction of the vascularized calvarial bone flap. *Plast. Reconstr. Surg.* 74:10, 1984.

44. McClean, D., and Buncke, H. Autotransplant of omentum to a large scalp defect with microsurgical revascularization. *Plast. Reconstr. Surg.* 49:268, 1972.

45. Miller, G., Anstee, E., and Snell, J. Successful replantation of an avulsed scalp by microvascular anastomoses. *Plast. Reconstr. Surg.* 58:133, 1976.

46. Mitz, V., and Peyronie, M. The superficial musculoaponeurotic system in the parotid and cheek area. *Plast. Reconstr. Surg.* 58:80, 1976.

47. Montgomery, W. Surgery of the frontal sinus. *Otolaryngol. Clin. North Am.* 4:97, 1971.

48. Munro, I., and Guyuron, B. Split rib cranioplasty. *Ann. Plast. Surg.* 7:341, 1981.

49. Nahai, F., Hurteau, G., and Vasconez, L. Replantation of an entire scalp and ear by micro-vascular anastomoses of only one artery and one vein. *Br. J. Plast. Surg.* 31:339, 1978.

50. Newman, M., and Travis, L. Frontal sinus fractures. *Laryngoscope* 83:1281, 1973.

51. Ohmori, K. Free scalp flap. *Plast. Reconstr. Surg.* 65:42, 1980.

52. Ohmori, K. Free scalp flap surgery. *Ann. Plast. Surg.* 5:17, 1980.

53. Orticochea, M. Four flap scalp reconstruction techniques. *Br. J. Plast. Surg.* 20:159, 1967.

54. Orticochea, M. New three-flap scalp reconstruction techniques. *Br. J. Plast. Surg.* 24:184, 1971.

55. Osborne, M. Complete scalp avulsion; report of cases: Experimental basis for production of free, hairbearing grafts from avulsed scalp itself. *Ann. Surg.* 132:198, 1950.

56. Pensler, J., McCarthy, J. The calvarial donor site: An anatomic study in cadavers. *Plast. Reconstr. Surg.* 75:648, 1985.

57. Pitanguy, I., and Ramos, A. S. The frontal branch of the facial nerve: The importance of its variations in face lifting. *Plast. Reconstr. Surg.* 38:352, 1966.

58. Riedel, K. Schenke Inaug. Dissertation, Jena, 1898.

59. Rish, B., Dillon, J., and Meinonsh, D. Cranioplasty: A review of 1070 cases of penetrating head injury. *Neurosurgery* 4:381, 1979.

60. Sasaki, G. H. Intraoperative sustained limited expansion (ISLE) as an immediate reconstructive technique. *Clin. Plast. Surg.* 14:563, 1987.

61. Schultz, R. Supraorbital and glabellar fractures. *Plast. Reconstr. Surg.* 45:257, 1980.

62. Sessions, R., et al. Current concepts of frontal sinus surgery: An appraisal of the osteoplastic flap fat obliteration. *Laryngoscope* 82:918, 1972.

63. Shehadi, S. Skull reconstruction with bone dust. *Br. J. Plast. Surg.* 23:227, 1970.

64. Spira, M., Daniel, R., and Agnes, J. Successful replantation of totally avulsed scalp with profuse regrowth of hair. *Plast. Reconstr. Surg.* 62:447, 1978.

65. Stock, Collins, and Davidson. Anatomy of the superficial temporal artery. *Head Neck Surg.* 2:466, 1980.

66. Stuzin, J. M., et al. Radiographic documentation of direct injury of the intracanalicular segment of the optic nerve in the orbital apex syndrome. *Ann. Plast. Surg.* 20:368, 1988.

67. Stuzin, J. M., et al. Anatomy of the frontal

branch of the facial nerve: The significance of the temporal fat pad. *Plast. Reconstr. Surg.* 83:265, 1989.

68. Tessier, P. Autogenous bone grafts taken from the calvarium for facial and cranial applications. *Clin. Plast. Surg.* 9:531, 1982.

69. Vallis, C. Surgical treatment of the receding hairline. *Plast. Reconstr. Surg.* 44:271, 1969.

70. Van Beek, A., and Zook, E. Scalp replantation by microsurgical revascularization. *Plast. Reconstr. Surg.* 61:774, 1978.

71. Vandervord, J. G., Watson, J. D., and Teasdale, G. M. Forehead reconstruction using a bipedicled bone. *Br. J. Plast. Surg.* 35:75, 1982.

72. Walton, R., and Krizek, T. The scalp flap on-lay: A method of managing large dural defects. *Plast. Reconstr. Surg.* 66:684, 1980.

73. Whited, R. Anterior table frontal sinus fractures. *Laryngoscope* 89:1951, 1979.

74. Wolfe, S. A. The utility of pericranial flaps. *Ann. Plast. Surg.* 1:146, 1978.

75. Wolfe, S. A. Discussion: Frontal cranioplasty: Risk factors, choice of cranial vault reconstructive material. *Plast. Reconstr. Surg.* 77:901, 1986.

76. Zins, G., and Whitaker, L. Membranous versus endochondral bone implications for craniofacial reconstruction. *Plast. Reconstr. Surg.* 72:778, 1983.

*James H. Carraway*

# 14

# Reconstruction of the Eyelids and Eyebrows and Correction of Ptosis of the Eyelid

## Reconstruction of the Eyelids and Eyebrows

### Anatomy and Physiology

The upper eyelids consist of three layers: skin, orbicularis muscle, and the tarsoconjunctival layer (Fig. 14-1). The tarsus is about 12 to 15 mm wide from the lid margin to its cephalad portion, where it is joined by Müller's muscle and the levator aponeurosis. The tarsus is approximately 2 mm thick and contains vertically oriented meibomian glands, which exit on the lid margin [1]. Although the tarsus is somewhat rigid, it is flexible enough to conform to the shape of the globe and the cornea. Medially and laterally, the tarsus becomes a series of fibrous strands that converge to form the medial and lateral canthal tendons (Fig. 14-2). On the medial part of the lid margin, the upper and lower punctae are located. The upper and lower lacrimal canaliculi, which continue from the lacrimal punctae, are located under the fibrous strands, which converge to become the medial canthal tendon. These canaliculi converge and run behind the medial canthal tendon under the lacrimal crest and empty into the lacrimal sac (Fig. 14-3).

The levator aponeurosis and Müller's muscle are closely approximated and are lined on the conjunctival surface with a thin layer of epithelium [5]. The levator aponeurosis transmits the force of pull from the levator muscle to the tarsal plate [1]. The final level of the lid depends on the action of the levator plus the length of Müller's muscle. If Müller's muscle is paralyzed or cut, 2 to 3 mm of ptosis occurs.

The lacrimal gland is situated just posterior and adjacent to the superior lateral orbital rim. The size of the gland is about $2.0 \times 1.5 \times 0.5$ cm with collecting ducts that carry tears to a small opening in the aponeurosis 4 to 5 mm above the tarsus in the upper lateral fornix. Approximately 1 ml of tear fluid is secreted daily under normal circumstances and may increase with emotional stimulation, use of certain drugs, or abnormal conditions of the eye and lids. The gland is held in place by fibrous attachments to the periosteum and orbital septum. The surgical importance of this gland is that it may be the site of tumor formation, or it may pro-

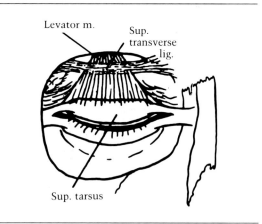

**Figure 14-5** *Superior transverse ligament varies from a filmy structure to a thick white band. It lies on top of the levator muscle at the point of insertion into the aponeurosis. It is suspended medially and laterally from the periorbitum of the lateral and medial orbital walls.*

tion of the levator muscle. In many cases, to approach the levator muscle it is necessary to divide or dissect this ligament away for access. It acts as a check ligament for the levator muscle.

## Pathology of Eyelid Lesions

The skin and epithelial appendages of the eyelids are subject to the development of benign and malignant skin tumors. Actinic exposure is the most common etiologic factor in development of the eyelid skin lesions. The most common malignant tumor seen is basal cell carcinoma. The glands of Zeis and Moll and the meibomian glands may also give rise to malignant tumors that appear to be variants of basal cell carcinoma. Lower lid tumors are most common, and the regions of highest occurrence are the medial and lateral canthal areas. Only about 10 percent of malignant tumors occur on the upper lid. Squamous cell carcinoma is much less common, with a reported frequency of less than 2 percent of all lid tumors [6]. Unlike basal cell carcinoma, these tumors can metastasize to lymph nodes of the face and neck area.

Recurrent basal cell carcinoma is an aggressive tumor and has a high recurrence rate after repeat excision. A study of recurrent basal cell carcinoma strongly suggested that the presence of irregularities in the peripheral palisade in more than 75 percent of the cords or nest of tumors or absence of infiltrates of small lymphocytes at the tumor base are significant in characterizing recurrent basal cell carcinoma [3]. In terms of surgical treatment, this finding suggests that the standard nodular basal cell with translucent pearly borders may be removed by surgical excision, radiation therapy, cryosurgery, or curettage, with a 5-year cure rate of 90 to 95 percent [2]. Recurrent basal cell carcinoma is treated more aggressively and monitored by careful pathologic evaluation to ensure adequate excision. Permanent sections show more clearly than do frozen sections the finer histopathologic detail at the border of the tumor, and therefore they are heavily relied on. When excising a recurrent basal cell carcinoma, the surgeon works closely with the pathologist in determining adequacy of excision, as recurrence after inadequate excision of a basal cell carcinoma can result in a "horrifying" basal cell tumor [7].

Lentigo maligna, the preinvasive stage of malignant melanoma, accounts for about 1 percent of all lid lesions and may be treated by simple excision [6]. Malignant melanoma is rare in eyelid skin but must be aggressively treated by excision as widely and deeply as indicated. Reconstruction may be a problem after such an excision. There is still controversy as to whether radical neck dissection should be carried out prophylactically, and it relates to the level of tumor invasion [10, 12].

The key to cure of malignant tumors of the eyelid is an accurate evaluation of the margin of an excised specimen. A word of advice to surgeons is to avail themselves of the microscopic studies of all lesions they have removed so that they may accurately assess the efficacy of their surgical excision.

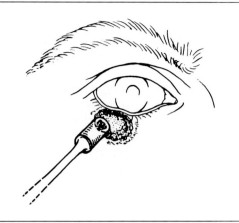

**Figure 14-6** *A 2- or 3-mm punch is used with local anesthesia for biopsy of lesions of the lid margin. No suturing is necessary.*

Only after adequate surgical excision of malignant tumors, as monitored by pathologic examination, is reconstruction performed.

## Biopsy and Shaving Techniques

To plan for adequate treatment of eyelid and other skin lesions, it is helpful and time-saving to have a preoperative pathologic diagnosis of the lesion. Two techniques of biopsy have been helpful to this author. Punch biopsy with a 2- or 3-mm round, disposable punch is an effective way to obtain a full-depth biopsy specimen of multiple layers of a lesion (Fig. 14-6). The technique is simple and involves initial infiltration of 1% lidocaine (Xylocaine) with epinephrine to the soft tissues of the lid adjacent to the lesion. After infiltration, the punch biopsy is used to remove a small section of the lesion. Small forceps and scissors are used to lift and cut the base of the biopsy specimen, and simple compression for a few minutes stops bleeding. This method gives ample material for diagnosis prior to the operative procedure. Suturing is not necessary, and healing is spontaneous over 5 to 7 days, leaving only a tiny crust, which sloughs.

The technique of "shaving" eyelid margin

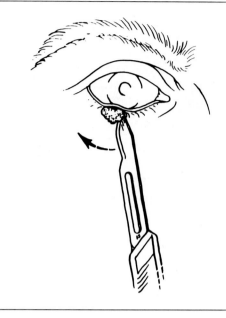

**Figure 14-7** *Lesions of the lid margin that require tissue diagnosis may be biopsied and removed by "shaving" with a No. 15 blade. The defect heals without notching, and the lashes usually return.*

lesions is useful and has been advocated by Smith and Nesi [11] (Fig. 14-7). This technique has the dual advantage of obtaining a biopsy specimen and sometimes eliminating the lesion in question [11]. If the lesion is malignant, definitive reexcision and reconstruction can be performed. This specimen is sent to the pathologist labeled as a shave excision so that it may be properly oriented in the paraffin mounting block. It is helpful to examine lesions of the lid margin and canthal areas using loupe magnification or microscopy. It is often possible using this method to determine accurately the extent of spread of the tumor rather than relying on the naked eye. Proper identification of the margin of an irregular basal cell tumor or recurrent, inadequately treated basal cell lesion allows more accurate excision of the tumor. Once the tumor has been identified and excised, frozen or permanent pathologic diagnosis can confirm adequate resection of these tumors.

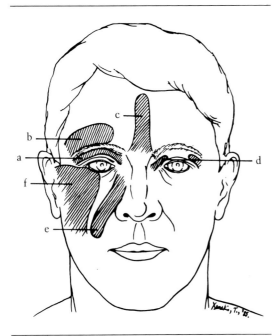

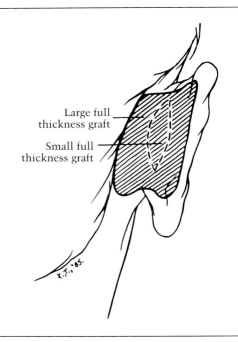

**Figure 14-8** *a = Bipedicled Tripier flap composed of skin and orbicularis muscle. b = Fricke flap laterally based on superficial temporal vessels. It is reliable but is thick skin. c = Midline forehead or glabellar flap. It is a reliable flap with thick skin. d = Medial and lateral skin–muscle flaps can be used to cover composite grafts for full-thickness lid reconstruction. e = Nasolabial flap, superiorly based, is used for lower lid reconstruction. f = Cheek flap, small or large, is used for lower lid and cheek reconstruction.*

**Figure 14-9** *Postauricular full-thickness grafts can be taken as a small ellipse. Up to 3 × 5 cm can be closed. The whole postauricular area can be removed for a large full-thickness graft and replaced with a split-thickness skin graft.*

### Lower Lid Reconstruction

Partial-thickness loss of the lower lid may occur with tumor, trauma, or burns as the etiologic factor. It could involve skin loss only or a combination of skin and muscle. In the event that there is enough skin in the adjacent area, primary closure of the defect may be possible. If the defect is horizontal, attempted closure of a large defect may result in ectropion.

If it is obvious that primary closure is not possible, local flap coverage or a full-thickness graft is necessary. There are numerous available local flaps that are useful, varying in quality and availability of skin (Fig. 14-8).

Adjacent eyelid skin is the best color match for use during coverage of defects around the eye. Lateral cheek skin is a good match in terms of texture and color. Glabellar and nasolabial skin are useful flaps on occasion, but the color and texture match are not always best for eyelid defects.

If primary closure and local flap coverage is not feasible, a graft may be used. Split-thickness grafts are easy to obtain and heal readily, but they also have a tendency to contract and give poor color match. If the split-thickness graft is taken from above the clavicle, the color match is usually better than if taken from elsewhere on the body. Thick split-thickness grafts from the upper inner arm are hairless and pliable, but the color match may not be good. If a large "unit" graft is necessary, this area may be choice simply because of the ample size of grafts that may be taken. It is usually best to use

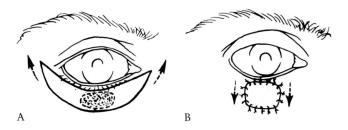

A                                    B

**Figure 14-10** *A. Full-thickness "unit" graft with the margins extending beyond the medial and lateral fissures tends to lend good support as the scar shortens in the horizontal direction. B. "Patch" graft with vertical lines in a lax lower lid may tend to cause contracture and downward pulling of the lid margin.*

full-thickness grafts for the lower lid when grafting is indicated. With full-thickness grafts there is little or no contracture, a good color match is usually possible, and donor areas are readily available. For small defects, skin from the upper lid "takes" readily and furnishes a good color match. Both upper lids may be used, however, and furnish up to about 4 × 4 cm of graft in some cases. If the defect to be covered also has orbicularis muscle loss, a composite muscle and skin

**Figure 14-11** *With partial-thickness excision of a skin lesion from a patient with a relaxed lower lid, a wedge excision of tarsus can be first performed to tighten the lower lid. A full-thickness graft overlay gives ample coverage and heals well over the tarsectomy closure.*

patch from the upper lid may be used as a graft. These composite grafts heal well.

Another excellent source for donor full-thickness skin is the postauricular area. Up to about 5 × 6 cm of full-thickness skin may be obtained (Fig. 14-9). There usually is an excellent color match. These grafts heal with some stiffness, which tends to lend additional support when they are used as grafts to the lower lid.

A helpful technique, especially with large defects of the lower lid, is to extend the medial and lateral fixation points of the graft beyond the medial and lateral palpebral fissure, which tends to lend support to the lower lid area by a sling-like effect (Fig. 14-10).

If a graft is to be placed on the lower lid and the lid margin is relaxed, it furnishes poor support and has a tendency to allow lid eversion postoperatively. In this case, a wedge excision of tarsus and lid margin may be indicated, and the graft may be placed directly over the closure with good graft "take" (Fig. 14-11).

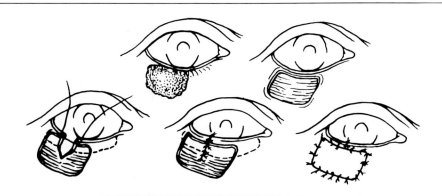

## Full-Thickness Defects

Tumors that involve the lid margin as well as skin are directly excised, preferably under magnification. To orient this specimen for pathologic sectioning, the specimen is dried with a sponge and an orienting mark placed on the designated margin for pathologic orientation with a marking pen. If the margins of the tumors are not sharply defined, frozen section may be necessary. If the frozen section is necessary to determine the adequacy of the excision, reconstruction of the lid is delayed until the report is completed. For excision of one-fourth to one-third of the lid margin, primary closure can usually be performed. The excision is vertically oriented in the tarsus so the shape of the defect is a pentagon (Fig. 14-12). Approximation of these vertical cut edges results in a straight lid margin without notching (Fig. 14-13).

The "extensile" approach to reconstruction of the lower lid defects is useful. It simply means that after excision of tumor the surgeon may take each step from the simple to the more complex to complete the reconstruction. After excision of the full thickness of the lid, a silk stitch is placed through the tarsal "gray" margin of the medial and lateral segments with subsequent crossing of the ends of the suture (Fig. 14-13A). By pulling on these sutures, one may determine if closure is possible. If it is seen that primary closure is not possible, the next step in the extensile approach is lateral canthotomy and closure (Fig. 14-13B). It is achieved by an incision in the lateral palpebral fissure with subsequent detachment of the lower limb of the lateral canthal tendon, which allows relaxation of the lateral portion of the lower lid and adjacent cheek skin. If there is only a millimeter or two of gap prior to canthotomy, closure is possible. With this procedure the lining is not a problem because the lateral conjunctiva of the fornix rotates in with the lower lid when it moves medially for closure. If lateral canthotomy does not allow closure of the gray margin, undermining of the cheek for a few centimeters laterally may be necessary. If there is still

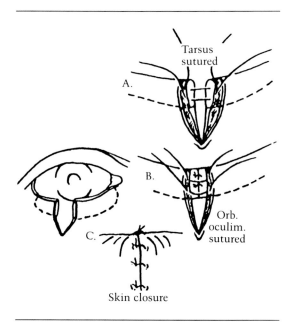

**Figure 14-12** *Closure of the tarsus and conjunctiva can be performed by "pull-out" sutures or by interrupted fine catgut sutures. The knot must be tied away from the conjunctiva to prevent irritation. The wound is closed in three layers to include the tarsus, conjunctiva, orbicularis muscle, and skin.*

difficulty advancing the wound edges for closure, a backcut at the end of the lower incision, usually 4 to 5 cm lateral to the canthal tendon, may be done with the angle of the cut toward the lateral canthus (Fig. 14-13C). Advancement of this flap along with rotation of the conjunctiva then generally allows closure of defects, in some cases up to nearly one-half of the lower lid. If there is a mucosal defect laterally, a small graft from the nasal septum may be necessary.

If the defect from the resection is one-half of the width of the lower lid, mobilization of a cheek rotation flap and cartilage graft is indicated (Fig. 14-13D). When designing an incision for a cheek flap, a straight lateral cut is not adequate, as it results in shortness of the lateral lower lid [9]. Instead, the incision from the lateral canthus must be directed

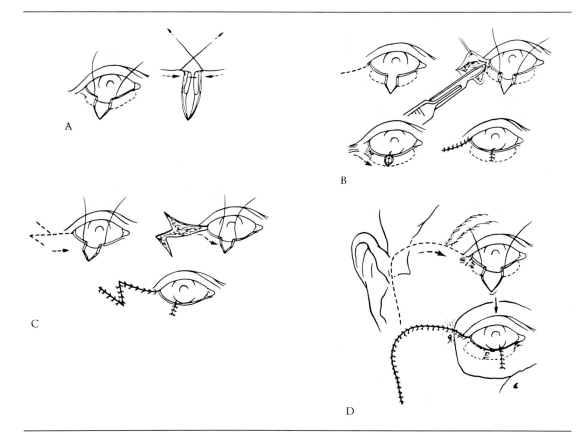

**Figure 14-13** A. After excision of one-fourth to one-half of the lower lid, "tag" sutures of fine silk can be placed in the tarsal margin under tension to see if closure is possible. B. If direct closure is not possible, exposure and cantholysis of the lateral canthal tendon may be performed to relax the lateral eyelid for closure of the defect directly. C. If lateral cantholysis is not adequate for closure, a skin flap may be designed with the incision extended onto the cheek or with a "back cut" of the flap as shown. D. If a small cheek advancement is not adequate, a large cheek flap may be designed and used. Defects up to complete lower lid loss may be reconstructed by this technique. The shaded area denotes a composite cartilage–mucosa graft. In the event of total lid reconstruction, a cartilage–mucosa graft large enough to reconstruct the whole conjunctival and tarsal layer must be used.

upward in an arch, laterally to the preauricular area, and then downward. Mobilization of the cheek flap is accomplished by wide undermining in the superficial subcutaneous layer.

After the undermining and achieving hemostasis, the size of the mucosal defect is estimated. One may proceed with a septal cartilage-mucosal composite graft to lend support to the newly reconstructed lateral canthal area. An easy method of removal of the cartilage graft is to cut a template of glove paper the size of the eyelid defect. This template is then placed on the cocainized septal mucosa. While it is attached to the moist mucous membrane, an incision is made with a scalpel (Fig. 14-14). The cartilage–mucosa graft is removed as a two-layered wafer and the cartilage thinned by splitting it with a No. 10 blade. This maneuver allows slight convex curvature of the cartilage side of the graft while the concave mucosal side conforms to the curved globe. The graft is sutured into the conjunctival defect of the lower lid. The cheek flap is completely dissected free for easy medial rotation into place. The lateral incision is then closed with a few subcutaneous 5-0 Vicryl sutures and the skin with 6-0 nylon. The deep dermis of the cheek flap is sutured to the lateral orbital rim periosteum with a permanent suture, and a small suction drain is placed under the cheek flap. For total or near-total loss of the lower lid, a larger cheek flap is indicated along with a composite septal mucosa–cartilage graft. The conjunctival defect is again estimated using a paper pattern, which is placed on the cocainized septal mucosa, and the composite graft is excised. In this instance there remains a border of exposed cartilage around this larger defect in the nasal septum that could create a problem of nonhealing. To avoid this problem, 1 to 2 mm of cartilage is ronguered away from the wound edges, allowing the mucosa to drop down to cover the remaining exposed edge of cartilage. A piece of Gelfoam cut to pattern is placed in the septal defect, and nasal gauze packing is placed in the nasal airway over the Gelfoam. The opposite nostril does not require packing. It may be necessary to cauterize bleeding vessels in the septal defect. Note also that the vertical height of the cartilage graft must be made larger than the area of defect to overcorrect in the vertical dimension. This step allows good support over time for the newly reconstructed lower lid.

When using reconstruction with a large cheek flap, it is important to achieve good hemostasis so as to prevent postoperative hematoma, which could compromise flap circulation. The initial anchoring of the cheek flap must be at the deep lateral canthal area with a permanent suture approximating the dermis of the flap to the lateral canthal tendon or periosteum of Whitnall's tubercle. At that point, deep 5-0 Vicryl sutures are placed along the subcutaneous tis-

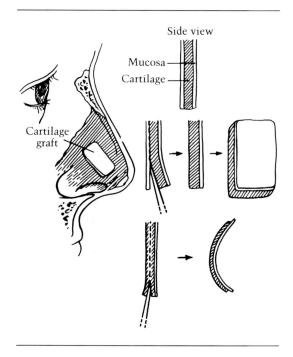

**Figure 14-14** *Composite cartilage–mucosa graft up to 1.5 × 2.5 cm can easily be obtained. The mucosa and cartilage are stripped away from the subperichondral space of the opposite side of the septum. Thinning the cartilage by shaving it to half-thickness results in the cartilage curving away from the shaved area. The mucosal side rests against the globe and conforms with its curved shape to the globe. A small flange of mucosa is left for suturing on the lid margin and in the fornix.*

sue plane. Skin closure is completed with 6-0 nylon. Because the circulation in this falp is excellent, total survival of these large cheek flaps as well as the composite graft can be anticipated.

In the case of small full-thickness defects of the medial canthal and lower lid area combined, a small flap based medially and utilizing the upper lid skin and muscle may be used in association with the small cartilage graft (Fig. 14-15). In this case, lateral canthotomy or cheek advancement is not necessary. A composite mucosa–cartilage graft is necessary to fill the defect. As previously described, the composite graft is cut to conform to the defect, and the medially

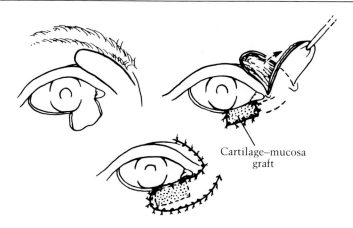

*Figure 14-15 Medially based skin–orbicularis muscle flap can be mobilized and used to cover a cartilage–mucosa graft. This flap is useful for medial lower lid full-thickness defects.*

based upper lid skin muscle flap is brought down over the graft.

Healing of these cartilage grafts is always good so long as they are completely covered by vascularized tissue. In the event of loss of the flap margin with exposure of the carti-

*Figure 14-16 For lateral defects, a larger unipedicle skin–orbicularis muscle flap can be used in full-thickness lid reconstruction. Up to about one-half of the lower lid can be reconstructed by this method.*

lage portion of the composite graft, the cartilage can simply be trimmed back so that the edges of the flap and mucosa close over the remaining cartilage graft.

In the event of a small horizontal defect laterally, which cannot be closed primarily, a laterally based flap of skin and orbicularis muscle may be used in a similar manner to cover a small composite mucosal cartilage graft (Fig. 14-16). The donor area may be closed primarily, and good healing is generally ensured.

In the event that the defect is a horizontal defect of the entire thickness of the lid, a

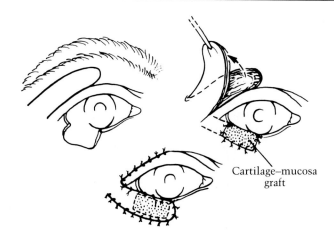

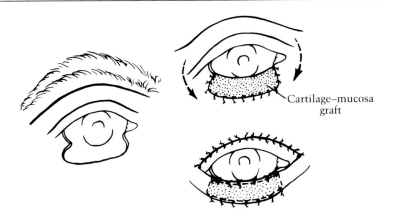

Cartilage–mucosa graft

**Figure 14-17** *Bipedicle Tripier flap of skin and orbicularis muscle can be used for total lower lid reconstruction to cover a cartilage–mucosa graft. The graft must be cut as widely as possible to give good support to the lower lid. Detachment of the lateral pedicles can be done in 10 days.*

composite graft may be utilized in conjunction with a bipedicled skin and muscle (Tripier) flap from the upper lid (Fig. 14-17). In this instance, the mucosal pattern is cut to the size of the defect. It must be cut accurately to prevent relaxation of the new lower lid due to excess graft length. After the graft is sutured in place using interrupted 6-0 chromic sutures, the bipedicled upper lid flap is sutured over the cartilage graft, and the upper edge of the flap is sutured to the upper edge of the mucosa. The medial and lateral limbs of the flap can then be "tubed" with one or two interrupted sutures. If the defect involves the inferior lacrimal punctum, the lacrimal canaliculus may sometimes be mobilized and redirected medially. If this step is necessary, a 1-mm Silastic tube may be placed in the lumen to maintain patency until healing is complete.

An alternate method, the Hughes technique, is used for reconstruction of the lower lid defect using tarsoconjunctiva from the upper lid in association with a full-thickness graft or local flap to cover the shaved inner layer. Good results can be achieved using this technique by surgeons trained in these methods. With this technique, the eye must remain closed for several weeks after the procedure is performed until it is time to detach the lower lid from the upper lid. Lid retraction and inversion can occur as a complication of this technique.

## Upper Lid

With partial-thickness defects of the upper lids, it is best to begin by measuring the size of the defect and the mobility of the adjacent tissues. If there is loss of the orbicularis muscle, it is best to replace it by moving adjacent muscle into the defect or by a composite graft of muscle and skin from the opposite upper lid. If only a skin defect is present, direct closure, local flap, or skin graft may be indicated.

Although adjacent local eyelid skin gives a good match for upper eyelid reconstruction in color and texture, a limited amount is available for donor use. An excellent flap for local coverage may come from adjacent lateral eyelid or temporal skin (Fig. 14-18). A flap up to 2 cm wide can be mobilized. Results of the flap as well as the donor scars are usually good.

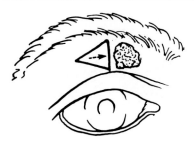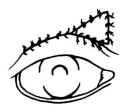

*Figure 14-18 Small defects around the upper and lower lid area can be handled by adjacent pedicle flaps advanced in V-Y fashion for closure. Care must be taken to free the pedicle for adequate mobility of the flap skin.*

The midline forehead and glabellar area are sources of donor flap skin, but the color and texture matches are not generally good. If primary closure or local flap coverage is not feasible, skin grafting of the defect is considered. The best donor source for color match and texture for upper lid defects is the same or opposite upper lid skin. If the defect is large, adequate amounts of opposite upper lid skin may not be available to cover it, and a skin graft from a remote source may be considered. In the event a full-thickness graft from a remote source is indicated, a

*Figure 14-19 The whole upper eyelid skin area may be replaced as a "unit" from split-thickness supraclavicular or medial upper arm skin. A full-thickness graft is usually too bulky for this area. This graft pattern design is especially useful for eyelid burns.*

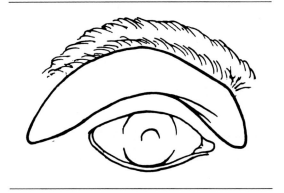

thin postauricular full-thickness graft is a good color match. If this skin is used, it is thinned as much as possible so it is pliable and is a closer match for the thin upper lid skin. A full-thickness skin graft can be taken from the postauricular area and grafted as a unit to the whole upper lid (Fig. 14-19). This unit graft can give a good cosmetic result. An alternate donor area for upper lid skin is a split-thickness graft from the inner upper arm. These grafts are cosmetically good, especially in women because the graft is lighter in color than a full-thickness graft from the neck or face, and cosmetics may be used postoperatively to help camouflage the difference.

If the full-thickness graft is used on part of the upper lid as a patch or to cover a round defect, it is best to do a zigzag incision and closure of the wound for healing without contracture of the scar. When reconstructing partial-thickness defects of the upper lid, remember that the pretarsal orbicularis muscle is responsible for lid closure and is preserved if possible.

If there is significant loss of muscle, an adjacent muscle flap from a higher point on the lid may be utilized for muscle reconstruction. Reinnervation of grafted muscle in the eyelid is the rule rather than the exception, and the muscle appears to function well after healing is complete.

Full-thickness defects of the upper lid can be treated in the same way as the lower lid defects. The difference is that, with the constant movement of blinking of the upper lid,

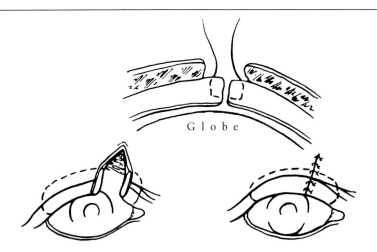

Globe

any rough or irregular area on the inner lid scratches and irritates the cornea, which may cause abrasion, infection, or perforation of the cornea. Therefore it is important to close the tarsal wound so the sutures do not go through the conjunctiva, where they can scratch the cornea (Fig. 14-20). This point is important for upper lid closure, which is performed using magnifying loupes.

The tarsal closure is usually performed with 6-0 chromic gut. As in the lower lid, a silk suture is placed into the gray line on the lid margin and left long so that it may be taped to the cheek for postoperative traction and immobilization of the upper lid. With tumor resection it is important to make a perpendicular cut at the lid margin, so closure results in an even lid margin (Fig. 14-21).

With traumatic lid lacerations the edge of the disrupted tarsus and skin are evenly cut with a scalpel so approximation is as perfect as possible.

*Figure 14-20 Closure of a defect or laceration of the upper tarsus must be performed with care. A suture must not exit through the conjunctiva, where it can irritate the corneal surface. This suturing technique may also be used when placing a cartilage–mucosa graft in the upper lid for reconstruction.*

If it is not certain that direct closure can be achieved, the lid margin may be sutured with 6-0 silk suture, pulling the two ends of the suture so they overlap, to test for ease of closure. If it is seen that closure cannot be achieved, it may then be necessary to do a lateral canthotomy to relax the lateral lid. To do this procedure it is necessary to make an incision laterally to cut the canthal tendon, thereby relaxing the lid closure.

*Figure 14-21 Pentagonal excision of an upper lid lesion results in closure without notching of the lid margin. If closure cannot be achieved directly, lateral canthotomy can relax the lid margin enough for it to be performed.*

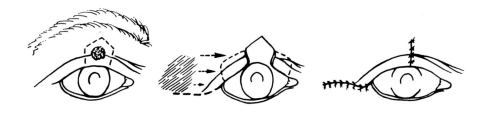

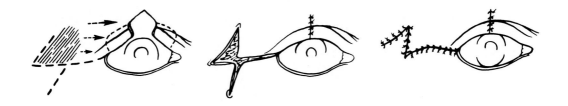

**Figure 14-22** *If direct closure with lateral canthotomy is not adequate to achieve closure, a superiorly based temporal skin advancement flap with rotation of the conjunctiva medially on its undersurface allows closure of defects of approximately one-half of the upper lid.*

After canthotomy, the upper lateral conjunctival mucosa may be rotated in a medial direction. If there is medial rotation of the mucosa, no mucosal defect will be present on the inner lid. The wound edge where the lateral canthal skin has been moved medially may be closed with a 6-0 silk suture, left

**Figure 14-23** *For defects of the upper lid that cannot be closed directly, a cartilage–mucosa graft covered with an adjacent pedicle flap provides excellent reconstruction. The defect resulting from transposition of the flap can be closed by direct means or skin-grafted if necessary. Full-thickness skin from the opposite upper lid is the best color match for coverage of this defect.*

long for easy retrieval.

In the event that lateral canthotomy alone does not allow closure of the defect, additional mobilization of the upper lateral canthal area and temporal skin is indicated. This technique includes extending the incision several centimeters laterally onto the temporal area and mobilizing the temporal skin at the subcutaneous level. The mucosa of the upper lateral fornix is left intact and stretches as it is rotated medially to cover the underside of the new lateral lid. If necessary, a back cut may be performed to allow greater ease of mobility of the temporal skin flap. It may be finalized by designing a Z-plasty from the opposite side of the incision (Fig. 14-22).

If closure by direct approximation, lateral canthotomy, or temporal flap does not appear to be feasible because of the location or size of the defect, a composite septal mu-

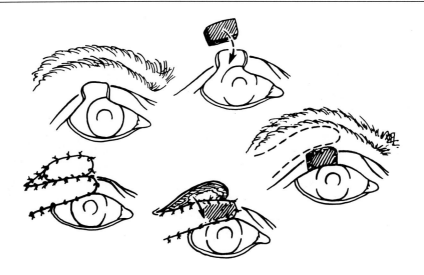

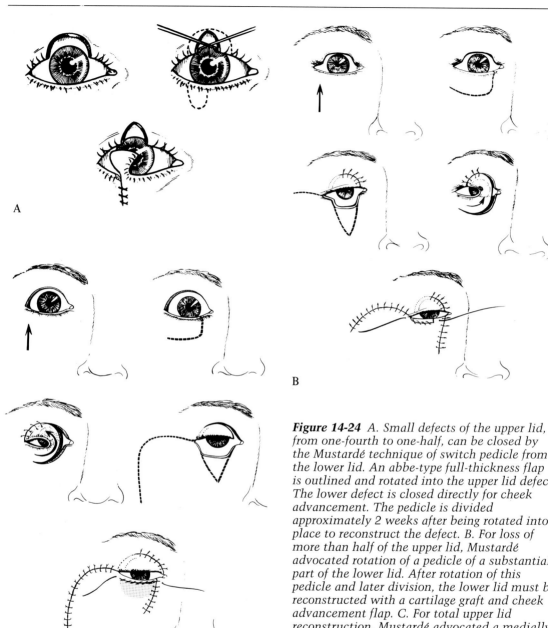

**Figure 14-24** A. Small defects of the upper lid, from one-fourth to one-half, can be closed by the Mustardé technique of switch pedicle from the lower lid. An abbe-type full-thickness flap is outlined and rotated into the upper lid defect. The lower defect is closed directly for cheek advancement. The pedicle is divided approximately 2 weeks after being rotated into place to reconstruct the defect. B. For loss of more than half of the upper lid, Mustardé advocated rotation of a pedicle of a substantial part of the lower lid. After rotation of this pedicle and later division, the lower lid must be reconstructed with a cartilage graft and cheek advancement flap. C. For total upper lid reconstruction, Mustardé advocated a medially or laterally based total lower lid full-thickness pedicle. The resulting full-thickness loss of the lower lid is reconstructed by way of a rotation advancement cheek flap with a large composite cartilage–mucosa graft.

cosal graft and a local pedicle flap may be used (Fig. 14-23). With this method, a mucosal graft is cut by laying a pattern of the defect on the nasal septal mucosa and cutting the graft to the proper size. The cartilage is thinned out and sutured in place to the medial and lateral edges of the conjunctiva in the defect.

After proper fixation of the cartilage graft, a pedicle flap is mobilized from the remaining upper eyelid skin and brought in place over the graft. The defect from which the pedicle graft was taken may be covered with a full-thickness graft from the opposite upper lid or postauricular area. Most defects of the upper lid can be reconstructed by methods that have been discussed, although alternate methods of reconstruction of the upper lid can be mentioned.

For full-thickness upper lid defects, Mustardé [9] advocated rotation of pedicle flaps of full-thickness lower lid tissue. The technique requires cutting through the full thickness of the tarsus on one side of the pedicle and leaving the other side attached as the base of the pedicle, which is rotated 180 degrees upward into the defect. This flap may be used with small defects or with total upper lid loss. After the lower lid is used to reconstruct the upper lid, the defect of the lower lid is reconstructed with a free cartilage–mucosa graft and rotation cheek flap. The base of the pedicle is later severed, allowing mobility of the newly reconstructed lids. Early in his writing Mustardé advocated a small pedicle width but more recently has advocated a wider pedicle attachment, which is more cumbersome but ensures greater viability of the pedicle during the healing period (Fig. 14-24).

Obviously, many types of procedures are acceptable for lid reconstruction, and it is good for the surgeon to have a knowledge of all of these techniques so that he or she may use them as indicated.

## Medical Canthal Reconstruction

Defects of the medial canthal area are almost always a result of tumor excision. The surgeon must be certain of complete excision before proceeding with reconstruction because the consequences of reconstruction over residual tumor in this area can be disastrous, resulting in extensive deep tumor infiltration. Once the decision is made for reconstruction, the method to be used must be based on a number of factors, including the size of the defect, if exposed bone is present, and if adequate local skin is available for flap coverage.

If there is a small amount of bone exposed in the base of the defect, split-thickness grafts "take" well. If the surgeon feels the need to watch for tumor recurrence for some time before reconstruction, this technique may be useful. It allows healing to progress, and the thin graft does not prevent detection of a recurrence. The graft may be excised later at the time of definitive reconstruction, and little is lost except for the split-thickness graft. Another possible indication for a split-thickness graft is when there is a large defect and coverage is needed awaiting delayed reconstruction, such as use of a skin expander of the forehead.

Many defects of the medial canthal area may be covered with full-thickness grafts obtained from the upper eyelid or postauricular area (Fig. 14-25A). Some authors have advocated preauricular grafts, but in my experience preauricular grafts tend to be lighter and not a good color match. Full-thickness grafts are capable of "take," even if the canthal tendon or a small amount of bone is in the base of the wound, because of the "bridging" effect of several millimeters over a relatively nonvascular area. After the graft has been cut and tailored to fit the defect, it is sutured and held in place with bolus sutures. These sutures are tied over the bolus, which remains in place for at least 6 to 7 days for complete healing. The cosmetic results are usually good, and the grafts nearly always heal completely.

If a larger graft is needed, up to 5 × 6 cm may be removed from the postauricular area. The postauricular defect may be primarily closed or replaced with a split-thickness graft.

For smaller defects in the medial canthal

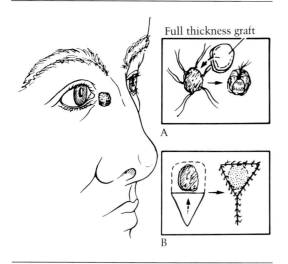

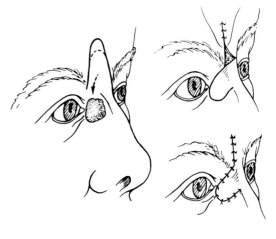

*Figure 14-25* A. Defects of the medial canthal area are easily reconstructed by full-thickness postauricular grafts, which give an excellent color match. Upper eyelid skin for the graft also provides an excellent color match. Preauricular grafts may be useful, but the color match is not always good. B. Defects of the medial canthal area can be closed by **V-Y** pedicle advancement flap with the blood supply to the pedicle based on subcutaneous tissue and muscle.

*Figure 14-26* Large defects of the medial canthal area can be reconstructed by glabellar flap up to several centimeters in width or length. The skin is thicker than the eyelid skin but may be defatted. The color match is usually good.

area, up to about 2 cm, a **V-Y** pedicle advancement flap based on the subcutaneous tissue may be used (Fig. 14-25B). The flap may come from the adjacent lid area, nasal dorsum, glabella, or lateral nasal area, the latter of which is the most common donor site. The **V-Y** flap is mobilized by making an incision around the periphery of the pedicle, with enough undermining to allow movement of the pedicle in the intended direction. If the pedicle base is undercut extensively, the subsequent lack of vascular supply may cause necrosis of the advanced pedicle. Mobility is usually not a problem with these small flaps, and the donor area is closed directly as the pedicle moves forward to fill the defect. Postoperatively, there may be some edema of the pedicle, which can be helped by massing the pedicle to flatten and soften it.

For large defects that cannot be covered

using other reconstructive techniques, a glabellar flap may be used (Fig. 14-26). If there has been a deep excision of tissue in the medial canthal area with exposed bone, the glabellar area is marked as a flap based on the angular and supratrochlear vessels of the opposite side of the nose. Once the flap has been mobilized, the skin of the glabellar and nasal dorsal area is freed from the attachments of nasal periosteum so the flap can be moved onto position easily. After the pedicle flap is moved in the new position, the donor area may be primarily closed with Vicryl 5-0 deep and nylon 6-0 on the skin. Mobility of the skin in this area allows redraping of the skin and usually results in a good cosmetic appearance. The flap may be thinned without endangering tissue viability. If the palpebral fissure has been removed, the glabellar flap may be split to recreate this fissure. Prior to this step, the glabellar skin flap is thinned to approximately the thickness of the eyelid skin. Large amounts of skin for lower lid and medial canthal defects can be obtained using a skin expander in the medial forehead area. This skin can be brought down into almost any position without fear of compromising the flap viability. The skin expansion must be calculated to give the amount of skin necessary for the reconstruction. The expander is placed in the subcutaneous space via a skin incision in the scalp and expanded over several weeks until the desired amount of skin is available.

If the lacrimal drainage apparatus is involved in the resection, it may be possible and desirable to reconstruct it. Often it is not necessary because there is a balance between the secretion and evaporation of the tears. More than 90 percent of the patients with excision of the lacrimal outflow system do well and usually remain free from symptoms of epiphora.

## Lower Lid Ectropion

*Cicatricial ectropion* is characterized by eversion and downward pull of the lower eyelid, causing the lid margin to fall away from the globe, where it usually rests. It may be caused by loss of skin due to burn, trauma, or a chronic dermatitis that causes skin retraction. A vertical scar running to the lid margin may also create downward pull on the lid causing ectropion.

If the ectropion is due to linear scar contracture, the best approach is by Z-plasty correction (Fig. 14-27). The Z-plasty angles are marked and the flaps transposed. Care must be taken to transect and release all of the deep scar to fully correct the ectropion before transposing the Z-plasty flaps. Multiple Z-plasties may be necessary in cases in which the scar is long.

With cicatricial ectropion due to skin loss, the skin must be replaced by a skin graft or local flap. There may also be associated laxity of the tarsal margin, which must be corrected by tarsal wedge excision. To correct this type of ectropion, the defect must be re-created by an incision along the infraciliary margin. The muscle and tarsal plate can be

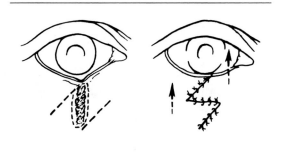

**Figure 14-27** *Scarring of the lower lid with vertical shortening and notching of the lid can be corrected by partial- or full-thickness Z-plasty of the lid margin.*

freed up, and the defect becomes larger as the dissection continues. It is then overcorrected so that no residual ectropion remains. Once the defect is re-created and hemostasis is achieved, the defect may be covered with a local flap or full-thickness graft (Fig. 14-28). Usually enough tissue is available

**Figure 14-28** *Ectropion due to scar can be corrected by release of the scar and re-creation of the defect. The resulting defect is treated with a full-thickness skin graft from the postauricular area. If laxity of the lid margin is present, tarsectomy should also be part of the procedure.*

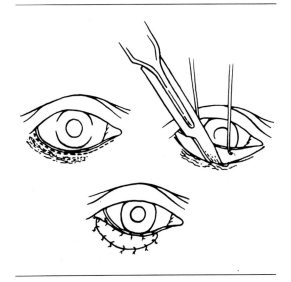

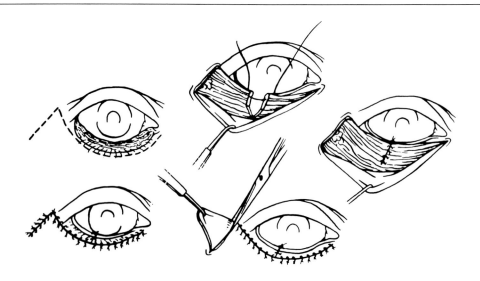

from the upper lid for a local flap about 1 cm in width. Sources of full-thickness graft skin include postauricular, upper eyelid, and supraclavicular areas.

Remote donor areas such as the groin are not good color matches but may need to be used when a large skin graft is required. The postauricular skin seems to give the best match for color and texture. Therefore if the defect is small, upper lid skin may be used for grafting. If the defect is large, a postauricular graft is the best choice. It is necessary to make certain that there is good support along the tarsal margin so that the postoperative relaxation and recurrent ectropion is not seen. When tarsal relaxation is present, a wedge tarsectomy with closure can be done with the graft placed directly on the closure. Whenever possible, the lateral and medial ends of the graft are carried beyond the points of insertion of canthal tendons to give a sling-like effect.

*Senile ectropion* results from laxity of the tarsus as well as the skin. Correction is aimed at tightening the tarsus and pulling up the skin laterally for support. The approach is via an infraciliary incision, exposing the tarsal plate for subsequent full-

**Figure 14-29** *The relaxed lower lid margin with ectropion due to senile changes is corrected by tightening the tarsal margin in a horizontal manner and lateral suspension of the lower lid skin. Removal of excess skin and the tarsal plate is part of this procedure. The lower lid tarsectomy is performed in the lateral third of the eyelid within several millimeters of the lateral palpebral fissure. This procedure is a modification of the Kuhnt-Simonowski technique.*

thickness wedge excision of the tarsus. After tarsal closure the skin is pulled up laterally for support (Fig. 14-29).

*Paralytic ectropion* results when the orbicularis muscle loses the ability to contract. Simple tightening procedures, such as wedge excision of the tarsus and lateral pull of the skin, suffice in the simpler cases. The defect is corrected by the same technique as used for senile ectropion. If a more extensive procedure is needed, a static or dynamic fascia sling may be suspended from the medial canthal tendon to the lateral orbital rim (Fig. 14-30).

In cases where more extensive support is needed, a dynamic fascia sling from the temporalis muscle fascia may be used (Fig. 14-31). Using a temporal incision about 2 cm

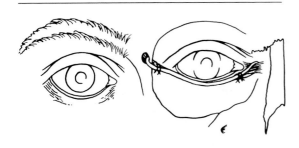

**Figure 14-30** *If the lid is markedly relaxed, a wedge tarsectomy can be bolstered with a full lower lid fascial sling suspended from the medial canthal tendon to the lateral orbital rim. This graft runs between the orbicularis muscle and the tarsal plate.*

behind the temporal hairline, a 1 cm wide strip of fascia is removed starting from the low point at the zygomatic arch to the upper point where it blends into the pericranium. The inferior part of the fascia sheet is incised and dissected away from the muscle up to the point where fascia is attached to the periosteum, leaving intact the connection from the muscle to the fascia. The muscle unit then has the strip of fascia connected to it as the distal part of the unit. A tunnel is dissected in the subcutaneous space to the lateral canthus and around both upper and lower lid margins to the medial canthus. The tension on the fascia sling is determined on the medial canthal area, where the final tightening is performed with enough tension to pull the lower eyelid and upper eyelid margins together. The fascia sling is tunneled between the orbicularis muscle and tarsus, as close to the lid margins as possible to give maximum support to the lid margins.

The wounds are closed and the eye patched for the first postoperative day. It may be several weeks before the pull of the levator muscle is able to overcome the tightness of the fascia sling. Therefore the upper eyelid remains ptotic until it is overcome. The patient is then sent to the physical therapy department for training for eyelid closure, which eventually becomes voluntary, mediated through the temporalis muscle.

## Entropion

*Entropion* is defined as the turning in of the upper or lower lid margin. The most common type is senile or spastic entropion. Congenital entropion is rare. Cicatricial entropion may occur after a surgical procedure or trauma to the eyelids. In the United States, we do not see disease-related entropion.

*Trichiasis* is defined as the condition in which the lashes are turned inward against the cornea. It is associated with entropion.

*Spastic* or *senile entropion* occurs when the orbital septum and the inferior retractors of the tarsal plate are relaxed enough to allow inversion of the lid, brought about by contraction of the orbicularis muscle (Fig. 14-32). With spastic entropion, the portion of the lower lid containing the tarsus and lashes rolls 180 degrees inward to settle in the lower fornix. The result is that the lashes are turned against the sclera, and the lower lid is shortened vertically owing to doubling inward on itself. There is conjunctival irritation, discomfort, tearing, and chronic inflammation. Bacterial conjunctivitis may occur as a result. Spastic entropion may occur when the orbital septum and inferior lid retractors are lax, and the skin and orbicularis muscle overlying the lid are redundant. With blinking, the orbicularis muscle and skin roll up and over the tarsal plate, pulling up the inferior portion and orbital septum and turning the lid inward. Once the lid turns inward, the irritation increases the spastic tone of the orbicularis muscle and maintains the inverted position of the eyelid.

Operative procedures described to correct this problem include horizontal shortening of the tarsal plate, tightening of the orbital septum [4], repositioning of the orbicularis

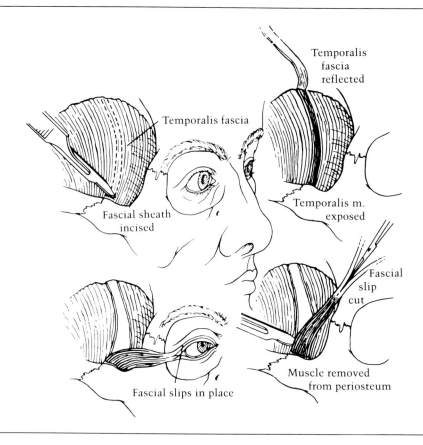

Temporalis fascia

Temporalis
fascia
reflected

Fascial sheath
incised

Temporalis m.
exposed

Fascial
slip
cut

Fascial slips in place

Muscle removed
from periosteum

**Figure 14-31** *For paralytic ectropion with lagophthalmos of the upper lid, a dynamic temporalis fascia and muscle suspension procedure can be used. The fascia overlying the temporalis muscle is detached inferiorly and brought up as a strip that is subsequently split to encircle the upper and lower lids. At the upper point it is reflected off the periosteum and left in continuity with the origin of the temporalis muscle fibers. With the fascia attached to the muscle, a muscle flap is mobilized. The whole unit is tunneled subcutaneously around the upper and lower lids between the orbicularis muscle and tarsus plates. It is attached medially to the canthal tendon. Contraction of the temporalis muscle aids in blinking.*

muscle [14], and excision of excess skin and muscle. The author's approach is to excise an inverted triangle from the tarsus and adjacent conjunctiva to the inferior fornix (Fig. 14-33). Closure of this incision in a horizontal direction tightens the inferior portion of the tarsal plate and orbital septum. With removal of the inverted triangle, the pretarsal muscle is left attached to the tarsal plate. Closure is performed with interrupted 6-0 chromic sutures. The next step is excision of a portion of skin and muscle, thereby reducing the bulk of the muscle, which rolls up over the lid margin causing inversion. This method has been effective and is simple to perform through a lower blepharoplasty incision.

If there is laxity of the lower lid as well, a full-thickness wedge excision of the tarsus and lid margin is performed (Fig. 14-34). In

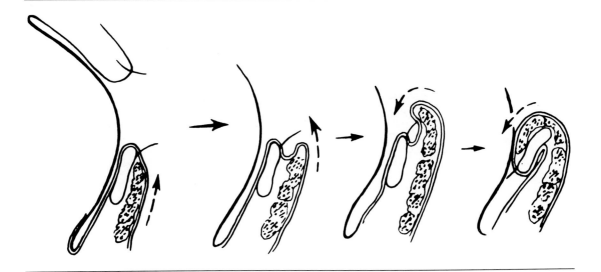

**Figure 14-32** *Senile entropion results when the relaxed lower orbital septum allows inversion of the lid and lash margins. It is initiated by spastic blinking with rolling of the orbicularis muscle over the tarsal margin.*

**Figure 14-33** *Correction of entropion involves shortening the lower part of the tarsus and conjunctiva by an inverted triangle incision. A. Eyelid shows outline of tarsal plate. B. Excision of base—down triangle from tarsus and conjunctiva. Closure of this triangle (C) prevents "flipping" of the tarsus to the inverted position. Excision of skin and muscle (D) prevents the orbicularis muscle from initiating the process of inversion. (E) Closure.*

this case, the lower part of the wedge must be wider than the upper part to tighten the lid on the horizontal direction. With this technique, as with the standard repair, excess skin and muscle are removed prior to closure of the incision. Postoperative treatment after surgical correction of entropion consists in application of cold saline compresses and antibiotic ophthalmic ointment.

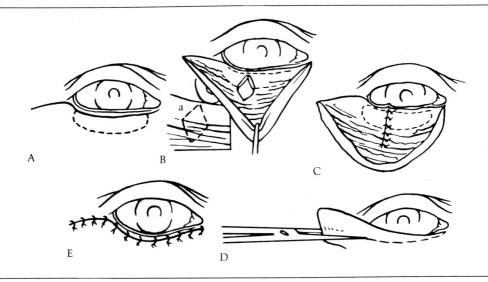

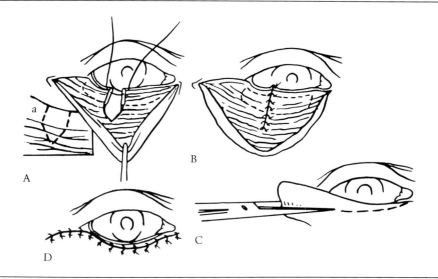

*Figure 14-34* Senile entropion combined with a lax lower lid can be corrected by excision of pentagon wedge from tarsal margin (A), closure of excision (B), excision of excess skin and muscle (C), and final closure (D). It is performed as in the simple procedure show in Figure 14-34.

*Congenital entropion* describes the condition of persistent inversion of the lower lid, which occurs from birth. With this condition the lid usually rests in a higher position than with senile entropion, and the lashes can directly irritate the cornea, causing conjunctivitis or corneal ulceration. With milder forms, the lower lid lashes may be turned toward the cornea but not actually lie against it. There is usually no spastic component to this condition. Surgical treatment of congenital entropion consists in removal of a strip of skin and muscle from the infraciliary area from the medial to the lateral canthus in an elliptical excision. Closure of the muscle layer and the skin completes the procedure. Postoperative treatment consists in topical application of antibiotic ointment.

*Cicatricial entropion* (Fig. 14-35) may be caused by trauma, surgical procedures, or infection. The most common infection that causes this disorder is trachoma, which is not seen in the United States. Most commonly, cicatricial entropion is produced by surgical or traumatic scarring with loss of tarsus and conjunctiva.

Entropion may be seen in the upper lid after some forms of ptosis repair. Overcorrection of ptosis with retraction of the tarsus with overlapping of the orbicularis can create entropion and trichiasis. With both of these conditions, the end result is irritation of the cornea.

To correct entropion of the upper lid secondary to overcorrected ptosis, one must first deal with the overcorrection. The problem is approached through a standard blepharoplasty incision, exposing the orbital septum and levator aponeurosis. In these cases there is often some scarring of the aponeurosis, particularly at the medial and lateral attachments. These scars must be released adequately so there is mobility of the upper lid. If free motion of the lid is not possible after lysis of these adhesions, the levator muscle or aponeurosis is released and a scleral graft placed in the defect to act as a spacer. The orbicularis muscle is then dissected away from the tarsus and sutured in a higher, more cephalad, upward position, pulling the inverted lashes away from the cornea. Vicryl 6-0 is used to suture the orbi-

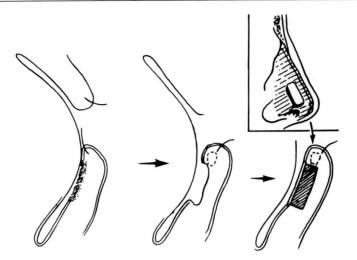

**Figure 14-35** *Cicatricial entropion secondary to partial loss of the lower lid, tarsus, and conjunctiva may be corrected by re-creating the defect surgically and placing a composite cartilage–mucosa graft in the defect.*

cularis muscle in the new position of the tarsus. The upper border of the orbicularis muscle is then sutured to the aponeurosis to "anchor" it into position. An intermarginal tarsorrhaphy suture is helpful for maintaining traction on the upper lid during this healing phase.

## Socket Problems

After enucleation of an eye, a spacer or spherical implant is placed in the muscle cone of the newly created defect. Closure of the muscles over the implant with conjunctival closure maintains some of the volume of the orbit lost by enucleation. An artificial prosthetic eye is placed in the socket anterior to the mucosal closure and is held in place by the upper and lower lids (Fig. 14-36). Some of the problems that may occur are a result of extrusion of the implant, contracture of the socket, and abnormalities of the lids including ptosis and ectropion. To correct these problems and achieve the best cosmetic result, treatment is based on correction of the defect.

If the implant is extruded or displaced downward, an abnormal appearance of the lids occurs. Downward displacement of the implant leads to excessive pressure along the lower part of the prosthesis, which transmits this pressure to the lower lid (Fig. 14-37). This pressure causes the prosthesis to come forward and stretch the lower lid with resulting lagophthalmos or ectropion. It is sometimes possible to correct the problem with a fascia sling [13]. This technique involves placing a strip of fascia lata between the tarsus and orbicularis layer of the lower lid suspended from the medial canthal tendon to a drill hole in the lateral orbital rim (Fig. 14-38). If the implant is extruded or displaced, the socket can be reconstructed with an implant of rib cartilage placed as a graft (Fig. 14-39). The cartilage graft stays in position and is not vulnerable to infection or extrusion, as an alloplastic implant can be. The rib cartilage graft is shaped slightly larger than the original implant, which tends to maintain the position and give a good cosmetic result. If the implant has previously extruded, subsequent replacement with an allograft material might again result in extrusion. In this instance, a new implant of rib cartilage is useful.

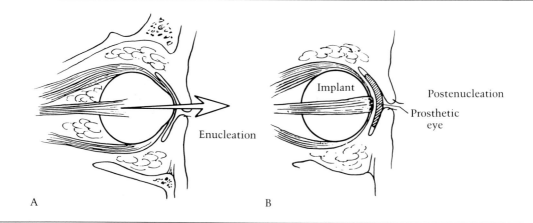

A                                    B

*Figure 14-36* A. Enucleation results in loss of volume in the orbit. B. Restoration to normal appearance is aided by placing an implant in the "muscle cone." The muscle transmits motion to the socket. The prosthetic eye is a flat, thin shell. The combination of prosthesis and implant add volume and normal appearance to a postenucleation socket.

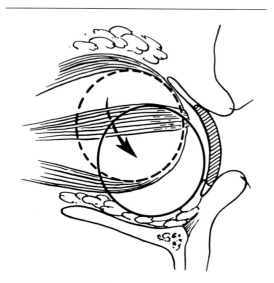

*Figure 14-37* If the implant drifts downward in the socket it may push the lower lid out, causing edema of the lower conjunctiva and a shallow fornix. The prosthesis may fall out. If so, correction is performed by a fascia sling to the lower lid. In more severe cases, the implant may be replaced by an autogenous cartilage graft, which maintains a better upward position.

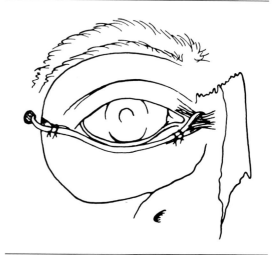

*Figure 14-38* If there is pressure of the prosthesis against the lower lid due to downward placement of the implant, the technique described by Vistnes to tighten the lower lid may produce good results. Fascia lata or temporalis fascia may be used. The fascia sling is tunneled between the orbicularis muscle and the tarsal plate from the lateral orbital rim to the medial canthal tendon.

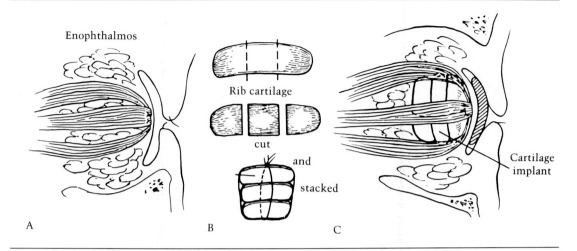

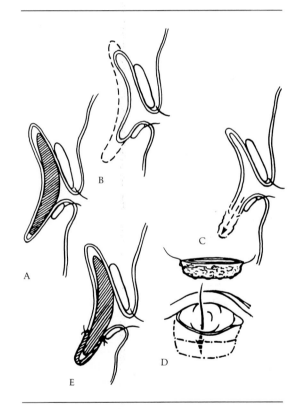

***Figure 14-39*** *For anophthalmic enophthalmos due to extrusion of an implant (A), a new implant of rib cartilage may be placed by cutting and stacking the cartilage graft (B). C. It is placed into the muscle cone and the conjunctiva closed over it. A prosthesis is placed in the socket, correcting the enophthalmos and allowing transmission of motion from the muscle cone to the prosthesis. If the enophthalmos correction is attempted by a larger prosthesis alone, it may result in laxity of the lower lid.*

***Figure 14-40*** *A. Normal prosthesis with extension in the upper and lower fornix. B. If a contracted socket occurs, it may be necessary to correct it surgically. C. Deepening of the inferior fornix is performed followed by placement of a boat-shaped postauricular full-thickness graft sutured into the defect. D. The prosthesis is then put in place as a "stent." Excellent healing without subsequent contracture of full-thickness grafts is usual after this procedure. E. Prosthesis in place in newly formed fornix.*

When dealing with the problem of contracture of the socket, the author has used postauricular full-thickness grafts to expand the socket. To measure the amount of graft needed, a defect is made by incising the mucosa of the fornix of the lid involved in the contracture (Fig. 14-40). The amount of defect created by this incision determines the measurement of the graft necessary to use. A pattern of glove paper may be used, and a postauricular graft is cut to this size. The graft is then sutured in place with the epidermal side facing the socket and the dermis adjacent to the defect. The prosthesis is then put in place as a spacer, and marginal tarsorrhaphy suture of 6-0 Prolene suture is used on two points of the lid. The lid margin is left closed for 2 weeks, at which time the intermarginal suture is removed to gain access to the prosthesis and to inspect the socket. At that point, if the graft is healed, the prosthesis is reinserted and left in place until a new prosthesis is fashioned by the ocularist.

## Reconstruction of the Eyebrows

Reconstruction of the eyebrows may be indicated after ablation due to trauma, tumor excision, or burns. Idiopathic alopecia of the eyebrows is another indication for reconstruction if this condition does not spontaneously reverse within a year of onset.

An eyebrow can be reconstructed using free hair-bearing scalp or pedicle flaps. Free grafts are usually reliable but deliver fewer hair follicles to the recipient area than a pedicle flap of hair-bearing scalp tissue. The "take" of grafts is generally good, but hair growth is sometimes sparse after healing. For bilateral alopecia of the eyebrows, grafting is a simpler procedure and probably is the procedure of choice if heavy brows are not essential. The grafting procedure is performed by selecting a hair-bearing area of scalp with the proper orientation of hair follicles (Fig. 14-41). Eyebrow strip grafts of 3 to 4 mm width can be taken.

A wider graft may have less chance of take. The use of two narrow strips, which are parallel with an intervening epithelial strip, is probably the safest way but requires a secondary procedure to remove the hairless skin strip. If heavier brows are required, two parallel strips with subsequent removal of the medial strip is the procedure of choice. The procedure may be done 4 to 6 weeks after the initial hair-bearing grafts are placed.

If there is scarring or irradiation of the

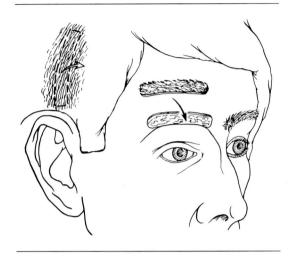

**Figure 14-41**  *The eyebrow can be reconstructed with a graft of hair-bearing scalp tissue. A graft up to 4 to 5 mm wide may "take" well. A parallel graft may be repeated at a later date. The hair follicles must be aligned so that they are pointing a few degrees to the upward outer direction.*

area, a pedicle graft of hair-bearing skin is based on a branch of the superficial temporal artery and vein enclosed in soft tissue to protect the vessels during transfer. A parallel cut in the direction of the growth of the hair follicles is made approximately 3 cm in length and 6 to 8 mm in width. After the skin incision is made, the incision is beveled away from the pedicle so that the base of the pedicle is wider than the skin portion. Doppler imaging may be used to locate the direction of the atrial segment leading up to the proposed donor area. Once the donor pedicle is isolated, the defect to be reconstructed is opened and the recipient area prepared. At that point, a subcutaneous tunnel from the base of the arterial pedicle to the defect is created; the pedicle flap is then pulled through the tunnel and sutured in the defect, and the donor area is closed primarily (Fig. 14-42).

The hairs that grow from these grafts or pedicles are sometimes difficult to control and may be "tamed" with mustache wax.

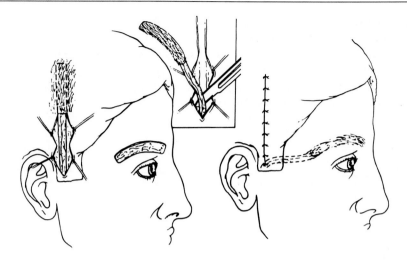

**Figure 14-42** *Vascularized pedicle flap of hair-bearing scalp can be mobilized on a branch of the superficial temporal artery. The donor area is closed primarily. This pedicle flap is moved via a subcutaneous tunnel to the defect.*

The hairs grow to full length and must be trimmed occasionally. Even with this problem, though, the acceptance of these grafts among patients is high, and the results are usually good.

# Correction of Ptosis of the Eyelid

*Ptosis* is defined as an abnormal drooping of the eyelid. The normal level of the eyelid is that position where it covers 1 to 2 mm of the upper limbus of the cornea. When dealing with ptosis patients, factors other than lid level must be considered, including the amount of levator function, the level of the ptotic lid, and the level of the opposite lid.

In the normal eyelid the orbicularis muscle and levator muscle act synergistically, allowing rapid opening and closing during the finely tuned movement of blinking. The levator muscle is skeletal muscle under voluntary control to a major extent, although certain neural reflexes come into play to give fine "tuning" to muscle function. The interposing structure between the levator muscle and the tarsal plate is the levator apo-neurosis, backed by Müller's muscle, which also adjusts the lid level to a small degree (2 to 3 mm). Müller's muscle is not under voluntary control but, rather, is smooth muscle innervated by the sympathetic part of the autonomic nervous system.

## Anatomy

Although most plastic surgeons are well versed on anatomy of the eyelids and orbit, it is worthwhile to emphasize a few important points related to ptosis repair. The levator muscle is 40 mm in length, with the origin in the muscle cone of the orbit. It is attached distally where the muscle fibers blend into fascia at the cephalad edge of the levator aponeurosis, which is 15 mm in length. The aponeurosis is mobile in a superoinferior direction and is attached laterally and medially to fascia bands known as "levator horns."

On the undersurface of the aponeurosis adjacent to the conjunctiva lies Müller's muscle, which in the event of dysfunction can give rise to ptosis. For example, Horner's syndrome includes ipsilateral ptosis of 2 to 3 mm due to paralysis of autonomically innervated Müller's muscle. On the other hand, paralysis or congenital lack of development of the levator muscle can cause ptosis, as can stretching of the aponeurosis. The superior transverse ligament of Whitnall is an important structure in some procedures for ptosis correction, as it overlies the levator muscle at its insertion into the aponeurosis. The tarsus is about 10 to 12 mm in length and has the pretarsal orbicularis oculi muscle attached to its anterior surface. Laterally and medially, the canthal tendons attach the tarsus to the medial and lateral walls of the orbit.

## Classification of Ptosis

Most authors classify ptosis on the basis of congenital or acquired dysfunction. With acquired ptosis, except the neurogenic and myasthenic types, muscle function is usually good to excellent. With congenital ptosis, the underdeveloped levator muscle often functions poorly. The following classification is relatively complete and encompasses most cases of ptosis [18].

Congenital ptosis
  Simple
  With lid anomalies
  With ophthalmoplegias
  Synkinetic (Marcus-Gunn)
Acquired ptosis
  Neurogenic
  Myogenic
  Traumatic
  Mechanical
  Pseudoptosis

Congenital ptosis is associated with myogenic dystrophic changes of the levator muscle resulting in poor levator function. A small percentage of these changes include two types: misdirected third cranial nerve (CN III) ptosis of the Marcus-Gunn type and blepharophimosis. Neurogenic ptosis includes CN III palsy, congenital or acquired, and Horner's cervical sympathetic nerve palsy. Myogenic ptosis includes "involutional," or senile, ptosis, acquired muscular dystrophy, progressive external ophthalmoplegia, and myasthenia gravis. Traumatic ptosis varies according to the location of the injury to the levator muscle or lid mechanism. Mechanical ptosis is due to a tumor, cyst, or enlarged lacrimal gland pushing down the eyelid. Pseudoptosis refers to the drooping lid skin of blepharochalasis and to the apparent ptosis seen in the postenucleation eyelid.

Before proceeding with surgery in the ptosis patient, it is wise to make a detailed evaluation of the history and development of the problem. Often the surgeon can isolate an unusual finding in the history or physical examination that sheds some additional light on the diagnosis. The following preoperative checklist is a useful guide to the work-up of ptosis.

## Preoperative Testing

Factors to be considered during preoperative testing are covered by the following measures.

1. Obtain the patient's history.
2. Perform a careful gross examination of the eyes.
3. Measure the supratarsal fold and symmetry.
4. Evaluate the lid contour.
5. Measure the ptosis (in millimeters).
6. Measure the difference between the two eyelids (width of the palpebral fissure).
7. Measure levator function (lid excursion with the brow static).
8. Check the visual acuity of each eye.

**9.** Check the extraocular muscle movements.

**10.** Check for Bell's phenomenon.

**11.** Check for jaw-winking motion.

**12.** Check for lagophthalmos and lid lag.

In addition to testing, attention must be paid to the details of previous problems, such as excessive tearing or dryness, allergy, or irritation. Taking photographs in downward, forward, and upward gaze is important. When evaluating late-onset ptosis, consider having the patient tested for myasthenia gravis by the Tensilon test. Horner's syndrome can be tested by stimulation with

***Figure 14-43*** *Fascia sling for correction of severe ptosis with poor levator function.*
*A. Incisions at the lid margin. B. Fascia is inserted between the orbicularis muscle and the tarsus at the lid margin. C. A reverdin needle is used to pull fascia to the upper brow level.*
*D, E. Crossover of the fascia sling pulls the lid to the desired level. Simple suture ties are used for fixation. F. Eyelid is at the desired level.*

10 percent phenylephrine hydrochloride solution, which corrects the ptosis.

***Classification of ptosis severity***

| | |
|---|---|
| Mild | 1–2 mm |
| Moderate | 3 mm |
| Severe | 4+ mm |

***Classification of levator function***

| | |
|---|---|
| Excellent | 12–15 mm |
| Good | 8–12 mm |
| Fair | 5–7 mm |
| Poor | 2–4 mm |

## Selection of the Correct Operation

For patients with absent function and severe ptosis, a frontalis sling is the procedure of choice (Fig. 14-43). The principle of this operation is direct attachment of the frontalis muscle at the brow to the lid margin by means of a fascia lata sling or strip. One must check the excursion of the frontalis muscle prior to placing a sling. Movement may be absent, but it usually is 10 to 15 mm

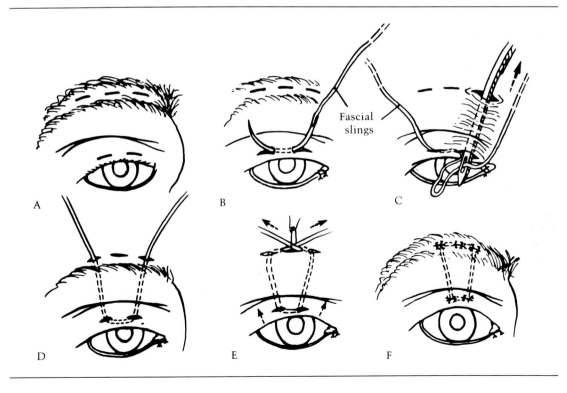

Fascial slings

A  B  C

D  E  F

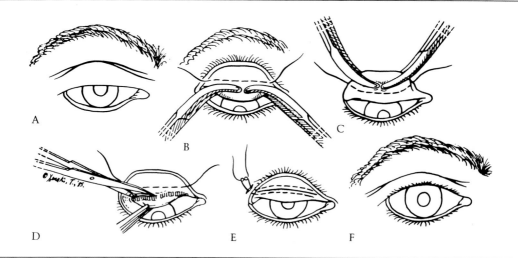

of excursion. Many techniques have been described, but the author uses a modified Fox technique [20]. A number of procedures have been advocated for treatment of mild ptosis. One technique—resection of the conjunctiva and Müller's muscle—elevates the lid in the presence of mild ptosis [24]. Combination of tarsal plate resection with müllerectomy and aponeurosectomy, popularized by Fasanella-Servat (Fig. 14-44), utilizes the posterior conjunctival approach [19]. In fact, to correct mild ptosis, separate or combined resection of the tarsal plate, Müller's muscle-conjunctiva, aponeurosis, or levator muscle has been used effectively. Each technique used must be one with which the surgeon is familiar, for each has its limitations and possible complications.

The author has used all of these techniques but has most often performed the Mustardé split-level tarsectomy for mild ptosis (Fig. 14-45). This technique is simple, noninvasive, and predictable. It also addresses the anterior skinfold, which the posterior conjunctival approach cannot do. Mustardé [23] used this technique in combination with a procedure that turns up, or "hitches," the levator aponeurosis for more severe cases of ptosis (Fig. 14-46).

For moderate ptosis with fair to good levator function, many procedures have been

*Figure 14-44* Fasanella-Servat procedure (for mild ptosis). A. Ptotic eyelid. B. Eversion of the lid, clamping the combined edge of the upper tarsus, conjunctiva, and Müller's muscle. C. Running crossover pull-out suture above the clamped area. D. Excision of tissue included in the clamped specimen. E. Tissue is excised, and the lid is shortened by excision of the tarsus, conjunctiva, and Müller's muscle, with tying of crossover stitches. F. Final position of eyelid.

*Figure 14-45* Mustardé's "split-level" tarsectomy. A. Planned resection of skin, muscle, and tarsus. B. Resected areas shown. C. "Split-level" closure of the eyelid for the desired level.

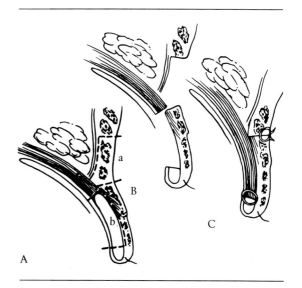

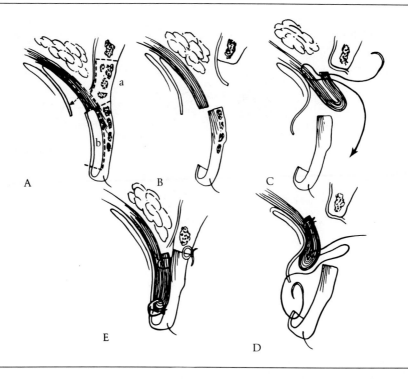

**Figure 14-46** *Mustardé's "split-level tarsectomy with hitch." It is the same as the split-level tarsectomy except for folding back the aponeurosis upon itself to preserve Müller's muscle function while shortening the levator complex. A. Dissection of the conjunctiva off the aponeurosis and Müller's muscle. Planned resection of skin and muscle (a, b). B. Skin and muscle area are resected with exposure of the aponeurosis and Müller's muscle. C. Turnback of aponeurosis and Müller's muscle on itself. D. Hitch-up of aponeurosis and Müller's muscle. E. Suturing of the lower margin of the aponeurosis to the upper tarsal border and closure of the skin.*

described that achieve good results. Some form of levator shortening procedure is used by most surgeons, depending on the procedure for which they were trained. Levator resection, levator "tucking" procedures, levator advancement, and aponeurosis shortening procedures have been advocated by various authors for treatment of moderate ptosis.

The aponeurosis approach to ptosis surgery has been advocated by Anderson, McCord, Jones, and others [16, 21]. The Anderson approach utilizes "tucking" sutures, which bring the aponeurosis down to the tarsus (Fig. 14-47). It is monitored by having the patient look up, thereby determining the level of correction, which requires that the patient be awake. This procedure requires some experience before accuracy of repair is consistently achieved. The McCord technique is performed by full-thickness excision of aponeurosis, Müller's muscle, and conjunctiva [22]. The formula for resection is related to the amount of levator function, with a greater resection done in the lid with poor levator function. Levator shortening is used by many surgeons for treatment of moderate ptosis. The conjunctival approach to levator shortening is popular and is performed by everting the lid to incise the conjunctiva and gain access to the aponeurosis. The aponeurosis is then transected and brought down, where it is shortened according to formula and reattached to the upper tarsus (Fig. 14-48). The anterior skin approach to

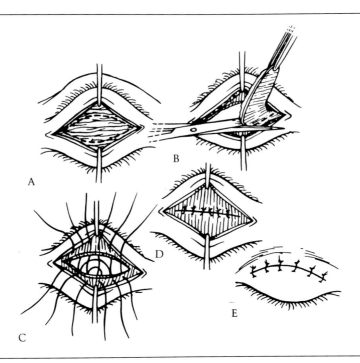

**Figure 14-47** *Aponeurosectomy (for mild ptosis). A. Exposure of the aponeurosis. B. Excision of the ellipse of the aponeurosis, Müller's muscle, and conjunctiva. C, D. Closure defect. E. Defect closed.*

levator shortening is similar and involves removal of a skin and muscle ellipse, a transverse incision of the aponeurosis, and dissection away from the conjunctiva. Advancement downward with resection and reattachment completes the procedure. Plication of the aponeurosis for ptosis has also been described (Fig. 14-49).

The author's surgical preference for treating moderate ptosis with fair to good levator function is a levator advancement procedure (Fig. 14-50) similar to that described by Jones et al. [21] and later Beard [17]. With the strong conviction that little or no levator muscle excision should be performed in muscle with limited function, an effort is made to save the full length of the muscle. The adhesions surrounding the muscle as well as the superior transverse ligament of Whitnall are dissected away from the muscle at the point of insertion of the levator into the aponeurosis. This maneuver allows subsequent detachment of the muscle at that point and advancement over the aponeurosis to the tarsal plate without dissec-

tion of the aponeurosis. Although the muscle is not resected, lifting the lid occurs as a result of advancement of the muscle downward to a lower point of attachment at the level of the tarsus. Levator function has been preserved and even improved in cases using this procedure. In addition, the technique is reversible, predictable, and teachable because of the anatomic precision of the operation. As with most levator shortening procedures, with absent to poor function the results are not as good as when there is some levator function.

Most surgeons prefer to use levator shortening as the first procedure, hoping to get a reasonably good result without having to resort to a fascia sling. If correction utilizing the patient's levator muscle function is possible, it can potentially give a more natural result.

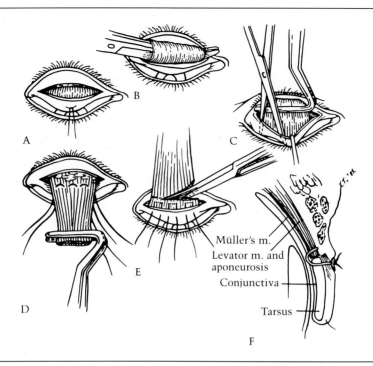

Müller's m.

Levator m. and
aponeurosis

Conjunctiva

Tarsus

***Figure 14-48*** *Standard (Blaskovic's)
transconjunctival levator shortening procedure.
A. Conjunctival incision to expose aponeurosis.
B. Dissection of aponeurosis. C. Cross clamping
of aponeurosis. D. Downward pull after
resection of lateral horns. E. Transection and
suturing of the levator muscle for the desired
lid level. F. Lateral view of the levator sutured
to tarsus.*

***Figure 14-49*** *Aponeurosis plication (for mild
ptosis). A. Incision to expose aponeurosis.
B. Exposed aponeurosis with plication sutures.
C. Plication sutures tied to desired level.
D. Lateral view of plicated aponeurosis.*

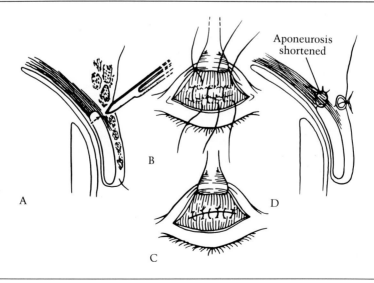

Aponeurosis
shortened

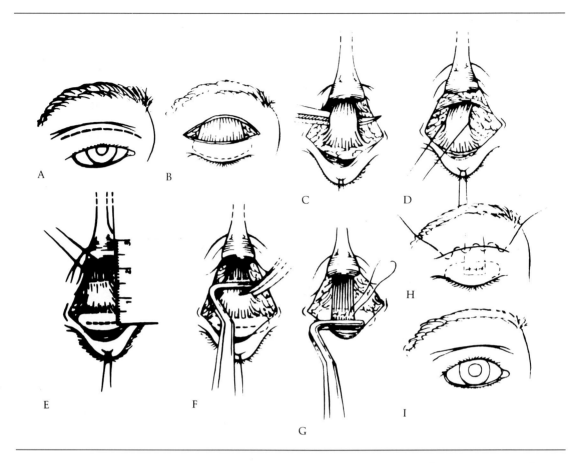

*Figure 14-50* Levator advancement procedure (for moderate ptosis with fair to good levator function). A. Incision in tarsal crease. B. Exposure of aponeurosis and Whitnall's ligament. C, D. Isolation of levator muscle after Whitnall's ligament has been dissected away. E. Marking of points on levator muscle and tarsus. F. Cross clamping of levator muscle at level of insertion into aponeurosis. G. Advancement of levator muscle to tarsal plate, with fixation by permanent sutures. H, I. Desired lid level achieved by advancement of 4 mm of levator muscle to the tarsus for each 1 mm of ptosis.

## Complications

The best results are obtained in those patients who have the least severe ptosis with the greatest amount of levator muscle function—and of course who are operated on by the most experienced surgeons. Selection of the proper operation for the patient is the most important part of the process, although skillful execution of the procedure is also of great importance.

Undercorrection is probably the most common complication and is not associated with corneal problems such as exposure or drying. Rather, the cosmetic appearance is less than desirable because some ptosis is still present in the operated eye. Short of another operative procedure, nothing corrects this problem. With overcorrection, the postoperative lid level is higher than normal and often leads to corneal exposure (especially during sleep), drying, and possible corneal erosion. If the overcorrection is mild, massage of the lid with gentle intermittent traction may be effective. If the procedure performed was tarsectomy or a similar operation, gentle separation of the suture line under topical anesthesia often corrects the problem by forcing the lid level down. If the overcorrection is severe, opening the defect in the aponeurosis and placing a scleral graft as a spacer may be necessary. This technique may allow the lid level to drop down to normal and overcome the corneal problems.

Lagophthalmos may result from removing a large amount of aponeurosis with subsequent adhesions preventing the downward motion of the eyelid. Usually time and massage take care of this problem, but in the interim the cornea must be protected from drying, especially at night, by artificial tears or ointment. If lagophthalmos persists and the lid level is normal, surgical exploration and lysis of adhesions may be indicated if severity of symptoms indicates it. Hematoma or excessive swelling may occur and may compromise the result by causing excessive fibrosis, chronic edema, loss of lid fold, or loss of the surgical correction. The best methods of prevention include absolute hemostasis, irrigation of the wound at the end of the procedure, and preventing the patient from "bucking" while coming out of anesthesia.

Loss of eyelashes may occur, probably due to dissecting too close to the lid margin during exposure of the tarsal plate. Once the loss occurs, there is no good procedure to correct it.

Entropion sometimes occurs as a result of removing too much tarsal plate or poor placement of the sutures, which reattach the levator muscle to it.

In summary, great care must be exerted to avoid the complications of ptosis surgery, as these problems may give rise to severe corneal symptoms or an unhappy patient. Moreover, they often require another operative procedure for correction.

## References

RECONSTRUCTION OF THE EYELIDS AND EYEBROWS

1. Anderson, R. L., and Beard, C. The levator aponeurosis attachments and their clinical significance. *Arch. Ophthalmol.* 95:1437, 1977.
2. Ansell, H. B. Treatment of cancer of the eyelids. *Cutis* 19:273, 1977.
3. Dellon, A. L. Histological study of recurrent basal cell carcinoma. *J. Plast. Reconstr. Surg.* 75:853, 1985.
4. Fox, S. A. Correction of a senile ectropion. *Arch. Ophthalmol.* 48:624, 1952.
5. Fox, S. A. *Ophthalmic Plastic Surgery* (4th ed.). Orlando: Grune & Stratton, 1963.
6. Henkind, P., and Friedman, A. Cancer of the Lids and Ocular Adnexa. In R. Andrade et al. (eds.), *Cancer of the Skin.* Philadelphia: Saunders, 1976. Pp. 1345–1371.
7. Jackson, R., and Adams, R. H. Horrifying basal cell carcinoma, a study of 33 cases in comparison of 435 non-horror cases and a report of four metastastic cases. *J. Surg. Oncol.* 5:43, 1973.
8. Jones, L. Anatomy of the tear system. *Int. Ophthalmol. Clin.* 13:3, 1973.
9. Mustardé, J. C. *Repair and Reconstruction in the orbital Region* (2nd ed.). Edinburgh: Churchill Livingstone, 1980. Pp. 133–147.
10. Polk, H., Cohn, T. D., and Clarkson, J. C. An Appriasal of Elective Regional Lymphadenectomy for Melanoma. In G. D. Zuidema and D. B. Skinner (eds.), *Current Topics in Surgical Research.* New York: Academic Press, 1969.
11. Smith, B. C., and Nesi, F. A. *Practical Techniques in Ophthalmic Plastic Surgery.* St. Louis: Mosby, 1981. Pp. 53–59.
12. Storm, F. K., et al. A prospective study of parotid metastases. *Am. J. Surg.* 134:115, 1977.
13. Vistnes, L., Iverson, R., and Laub, D. The anophthalmic orbit. *J. Plast. Reconstr. Surg.* 52:346, 1973.
14. Wheeler, J. M. Spastic ectropion correction by orbicularis muscle transplantation. *J. Am. Ophthalmol. Soc.* 36:157, 1938.
15. Zide, B. M., and Jelks, G. W. *Surgical Anatomy of the Orbit.* New York: Raven Press, 1985. Pp. 21–31.

CORRECTION OF PTOSIS OF THE EYELID

16. Anderson, R. L., and Dixon, R. S. Aponeurotic

ptosis surgery. *Arch. Ophthalmol.* 97:1123, 1979.

17. Beard, C. *Ptosis.* St. Louis: Mosby, 1981.

18. Beyer, C. H. *Advances in Ophthalmological Plastic and Reconstructive Surgery* (Vol. 1). Elmsford, NY: Pergamon, 1982. Pp. 13–18.

19. Fasanella, R. M., and Servat, T. Levator resection for minimal ptosis, another simplified operation. *Arch. Ophthalmol.* 65:493, 1961.

20. Fox, S. A. *Surgery of Ptosis.* Orlando: Grune & Stratton, 1968.

21. Jones, L. T., Quickert, M. H., and Wobig, J. L. The cure of ptosis by aponeurotic repair. *Arch. Ophthalmol.* 93:629, 1975.

22. McCord, D. D., Jr. An external minimal ptosis procedure—external tarso-aponeurosectomy. *Trans. Am. Acad. Ophthalmol. Otolaryngol.* 70:683, 1975.

23. Mustardé, J. C. *Repair and Reconstruction in the Orbital Region* (2nd ed.). Edinburgh: Churchill Livingstone, 1980. Pp. 316–325.

24. Putterman, A. M., and Urisf, M. J. Müller's muscle conjunctival resection: A method for treatment of blepharoptosis. *Arch. Ophthalmol.* 92:619, 1975.

# 15

Burt Brent

# Reconstruction of the Ear

Reconstruction of the auricle is a challenging discipline that prompts innovation and creativity while simultaneously demanding strict adherence to basic principles of plastic surgery and tissue transfer. Because limitation of space prevents the inclusion of all techniques, the material for this chapter has been carefully selected to provide the reader with guidelines for practical surgical techniques and sound patient management in auricular surgery. It is based on the author's 15-year experience in reconstructing 500 auricles with autogenous tissues.

## Total Construction of the Microtic Ear

### SURGICAL CONSIDERATIONS AND LIMITATIONS

Total construction of the auricle is one of the greatest challenges that confronts the plastic surgeon. Comprised of a delicately convoluted cartilage frame covered by a fine skin envelope, the ear is a difficult structure to draw or sculpt, let alone surgically reproduce. Generally, alloplastic frameworks are not well tolerated [11, 16, 26, 65], and contralateral auricular cartilage is inadequate for a total ear framework. At this time, autogenous costal cartilage remains the most

reliable tissue for an underlying framework support.

Although costal cartilage can be carved to form a delicate framework, it must be remembered that the volume and detail of the furnished three-dimensional framework are limited by the two-dimensional skin flap under which it is placed. Furthermore, because the retroauricular-mastoid skin that covers the framework is somewhat thicker than normal, delicate anterolateral auricular skin, it blunts the details of a carved framework. Hence the plastic surgeon's aim is to achieve accurate representation—that being to create an acceptable facsimile of an ear that is the proper size, in the proper position, and properly oriented to other facial features.

### PREOPERATIVE CONSULTATION

During the initial consultation, surgical expectations and psychological considerations are discussed with the patient and the family, emphasizing the earlier stated goals of the reconstruction. The age at which to begin the reconstruction is influenced strongly by psychological considerations. Microtia creates significant emotional disturbances in most of its unfortunate possessors. This deformity, which conceivably can be concealed by a long hair style, is by no means

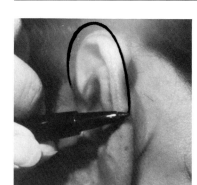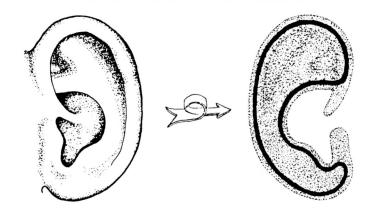

overlooked by the youngster's peers. It is this factor that prompts surgical consideration at an early age [24].

The ear is approximately 85 percent grown by age 4 [18, 20] and the rib cartilages are of reasonable size to permit fabrication of an adult-sized framework at age 6. Therefore reconstruction can be initiated before the child is psychologically traumatized by his peers' cruel ridicule and the family's overprotective concern [4, 6].

The consensus discourages middle ear surgery [6, 40] except for severe bilateral hearing deficits, which are limited almost exclusively to bilateral microtia. In those rare cases, a team approach is planned with a competent otologist [6, 10], and the auricular reconstruction precedes the middle ear surgery because once an attempt is made to "open" the ear the chances of attaining a satisfactory auricular construction are severely compromised because the invaluable virgin skin is scarred.

During the consultation, the previously stated surgical limitations must be fully explained and emphasized to the family. This process is best culminated by showing the parents photographs of the surgeon's *average* results, so they retain realistic expectations. Likewise, accompanying surgical discomforts and inconveniences are described, in-

*Figure 15-1* Planning the auricular framework from a reversed film pattern traced from the opposite, normal ear.

cluding the expected chest pain, duration of dressings, and limited activities for 4 to 6 weeks.

Finally, risks and possible complications of the surgery are discussed thoroughly, including pneumothorax, cartilage-graft loss secondary to infection, skin flap necrosis, and hematoma. It is stressed that with proper precautions these risks are less severe than the emotional trauma created by an absent ear.

PLANNING AND PREPARATION
The result of a total ear reconstruction depends not only on a surgeon's meticulous surgical technique but on careful preoperative planning. It is essential that one practices carving techniques on a volume of human cadaver cartilage prior to any live-patient application. An acrylic or plaster replica of a normal ear serves as an excellent model for practice carvings.

During the patient's second office consultation, preoperative study photographs are obtained, and a radiographic pattern is traced from the opposite, normal ear (Fig. 15-1). This pattern is reversed, and a framework pattern is designed for the new ear. After sterilization,

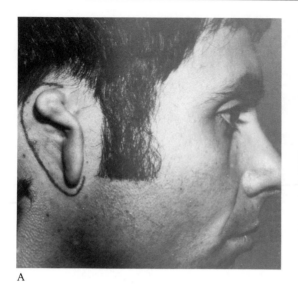

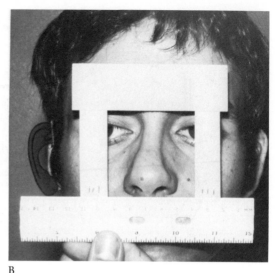

A                                                                B

**Figure 15-2** *Location and orientation of the ear. A. Although normal in configuration, the earlobe is usually displaced anteriorly and superiorly. Note that the axis of the ear should be roughly parallel to the nose. B. The inferior border of the proposed ear is determined by taping the film pattern to the head and comparing its height to the opposite, normal ear.*

these patterns serve as guidelines for framework fabrication at the time of surgery.

The reconstructed ear's location is predetermined by taping the reversed film pattern to the proposed reconstruction site and then comparing its height from the front view with that of the opposite, normal ear (Fig. 15-2B). From the side, it should be noted that the ear's axis is roughly parallel to the nasal profile [3, 9, 21] (Fig. 15-2A). Finally, one notes and records the distance between the lateral canthus and the normal ear's helical root.

FIRST STAGE OF RECONSTRUCTION
Almost invariably, the first stage "foundation" when correcting microtia involves fabricating and inserting the cartilaginous ear framework. Because resulting scars can be a

significant handicap, a preliminary procedure is rarely employed.

As when constructing a house, the cartilage graft serves as a foundation and should be built and become well established under ideal conditions. By implanting a cartilage graft as the first surgical stage, one takes advantage of the optimal elasticity and circulation of an unviolated, virgin skin "pocket."

For these reasons, initial lobule rotation or vestige division is avoided, as the resulting scars cannot help but inhibit the circulation and restrict the skin's elasticity, which in turn diminishes its ability to safely accommodate a three-dimensional cartilage graft [4–6].

Usually, a first stage reconstruction entails implantation of the supportive framework, for which a wide variety of autogenous, homogenous, heterogenous, and alloplastic materials have been used [1–3, 11–17, 19, 21, 23, 26–29, 30–41, 45–53]. Homogenous cartilage undergoes absorption readily [31, 49], and Silastic frameworks suffer a high incidence of extrusion [11, 16, 26]. Initially, Cronin minimized this problem by providing fascia lata [15] or galeal and fascial flaps [19, 27, 41] for extraautogenous rim coverage, but later, when he found

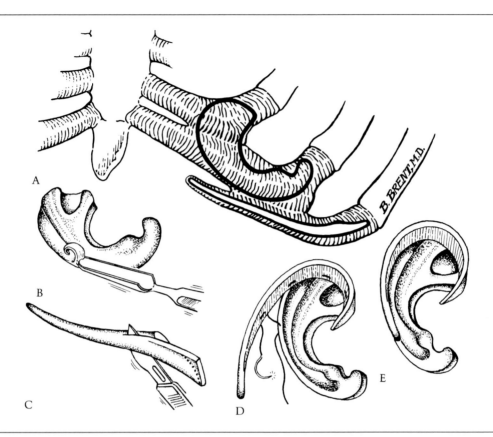

that the alloplastic frames still extruded, he discontinued their use.

To date, autogenous cartilage has produced the most reliable, lasting result with, comparatively, the fewest complications [4, 6, 38]. Furthermore, rib cartilage provides the most substantial source for fabricating a total ear framework. Although contralateral conchal cartilage has been used for this purpose [58, 60], it seems best to reserve auricular cartilage for repairing partial ear defects, for which considerably less tissue bulk is needed.

*Obtaining Rib Cartilage*
Rib cartilages are obtained en bloc from the side contralateral to the ear being constructed so as to utilize natural rib configuration (Fig. 15-3A). The rib cartilages are removed through a horizontal or slightly oblique incision that is made just above the costal margin. After division of the rectus

**Figure 15-3** *Fabricating an ear framework from costal cartilage. A. Donor site: the contralateral thorax. The helical rim is obtained from a "floating" rib cartilage, the main pattern from the synchondrosis of two cartilages.*
*B. Sculpting the main block. C. Thinning the "floating" rib cartilage to produce a delicate helical rim. D. Affixing the rim to the main framework block. E. Completed framework.*

muscle, the film pattern is placed on the exposed cartilages to determine the necessary extent of rib resection.

The helical rim is fashioned separately with cartilage from the first free-floating rib (Figs. 15-3C, D). Excision of this cartilage facilitates access to the synchondrotic region of ribs 6 and 7, which supplies a sufficient block to carve the framework body. Extraperichondrial dissection is preferable for obtaining an unmarred specimen.

In cases where the delicate pleura is en-

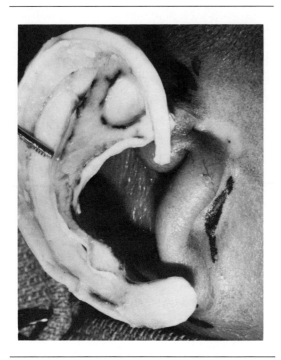

**Figure 15-4** *Ear framework, sculpted from rib cartilage as per the method outlined in Fig. 15-3. Note the marked site for the preauricular incision.*

tered during this dissection, there is no great reason for concern, as a leak in the lung has not been produced. However, when a pleural tear is discovered, a rubber catheter is inserted well into the chest through the pleural opening; the chest wound is then closed in layers by the assistant while the surgeon fabricates the framework, thus conserving operative time. When skin closure is complete, the catheter is attached to suction, the lung is expanded, and the catheter is rapidly withdrawn. As a final precaution, each patient undergoes portable upright chest radiography in the operating room.

### Framework Fabrication

Generally speaking, a novice at ear reconstruction has the tendency to become preoccupied with carving framework details. As experience is gained, it becomes evident that a reconstruction's shortcomings arise not from lack of framework detail but from the shortage of skin needed to cover the framework and to permit fine detail.

The surgeon's realistic aim is to fabricate a framework with an exaggerated rim and distinct details of the antihelical complex (Fig. 15-4). It is achieved with scalpel blades and a rounded wood-carving chisel. To minimize possible chondrocytic damage, the use of power tools for sculpting is strictly avoided: One must keep in mind that cartilage sculpting differs from basic wood-carving in that a good long-term result ultimately depends on living tissue.

The basic ear silhouette is carved from the previously obtained cartilage block (see Fig. 15-3B). It is necessary to thin little if any of the basic form for a small child's framework, although thinning is essential for framework fabrication in most older patients. When thinning is necessary, care is taken to preserve the perichondrium on the lateral outer aspect of the framework to facilitate its adherence, "take," and subsequent nourishment. Because warping must be taken into consideration [46] one sculpts and thins the cartilage to cause a deliberate warping in a favorable direction. This measure allows one to produce the acute flexion necessary to create a helix, which is fastened to the framework body with horizontal mattress sutures; the knots are buried on the frame's undersurface.

### Framework Implantation

A cutaneous pocket is created with meticulous technique to provide an adequate recipient vascular covering for the framework. Because several hours lapse during the rib removal and framework fabrication, the auricular region is prepared and scrubbed just prior to creating the cutaneous pocket.

Through a small incision anterior to the auricular vestige (see Fig. 15-4), a thin flap is raised by sharp dissection, taking care to preserve the subdermal vascular plexus. In order to evaluate the flap's vascular status and to ensure hemostasis, epinephrine-containing solutions are avoided. With great care, one dissects the skin from the gnarled, native cartilage remnant, which then is excised and discarded. Finally, the pocket is completed by dissecting 1 to 2 cm peripherally to the projected framework markings (Fig. 15-5A).

Insertion of the framework into the cutaneous pocket takes up the valuable skin slack that was created when the native cartilage remnant was removed (Fig. 15-5B). The framework displaces this skin centrifugally in an advantageous posterosuperior direction so as to displace the hairline just behind the rim. This principle of anterior incision and centrifugal skin relaxation, introduced by Tanzer [33], permits advantageous use of the hairless skin for microtia.

Tanzer initially suggested the use of bolster sutures to coapt the skin flap to the underlying framework [33, 37]. It seems far safer, however, to do this step with suction, which simultaneously prevents fluid collection and minimizes the risk of flap necrosis along the helical margin.

To attain skin coaption via suction, one uses a silicone catheter or fashions a perforated drain from an infusion catheter with the needle inserted into a rubber-topped vacuum tube [22] (Fig. 15-5E), the tubes being retained on a rack to observe changes in the quantity and quality of drainage. Although a dressing is applied that accurately conforms to the convolutions of the newly created auricle (Fig. 15-5D), firm pressure is dangerous and unnecessary; it must be avoided. Hemostasis and skin coaptation are provided by the suction drain [4, 6, 7] (Fig. 15-5C).

*Postoperative Management*

Attentive postoperative management is imperative for a successful ear reconstruction that remains unhampered by disastrous complications. The newly constructed auricle is scrutinized frequently and carefully for signs of infection or vascular compromise.

Usually early infection manifests by neither auricular pain nor fever but through local erythema, edema, subtle fluctuance, drainage, or a combination of the above. Hence frequent observations and the immediate institution of aggressive therapy can deter an overwhelming infection.

Immediately on suspecting an infection, an irrigation drain is introduced below the flap, and continuous antibiotic drip irrigation is begun. Appropriate adjustments are made in both the antibiotic drip irrigation and the systemic therapy when sensitivities are available from the initial culture. Cronin has salvaged Silastic-frame reconstructions impressively by this technique [14], and I have had excellent success managing the occasional infection in cartilage-graft reconstructions (less than a 1 percent incidence).

Skin flap necrosis results from excess tension in an inadequately sized pocket, tight bolster sutures, or damage to the subdermal vascularity during the flap dissection. This complication is best avoided by meticulous technique; however, once skin necrosis becomes evident, appropriate steps must be taken without delay.

Although at times a small local flap is required to cover exposed cartilage, *small* localized ulcerations may heal with good local wound care. Such care consists in keeping the wound covered with antibiotic ointment to prevent cartilage desiccation and using restraints to prevent the patient from lying on the ear during sleep.

Major skin flap necrosis merits a more aggressive approach if the framework is to be salvaged. The necrotic skin is excised early, and the framework is covered by transposing a local skin flap or using a small fascial flap and skin graft.

Once initially healed, no specific care is necessary for an ear constructed with autogenous tissues. To avoid flattening of the helical rim, the patient is instructed to sleep on the opposite side. A soft pillow ensures protection should he turn while asleep.

At 2½ to 3 weeks postoperatively the patient may return to school; however, run-

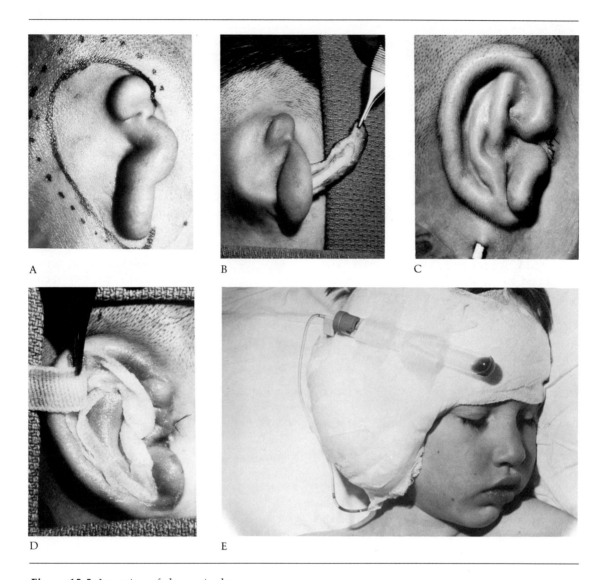

A

B

C

D

E

**Figure 15-5** *Insertion of the auricular framework. A. Solid line indicates the proposed implantation site. The surgeon must dissect more peripherally than indicated by the dotted line here. B. Insertion of cartilage framework. C. Implanted framework immediately after the operation. Note that the skin coaption has been obtained by a suction-catheter. The lobule will be rotated at the next surgical stage (see Fig. 15-6). D. Packing convolutions of the new ear with Vaseline gauze. E. Suction system, consisting of a silicone catheter and a rubber-topped vacuum tube.*

ning and sports are discouraged an additional 3 weeks while the chest wound heals. Such a schedule is appropriate after any major surgical procedure where wound strength is essential.

The ear itself withstands trauma well because it, like the opposite, normal ear, houses a framework of autogenous cartilage. To date, I have witnessed numerous reconstructed ears' traumatic episodes (e.g., baseball and soccer blows, a bee sting, and a dog bite). They have all healed well.

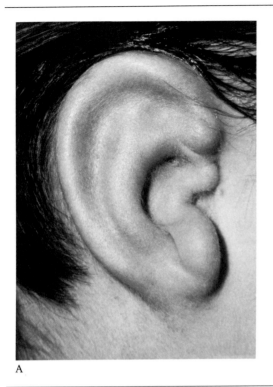

A

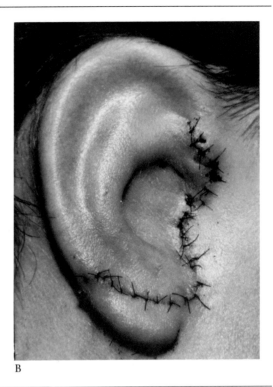

B

**Figure 15-6** *Second surgical stage. A. Healed ear construction several months after placing the cartilage framework. B. Lobule transposition and excision of unusable vestigial tissues.*

## OTHER STAGES OF AURICULAR CONSTRUCTION

Major stages in auricular construction subsequent to the initial framework implantation are lobule rotation, "elevation" of the ear, deepening of the concha, and formation of a tragus. These stages can be planned independently or in various combinations, depending on which schedule best achieves the desired end result.

### Rotation of the Lobule

Earlobe transposition is best performed as a secondary procedure in my experience, as it seems easier to judge placement of the earlobe and to "splice" the lobule correctly into position with reference to a well established, underlying framework. Although I have occasionally transposed the lobule simultaneously with implantation of the cartilage graft, it has been safer and far more accurate to transpose the lobule as a secondary procedure [4, 6].

The "rotation" or repositioning of this normal but displaced structure is accomplished essentially by Z-plasty transposition of a narrow, inferiorly based triangular flap (Fig. 15-6).

### Tragal Construction and Conchal Definition

One can form the tragus, excavate the concha, and mimic a canal in a single operation. This sequence is accomplished by placing a thin elliptically shaped chondrocutaneous

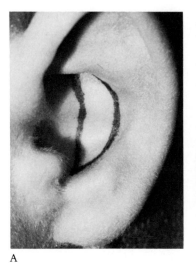

A

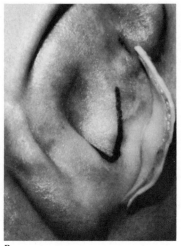

B

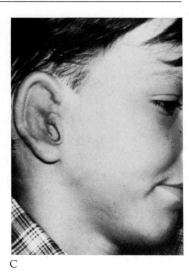

C

*Figure 15-7* Tragus construction with composite graft. A. Donor site in contralateral concha's anterior surface. B. Chondrocutaneous composite graft. A J-shaped incision outlines the proposed posterior tragal margin and intertragal notch. C. Completed repair.

composite graft underneath a J-shaped incision in the conchal region [4, 6] (Fig. 15-7). The main limb of the J is placed at the proposed posterior tragal margin; the crook of the J represents the intertragal notch (Fig. 15-7B). Extraneous soft tissues are excised underneath this tragal flap to deepen the concha; this excavated region resembles a meatus when the newly constructed tragus casts a shadow on it [4, 6] (Fig. 15-7C).

It is advantageous for one to harvest the composite graft from the normal ear's anterolateral conchal surface owing to the paucity of subcutaneous tissue between the delicate anterolateral skin and adjacent cartilage (Fig. 15-7A). This technique is particularly advantageous when a prominent concha exists in the normal donor ear, as closure of the donor site facilitates an otoplasty, which often is needed to gain frontal symmetry.

### Detaching the Posterior Auricular Region

Auricular elevation with skin grafting is done solely to eliminate the cryptotic appearance by defining the ear through creating a sulcus. This procedure does not project a framework that has been carved with insufficient depth.

The posterior auricular margin is defined by separating the ear from the head and covering its undersurface with a thick, split skin graft. This procedure is not attempted until the edema has markedly subsided and the auricular details have become well defined. At this point, an incision is made several millimeters behind the rim, taking care to preserve a protective, connective tissue layer on the cartilage framework (Fig. 15-8). One then advances the retroauricular skin into the newly created sulcus so that the only graft requirement is on the ear's undersurface (Fig. 15-8C,D). To secure the graft, the sutures are left long and tied over a gauze bolster (Fig. 15-8F).

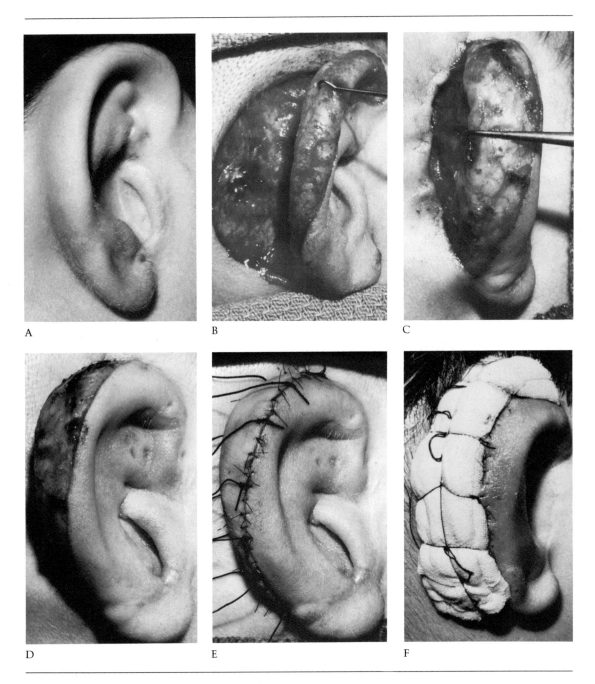

A

B

C

D

E

F

**Figure 15-8** *Separating the ear from the head.
A. Healed auricular construction. B. Sharply
lifting the ear from its fascial bed. Note that
connective tissue has been carefully preserved
over the cartilage frame. C, D. Advancing*
*retroauricular skin into newly created
auriculocephalic sulcus. This maneuver
decreases the size and visibility of the skin
graft. E. Skin graft applied to the ear's back
surface. F. Tie-over bolster dressing.*

## Managing the Hairline

A persistent problem, scalp hair on the reconstructed rim, has largely been eliminated in microtia by the anterior incision–centrifugal relaxation principle [33]. The hairline, however, remains a perplexing problem in major acquired auricular deformities.

Although the "scalp roll" and free graft provide a hairless skin cover [25, 40], this new cover lacks the elasticity of virgin skin. Instead, it is preferable to first implant the framework and later eradicate any undesirable hair. Removal can be done with electrolysis or by replacing the follicular skin with a graft.

Prior to placing an ear framework, if one predicts a tight pocket and a hairline that will cover half of the new ear, a primary fascial flap is considered [5]. Although a big operation, a fascial flap represents "two operations in one," i.e., simultaneously placing an ear framework and dealing with the low hairline. Furthermore, the fascial flap advantageously overcomes skin shortages [7].

## Total Ear Reconstruction in the Acquired Deformity

Total auricular reconstruction of the acquired deformity presents special problems not encountered in microtia. These problems merit separate consideration.

The lack of skin coverage is much more critical than in microtia, as an existing meatus precludes use of the anterior incision, and extra skin, as usually gained by removing the crumpled microtic cartilage, is not available. This factor compounds the previously mentioned hairline problem. If one can use the existing skin, the cutaneous pocket is best developed by incisions above, below, or above and below the proposed auricular site. If the local tissues are heavily scarred or restrict the surgeon from developing an ample skin pocket, one must supplement the repair with fascial flap coverage [7, 8].

Prior to use of the temporoparietal fascial flap [7, 41], acquired ear losses and secondary reconstructions were managed by first excising the scar, skin-grafting the defect, and then waiting for the graft to mature before implanting a new cartilage framework [36, 64].

The above method is often beset with compromises in that skin-grafted tissues have limited elasticity as a cutaneous pocket; therefore a detailed framework with depth cannot be introduced without significant tension [4]. The fascial flap permits one to surpass this skin coverage dilemma, just as the myocutaneous flap permits one to resolve coverage problems in breast reconstruction; that is the temporoparietal fascial flap provides an instantaneous abundance of thin, vascularized tissue that in turn permits a framework of any size or thickness to be covered easily [7].

When the superficial temporal vessels are not patent, the flap width is increased and the postauricular vessels are included, if present. As extra security, one can incorporate the middle temporal artery by reflecting the deep, investing muscle fascia over the framework.

## Auricular Prostheses

The auricular prosthesis is reserved for instances in which surgical reconstruction is impractical or contraindicated, or for cases in which an experienced surgeon is unavailable. For the most part, an auricular prosthesis has no practical value for children, but it is worthwhile for older patients who have undergone ablative cancer surgery [42, 44]. Even so, many adults find the prostheses undesirable after a short trial, as there is the constant fear of it becoming dislodged at an embarrassing moment and the psychological discomfort of wearing an "artificial part."

Additional problems that arise from local skin irritation caused by the adhesive glue frequently necessitate discontinuance of the prosthesis for a period of time, which also causes the patient embarrassment. Furthermore, obvious color contrast calls attention to the prosthetic ear during climatic changes where the prosthetic part remains a constant color while the surrounding skin varies as the patient passes from indoor to outdoor environmental surroundings.

When an auricular prosthesis has been elected for the younger patient, a trial period should ensue, with the realization that surgical reconstruction may be desired later. It is wise to avoid preliminary excision of the microtic lobule or other remnants merely to "gain an improved surface for adherence of the prosthesis," as has been advocated [43]. Should the patient desire surgical reconstruction later, which has often been my experience, the missing lobule, shortage of skin, and existing scar become significant handicaps.

## Acute Auricular Trauma

Because of the delicate nature of the auricle, it is exceptionally vulnerable to various types of trauma for which the plastic surgeon frequently is summoned to the emergency room. Initially, block anesthesia is administered that promptly relieves the patient's discomfort and permits proper cleansing, evaluation, and repair of the injury. I prefer 0.5% xylocaine with 1:200,000 epinephrine, the latter being omitted only if there are long, thin pedicles of tissue resulting from the injury.

OTOHEMATOMA
A common injury in contact sports, otohematoma must be treated aggressively to avoid multiple recurrences [70, 75]. Whereas mere needle aspiration is almost invariably followed by recurrent fluid collection, a small incision permits evacuation of the hematoma under direct vision. Conforming, compressive gauze bolsters are placed on either side of the auricle and are maintained

for 7 to 10 days by horizontal mattress sutures (4-0 nylon), which traverse the bolsters as well as the ear (Fig. 15-9).

AMPUTATED EAR
Until the 1970s, subcutaneous "banking" of the filleted cartilage seemed the only worthwhile method of handling auricular avulsion [74, 78]. When employing this technique, the salvaged cartilage is commonly placed under the intact, retroauricular skin. Although logical, I have found this procedure futile, as the flimsy ear cartilage almost invariably flattens underneath the snug, discrepant two-dimensional skin cover.

Unless a highly vascularized recipient area is first prepared [67, 72, 73], almost invariably the replanting of large composite parts is doomed to fail [68, 69, 71]. Even microvascular repair only offers occasional successful ear salvage because the ear itself lacks suitable vessels [76, 77]. However, dermabrading, reattaching, and temporarily "pocketing" the amputated part underneath a retroauricular flap [80] seems to offer an approach that offers variable success.

Of course there are other valid alternatives for salvaging amputated ears [79]. Several successful cases have been reported where the posteromedial skin was removed from the amputated part, and the cartilage was then "fenestrated," thus increasing the reattached ear's recipient vascular surface [67]. The anterolateral auricular skin is then nourished through the cartilage fenestrations by means of direct contact with a vascular bed that is prepared when a retroauricular flap is raised.

Finally, in selected cases where the wounds are clean, the scalp is intact, and the patient's general condition is stable, one might be tempted to remove the amputated ear's skin and cover the filleted cartilage immediately with a fascial flap and skin graft. Because of routinely poor results with filleted ear cartilages that have been subcutaneously banked, I prefer to utilize Baudet's fenestration tech-

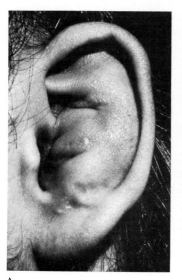
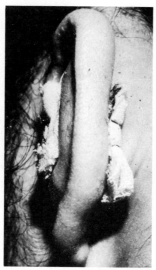
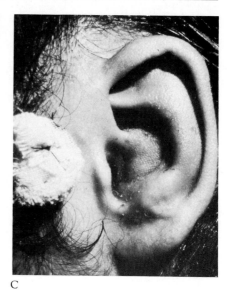

A           B           C

***Figure 15-9*** *Management of acute otohematoma. A. Recurrent conchal hematoma, after several aspiration attempts. B. Through-and-through bolster sutures, after surgical evacuation of the hematoma. C. Auricle, after removal of compression sutures at 10 days.*

nique initially [67] and to reserve the fascia for secondary reconstruction should this effort fail.

ACUTE AURICULAR BURNS

The protruding, delicate nature of the auricle makes it particularly susceptible to thermal trauma. Often direct thermal injury results in a full-thickness loss that is confined to the helical rim. Usually such an injury heals by "autoamputation," a spontaneous separation of the eschar.

A far more dreaded complication is chondritis, which follows infection or external trauma to the burned tissue. The latter, which results predominantly from pillow pressure or friction, can be prevented by substituting a rolled sheet or doughnut-shaped support for the offending pillow [81, 84].

Characterized by tenderness, erythema, warmth, and induration, chondritis occurs most commonly between the third and fifth week postburn [83]. This severe complication is largely circumvented by sound wound management, which includes the aforementioned avoidance of pressure and friction, frequent soap and water cleansing [81], and the liberal use of topical antibiotics [81, 83, 85]. With early tangential excision or dermabrasion of the involved tissue and skin grafting, the incidence of infection is lessened and prompt wound healing is facilitated [84].

However, once chondritis is diagnosed, aggressive steps must be taken to eradicate the infection and prevent subsequent severe deformity. Local instillation of antibiotic solution combined with warm compresses has offered a hopeful remedy [80, 82], but if this therapy fails, incision, drainage, and adequate chondrectomy must be performed. When the latter becomes necessary, incisions are planned judiciously to permit later reconstruction, and the helical cartilage is preserved when feasible.

Frequently, postburn reconstruction must be preceded by resurfacing, as the healed auricular skin often consists of thin, friable scar tissue. Full-thickness skin grafts are preferable for this purpose, followed by a long waiting period prior to cartilage implantation. Most often, the only way to obtain suitable coverage is via a fascial flap [7].

## Reconstruction of Acquired Partial Defects

Most auricular deformities one encounters in everyday practice are acquired *partial* defects. They present the surgeon with an unlimited variety of unique problems whose reconstructions are influenced by the etiology, location, and nature of each residual deformity.

### UTILIZATION OF RESIDUAL TISSUES

When managing acute auricular trauma, initial meticulous reapproximation of tissues and appropriate wound care greatly facilitates the reconstructive task ahead. Likewise, the innovative utilization of residual local tissues in a posttraumatic deformity greatly simplifies the reconstruction and contributes to a pleasing outcome.

### STRUCTURAL SUPPORT

*Contralateral Conchal Cartilage*

A variety of tissues are available to provide the structural support required for an auricular reconstruction. Although the quantity of cartilage needed to fabricate a total ear framework necessitates the use of costal cartilage [4, 6, 33], rarely is one compelled to employ this tissue in a *small*, partial auricular reconstruction. Because it is often possible to utilize an auricular cartilage graft, which is obtained most frequently from the contralateral concha under local anesthesia, the correction of partial losses is less extensive than the procedures to correct total auricular losses. Auricular cartilage, used as an orthotopic graft in ear reconstruction, is superior to costal cartilage in that it provides a delicate, flexible, thin support [55, 59, 62, 63].

The conchal cartilage graft can be obtained by a posteromedial incision, as described by Adams [54] and Gorney et al. [61], or through an anterolateral approach, which I use frequently [56]. The latter, performed through an incision several millimeters inside the posterior conchal wall–inferior crus contour line, is a simple method of obtaining a precise cartilage graft with direct visual exposure (Fig. 15-10B).

*Ipsilateral Conchal Cartilage*

For certain partial reconstructions, it is more advantageous to employ an ipsilateral than a contralateral conchal cartilage graft. However, it is imperative that an intact antihelical strut be present to permit removal of an ipsilateral conchal cartilage graft without subsequent collapse and further deformity of the ear.

An ipsilateral conchal cartilage graft is particularly advantageous when a retroauricular flap is being raised to repair a major defect in the helical rim (Fig. 15-11). Elevation of the flap provides the required conchal cartilage exposure without the necessity of an additional incision, and removal of this cartilage graft subsequently lowers the ear closer to the mastoid region. In effect, it produces a relative gain in length, thereby enabling the flap to cover the cartilage graft once it is spliced onto the rim (Fig. 15-11B,C) and eliminating the need for a skin graft in the flap's donor bed.

Furthermore, the ipsilateral concha is used occasionally as a composite flap of skin and cartilage (see Fig. 15-13H). This innovative technique, proposed by Davis [106], is applicable to defects of the upper third of the auricle; again, it is employed only when the antihelical support remains intact.

*Chondrocutaneous Composite Graft*

In certain conditions, a composite graft can effectively provide the supportive tissue required for a reconstruction [86–90]. The success of these grafts is greatly enhanced by removing a portion of the posteromedial skin and cartilage, thus converting part of the

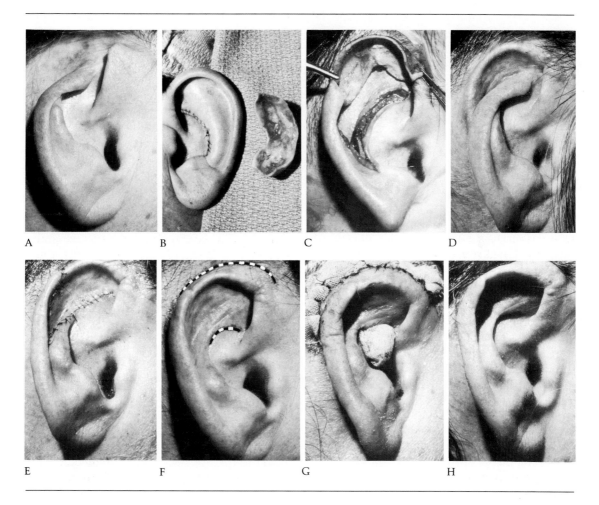

A           B           C           D

E           F           G           H

**Figure 15-10** *Reconstruction of a major defect of the superior third of the auricle with an auricular cartilage graft. A. Postsurgical deformity. B. Contralateral conchal cartilage graft is removed via an anterolateral approach; note the inconspicuous incision. C, D. Cartilage graft prior to and 6 weeks after implantation. E. The helical component is transposed to a suitable position on the rim. F, G. Incisions are planned to create "valise-handle," elevation, skin grafting, and employment of a T-shaped tie-over dressing. H. Final result. A well defined inferior crus has resulted from the intentionally created "valise handle." (From B. Brent. The acquired auricular deformity: A systematic approach to its analysis and reconstruction. Plast. Reconstr. Surg. 59:475, 1977.)*

"wedge" to a full-thickness skin graft that is readily vascularized by a recipient advancement flap mobilized from the loose retroauricular skin adjacent to the defect (Fig. 15-12). A strut of helical cartilage is preserved within the graft to maintain contour and support (Fig. 15-12C).

## SPECIFIC REGIONAL DEFECTS
### External Auditory Canal
It is more efficacious to prevent stenosis of the canal than to be faced with treating it once it has occurred [92, 94]. Careful realignment of severed tissues followed by insertion of an acrylic mold prevents stenosis, provided the patient retains the obturating device faithfully for at least 6 months.

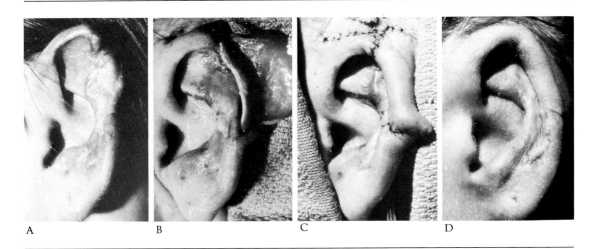

A              B              C              D

*Figure 15-11* *Helical rim reconstruction with an auricular cartilage graft. A. Traumatic deformity of the helical rim. B. Development of a flap composed of retroauricular and medioauricular skin; an ipsilateral conchal cartilage graft has been spliced onto the rim (see text for further explanation). C. The flap is advanced over the cartilage graft. No attempt has been made to excise the "dog ear," which is removed later when the ear is elevated from the head with a skin graft. D. Final result. (From B. Brent. The acquired auricular deformity: A systematic approach to its analysis and reconstruction. Plast. Reconstr. Surg. 59:475, 1977.)*

Stenosis is best treated by a full-thickness graft carefully applied over an acrylic mold, provided a reasonable recipient vascular bed can be prepared [91]. Occasionally, multiple Z-plasties can be utilized to relieve webbing of the orifice [96], and at times a local flap is necessary to line the canal and break up the contracture [93, 95].

*Helical Rim*
Acquired losses of the helical rim may vary from small defects to major portions of the helix [98, 100]. The former, which usually result from tumor excisions or minor traumatic injuries, are best closed by advancing the helix in both directions, as described by Antia and Buch [97]. The success of this excellent technique depends first on freeing the entire helix from the scapha via an incision in the helical sulcus that extends through the cartilage but not through the skin on the ear's back surface. Second, the posteromedial auricular skin is undermined, dissecting just superficial to the perichondrium until the entire helix is hanging as a chondrocutaneous component of the loosely mobilized skin (Fig. 15-13A). Extra length can be gained by a V-Y advancement of the crus helix (Fig. 15-13B), and surprisingly large defects can be closed without tension (Fig. 15-12F, G).

Although originally described for upper third auricular defects [97] (Fig. 15-13A, B), this technique is even more effective for middle third defects (Fig. 15-12E, G) and is equally applicable for repairing earlobe losses (Fig. 15-14E–H).

Reconstruction of large helical defects requires a more sophisticated procedure that recreates the absent rim using an auricular cartilage graft covered by an adjacent flap, as previously described in the text (see Fig. 15-11). Although advancement flaps of local soft tissues have also been employed to provide helical contour [99, 101, 102], these flaps often suffer a disappointing long-term

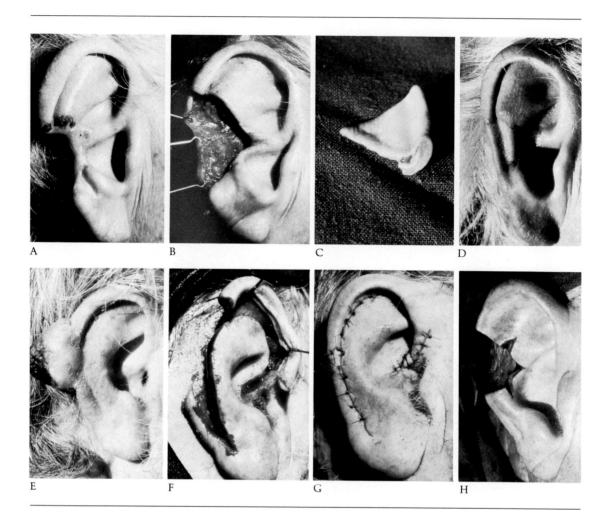

**Figure 15-12** *Repair of defects of the middle third of the auricle. A. Status after resection of chondrodermatitis in an 83-year-old patient. B, C. Residual diseased tissue is excised, and a retroauricular flap is advanced to serve as a recipient bed for the specially prepared composite graft that is illustrated. Survival of the contralateral composite graft has been enhanced by removing the medial auricular skin and cartilage while preserving a cartilage strut in the helical rim for contour and support (see text for further explanation). D. Final result. E. Large keratoacanthoma. F, G. Excision of the lesion and preparation and advancement of helical flaps. Note the extent of dissection to mobilize the helix; a small Z-plasty was used to ensure a clean splice. H. Alternate method of closure by V wedge. This closure is facilitated by excision of "accessory triangles," as illustrated. (From B. Brent. The acquired auricular deformity: A systematic approach to its analysis and reconstruction. Plast. Reconstr. Surg. 59:475, 1977.)*

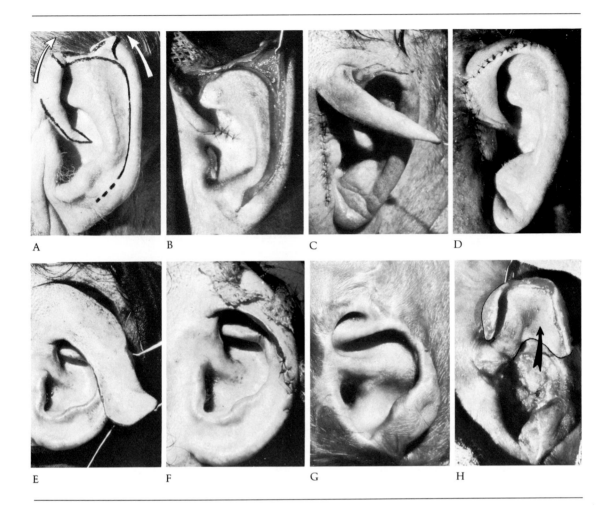

A    B    C    D

E    F    G    H

**Figure 15-13** *Four techniques for repairing upper third auricular defects using local flaps. A, B. Advancement of chondrocutaneous helical flaps (after Antia and Buch [107]). Note the extra length gained by V-Y advancement of the crus heliz. C, D. The preauricular flap is transposed to repair a minor rim defect. E, F. The banner flap is raised from the auriculocephalic sulcus (after Crikelair [115]). G, H. An upper helicoscaphal thermal loss with a large residual concha favors transposition of a chondrocutaneous conchal flap to recreate the upper third of the auricle (after Davis [116]). Both the donor bed and the raw surface of the newly created rim are to be grafted. (From B. Brent. The acquired auricular deformity: A systematic approach to its analysis and reconstruction. Plast. Reconstr. Surg. 59:475, 1977.)*

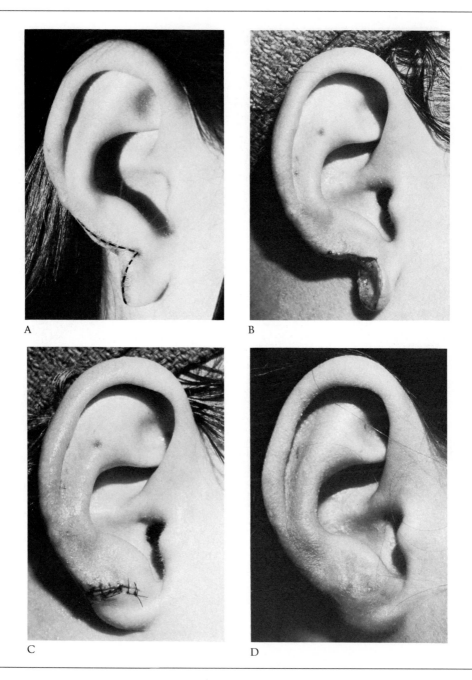

**Figure 15-14** *Repair of minor posttraumatic earlobe losses. A–D. Dog-bite injury treated by merely "freshening the edges" of the residual tissue and settling for a slightly smaller but pleasing earlobe.*

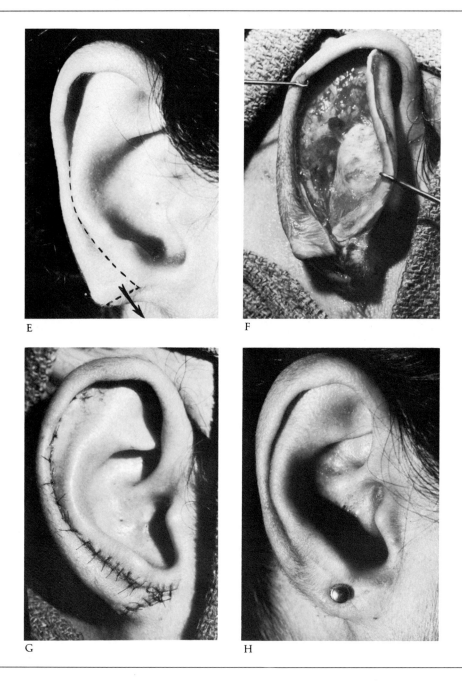

E

F

G

H

**Figure 15-14** *(continued) E–H. Minor earlobe deficiency corrected by downward advancement of a helical flap. (From B. Brent. The acquired auricular deformity: A systematic approach to its analysis and reconstruction. Plast. Reconstr. Surg. 59:475, 1977.)*

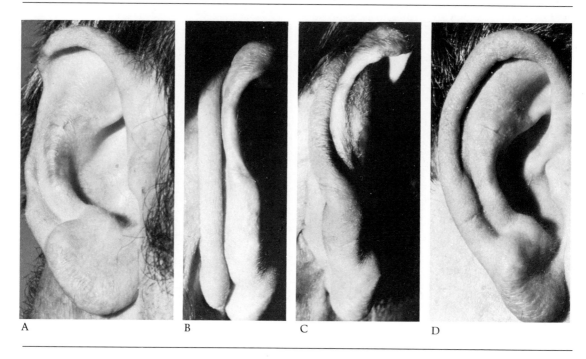

A               B               C               D

***Figure 15-15*** *Helical reconstruction with a thin-calibered tube. A. Burn deformity of the helix. B, C. Construction and migration of a tube formed in the auriculocephalic sulcus. D. Final result. (From B. Brent. The acquired auricular deformity: A systematic approach to its analysis and reconstruction.* Plast. Reconstr. Surg. *59:475, 1977.)*

result unless a strut of cartilage has been incorporated into the repair.

Another sophisticated method of helical reconstruction is the use of thin-calibered tubes, which can successfully create a fine, realistic helical rim when meticulous technique is utilized in conjunction with careful case selection (Fig. 15-15). Minor burns often destroy the helical rim yet leave the auriculocephalic sulcus skin intact, thereby providing a superb site for tube construction [103, 104] and minimizing tube migration, risk of failure, and secondary deformity.

### Upper Third Auricular Defects

Upper third defects may be reconstructed by five major methods. Usually, minor losses are confined to the rim and are repaired either by helical advancement, as previously described (see Fig. 15-13A,B), or by a readily accessible preauricular flap (see Fig. 15-13C,D). Intermediate losses of the upper third are repaired with a banner flap, as described by Crikelair [105]. This flap, based anterosuperiorly in the auriculocephalic sulcus (see Fig. 15-13E,F), is used in conjunction with a small cartilage graft to ensure a good long-term result.

Major losses in the superior third are most successfully reconstructed with a contralateral conchal cartilage graft, as classically described in 1955 by Adams [54] (see Fig. 15-10). When utilizing this technique, it is imperative that the cartilage graft be anchored to the cartilaginous remnant of the helical root by means of a suture placed through a small incision at that point. This step prevents the cartilage graft from "drifting" and ensures helical continuity.

Should the existing skin be unfavorable for the above technique, the entire concha may be rotated upward as a chondrocuta-

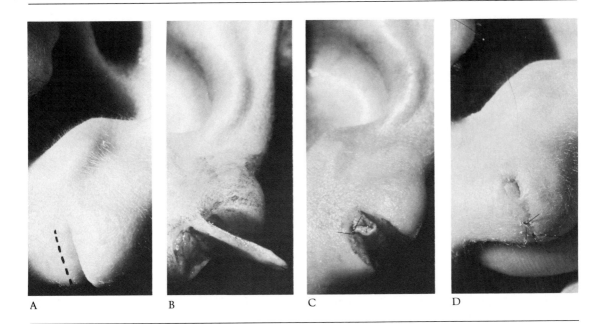

A            B            C            D

neous composite flap on a small anterior pedicle of the crus helix, as previously described [106]. Technically, it is a demanding procedure and is restricted to individual instances in which a large concha exists (see Fig. 15-13G,H).

*Middle Third Auricular Defects*
Major middle third auricular defects are usually repaired with a cartilage graft that is either inserted via Converse's tunnel procedure [12] or covered by an adjacent skin flap (see Fig. 15-11). Occasionally, conditions favor a specially prepared composite graft, as described previously (see Fig. 15-12). Middle third auricular tumors are excised and closed by either a wedge resection with accessory triangles (see Fig. 15-12H) or a helical advancement, as previously described (see Fig. 15-12E–G).

*Lower Third Auricular Defects*
Lower third losses that encompass more than earlobe tissue are an especially complex challenge and must include a cartilage graft to provide the support necessary to ensure long-term contour. Preaux has de-

***Figure 15-16*** *Repair of a traumatic earlobe cleft. A–C. Earring tear repaired by creating a thin flap from one edge of the cleft and rolling it into the apex of the wedge repair (after Pardue [123]). D. The other edge is then denuded, and closure is made around the skin-lined channel, which remains patent for future earring use. (From B. Brent. The acquired auricular deformity: A systematic approach to its analysis and reconstruction.* Plast. Reconstr. Surg. *59:475, 1977.)*

scribed an impressive technique for repairing lower third defects by means of a superiorly based flap doubled on itself [111]. In my experience, however, contour and support are created and maintained with less risk by primarily inserting a contralateral conchal cartilage graft subcutaneously in the proposed site of reconstruction [57].

*Acquired Earlobe Deformities*
Traumatic clefts and keloids that result from ear piercing are the most common acquired defects of the earlobe. Cleft earlobes, usually caused by dramatic extraction of earrings, can be repaired most efficiently by means of

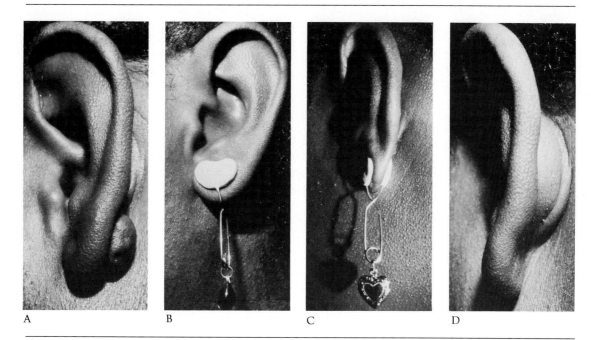

A        B              C                D

**Figure 15-17** *Control of postexcisional keloid recurrence with spring-pressure earrings. A. Earlobe keloid secondary to lobule-piercing. B, C. Spring-pressure earring. D. Lack of recurrence at 15 months after excision and sole treatment by spring-pressure earring. (From B. Brent. The role of pressure therapy in management of earlobe keloids: Preliminary report of a controlled study.* Ann. Plast. Surg. *1:579, 1978.)*

Pardue's ingenious adjacent flap [110], which is rolled into the apex of the wedge repair, thereby maintaining a tract lined with skin. The latter permits further use of earrings (Fig. 15-16).

Another common occurrence in everyday practice is the earlobe keloid, which heretofore has been treated, with varying degrees of success, by irradiation and steroid injections [115, 116, 118]. Because there is strong evidence that pressure plays an important role in keloid therapy [117, 119] a light pressure-spring earring device may be worth a trial in reducing postexcisional recurrence of earlobe keloids [114] (Fig. 15-17).

Effective techniques for actual reconstruc-

tion of the earlobe have been described by Zenteno Alanis [113], Brent [107], and others [108, 109, 112]. Before undertaking any of these sophisticated techniques, it is advisable to carefully assess residual local tissues and contemplate a simple repair (see Fig. 15-14A,D) or employment of the helical advancement principle so as to move available tissue downward (see Fig. 15-14E–H).

## References
TOTAL EAR RECONSTRUCTION

1. Bărinka, L. Congenital malformations of the auricle and their reconstruction by a new method. *Acta Chir. Plast.* 8:53, 1966.
2. Brent, B. Ear reconstruction with an expansile framework of autogenous rib cartilage. *Plast. Reconstr. Surg.* 53:619, 1974.
3. Brent, B. Reconstruction of ear, eyebrow, and sideburn in the burned patient. *Plast. Reconstr. Surg.* 55:312, 1975.
4. Brent, B. The correction of microtia with autogenous cartilage grafts. I. The classic deformity. *Plast. Reconstr. Surg.* 66:1, 1980.

5. Brent, B. The correction of microtia with autogenous cartilage grafts. II. Atypical and complex deformities. *Plast. Reconstr. Surg.* 66:13, 1980.

6. Brent, B. Total Auricular Construction with Sculpted Costal Cartilage. In B. Brent (ed.), *The Artistry of Reconstructive Surgery.* St. Louis: Mosby, 1987. Pp. 113–127.

7. Brent, B., and Byrd, H. S. Secondary ear reconstruction with cartilage grafts covered by axial, random, and free flaps of temporoparietal fascia. *Plast. Reconstr. Surg.* 72:141, 1983.

8. Brent, B., et al. Experience with the temporoparietal fascial free flap. *Plast. Reconstr. Surg.* 76:177, 1985.

9. Broadbent, T. R., and Mathews, V. L. Artistic relationships in surface anatomy of the face: Application to reconstructive surgery. *Plast. Reconstr. Surg.* 20:1, 1957.

10. Broadbent, T. R., and Woolf, R. M. Bilateral Microtia. A Team Approach to the Middle Ear. In R. C. Tanzer and M. T. Edgerton (eds.), *Symposium on Reconstruction of the Auricle.* St. Louis: Mosby, 1974. P. 168.

11. Carroll, D. B. Experiences with Silastic Implants and Autogenous Cartilage in the Treatment of Microtia. In R. C. Tanzer and M. T. Edgerton (eds.), *Symposium of Reconstruction of the Auricle.* St. Louis: Mosby, 1974. P. 69.

12. Converse, J. M. Reconstruction of the auricle. *Plast. Reconstr. Surg.* Parts I and II. 22:150, 230, 1958.

13. Converse, J. M. Construction of the auricle in congenital microtia. *Plast. Reconstr. Surg.* 32:425, 1963.

14. Cronin, T. D. Use of a Silastic frame for total and subtotal reconstruction of the external ear: Preliminary report. *Plast. Reconstr. Surg.* 37:399, 1966.

15. Cronin, T. D. Use of a Silastic Frame for Construction of the Auricle. In R. C. Tanzer and M. T. Edgerton (eds.), *Symposium on Reconstruction of the Auricle.* St. Louis: Mosby, 1974. P. 33.

16. Curtin, J. W., and Bader, K. F. Improved techniques for the successful silicone reconstruction of the external ear. *Plast. Reconstr. Surg.* 44:372, 1969.

17. Dupertius, S. M., and Musgrave, R. H. Experiences with the reconstruction of the congenitally deformed ear. *Plast. Reconstr. Surg.* 23:361, 1959.

18. Farkas, L. Growth of Normal and Reconstructed Auricles. In R. C. Tanzer and M. T. Edgerton (eds.), *Symposium on Reconstruction of the Auricle.* St. Louis: Mosby, 1974. P. 24.

19. Fox, J. W., and Edgerton, M. T. The fan flap: An adjunct to ear reconstruction. *Plast. Reconstr. Surg.* 58:663, 1976.

20. Fukuda, O. The microtic ear: Survey of 180 cases in 10 years. *Plast. Reconstr. Surg.* 53:458, 1974.

21. Gorney, M., Murphy, S., and Falces, E. Spliced autogenous conchal cartilage in secondary ear reconstruction. *Plast. Reconstr. Surg.* 47:432, 1971.

22. Kaye, B. L. "Home-made" suction drain for small areas. *Plast. Reconstr. Surg.* 52:447, 1973.

23. Kirkham, H. L. D. The use of preserved cartilage in ear reconstruction. *Ann. Surg.* 111:896, 1940.

24. Knorr, N. J., Edgerton, M. T., and Barberie, M. Psychologic Factors in Reconstruction of the Ear. In R. C. Tanzer and M. T. Edgerton (eds.), *Symposium on Reconstruction of the Auricle.* St. Louis: Mosby, 1974. P. 183.

25. Letterman, G. S., and Harding, R. L. The management of the hairline in ear reconstruction. *Plast. Reconstr. Surg.* 18:199, 1956.

26. Lynch, J. B., et al. Our experiences with Silastic ear implants. *Plast. Reconstr. Surg.* 49:283, 1972.

27. Ohmori, S., and Nakai, H. A refined approach to Silastic ear reconstruction: Preliminary report. Presented at the annual meeting of the American Society of Plastic and Reconstructive Surgeons, Boston, September 1976.

28. Ohmori, S., Matsumoto, K., and Nakai, H. Follow-up study on reconstruction of microtia with a silicone framework. *Plast. Reconstr. Surg.* 53:555, 1974.

29. Pierce, G. W. Reconstruction of the external ear. *Surg. Gynecol. Obstet.* 50:601, 1930.

30. Spina, V., Kamakura, L., and Psillakis, J. M. Total reconstruction of the ear in congenital microtia. *Plast. Reconstr. Surg.* 48:349, 1971.

31. Steffensen, W. H. Comments on reconstruction of the external ear. *Plast. Reconstr. Surg.* 16:194, 1955.

32. Steffensen, W. H. A method of total ear reconstruction. *Plast. Reconstr. Surg.* 36:97, 1965.

33. Tanzer, R. C. Total reconstruction of the external ear. *Plast. Reconstr. Surg.* 23:1, 1959.

34. Tanzer, R. C. An analysis of ear reconstruction. *Plast. Reconstr. Surg.* 31:16, 1963.

35. Tanzer, R. C. Total reconstruction of the auricle: A 10-year report. *Plast. Reconstr. Surg.* 40:547, 1967.

36. Tanzer, R. C. Secondary reconstruction of microtia. *Plast. Reconstr. Surg.* 43:345, 1969.

37. Tanzer, R. C. Total Reconstruction of the auricle: The evolution of a plan of treatment. *Plast. Reconstr. Surg.* 47:523, 1971.

38. Tanzer, R. C. Correction of Microtia with Autogenous Costal Cartilage. In R. C. Tanzer and M. T. Edgerton (eds.), *Symposium on Reconstruction of the Auricle.* St. Louis: Mosby, 1974. P. 46.

39. Tanzer, R. C., and Chaisson, R. A protective guard for use during reconstruction of the auricle. *Plast. Reconstr. Surg.* 53:236, 1974.

40. Tanzer, R. C., Converse, J. M., and Brent, B. Deformities of the Auricle. In J. M. Converse (ed.), *Reconstructive Plastic Surgery* (2nd ed.). Philadelphia: Saunders, 1977. P. 1671.

41. Tegtmeier, R. E., and Gooding, R. A. The use of a fascial flap in ear reconstruction. *Plast. Reconstr. Surg.* 60:406, 1977.

EAR PROSTHESES

42. Bulbulian, A. H. *Facial Prosthetics.* Springfield, IL: Thomas, 1973.

43. Simons, J. N. The Role of the Prosthesis in Correction of Ear Deformities. In R. C. Tanzer and M. T. Edgerton (eds.), *Symposium on Reconstruction of the Auricle.* St. Louis: Mosby, 1974. P. 178.

44. Snow, R. S. An improved ear prosthesis in silicone rubber incorporating an adhesive surface. *Br. J. Plast. Surg.* 28:289, 1975.

CARTILAGE AND
PERICHONDRIAL GRAFTING

45. Brent, B., and Ott, R. The perichondrocutaneous graft. *Plast. Reconstr. Surg.* 62:1, 1978.

46. Gibson, T., and Davis, W. B. The distortion of autogenous cartilage grafts: Its cause and prevention. *Br. J. Plast. Surg.* 10:257, 1957.

47. Hagerty, R. F., et al. Characteristics of fresh human cartilage. *Surg. Gynecol. Obstet.* 110:3, 1960.

48. Hagerty, R. F., et al. Human cartilage grafts stored in air. *Surg, Gynecol. Obstet.* 110:433, 1960.

49. Hagerty, R. F., et al. Viable and nonviable human cartilage homografts. *Surg. Gynecol. Obstet.* 125:485, 1967.

50. Ohlsén, L. Cartilage formation from free perichondrial grafts: An experimental study in rabbits. *Br. J. Plast. Surg.* 29:262, 1976.

51. Skoog, T., and Johansson, S. H. The formation of articular cartilage from free perichondrial grafts. *Plast. Reconstr. Surg.* 57:1, 1976.

52. Skoog, T., Ohlsén, L., and Sohn, S. A. The chondrogenic potential of the perichondrium. *Chir. Plast.* 3:91, 1975.

53. Sohn, S. A., and Ohlsén, L. Growth of cartilage from a free perichondrial graft placed across a defect in a rabbit's trachea. *Plast. Reconstr. Surg.* 53:55, 1974.

GRAFTS OF CONCHAL CARTILAGE

54. Adams, W. M. Construction of upper half of auricle utilizing composite concha cartilage graft with perichondrium attached to both sides. *Plast. Reconstr. Surg.* 16:88, 1955.

55. Brent, B. The acquired auricular deformity: A systematic approach to its analysis and reconstruction. *Plast. Reconstr. Surg.* 59:475, 1977.

56. Brent, B. The versatile cartilage autograft: Current trends in clinical transplantation. *Clin. Plast. Surg.* 6:163, 1979.

57. Brent, B. Auricular Repair with a Conchal Cartilage Graft. In B. Brent (ed.), *The Artistry of Reconstructive Surgery.* St. Louis: Mosby, 1987. P. 107.

58. Davis, J. Repair of Severe Cup Ear Deformities. In R. C. Tanzer and M. T. Edgerton (eds.), *Symposium on Reconstruction of the Auricle.* St. Louis: Mosby, 1974. P. 134.

59. Falces, E., and Gorney, M. Use of ear cartilage grafts for nasal tip reconstruction. *Plast. Reconstr. Surg.* 50:147, 1972.

60. Gorney, M. The Ear as a Donor Site. In R. C. Tanzer and M. T. Edgerton (eds.), *Symposium on Reconstruction of the Auricle.* St. Louis: Mosby, 1974. P. 106.

61. Gorney, M., Murphy, S., and Falces, E.

Spliced autogenous conchal cartilage in secondary ear reconstruction. *Plast. Reconstr. Surg.* 47:432, 1971.

62. Stark, R. B., and Frileck, S. P. Conchal cartilage grafts in augmentation rhinoplasty and orbital floor fracture. *Plast. Reconstr. Surg.* 43:591, 1969.

## ACQUIRED AURICULAR DEFORMITY, GENERAL

63. Brent, B. The acquired auricular deformity: A systematic approach to its analysis and reconstruction. *Plast. Reconstr. Surg.* 59:475, 1977.

64. Tanzer, R. C. The reconstruction of acquired defects of the ear. *Plast. Reconstr. Surg.* 35:355, 1965.

65. Tanzer, R. C., and Edgerton, M. T. (eds.). *Symposium on Reconstruction of the Auricle.* St. Louis: Mosby, 1974.

66. Tanzer, R. C., Converse, J. M., and Brent, B. Deformities of the Auricle. In J. M. Converse (ed.), *Reconstructive Plastic Surgery* (2nd ed.). Philadelphia: Saunders, 1977. P. 1724.

## ACUTE AURICULAR TRAUMA

67. Baudet, J., Tramond, P., and Goumain, A. A propos d'un procédé original de réimplantation d'un pavillon de l'oreille totalement séparé. *Ann. Chir. Plast.* 17:67, 1972.

68. Clemons, J. E., and Connelly, M. V. Reattachment of a totally amputated auricle. *Arch. Otol.* 97:269, 1973.

69. Grabb, W. C., and Dingman, R. O. The fate of amputated tissues of the head and neck following replacement. *Plast. Reconstr. Surg.* 49:28, 1972.

70. Kellerher, J. C., et al. The wrestler's ear. *Plast. Reconstr. Surg.* 40:540, 1967.

71. McDowell, F. W. Successful replantation of a severed half ear. *Plast. Reconstr. Surg.* 48:281, 1971.

72. Mladick, R. A., and Carraway, J. H. Ear reattachment by the modified pocket principle. *Plast. Reconstr. Surg.* 51:584, 1973.

73. Mladick, R. A., et al. The pocket principle, a new technique for the reattachment of a severed ear part. *Plast. Reconstr. Surg.* 48:219, 1971.

74. Musgrave, R. H., and Garrett, W. S. Management of avulsion injuries of the external ear. *Plast. Reconstr. Surg.* 40:534, 1967.

75. Ohlsén, L., Skoog, T., and Sohn, S. A. The pathogenesis of cauliflower ear. *Scand. J. Plast. Reconstr. Surg.* 9:34, 1975.

76. Pennington, D. G., Lai, M. F., and Pelly, A. D. Successful replantation of a completely avulsed ear by microvascular anastomosis. *Plast. Reconstr. Surg.* 65:820, 1980.

77. Salyapongse, A., Mann, L. P., and Suthunyarat, P. Successful replantation of a totally severed ear (by the Baudet technique). *Plast. Reconstr. Surg.* 64:706, 1979.

78. Sexton, R. P. Utilization of the amputated ear cartilage. *Plast. Reconstr. Surg.* 15:419, 1955.

79. Spira, M. Early Care of Deformities of the Auricle Resulting from Mechanical Trauma. In R. C. Tanzer and M. T. Edgerton (eds.), *Symposium on Reconstruction of the Auricle.* St. Louis: Mosby, 1974. P. 204.

## ACUTE AURICULAR BURNS

80. Apfelberg, D. B., et al. Treatment of chondritis in the burned ear by the local instillation of antibiotics. *Plast. Reconstr. Surg.* 53:179, 1974.

81. Carroll, D. B. Early Treatment of Burned Ears. In R. C. Tanzer and M. T. Edgerton (eds.), *Symposium on Reconstruction of the Auricle.* St. Louis: Mosby, 1974. P. 191.

82. Collentine, G., Waisbren, B. A., and Mellendor, J. Treatment of burns with intensive antibiotic therapy and exposure. *J.A.M.A.* 200:939, 1967.

83. Dowling, J. A., Foley, F. D., and Moncrief, J. A. Chondritis in the burned ear. *Plast. Reconstr. Surg.* 42:115, 1968.

84. Grant, D. A., Finley, M. L., and Coers, C. R. Early management of the burned ear. *Plast. Reconstr. Surg.* 44:161, 1969.

85. Moyer, C. A., et al. Treatment of large human burns with 0.5% silver nitrate solution. *Arch. Surg.* 90:812, 1965.

## COMPOSITE GRAFTS

86. Aragamaso, R. V. An ideal donor site for the auricular composite graft. *Br. J. Plast. Surg.* 28:219, 1975.

87. Dufourmentel, C., and LePesteur, J. Les greffes auriculaires composées dans la reconstruction de l'étage inférieur de la pyramide nasale: A propos de 43 greffes. *Ann. Chir. Plast.* 18:199, 1973.

88. Nagel, F. Reconstruction of a partial auricular loss. *Plast. Reconstr. Surg.* 49:340, 1972.

89. Pegram, M., and Peterson, R. Repair of partial defects of the ear. *Plast. Reconstr. Surg.* 18:305, 1956.

90. Symonds, F. C., and Crikelair, G. F. Auricular composite grafts in nasal reconstruction: A report of 36 cases. *Plast. Reconstr. Surg.* 37:433, 1966.

AUDITORY CANAL

91. Conley, J. J. Atresia of the external auditory canal occurring in military service. *Arch. Otol.* 43:613, 1946.

92. Gingrass, R. P., and Pickrell, K. L. Techniques for closure of conchal and external auditory canal defects. *Plast. Reconstr. Surg.* 41:568, 1968.

93. Macomber, W. B., Wang, M. K., and Lueders, H. W. Reconstruction of the traumatically stenosed external auditory canal. *Plast. Reconstr. Surg.* 22:168, 1958.

94. Owens, N. An effective method for closing defects of the external auditory canal. *Plast. Reconstr. Surg.* 23:381, 1959.

95. Pennisi, V. R., Klabunde, E. H., and Pierce, G. W. The preauricular flap. *Plast. Reconstr. Surg.* 35:552, 1965.

96. Steffensen, W. H. A method of correcting atresia of the ear canal. *Plast. Reconstr. Surg.* 1:329, 1946.

HELICAL RECONSTRUCTION

97. Antia, N. H., and Buch, M. S. Chondrocutaneous advancement flap for the marginal defect of the ear. *Plast. Reconstr. Surg.* 39:472, 1967.

98. Argamaso, R. V., and Lewin, M. L. Repair of partial ear loss with local composite flap. *Plast. Reconstr. Surg.* 42:437, 1968.

99. Cronin, T. D. One stage reconstruction of the helix: Two improved methods. *Plast. Reconstr. Surg.* 9:547, 1952.

100. Fan-Hu, K., Hung-Yin, C., and Chu-Jen, H. Experience in the plastic repair of the burned ear. *Chin. Med. J.* 85:47, 1966.

101. Kazanjian, V. H., and Converse, J. M. (eds.). Traumatic Deformities of the Auricle. In *Surgical Treatment of Facial Injuries* (3rd ed.). Baltimore: Williams & Wilkins, 1974. Pp. 1300–1301.

102. Lewin, M. L. Formation of the helix with a postauricular flap. *Plast. Reconstr. Surg.* 5:432, 1950.

103. McNichol, J. W. Total helix reconstruction with tubed pedicles following loss by burns. *Plast. Reconstr. Surg.* 6:373, 1950.

104. Steffanoff, D. N. Auriculo-mastoid tube pedicle for otoplasty. *Plast. Reconstr. Surg.* 3:352, 1948.

UPPER AURICULAR RECONSTRUCTION

105. Crikelair, G. F. A method of partial ear reconstruction for avulsion of the upper portion of the ear. *Plast. Reconstr. Surg.* 17:438, 1956.

106. Davis, J. Reconstruction of the Upper Third of the Ear with a Chondrocutaneous Composite Flap Based on the Crus Helix. In R. C. Tanzer and M. T. Edgerton (eds.), *Symposium on Reconstruction of the Auricle.* St. Louis: Mosby, 1974. P. 247.

LOWER AURICULAR AND
EARLOBE RECONSTRUCTION

107. Brent, B. Earlobe construction with an auriculomastoid flap. *Plast. Reconstr. Surg.* 57:389, 1976.

108. Guerrero-Santos, J. Correction of hypertrophied earlobes in leprosy. *Plast. Reconstr. Surg.* 46:381, 1970.

109. Paletta, F. X. *Pediatric Plastic Surgery, Vol. I: Trauma.* St. Louis: Mosby, 1967. P. 209.

110. Pardue, A. M. Repair of torn earlobe with preservation of the perforation for an earring. *Plast. Reconstr. Surg.* 51:472, 1973.

111. Preaux, J. Un procédé simple de reconstruction de la partie inférieure du pavillon d l'oreille. *Ann. Chir. Plast.* 16:244, 1971.

112. Subba Rao, Y. V., and Venkaleswara Roa, P. A quick technique for earlobe reconstruction. *Plast. Reconstr. Surg.* 41:13, 1968.

113. Zenteno Alanis, S. A new method for earlobe reconstruction. *Plast. Reconstr. Surg.* 45:254, 1970.

AURICULAR TUMORS AND KELOIDS

114. Brent, B. The role of pressure therapy in management of earlobe keloids: Preliminary report of a controlled study. *Ann. Plast. Surg.* 1:579, 1978.

115. Converse, J. M., and Stallings, J. O. Eradication of large auricular keloids by excision, skin grafting and intradermal injection of triamcinolone acetonide solution. *Plast. Reconstr. Surg.* 49:461, 1972.

116. Cosman, B., and Wolff, M. Bilateral earlobe keloids. *Plast. Reconstr. Surg.* 53:540, 1974.

117. Ketchum, L. D.. Cohen, I. K., and Masters, F. W. Hypertrophic scars and keloids. *Plast. Reconstr. Surg.* 53:140, 1974.

118. Ramakrishnan, K. M., Thomas, K. P., and Sundararajan, C. R. Study of 1,000 patients with keloids in South India. *Plast. Reconstr. Surg.* 53:276, 1974.

119. Snyder, G. B. Button compression for keloids of the lobule. *Br. J. Plast. Surg.* 27:186, 1974.

# 16

*Fritz E. Barton, Jr.*

# Nasal Reconstruction

The nasal lobule occupies the geometric center of the face, and this central location, combined with its projection from the plane of the face and relatively soft chondrocutaneous composition, makes it vulnerable to injury. Moreover, the nose is one of the most common sites of cutaneous malignancy, especially basal cell carcinoma.

From a historic standpoint, the development of nasal reconstruction procedures followed three courses: (1) the Indian method, utilizing a midline forehead flap; (2) the French method, employing lateral cheek flaps; and (3) the Italian method, involving a brachial flap. Most procedures available today are variations on these basic themes.

## Anatomy

Thorough familiarity with the anatomy of the nose is a prerequisite for reconstruction. Cottle [15] defined the lobule of the nose as comprising the tip, alae, columella, and membranous septum. The entrance to the vestibule is the sill. The soft triangle spans the junction of the ala with the columella on either side (Fig. 16-1A).

When viewed from the basal projection, the nostril normally comprises one-half to two-thirds of the total height of the lobule [66] (Fig. 16-1B). The soft tissue dome of the tip extends above the apex of the nostril to complete the projection of the lobule.

The lateral crus of the alar cartilage does not extend into the alar wing but, rather, courses obliquely up to define the lateral edge of the nasal tip. This anatomic peculiarity leaves the arch of the nostril susceptible to cicatricial distortion and collapse.

The nose can be divided into thirds according to the underlying skeletal structure. The proximal one-third of the nose rests on the nasal bones; the middle one-third lies over the upper lateral cartilages; and the distal one-third or lobule includes the nasal tip with its paired alar cartilages and membranous septum.

## Planning Reconstruction

When planning a nasal reconstruction it is helpful to conceptualize the nose as composed of three primary layers: lining, skeletal support, and skin cover. Historically, reconstructive procedures concentrated on achieving external form with little regard for the patency of the airway, an approach that often resulted in a constricted nostril and internal nasal valve. The functional purpose of the nose is to provide a humidified airway, and this goal must be kept in mind when planning the reconstruction.

**491**

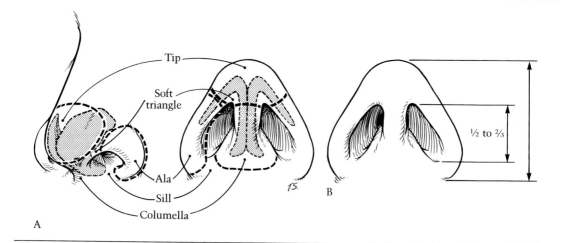

## Skin Cover

When planning surface reconstruction of the nose it is wise to remember the regional "aesthetic units" originally described by Gonzalez-Ulloa and Stevens [32] and redefined by Millard [52] (Fig. 16-2). These units are bound by the normal soft tissue creases and lines where a change in contour produces shadow definition of the nose. Junctures of skin grafts or flaps used for resurfacing the nose should correspond to these margins whenever possible.

The appropriate cutaneous cover for the nose matches or approximates the surrounding normal nasal skin in thickness, texture, and color. In addition, the vascularity of the recipient bed and the possible need for simultaneous nasal lining must also be considered. When lining is present, the operative plan is simplified; skin cover and skeletal support can usually be provided in a single step to produce the most aesthetic reconstruction.

### SKIN GRAFTS

The skin over the upper two-thirds of the nose is generally thin and mobile and has few sebaceous glands. Defects in this area repaired with full-thickness skin grafts yield excellent results. The skin of the lobule, on the other hand, is relatively thick and seba-

*Figure 16-1* *Anatomy of the nasal lobule.*
*A. Subunits of the lobule and alar cartilages.*
*B. Proportions of the nostril to the overall height of the lobule.*

ceous, especially in male subjects, and full-thickness skin grafts here are less desirable.

Full-thickness skin grafts for nasal resurfacing may be harvested from a number of donor sites. Gonzalez-Ulloa [31] measured the differing thickness of the skin over the body and suggested potential donor sites of skin grafts to the nose that were similar in thickness to the skin that was to be replaced. The varying skin thicknesses and

*Figure 16-2* *Aesthetic junction lines of the nose.*

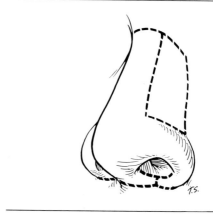

textures allow selection of donor areas that are best suited to the nasal skin requirements. Considerations of scar visibility and size limitation also come into play when choosing a donor site for a full-thickness graft to the nose.

The most common source of full-thickness skin for the nose is the postauricular area. Grafts up to 4 × 5 cm in diameter can be harvested while allowing primary closure of the donor site behind the ear. These grafts are relatively thin and neovascularize quickly and reliably.

Thicker skin may be obtained from the nasolabial fold, the preauricular area, and the supraclavicular area. Because they are on the anterior surface of the body, these donor sites are more conspicuous; moreover, skin grafts from these areas are thicker and so are less reliable in their "take."

Split-thickness skin grafts undergo significantly more secondary bed contraction and tend to have a smooth, white appearance upon healing that contrasts noticeably with the relatively ruddy complexion of the central face. Grafts of split skin are therefore reserved for compromise situations, such as to provide a platform on which to set a nasal prosthesis.

COMPOSITE GRAFTS

Small through-and-through defects of the nasal ala may be managed with composite grafts of auricular tissue [6, 28, 38] obtained from the earlobe [22], helical rim [6, 28], or root of the helix [1] (Fig. 16-3).

Composite grafts of skin and fat from the earlobe can be used to satisfactorily repair small defects of the lateral ala or base of the columella [22], especially in children. They are most applicable in cases in which there is adequate skeletal support and where the primary reconstructive goal is to fill the soft tissue contour. Composite chondrocutaneous grafts from either the helical rim or the root have been recommended for small through-and-through defects of the nostril rim [1, 6, 28, 38].

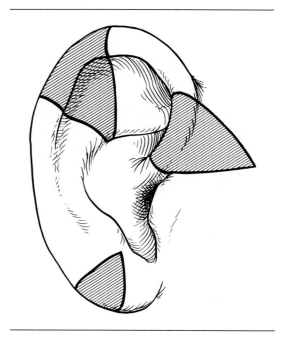

**Figure 16-3** *Sources of auricular composite grafts for nasal reconstruction.*

The traditional auricular composite graft used for nasal reconstruction is a wedge-shaped section of helical rim that includes two layers of skin separated by cartilage. Unlike skin grafts, composite grafts meet their recipient bed only along the perimeter, where their raw edges are in direct contact with the margins of the defect. Revascularization and graft "take" in these circumstances is less than optimal and places severe restrictions in the size of the graft used for the reconstruction.

In general terms, any grafted tissue more than 5 mm distant from a vascular bed is at significant risk of necrosis. Auricular composite grafts used for reconstruction of the alar rim should be no larger than 1.5 cm in diameter, so the center of the graft is never more than 5 to 8 mm away from a blood supply.

The clinical appearance of a healing composite graft was recorded by McLaughlin [46], who noted an initial dead-white color followed some 6 hours later by a pale pink tinge as a result of erythrocyte invasion. At 12 to 24 hours the graft becomes cyanotic from venous congestion, but if the procedure has been successful the cyanosis gradually turns into a healthy pink color within 3 to 7 days.

Various manipulations have been suggested to enhance the survival of composite auricular grafts. Postoperative cooling decreases the metabolic rate of the grafted tissue until secondary revascularization has taken place [9], and external application of ice compresses to lower the graft temperature by 5° to 10°C for a period of 72 hours is reportedly useful [61].

Another method of improving the "take" of a composite graft is to increase the area of vascular contact by using a turn-down flap of nasal skin for lining and applying a two-layer composite of skin and cartilage onto this raw bed [3]. Large full-thickness skin grafts covering as much as one-half of the nose augmented by narrow three-tiered composites along the rim have been reported to "take" successfully [2, 61].

LOCAL NASAL FLAPS

The relative laxity of the soft tissues in the upper two-thirds of the nose and glabellar area spurred the development of several designs of local flaps of nasal skin for reconstruction (Fig. 16-4).

The simplest and most popular is the *banner flap* described by Elliott [23]. It is a triangular flap with its base toward the nasal bridge that is transposed 90 degrees inferiorly to cover small defects of the dorsum (Fig. 16-4A). The donor site is closed primarily. As originally described, the banner flap can be used for defects up to 1.2 cm in diameter. However, by basing the flap on the side of the nose opposite the defect the flap reach is correspondingly increased, and larger wounds averaging 2 cm in diameter can be effectively covered [41].

Defects larger than 2 cm may be repaired with *bilobed flaps,* which use the secondary lobe of the flap to close the defect left by the primary lobe, which in turn is used in the reconstruction [44, 70] (Fig. 16-4B). An alternative to the bilobed flap technique is the *dorsal nasal flap* [39, 56, 62, 63], which is essentially a rotation advncement flap of the entire skin of the nasal dorsum (Fig. 16-4C). The dog-ear in the glabella is resected and the scar concealed in the vertical frown line. Initially described by Rieger [62] as a random skin flap with a wide pedicle encompassing one whole side of the nose, the flap can also be based on a branch of the angular artery that enters the skin of the nasal radix just below the medial canthal tendon [40]. This frontonasal flap can then be elevated on its narrow vascular pedicle for greater mobility.

The dorsal nasal flap provides good coverage of defects in the dorsum of the nose up to 2 cm in diameter. It is particularly useful for lesions of the tip, although it does not extend comfortably down onto the columella. Its advantage over other, smaller flaps of nasal skin is that it provides a single unit of closely matching tissue while it leaves scars that coincide with "aesthetic unit" junctions.

NASOLABIAL CHEEK FLAPS

European surgeons of the nineteenth century recognized the potential of paranasal skin redundancy as a source of tissue for nasal reconstruction. This skin laxity is usually exploited in one of three ways: as cheek advancement flaps, nasolabial transposition flaps, or subcutaneous pedicle flaps (Fig. 16-5).

*Cheek advancement* flaps based on the subdermal blood supply are especially useful for defects of the lateral nasal dorsum and nasal tip. When the inferior border of the incision is placed along the alar crease, the paranasal skin can be advanced medially onto the nasal wall to reach the midline. A compensatory Burow's triangle is excised from the alar base and nasolabial area (Fig. 16-5A). It is best not to carry the skin of the ala proper with a cheek advancement flap, as its subdermal blood supply tends to

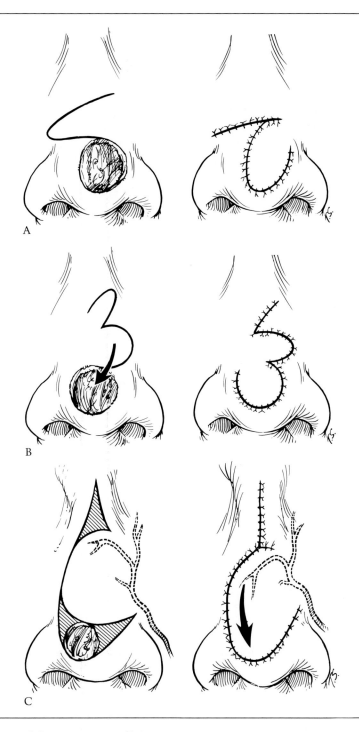

**Figure 16-4** *Local nasal flaps. A. Banner flap.*
*B. Bilobed flap. C. Dorsal nasal flap.*

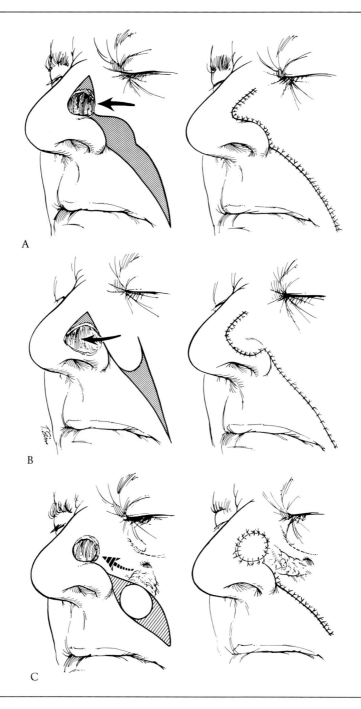

**Figure 16-5** *The cheek as a tissue donor in nasal reconstruction. A. Cheek advancement flap. B. Superiorly based nasolabial transposition flap. C. Nasolabial island subcutaneous-pedicle flap.*

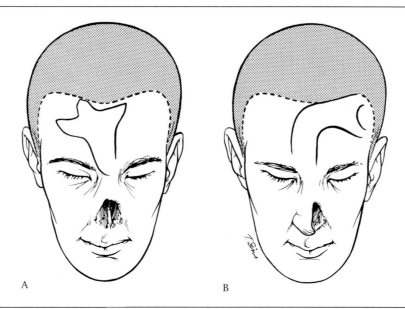

**Figure 16-6** *Midline forehead flap designs. A. Bilateral gull-wing (Millard). B. Oblique unilateral gull-wing.*

be poor. Moreover, the resultant scar violates nasal aesthetic units and may be noticeable [33, 45].

*Nasolabial transposition* flaps based either superiorly or inferiorly are of particular value for reconstruction of the alar wing. The superiorly based pedicle technique is most popular (Fig. 16-5B). Defects as large as 2.5 cm can be satisfactorily repaired in one operation, tailoring the flap to a thin layer of subcutaneous tissue and skin before transposition. A preliminary delay is advised, however, if the distal end of the flap is to be folded under for nasal lining.

Several authors [4, 21, 24, 34, 55] have used nasolabial skin carried on *subcutaneous pedicles,* primarily for reconstruction of the lateral nasal wall above the ala. The subcutaneous vascular pedicle is based over the infraorbital foramen [34], and the skin island from the nasolabial fold is easily transferred superiorly onto the area of the defect (Fig. 16-5C). The defect created by elevation of the flap is then closed by direct advancement of the redundant skin of the cheek.

MIDLINE FOREHEAD FLAP

The midline forehead flap has been the mainstay of nasal reconstructive surgery since it was first developed in India during the late eighteenth century. The flap may be elevated safely either on a single supratrochlear vessel or on an extension of the angular artery at the root of the nose [43]. Although the midline forehead flap has been raised as a skin island [13], it is more commonly transferred with the dermal pedicle intact in a two-stage operation. A delay procedure is necessary only in the event a lining graft needs to be applied to its undersurface when the reconstruction so demands it.

When intended for reconstruction of the lobule, the paddle of the midline forehead flap can be designed in the shape of a "gull wing" [51] (Fig. 16-6A). The entire lower half of the nose can thus be constructed from a single forehead flap while closing the donor defect primarily.

Closure of the donor site may be a problem when wide midline forehead flaps are used to resurface large nasal defects. A variety of maneuvers have been described to try to avoid grafting in the donor area, such as scoring the undersurface of the galea, bilat-

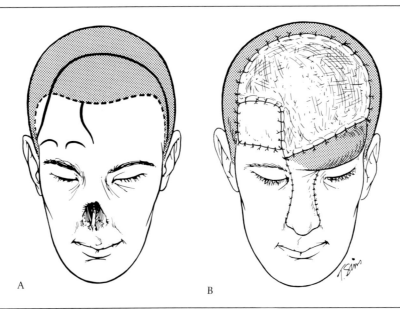

A                    B

*Figure 16-7 Scalping flap. A. Preliminary flap design. B. Flap transferred to nose with full-thickness skin graft to forehead donor site and single-thickness skin graft to scalp.*

eral forehead advancement flaps, and bilateral temporal rotation flaps.

Preliminary skin expansion also facilitates elevation of a large paddle while the defect is still closed primarily [13]. Skin expanders are most applicable when lining is already present and skeletal support can be added upon flap transfer. They are less useful for the repair of through-and-through nasal defects that must have chondrocutaneous grafts built into the flap lining, as expansion may distort the fine detail of the future nostril.

Another common problem with the midline forehead flap technique is insufficient length to comfortably reach the nasal lobule. For flaps that are too short because of narrow foreheads, the flap pedicle can be back cut deep into the nasal radix, provided the supratrochlear and angular collateral vessels are not disturbed. Alternately, the flap can be angled to follow the hairline, basing the pedicle on the supratrochlear vessels contralateral to the defect and extending the paddle along the hairline on the same side of the face as the reconstruction [5, 19, 65] (Fig. 16-6B). This modification in flap design not

only effectively lengthens the reach of the midline forehead flap but also minimizes twisting of the pedicle during transfer.

SCALPING FLAP

A number of procedures have been described using the superficial temporal vessels to carry forehead skin to the nose. The most useful is the scalping flap technique [10].

A segment of forehead skin large enough to reconstruct the entire surface of the nose can be carried undelayed based on the anterior half of the scalp that is supplied by the superficial temporal artery. The flap pedicle is usually placed on the side opposite the defect (Fig. 16-7).

Sometimes only surface coverage is required for the reconstruction. In this case the paddle on the forehead can be dissected in the subcutaneous plane, leaving the frontalis muscle intact to be covered later with a full-thickness graft [11, 12]. Alternatively, the skin may be expanded at a preliminary

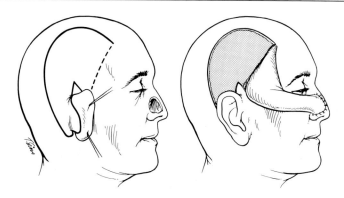

***Figure 16-8*** *Temporomastoid (Washio) flap.*

operation and the wound sutured primarily.

The scalping flap is transferred in a single stage, and the cranial periosteum is left to granulate by secondary intention or is protected with a temporary split-thickness graft. After the skin paddle is completely revascularized on the nose, the pedicle is divided and the anterior scalp replaced. The advantages of the scalping flap technique are the rich vascular supply of the broad skin paddle and the lack of incisions on the central forehead.

TEMPOROMASTOID FLAP

The temporomastoid flap represents a variation in the use of the superficial temporal vessels for nasal reconstruction. Skin from the postauricular and mastoid area is carried on the vascular loop between the superficial temporal vessels and the postauricular artery [68] (Fig. 16-8).

The flap can be transferred undelayed even when it incorporates conchal cartilage for alar support [57, 58]. The pedicle is divided and returned to its donor area after several weeks, during which time the paddle is revascularized in the recipient bed.

The advantage of the temporomastoid procedure is twofold: It avoids forehead scarring, and it places the incisions in hairbearing scalp where they are easily concealed. The technique is especially useful in chil-

dren and young adults who have minimal forehead laxity. A disadvantage of the temporomastoid flap is that it transfers thin, nonsebaceous skin to the nasal lobule.

DISTANT FLAPS

When there are no flap donor sites available in the head and neck area for nasal reconstruction, the transfer of tissue from greater distances may be considered. The classic example of distant tissue transfer is the *Tagliacozzi method* of nasal reconstruction with skin from the arm. The original Tagliacozzi flap was based distally and required delay, but the modern technique uses a proximally based flap that encompasses the axial vessel to the medial arm skin [16, 20, 36, 47, 53, 67]. A delay procedure is not necessary. After transfer, the upper extremity is immobilized for approximately 3 weeks until the pedicle is divided. Although the brachial flap technique furnishes soft, pliable skin with a thin subcutaneous layer, this skin is also less sebaceous and lighter in pigment than that of the nose.

Another useful option in nasal reconstruction by distant tissue transfer is the *free dorsalis pedis flap*, which can be taken with its accompanying second metatarsal to fashion a cantilever bone graft [54]. The dorsal foot skin has minimal subcutaneous tissue and conforms well to the nasal skeleton.

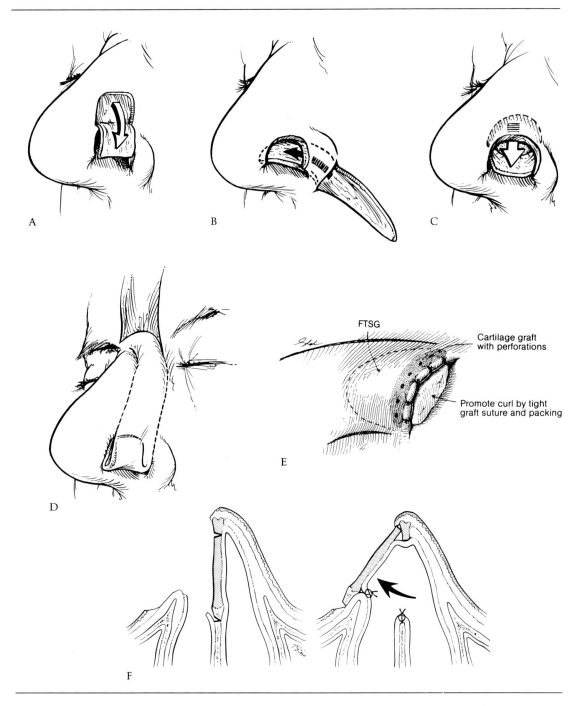

**Figure 16-9** *Methods for reconstructing the nasal lining. A. Turn-down flap from the wound margin. B. Nasolabial flap burrowed under the alar base and inverted. C. Bipedicled advancement of the superior nasal mucosa. D. Infolded end of coverage (midline forehead) flap. E. Composite chondrocutaneous graft. F. Chondromucosal septal flap.*

## Lining

The importance of airway caliber and the need to restore lining for the nose went largely ignored during the early days of nasal reconstruction. In the presence of intact lining the repair of nasal defects is relatively uncomplicated, as skeletal support and external coverage can be provided simultaneously. When nasal lining is deficient, however, the reconstruction becomes much more complex.

There are six common alternatives for replacing the internal surface of the nostril in through-and-through defects: (1) turn-down flaps of nasal skin based on the margin of the defect; (2) nasolabial flaps tunneled subcutaneously; (3) inferior advancement of remaining nasal lining; (4) infolded tips of other flaps; (5) skin grafts applied to the undersurface of coverage flaps; and (6) chondromucosal flaps from the nasal septum (Fig. 16-9).

Perhaps the most common source of lining for the nose is *turn-down flaps* based on the wound edge [35] (Fig. 16-9A). These flaps can be surprisingly healthy, but one must guard against airway constriction by the thick, inverted skin of the lobule.

A variation of this method uses *skin from the nasolabial or cheek area* tunneled subcutaneously, with its raw surface to the outside (Fig. 16-9B). External cover by any of the methods discussed above is affixed directly onto the lining flap. The same precautions regarding bulky tissue on the inside of the nose apply here.

When the lining defect is confined to the area of the nostril rim, it may be possible to advance a *bipedicled flap* of vestibular skin and mucosa from just above the defect to line the reconstructive area [8] (Fig. 16-9C), leaving a secondary lining defect farther up the nose. Cartilage grafts may be incorporated in the flap at the time of advancement with no ill effects.

It is also possible to replace lining by *infolding the tip* of the primary reconstructive flap (Fig. 16-9D), but only when the deficiency is small and located near the alar rim

[17, 25, 27, 42, 59, 64]. This method unfortunately tends to yield lining that is bulky and vascularly unreliable, especially if carried high into the nasal vault.

Defects in the nasal lining proximal to the alar rim are less critical and can be repaired either with a skin graft applied directly onto the primary reconstructive flap before transfer or with a chondromucosal septal flap.

Preliminary *skin grafts* placed on the undersurface of coverage flaps comprise a reliable method of reconstruction for major lining deficiencies [26, 48] (Fig. 16-9E). They are usually combined with forehead flaps and may incorporate cartilage in a multilayered template. Grafting is usually performed at the initial stage before transfer to the nose. After the composite graft is well established on the underside of the forehead flap (usually a period of 3 to 4 weeks), the laminated complex is mobilized and sutured on the nose, providing an already healed three-layered reconstruction. The flap pedicle is divided in the usual manner some 3 weeks later.

*Chondromucosal flaps of nasal septum* are based on the contralateral dorsal attachment of nasal mucosa to the septum [18, 29, 37, 49, 50, 60, 69] (Fig. 16-9F). These flaps are especially useful for restoring lining as well as skeletal support in the area of the upper lateral cartilages; they do not reach down far enough to line the nostril rim. One must take care to maintain a stable L-strut to prevent collapse of the lobule.

## Skeletal Support

Skeletal support to the nose, if inadequate, is preferably furnished at the same time as external coverage, so the soft tissues heal in their final, fully expanded shape. Once allowed to contract during the healing process, it is difficult to stretch the skin and subcutaneous tissues to accommodate subsequent cartilage placement.

Skeletal support of the nose can be conceptually divided into two components: rigid

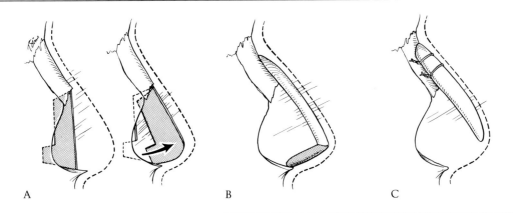

A                          B                          C

*Figure 16-10* Methods for reconstructing skeletal support to the nose. A. Septal hinge flap (Millard). B. *L* strut. C. Cantilever bone graft.

midline support and flexible lateral airway support. Most structural defects involve only cartilage: From a skeletal standpoint these defects are considered "subtotal." When the rigid nasal bones and nasal processes of the maxilla are absent, the defect as well as the reconstruction become much more complex and are termed "total" [48].

Three common methods of reconstituting the projection of the quadrangular nasal septum in subtotal nasal reconstruction are (1) septal hinge, (2) L-strut, and (3) cantilever bone graft (Fig. 16-10).

When only the septal angle is missing and the anterior nasal spine remains, the *septal hinge flap* [49, 51] is a simple and efficient technique to restore approximately 1 cm of nasal projection. Based on the soft tissue attachments at the junction of the cartilaginous septum with the nasal bones, the chondromucosal septal flap is rotated superiorly and set on the anterior nasal spine (Fig. 16-10A).

*Figure 16-11* Columellar reconstruction with a transnasal nasolabial flap (daSilva).

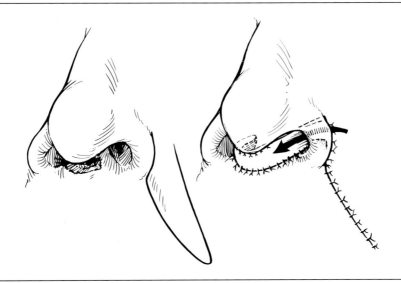

When one cannot advance a sufficient length of septum to form a new nasal angle and support the tip, bone grafts of either the L-*strut* [7, 28, 30] (Fig. 16-10B) or *cantilever* [14, 48] type (Fig. 16-10C) are best. Because reconstruction of the nasal lobule often involves asymmetric soft tissue forces, the cantilever bone graft is the most stable and reliable.

Many sources of bone for nasal grafting have been proposed. The classic donors are the rib and iliac crest, although membranous calvarial bone is an alternative when a sufficiently large and straight piece can be harvested.

## Columella

The columella can be one of the most difficult elements to restore because of its location just at the limits of reach of all available soft tissue flaps. Undoubtedly, the best columellar reconstructions are the results of extensions of forehead flaps used for the lobule.

Isolated columellar defects in adults are best repaired with a superiorly based nasolabial flap temporarily burrowed under the nasal ala [17]. This tunnel technique effectively shortens the flap and makes it much more reliable. The procedure requires a secondary division of the pedicle and reinset of the alar base (Fig. 16-11).

For small defects of the columella, especially in children, a composite graft of skin and subcutaneous fat from the earlobe may be useful.

## References

1. Argamaso, R. V. An ideal donor site for the auricular composite graft. *Br. J. Plast. Surg.* 28:219, 1975.
2. Avelar, J. M., Psillakis, J. M., and Viterbo, F. Use of large composite grafts in the reconstruction of deformities of the nose and ear. *Br. J. Plast. Surg.* 37:55, 1984.
3. Baker, D. C. Massive chondrocutaneous grafts for nasal reconstruction. Presented at the 63rd Annual Meeting of the American Association of Plastic Surgeons, Chicago, May 1984.
4. Barron, J. N., and Emmett, A. J. J. Subcutaneous pedicle flaps. *Br. J. Plast. Surg.* 18:51, 1965.
5. Barton, F. E., Jr. Aesthetic aspects of partial nasal reconstruction. *Clin. Plast. Surg.* 8:77, 1981.
6. Brown, J. B., and Cannon, B. Composite free grafts of skin and cartilage from the ear. *Surg. Gynecol. Obstet.* 82:253, 1946.
7. Brown, J. B., and McDowell, F. *Plastic Surgery of the Nose.* St. Louis: Mosby, 1951. Pp. 320–326.
8. Burget, G. C., and Menick, F. J. Nasal reconstruction: Seeking a fourth dimension. *Plast. Reconstr. Surg.* 78:145, 1986.
9. Conley, J. J., and Von Fraenkel, P. H. The principle of cooling as applied to the composite graft in the nose. *Plast. Reconstr. Surg.* 17:444, 1956.
10. Converse, J. M. New forehead flap for nasal reconstruction. *Proc. R. Soc. Med.* 35:811, 1942.
11. Converse, J. M. Reconstruction of the nose by the scalping flap technique. *Surg. Clin. North Am.* 39:335, 1959.
12. Converse, J. M. Clinical applications of the scalping flap in reconstruction of the nose. *Plast. Reconstr. Surg.* 43:247, 1969.
13. Converse, J. M., and Wood-Smith, D. Experience with the forehead island flap with a subcutaneous pedicle. *Plast. Reconstr. Surg.* 31:521, 1963.
14. Converse, J. M., et al. Corrective and Reconstructive Surgery of the Nose. In J. M. Converse (ed.), *Reconstructive Plastic Surgery* Vol. 2 (2nd ed.). Philadelphia: Saunders, 1977.
15. Cottle, M. H. *Corrective Surgery of the Nasal Septum and the External Pyramid—Study Notes and Laboratory Manual.* Chicago: American Rhinolaryngological Society, 1960.
16. Daniel, R. K., Terzis, J., and Schwarz, G. Neurovascular free flaps—a preliminary report. *Plast. Reconstr. Surg.* 56:13, 1975.
17. DaSilva, G. A new method of reconstructing the columella with a naso-labial flap. *Plast. Reconstr. Surg.* 34:63, 1964.
18. DeQuervain, F. Ueber patielle seitliche rhinoplastik. *Zentralbl. Chir.* 29:297, 1902.
19. Dhawan, I. K., Aggarwal, S. B., and Hariharan, S. Use of an off-midline forehead flap for the

repair of small nasal defects. *Plast. Reconstr. Surg.* 53:537, 1974.

20. Dolmans, S., Guimberteau, J. C., and Baudet, J. The upper-arm flap. *J. Microsurg.* 1:162, 1979.

21. Dufourmentel, C., and Talaat, S. M. The kite flap. In *Transactions of the Fifth International Congress of Plastic and Reconstructive Surgery.* Melbourne: Butterworths, 1971. P. 1223.

22. Dupertuis, S. M. Free earlobe graft of skin and fat. *Plast. Reconstr. Surg.* 1:135, 1946.

23. Elliott, R. A., Jr. Rotation flaps of the nose. *Plast. Reconstr. Surg.* 44:147, 1969.

24. Emmett, A. J. J. The closure of defects by using adjacent triangular flaps with subcutaneous pedicles. *Plast. Reconstr. Surg.* 59:45, 1977.

25. Georgiade, N. G., Mladick, R. A., and Thorne, F. L. The nasolabial tunnel flap. *Plast. Reconstr. Surg.* 43:463, 1969.

26. Gillies, H. A new free graft applied to the reconstruction of the nostril. *Br. J. Surg.* 30:305, 1943.

27. Gillies, H. The columella. *Br. J. Plast. Surg.* 2:192, 1950.

28. Gillies, H. D. *Plastic Surgery of the Face.* London: Oxford Medical Publishers, 1920.

29. Gillies, H. D., and Millard, D. R. *The Principles and Art of Plastic Surgery.* Boston: Little, Brown, 1957. P. 230.

30. Gillies, H. D., and Millard, D. R., Jr. *The Principles and Art of Plastic Surgery.* Boston: Little, Brown, 1957. P. 576.

31. Gonzalez-Ulloa, M. Restoration of the face covering by means of selected skin in regional aesthetic units. *Br. J. Plast. Surg.* 9:212, 1956.

32. Gonzalez-Ulloa, M., and Stevens, E. Reconstruction of the nose and forehead by means of regional aesthetic units. *Br. J. Plast. Surg.* 13:305, 1960.

33. Hagerty, R. F., and Smith, W. S. The nasolabial cheek flap. *Am. Surg.* 24:506, 1958.

34. Herbert, D. C., and Harrison, R. G. Nasolabial subcutaneous pedicle flaps. I. Observations on their blood supply. *Br. J. Plast. Surg.* 28:85, 1975.

35. Ivy, R. H. Repair of acquired defects of the face. *J.A.M.A.* 84:181, 1925.

36. Kaplan, E. N., and Pearl, R. M. An arterial medial arm flap—vascular anatomy and clinical applications. *Ann. Plast. Surg.* 4:205, 1980.

37. Kazanjian, V. H., and Converse, J. M. *The Surgical Treatment of Facial Injuries.* Baltimore: Williams & Wilkins, 1949. Pp. 349–353.

38. Konig, F. On filling defects of the nostril wall. *Berl. Klin. Wochenschr.* 39:137, 1902.

39. Lipshutz, H., and Penrod, D. S. Use of complete transverse nasal flap in repair of small defects of the nose. *Plast. Reconstr. Surg.* 49:629, 1972.

40. Marchac, D., and Toth, B. The axial frontonasal flap revisited. *Plast. Reconstr. Surg.* 76:686, 1985.

41. Masson, J. K., and Mendelson, B. C. The banner flap. *Am. J. Surg.* 134:419, 1977.

42. Mazzola, R. F., and Marcus, S. History of total nasal reconstruction with particular emphasis on the folded forehead flap technique. *Plast. Reconstr. Surg.* 72:408, 1983.

43. McCarthy, J. G., et al. The median forehead flap revisited: The blood supply. *Plast. Reconstr. Surg.* 76:866, 1985.

44. McGregor, J. C., and Soutar, D. S. A critical assessment of the bilobed flap. *Br. J. Plast. Surg.* 34:197, 1981.

45. McLaren, L. R. Nasolabial flap repair for alar margin defects. *Br. J. Plast. Surg.* 16:234, 1963.

46. McLaughlin, C. R. Composite ear grafts and their blood supply. *Br. J. Plast. Surg.* 7:274, 1954.

47. Meldelson, B. C., et al. Flaps used for nasal reconstruction: A perspective based on 180 cases. *Mayo Clin. Proc.* 54:91, 1979.

48. Millard, D. R., Jr. Total reconstructive rhinoplasty and a missing link. *Plast. Reconstr. Surg.* 37:167, 1966.

49. Millard, D. R., Jr. Hemirhinoplasty. *Plast. Reconstr. Surg.* 40:440, 1967.

50. Millard, D. R. The versatility of a chondromucosal flap in the nasal vestibule. *Plast. Reconstr. Surg.* 50:580, 1972.

51. Millard, D. R., Jr. Reconstructive rhinoplasty for the lower half of a nose. *Plast. Reconstr. Surg.* 53:133, 1974.

52. Millard, D. R., Jr. Aesthetic reconstructive rhinoplasty. *Clin. Plast. Surg.* 8:169, 1981.

53. Newsom, H. T. Medial arm free flap. *Plast. Reconstr. Surg.* 67:63, 1981.

54. Ohmori, K., Sekiguchi, J., and Ohmori, S. Total rhinoplasty with a free osteocutaneous flap. *Plast. Reconstr. Surg.* 63:387, 1979.

55. Ohtsuka, H., Shioya, N., and Asano, T. Clin-

ical experience with nasolabial flaps. *Ann. Plast. Surg.* 6:207, 1981.

56. Olbourne, N. A., and Kraaijenhagen, J. H. Rotation flap for distal nasal defects. *Br. J. Plast. Surg.* 28:64, 1975.

57. Orticochea, M. A new method for total reconstruction of the nose: The ears as donor areas. *Br. J. Plast. Surg.* 24:225, 1971.

58. Orticochea, M. Refined technique for reconstructing the whole nose with the conchas of the ears. *Br. J. Plast. Surg.* 33:68, 1980.

59. Ortiz-Monasterio, F. Labat and the three-lobed forehead flap [letter]. *Plast. Reconstr. Surg.* 73:705, 1984.

60. Rawat, S. S., and Sharma, K. One-stage repair of full-thickness alar defects. *Br. J. Plast. Surg.* 28:317, 1975.

61. Rees, T. D., et al. Composite grafts. In *Transactions of the Third International Congress of Plastic and Reconstructive Surgery.* Washington, DC: Excerpta Medica, 1963.

62. Rieger, R. A. A local flap for repair of the nasal tip. *Plast. Reconstr. Surg.* 40:147, 1967.

63. Rigg, B. M. The dorsal nasal flap. *Plast. Reconstr. Surg.* 52:361, 1973.

64. Santos, O. A., and Pappas, J. C. Repair of nostril defect with a contralateral nasolabial flap. *Plast. Reconstr. Surg.* 57:704, 1976.

65. Sawhney, C. P. A longer angular midline forehead flap for the reconstruction of nasal defects. *Plast. Reconstr. Surg.* 58:721, 1976.

66. Sheen, J. H. *Aesthetic Rhinoplasty.* St. Louis: Mosby, 1978.

67. Song, R., et al. The upper arm free flap. *Clin. Plast. Surg.* 9:27, 1982.

68. Washio, H. Retroauricular temporal flap. *Plast. Reconstr. Surg.* 43:162, 1969.

69. Young, L., and Weeks, P. M. Reconstruction of a large unilateral nasal defect. *Ann. Plast. Surg.* 1:485, 1978.

70. Zimany, A. The bilobed flap. *Plast. Reconstr. Surg.* 11:424, 1953.

# 17

*Daniel C. Baker*

# Reconstruction of the Paralyzed Face

In a society that places a premium on beauty and facial symmetry, an individual with facial paralysis suffers from functional, emotional, and social handicaps. One's goals in correcting facial paralysis are to achieve normal appearance at rest; symmetry with voluntary motion; control of the ocular, oral, and nasal sphincters; symmetry with involuntary emotion and controlled balance when expressing emotion; and no significant functional deficit secondary to the reconstructive surgery.

The treatment of facial paralysis is not in the realm of any one specialty. The intracranial, intratemporal, and extratemporal lesions of the facial nerve require the skill and cooperation of the neurosurgeon, neurologist, ophthalmologist, otolaryngologist, and plastic surgeon. It is only through the close interchange of ideas among these specialists that advances in facial rehabilitation will continue to occur.

Some of the treatment methods for facial paralysis are controversial, and some are still being evolved and developed. The surgeon must employ a number of concepts depending on the cause, time interval, and wound characteristics, as well as the availability of and necessity for neuromuscular substitution.

Patterns of facial paralysis vary in degree of involvement and duration, and no single surgical method can restore a complex combination of axonal and muscular degeneration. Careful preoperative selection of patients based on sound judgment of what can and cannot be achieved by the proposed surgical technique is paramount to a successful operation and a satisfied patient. A multiple or combined surgical approach often yields maximal results. The fact that the totally paralyzed face can never be made normal by any of the current methods of reconstruction does not detract from the measured and recognized success of these techniques.

Although much of the current progress has its origins in the past, the fundamental advances that have been made are associated with nerve–muscle physiology and rehabilitation of the neuromuscular system. Nerve grafts, crossovers, muscle transfers, free muscle and nerve–muscle grafts, and microneurovascular muscle transfers are the principal methods being developed. All of these techniques concentrate on dynamic reconstruction. Static methods comprise the well known techniques of fascia lata suspension and various rhytidoplasties [9, 10].

## Etiology, Classification, and Evaluation

Facial paralysis usually represents a manifestation of any number of disorders or abnormalities, the differential diagnosis of which has been extensively reviewed by May [23]. The various etiologic factors involved may be broadly classified into three major groups: intracranial, intratemporal, and extracranial.

*Central or intracranial region*
  Vascular abnormalities
  Central nervous system degenerative diseases
  Tumors of the intracranial cavity
  Trauma to the brain
  Congenital abnormalities and agenesis
*Temporal bone region*
  Bacterial and viral infections
  Cholesteatoma
  Trauma
    Longitudinal and horizontal fractures of the temporal bone
    Gunshot wounds
  Tumors invading the middle ear, mastoid, and facial nerve
  Iatrogenic causes
*Parotid gland region*
  Malignant tumors of the parotid gland
  Trauma (lacerations and gunshot wounds)
  Iatrogenic causes
  Primary tumors of the facial nerve
  Malignant tumors of the ascending ramus of the mandible, pterygoid region, and skin

Any plan to correct facial weakness or paralysis must begin with an analysis of the degree of weakness present and the status of the involved neural and muscular elements. A careful history is obtained, including the onset and duration of the condition and the recovery, if applicable. Additionally, the physician examines the face at rest and in motion, noting muscular tone and symmetry and analyzing the various mimetic muscles. Electrical testing must be performed to establish a physiologic baseline of neuromuscular status, which can then serve as a guideline for diagnostic and prognostic evaluation. The most popular tests are chronaxial level measurement, electromyography, nerve excitability (conduction) test, and electroneurography.

Although these tests do provide a physiologic baseline, certain subliminal responses of nerve and muscle may go unnoticed. For example, such tests do not always reveal the complete anatomic status of the facial nerve and mimetic muscles or their potential for rehabilitation. Researchers have demonstrated this fact by comparing electrical testing to direct inspection of the nerve and muscles at surgery, along with electron microscopic findings of biopsy specimens obtained from 32 patients with facial paralysis of 2 to 50 years' duration. In general, the electrical tests underevaluated the status of the facial nerve and mimetic muscles. Despite adverse electrical tests, for example, good results were obtained with facial nerve grafting and crossover in some patients with long-standing paralysis. Lacrimation, salivation, stapedial reflex, taste, audiometric, and vestibular tests (together with tomographic, angiographic, and neurologic investigation) add valuable information about intratemporal lesions [24].

Ideally, the goals of rehabilitation of the paralyzed face are to achieve the following goals: normal appearance at rest; symmetry with voluntary motion; restoration of oral, nasal, and ocular sphincter control; symmetry with involuntary motion and controlled balance when expressing emotion; and no loss of other significant functions. No surgical technique can accomplish all of these goals, and no single routine approach is suitable for all patients. The choice of a corrective procedure requires a detailed analysis of the cause, duration, extent of deformity, and the patient's overall prognosis. Dynamic reconstruction and neural reconstitution are almost always preferred to static methods, except under special circumstances.

## Direct Nerve Repair and Grafting

The most effective means of rehabilitating the paralyzed face is to reestablish the neural pathway by direct suture or autogenous nerve grafting. Each of these approaches requires adequate mimetic muscle function. Usually no difficulty is encountered when reinnervating facial musculature for up to 1 year, and good results have been seen as late as 2 and 3 years after loss of facial movement [9, 10].

Despite statements to the contrary, facial nerve repair and grafting are best done immediately in cases of clean traumatic injuries or ablative procedures for cancer. Although many researchers believe that repair done prior to 3 weeks after injury results in excess scar tissue at the juncture site, this theory has been disproved by the experiments of Hastings and Peacock [20], who demonstrated no difference in the amount of scar tissues at juncture sites in nerves repaired at various intervals. After scarring, fibrosis, and atrophy have complicated the healing process, nerve repair is more difficult.

Direct nerve suture is indicated in any instance in which the main trunk can be reapproximated with no tension, as is the case for lacerations, iatrogenic injuries, and certain benign conditions. After an ablative procedure for cancer, however, immediate facial nerve grafting is used to overcome loss of the main trunk and peripheral branches. At present, 95 percent of properly selected patients are expected to have some return of movement after grafting. Patients at high risk, however, including those who require extensive ablation (e.g., those who are undergoing "superradical parotidectomy") and those with poor tissue beds, are seldom good candidates for nerve grafts. Obviously, if the distal part of the facial nerve including the mimetic muscles is ablated, nerve grafting is unrealistic. Muscle transposition is the preferred treatment in such cases.

The cervical plexus at the C3 and C4 levels from the ipsilateral or contralateral side is most frequently used for facial nerve autografting (Fig. 17-1), and it has proved to be convenient and adaptable for the head and neck surgeon. Four branches can usually be obtained and sutured to the terminal branches of the temporal, zygomatic buccal, and mandibular division (Fig. 17-2). The diameters of this nerve usually accommodate the counterparts in the face, with some minor inequities. The graft must lie in a healthy, well vascularized area free of scar tissue. There must be no tension on the junctures. Because of slight shrinkage, a graft about 20 percent longer than the defect is used. When treating long-standing facial paralysis, it is important to resect fibrotic tissue in addition to any neuroma of the proximal stump. The sural nerve is also a popular donor for nerve grafts.

The basic techniques of neurorrhaphy have evolved through the stages of gross approximation to their current sophisticated level, in which fascicular repair is accomplished with the use of fine atraumatic sutures and the operating microscope (Fig. 17-3). Several sutureless methods have been advocated, e.g., plasma clot method, micropore adhesive tape method, and tubular union. Most adhesive nonsuture techniques, however, have been abandoned because of foreign body reaction, increased fibrosis, and inferior results in comparison to suture techniques.

The classic technique of nerve repair is to place a number of sutures about the circumference of the nerve to achieve tight union of the epineural layers. This technique is simple and has yielded a high success rate, especially for repair and grafting of the facial nerve. Some surgeons believe, however, that the technique has several disadvantages: There is no control of behavior of the fascicles, which could be important in a multifascicular nerve; the outer layers of the epineurium proliferate intensively, contributing to the scar tissue at the neurorrhaphy site; and the sutures themselves cause a foreign body reaction, varying with material,

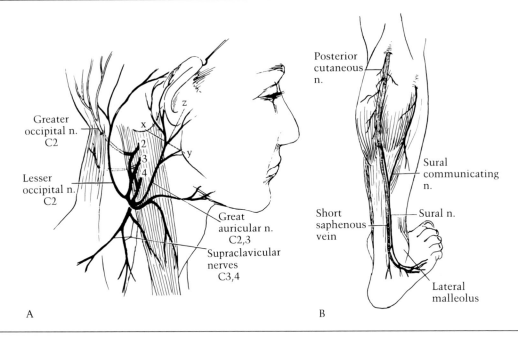

**Figure 17-1** *A. A cervical plexus graft from the ipsilateral side of the neck is preferred (contralateral if nodes are involved). Usually a 9- to 12-cm graft can be obtained with a main trunk and four or five branches of good physical match. B. For cross-face nerve grafting, a sural nerve graft 30 to 40 cm length is obtained. (This and all figures in this chapter are from D. C. Baker and J. Conley. Facial nerve grafting: A thirty year retrospective review. Clin. Plast. Surg. 6:343, 1979.)*

size, and amount. According to Millesi, the amount of scar tissue formation and the width of the gap that can form between two joined nerves is directly related to the amount of tension at the suture site.

Millesi [26–28] advocated fascicular or interfascicular nerve repair to achieve maximal exactness of coaptation with minimal surgical trauma. He stated that this technique is possible only if one condition is fulfilled: There must be no tension at the line of coaptation. After resecting a strip of epineurium, a few fine stitches (10-0 or 11-0 nylon) are used to approximate corresponding fascicles or fascicle groups. One stitch is usually sufficient to keep the two ends together until fibrin clotting occurs.

Fascicular coaptation is performed if the nerve consists of several large fascicles, whereas interfascicular coaptation is used for nerves consisting of many fascicles. Millesi believed in addition that resection of the epineurium results to reduction of the nutrient supply.

In addition to scar tissue production, an-

other advantage of fascicular coaptation, as stated by Millesi, is that corresponding fascicles or fascicle groups are united, and the outgrowth of axons in the wrong direction is thereby reduced. The spatial orientation of the facial nerve, however, is still a matter of dispute. Sunderland believed that the nerve fibers are more or less diffusely distributed, whereas Miehlke [25], May [24], and Apfelberg and Gingrass [4] noted that discrete fasciculi may be present proximal to the stylomastoid foramen. Theoretically, if a fascicular pattern exists, nerve grafting of individual fasciculi would result in selective facial muscle reinnervation and significantly less

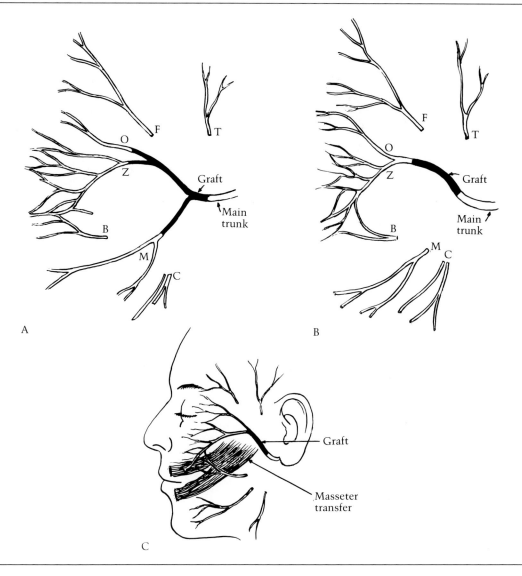

**Figure 17-2** *Variations in nerve grafting.*
*A. Main trunk and three peripheral branches.*
*B. A single graft is interposed between the main*
*trunk and the dominant peripheral division (it*
*can be confirmed by electrical testing on the*
*operating table). Good return of movement*
*could still be anticipated with this single graft*
*because of numerous interconnections with*
*other divisions of the facial nerve. C. If a single*
*graft is used, we usually combine*
*reconstruction with an immediate masseter*
*muscle transposition, which immediately*
*rehabilitates the lips and commissure and*
*creates an ideal situation for myoneurotization.*

mass action. This theory has not yet been
proved.

A composite experience [9, 10] with more
than 170 autogenous facial nerve grafts involved the use of 6-0 atraumatic silk in an
early group with and without loupe magnification, an epineural technique on the main
trunk, and a single through-and-through suture in the peripheral branches. This experience established the efficacy of the tech-

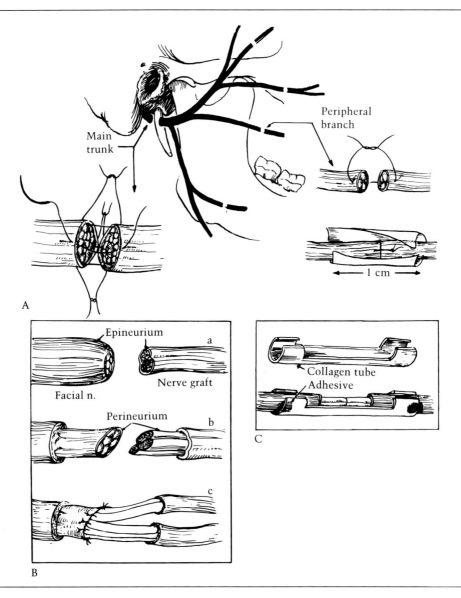

A

B

C

nique and proved the high regenerative and adaptive capacities of the facial nerve. At present, with the use of finer suture materials and $4\times$ loupe magnification, 95 percent of optimally selected patients can expect some return of movement.

The timing of repair is of utmost importance, the ideal situation being at the time of the primary ablative procedure. Factors that influence the success of repair include

**Figure 17-3** *Techniques of nerve grafting. A. There are several epineural sutures in a main trunk and a single suture in the peripheral branch. If a Silastic sleeve is used, it must be nonconstrictive and not more than 1 cm in length (this technique is controversial and probably unnecessary if good end-to-end approximation is obtained). B. Millesi technique of interfascicular repair. Theoretically it enhances return and minimizes mass movement, but these results have not been demonstrated clinically. C. Collagen adhesives are rarely employed at present.*

tension, the character of the wound and scar tissue, the length of the graft, the patient's age, and the time lag to repair. Clinical and experimental work by Conley [11] and Miehlke [25] has also demonstrated no difference in the functional results between patients who had undergone a full course of postoperative irradiation and those who had not.

The time interval for return of facial movement varies from 6 to 24 months, depending on the length of the graft. Initially there is improvement in the tone of the paralyzed face, and movement usually appears in the middle third of the face about the oral commissure. This movement gradually extends to include muscles about the mouth, cheek, and orbit. Only rarely is there satisfactory return of movement to the forehead and lower lip. The quality of return is always mass movement with associated weakness and recognizable dyskinesia, although this situation can be improved with concentration and exercise before a mirror. There is always a deficit in emotional expression, but movement on intention and command may be almost normal.

## Cross-Face Nerve Grafting (Faciofacial Anastomoses)

Cross-face nerve grafting was introduced by Scaramella in 1970 at the Second International Symposium on Facial Nerve Surgery held in Osaka, Japan [35]. He presented a case in which the intact buccal ramus on the nonparalyzed side had been sutured to the paralyzed stem of the facial nerve with a sural nerve graft. The patient had gained symmetry and some degree of active movement. This technique has been further expanded and developed by Anderl [1–3], Fisch [13], Freilinger [14], Samii [34], and Smith [37].

The procedure is based on cross-innervation from the nonparalyzed side by means of sural nerve grafts that connect the reservoir of peripheral healthy facial nerve fascicles to the corresponding branches of specific mus-

cle groups on the paralyzed side (Fig. 17-4). The Millesi technique of fascicular repair is used, and the lengths of the grafts vary from 6 to 8 cm. Anderl favored a two-staged procedure, allowing the nerve axons to grow to the opposite side, then resecting the neuroma to demonstrate the success of the axon regrowth before suturing the graft to the paralyzed side. Smith and Samii, on the other hand, repaired both junctures simultaneously. There are no conclusive data showing significant differences in the final result, although most authors prefer a two-stage procedure. There is also disagreement as to whether reversal of the nerve graft ensures that all axons entering tubules on the innervated side present to the opposite end of the graft or nonreversal permits axon outgrowth and neurotization through nerve branches along the way.

Although there was initially great enthusiasm for this technique, it took almost 10 years for others to gain enough experience with cross-face nerve grafting to discover that it has limited applications (except when combined with microneurovascular muscle transfers) and that the overall results were disappointing when compared to those obtained with classic procedures.

OPERATIVE TECHNIQUE
In the first stage an incision is made lateral to the nasolabial fold on the nonparalyzed side of the face to identify the buccal branches of the facial nerve. A nerve stimulator is used to map the branches supplying the elevators, upper lip, and orbicularis oris. A dominant branch of cross section similar to that of the sural nerve graft is divided and microsurgical anastomosis performed. Sometimes the fascicles of the sural nerve are separated and each fascicle anastomosed to a buccal branch. With early paralysis, if the orbicularis oculi is to be reinnervated, another graft can be anastomosed to a branch of the zygomatic or temporal nerve. Often a separate incision is required. These long grafts are then pushed through a subcuta-

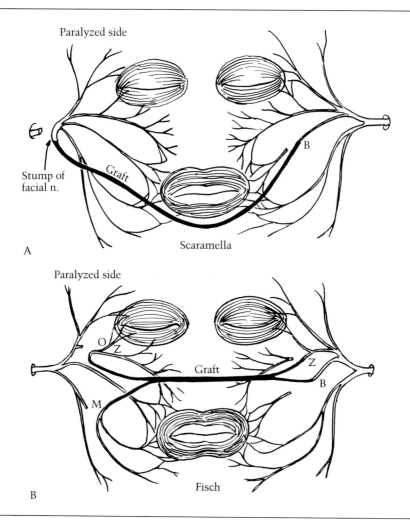

Paralyzed side

Stump of
facial n.

Graft

Scaramella

A

Paralyzed side

O Z

Graft

Z

B

M

Fisch

B

neous tunnel in the upper lip to the para-lyzed side and anchored in the dermis near the tragus. A silver clip in proximity to the distal end is helpful for identifying the nerve at the second stage. Sacrifice of facial nerve branches on the normal side does not pro-duce significant paralysis and may even be beneficial in equalizing the two sides.

The second stage usually is performed 9 to 12 months later after a positive Tinel's sign has been followed to the distal end of the graft. Neuromas are removed, and the graft is sutured to the corresponding branches of

**Figure 17-4** *A. Scaramella's technique of cross-face nerve graft. This graft may also be passed over the upper lip. B. Fisch's technique. C. Anderl's modifications. In our experience the frontal and marginal mandibular functions return in only 15 percent of patients, even with primary nerve grafting. D. We prefer to anastomose the entire lower division of the normal side with the main trunk of the paralyzed side. Exposure is easily obtained with standard parotid incisions. The graft may be passed over the upper lip.*

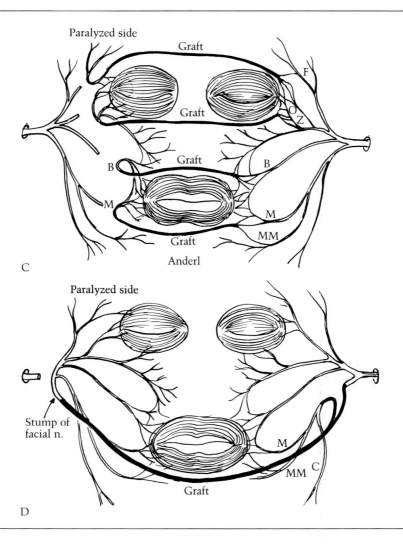

**Figure 17-4** *(Continued)*

the facial nerve on the paralyzed side (or to nerve of a vascularized muscle).

The concept of cross-face nerve grafting is ingenious, and its theoretical advantage is facial reanimation through specific nerve branches to specific mimetic muscle groups. The primary disadvantage, aside from the need for specialized techniques and long operating time, is the period required for return of function. The facial muscles undergo further atrophy during the time required for axonal growth through the long nerve grafts.

Technical difficulties have been encountered using the techniques of Scaramella [36], Fisch [13], and Anderl [3] in identifying the distal branches of the facial nerve because of the intimate plexus formation with the trigeminal nerve, which varies considerably and cannot be standardized. Suturing the sensory nerve branches of the infraorbital, buccal, zygomaticofacial, and mental nerves to branches of the facial nerve has been reported [3]. Perhaps the greatest disadvantage of this technique, as noted by Samii [34] and Anderl [3], is that only 50 percent of all nerve fibers of the facial nerve can be used from the normal side, and they are joined to about 50 percent of the paralyzed side, thereby limiting the amount of axonal input. In general, the distinct disadvantages include the following.

1. There is surgical intrusion on the normal side of the face with sacrifice of some axonal input, although the resulting deficits are minimal.
2. Highly specialized techniques are required, as is a longer operating time (and often two operative stages).
3. There are two suture lines for each nerve graft, increasing the probability of a greater loss of spouting axons.
4. A longer time is required for reinnervation from these long grafts, during which there may be further muscle atrophy.
5. The greatest disadvantage is the reduced axonal input to accomplish powerful reinnervation if one is not to sacrifice too much on the normal side.
6. Because of the intimate plexus formation of the trigeminal nerve with the facial nerve, technical difficulties may be encountered when identifying distal branches of the facial nerve.
7. The results of this method are not free of the mass movements (synkinesis) associated with other methods of rehabilitation.

Samii [34] reported on ten cases; five showed symmetric position of the face in repose, one demonstrated good facial movement, and the others evidenced some degree of movement. Anderl [1,2] reported on 15 patients, five of whom demonstrated good symmetry with some degree of movement. More recently, Anderl [3] emphasized that if cross-face nerve grafting is performed later than 6 months after onset of paralysis, the results are unacceptable in most cases. In a review of 20 patients by Ba Huy et al. [5], only 25 percent of patients obtained a satisfactory result with good symmetry during spontaneous and emotional mimics. The au-

thors have since abandoned the technique in favor of the easier XII–VII anastomosis.

The present consensus among surgeons operating on patients with facial paralysis is that the cross-face nerve graft is only another alternative to the classic procedures of hypoglossal facial nerve crossover and muscle transposition. The alternative proposed by Fisch [13] of performing an immediate hypoglossal nerve crossover to restore tone and maintain muscular bulk and then to perform a cross-face nerve graft for more controlled movement is gaining in popularity. Another application, which consists in reinnervating a free muscle graft [15] or combining a cross-face nerve graft with masseter and temporalis transfers [14], has not gained acceptance.

## Nerve Crossovers

Nerve crossovers employing the glossopharyngeal, accessory, phrenic, and hypoglossal nerves have been used for more than a half-century. These techniques generally are used when direct suture or grafting is not feasible, as in the case of an obliterated central facial nerve segment with intact peripheral nerve segments and adequate mimetic muscles. They are particularly applicable to facial paralysis resulting from intracranial lesions or disorders of the temporal bone.

Nerve crossover techniques are advantageous because they are simple, require only a single suture line, and serve as a powerful source of reinnervation. All of these techniques have been severely criticized because they result in associated, uncoordinated movements and in loss of function of the donor nerve. Extensive clinical experience, however, has demonstrated that many of these criticisms are overemphasized, particularly with regard to the hypoglossal-facial nerve crossover, which is the most popular crossover operation in use today.

Experience with almost 200 cases of hypoglossal nerve crossover used for various causes of facial paralysis yielded the following results: 22 percent of patients had minimal atrophy of the tongue, 53 percent had moderate atrophy, and 25 percent had severe atrophy [6, 7, 9, 10]. Patients who had undergone hypoglossal nerve crossover performed immediately as part of the ablative procedure were much more satisfied than those who underwent delayed crossover. Perhaps because of their overriding concern about the success of their cancer program, patients in the "immediate" group complained little about interference with chewing, swallowing, and speaking. Only 3 percent complained about mastication, 2 percent about swallowing, and 2 percent about speech.

Ninety-five percent of all patients had some type and quality of movement, and 77 percent in the "immediate" group were classified as good, compared with 41 percent in the delayed group. In patients with good return of movement, about 15 percent had hypertonia with overproduction of movement with eating, swallowing, and talking. Some patients were able to develop and refine this movement to obtain normal smiling and involuntary closing of the eye.

Hypoglossal nerve crossover is a valuable technique, particularly when used as an integral part of the primary ablative operation for regional cancer. It provides excellent facial tone and normal appearance at rest, allows protection of the eye, and permits intentional movement of the face controlled by movements of the tongue. Its disadvantages include minimal to moderate intraoral dysfunction, mass movement, and occasional hypertonia in the face (particularly in association with the act of chewing). The hypoglossal nerve crossover technique is not used to treat moderate general facial paresis, segmental paralysis, or regional paralysis [8].

## Muscle Transfers

Transfer of muscle to the paralyzed face (Fig. 17-5) is usually done under three circumstances: (1) in the absence of mimetic muscles after long-standing atrophy; (2) as an adjunct to the mimetic muscles to provide new muscle and myoneurotization; and (3) occasionally in combination with a nerve graft or crossover implanted in the transposed muscle. Although most of the available muscles about the head and neck have been transposed in whole or in part, by far the most popular muscle transposition techniques involve the masseter and temporalis muscles [6, 7, 9, 10].

The basic technique of masseter transfer, first delineated by Lexer in 1908, is still used today. However, Lexer's original description of the procedure entailed rotating the anterior half of the muscle, a step that would introduce the possibility of transecting the nerve supply, as demonstrated by de Castro Correia and Zani [12]. This muscle is ideally suited to give motion to the lower half of the face (Fig. 17-6). Commonly, three muscle slips are sutured to the dermis of the lower lip, oral commissure, and upper lip. Overcorrection must be accomplished; if some mimetic muscles remain, the slips can be interdigitated with them. Postoperative immobilization and a liquid diet are instituted for about 10 days to allow healing. Chewing is then begun gradually, after which the patient is taught to practice control of facial movements before a mirror. Masseter transfer has proved to be a valuable technique in certain cases of radical parotidectomy in which a nerve graft did not prove advantageous (Fig. 17-7). Transposing the masseter with interdigitation into the freshly denervated mimetic muscles provides maximum myoneurotization of all the muscles in the middle third of the face (Fig. 17-8).

For facial rehabilitation, the temporalis muscle has enjoyed more popularity than the masseter because of its position, its facility for greater excursion of movement, and its adaptability to the orbit. Numerous ingenious techniques using various slings about the orbit and mouth have been described, as has been transposition of the muscle insertion with the coronoid process to the middle third of the face (Fig. 17-9). The technique that is now most widely em-

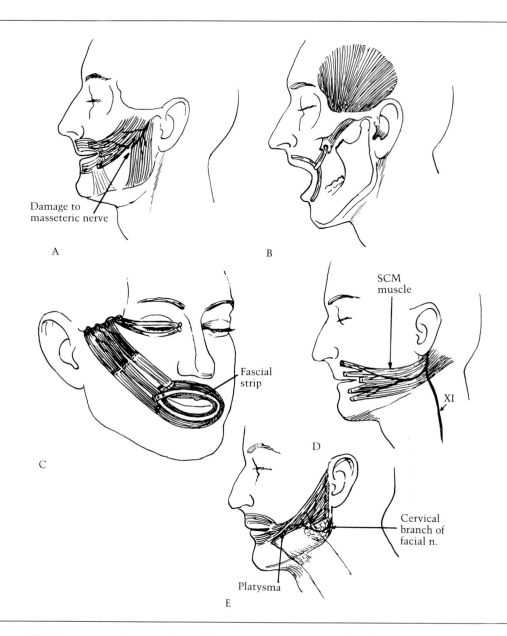

**Figure 17-5** *Some types of regional muscle transposition. A. Lexer's original technique risked transecting the nerve supply to the masseter muscle. B. McLaughlin procedure, attaching the coronoid process to the circumoral fascia lata suspension. Movement is not at the melolabial crease. C. Original technique of temporalis transfer with fascial strips or superficial temporal fascia turned down to obtain length. D. Sternocleidomastoid transposition. Movement is more unnatural, in the wrong direction, and muscle is bulky. E. Platysma transposition. Muscle is thin and delicate, and it does not provide much power; pull is in the wrong direction.*

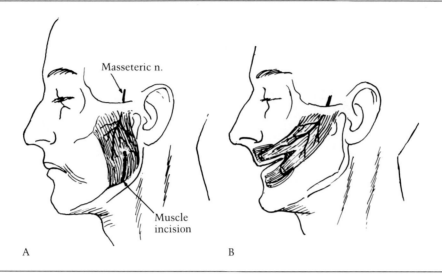

**Figure 17-6** *A. We recommend transferring the entire masseter muscle. Incision need only be several centimeters to avoid damage to the nerve. B. Anterior portion of the muscle is sutured to the orbicularis oris and to the dermis anterior to the melolabial fold. The posterior portion of the muscle is sutured to the lower lip and commissure.*

ployed involves transfer and suturing of the muscle with its fascial extensions to the eyelids, ala of the nose, oral commissure, and upper and lower lips. The depression in the temporal area can be corrected by inserting a carved block of soft silicon. Although Rubin [32, 33] has indicated that the muscle is not long enough to go down to the mouth or reach the medial canthus without the fascial attachment, the full muscle can be taken without difficulty to the canthi and commissure with a border of epicranium and suture slips. The technique has several advantages, one of which is that the muscle provides bulk in the severely atrophic face. Furthermore, there is direct muscular insertion on the structures to be moved, and the possibility of myoneurotization is enhanced.

Because the impulse for muscle movement in temporalis and masseter transfers originates from the trigeminal nerve, facial movement is not physiologic. A facial nerve graft with nerve implantation into the transposed muscle to achieve specific innervation from the facial nerve can therefore be performed. Cross-face nerve grafts with muscle implantation have also been done, as have cross-face nerve grafts to the masseteric nerve at the foramen ovale [14]. The results of these procedures have not yet been sufficiently evaluated to justify their routine use.

## Free Muscle Grafts

In 1971 Thompson [39] reported on the successful transplantation of free autogenous muscle grafts in humans, and in 1974 he established its clinical application for the treatment of unilateral facial paralysis [40]. Since then, other investigators have reported success with free muscle grafts. According to Thompson, the success of this procedure depends on three factors: (1) the muscle belly selected for transplantation must be denervated 14 days prior to transplantation; (2) a full length of muscle fiber must be preserved; and (3) the denervated muscle must be placed in direct contact with normal, fully innervated, vascularized skeletal muscle at the recipient site before neurotization can occur. Thus at least two operations are

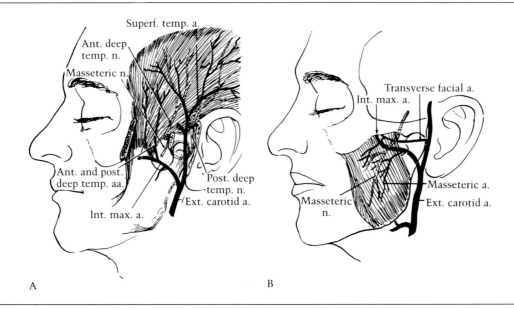

A                                                    B

*Figure 17-7* A. Neurovascular supply of the temporalis muscle. B. Neurovascular supply of the masseter muscle; note the oblique direction of the nerve.

required with an interval of 14 days between them. The technique consists in placing denervated muscle in contact with normal muscle on the nonparalyzed side of the face. The transplanted muscle tendon is then sutured to the appropriate area to obtain movement (e.g., the zygomatic arch for the oral sphincter and the lateral canthal tendon for the eye sphincter).

Thompson reported that of 54 patients treated for oral sphincter reconstruction, 90 percent had good results and 10 percent showed satisfactory improvement. Of these 54 patients, 17 percent required another surgical procedure to tighten the tendon sling. Among 62 patients who underwent reconstruction for paralyzed eyelids, 48 percent had good results and 45 percent satisfactory results. Secondary operations to adjust tension or perform tenolysis were required in 22 percent of the 62 patients. The advantage of this technique is that movement is controlled by the normal side of the face.

Despite the successful reports of Thompson [40] and Hakelius [15], considerable skepticism exists about the reproducibility of free muscle grafting for reconstructive surgery.

Watson's attempt to reproduce Thompson's experiments in dogs proved unsuccessful, and it is still uncertain which factors are responsible for the survival of free muscle grafts. In addition to this uncertainty and reports that grafts have become fibrotic, other disadvantages include the multiple stages required, the high incidence of reoperation, and the intrusion on the nonparalyzed side of the face.

### Nerve–Muscle Pedicle Techniques

From previous work involving reinnervation of paralyzed vocal cords, Tucker [41] has extended the nerve–muscle pedicle technique to the treatment of facial paralysis. This technique involves transplanting an intact motor nerve with an attached small block of donor muscle from the point of nerve entry, after which this pedicle is sutured to the

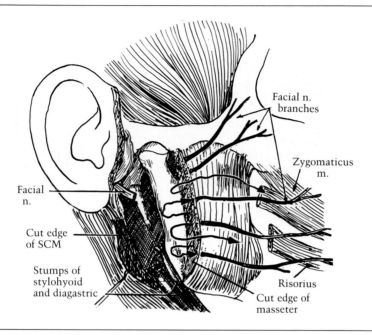

**Figure 17-8** *Ideal circumstances for myoneurotization. Freshly denervated mimetic muscles (vascular supply intact) come in contact with transposed masseter muscle (neurovascular supply intact). Raw, living muscle is interdigitated with raw living muscle.*

muscle to be innervated. If most of the motor endplates are preserved, the pedicle is prevented from degenerating, and reinnervation of the recipient muscle takes place within 2 to 8 weeks (as demonstrated by experimental work in rabbits). The ansa hypoglossi nerve is used with muscle pedicles from the anterior belly of the omohyoid, the sternohyoideus, and the sternothyroideus. These pedicles can reach to be implanted in the levator anguli oris and the orbicularis oris, but they cannot reach to the eye. For reconstruction of the orbicularis oculi, Tucker recommended a temporalis muscle pedicle. Minimal clinical experience has been amassed on this technique; in theory, however, it could rehabilitate the face without loss of function, perhaps doing so within a shorter period of time than some other currently used techniques.

## Static Methods of Reconstruction

The static methods of reconstruction of the paralyzed face are the well known techniques of suspension with fascia lata, tendon, or alloplastic materials. Various rhytidoplasties and stabilization with dermal flaps have also been used. Reactivation of the facial muscles by neural reconstitution or muscle transposition supersedes any type of rehabilitation by suspension or skin stretching, except perhaps in the elderly or debilitated patient. These techniques can, however, be complementary.

## Microneurovascular Muscle Transfers

One contribution to reanimation of the paralyzed face is the microneurovascular muscle transfer combined with cross-face nerve graft, ipsilateral nerve graft, or split hypoglossal anastomoses. This technique provides new, vascularized muscle to the face that can produce pull in various directions and accomplish more normal facial anima-

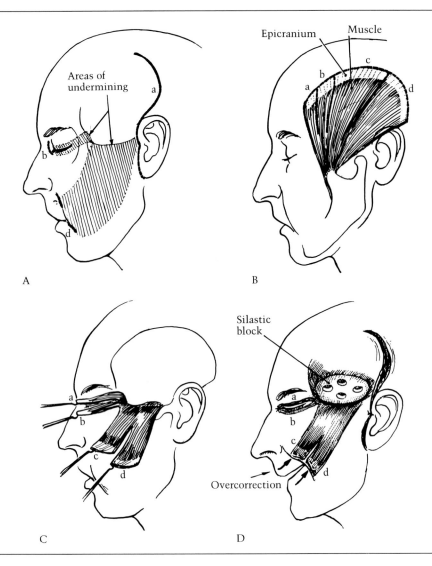

A

B

C

D

**Figure 17-9** *A. Temporalis transposition. Preauricular incision with extension into the scalp. Shaded areas represent undermined tunnels. B. Several centimeters of epicranium are left attached to the temporalis muscle. The entire muscle is elevated, and four or five incisions are made for the slips to be inserted. C. Muscle slips are transposed to the upper and lower eyelids, upper lip and melolabial fold, lower lip and commissure. D. Overcorrection is essential. The muscle is sutured anterior to the melolabial fold and interdigitated with the orbicularis oris muscle in the upper lip.*

tion. The indications for its use are similar to those for regional muscle transfer; the advantage over the latter technique is that the transferred muscle can be reinnervated by a cross-face nerve graft, thereby enhancing control of voluntary facial movement. Despite the success and enthusiasm for this technique, its limitations must be kept in mind and the indications for its use clear. At present, it is merely another alternative in the surgeon's armamentarium of facial reanimation procedures.

HISTORY

Harii [18] was the first to report a successful microvascular transfer of the gracilis muscle to provide elevation of the oral commissure. In the first case, performed in 1973, the motor nerve to the temporalis muscle was employed. In subsequent cases a cross-face nerve graft was anastomosed to the transferred muscle at the second stage. Harii's report on 18 cases demonstrated encouraging results [17]. Two of the major drawbacks were excessive bulk of the transferred muscle and excessive movement. In 1980 O'Brien et al. reported on their experience with favorable results [29].

In 1982 Tolhurst reported on seven cases using the extensor digitorum brevis muscle, with only two satisfactory results. The experience of Harii and O'Brien et al. using the extensor digitorum brevis as a donor muscle was similarly disappointing, and most surgeons no longer use it for facial paralysis reconstruction.

Terzis and Manktelow reported on the use of pectoralis minor muscle for facial reanimation, and Harrison [19] used it as a donor muscle in ten patients with 50 percent excellent results, 30 percent good results, and two failures. The advantages of this muscle are its small, flat configuration, minimal functional loss, and acceptable donor scar. Buncke reported on the successful use of serratus anterior muscle for facial reanimation. More recent reports by Manktelow [22], O'Brien et al. [30], and Harii seem to favor the gracilis as the donor muscle of choice.

CHOICE OF DONOR MUSCLE

The ideal donor muscle provides the following.

*1.* Excursion equal to the normal side of the face

*2.* Reliable vascular and nerve pattern of a size similar to that of the recipient

*3.* Removal of the muscle leaving no functional deficit

*4.* Location distant enough from the face to allow two operating teams to work simultaneously

Numerous muscles have been used for transplantation to the face [38]. The following are those most commonly in use at present.

*1. Gracilis muscle* has a predictable and adequate neurovascular pedicle with adequate bulk but excessive length [16]. Because various portions are supplied by different fascicles, the muscle can be split longitudinally and cut transversely to produce the required size muscle needed for transfer. The initial work of Harii [17, 18] utilized the entire gracilis muscle with the resulting facial bulk and distortion. With the refinements of Manktelow [22], a single fascicle supplying the anterior third of the muscle can be taken with the desired length and bulk.

*2. Pectoralis minor muscle* had adequate weight but excessive length, and its flat shape facilitates insertion in the face. However, as Manktelow [21] pointed out, the neurovascular pedicle is complex and variable, and its motor supply may present significant problems in reinnervation. In addition, the proximity of the upper chest makes simultaneous two-team dissection difficult. Nevertheless, Terzis [38] has been encouraged with the results of using this muscle for facial reanimation.

*3. Latissimus dorsi muscle* and *serratus muscle* have a predictable neurovascular pedicle and longitudinal intramuscular pattern. The latissimus dorsi muscle can be segmentally separated similar to the gracilis to reduce its bulk. The nerve to the serratus is short [16], and usually the lower four segments are utilized. It also requires segmental separation to reduce its bulkiness.

**4.** *Rectus abdominus muscle* is bulky and long but like the previously discussed muscle segments, can be transferred. It has a long, predictable vascular supply and a laterally based segmental nerve supply.

**5.** *Platysma muscle* is a thin facial muscle supplied by the facial artery and cervical branch of the facial nerve. Because of its weight and thinness, Terzis [38], has utilized it for reconstructing the orbicularis oculi.

All of the aforementioned muscles leave minimal or no functional deficit when sacrificed. As operative techniques are refined, the emphasis is toward harvesting well innervated pieces of muscle that have the correct functional length to replace the appropriate facial muscles. There are numerous muscles with a predictable neurovascular supply from which such pieces of muscle may be taken.

OPERATIVE TECHNIQUE
The operative procedure is usually divided into two stages unless the ipsilateral facial nerve can be utilized or the hypoglossal is split and anastomosed. The first stage consists in a classic cross-face nerve graft. If the muscle transfer is to reanimate both eye and mouth, two cross-face nerve grafts are required. Tinel's sign is followed, and about 9 to 12 months later the vascularized muscle is transferred and its neural element anastomosed to the distal end of the cross-face nerve graft.

For the second stage the two-team approach is best: One team prepares the facial nerve graft and recipient vessels (usually the superficial temporal or facial), and the other harvests and prepares the donor muscle on its neurovascular pedicle. It is important to carry out fascicular nerve stimulation of the donor muscle to determine which portion of the muscle each fascicle supplies. Usually the anterior one-third of the gracilis is utilized.

According to Manktelow [21], the zygomaticus major is the single facial muscle that most nearly produces a normal smile. It is approximately 5 cm in length and produces a maximum shortening of 1.5 to 2.0 cm in the normal face. With preoperative observation, the excursion of the oral commissure and shape of the patient's smile can be recorded, and an attempt is made to stimulate the normal side with the transferred muscle. The muscle usually runs from the oral commissure to the body of the zygoma along the normal course of the zygomaticus major. A functioning muscle length of 5 to 6 cm is generally required.

The transferred muscle is sutured into the commisssure and can be interdigitated with any remaining facial muscles in the upper and lower lip, nasolabial fold, and alar base. The site of the muscle's origin depends on the direction of pull desired, usually between the zygomatic arch and tragus.

Determining the correct tension at which the muscle is to be inserted has not yet been demonstrated. Manktelow [22] placed the muscle in enough tension so that under anesthesia it was tight enough to place the paralyzed oral commissure in balance with the normal side. Microvascular anastomoses of artery and vein are completed along with fascicular nerve repair. Overlying skin closure avoids tension on the vascular anastomoses, and drains are kept distant.

RESULTS
The reports of Harrison [19], Harii et al. [17, 18], O'Brien et al. [30], and Manktelow [22] have been encouraging, with most of the results good to excellent. Of the 40 patients studied by O'Brien et al., 35 obtained good symmetry at rest and reasonably active lifting of the angle of the mouth and cheek. In addition, 19 patients obtained independent movements of the face despite the fact that both sides of the face were supplied by the same facial nerve. No satisfactory explanation has been determined for this phenomenon.

It is important to emphasize that movement of the face after microneurovascular muscle transfer is never normal. As pointed out by Rayment [31], it is simplistic to use one reinnervated muscle along one vector to reanimate the oral commissure and upper lip, an area that normally has ten muscles acting on it along different vectors. Patients do learn to produce a definitive smile, but the ability to produce the involuntary, spontaneous "flash" smile rarely returns. Therefore during speech some asymmetry of the face is usually evident. It is also difficult to obtain independent movements in the eye and mouth [22].

Rayment [31] analyzed the problem of poor symmetry of synergistic facial movement in patients who have had successful reinnervation of transplanted muscle. He explained that the adequacy of reinnervation of muscle is directly related to the number of axons that manage to cross the sural nerve graft to the muscle—different ratios of axons to muscle fibers exist for different muscles. Normal facial muscles have about 25 muscle fibers innervated by one axon, whereas gracilis and pectoralis minor muscles have about 150 to 200 muscle fibers to each axon. Muscles with a smaller ratio of muscle fibers to axons, e.g., facial muscles, are capable of producing a wide variety of finely tuned movements [31]. The facial muscles have been described as being "intelligent" and the gracilis and pectoralis minor muscles as "stupid" [38].

With cross-face nerve grafting, even with the most meticulous technique, it has been demonstrated that only 20 to 50 percent of axons cross the nerve graft [19]. The different muscle fiber to axon ratio would explain the poor success of cross-face nerve grafting alone in contrast to combining it with microvascular muscle transfer (muscles requiring few axons to reinnervate a large number of muscle fibers).

INDICATIONS, ADVANTAGES,
AND DISADVANTAGES
Microneurovascular muscle transfer is another alternative for facial reconstruction to alleviate paralysis. Some of the best candidates for this technique are patients with a regional paralysis, especially involving the elevators of the lip, and when the ipsilateral facial nerve is intact, as after trauma or extensive facial tumor resections where the facial muscles have been ablated. Young patients with congenital paralysis or those who have had surgery for an intracranial tumor are well suited to this technique. Old or infirm patients with facial paralysis more often prefer a simple, pragmatic approach to facial reanimation, such as regional muscle transfers.

The main advantage of the technique is that facial movement is provided and controlled by the contralateral facial nerve, providing for better symmetry and perhaps a more definitive smile. Many disadvantages, however, still exist: (1) There are at least two operative stages with a long surgical time. (2) There are two donor site scars. (3) Usually 2 years elapse before return of facial movement. (4) Complete eyelid closure, forehead movement, oral sphincter, and depressor lip function are almost never restored. (5) The technique is not free of synkinesis and deficit of involuntary emotional expression, common to most other rehabilitative techniques.

## References

1. Anderl, H. Reconstruction of the Face Through Cross-Facial Nerve Transplantation in Facial Paralysis. In J. M. Converse (ed.), *Reconstructive Plastic Surgery* (2nd ed.). Philadelphia: Saunders, 1977.
2. Anderl, H. (moderator). Rehabilitation of the Face by VIIth Nerve Substitution (panel discussion no. 6). In U. Fisch (ed.), *Facial Nerve Surgery*. Birmingham, AL: Aesculapius, 1977.
3. Anderl, H. Cross Face Grafting in Facial Palsy. In M. Portman (ed.), *Facial Nerve*. New York: Masson, 1985.
4. Apfelberg, D. B., and Gingrass, R. P. Experimental unicular nerve grafting of the facial nerve. *Plast. Reconstr. Surg.* 55:195, 1975.
5. Ba Huy, P. T., Monteil, J. P., and Rey, A. Re-

sults of Twenty Cases of Trans Facio-Facial Anastomosis as Compared with Those of XII–VII Anastomoses. In M. Portman (ed.), *Facial Nerve.* New York: Masson, 1985.

6. Baker, D. C. Hypoglossal-Facial Nerve Anastomosis: Indications and Limitations. In M. Portman (ed.), *Facial Nerve.* New York: Masson, 1985.

7. Baker, D. C. Reanimation of the Paralyzed Face: Nerve Crossover, Cross-Face Nerve Grafting, and Muscle Transfers. In Chretien et al. (eds.), *Head and Neck Cancer.* Philadelphia: B. C. Decker, 1985.

8. Baker, D. C. Hypoglossal-Facial Nerve Anastomoses. In B. Brent (ed.), *The Artistry of Reconstructive Surgery.* St. Louis: Mosby, 1987.

9. Baker, D. C., and Conley, J. Facial nerve grafting: A thirty year retrospective review. *Clin. Plast. Surg.* 6:343, 1979.

10. Baker, D. C., and Conley, J. Regional muscle transposition for rehabilitation of the paralyzed face. *Clin. Plast. Surg.* 6:317, 1979.

11. Conley, J. J. *Salavary Glands and the Facial Nerve.* Stuttgart: Georg Thieme Verlag, 1975.

12. De Castro Correia, P., and Zani, R. Masseter muscle rotation in the treatment of inferior facial paralysis. *Plast. Reconstr. Surg.* 52:370, 1973.

13. Fisch, U. Facial nerve grafting. *Otolaryngol. Clin. North Am.* 7:517, 1974.

14. Freilinger, G. A new technique to correct facial paralysis. *Plast. Reconstr. Surg.* 56:44, 1975.

15. Hakelius, L. Free muscle grafting. *Clin. Plast. Surg.* 6:301, 1979.

16. Hamilton, S. G., Terzis, J. K., and Carraway, J. T. Surgical Anatomy of the Facial Musculature and Muscle Transplantation. In J. K. Terzis (ed.), *Reconstructive Microreconstruction of Nerve Injuries.* Philadelphia: Saunders, 1987.

17. Harii, K. Microneurovascular free muscle transplantation for reanimation of facial paralysis. *Clin. Plast. Surg.* 6:361, 1979.

18. Harii, K., Ohmori, K., and Torii, S. Free gracilis muscle transplantation with microneurovascular anastomoses for the treatment of facial paralysis. *Plast. Reconstr. Surg.* 57:133, 1976.

19. Harrison, D. H. The pectoralis minor vascularized muscle graft for the treatment of unilateral facial palsy. *Plast. Reconstr. Surg.* 75:206, 1985.

20. Hastings, J. C., and Peacock, E. E. Effect of injury, repair, and ascorbic acid deficiency on collagen accumulation in peripheral nerves. *Surg. Forum* 24:516, 1973.

21. Manktelow, R. T. Discussion of the pectoralis minor vascularized muscle graft for the treatment of unilateral facial palsy. *Plast. Reconstr. Surg.* 75:214, 1985.

22. Manktelow, R. T. Free Muscle Transplantation for Facial Nerve Paralysis. In J. K. Terzis (ed.), *Microreconstruction of Nerve Injuries.* Philadelphia: Saunders, 1987.

23. May, M. Facial paralysis: Differential diagnosis and indications for surgical therapy. *Clin. Plast. Surg.* 6:275, 1979.

24. May, M. *The Facial Nerve.* New York: Thieme, 1986.

25. Miehlke, A. *Surgery of the Facial Nerve.* Philadelphia: Saunders, 1973.

26. Millesi, H. Facial Nerve Suture. In U. Fisch (ed.), *Facial Nerve Surgery.* Birmingham, AL: Aesculapius, 1977. P. 209.

27. Millesi, H. Technique of Free Nerve Grafting in the Face. In L. R. Rubin (ed.), *Reanimation of the Paralyzed Face.* St. Louis: Mosby, 1977.

28. Millesi, H. Nerve suture and grafting to restore the extratemporal facial nerve. *Clin. Plast. Surg.* 6:333, 1979.

29. O'Brien, B. M., Franklin, J. D., and Morrison, W. A. Cross-facial nerve grafts and microneurovascular free muscle transfer for long established facial palsy. *Br. J. Plast. Surg.* 33:202, 1980.

30. O'Brien, B. Mc., and Morrison, W. Facial Palsy. In *Reconstructive Microsurgery.* London: Churchill Livingstone, 1987.

31. Rayment, R., Poole, M. D., and Rushworth, G. Cross-facial nerve transplants: Why are spontaneous smiles not restored? *Br. J. Plast. Surg.* 40:592, 1987.

32. Rubin, L. The Moebius syndrome: Bilateral facial diplegia. *Clin. Plast. Surg.* 3:625, 1976.

33. Rubin, L. *Reanimation of the Paralyzed Face.* St. Louis: Mosby, 1977.

34. Samii, M. Rehabilitation of the Face by VIIth Nerve Substitution (panel discussion no. 6). In U. Fisch (ed.), *Facial Nerve Surgery.* Birmingham, AL: Aesculapius, 1977.

35. Scaramella, L. F. Preliminary report on facial nerve anastomosis. Read before the Second International Symposium on Facial Nerve Surgery, Osaka, Japan, 1970.

36. Scaramella, L. F. On the repair of the injured facial nerve. *Ear Nose Throat J.* 58:45, 1979.

37. Smith, J. W. A new technique of facial reanimation. In J. T. Hueston (ed.), *Transactions of the Fifth International Congress of Plastic and Reconstructive Surgery.* Melbourne: Butterworths, 1971.

38. Terzis, J. K. *Reconstructive Microreconstruction of Nerve Injuries.* Philadelphia: Saunders, 1987.

39. Thompson, N. Autogenous free grafts of skeletal muscle: A preliminary experimental and clinical study. *Plast. Reconstr. Surg.* 48:11, 1971.

40. Thompson, N. A review of autogenous skeletal muscle grafts and their clinical applications. *Clin. Plast. Surg.* 1:349, 1974.

41. Tucker, H. M. Restoration of selective facial nerve function by the nerve-muscle pedicle technique. *Clin. Plast. Surg.* 6:293, 1979.

# 18

# Intraoral Tumors and Radical Neck Dissection for Oral Cancer

It is imperative, if one is to communicate meaningfully about head and neck malignancy, that the T, N, and M classification be understood and memorized [23].

## TNM Classification

T = extent of the primary tumor
N = state of regional lymph nodes
M = metastases

The number appended to each component indicates the state of the disease in relation to that component.

TNM PRETREATMENT
CLINICAL CLASSIFICATION

| | |
|---|---|
| T | Primary tumor |
| $T_{is}$ | Preinvasive cancer (carcinoma in situ) |
| $T_0$ | No evidence of primary tumor |
| $T_1$ | Tumor 2 cm or less in greatest dimension |
| $T_2$ | Tumor more than 2 cm but not more than 4 cm |
| $T_3$ | Tumor more than 4 cm |
| $T_4$ | Tumor with extension to bone muscle, skin, antrum, neck, etc. |
| $T_x$ | Minimum requirements to assess primary tumor cannot be met |

| | |
|---|---|
| N | Regional lymph nodes |
| $N_0$ | No evidence of regional lymph node involvement |
| $N_1$ | Evidence of involvement of movable homolateral regional lymph nodes |
| $N_2$ | Evidence of involvement of movable contralateral or bilateral regional lymph nodes |
| $N_3$ | Evidence of involvement of fixed regional lymph nodes |
| $N_x$ | Minimum requirements to assess the regional nodes cannot be met |

| | |
|---|---|
| M | Distant metastases |
| $M_0$ | No evidence of distant metastases |
| $M_1$ | Evidence of distant metastases |
| $M_x$ | Minimum requirements to assess the presence of distant metastases cannot be met |

| | |
|---|---|
| $p^{TNM}$ | Postsurgery histopathologic classification |
| $p^T$ | Primary tumor—categories correspond to the T categories |
| $p^N$ | Regional lymph nodes—categories correspond to the N categories |
| $p^M$ | Distant metastases—categories correspond to the M categories |

One of the primary functions of the TNM system is to allow staging of disease. This system provides the means to accumulate more accurate statistics if applied correctly.

STAGING

| | | | |
|---|---|---|---|
| Stage 1 | $T_1$ | $N_0$ | $M_0$ |
| Stage 2 | $T_2$ | $N_0$ | $M_0$ |
| Stage 3 | $T_3$ | $N_0$ | $M_0$ |
| Stage 4 | $T_1\ T_2\ T_3\ T_4$ | $N_1$ | $M_0$ |
| | Any T | $N_{01}\ N_1$ | $M_0$ |
| | Any T | $N_2\ N_3$ | $M_0$ |
| | | Any N | $M_1$ |

Although these categories are convenient forms of shorthand, they can be applied only if assessment is accurate. This statement particularly applies to estimate of size, which can be grossly inaccurate particularly in the appreciation of depth of involvement. One must be careful to avoid laying down hard and fast rules of therapy based on the TNM classification. The treatment of each tumor is decided on as a result of the surgeon's experience in the field and appreciation of the biologic behavior of that particular tumor. Obviously, as statistics build up, efficacious treatment trends emerge.

Intraoral tumors are best grouped into the areas involved: tongue, floor of mouth, alveolus (lower), alveolus (upper), palate, buccal, tonsillar fossa, jaws. With some more extensive tumors, the exact location of origin is difficult or impossible to determine.

## Intraoral Cancer

The incidence of this disease varies greatly from one part of the world to another; it accounts for 5 percent of all cancers in the United States [21] and 50 percent in India [94]. This difference is the result of cultural variations, e.g., the excellent oral hygiene in the United States, the high incidence of denture wearing and dental caries in the United Kingdom, and the betel chewing of India.

ETIOLOGIC FACTORS
*Tobacco*
The incidence of intraoral cancer increases as the magnitude and length of tobacco use increases [123]; patients smoking one pack of cigarettes or five or more cigars or pipes per day have an incidence six times that of nonsmokers [97]. It is of interest to note that successfully treated intraoral cancer patients who continue to smoke have a 40 percent chance of developing a new lesion compared with 6 percent of nonsmokers [69]. Smokers have lower 5-year survival statistics [69, 97].

Holding chewing tobacco or snuff against the mucosa produces the typical variant of verrucous carcinoma [109]. It appears that national incidences of snuff-induced oral cancer are directly related to the content of nitrosamines in the snuff [45]. As mentioned above, the habit of chewing "the betel" (tobacco leaf, betel leaves, powdered betal nut, and slaked lime) causes a high incidence of intraoral carcinoma; in this situation tobacco is probably the significant substance [59, 94]. Hard palate cancer can be caused by the bizarre practice of reversed cigar smoking, as done in India and parts of South America [59, 82].

*Alcohol*
Heavy alcohol consumption is associated with a sixfold increase in acrodigestive cancer compared with that in nondrinkers [48]. Carcinoma of the floor of the mouth is particularly associated with alcoholism [87]. Moreover, the tumor stage is frequently more advanced. For oral cancer, this figure increases to 15 times when alcohol and tobacco are combined [84].

*Other Factors*
It is difficult to prove that dietary deficiencies play a part in oral cancer causation, but they could be part of its relation with excessive alcohol intake, e.g., riboflavin [122]. Denture wearing and poor oral hygiene certainly seem to be associated factors. The Plummer-Vinson syndrome of iron deficiency in women over middle age results in atrophic intraoral mucosal changes and a significantly higher incidence of intraoral cancer in this group than in the general population [124].

PATHOLOGY
Intraoral malignant lesions are predominantly (more than 90 percent) squamous carcinoma. The other tumors are melanoma, lymphoma, sarcoma, and, perhaps most frequently, malignancy of the minor salivary glands: mucoepidermoid and adenoid cystic carcinoma.

## Leukoplakia

Leukoplakia, literally "a white patch," is a premalignant lesion. The description indicates thickening of the superficial mucosal layer. The rete ridges of the basal layer extend into the submucosa (acanthosis). As more dysplasia of the cells occurs, the spectrum moves toward malignancy; the lesion essentially remains premalignant, although this state may be difficult to differentiate histologically. The occurrence of erythema around the white patch is suggestive of significant change and merits biopsy [62, 90]. In one large series where pure leukoplakia was biopsied, the incidence of in situ carcinoma was 1.8 percent and invasive carcinoma 8.1 percent [117]. *If in doubt, biopsy is justified.*

## Squamous Carcinoma

Squamous carcinoma is typically an ulcerated lesion with indurated edges. It may project from the surface (exophytic) or infiltrate deeply (endophytic). Verrucous carcinoma is a particular lesion that is raised above the surface having multiple papillae. More than one tumor may be present at the same time or at intervals.

In the past it was typical to grade squamous carcinoma as high or low grade, well or poorly differentiated lesions, but this grading is subjective and of limited value [51]. the variation between tumors showing well differentiated epithelial pearls, low pleomorphism, and few mitosis and those with poor differentiation, extensive pleomorphism, and abundant mitosis is considerable. Many lesions contain variable patterns. Probably more important in terms of treatment and prognosis are the size of the tumor and the depth of penetration.

## Metastatic Lesions

Intraoral cancer metastasizes to neck nodes. A convenient division of nodal areas was suggested by Strong and Spiro [111]: The submandibular area is level I; upper, middle, and lower jugular nodes are levels II, III, IV, respectively; and the posterior triangle is

level V. In level I are metastases from the floor of the mouth, the lip, and the anterior cheek mucosa. In level II the metastases are from tongue, tonsil, retromolar triangle, and posterior gingiva. These upper levels spread to lower areas. The posterior triangle is rarely involved independently with spread from an intraoral lesion. Large lesions metastasize more frequently than small ones. A significant number of people have neck node involvement at time of the initial consultation. Lip and palate carcinoma have a lower incidence of metastases than do other intraoral lesions. A positive neck node reduces the prognosis by 50 percent compared to a lesion without metastatic spread [105]. Multiple nodal involvement, especially low in the neck, or extracapsular spread greatly diminishes the chance of tumor eradication [92].

## Distant Metastases

Tumors of the intraoral cavity do not show widespread metastases until late in the disease course. The main areas involved are lungs and bone. Metastasis usually occurs with disease remaining in the head and neck region.

## TREATMENT

The site and size of the lesion determines the treatment choice. Small lesions (stage 1) can be excised or irradiated. In terms of patient convenience, anterior lesions are excised and posterior lesions may be irradiated. Stage II and III lesions usually receive combined therapy. Irradiation may be done pre- or postoperatively; the latter is more popular and can be given in larger doses, 4 to 6000 rad [47, 60].

Postoperative radiotherapy is given after excision of large primaries ($T_3$ or $T_4$), with extensive nodal metastases ($N_2$ or $N_3$), or when excision is incomplete. The commencement of therapy must not be delayed longer than healing of the surgical wound. If possible, the primary tumor is excised through the mouth. If it is too large or is situated posteriorly, the lip is split and the cheek and upper neck flap are elevated using a buccal sulcus incision. If this incision is insufficient for exposure, the mandible is split in the midline, and through an incision in the floor of the mouth it is swung back to give excellent exposure—the *mandibular swing.* Early mandibular involvement, e.g., in squamous cell carcinoma of the alveolus, may allow localized resection of the mandible, with preservation of the lower border. More significant involvement calls for resection of the involved area as a *total* mandibular block. In this situation, the inferior dental nerve must be biopsied to eliminate any tumor spread along the nerve. Involvement of skin requires full-thickness resection of all layers including the mandible, if involved. In the upper alveolus and palate, the underlying bone is frequently removed, the extent depending on the involvement: It can range from removal of the alveolus to partial or total maxillectomy. In the latter cases a Weber-Ferguson incision may be necessary. It is rarely necessary to use the classic subciliary extension. More extensive procedures may be required to effect complete eradication of the tumor, among which are infratemporal fossa resection and removal of orbital contents.

## Nerve Involvement

Symptoms of numbness over the trigeminal area, facial palsy, and facial pain suggest nerve involvement. The symptoms are usually due to invasion and extension along the epineural spaces, frequently referred to as perineural lymphatic invasion. It is an adverse prognostic sign. For extensive tumors in the infratemporal fossa with signs of trigeminal involvement, it is recommended that the first step in surgical treatment be a temporal craniotomy. The trigeminal ganglion is exposed in Meckel's cave and is biopsied. If the specimen contains tumor, the lesion is considered unresectable, as the tumor is now intracerebral. It is ascertained prior to surgery if the patient would wish a resection after this diagnosis. We advise against it because of the resulting functional and cosmetic deformity in an incurable situation.

## Neck Dissection

Neck dissection becomes more complex, as a degree of conservation has crept into surgical management of the neck. Despite claims to the contrary by radiotherapists [86, 121], when possible a clinically positive neck should always undergo node dissection.

Some recommend a standard radical neck dissection in any involved neck [61], whereas other authorities use a modified dissection only in selected cases [13]. It is important to realize that 50 percent of positive necks have a recurrence in the neck after having had radical dissection alone [35]. Although not absolutely necessary, it is beneficial, when possible, to resect the primary and the neck nodes as one block specimen. If for the exposure to the primary lesion a lip cheek flap is used in the presence of an $N_0$ neck, a modified neck dissection or a supraomohyoid dissection may be used. In the short, thick neck of a patient who may well develop a metastasis, which would be difficult to detect early, a prophylactic neck dissection is advocated. Unreliable patients, who may not return for follow-up, are treated in a similar fashion. About one-third of clinical $N_0$ necks have microscopic nodal involvement. If the dissection contains positive nodes, postoperative radiotherapy (5000 rad) is given.

## Chemotherapy

Some drugs with an antitumor effect, e.g., methotrexate, bleomycin, cisplatinum (cisdiamino-dichloroplatinum), induce a short remission alone or in conjunction with external irradiation in 70 percent of patients with untreated tumors that are advanced and judged to be untreatable [11, 52, 80, 120]. It is important to realize that preoperative chemotherapy may reduce tumor size considerably, but the resection is based on the pretreatment tumor dimensions.

## Special Areas

### TONGUE

Although the main incidence of tongue carcinoma is in the 60-year-old group, it can occur in young adults and even in adolescents [18]. The tongue is the most common site for intraoral malignancy. Probably owing to increased alcohol and tobacco consumption, the incidence in women has increased to 26 percent [107].

The site of most tongue cancers is the anterior two-thirds on the lateral borders or the ventral surface. It is rare to have a lesion in the midline or on the dorsum. Just over one-third of tongue cancers arise behind the circumvallate papillae.

The lesion is painless and thus is often neglected. Pain, difficulty with speech, and difficulty swallowing are late symptoms. The lesion arises as an ulcer with indurated edges on the lateral border of the anterior two-thirds of the tongue. Progression involves an increase in size and depth with eventual involvement of the tongue muscles. It is frequently larger to palpation than inspection. Locally it spreads to the floor of the mouth and with continued growth invades the mandible. Restricted tongue movement indicates extensive muscle infiltration.

The usual presentation is that of a $T_2$ tumor (2.1 to 4.0 cm). The oral tongue shows 30 percent lymph node metastasis on presentation. In one series, 5 percent had bilateral involvement, and 60 percent had involvement of the tongue base; of that 60 percent, 29 percent had bilateral neck disease [54]. The most frequently involved nodes are the submandibular, subdigastric, and midjugular. Involvement of submental, low jugular, and posterior triangle nodes is rare.

### Treatment

For $T_1$ lesions surgery and irradiation are equally effective. Wedge resection is simple, can be performed under local anesthesia, and causes little or no morbidity. If the chosen treatment is radiotherapy, the current preference is for local implantation of radioactive sources, e.g., radium needles or iridium 192 wire [15, 85]. It is now more popular to place hollow nylon tubes and then after-load the tubes with the radioactive wires [78]. There may be much tongue swelling, and a tracheostomy may be necessary; but a high dose of radiation can be delivered (up to 10,000 rad) by this method.

With large lesions, e.g., $T_2$, removal is by partial glossectomy through the mouth. Should this exposure be too limited, the lower lip is split and the cheek lifted as a flap by an incision through the buccal sulcus. If there is mandibular involvement, upper or total block mandibular resection is performed depending on the degree of invasion. Neck dissection is undertaken with $T_2$ to $T_3$ lesions with $N_0$ necks [106]. Some recommend radiotherapy to the neck in this situation rather than surgery [3, 68]. Extensive lesions requiring mandibulectomy are given 5000 rad of radiation as soon as the wounds are adequately healed. With more extensive involvement, a chemotherapy regimen may be added.

### Results

The reported overall 5-year cure rate is 49.1 percent [107]. The corresponding figure for irradiation alone is 45 percent [57]. Ninety percent of $T_1$ lesions can be controlled by partial glossectomy [118] or interstitial radiotherapy [24, 78]. The two factors that influence prognosis are size of lesion and presence of nodal involvement. One series reported the 5-year cure rate for stage I disease to be 69.2 percent, stage II 52.7 percent, and stage III 36.6 percent [107]. In another series of cancer of the tongue and base of the tongue, 71 percent of patients were treated surgically and 82 percent with surgery plus radiotherapy. The overall 5-year survival rate was 42 percent. For stage I and II disease it was 71 percent for the oral tongue and 33 percent for the tongue base. For stages III and IV disease the corresponding results were 31 percent and 16 percent, respectively [20]. What can improve on these figures is not a new surgical or radiotherapeutic technique but earlier presentation of the patient.

FLOOR OF THE MOUTH

Carcinoma of the floor of the mouth occurs most frequently around the age of 60, and its incidence approaches that of tongue carcinoma. The male/female ratio is between 3:1 and 4:1 [37]. The causative factors seem to be alcohol and tobacco consumption.

The site of most occurrences is usually anterior, although it may be in the midline. By the time the patient presents, it is not unusual to find submandibular lymph node enlargement due to metastasis. The submandibular gland itself may be distended owing to blockage of Wharton's duct.

The lesion begins as an inflamed superficial ulcer, sometimes with associated leukoplakia. As the condition progresses, the ulcer deepens. The edges become more distinct, and it may involve the base of the tongue and the lingual aspect of the alveolus. In fewer than 50 percent of cases, it is localized to the floor of the mouth on first presentation [42, 49]. Further spread may be to the retromolar trigone and tonsillar pillar. In a study of 320 patients, 27 percent of the lesions were stage I, 22 percent stage II, 26 percent stage III, and 25 percent stage IV [93].

Bimanual palpation indicates deep infiltration. There may be penetration to involve neck skin. Adherence to the mandible usually indicates periosteal involvement; mandibular invasion is a late stage of the condition, and it is probably best picked up preoperatively at an early stage by bone scans and other radiographs. Lymph node involvement at presentation varies from 39 to 63 percent [8, 29, 42, 49]. The submandibular nodes are most frequently involved, followed by the jugulodigastric, the mid-jugular, and rarely the submental, low jugular, and posterior triangle nodes. Stage I tumors are seen in 20 percent of patients, and approximately 50 percent have stage III or IV

disease. A submandibular mass causing confusion between gland enlargement due to duct obstruction or nodal enlargement due to tumor metastasis can be differentiated by fine needle aspiration.

*Treatment*

Small lesions are most conveniently treated by excision, although radiotherapy is equally effective. The defect is reconstructed by direct suture, skin grafting, or spontaneous healing. Any of these procedures may result in stenosis of the submandibular duct and resultant enlargement of the submandibular gland. Radiotherapy is usually given as a combination of external irradiation and interstitial implantation [78]. When large cancers remain localized to the floor, they may be removed through a perioral approach. Even by this approach, the inner cortex of the mandible or the alveolus can be resected in continuity.

$T_3$ or $T_4$ lesions require a lip split, cheek flap procedure for exposure. Usually the base of the tongue and a portion of the mandible (partial or total segment) are also excised. Maintenance of the lower border of the mandible [40] or immediate osseous reconstruction with a composite free flap greatly diminishes the aesthetic and functional defect following these resections, especially in the midline. For the $N_0$ neck, observation may be chosen, which can be difficult if the submandibular glands become enlarged. A biopsy may be necessary. If a cheek flap is being used, it is convenient to proceed with an incontinuity neck dissection. Others choose to irradiate the neck instead of performing a dissection. When the neck is clinically positive, a neck dissection is performed. In bilateral cases the dissections are staged. In our hands and in others, there has been considerable morbidity with simultaneous bilateral neck dissection [70]. Extensive nodal involvement or large primary tumors necessitate combined surgery, radiotherapy, and chemotherapy.

*Results*

Stage I and II lesions have 70 to 90 percent 5-year cure rates with excision and interstitial radiotherapy. Large lesions have a much poorer prognosis, ranging from 30 to 60 percent. Fortunately, fewer of these cases are being seen because patients present at an earlier stage. The overall 5-year survival rate has been reported as 65 percent [93].

LOWER ALVEOLUS–GINGIVA

The lower alveolus is the third most common site of intraoral cancer. It rarely occurs in individuals below 50 years of age. Men are affected two to three times more often than women [72]. The ratio of lower alveolus carcinoma to that occurring in the upper alveolus is reported to be 80 percent to 20 percent; of the former, 60 percent lie behind the bicuspid teeth [19]. These authors showed tobacco to be high on the list of causes: 94 percent of the men were smokers, whereas only 48 percent of the women smoked. There is a tendency for multiple lesions to develop in these patients.

The presentation is one of ulceration with or without pain. Denture wearers may be unable to wear their prosthesis because of tumor bulk or pain. Frequently referral is from a dentist, as patients often consult the dentist in the first instance.

The lesion usually arises on the alveolar ridge rather than on the lingual or buccal areas. The spread is lateral rather than deep initially. If there is a carious tooth with a resulting cavity in the alveolus, there can be bony invasion at an early stage. When the cancellous bone is invaded, the neurovascular bundle is at risk. This situation opens an avenue for tumor extension along the nerve without related bony involvement. It is interesting to note that the number of small alveolar tumors are increasing, indicating earlier referrals, but the amount of bone and adjacent structure involvement remains the same [19].

Regional node metastasis is more common with carcinoma of the lower alveolus than of the upper alveolus. Nodal involvement is most common in the jugulodigastric, submaxillary, and mid-jugular regions. It is rare in the lower jugular, submental, and posterior triangle areas.

*Treatment*

For $T_1N_0$ lesions, a localized excision with marginal mandibular resection can be accomplished through the mouth. This technique is efficacious from the point of view of tumor excision, and there is much less deformity than with block mandibular resection [116]. More extensive lesions with more significant mandibular involvement require a lip split, cheek flap, and segmental mandibular resection.

In the upper jaw a partial maxillectomy is performed through a modified Weber-Ferguson incision. With more invasive lesions that have broken into the maxillary antrum, total maxillectomy is indicated.

With an $N_0$ neck and a large tumor requiring a cheek flap, it is convenient to perform an elective neck dissection. Palpable nodes make this procedure mandatory.

Small tumors may be treated with external beam irradiation. This therapy is not advised for large invading tumors, as osteoradionecrosis may occur. After large tumors have been resected, or in the case of a positive neck, irradiation is employed.

*Results*

A 20-year review by Cady and Catlin [19] showed that the 5-year survival rate increased from 35 to 64 percent. This increase is probably due to increasingly earlier diagnosis. For localized disease, the survival rate increased to 80 percent; when level 1 nodes were involved, survival was 54 percent compared to 35 percent survival when there was involvement of nodes at all levels.

MacComb and Fletcher [57] showed, in 101 patients with lower alveolar cancers, that 48 percent were disease-free during the observation time. With stage I disease survival was 78 percent, with stage II 64 percent, with stage III 35 percent, and with stage IV 15 percent. These results were better than those achieved by radiation therapy.

## RETROMOLAR TRIGONE

The retromolar trigone is an indefinite area covered under the terms posterior floor of mouth, posterior alveolus, and anterior pillar of fauces. The main points of significance about this region are that diagnosis may be delayed, it is less accessible, and reconstruction is somewhat more difficult.

## BUCCAL MUCOSA

Squamous carcinoma of the buccal mucosa is a disease of the elderly, i.e., those over 65. It accounts for only 10 percent of intraoral cancers. The male/female ratio is 3:1 [28]. There is a high incidence of carcinoma of the buccal mucosa in India, where it occurs at an earlier age than in the West [98]. In the southern United States a similar picture is seen in "snuff dippers," who develop due to tobacco chewing [109]. Other causative factors are trauma from the teeth, leukoplakia, alcohol, and tobacco.

The lesions begin as flat, erythematous, roughened areas, later becoming ulcerated; finally the base is indurated. Pain is not common but, when present, is a poor prognostic sign. The lesion may erode the cheek, involve the oral commissure, or spread onto the upper or lower alveolus. Eleven percent of these patients have stage I lesions and 26 percent stage II. Involved cervical nodes are present initially in 37 to 44 percent [28]. The submandibular nodes are usually involved, but there may be direct spread to the jugulodigastric, preparotid, and mid-jugular nodes. Lower cervical, submental, and posterior triangle nodes are rarely involved.

## Treatment

For early small lesions, excision and radiotherapy are equally effective. Large, indurated lesions may require full-thickness resection of the cheek with a variety of flap reconstructions [6, 28]. Maxillectomy and mandibulectomy are indicated if invaded by tumor. Radical neck dissection is recommended for the involved neck or in the $N_0$ neck when it is encroached on by the resection of the primary tumor. Postoperative irradiation is recommended in patients with incomplete resection and stage III and IV disease.

## Results

In one series that contained 65 percent of $T_1$ and $T_2$ tumors, the 5-year cure rate was 70 percent [57]. Salvage was as follows: stage I, 92 percent; stage II, 86 percent; stage III, 65 percent; stage IV, 15 percent.

In another study, the 5-year cure rate was 51 percent. In this group 21 percent had required further treatment for recurrence. Among patients with $N_0$ disease, 56 percent were salvaged; whereas among those with involved cervical nodes, only 23 percent were alive at 5 years [74].

## PALATE

Squamous carcinoma of the palate is a disease of older patients (over 65). Most (80 percent) are men [81]. The condition is infrequent in the Western world. The causative agents are tobacco and alcohol, and in India there is a thermal element due to reversed smoking [82]. Often there is associated leukoplakia.

The patient notices a swelling on the palate, and there may be bleeding, occasionally pain, or problems with denture fitting. Palatal cancers may be ulcerated or exophytic; bone invasion is a late occurrence [81]. The palatal bone, nasal cavity, or maxillary antrum may be invaded, which is best assessed by computed tomographic (CT) scanning. There may be lateral spread to the buccal sulcus and cheek. Advanced tumors are associated with pain, a foul smell, and difficulty swallowing. Nodal involvement is seen in 16 percent of hard palate cancers and 37 percent of soft palate lesions [50]. The submandibular and upper jugular groups are most often involved. Rarely are the retropharyngeal nodes affected, except with posterior palatal lesions.

*Treatment*
Resection with underlying bone through the mouth is advocated. Radiotherapy may cause bone exposure and necrosis. With more extensive lesions, a partial hemimaxillectomy is performed through a Weber-Ferguson incision and the defect reconstructed with a skin graft and a prosthesis. More extensive lesions require total hemimaxillectomy. So long as the inferior periorbitum (Lockwood's ligament) is not breached, there is no change in position of the eye and no double vision. Cervical node involvement requires neck dissection, which includes the parotid region. Radiotherapy is given for large tumors, incompletely excised tumors, and after neck dissection.

*Results*
The 5-year survival rate is reportedly 31 percent [18]. In another report, radiotherapy plus surgery or radiotherapy alone gave a 40 percent 3-year survival rate [50]. If the lesion is smaller than 3 cm, the salvage rate is 56 to 86 percent. Ratzer et al. [81] stated that only 8 percent with involved neck nodes on admission were alive and well over the long term.

TONSIL
In the oropharyngeal area, the most frequent site for squamous carcinoma is the tonsil. Because the condition presents late (60 to 80 percent are stage III or IV), the overall prognosis is poor. The lesion presents as an indurated ulcer, and there may be pain. About 76 percent of patients present with nodal involvement and in 11 percent it is bilateral [44]. Local areas may be invaded, with the soft palate, pharynx, and tongue being equally involved. With large lesions, tongue involvement is common. Spread is to the jugulodigastric, mid-jugular, submandibular, lower jugular, and posterior triangle nodes.

*Treatment*
Stage I and II lesions are resected and closed directly with local flaps or distant flaps, as indicated. Neck dissection is performed because of the likelihood of nodal involvement. Stage III and IV lesions require wide local resection with appropriate reconstruction, neck dissection, and postoperative radiotherapy.

*Results*
The overall 5-year survival is 24 to 57 percent. With a negative neck, the 5-year survival ranges from 42 to 70 percent. In the presence of a positive neck, the figures range from 0 to 50 percent.

NONSQUAMOUS CARCINOMA
Nonsquamous carcinomas account for fewer than 10 percent of intraoral cancers, but more than one-half of malignant tumors on the palate fall into this group. They are tumors of the minor salivary glands, malignant melanomas, sarcomas, and lymphomas.

*Minor Salivary Gland Tumors*
Minor salivary gland tumors have the same pathology as tumors of the major glands: mucoepidermoid cancer, adenoid cystic carcinoma, and adenocarcinoma. Of the swellings of these minor glands, 85 percent are malignant; and most of these lesions are adenoid cystic carcinomas [108]. The most common site of origin is the palate. The average age is during the sixth decade, men and women being equally affected.

These lesions present as enlarging symptomless masses under the mucosa. Pain is not infrequent, particularly with recurrences. They are slow-growing and may have been present for many months or years before the patient seeks treatment.

The preferred treatment is surgery. Small lesions can be resected through the mouth; if the maxilla is involved, it is resected en bloc. Neck node involvement is not common, occurring in fewer than 25 percent of patients. Thus dissection is performed only for positive nodes or where resection of the primary tumor encroaches on the neck.

Minor salivary gland tumors may respond to radiotherapy, so it is given when resection has been incomplete. Chemotherapy appears to be of no value.

The 10-year survival rate is around 40 percent, but patients can live for many years with recurrent adenoid cystic carcinoma and remain active and well, even with distant metastases.

*Malignant Melanoma*
Fewer than 10 percent of malignant melanomas originate in the mucosa, and 25 to 50 percent of these lesions are intraoral [27, 91]. They usually occur in the 60- to 70-year age group, and the male/female ratio is 2:1. Most of the lesions are on the hard and soft palates [41].

Intraoral pigmentation is common in black patients; it is rare in whites and, if present, must be examined carefully. The lesions are flat or slightly raised and are frequently speckled with light and dark areas. They may show considerable local spread at the time of initial presentation.

Wide resection is recommended with neck dissection for involved nodes or when resection of the primary lesion encroaches on the neck. Elective neck dissection is not advised. The survival is depressing: Only 10 to 15 percent of patients are alive 5 years after adequate surgery. Irradiation and chemotherapy have little to offer.

## Reconstruction
Resection of intraoral tumors may have a significant effect on appearance and function. Sacrifice of the tongue interferes with speech and swallowing; mandibular resection causes chewing problems, and if it is in the symphyseal area there is drooling and an

"Andy Gump" deformity. Lip resection may also cause drooling and speech articulation disorders. Maxillectomy may make speech unintelligible; if the floor of the orbit is sacrificed with the overlying periorbita, there may be dystopia of the globe and double vision. Resection in the pterygoid fossa area may produce trismus.

Reconstructing complex defects often necessitates complex and staged techniques, and judgment is required as to when it should be done. One must take into consideration the patient's age and state of health, the biology of the tumor and whether it is primary or recurrent, the likelihood of further recurrence, the ultimate prognosis, and the experience of the reconstructive surgeon with these techniques. There are a few *essential* goals: restoration of swallowing, intelligible speech, prevention of drooling, avoidance of salivary fistulas. Moreover, an acceptable aesthetic result must be achieved if possible.

The techniques used for reconstruction of defects following excision of intraoral cancer have been extensively covered in other publications [26, 67]. It is important to remember that radiotherapy is prejudicial to successful reconstruction. In this situation, the importation of well vascularized tissue is almost mandatory.

SMALL DEFECTS
Floor-of-mouth defects may be closed directly, especially when the alveolus has been sacrificed. In selected cases this technique gives a rapid, complication-free reconstruction. If, however, there is significant tongue tethering, it can interfere with speech and perhaps with swallowing. Direct approximation is ideally suited for the tongue and buccal mucosa.

Tongue flaps of varying design can be utilized [36, 89], but once again care must be taken not to tether the tongue. A posteriorly based lateral flap to reconstruct a tonsillar defect can be most useful [22].

## LARGE DEFECTS

In many areas, side-of-tongue defects and floor-of-mouth defects without exposure of bone and buccal mucosa can be reconstructed with split skin grafts. Tie-over dressings are messy, and thus the "quilting" technique [66] is recommended with stab drainage incisions of the graft between the quilting sutures. With the anterior midline floor-of-mouth flap, cover is essential; otherwise the tongue is pulled forward by scarring. The tongue displacement results in severe functional defects in phonation and swallowing. This situation can be prevented by reconstructing the defect with one or (more usually) two nasolabial flaps tunneled through the cheeks and laid into the floor of the mouth [25, 125]. The pedicles are divided at 10 to 14 days. If teeth are present, bite blocks are inserted to prevent premature pedicle division. To further ensure tongue mobility with large resections, any raw area on the undersurface of the tongue is resurfaced with a "quilted" split-thickness skin graft.

For large defects, distant pedicled skin flaps have been used: (1) the forehead flap based on the superficial temporal vessels [65]; (2) cervical apron flap on the facial vessels [126]; (3) deltopectoral flap on the internal mammary perforators [5]; (4) pectoralis major myocutaneous flap on the acromiothoracic axis [1, 2, 46]; (5) trapezius myocutaneous flap on the transverse cervical vessels [64]; (6) latissimus dorsi myocutaneous flap on the lateral thoracic vessels [75, 79]; (7) platysma myocutaneous flap on the facial vessels [38]; and (8) sternomastoid myocutaneous flap from the occipital vessels [55, 76].

The *most reliable distant pedicled flaps* are prepared from the forehead, deltopectoral muscle, cervical apron, pectoralis major myocutaneous muscle, trapezius muscle, and latissimus dorsi muscle. *Less reliable flaps* are obtained from the sternomastoid muscle and the platysma muscle.

The flaps most frequently used for intraoral reconstruction are from the deltopectoral and pectoralis major myocutaneous muscles. The latter is good for providing bulk, especially after large resections of tongue. The next best choices are trapezius and cervical flaps. The forehead flap, although reliable and much used in the past, is rarely used now because of the unaesthetic donor defect, which is split-skin-grafted. The latissimus is not suitable for intraoral reconstruction, and the platysma and sternomastoid muscles are less reliable especially after neck dissection.

Bone may be carried with the trapezius flap (spine of scapula) [77], the latissimus dorsi (ribs on the serratus anterior branch) [4], serratus anterior (ribs), pectoralis major (ribs) [30], pectoralis major (sternum) [39], and sternomastoid (clavicle) [96]. The *reliability* of these flaps, in descending order, is as follows: trapezius, latissimus/serratus anterior, pectoralis (ribs), pectoralis major (sternum), and sternomastoid.

These flaps are used for mandibular reconstruction, either unilaterally or bilaterally. The trapezius flap is by far the best, with or without a skin island. The latissimus flap with ribs gives the advantage of wide separation of the soft tissue and bone, which allows more flexibility in the reconstruction. With the other flaps, the blood supply to the bone is precarious. A method that must be mentioned is use of vascularized skull on the superficial temporal vessels and galea [31], which has been utilized for palate alveolus and mandible reconstruction. The reconstruction can be covered by a skin graft on the galea.

## FREE TISSUE TRANSFER

### Mucosal Replacement

Mucosal replacement may well be the preferred method of "instant" reconstruction. Many flaps have been used for the lining, but those that provide the best replacement are the radial forearm flap [102], ulnar forearm flap [56], scapular flap [33], lateral arm flap [88], and dorsalis pedis flap [53, 63]. Of these flaps, at the moment, the radial and ulnar forearm flaps and the scapular flap are the favorites, although some of the others have their advocates. There has been some popularity for the use of jejunal patches [83], but unfortunately the jejunal mucosa may be somewhat exuberant and may continue to produce mucus. Small doses of radiotherapy have been given to flatten the mucosa and reduce secretions.

### Mucosa and Bone Replacement

The flaps that can carry bone and replace primarily mandible [30] are the radial forearm flap [104], scapular flap [113], dorsalis pedis flap [58], and iliac flap based on the deep circumflex iliac vessels [112]. Those most commonly used are the scapular flap and the radial forearm flap.

### OTHER RECONSTRUCTIVE MEASURES

Postmaxillectomy defects are skin-grafted, and a dental prosthesis is placed in the defect. Most patients are happy with the results and do not ask for further reconstruction. Simply filling the maxillary defect gives a good result from many points of view [9]; however, it is unlikely to aid dental rehabilitation and may in fact make matters worse because of the softness of the reconstruction. Probably a vascularized cranial bone graft gives the best results.

Late mandibular reconstruction can be performed with conventional free bone grafts of rib or iliac crest or with a metal tray filled with cancellous bone [16]. These grafts are prone to resorption in the case of bone and to exposure in the case of trays and metallic implants. These problems are particularly significant in postradiotherapy patients. The best and most secure results are obtained by free vascularized bone transfers. Unfortunately, many of these patients wear dentures for appearance, but the dentures are not functional. The increasing use of osseointegration may reverse this unsatisfactory situation.

## Complications

Some of the complications are the same as those of any surgical procedure: infection, hematoma, skin necrosis. In this anatomic area, however, salivary fistula may occur as well and be difficult to deal with in the irradiated patient. The incidence of complications is increased when a simultaneous neck dissection is performed. If the carotid artery is exposed in the wound, especially if it is bathed in saliva and there has been previous irradiation, there is a considerable risk of catastrophic hemorrhage. Immediate cover with a muscle flap is advocated, which may be performed prophylactically at the time of neck dissection [101].

Because many patients have had a high alcohol intake, they must be observed postoperatively for delerium tremens. Parenteral vitamin B complex is administered when indicated.

Operative mortality is low but can be as high as 18 percent in elderly patients having extensive resection [20].

## Neck Dissection

There is much confusion about the terminology associated with neck dissection. For accurate record-keeping and publications, this problem needs to be clarified [7]. Definitions are therefore listed below.

*Suprahyoid neck dissection:* Submandibular gland and adjacent lymph nodes as well as submental and facial vessel lymph nodes are removed.

*Supraomohyoid neck dissection:* Contents of the suprahyoid triangle, jugulodigastric, and mid-jugular lymph nodes together with nodes from the posterior triangle along the accessory chain are removed. (This procedure is a staging operation in a clinically negative neck with a suspicion of metastasis rather than a therapeutic procedure. If the jugular nodes are negative, involvement of the accessory group is unlikely.)

*Modified radical neck dissection:* The internal jugular, accessory nerve, and sternomastoid muscle are spared.

*Functional neck dissection:* The accessory nerve alone is spared.

*Radical neck dissection* [61]: All structures mentioned above are sacrificed. In addition, other structures such as skin, strap muscles, and external carotid may be resected. (This procedure is probably too radical to be an elective operation. It does not remove all the nodes, has significant morbidity, and is associated with an appreciable recurrence rate.)

The latter two points should be addressed. To increase the number of nodes removed, specific drainage areas must be considered. Any lesion draining to the parotid area must have that area of drainage removed. The same goes for the postauricular, occipital, facial vessel, retropharyngeal, thyroid, and perithyroid nodes.

The justification for the functional dissection, which reduces shoulder morbidity by preserving the accessory nerve, is that accessory nodal involvement is low and recurrence in this area is not increased. The accessory nerve can be preserved in all elective dissections but is sacrificed when the tumor is in close proximity.

## MODIFIED RADICAL NECK DISSECTION

The modified neck dissection is more time-consuming than the more radical procedures and is accomplished by retraction of the sternomastoid or preferably by dividing its lower end and elevating it for exposure [13, 14, 99]. At completion of the procedure, it is sutured back in place. This latter technique is advocated as being easier and quicker. The modified technique has taken over as the treatment of choice for elective procedures. Despite statements to the contrary [34], shoulder dysfunction results when the accessory nerve is sacrificed, causing drooping,

heaviness, pain, and decreased range of movement [71]. These symptoms do not occur in every patient, but they do become more significant as age increases. This situation is much improved in patients having a modified neck dissection. Preservation of the sternomastoid muscle reduces the cosmetic defect, and the intact internal jugular vein minimizes head and neck edema [95]. Necks with problems bilaterally must be staged if both internal jugular veins are to be removed (rarely indicated). Simultaneous bilateral neck dissection calls for the preservation of at least one internal jugular vein. Failure to provide such salvage leads to massive edema, cyanosis, and extreme discomfort; this situation improves, but frequently the edema and cyanosis do not resolve completely.

## RULES OF NECK DISSECTION

1. Perform an elective neck dissection for large tumors ($T_3$ and $T_4$), in cases where the primary lesion is easier to resect with the neck, in obese patients, and in unreliable follow-up patients.

2. Modified dissection is suitable for clinical $N_0$ or $N_1$ necks and for the pathologic $N_1$ neck without extracapsular spread.

3. Bilateral dissection, either therapeutic or elective, is appropriate for lesions close to the midline and is usually staged.

4. Multiple nodal involvement, a node more than 3 cm in size, or extracapsular spread calls for postoperative radiation therapy at no later than 6 weeks (5000 rad in 5 weeks or 6000 rad in 6 weeks).

5. High numbers of false-positive results on clinical examination may be due to submandibular gland enlargement caused by blockage of Wharton's duct.

6. Rarely are posterior triangle nodes involved in an $N_0$ neck.

7. Incontinuity resection with the primary tumor is performed when anatomically convenient. Pathologically, it is not necessary, as in-transit metastases rarely occur [119].

## NECK DISSECTION PROCEDURE

The patient is placed supine with a sandbag under the shoulders to extend the neck. The chin is turned to the contralateral side. The skin incision is frequently modified by the incontinuity resection of the primary tumor. The usual incision is the standard Y, although the vertical limb is S-shaped to avoid a straight line. In bilaterally involved necks, or with severe radiotherapy change, the McFee incision is advised. The flaps are raised above or deep to the platysma and, when possible, sutured to surrounding skin, which gives good unencumbered exposure.

The lower end of the sternomastoid is then identified and sharply incised from the clavicle. The internal jugular is dissected out, double-ligated, and divided. The posterior boundary of the dissection, the anterior edge of the trapezius, is located. The dissection is now begun. It is effected most elegantly and efficiently using the scalpel, which is changed frequently; a dull blade is a dangerous surgical instrument. The contents of the posterior triangle are lifted from posterior to anterior, and the numerous vessels are located and ligated. When doing this step, care is taken to carefully elevate the prevertebral fascia, not to dissect deep to the trapezius, and not to go behind the clavicle, where the subclavian vessels may be injured.

The accessory nerve is identified, as are the branches of the brachial plexus. The accessory nerve exits from the posterior border of the sternomastoid within its top half and passes into or under the trapezius 2 to 4 cm above the clavicle [103].

Inferiorly, the posterior belly of the omohyoid is divided and lifted with the specimen. The transverse cervical vessels are divided, as is the external jugular vein. As the specimen is elevated, care is taken not to dissect deeply and injure the phrenic nerve as it lies on the scalenus anterior.

Progressing medially, the sternomastoid muscle is lifted, and the internal jugular vein is reached. At this point, care is exercised in order not to delve too deeply lateral to the vein. Failure to observe this caution may result in damage to major lymph channels; on the left side it can produce a full-blown thoracic duct syndrome. Should the latter occur, the lymph vessels are ligated to prevent formation of a lymph fistula. The internal jugular vein can be elevated with impunity because it has no posterior branches. As this step is performed, the common carotid and the vagus nerve are exposed.

The specimen can then be rapidly dissected, dividing branches of the cervical plexus. The carotid bifurcation and the hypoglossal nerve are exposed. The ansa hypoglossi is transected as it runs into the specimen. Medially, loose areolar tissue is dissected from the strap muscles to the midpoint of the neck with division of the thyroid veins. In addition, the anterior body of the omohyoid is peeled off the infrahyoid muscles and divided at the hyoid bone. This point is the medial limit of the dissection. The external carotid may or may not be divided depending on the preference of the operator. Before dividing it, a branch is sought, which confirms that the vessel is indeed the external carotid rather than the internal carotid artery.

The dissection continues up and over the hypoglossal nerve. Small veins are divided in this area. The next superior landmark is the central tendon of the digastric muscle.

The next move is posteriorly; the upper limit, the transverse process of the atlas, is identified, and the sternomastoid muscle is sharply excised from the mastoid process. As this step is completed, the posterior belly of the digastric muscle can be seen to lie anterior and deep. It may be mistaken for a large vein. The muscle may be left intact or divided. At this point, the occipital artery may be divided. The lower pole of the parotid is cut through, accompanied by some bleeding, as the retromandibular vein is sometimes divided.

Moving medially over the posterior belly of the digastric, the upper end of the jugular is encountered; it is then dissected out, double-ligated, and divided. Note that 1.5 to 2.0 cm of the vein lies cranial to this area. The cervical branch of the facial nerve is sought and preserved by dissecting it free and retracting it superiorly. The inferior border of the mandible is located, and the facial vessels are divided. The submandibular gland is elevated with the specimen. Care is taken not to injure the lingual nerve, which lies deep and medially. Wharton's duct is divided. The dissection continues up and over the lateral edge of the myelohyoid muscle with excision of the submental contents. If the posterior belly of the digastric muscle was divided, the anterior belly is also divided.

If hypotension has been used, the pressure is allowed to come up to normal levels, and hemostasis is effected. The lower neck is reexamined for any escape of lymph. A red rubber catheter drain with many holes in it is placed in position for attachment to wall suction. This method is more effective than the commercially available self-contained systems. The wound is closed in layers without dressings, which allows ease of observation of the neck by nurses and can result in early detection of hematoma.

## MODIFIED NECK DISSECTION PROCEDURE

The modified neck dissection is performed as described above, but the accessory nerve, internal jugular vein, and sternomastoid muscle are preserved. The dissection may be done with the sternomastoid intact, working posterior below and anterior to the muscle. Alternatively, the sternomastoid is divided at the clavicle and turned up to facilitate exposure; this method is easier and quicker, and it is recommended.

## SUPRAOMOHYOID DISSECTION PROCEDURE

The supraomohyoid dissection includes the submandibular anterior triangle and submental triangle. The limits are the mandible superiorly, the contralateral submental triangle medially, the strap muscles as they proceed downward to join the medial edge of the sternomastoid, and the retracted medial edge of the sternomastoid to allow removal of internal jugular nodes up to the base of skull in the posterior margin.

## SPECIAL OBSERVATIONS

### Facial Nerve

The reader is referred to the study of Nelson and Gingrass [73] in which they stimulated the nerve during surgery to map its course. There are several cranial branches below the mandible, lying in the fatty fibrous tissue between the submandibular gland and the platysma, that must be raised with the platysma and actively identified. (The sacrifice of one branch is probably of little import.)

### Accessory Nerve

Below the skull base, the accessory nerve is associated with the internal jugular vein. It then reaches the anterior border of the sternomastoid muscle, passing into its substance. It emerges above the midpoint of its posterior border and then runs through the posterior triangle and into the trapezius 2 to 4 cm above the clavicle.

### Extension of Neck Dissection to Parotid Area

If parotid nodes are to be removed, the operation is performed in continuity through a preauricular incision that joins the neck incisions. If the sternomastoid muscle is being divided from its origin, the dissection is carried medially and superiorly to expose the facial nerve trunk. If the sternomastoid is preserved, the dissection is made medially and superiorly to the anterior edge of the muscle. A standard superficial parotidectomy is performed. It is often convenient because of the good exposure to also remove the deep lobe of the parotid. In some cases, this technique is positively indicated. Removal of the ear or petrous temporal bone (core resection, subtotal or total) simply involves a superior extension of the skin excision and the dissection. Intracranial resection is completed with the help of a neurosurgeon.

## Clinically Negative Neck

In one large series, on pathologic examination a single involved node was found in 9 percent, multiple positive nodes in 16 percent, and extracapsular invasion in 7 percent. Oral tumors most commonly spread to submental, submandibular, and jugulodigastric nodes. Lower jugular nodes were never involved; mid-jugular nodes were involved in 18 percent of patients with oral tongue tumors and 12.5 percent of those with retromolar trigone tumors. Posterior cervical nodes were involved by tongue base tumors. Surgery, which was used in only 69 percent, consisted in various types of modified neck dissection; 29 percent of patients had postoperative radiotherapy, and 2 percent had preoperative radiotherapy. If the nodes were pathologically negative, the recurrence rate with surgery alone was 8 percent and with surgery plus radiotherapy 3 percent. With pathologically positive nodes, the figures were 20 percent and 15 percent, respectively. In a prospective randomized trial in the $N_0$ neck, there was no difference in salvage between those treated by elective radical neck dissection plus observation and radical neck when and if indicated. Approximately one-half of the patients were spared neck dissection [114].

## Positive Neck with an Unknown Primary Lesion

When a patient presents with a neck mass and no obvious primary lesion, the following investigations are performed.

General examination
Careful head and neck and intraoral examination
Endoscopy (flexible and rigid) looking particularly at the nasopharynx and larynx
Chest radiography
Sinus radiography
Bronchoscopy and esophagoscopy as indicated
Mammography as indicated
Fine needle aspiration
Blind biopsies of base of tongue and nasopharynx

Most primary lesions located in these patients lie in the larynx or nasopharynx, or intraorally, especially the tongue base and tonsillar fossa. Treatment is by modified or radical neck dissection. Some advocate irradiation of the nasopharynx and neck. The necessity of the latter is based on the N value.

## RECURRENCE RATES AND COMPLICATIONS OF NECK DISSECTION

Recurrence varies from a low of 20 percent [12] to 35 percent or more [11]. Although Strong [110] reported a recurrence rate of 36.5 percent with metastasis at one level and 71.3 percent with multilevel involvement, Skolnik et al. [100] found no variation between these two groups.

Although improvement in the recurrence rate for stage III and IV squamous carcinomas treated with neck dissection and irradiation has been reported [115], others disagree. In addition, preservation or sacrifice of the accessory nerve does not alter results [17, 32]. Despite the latter findings, postoperative irradiation is advocated, as stated earlier.

The complications of neck dissection are hemorrhage, infection, flap necrosis, carotid exposure, and lymph fistula. Postoperative bleeding must be explored; frequently there is a generalized ooze rather than a single bleeding point. In the latter case, bleeding is usually in the posterior triangle. Infection is treated by drainage, if indicated, and the appropriate antibiotics.

Flap necrosis usually occurs in the irradiated neck; if it is extensive with carotid exposure, immediate cover with a well vascularized flap is indicated. Failure to cover the area may result in massive carotid bleeding and death of the patient.

A lymph fistula usually occurs on the left neck and is handled conservatively with drainage. Failure of the patient to improve calls for exploration and closure of the fistula by oversewing or ligation.

## References

1. Ariyan, S. The pectoralis major myocutaneous flap: A versatile flap for reconstruction in the head and neck. *Plast. Reconstr. Surg.* 63:73, 1979.
2. Baek, S. M., et al. The pectoralis major myocutaneous island flap for reconstruction of the head and neck. *Head Neck Surg.* 1:293, 1979.
3. Bagshaw, M. A., and Thompson, R. W. Elective irradiation of the neck in patients with primary carcinoma of the head and neck. *J.A.M.A.* 217:456, 1971.
4. Bailey, B. N., and Godfrey, A. M. Latissimus dorsi muscle free flaps. *Br. J. Plast. Surg.* 35:47, 1982.
5. Bakamjian, V. Y. A two-stage method for pharyngoesophageal reconstruction with a primary pectoral skin flap. *Plast. Reconstr. Surg.* 36:173, 1965.
6. Bakamjian, V. Y. The surgical management of cancers of the cheek. *J. Surg. Oncol.* 6:255, 1974.
7. Ballantyne, A. J. Modified neck dissection. *Recent Adv. Plast. Surg.* 3:169, 1985.
8. Ballard, B. R., et al. Squamous-cell carcinoma of the floor of the mouth. *Oral Surg. Oral Med. Oral Pathol.* 45:568, 1978.
9. Baudet, J., et al. Reconstruction after radical hemimaxillectomy using a free multidimensional latissimus dorsi myocutaneous flap. *Eur. J. Plast. Surg.* 9:60, 1986.
10. Blair, V. P., and Brown, J. B. The treatment of cancerous or potentially cancerous cervical lymph-nodes. *Ann. Surg.* 98:650, 1933.
11. Blum, R. H., Carter, S. K., and Agre, K. A clinical review of bleomycin—a new antineoplastic agent. *Cancer* 31:903, 1973.
12. Bocca, E. Conservative neck dissection. *Laryngoscope* 85:1511, 1975.
13. Bocca, E., and Pignataro, O. A conservation technique in radical neck dissection. *Ann. Otol. Rhinol. Laryngol.* 76:975, 1967.
14. Bocca, E., Pignataro, O., and Sasaki, C. T. Functional neck dissection: A description of operative technique. *Arch. Otolaryngol.* 106:524, 1980.
15. Botstein, C., Silver, C., and Ariaratnam, L. Treatment of carcinoma of the oral tongue by radium needle implantation. *Am. J. Surg.* 132:523, 1976.
16. Boyne, P. J., and Zarem, H. Osseous reconstruction of the resected mandible. *Am. J. Surg.* 132:49, 1976.
17. Brandenburg, J. H., and Lee, C. Y. The eleventh nerve in radical neck surgery. *Laryngoscope* 91:1851, 1981.
18. Byers, R. M. Squamous cell carcinoma of the oral tongue in patients less than thirty years of age. *Am. J. Surg.* 130:475, 1975.
19. Cady, B., and Catlin, D. Epidermoid carcinoma of the gum: A 20-year surgery. *Cancer* 23:551, 1969.
20. Callery, C. D., Spiro, R. H., and Strong, E. W. Changing trends in the management of squamous carcinoma of the tongue. *Am. J. Surg.* 148:449, 1984.
21. *Cancer Facts and Figures, 1978.* New York: American Cancer Society, 1977. P. 3.
22. Chambers, R. G., Jaques, L. D., and Mahoney, W. D. Tongue flaps for intraoral reconstruction. *Am. J. Surg.* 118:783, 1969.
23. Chandler, J. R., et al. Clinical staging of cancer of the head and neck: A new "new" system. *Am. J. Surg.* 132:525, 1976.
24. Chu, A., and Fletcher, G. H. Incidence and causes of failures to control by irradiation the primary lesions in squamous cell carcinomas of the anterior two-thirds of the tongue and floor of the mouth. *Am. J. Roentgenol. Radium Ther. Nucl. Med.* 117:502, 1973.
25. Cohen, I. K., and Edgerton, M. T. Transbuccal flaps for reconstruction of the floor of the mouth. *Plast. Reconstr. Surg.* 48:8, 1971.
26. Conley, J., and Dickinson, J. T. (eds.). *Plastic and Reconstructive Surgery of the Face and Neck; Proceedings* (Vol. 2). New York: Grune & Stratton, 1972.
27. Conley, J., and Pack, G. T. Melanoma of the mucous membranes of the head and neck. *Arch. Otolaryngol.* 99:315, 1974.
28. Conley, J., and Sadoyama, J. A. Squamous cell cancer of the buccal mucosa: A review of 90 cases. *Arch. Otolaryngol.* 97:330, 1973.
29. Correa, J. N., Bosch, A., and Marcial, V. A. Carcinoma of the floor of the mouth: Review of clinical factors and results of treat-

ment. *Am. J. Roentgenol. Radium Ther. Nucl. Med.* 99:302, 1967.

30. Cuono, C. B., and Ariyan, S. Immediate reconstruction of a composite mandibular defect with a regional osteomusculocutaneous flap. *Plast. Reconstr. Surg.* 65:477, 1980.

31. Cutting, C. B., and McCarthy, J. G. Comparison of residual osseous mass between vascularized and nonvascularized onlay bone transfers. *Plast. Reconstr. Surg.* 72:672, 1983.

32. DeSanto, L. W., et al. Neck dissection: Is it worthwhile? *Laryngoscope* 92:502, 1982.

33. Dos Santos, L. F. Retalho escapular: un novoretalho libre microcirurgico. *Rev. Bras. Cir.* 70:133, 1980.

34. Ewing, M. R., and Martin, H. Disability following "radical neck dissection": An assessment based on the postoperative evaluation of 100 patients. *Cancer* 5:873, 1952.

35. Farr, H. W., and Arthur, K. Epidermoid carcinoma of the mouth and pharynx 1960–1964. *J. Laryngol. Otol.* 86:243, 1972.

36. Friedman, M., and Rosenberg, M. Anterior glossectomy—reconstruction with a posterior tongue rotation flap. *Head Neck Surg.* 9:353, 1987.

37. Fu, K. K., Lichter, A., and Galante, M. Carcinoma of the floor of mouth: An analysis of treatment results and the sites and causes of failures. *Int. J. Radiat. Oncol. Biol. Phys.* 1:829, 1976.

38. Futrell, J. W., et al. Platysma myocutaneous flap for intraoral reconstruction. *Am. J. Surg.* 136:504, 1978.

39. Green, M. F., et al. A one-stage correction of mandibular defects using a split sternum pectoralis major osteo-musculocutaneous transfer. *Br. J. Plast. Surg.* 34:11, 1981.

40. Guillamondegui, O. M., and Jesse, R. H. Surgical treatment of advanced carcinoma of the floor of the mouth. *A.J.R.* 126:1256, 1976.

41. Hamaker, R. C., and Conley, J. Melanoma of the Head and Neck. In I. M. Ariel (ed.), *Malignant Melanoma.* New York: Appleton-Century-Crofts, 1981.

42. Harrold, C. C., Jr. Management of cancer of the floor of the mouth. *Am. J. Surg.* 122:487, 1971.

43. Hedd, D. P., et al. Cancer of the floor of the mouth in Connecticut, 1935–1959. *Cancer* 21:97, 1968.

44. Henk, J. M. Results of radiotherapy for carcinoma of the oropharynx. *Clin. Otolaryngol.* 3:137, 1978.

45. Hoffmann, D., and Adams, J. D. Carcinogenic tobacco-specific N-nitrosamines in snuff and in the saliva of snuff dippers. *Cancer Res.* 41:4305, 1981.

46. Hueston, J. T., and McConchie, I. H. A compound pectoral flap. *Aust. N.Z. J. Surg.* 38:61, 1968.

47. Jesse, R. H., and Lindberg, R. D. The efficacy of combining radiation therapy with a surgical procedure in patients with cervical metastasis from squamous cancer of the oropharynx and hypopharynx. *Cancer* 35:1163, 1975.

48. Kissin, B., et al. Head and neck cancer in alcoholics: The relationship to drinking, smoking, and dietary patterns. *J.A.M.A.* 224:1174, 1973.

49. Kolson, H., et al. Epidermoid carcinoma of the floor of the mouth: Analysis of 108 cases. *Arch. Otolaryngol.* 93:280, 1971.

50. Konrad, H. R., Canalis, R. F., and Calcaterra, T. C. Epidermoid carcinoma of the palate. *Arch. Otolaryngol.* 104:208, 1978.

51. Krishnamurthi, S., Shanta, V., and Udayachander. Stromal interference in radioresponse of squamous carcinoma of the oral cavity. *Clin. Radiol.* 15:246, 1964.

52. Lane, M., et al. Methotrexate therapy for squamous cell carcinomas of the head and neck: Intermittent intravenous dose program. *J.A.M.A.* 204:561, 1968.

53. Leeb, D. C., Ben-Hur, N., and Mazzarella, L. Reconstruction of the floor of the mouth with a free dorsalis pedis flap. *Plast. Reconstr. Surg.* 59:379, 1977.

54. Lindberg, R. Distribution of cervical lymph node metastases from squamous cell carcinoma of the upper respiratory and digestive tracts. *Cancer* 29:1446, 1972.

55. Littlewood, M. Compound skin and sternomastoid flaps for repair in extensive carcinoma of the head and neck. *Br. J. Plast. Surg.* 20:403, 1967.

56. Lovie, M. J., Duncan, G. M., and Glasson, D. W. The ulnar artery forearm free flap. *Br. J. Plast. Surg.* 37:486, 1984.

57. MacComb, W. S., Fletcher, G. H., and Healey, J. E., Jr. Intra-Oral Cavity. In W. S. MacComb and G. H. Fletcher (eds.), *Cancer of the Head and Neck.* Baltimore: Williams & Wilkins, 1967. P. 122.

58. MacLeod, A. M., and Robinson, D. W. Re-

construction of defects involving the mandible and floor of mouth by free osteocutaneous flaps derived from the foot. *Br. J. Plast. Surg.* 35:239, 1982.

59. Mahboubi, E. The epidemiology of oral cavity, pharyngeal and esophageal cancer outside of North America and Western Europe. *Cancer* 40(suppl 4):1879, 1977.

60. *Manual for Staging of Cancer, 1977.* Chicago: American Joint Committee on Cancer Staging and End Results Reporting, 1977.

61. Martin, H., et al. Neck dissection. *Cancer* 4:441, 1951.

62. Mashberg, A., Morrissey, J. B., and Garfinkel, L. A study of the appearance of early asymptomatic oral squamous cell carcinoma. *Cancer* 32:1436, 1973.

63. McCraw, J. B., and Furlow, L. T., Jr. The dorsalis pedis arterialized flap: A clinical study. *Plast. Reconstr. Surg.* 55:177, 1975.

64. McCraw, J. B., Magee, W. P., Jr., and Kalwaic, H. Uses of the trapezius and sternomastoid myocutaneous flaps in head and neck reconstruction. *Plast. Reconstr. Surg.* 63:49, 1979.

65. McGregor, I. A. The temporal flap in intraoral cancer: Its use in repairing the postexcisional defect. *Br. J. Plast. Surg.* 16:318, 1963.

66. McGregor, I. A. "Quilted" skin grafting in the mouth. *Br. J. Plast. Surg.* 28:100, 1975.

67. McGregor, I. A., and McGregor, F. M. *Cancer of the Face and Mouth: Pathology and Management for Surgeons.* Edinburgh: Churchill Livingstone, 1986.

68. Million, R. R. Elective neck irradiation for $T_xN_0$ squamous carcinoma of the oral tongue and floor of mouth. *Cancer* 34:149, 1974.

69. Moore, C. Cigarette smoking and cancer of the mouth, pharynx, and larynx: A continuing study. *J.A.M.A.* 218:553, 1971.

70. Moore, O. S., and Frazell, E. L. Simultaneous bilateral neck dissection: Experience with 151 patients. *Am. J. Surg.* 107:565, 1964.

71. Nahum, A. M., Mullally, W., and Marmor, L. A syndrome resulting from radical neck dissection. *Arch. Otolaryngol.* 74:424, 1961.

72. Nathanson, A., Jakobsson, P. A., and Wersall, J. Prognosis of squamous-cell carcinoma of the gums. *Acta Otolaryngol. (Stockh.)* 75:301, 1973.

73. Nelson, D. W., and Gingrass, R. P. Anatomy of the mandibular branches of the facial nerve. *Plast. Reconstr. Surg.* 64:479, 1979.

74. O'Brien, P. H., and Catlin, D. Cancer of the cheek (mucosa). *Cancer* 18:1392, 1965.

75. Olivari, N. The latissimus flap. *Br. J. Plast. Surg.* 29:126, 1976.

76. Owens, N. A compound neck pedicle designed for the repair of massive facial defects: Formation, development and application. *Plast. Reconstr. Surg.* 15:369, 1955.

77. Panje, W., and Cutting, C. Trapezius osteomyocutaneous island flap for reconstruction of the anterior floor of the mouth and the mandible. *Head Neck Surg.* 3:66, 1980.

78. Pierquin, B., et al. The place of implantation in tongue and floor of mouth cancer. *J.A.M.A.* 215:961, 1971.

79. Quillen, C. G., Shearin, J. C., Jr., and Georgiade, N. G. Use of the latissimus dorsi myocutaneous island flap for reconstruction in the head and neck area: Case report. *Plast. Reconstr. Surg.* 62:113, 1978.

80. Randolph, V. L., et al. Combination therapy of advanced head and neck cancer: Induction of remissions with diamminedichloroplatinum (II), bleomycin and radiation therapy. *Cancer* 41:460, 1978.

81. Ratzer, E. R., Schweitzer, R. J., and Frazell, E. L. Epidermoid carcinoma of the palate. *Am. J. Surg.* 119:294, 1970.

82. Reddy, C. R. R. M. Carcinoma of hard palate in India in relation to reverse smoking of chuttas. *J. Natl. Cancer Inst.* 53:615, 1974.

83. Robinson, D. W., and MacLeod, A. Microvascular free jejunum transfer. *Br. J. Plast. Surg.* 35:258, 1982.

84. Rothman, K., and Keller, A. The effect of joint exposure to alcohol and tobacco on risk of cancer of the mouth and pharynx. *J. Chronic Dis.* 25:711, 1972.

85. Saxena, V. S. Cancer of the tongue: Local control of the primary. *Cancer* 26:788, 1970.

86. Schneider, J. J., Fletcher, G. H., and Barkley, H. T., Jr. Control by irradiation alone of nonfixed clinically positive lymph nodes from squamous cell carcinoma of the oral cavity, oropharynx, supraglottic larynx, and hypopharynx. *Am. J. Roentgenol. Radium Ther. Nucl. Med.* 123:42, 1975.

87. Schultz-Coulon, H. J., and Schmidt, W. Zur Bedeutung des Alkoholabusus fur Atiologie, Verlauf und Prognose von malignen Mundschleimhaut- und Oropharynxtumoren. *HNO* 30:9, 1982.

88. Schusterman, M., et al. The lateral arm

flap—an experimental and clinical study. In H. B. Williams (ed.), *Transactions of the 8th International Congress of Plastic and Reconstructive Surgery.* Montreal: International Congress of Plastic and Reconstructive Surgery, 1983.

89. Sessions, D. G., Dedo, D. D., and Ogura, J. H. Tongue flap reconstruction in cancer of the oral cavity. *Arch. Otolaryngol.* 101:166, 1975.

90. Shafer, W. G., and Waldron, C. A. Erythroplakia of the oral cavity. *Cancer* 36:1021, 1975.

91. Shah, J. P., Huvos, A. G., and Strong, E. W. Mucosal melanomas of the head and neck. *Am. J. Surg.* 134:531, 1977.

92. Shah, J. P., et al. Carcinoma of the oral cavity: Factors affecting treatment failure at the primary site and neck. *Am. J. Surg.* 132:504, 1976.

93. Shaha, A. R., Spiro, R. H., Shah, J. P., and Strong, E. W. Squamous carcinoma of the floor of the mouth. *Am. J. Surg.* 148:455, 1984.

94. Shanta, V., and Krishnamurthi, S. A study of aetiological factors in oral squamous cell cancer. *Br. J. Cancer* 13:381, 1959.

95. Short, S. O., et al. Shoulder pain and function after neck dissection with or without preservation of the spinal accessory nerve. *Am. J. Surg.* 148:478, 1984.

96. Siemssen, S. O., Kirkby, B., and O'Connor, T. P. Immediate reconstruction of a resected segment of the lower jaw, using a compound flap of clavicle and sternomastoid muscle. *Plast. Reconstr. Surg.* 61:724, 1978.

97. Silverman, S., Jr., and Griffith, M. Smoking characteristics of patients with oral carcinoma and the risk for second oral primary carcinoma. *J. Am. Dent. Assoc.* 85:637, 1972.

98. Singh, A. D., and von Essen, C. F. Buccal mucosa cancer in South India: Etiologic and clinical aspects. *Am. J. Roentgenol. Radium Ther. Nucl. Med.* 96:6, 1966.

99. Skolnik, E. M., et al. Preservation of XI cranial nerve in neck dissections. *Laryngoscope* 77:1304, 1967.

100. Skolnik, E. M., et al. Evolution of the clinically negative neck. *Ann. Otol. Rhinol. Laryngol.* 89:551, 1980.

101. Smithdeal, C. D., Corso, P. F., and Strong, E. W. Dermis grafts for carotid artery protection: Yes or no? A ten year experience. *Am. J. Surg.* 128:484, 1974.

102. Song, R., et al. The forearm flap. *Clin. Plast. Surg.* 9:21, 1982.

103. Soo, K-C., et al. Anatomy of the accessory nerve and its cervical contributions in the neck. *Head Neck Surg.* 9:111, 1986.

104. Soutar, D. S., et al. The radial forearm flap: A versatile method for intra-oral reconstruction. *Br. J. Plast. Surg.* 36:1, 1983.

105. Spiro, R. H., and Frazell, E. L. Evaluation of radical surgical treatment of advanced cancer of the mouth. *Am. J. Surg.* 116:571, 1968.

106. Spiro, R. H., and Strong, E. W. Epidermoid carcinoma of the mobile tongue: Treatment by partial glossectomy alone. *Am. J. Surg.* 122:707, 1971.

107. Spiro, R. H., and Strong, E. W. Surgical treatment of cancer of the tongue. *Surg. Clin. North Am.* 54:759, 1974.

108. Spiro, R. H., et al. Tumors of minor salivary origin: A clinicopathologic study of 492 cases. *Cancer* 31:117, 1973.

109. Stecker, R. H., Devine, K. D., and Harrison, E. G., Jr. Verrucose "snuff dipper's" carcinoma of the oral cavity: A case of self-induced carcinogenesis. *J.A.M.A.* 189:838, 1964.

110. Strong, E. W. Preoperative radiation and radical neck dissection. *Surg. Clin. North Am.* 49:271, 1969.

111. Strong, E. W., and Spiro, R. H. Cancer of the Oral Cavity. In J. Y. Suen and E. N. Myers (eds.), *Cancer of the Head and Neck.* New York: Churchill Livingstone, 1981. P. 301.

112. Taylor, G. I. Reconstruction of the mandible with free composite iliac bone grafts. *Ann. Plast. Surg.* 9:361, 1982.

113. Teot, L., et al. The scapular crest pedicled bone graft. *Int. J. Microsurg.* 3:257, 1981.

114. Vandenbrouck, C., et al. Elective versus therapeutic radical neck dissection in epidermoid carcinoma of the oral cavity: Results of a randomized clinical trial. *Cancer* 46:386, 1980.

115. Vikram, B., et al. Elective postoperative radiation therapy in stages III and IV epidermoid carcinoma of the head and neck. *Am. J. Surg.* 140:580, 1980.

116. Wald, R. M., Jr., and Calcaterra, T. C. Lower

alveolar carcinoma: Segmental versus marginal resection. *Arch. Otolaryngol.* 109:578, 1983.

117. Waldron, C. A., and Shafer, W. G. Leukoplakia revisited: A clinicopathologic study of 3256 oral leukoplakias. *Cancer* 36:1386, 1975.

118. Whitehurst, J. O., and Droulias, C. A. Surgical treatment of squamous cell carcinoma of the oral tongue: Factors influencing survival. *Arch. Otolaryngol.* 103:212, 1977.

119. Willis, R. A. *The Spread of Tumours in the Human Body* (3rd ed.). London: Butterworths, 1973.

120. Wittes, R. E., et al. cis-Dichlorodiammineplatinum (II) in the treatment of epidermoid carcinoma of the head and neck. *Cancer Treat. Rep.* 61:359, 1977.

121. Wizenberg, M. J., et al. Treatment of lymph node metastases in head and neck cancer: A radiotherapeutic approach. *Cancer* 29:1455, 1972.

122. Wynder, E. L., and Klein, U. E. The possible role of riboflavin deficiency in epithelial neoplasia. *Cancer* 18:167, 1965.

123. Wynder, E. L., and Stellman, S. D. Comparative epidemiology of tobacco-related cancers. *Cancer Res.* 37:4608, 1977.

124. Wynder, E. L., et al. Environmental factors in cancer of the upper alimentary tract: A Swedish study with special reference to Plummer-Vinson (Paterson-Kelly) syndrome. *Cancer* 10:470, 1957.

125. Zarem, H. A. Current concepts in reconstructive surgery in patients with cancer of the head and neck. *Surg. Clin. North Am.* 51:149, 1971.

126. Zovickian, A. Preservation of facial contour after resection of mandible using cervical skin flaps. *Plast. Reconstr. Surg.* 21:433, 1958.

# 19

*John E. Woods*

# Primary Tumors of the Salivary Glands and Neck

## Tumors of the Salivary Glands

The paired parotid, submaxillary, and sublingual glands provide the major portion of salivary flow to the oral cavity through their respective ducts. Additionally, there are hundreds of minor salivary glands distributed throughout the tongue, tonsils, pharynx, palate, nasal cavity, paranasal sinuses, larynx, trachea, ear canal, and lacrimal glands.

INCIDENCE

Tumors, benign or malignant, may occur in any of these glands and have similar clinical and histologic patterns. They constitute approximately 6 percent of all head and neck tumors [36].

The parotid gland is the site of tumor occurrence in 75 to 85 percent of patients, the minor salivary glands in 10 to 20 percent, and the submaxillary glands in 5 to 8 percent. The sublingual glands are rarely affected [14, 24].

There is no sexual predilection in whites, but in Africa women are more frequently involved. The incidence of salivary gland tumors increases with age, the average age at diagnosis being 48 years for patients with benign tumors and 57 years for those with malignant tumors. Fewer than 2 percent of major salivary gland tumors occur in children 16 years or younger.[8]

Interestingly, the incidence of breast cancer is significantly higher in patients with salivary gland tumors.[7] Malignant salivary gland tumors have also been seen with greater than the expected frequency in patients subjected to radiation [6, 32].

Among parotid tumors 60 to 75 percent are benign, whereas in the submaxillary and minor salivary glands benign tumors constitute 40 to 50 percent and 20 to 25 percent, respectively.

CLINICAL FINDINGS

Salivary gland tumors are almost invariably diagnosed by palpation of a mass, though occasionally tumors reach visibility before they are recognized as such. Pain or nerve deficits are uncommon and are almost always associated with malignancy.

Palpation alone, although helpful, is not sufficient to distinguish accurately between benign and malignant tumors. Additionally, the examiner must be alert to the possibility that a parotid or submaxillary mass may represent metastatic nodes from a primary cutaneous malignant melanoma, squamous cell carcinoma, or, rarely, malignancy at a

*551*

distant site. Lymphoma may also present first in the parotid gland.

A complete examination of the head and neck area is appropriate when a salivary gland tumor is suspected. Any mass in the preauricular or infraauricular area in the region of the tail of the parotid, unless distinctly attached by a visible pore to the skin, is considered a tumor until proved otherwise. Intraoral examination occasionally reveals a bulge in the lateral pharyngeal area when there is retromandibular tumor extension. Examination for submaxillary tumors is always bimanual, with one index finger in the floor of the mouth, palpating for tumor, gland, or lymph nodes against the external examining fingers. Minor salivary tumors are most commonly detected as enlarging submucosal masses anywhere in the upper aerodigestive tract.

DIAGNOSTIC ADJUNCTS

Sialography is rarely if ever necessary inasmuch as it contributes little if anything to decision-making with respect to treatment. Plain radiographs are occasionally useful for detecting stones but otherwise are only rarely helpful.

Computed tomography (CT), magnetic resonance imaging, or both are considered when there is a question as to the extent of tumor with more advanced disease. These procedures may be useful when planning the appropriate surgical approach.

Fine needle biopsy is an established and acceptable technique, though it is rarely necesary when accurate frozen section diagnosis is available. Incisional biopsy is to be condemned as inappropriate with its risk of injury to the facial nerve and possible seeding of tumor cells.

CLASSIFICATION AND STAGING

Four clinical variables are considered when staging classifications of salivary gland tumors: (1) tumor size, (2) local extension of the tumor, (3) spread to regional nodes, and (4) distant metastases. The classification and

**Table 19-1** *Malignant salivary gland classification: American Joint Committee (1983)*

| Primary tumor | Size (cm) | Local extension* |
|---|---|---|
| $T_1$ | ≤2.0 | No |
| $T_2$ | 2.1–4.0 | No |
| $T_3$ | 4.1–6.0 | No |
| $T_{4a}$ | 6.0 | No |
| $T_{4b}$ | Any | Yes |

*Local extension means involvement of skin, soft tissue, bone, or facial or lingual nerves.

staging of tumors limited to the major salivary glands of the American Joint Committee on Cancer are shown in Tables 19-1 and 19-2.

PATHOLOGY

Although the incidence of the different tumor types seen in salivary glands differs with anatomic location, morphologically these lesions are generally similar. Most seem to be epithelial in origin.

*Benign Tumors*

Pleomorphic adenomas (mixed tumor) are slow-growing tumors that are occasionally lobulated or cystic and may have a thin capsule. They constitute 90 percent of benign tumors [17, 35, 36]. They are composed of varying proportions of epithelial and mesenchymal elements and are most commonly seen in the superficial portion of the parotid gland (Fig. 19-1). Their peak incidence is dur-

**Table 19-2** *Staging of malignant salivary gland tumors: American Joint Committee (1983)*

| Stage | T status | M and N status |
|---|---|---|
| 1 | $T_1$ or $T_2$ | $N_0M_0$ |
| 2 | $T_3$ | $N_0M_0$ |
| 3 | $T_1$ or $T_2$ | $N_1M_0$ |
|   | $T_{4a}$ or $T_{4b}$ | $N_0M_0$ |
| 4 | $T_3$ | $N_1M_0$ |
|   | $T_{4a}$ or $T_{4b}$ | $N_1M_0$ |
|   | Any T | Any N $M_1$ |

ing the fifth decade of life, and they are more common in women [28]. Recurrence is often seen after inadequate resection.

Adenolymphoma (papillary cystadenoma lymphomatosum) nearly always occurs in the parotid gland, where it may constitute 5 to 20 percent of benign tumors [43]. It occurs predominantly in men (80 to 90 percent) [28] and is bilateral in 10 percent of patients. It may be cystic and is often multiple in the same gland. It rarely if ever recurs.

Monomorphic adenoma and oxyphilic adenoma (oneocytoma) are rare tumors, the former being more common in the minor than in the major salivary glands. Other rare benign tumors include basal cell adenoma, glycogen-rich adenoma, and sebaceous lymphadenoma.

Lymphangioma (including cystic hygroma) and hemangioma are the most common parotid masses in children and frequently involute spontaneously, often requiring no treatment.

*Malignant Tumors*

Major and minor salivary gland malignancies may invade locally, involving muscle, bone, and nerves. They may also spread by lymphatics or hematogenously.

Mucoepidermoid carcinomas occur with the greatest frequency [43] and may be further classified as low or high grade. The former constitute 50 to 60 percent of the group and generally have an excellent prognosis. High grade mucoepidermoid carcinomas are more likely to recur locally and to metastasize.

Adenocystic carcinoma (cylindroma) is the most common malignancy in the submaxillary and minor salivary glands [35, 36]. It is slow-growing and apt to recur, often after many years, with subsequent further recurrences after resection. It is especially prone to invade adjacent nerves. Metastases are relatively common to the lung, brains, bone, and skin. The course is often long but relentless, causing death only after many years.

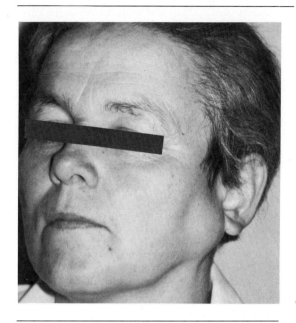

**Figure 19-1** *A 46-year-old woman with the typical appearance of a sizable benign mixed tumor of the left parotid.*

Adenocarcinomas are the next most frequently encountered malignancies in minor salivary glands (Fig. 19-2). They are locally invasive and firm to palpation, occurring most commonly in patients over age 60. They not infrequently produce facial paralysis when in the parotid gland.

Acinic cell carcinoma is a low grade tumor that occurs primarily in the parotid and seems to arise from the acini. About 15 percent metastasize to cervical lymph nodes.

Malignant mixed tumors are commonly seen during the seventh and eighth decades of life and arise in many instances from a long preexistent pleomorphic adenoma in the parotid gland. Primary malignant mixed tumors also occur but more rarely [5]. Malignancies arising from a previous benign pleomorphic adenoma are predominantly epithelial in type and frequently metastasize, though both adenocarcinoma and squamous cell carcinoma types are recognized. There is a great deal of confusion among authors

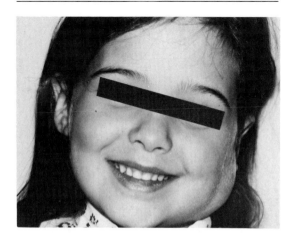

**Figure 19-2** *A 4-year-old patient demonstrates an unusual condition: an adenocarcinoma of the parotid gland that required sacrifice of the facial nerve. The patient has subsequently experienced spontaneous regeneration with much return of function.*

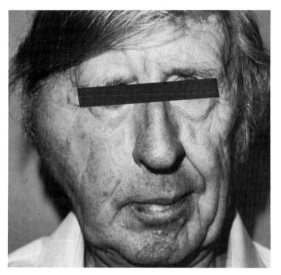

**Figure 19-3** *A 68-year-old man with an advanced neglected squamous cell carcinoma of the right parotid gland and facial paralysis, as noted by the disappearing right nasolabial fold and beginning sag of the right corner of the mouth.*

with regard to malignant mixed tumors, but they are generally acknowledged to be aggressive locally with a propensity to metastasize.

Squamous cell carcinoma is an aggressive malignancy that constitutes 5 to 10 percent of malignant parotid and submaxillary gland tumors (Fig. 19-3). It may be primary in the glands, but when skin is involved it may be difficult to distinguish from extension or metastatic spread from a primary squamous cell carcinoma of the skin.

Other malignancies include highly undifferentiated tumors that cannot be assigned to a more definite morphologic classification and, rarely, malignant melanoma, which is primary in the parotid gland [44]. Metastatic tumors from as widely disparate sites as breast, kidney, prostate, and elsewhere also occur. Lymphomas may also first manifest in the parotid gland.

TREATMENT

For benign tumors of the parotid, the treatment is superficial parotidectomy with spar-

ing of the facial nerve [42]. The deep portion of the gland is removed only if the tumor resides therein. For multiple recurrences of mixed tumor, local resection is carried out; radiation therapy may be considered after all gross disease has been removed.

Hemangiomas and lymphangiomas in children may be followed in anticipation of their involution. If disproportionate, aggressive, continued growth occurs after 2 to 3 years, parotidectomy to include the hemangioma is occasionally appropriate. Sparing of the facial nerve is usually possible in experienced hands.

Malignant tumors of the parotid glands may be treated by total conservative parotidectomy with sparing of the facial nerve, where the nerve is not enveloped by tumor [39]. Even when tumor is adherent to nerve, removal of all gross tumor and gland is acceptable so long as tumoricidal doses (5000 to 6000 rad) of radiation are given postoperatively. For small tumors separated by normal tissue from nerve branches, total parotidectomy may suffice [39].

If the tumor envelopes the facial nerve, the nerve is sacrificed. When contiguous structures such as muscle and bone are involved, they must be sacrificed with sufficient normal adjacent tissue to ensure free margins. Here again adjunctive radiation therapy may be considered.

Neck dissection is appropriate for high grade tumors or when clinically suspicious nodes are present. There is an increasing trend toward functional neck dissection, sparing the sternocleidomastoid muscle, internal jugular vein, and spinal accessory nerve if gross disease is not present or distant from these structures.

Submaxillary gland malignancies are removed along with all node-bearing tissue in the digastric triangle, with neck dissection as indicated for parotid malignancies. Minor salivary gland malignant tumors are removed with a margin of normal surrounding tissue.

*Technique*
The key to safe removal of a parotid tumor is identification and preservation of the facial nerve and its branches (Fig. 19-4). It is most easily accomplished using the mastoid process, with its proximity to the stylomastoid foramen, as the anatomic key. Dissection of the posterior aspect of the parotid gland away from the auditory canal, mastoid process, and anterior border of the sternocleidomastoid muscle provides a wide gutter in which the nerve may be readily identified as it penetrates the gland directly medial and opposite to the midpoint of the mastoid process, as described elsewhere in detail [41].

The key to safe removal of the submaxillary gland is an incision two fingerbreadths below the mandible, with incision of the platysma and cervical fascia over the gland. Dissection following the gland is carried upward to the border of the mandible, where the mandibular branch of the facial nerve is

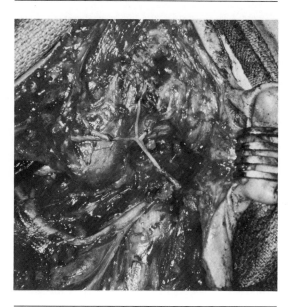

**Figure 19-4** *Intraoperative view of total parotidectomy. Note the clear dissection of the five branches of the facial nerve starting with the temporal (superiorly and posteriorly), zygomatic, and buccal, all branches of the upper division in this patient. The marginal mandibular branch and the cervical branches are seen off the lower division. All superficial and deep parotid glandular tissue has been removed.*

identified and preserved. Contents of the triangle are carried down after ligation of the anterior facial vein and artery, and the lingual and hypoglossal nerves are identified and preserved by retracting the posterior border of the myohyoid muscle anteriorly. This maneuver exposes the lingual nerve high up under the mandible and the hypoglossal nerve 1 to 2 cm inferiorly, which is often obscured to a degree by overlying veins. The facial artery is divided inferiorly, and the digastric triangle contents are readily removed.

PROGNOSIS
For benign salivary tumors the prognosis is excellent, though inadequately excised mixed tumors may result in multiple recur-

**Table 19-3** *Malignant parotid tumor:*
*5-year actuarial survival*

| Tumor type | Survival (%) |
| --- | --- |
| Mucoepidermoid | 96.7 |
| Adenocarcinoma | 68.5 |
| Acinic cell | 94.1 |
| Adenoid cystic | 71.2 |
| Squamous cell | 48.8 |
| Malignant mixed | 26.6 |
| Undifferentiated | 43.0 |

rences. The latter entail eventual facial nerve injury or sacrifice.

The 5-year survival for malignant parotid tumors is shown in Table 19-3. In a more recent study of patients with malignant tumor measuring less than 3 cm in diameter, all survived without evidence of disease. In tumors larger than 3 cm, the death rate was 32 percent with an additional 13 percent of patients alive with disease [39]. Prognosis in patients with malignant tumors of the submaxillary gland is distinctly worse, with about 80 percent of patients dying as a result of the disease [28, 35]. Curability of minor salivary gland malignancies relates to size, local excision, histology, and nodal metastases, with 45 percent and 21 percent of patients surviving at 5 and 15 years, respectively [28, 36].

## Thyroid Tumors
Although surgical conditions of the thyroid are the appropriate concern of endocrine surgeons, a knowledge of thyroid pathology is important to those dealing with other neoplastic conditions of the head and neck. Thyroid neoplasms fall into benign and malignant categories with expected variations in each group.

### BENIGN NEOPLASMS
Benign adenomas are encapsulated, usually cellular nodules that are found in otherwise normal thyroid glands. Aside from their po-

tential for autonomous growth, they may rarely undergo malignant transformation. They are to be distinguished from colloid nodules, which are encapsulated areas of hyperplasia found in adenomatous goiters, which are not true neoplasms. The classification of true adenomas includes the following [13].

*Embryonal adenoma:* resembles the embryonic thyroid prior to development of follicles
*Fetal adenoma:* has small acini and abundant interacinar loose ground substance; is similar to the fetal thyroid
*Hurthle cell adenoma:* has a trabecular pattern of large, pale acidophilic cells
*Follicular adenoma:* composed of a mixture of micro- and macro-follicles with a predominance of the former

The chief importance of benign adenomas lies in their differentiation from thyroid carcinoma. Scintiscanning, fine needle aspiration, and core needle biopsy are helpful, but surgical excision is necessary for certain diagnoses. Follicular adenomas occasionally become hyperactive, producing thyrotoxicosis.

### MALIGNANT NEOPLASMS
Although thyroid cancer has been thought to be uncommon, autopsy studies have revealed an incidence of up to 13 percent [29]. Many of these lesions are small papillary cancers, and overt thyroid cancer remains uncommon, especially as a cause of death [2].

There has been increasing evidence that the risk of thyroid cancer is greater in patients who have previously received radiation to the head and neck region [10]. More than a million patients may have undergone such therapy for highly varied indications 20 to 30 years ago. If a thyroid nodule is palpated in such a patient, surgery is indicated, as the chance of malignancy under these circumstances is 25 to 40 percent [16].

**Table 19-4** *Classification of thyroid cancers*

| Cellular origin | Histology | | Pathology | |
| | Type | %* | State | % |
| --- | --- | --- | --- | --- |
| Follicular | Papillary | 62 | Occult (1.5 cm diameter) | 35 |
| | | | Intrathyroid | 50 |
| | | | Extrathryoid (thyroid capsule breached) | 15 |
| | Follicular | 18 | Angioinvasion | |
| | | | Minimal | 50 |
| | | | Moderate or marked | 50 |
| | Anaplastic | 14 | | |
| Parafollicular (C) | Medullary | 6 | | |
| Lymphoreticular | | <1 | | |

*Percentages are the relative incidence among 1181 cases at the Mayo Clinic, 1926 through 1960.
*Source:* A. J. Edis. Surgical treatment for thyroid cancer. *Surg. Clin. North Am.* 57:533, 1977.

The frequency with which thyroid nodules are encountered in the general population (5 to 10 percent) makes it important to determine which ones should be removed and which may be followed by observation only. It has been estimated that only about 5 percent of nodular goiters harbor malignancy [38].

Certain factors increase the likelihood of cancer. They include (1) age, with a 50 percent incidence of malignancy in thyroid nodules in children under 14 years of age; (2) sex—cancer is more common in males; (3) increasing size of a nodule; (4) a previous history of radiation exposure to the head and neck; and (5) a family history of thyroid cancer.

Physical findings of concern include the finding of a solitary nodule, rather than a multinodular goiter. Firm nodules are more likely to be cancerous, as are fixed nodules. The presence of cervical lymphadenopathy in association with a thyroid is highly suggestive of malignancy. Recurrent nerve paralysis with a fixed vocal cord and a thyroid mass is virtually diagnostic of cancer.

The most important development in diagnosis of thyroid cancers in recent years has been fine needle aspiration. Scintiscanning and ultrasonography, although useful, have yielded in importance to the ease and accuracy of fine needle aspiration in experienced hands. The number of thyroid operations is reduced substantially wherever this technique is employed [13].

Thyroid malignancies may be classified as to their cellular origin: follicular, parafollicular, or lymphoreticular [12]. Table 19-4 outlines their classification.

*Tumors of Follicular Origin (Papillary, Follicular, and Anaplastic Carcinomas)*
Papillary carcinomas containing characteristic papillary follicles are by far the most common and are generally indolent and slow-growing. Lymph node metastases occur in approximately 50 percent of patients and distant spread in fewer than 5 percent [45]. Paradoxically, curability is not related to nodal spread but, rather, to invasion of the capsule. Intrathyroid tumors are generally curable.

Acceptable treatment is ipsilateral total thyroid lobectomy and contralateral near-total lobectomy, sparing a small amount of thyroid tissue to conserve at least one parathyroid gland. Lymph nodes above and below the isthmus and from the tracheoesophageal grooves are removed in continuity with the thyroid specimens. Lateral neck dissection is carried out only if such nodes are palpably enlarged [13]. Functional neck dissection, preserving the sternocleidomastoid muscle and the internal jugular vein, is usually appropriate.

Suppressive therapy with thyroid hormone is employed for the remainder of the patient's life. Adjunctive therapy with radioactive iodine after thyroid deprivation is routinely employed at some institutions to ablate any remnants of thyroid. This combined form of therapy yields a high cure rate. Extrathyroid extension is associated with a lower chance of survival.

Follicular carcinoma is characterized by the presence of well differentiated thyroid follicles containing varying amounts of colloid. It rarely invades lymph nodes, spreading instead to adjacent blood vessels and from there to distant sites such as lung and bones. In the absence of angioinvasion, survival is essentially the same as for a normal population, being halved when such invasion is present [45]. The treatment of follicular thyroid cancer follows the same principles outlined for papillary carcinoma.

Anaplastic carcinoma grows rapidly, directly invading adjacent structures and spreading by the bloodstream to distant sites. Death occurs within 36 months in almost all patients [45]. Preservation of the airway may be possible by debulking, and external radiation therapy may be useful for limited palliation. More commonly, the surgeon's role is limited to making the diagnosis by biopsy.

*Tumors of Parafollicular Origin*
Medullary thyroid carcinomas (MTCs) are composed of small, rather uniform cells of the calcitonin-secreting (parafollicular) cells of the thyroid gland. Having their embryologic origin from neutral ectoderm in common with other APUD cells found distributed throughout the adult endocrine system [30], they are not uncommonly associated with tumors of the adrenal medulla and parathyroid glands. This clinical combination is known as type II multiple endocrine neoplasia syndrome. Therefore with proved MTC it is important preoperatively to look for associated endocrine disease.

In patients with familial MTC, the disease is usually bilateral; and lymph node involvement is present in 35 to 50 percent of patients [33]. Prognosis for patients without nodal metastases is similar to that of the normal population, but survival is only about 40 percent when nodes are involved [45]. Treatment is total thyroidectomy and, if nodal biopsy reveals metastatic involvement, functional neck dissection.

*Tumors of Lymphoreticular Cell Origin*
Lymphosarcomas are small cell tumors of the thyroid gland that are typically large, rapidly growing goiters. They are most common in older women. When feasible, thyroidectomy is the treatment followed by irradiation of the neck. If resection is not possible, irradiation is employed.

Prognosis is good if the disease is confined to the gland. With extraglandular extension, the outlook is usually poor [40].

*Metastatic Lesions*
Carcinomas metastatic to the thyroid are uncommon, with only 14 cases being described in a series of 20,000 patients undergoing thyroid surgery over 23 years [47].

## Carcinoma of the Larynx
Overwhelmingly, the most common neoplastic condition of the larynx is squamous cell carcinoma. It is of particular importance because of the potential loss of voice with total laryngectomy. Fortunately, with advances in technique and earlier diagnosis of the condition, voice conservation procedures are possible in most cases. In one large institutional practice, only 15 percent of patients required total laryngectomy [31].

Diagnosis is primarily by indirect, fiberoptic, and suspension laryngoscopy. The therapeutic approach is determined by a critical assessment of the extent of tumor. The approach varies from one institution to another: Irradiation used in all cases by some, who reserve surgery for failures. Others irradiate small cancers, utilizing surgery for

**Table 19-5** *Surgical options for laryngeal cancer*

*Note:* Surgery of the larynx for cancer breaks down logically into the following categories, which address increasing tumor volumes and present increasing degrees of disability. The addition of modified radical or bilateral neck dissections is an independent consideration that depends on the presence of disease in the neck.

I. Requires no external operation: completed simultaneously with the biopsy. Voice remains normal.
   A. Vocal cord stripping for premalignant lesions
   B. Transoral cordectomy for small cordal cancers
      1. Sharp dissection
      2. Dissection and cautery
      3. Laser excision
II. Preserves airway and voice but voice is modified. For glottic lesions on mobile cords.
   A. Laryngofissure and cordectomy
   B. Vertical hemilaryngectomy
   C. Frontolateral partial laryngectomy
III. Preserves airway and voice but swallow is modified. For supraglottic lesions without glottic involvement.
   A. Supraglottic laryngectomy
   B. Extended supraglottic laryngectomy
IV. Requires permanent tracheotomy but preserves voice. For cancers large enough to fix the vocal cord.
   A. Near-total laryngectomy (for intrinsic laryngeal cancer)
   B. Near-total laryngopharyngectomy (for extrinsic or piriform cancer)
V. Requires a permanent tracheotomy and sacrifices voice.
   A. Total laryngectomy
   B. Total laryngectomy with partial pharyngectomy
   C. Total laryngopharyngectomy with pharyngeal reconstruction
      1. Skin flap
      2. Visceral transposition
      3. Free transplant and microvascular anastomosis

large lesions and a combination of modalities for far-advanced cancers. A third approach is entirely surgical using the conservational approach for small tumors and reconstructive operations followed by speech therapy for larger ones. Perhaps the most appropriate approach is one that individualizes case by case, using irradiation in some instances and surgery in others [31]. The treatment of laryngeal carcinoma is not for the occasional operator.

The debate over radiation versus surgery is influenced by a number of factors. The advantages of radiation are the avoidance of an invasive procedure, avoidance of a temporary tracheostomy, and often preservation of a better voice. The major problem with radiation therapy is that of tumor persistence and undetected progression. This progression may be difficult to detect even with careful follow-up, with the only indication being subtle fixation of a previously mobile cord.

Thus radiation failures may result in the ultimate loss of voice by total laryngectomy, whereas conservation therapy performed initially with the securing of frozen section tumor-free margins yields high cure rates [25] while preserving the voice. In addition, there is the long-term hazard of subsequent tumor formation of the site of radiation damage [20, 23].

The surgical options for laryngeal carcinoma have been outlined by Pearson and Donald, as shown in Table 19-5 [31]. These investigators classified the procedures according to the operative approach demanded by increasing tumor volumes.

The approaches in *category I* for premalignant lesions and small cordal cancers are vocal cord stripping and transoral cordectomy, respectively. For glottic lesions on mobile cords in *category II* the procedures employed are laryngofissure and cordectomy, vertical laryngectomy, or frontolateral partial laryngectomy. These procedures preserve the airway but modify the voice. *Category III* procedures, for supraglottic lesions without glottic involvement, which preserve airway and voice but modify swallowing, include supraglottic and extended supraglottic laryngectomy.

For cancers large enough to fix the vocal cord, *category IV* procedures are near-total laryngectomy (for intrinsic laryngeal cancer) and near-total laryngopharyngectomy (for extrinsic or piriform cancer). These techniques preserve the voice but require permanent tracheostomy. *Category V* techniques, for more advanced cancers, require a permanent tracheostomy with sacrifice of the voice and include total laryngectomy with or without partial pharyngectomy or total laryngopharyngectomy with pharyngeal reconstruction by any of several methods available. The sacrifice of voice is temporary. Most patients recover communication through esophageal speech or tracheoesophageal puncture plus implantation of a valved plastic prosthesis.

Unilateral or bilateral modified or radical neck dissection is carried out depending on the presence of disease in the neck. The prognosis for laryngeal carcinoma overall is excellent when conservation principles are employed. Kennedy and Krause reported an 84 percent 5-year survival rate, which is typical [22]. After irradiation failure the salvage rate may be as low as 26 percent for lesions that were initially $T_1N_0M_0$ or $T_2N_0M_0$ prior to irradiation.

Vocal rehabilitation after total laryngectomy has been summarized by Pearson and Donald (Table 19-6) [1, 3, 19, 37]. Among the techniques shown, esophageal speech remains the most effective rehabilitative measure and may be surprisingly good. The success of rehabilitation varies to a significant

**Table 19-6** *Vocal rehabilitation techniques for the laryngectomee*

I. Nonsurgical techniques
  A. Esophageal speech
  B. Mechanical speaking aids
    1. Stoma-driven transoral reed
    2. Battery-driven transcervical vibrator
    3. Miscellaneous electromechanical devices
II. Surgical techniques
  A. Multistaged reconstruction (e.g., Asai laryngoplasty)
  B. Single-stage reconstruction
    1. External fistula (e.g., Taub air bypass method)
    2. Internal fistula
      a. Without prosthesis
        (i) Tracheoesophageal fistula (e.g., Amatsu TE shunt)
        (ii) Tracheopharyngeal fistula (e.g., Staffieri neoglottis)
      b. With prosthesis (e.g., Blom-Singer duckbill)

degree with the patient, the teacher, and the institution.

## Hypopharyngeal and Cervical Esophageal Tumors

As in the larynx, tumors of the hypopharynx and cervical esophagus are overwhelmingly squamous cell carcinoma. They carry with them an increasingly ominous prognosis as their location progresses downward from the base of the tongue toward the stomach.

These cancers are biologically agressive, with rapid local mucosal and submucosal spread and a propensity toward regional and even distant metastases. Multicentric disease and skip areas are common. Because symptoms of early disease are minimal, tumors are often large before they are discovered and may in fact be suspected only when sizable cervical metastases are noted.

Aside from postcricoid carcinoma, these types of cancer occur predominantly in men with a history of heavy alcoholic intake. The peak age incidence is 40 to 60 years

Female patients with postcricoid carcinoma commonly exhibit Plummer-Vinson syndrome with anemia, achlorhydria, and mucosal atrophy. Diagnosis is often possible with simple indirect laryngoscopy, though esophageal swallow, esophagoscopy, and direct laryngoscopy supplemented with CT scanning are important for delineating the extent of the disease.

Treatment of carcinoma of this type is complicated by early spread to contiguous structures and the presence of nodal metastases in a large percentage of patients. The dismal results achieved with radiation therapy [34] leave little argument with surgery as the treatment of choice. The operative approach is en bloc resection of the tumor, almost always including the larynx or hemilarynx. Bilateral neck dissections are often carried out even in the absence of palpable cervical nodes. Simultaneous neck dissections may be performed with sparing of the internal jugular vein on the side where disease is less extensive. In the absence of gross metastatic disease the sternocleidomastoid muscles may be spared as well. These muscles offer protection to the carotid arteries in the face of radiation damage.

Adjunctive postoperative irradiation may increase survival [11] and is perhaps preferred to preoperative irradiation, which not only makes the extent of tumor less easy to define but increases the postoperative complication rate substantially.

Reconstruction of a conduit may be accomplished by several methods, including those of Wookey, which employs cervical skin flaps (largely of historical interest) [46], the deltopectoral flap approach popularized by Bakamjian [9], the pectoralis major myocutaneous flap reconstruction [27], and the gastric pull-up procedure. With continuing advances in technique and expertise in microvascular free jejunal transfer, this approach seems to be the preferred method in many cases. In experienced hands there is a high success rate [26].

The prognosis for hypopharyngeal and cervical esophageal cancer treated with an aggressive surgical approach and adjunctive irradiation is in the 30 to 40 percent range for 5-year survival.

## Miscellaneous Tumors of the Neck

Cervical nodal masses may be detected without any evidence of a primary lesion in the upper aerodigestive tract. After a careful search has been made for such a primary lesion, including sinus radiographs, CT scanning, and fiberoptic examination, a surgical approach may be made, anticipating radical neck dissection. Occasionally, the mass proves to be a lymphoma, in which case resection of the lesion is all that is indicated in anticipation of appropriate work-up and therapy as dictated by the findings.

Commonly, the mass represents metastatic disease from the upper aerodigestive tract that is nearly always squamous cell carcinoma and requires neck dissection. Much less commonly the type of metastatic disease noted indicates a primary site below the clavicles. The histologic type often yields a high index of suspicion to a particular anatomic site. An appropriate search for the primary is then carried out.

### PRIMARY BRANCHIOGENIC CARCINOMA

Squamous cell carcinoma may rarely occur in a branchial cleft cyst [4]. This diagnosis is presumed only after a thorough search for another primary site is negative, as indicated above, and only when the site is appropriate for a branchial cleft cyst. There is some question as to whether this entity exists. Standard neck dissection is usually curative.

### CAROTID BODY TUMORS

Carotid body tumors, also known as chemodectomas, occur most commonly at the bifurcation of the carotid artery. They are only rarely malignant, and metastasis is uncommon.

The history is usually one of a slowly enlarging, painless upper cervical mass located just inferior to the angle of the jaw. The mass is firm and rubbery in consistence and pulsatile to palpation. It can usually be translocated in the transverse but not the vertical orientation. Diagnosis is confirmed by angiography.

Though there is a certain hazard to the cerebral circulation with resection, in our experience the risk is minimal. The tumor is nearly always resected with minimal difficulty and morbidity if the appropriate plane is followed and a meticulous dissection is carried out [21].

SARCOMA

Though not common in the head and neck areas, sarcomas do occur in all the generally accepted categories, including fibrosarcoma, chondrosarcoma, osteogenic sarcoma, angiosarcoma, leiomyosarcoma, liposarcoma, rhabdomyosarcoma, and a more recently accepted group of tumors (with subtypes) known as malignant fibrous histiocytoma (MFH).

Malignant fibrous histiocytoma, with its fibrous, myxoid, and other subtypes, is the most frequently occurring malignant soft tissue tumor. This large number is in part due to the fact that some tumors previously classified as fibrosarcomas or leiomyosarcomas are now designated MFH, fibrous subtype, and some liposarcomas are now designated MFH, myxoid subtype.

As a group, sarcomas spread hematogenously. Hence in the absence of known distant metastases, en bloc local resection is carried out. Regional node dissections are performed only when there is clinically suspicious adenopathy [18].

The exception to the above is rhabdomyosarcoma, which is most commonly seen in children and the elderly. The treatment of embryonal rhabdomyosarcoma in children by surgical resection, followed by chemotherapy and radiation therapy (4500 to 7000 rad), has resulted in significantly improved 5-year survival [15].

Prognosis is perhaps best judged by the degree of differentiation. Patients with poorly differentiated (high grade) sarcomas fare much worse than those with well differentiated (low grade) sarcomas, regardless of the specific type.

## References

1. Amatsu, M. A new one stage surgical technique for postlaryngectomy speech. *Arch. Otol. Rhinol. Laryngol.* 220:149, 1978.
2. American Cancer Society. 1976 Cancer facts and figures based on rates from the NCI: Third National Cancer Survey. *CA* 26:150, 1976.
3. Asai, R. Laryngoplasty after total laryngectomy. *Arch. Otol.* 95:114, 1972.
4. Batsakis, J. G. *Tumors of the Head and Neck.* Baltimore: Williams & Wilkins, 1974.
5. Batsakis, J. G. Tumors of the Major Salivary Glands. In *Tumors of the Head and Neck.* Baltimore: Williams & Wilkins, 1974. P. 8.
6. Belsky, J. L., et al. Salivary gland tumors in atomic bomb survivors, Hiroshima–Nagasaki, 1957–1970. *J.A.M.A.* 219:864, 1972.
7. Berg, J. W., Hutter, R. V. P., and Foote, F. W., Jr. The unique association between salivary gland cancer and breast cancer. *J.A.M.A.* 204:771, 1968
8. Castro, E. B., et al. Tumors of the major salivary glands in children. *Cancer* 29:312, 1972.
9. Daniel, R. K., Cunningham, D. M., and Taylor, G. I. The deltopectoral flap: An anatomical and hemodynamic approach. *Plast. Reconstr. Surg.* 55:275, 1975.
10. DeGroot, L. J., et al. *Radiation-Associated Thyroid Carcinoma.* New York: Grune & Stratton, 1977.
11. Donald, P. J., Hayes, R. H., and Dhaliwal, R. Combined Rx for pyriform sinus cancer using postoperative irradiation. *Otolaryngol. Head Neck Surg.* 88:738, 1980.
12. Edis, A. J. Surgical treatment for thyroid cancer. *Surg. Clin. North Am.* 57:533, 1977.
13. Edis, A. J. Surgery of the Thyroid Gland. In J. M. Lorré (ed.), *Head and Neck Surgery.* Philadelphia: Harper & Row, 1981. Pp. 30–48.
14. Eneroth, C. M. Salivary gland tumors in the parotid gland, submandibular gland, and the palate region. *Cancer* 27:1415, 1971.
15. Exelby, P. R. Management of embryonal rhabdomyosarcoma in children. *Surg. Clin. North Am.* 54:849, 1974.

16. Favus, M. J., et al. Thyroid cancer occurring as a late consequence of head-and-neck irradiation: Evaluation of 1,056 patients. *N. Engl. J. Med.* 294:1019, 1976.

17. Frazell, E. L. Clinical aspects of tumors of the major salivary glands. *Cancer* 7:637, 1954.

18. Gaisford, J. C., and Hanna, D. C. Sarcomas of the head and neck. *Plast. Reconstr. Surg.* 29:250, 1962.

19. Griffiths, C. M. Neoglottic reconstruction after total laryngectomy. *Arch. Otolaryngol.* 106:77, 1980.

20. Harwood, A. R., et al. Radiotherapy of early glottic cancer. *Laryngoscope* 90:465, 1980.

21. Irons, G. B., Weiland, L. H., and Brown, W. L. Paragangliomas of the neck: Clinical and pathologic analysis of 116 cases. *Surg. Clin. North Am.* 1:575, 1977.

22. Kennedy, J. T., and Krause, C. J. Survival rates in conservation surgery of the larynx. *Arch. Otolaryngol.* 99:274, 1974.

23. Lawson, W., and Som, M. Second primary cancer after irradiation of laryngeal cancer. *Ann. Otol.* 84:771, 1975.

24. Leading article. Salivary gland tumours. *Lancet* 1:655, 1969.

25. Lillie, J. C., and DeSanto, L. W. Transoral surgery of early cordal carcinoma. *Trans. Am. Acad. Ophthalmol. Otolaryngol.* 77:92, 1973.

26. McConnel, M. S., et al. Free jejunal grafts for reconstruction of pharynx and cervical esophagus. *Arch. Otolaryngol.* 107:476, 1981.

27. McCoy, F. J. Immediate Reconstruction of Pharynx and Cervical Esophagus with Pectoralis Major Myocutaneous Flap Following Laryngopharyngectomy. In F. J. McCoy (ed.), *Year Book of Plastic and Reconstructive Surgery.* Chicago: Year Book, 1983. Pp. 88–89.

28. McKenna, R. J. Tumors of the major and minor salivary glands. *Ca. J. Clin.* 34:24, 1984.

29. Nishiyama, R. H., Ludwig, G. K., and Thompson, N. W. The Prevalence of Small Papillary Thyroid Carcinomas in 100 Consecutive Necropsies in an American Population. In L. J. DeGroot (ed.), *Radiation-Associated Thyroid Carcinoma.* New York: Grune & Stratton, 1977. P. 123.

30. Pearse, A. G. E., and Takor, T. T. Embryology of the diffuse neuroendocrine system and its relationship to the common peptides. *Fed. Proc.* 38:2288, 1979.

31. Pearson, B. W., and Donald, P. J. Larynx. In *Head and Neck Cancer: Management of the Difficult Case.* Philadelphia: Saunders, 1984. Pp. 95–96.

32. Sener, S. F., and Scanlon, E. F. Irradiation-induced salivary gland neoplasia. *Ann. Surg.* 191:304, 1980.

33. Sizemore, G. W., Carney, J. A., and Heath, H., III. Epidemiology and medullary carcinoma of the thyroid gland: A 5-year experience (1971–1976). *Surg. Clin. North Am.* 57:633, 1977.

34. Som, M. L., and Nussbaum, M. Surgical therapy of carcinoma of the hypopharynx and cervical esophagus. *Otolaryngol. Clin. North Am.* 2:631, 1969.

35. Spiro, R. H., Hajdu, S. I., and Strong, E. W. Tumors of the submaxillary gland. *Am. J. Surg.* 132:463, 1976.

36. Spiro, R. H., et al. Tumors of minor salivary origin: A clinicopathologic study of 492 cases. *Cancer* 31:117, 1973.

37. Taub, S., and Bergner, L. H. Air bypass voice prosthesis for vocal rehabilitation of laryngectomees. *Am. J. Surg.* 125:748, 1973.

38. Thompson, N. W., Nishiyama, R. H., and Harness, J. K. Thyroid carcinoma: Current controversies. *Curr. Probl. Surg.* 15:1, 1978.

39. Woods, J. E. Parotidectomy: Points of technique for brief and safe operation. *Am. J. Surg.* 145:678, 1983.

40. Woods, J. E. The facial nerve in parotid malignancy. *Am. J. Surg.* 146:493, 1983.

41. Woods, J. E. Parotidectomy versus limited resection for benign parotid masses. *Am. J. Surg.* 149:749, 1985.

42. Woods, J. E., Chong, G. C., and Beahrs, O. H. Experience with 1,360 primary parotid tumors. *Am. J. Surg.* 130:460, 1975.

43. Woods, J. E., et al. Pathology and surgery of primary tumors of the parotid. *Surg. Clin. North Am.* 57:565, 1977.

44. Wookey, H. The surgical treatment of carcinoma of the pharynx and upper esophagus. *Surg. Gynecol. Obstet.* 75:499, 1949.

45. Woolner, L. B., et al. Primary malignant lymphoma of the thyroid: Review of forty-six cases. *Am. J. Surg.* 111:502, 1966.

46. Woolner, L. B., et al. Thyroid Carcinoma: General Considerations and Follow-Up Data on 1,181 Cases. In S. Young and D. R. Inman (eds.), *Thyroid Neoplasia.* London: Academic Press, 1968. P. 51.

47. Wychulis, A. R., Beahrs, O. H., and Woolner, L. B. Metastasis of carcinoma to the thyroid gland. *Ann. Surg.* 160:169, 1964.

# 20

## Aesthetic Surgery of the Eyelids and Periocular Region

*Ulrich T. Hinderer*

The ocular region is the most important site of expression of human emotions and plays an outstanding role in interpersonal communication. Local, systemic, and endocrine disorders as well as adverse life conditions may alter the appearance of the ocular region. Aging usually shows first at the palpebral and periorbital region.

Treatment of ocular region changes has evolved over the last few decades—since the basic surgical technique of palpebral skin excision and treatment of eyelid bags described by Castañares in 1951 [14]—toward a selective approach to the correction of each of the eyelid structures affected by the process of aging. Various techniques are now available for the correction of these structures—skin, orbicularis muscle, septum orbitale, canthal ligaments, eyelid retractors, and tarsal plates—which are combined according to individual needs. Improvement of the eyelid unit is incomplete without restoration of the tension of the periorbital region if it is decreased—the frame in which the eyelids are inserted [36]. The palpebral and the periorbital regions are regarded as an entity.

A precise preoperative evaluation is essential. For some patients, mainly those with asymmetries or who are having secondary surgeries, a quantitative appraisal can be of great value as a complement to a careful qualitative evaluation.

Surgery itself, if not properly performed, may change the expression or impair function, resulting in important complications that are difficult to repair without aesthetic sequelae. An apparently insignificant removal of tissue may later become conspicuous. Careful surgery is therefore of utmost importance, and the beginner must start with simple techniques. Experience then allows safety in the performance of advanced techniques.

### Preoperative Evaluation
GENERAL CONDITION

A thorough clinical history and physical examination are mandatory to assess the local implications of organic or systemic alterations (renal, cardiac, or chronic liver diseases; diabetes or thyroid disorders; allergies; and coagulation alterations). The clinical findings rarely contraindicate surgery, but they are taken into account so as to institute necessary treatment. The use of aspirin or anticoagulants is discontinued for 2 weeks before surgery. The patient's personality, motivations for surgery, and other factors related to his or her life are considered, as the surgical improvement is expected to be matched by a favorable psychic result.

## EYE FUNCTION

Visual acuity, intraocular pressure, and the function of the intrinsic muscles must be assessed to detect cases of unilateral blindness (of which even the patient may be unaware), glaucoma, strabismus, retinal detachment, or other sight impairment. The assistance of an ophthalmologist may be advisable for diagnosis and advice.

## FRAME OF THE EYELIDS

The patient requesting aesthetic surgery of the eyelids for aging wants to look younger and better. Patients in their thirties are frequently experiencing a descent of the eyebrow and hooding of the upper part of the superior palpebral region. This problem cannot be adequately corrected by blepharoplasty alone. A browlift is needed to reduce the amount of skin to be resected from the upper eyelid and to avoid extension of the scar into the thicker lateral periorbital skin. By the time the average person reaches his or her forties the facial skin also loses its elasticity. The forehead, periorbital soft tissues, and cheeks descend, producing deeper nasolabial folds. Consequently, the tension of the forehead and periorbital and facial tissues should be restored in addition to blepharoplasty. Most patients agree with this assessment if, in front of a mirror, they are given a well grounded explanation. Evaluation is therefore extended to the following areas.

1. Forehead (ptosis, width, and wrinkles). Horizontal wrinkles are caused by the frontalis muscle; transverse wrinkles at the root of the nose by the procerus muscle; glabellar frowns by the corrugator supercilii muscle; and crow's feet by the orbicularis muscle.
2. Shape and position of the eyebrow. The descent of the medial brow causes an angry look, and descent of the tail a concerned or sad appearance. Excessive elevation expresses astonishment. Descent of the entire brow provides an aged or tired look; a low medial brow with excessive lateral elevation confers a somewhat diabolic appearance. Brow mobility is checked for possible paresia of the frontal branch causing unilateral brow ptosis; a unilateral elevation with increased transverse forehead wrinkles may result from hyperactivity of the frontalis muscle to compensate for ptosis of an upper lid.
3. Cheeks and depth of the nasolabial folds, as ptosis increases the traction on the lower eyelids.
4. Upper orbital rim. A low lateral upper orbital rim may enhance a "sunken eye" appearance or provide a triangular shape of the upper palpebral region, also increasing "hooding."

## QUALITATIVE EVALUATION OF THE PALPEBRAL REGION

The main alterations of the palpebral tissues produced by the aging process, which vary in degree depending on constitutional-hereditary factors influenced by personal mimic expression habits and by general health, are evaluated with regard to each eyelid structure.

### Skin and Subcutaneous Tissue

Ptosis with folding and wrinkling of the skin is due to a decrease in thickness and to distention of the elastic fibers. The thin skin of the eyelids has all the cutaneous elements and may therefore show the pathologic alterations of the skin in other regions. These changes are recorded, as are the locations of folds and wrinkles and the adherence of the pretarsal skin to the tarsus [105]. Edema due to general or local causes easily occurs in the subcutaneous tissue, producing puffiness. The skin above the superior palpebral sulcus is approximately twice as thick as that below [56].

The levator aponeurosis, the septum, and

the orbicularis fascia fuse to form a conjoint preseptal fascia adhered inferiorly to the tarsal plate. If there is high fusion, the eye appears hollow; low fusion over the tarsal plate may result in a low supratarsal fold [105]. The site of insertion of the expansion of the aponeurosis of the levator muscle to the dermis determines the distance of the supratarsal fold from the ciliary border. According to Sheen [100], this distance is usually 10 mm measured at the mid-pupillary line. Rees stated that the average distance is 6 to 8 mm, which may be increased to 8 to 13 mm in the deep-set eye. At surgery the author prefers to place the fold at 8-mm distance. The location of the supratarsal fold is best determined as suggested by Sheen [100] (Fig. 20-1).

Approximately 70 percent of Asians lack a supratarsal fold due to the absence of endings of the aponeurosis of the levator muscle in the dermis. They also have a greater amount of fat in the subcutaneous tissue, between the orbicularis muscle and the septum (preseptal space), and in the preaponeurotic space in front of the levator aponeurosis. Epicanthal folds are also frequently present.

*Orbicularis Oculi Muscle*
Some anatomic facts must be remembered: The palpebral (pretarsal and preseptal) orbicularis, responsible for the voluntary and involuntary and the spontaneous and reflex closure of the eyelid, contributes to the formation of the medial canthal ligament and is attached to the diaphragma lacrimalis and the crista lacrimalis. It contributes to the tear collection and provides a lacrimal pump mechanism.

Laterally, the upper and lower lid pretarsal orbicularis join, forming a raphe, which is attached to the lateral canthal skin and contributes to the lateral canthal ligament. The orbital part depresses the eyebrow with its lateral segment and forms by divergent fibers the corrugator muscle, which inserts at the medial orbital region and intertwines

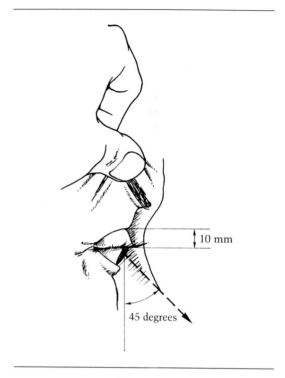

**Figure 20-1** *Sheen's [100] test for determination of the supratarsal fold. The eyebrow is elevated enough to compensate for the excessive skin, and the patient is requested to assume a 45 degree downward gaze. The height of the fold from the eyelid rim can be measured in this position.*

with the vertical fibers of the frontalis muscle. At the palpebromalar sulcus some connective fibers join the limits of the orbicularis muscle and the zygomatic muscle, inserting into the underlying periosteum. Toward the nose, the orbicularis muscle is continued by a fibrous tissue layer that connects with the levator alae nasi and the quadratus levator labii superioris. Deep bluish nasopalpebral furrows are due to a wide gap [92].

With aging, the orbicularis muscle relaxes, becomes hypotonic, and descends. This phase may cause diminished adaptation of the lower eyelid to the globe, with a tendency to epiphora, and a fold hanging over the palpebromalar crease. The tonus of the orbicularis is always checked (Fig. 20-2).

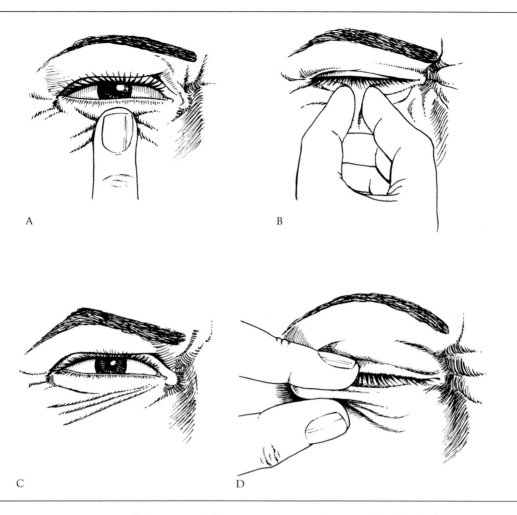

A

B

C

D

**Figure 20-2** *A. Assessment of the tonus of the orbicularis muscle [49]. With the examiner's index finger on the lower eyelid, the patient is asked to close the eyelid tightly, which helps to evaluate the tension of the orbicularis muscle and whether a fold involves only the skin or both skin and muscle. B. "Pinch" test [34]. Similar to the previous test, the skin is pinched with thumb and index finger, and a forceful contraction of the orbicularis is then opposed against the resistance of the examiner's pinch. C. Squint test for evaluation of hypertrophic orbicularis fibers [66, 67]. Intense muscular activity due to mimic expression or frequent squinting due to exposure to strong light or sun may cause hypertrophy of palpebral muscle fibers, producing an oblique lateral and downward thickening. It can be checked by asking the patient to squint as if looking at a strong light source. The test also serves for evaluation of the pretarsal orbicularis muscle. D. "Squinch" test for evaluation of festoons [34]. With advanced age and due to major relaxation of the orbicularis, festoons may appear at the preseptal and orbital areas. With tight contraction of the orbicularis the festoons may efface, reappearing when the muscle relaxes. If the festoons also contain orbital fat, the position of the festoon changes.*

*Supporting Structures of the Eyelids*

The supporting structures of the eyelids are formed, first, by a fibrous diaphragm formed by the tarsal plates attached to the periosteum of the orbital margins through the septum orbitale, both medially and laterally by the pretarsal and preseptal parts of the orbicularis muscle, and by the bony insertions of the canthal ligaments. Second are the eyelid retractors (represented in the upper eyelid by the superior rectus muscle, levator palpebrae, sympathetic Müller's muscle, and associated aponeurosis and fascias, and in the lower eyelid by the aponeurosis, which corresponds to the upper eyelid's levator muscle and the lesser developed sympathetic tarsalis inferior muscle, connected to the tendon sheet of the inferior rectus muscle. Thus attached to the tarsal plate, the capsulopalpebral head of the inferior rectus muscle contributes to stabilize the lower lid and retracts the lid when the eye rotates downward. The eyelid retractors act as antagonists to the protracting action of the orbicularis muscle [52, 53].

In the aging eyelid relaxation of the supporting structures may cause the following alterations.

1. Involutional ectropion with separation of the rim from the globe.
2. Elongation of the lower eyelid rim (loss of resilience and thinning of the tarsal plates).
3. Descent of the lateral canthus (elongation of the lesser developed lateral canthal ligament with lateral downward slanting of the palpebral fissure).
4. Acquired ptosis (stretching, detachment, or disruption of the multiple flimsy fibrous attachments of the levator aponeurosis into the top of the tarsal plate, mostly due to excessive muscular pull to elevate heavy eyelids or caused by trauma [83]. During surgery excessive traction is avoided to prevent iatrogenic ptosis. Dehiscence can be diagnosed by having the patient gaze upward while holding the lashes down: The eyelid pull of the levator occurs above the upper border of the tarsus [121]. A dysfunction of the sympathetic innervated Müller's muscle (Horner's syndrome) may be assessed by instillation of several drops of 10% phenylephrine hydrochloride solution, which corrects the mild unilateral ptosis.
5. Shallow lower fornix (laxity of lower lid retractors), or entropion, mainly caused by deinsertion of the lower lid retractors, occasionally associated with deepening of the fornix [86, 97, 98] (Fig. 20-3).

*Orbital Fat Tissue*

Intraorbital fat constitutes a cushion-like shock absorber for the eyeglobe. It prolapses through five foramina between the periorbita, globe, oblique muscles, and arcuate expansion, producing eyelid bags in two pockets in the upper and three in the lower eyelid, as described by Castañares in 1951 [14, 18, 19, 21]. Eyelid bags are often hereditary or idiopathic and in these cases may appear in the young person.

Four factors contribute to the appearance of eyelid bags: augmentation of the intraorbital pressure, such as by increase of the fat volume; weakness of the septum orbitale and of the fibrous supporting structures; descent of the eyeglobe due to laxity of the multiple orbital muscular-fascial structures, such as Lockwood's ligament, the hammock on which the globe rests [123]; and relaxation of both orbicularis and skin. A lateral upper eyelid fat pad may be encountered attached to the superior lateral orbital rim, adherent to the underside of the orbicularis muscle [82], thereby contributing to heaviness of the upper lid (Fig. 20-4).

*Lacrimal Gland and Function*

Some patients exhibit a displaced lacrimal gland with puffiness of the lateral aspect of the upper eyelid [107], which occurs more frequently in men, usually bilaterally. Occasionally hypertrophy of the larger orbital portion is also found (Fig. 20-5B).

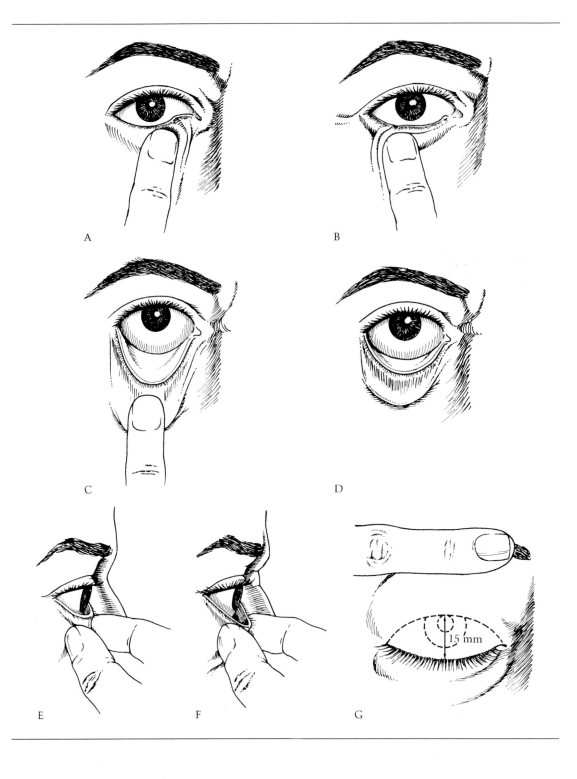

A

B

C

D

E          F          G

15 mm

*Figure 20-3* A, B. Tension test for the canthal ligaments [49]. The rim of the lower eyelid is moved in a medial and lateral direction, checking its extent of displacement of the canthus. C, D. Flowers' "eyelid retraction test" [29]. Relaxation of the fibrous supporting structures of the eyelids and the tone of the orbicularis muscle can be checked by gentle pulling on the lower eyelid downward, away from the globe, and releasing it. "In many lids— sometimes in surprisingly young people—the lid will go back to contact the globe either very slowly or not at all until the eye is blinked. This means that the main thing holding the lid in contact with the globe is a 'water seal'" [29]. E, F. Schaefer's "lid retraction test" for evaluation of the lower eyelid retractors [99]. This test is especially indicated in patients with involutional entropion due to disruption or distention of the aponeurosis of the capsulopalpebral head. The lower eyelid is grasped with the index finger and thumb just below the lash border centrally and is withdrawn from the globe. Normally the lid withdraws 3 to 5 mm, but this distance increases in patients with involutional entropion up to 10 or 12 mm and in patients with marked lid relaxation up to 25 mm. When pulling the eyelid rim from the globe, the separation should be less than 8 mm [112]. G. "Levator excursion" test [110]. With the brow immobilized, the excursion of the lid margin is measured from the eyes-down to the eyes-up position. The normal excursion is about 15 mm; in ptotic eyelids it is 0 to 12 mm.

*Figure 20-4* Evaluation of palpebral bags. Moderate pressure applied over the closed eye helps to determine the compartments described by Castañares [14] and the volume of protruding fat.

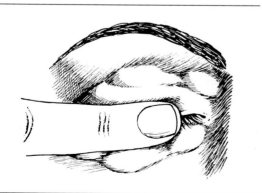

Epiphora may result from excess tear production or a decrease in transportation, mainly caused by obstruction or anomalies of the position of the eyelid due to aging or trauma. A decrease in tear production may cause "dry eye syndrome," or keratoconjunctivitis sicca, which may be complicated by xerophthalmia and corneal ulcers. However, in some patients the palpebral Krause glands may compensate for the lack of corneal moistening. Patients with scleral show or exophthalmos causing alterations of tear drainage may show a major tendency to a dry eye syndrome [89]. In the dry-eye patient skin excision must be conservative [113], and the patient is informed of a possible increase in irritation after surgery. The use of polyvinyl pyrrolidone or methylcellulose derivatives is then indicated postoperatively.

In addition to evaluation of the conjunctiva for alterations or conjunctivitis (to be treated before surgery), a Schirmer test (Fig. 20-5A) is always performed in patients with a history of frequent irritation with soreness, burning, itching, or foreign body sensation. It is also done in patients with epiphora, as basic secretion may be deficient but reflex tearing from the lacrimal gland is preserved [37]. A fluorescein dye test is useful for diagnosing abrasions or ulcers: A fluorescein strip is placed in the lower fornix, the eye is closed, and the cornea is examined for staining.

*Lower Orbital Rim*
Deep setting of the lower eyelid may be increased by major protrusion of the inferior orbital rim [90], which is evaluated by palpation.

QUANTITATIVE EVALUATION OF THE PALPEBRAL AND PERIORBITAL REGION
A quantitative telephotographic evaluation (Fig. 20-6) is performed whenever an asymmetry is encountered as well as before secondary blepharoplasties for unfavorable results [44]. Together with postoperative photographs, it provides a more objective

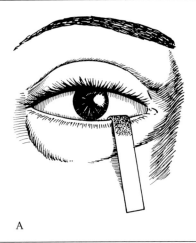

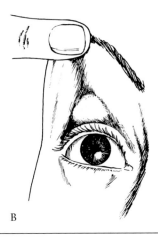

A                                                    B

judgment of the postoperative result and constitutes a psychologically valuable document that clearly demonstrates the results achieved with the operation. Such a record may be important, as patients have a short memory of their preoperative status. The pre- and postoperative frontal photographs are taken under the same conditions, with the patient's head in an upright position and the frontalis and orbicularis muscles relaxed. The camera lens is at the same level as the patient's eyes. A cephalostat can be used for greater accuracy.

Black-and-white life-size enlargements (with a transverse eye aperture of approximately 30 mm) permit one to draw lines and to take measurements, which have proved useful as guides.

*"Scleral show"* (see Fig. 20-6, line 1). With preectropion conditions, the visibility of the sclera, normally not more than 1 mm, increases.

*Aperture of the eyelid (vertical palpebral fissure)* (lines 2 and 3). These lines are drawn at the medial and lateral limits of the cornea. The vertical width of the palpebral fissure is approximately 9 mm (between 7 and 11 mm). The upper palpebral rim should be symmetric on both sides approximately 1 mm below the limbus. The vertical lateral

**Figure 20-5**  *A. Schirmer test. In a moderately illuminated room to reduce reflex secretion [91] or after topical anesthesia of the conjunctiva to eliminate this reflex secretion [37], the conjunctiva is gently dried and a sterile filter paper strip (5 × 35 mm) is hung over the lower eyelid rim toward the fornix at the junction of the central and medial thirds, maintained 5 minutes, and the moistened area then measured. A value of 15 mm or more is normal; values below 10 mm are found in keratoconjunctivitis sicca and Sjögren's syndrome [37]. The result may vary in the same patient and should therefore be repeated. B. Evaluation of the lacrimal gland [49]. In patients with puffiness of the lateral aspect of the upper eyelid, the eyebrow is strongly pulled upward, which helps to define the limits of a ptotic or hypertrophic lacrimal gland. With ptosis, the lacrimal gland is displaced under the orbital rim. Moderate pressure on the closed eyelid helps to differentiate the lacrimal gland from protruding fat from the central compartment.*

aperture is increased in preectropion conditions with respect to the medial aperture. However, in patients with ptotic or heavy upper eyelids or with hypertrophy of the lacrimal gland, the vertical lateral aperture is reduced. With exophthalmos, both are increased.

*Transverse axial line's angle (TALA)* (4). The lateral and medial canthi of each eye are connected with a line that is prolonged over

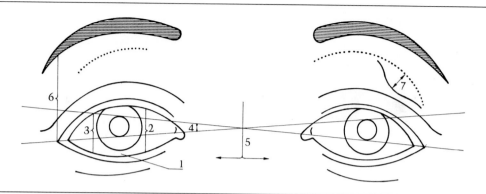

**Figure 20-6** *Hinderer's measurements for quantitative evaluation of the palpebral and periorbital regions [46] (see text). 1 = scleral show; 2, 3 = vertical aperture of the eyelid (medial and lateral); 4 = transverse axial lines' angle (TALA); 5 = intersection of the axial lines; 6 = vertical distance between lateral canthus and tail of the eyebrow; 7 = lateral upper orbital rim determined by palpation.*

the dorsum of the nose. The TALA is positive when the lateral canthi are above the level of the medial canthi and is negative when the lateral canthi are below this level. The lateral upward slant of the palpebral fissure, considered attractive in Caucasians, is characteristic of the young eye. This inclination may be constitutionally reversed, producing a sad and aged appearance. It also forms part of some congenital malformations. With age, and caused by a relaxation of the lateral canthal ligament and the neighboring septum fibers, the TALA may tend to become negative. However, this situation is not the rule, as there are individual and racial variations.

*Intersection of both transverse axial lines* (point 5). The intersection can be shifted to either the right or the left of midline, revealing asymmetries of the palpebral regions and the orbits.

*Vertical distance from the lateral canthus to the tail of the eyebrow* (line 6). This distance varies in proportion to the descent of both.

## Planning Surgery
PATIENT INFORMATION

The planning of the operation is discussed with the patient prior to surgery. Detailed information is provided regarding the location and extension of scars, their eventual visibility, and their possible evolution. The patient's sensitivity to a detectable scar is determined. Eyelid scars are usually inconspicuous so long as they do not surpass the eyelid skin, extending to the nose or to the thicker lateral palpebral skin.

SELECTION OF TECHNIQUE

Selection of technique depends on the degree of relaxation and ptosis of each eyelid structure. The indications, as seen by the author, are summarized in Tables 20-1 to 20-4. In addition, for lateral downward slant of the palpebral fissure (caused by aging, congenital malformations, or trauma, blepharoplasty with browlift (supraciliary or preferably forehead) is usually done.

## General Surgical Management
PREPLANNING THE INCISIONS

According to Rogers [95], premarking was suggested by Ambroise Paré during the fourteenth century to avoid insufficient or excessive skin removal. I have used preplanning with the patient in a sitting position since 1955 for better achievement of symmetry. The horizontal position on the table

**Table 20-1** *Repair of the soft tissue frame of the eyelids*

| Problem | Procedure |
|---|---|
| Brow ptosis, asymmetric, and hooding of upper eyelid | Supraciliary browlift |
| Forehead-brow ptosis (wrinkles and glabellar frowns) and | Forehead lift |
| Periorbital tissue ptosis, crow's feet, deep palpebromalar sulcus, cheek ptosis, deep nasolabial folds or postoperative "round eye" | Upper face rhytidectomy: sub-SMAS "blepharo-periorbitoplasty" or subperiosteal "mask lift" |

reduces the downward gravitational displacement of the palpebral tissues seen in the erect position.

*Preplanning a Browlift*

For browlift, the future shape and position of the eyebrow is discussed with the patient sitting in front of a mirror. A line is drawn at the upper row of hair (subtotal length of the brow, lateral two-thirds, or tail). The skin above the eyebrow is plicated with delicate angulated forceps or between thumb and index finger for marking of reference points. A gently curved upper incision line can then be marked. The highest point is usually at the limit of the medial and lateral thirds of the eyebrow. When the hair implantation is irregular, some hair is included within the area to be excised. If the eyebrows are excessively wide, the patient is instructed not to pluck the eyebrows for a few weeks prior to surgery to facilitate more precise partial excision. I do not prolong the lower incision horizontally for a few millimeters beyond the tail of the eyebrow. If it is required, the indication is to perform a forehead-temporal browlift. The difference in length of the upper and lower incision lines can be easily compensated if suturing starts from both ends and progresses medially.

More exact planning of the upper incision has been proposed by Connell [22]: The edge of the supraorbital rim is indicated by three or more marking pencil dots. As the eyebrow is elevated, the supraorbital ridges are again indicated by skin dots. The distance

**Table 20-2** *Repair of the bony frame of the eyelids*

| Problem | Procedure |
|---|---|
| Low lateral upper orbital rim with "sunken eye" appearance or triangular shape of upper eyelid | Ostectomy through blepharoplasty approach, supraciliary browlift approach, or forehead lift approach |
| Protrude lower orbital rim with depressed lower eyelid | Ostectomy |

**Table 20-3** *Repair of upper eyelids*

| Problem | Procedure |
|---|---|
| Redundant wrinkled skin | Skin–orbicularis excision blepharoplasty |
| Bags | Fat removal |
| Asian "single" eyelid; supratarsal fold less than 8 mm from the ciliary border | Supratarsal fixation |
| Acquired ptosis | Levator shortening with supratarsal fixation |
| Ptosis of the lacrimal gland | Additional dacryoadenopexy |

**Table 20-4** *Repair of the lower eyelids*

| Problem | Procedure |
|---|---|
| Skin redundance, wrinkling | |
|     Moderate | Skin–orbicularis excision |
| | Skin flap blepharoplasty |
|     Severe | Skin flap–muscle suspension blepharoplasty |
|       and | |
|     Hypotony of orbicularis | Skin flap-muscle suspension blepharoplasty |
|       and | |
|     Eyelid rim elongation | Skin flap-muscle suspension blepharoplasty with wedge excision of the tarsal plate |
|     Entropion | Skin flap-muscle suspension blepharoplasty with wedge excision of the tarsal plate and eyelid retractors-tarsal plate-preseptal orbicularis sutures |
| Lateral downward slant of the palpebral fissure | Blepharocanthoplasty with browlift |

between these dots indicates the eyebrow elevation needed at each part of the eyebrow. Remember that the ratio of scalp excision for elevation of the brow is approximately 2:1 instead of the (almost) 1:1 ratio for supraciliary browlifts.

PLANNING THE UPPER EYELID EXCISION. With the eyelid closed (Fig. 20-7A,B), moderate tension is applied to the supraciliary region so as to stretch the pretarsal skin. Pointing of the eyelashes should be the same on both sides. The lower incision follows a curved line of inferior concavity with its apex approximately 8 mm from the lash line, coinciding usually with the most inferior palpebral wrinkle. The medial end of this incision is extended 1 to 2 mm in the horizontal direction but remains within the limits of the eyelid skin. The lateral extension curves slightly upward from a level approximately 1 mm lateral to the canthus and approximately 3 mm above it, thereby leaving a skin bridge wide enough to ensure lymphatic drainage. The elevation achieved by an eventual browlift or foreheadlift must be taken into account when marking the width of upper eyelid skin to be removed by blepharoplasty.

For marking of the upper incision, the patient looks straight forward. Several reference points are marked corresponding to the level of the lower marking. With the eyes closed, the width of the palpebral skin to be removed is rechecked using delicate angulated forceps. The forceps closure just pulls taut the eyelid skin but does not elevate the palpebral margin or evert the lashes. The reference points are then united.

PLANNING THE LOWER EYELID SKIN EXCISION. The patient is requested to look upward. The upper incision (Fig. 20-7C–E) begins at the level of the punctum, follows the ciliary margin at a distance of approximately 2 mm, and extends horizontally past the canthus for a few millimeters on one of the horizontal "crow's feet." Using delicate angulated forceps and with the patient looking upward, the skin is plicated and several reference points are marked. The plication tenses the skin but does not lower the palpebral margin or evert the lashes. The marking line is completed by joining the reference points.

In blepharoplasties without undermining, the skin excision corresponds exactly to the marking. In skin flap or skin–muscle flap suspension blepharoplasties, usually an extra strip of skin has to be excised owing to

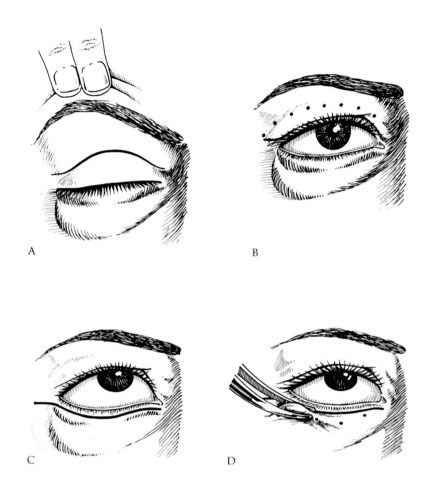

A                    B

C                    D

*Figure 20-7* Preplanning eyelid skin excision [40]. A, B. At the upper eyelid. C, D. At the lower eyelid.

the more extensive upward displacement achieved. In this case the marks serve as a guideline for a more regular excision performed parallel to the marking.

ANESTHESIA

Blepharoplasty is performed by many surgeons under local anesthesia and sedation.

The traction on orbital fat may be painful, requiring deep sedation. Local anesthesia with mild diazepam (Valium) sedation is occasionally used and always when ptosis is corrected simultaneously. However, as stated by Ellenbogen and Swara [26], amounts of diazepam above 10 mg may cause dysconjugate gaze from the drug's muscle-relaxing effect. In most patients, neuroleptic analgesia is preferred complemented with submuscular lidocaine-epinephrine infiltration to facilitate dissection and to achieve a more bloodless field; general anesthesia with intubation is used when a rhytidectomy is performed as well. The recovery must be without excitement, vomiting, or hypertension to avoid postoperative bleeding.

## PREVENTING DESICCATION OF THE CORNEA

During surgery the cornea must be protected from the heat of the lamp, trauma due to instruments or gauze, and dryness caused by constant irrigation with saline solution. A protective ointment is applied at the beginning and at the end of surgery.

## SEQUENCE OF SURGICAL STEPS

Browlift is done prior to the upper blepharoplasty and this before the lower blepharoplasty so as to avoid excessive excision of skin of the upper and lower eyelids.

## TREATMENT OF EYELID BAGS

### Transpalpebral Fat Removal

For better identification of the fat compartments, gentle digital pressure is applied to the closed eye. For skin flap blepharoplasties, the orbicularis muscle is split at the site of the bags in the direction of its fibers, the septum orbitale is opened, and the protruding fat is grasped with a forceps; the excess is then cut off, and the stumps are coagulated without touching the forceps, which serve to dissipate the heat. However, blood vessels at the base may be coagulated individually with fine bipolar forceps and the fat stripped off.

Excessive traction on the fat from one compartment may reduce the fat from neighboring pockets through their continuity with the deeper fat, sometimes leaving unsightly depressions. If a muscular flap technique is used, the protruding fat is removed through a large horizontal incision of the septum.

If there is also fat extending from the central third into the lateral third of the upper eyelid, it can be differentiated from the lacrimal gland by its texture and yellow coloration. According to Owsley [82] and Wilkinson [122], a lateral upper fat pad is occasionally found above the septum adherent to the orbicularis and extending over the orbital rim, which is also removed. In patients not requiring skin incisions, Ortiz-Monasterio and Krugman [80] removed the protruding fat through minimal stab incisions.

### Transconjunctival Removal of Lower Eyelid Bags

In young people with eyelid bags but without skin excess on eyelid wrinkles, fat removal from the lower eyelids may be performed through the conjunctival approach (Figs. 20-8 and 20-9). This procedure was first reported by Bourguet during the 1920s [12], was popularized by Tessier during the 1950s [114], and is used by several authors today [69, 115].

Identification of the inferior oblique muscle is required to avoid its injury in patients in whom a major quantity of fat must be removed [119]. This approach can also give access to the orbital rim. Care must be taken to not remove an excessive quantity of fat, producing enophthalmos with the appearance of a "sunken eye."

Despite the fact that this approach partially transects the inferior tarsalis muscle and aponeurosis, impairment of the lid retractor function has not been observed, probably owing to reestablishment of its continuity when suturing or by scar tissue.

### Reinsertion of Fat

Protruding orbital fat tissue is usually removed. However, in moderate bags, the fat tissue may be reinserted by restoring the

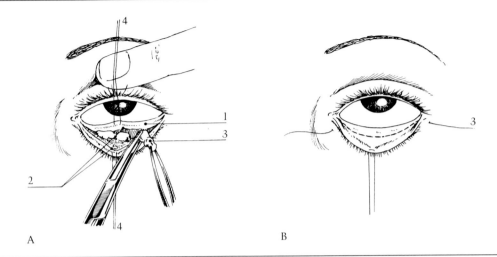

A                                              B

tension of the orbicularis muscle and the skin as achieved by a "skin flap–muscle suspension blepharoplasty" or a "blepharo-periorbitoplasty" [51]. Cardoso suggested [13] insertion of vertical plication sutures of the lower preseptal orbicularis for reinserting the protruding fat.

Except for large bags or with exophthalmos, a new procedure has been devised by de la Plaza [84] that consists in placing the fat tissue back into the orbital cavity, achieving the retention by suturing the capsulopalpebral aponeurosis, especially if distended, to the periosteum of the lower orbital rim.

*Figure 20-8* *Transconjunctival removal of lower eyelid bags. A. A traction suture is placed at the lower eyelid margin to evert it. Two traction sutures (4) are placed on the conjunctiva of the fornix (1) and above to facilitate a transverse incision through the conjunctiva (2) and downward dissection, taking care not to injure the inferior oblique muscle. Gentle pressure applied to the eyeball aids removal of the fat pads (3) and stump coagulation. B. Conjunctival closure is performed with a removable 6-0 Ethilon suture entering and emerging through the skin. The suture is fastened to the skin with adhesive tape strips and is removed after 1 week.*

*Figure 20-9* *Large eyelid bags in a young girl with exophthalmos, removed through a transconjunctival approach. Malar augmentation has also been performed.*

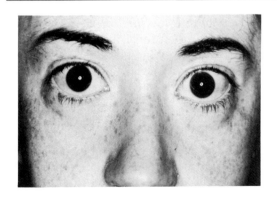
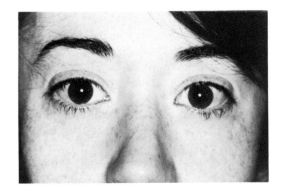

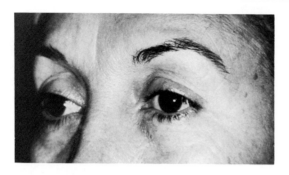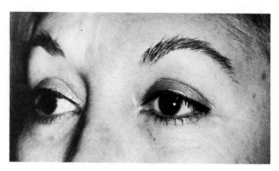

**Figure 20-10** *Skin flap blepharoplasty and rhytidectomy in a patient with lower eyelid bags and depressed upper eyelids. Improvement was obtained by removing a downward-slanted upper lateral orbital rim and fat transplantation from the lower eyelid into the upper eyelid.*

*Fat Tissue Grafts*

The volume of intraorbital fat may decrease with age. The eyeball then displaces deeper into the orbit, and the upper palpebral region has a concave depression. In other patients distention of the intraorbital musculofascial system holding the eyeglobe may cause a minimal descent of the eyeglobe—enough, together with the decreased tension of the orbicularis muscle, of the septum and skin to produce eyelid bags in the lower eyelid combined with a depression at the medial upper eyelid.

In these patients the protruding orbital fat of the lower eyelid is excised, reinserting it through a stab wound into the medial and/ or central compartments of the upper eyelid (Fig. 20-10). Uchida [116] used fat tissue grafts from the forearm to treat the hollow Asian eyelid, and Loeb [68] recommended use of submental fat grafts in Caucasian patients.

PREVENTION OF POSTOPERATIVE
"ROUND-EYE" APPEARANCE
AND ECTROPION

Skin removal is evaluated after redraping the skin without tenting. Several measures may help to prevent excessive removal: If general anesthesia is used, the cheeks are put under moderate tension to reproduce the gravitational effect in erect position, or the head is elevated [68]; light pressure on the closed eye somewhat elevates the lower eyelid rim [87]. The patient operated on under local anesthesia is invited to open his mouth and to look upward.

The septum is not sutured, as there is no difference in result [114] and eventual infolding and shortening are prevented, as are incarcerations of orbital structures such as the inferior oblique tendon, which would result in a torsional diplopia [118].

Skin flaps must be widely undermined to avoid upward "angulation" of the anesthetized or weakened orbicularis fibers, which, when the tonus recovers, may displace the lid downward, as mentioned by Edgerton [25]. Edgerton resects the skin, with the patient looking straight forward, at 1 mm above the limbus.

Adhesive paper tapes applied obliquely and toward the temple support the lid and reduce the tendency to edema and ecchymosis, as suggested by Lewis [63]. If, despite these precautions, a tendency to a round-eye appearance is noted at the end of surgery, a Frost suture in the lower eyelid and taped to the forehead skin is used for 2 to 3 days.

SUTURING

Ethilon 6-0 or Mirafil 6-0 is used for a running intradermal suture on the upper eyelid and for interrupted stitches on the lower eyelid. Steri-Strips are applied for superficial skin adaptation on the upper eyelids and at the canthal region. This measure allows early postoperative removal of the interrupted sutures (second or third postoperative day), thereby preventing epithelial tunnels. The intradermal suture is removed after 1 week.

POSTOPERATIVE CARE

To avoid claustrophobia, cold compresses moistened with camomile, which has a mild antiphlogistic and antiseptic action, are used during the first postoperative day, as suggested by the author in 1969 [40]. The patient may remove them whenever he wishes. Desiccation of the cornea and crust formation along the incision line and the stitches are prevented. Ice packs may be used in addition to elevation of the head, antiinflammatory enzymes, diuretics, and limitation of salt intake if there is a tendency to edema.

Usually, the eyelids do not close at the end of surgery due to hypotony of the orbicularis caused by the anesthetic drugs and by edema. A separation of 1 mm or at most 2 mm may occur during the first hours, after which the orbicularis begins to recover its tone; later the eyes usually close and remain closed during sleep. If complete closure is delayed, the following treatment is used: tight closure exercises of the eyes to recover the orbicular tonus; gentle upward and outward massage with a lubrificating ointment of the lower eyelids 1 week after surgery; instillation of artificial tears; taping or use of a gauze moistened with camomile solution at night, especially if the preoperative evaluation revealed a weakness of the superior rectus muscle, which prevents upward deviation of the globe during sleep, thus exposing the cornea when a postoperative lagophthalmos has occurred.

Female patients are instructed to avoid wearing makeup during the 2 weeks after surgery. Later, they must remove it as gently as possible.

## Surgical Techniques
UPPER EYELIDS
*Skin–Orbicularis*
*Excision Blepharoplasty*
For the skin–orbicularis excision blepharoplasty the skin is excised with a thin layer of orbicularis muscle at the site of the preplanned excision.

*Supratarsal Fixation*
The performance of supratarsal fixation (Fig. 20-11) originated from the trend to create a supratarsal fold to "westernize" the Asian "single eyelid." Shirakabe [104] reported that 21 technical variations were published in the Japanese literature following Mikamo's first publication in 1896 and before reports began to appear in the Western literature by Sayoc [96], Millard [73], Fernandez [27], Uchida [116], Khoo Boo-Chai [9, 10, 11], and others [103]. Treatment was extended to the Caucasian eyelid by Flowers (anchor blepharoplasty) [28, 29] and Sheen [100, 101] for achievement of better definition or of upper displacement of low folds.

The principles of the various techniques are based on, or combine, several technical steps.

1. External fixation through the lid and conjunctiva, as practiced by many Asian authors for treatment of "single" eyelids.
2. Clearance of fat, fascia, and a strip of pretarsal orbicularis from the pretarsal space [9, 27–29, 73, 96]. Apart from the Asian eyelid, this procedure may also be indicated for patients with heavy pretarsal eyelids or to achieve skin–tarsal adhesions in patients with excessively lax or wrinkled pretarsal skin [105].
3. Electrocoagulation to provoke skin–orbicularis adhesion, used by Rogers [94].
4. Orbicularis strip excision without tarsal or levator fixation [5].
5. Dermal-tarsal fixation [73, 96].
6. Dermal-levator-tarsal fixation [28, 29].
7. Dermal-levator aponeurosis edge fixation [9, 27].

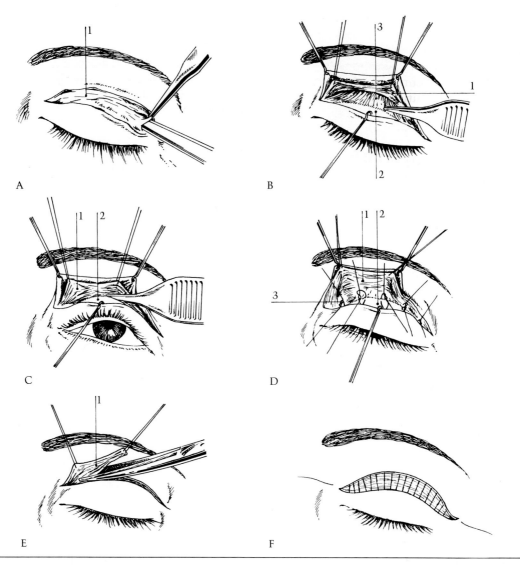

**Figure 20-11** Supratarsal fixation. A. After preplanned skin excision with the lower marking at 8 mm from the lash line at the midpupillary line, the orbicularis muscle (1) is undermined medially, transected along the lower skin margin, and the orbicularis above it elevated. B. The septum is incised and the excess fat removed. Care has to be taken not to injure the levator aponeurosis. The presence of the supratarsal arterial arcade, which lies on Müller's muscle, indicates that the aponeurosis has been severed, a defect that must be sutured. In heavy pretarsal eyelids, the upper pretarsal space is cleared of fat and fascia, and a small pretarsal orbicularis strip is removed. B, C. The lower edge of the levator aponeurosis (3) is identified. D. The border of the pretarsal orbicularis (or, if preferred, of the lower dermis) is sutured with 6-0 Vicryl to the edge of the levator aponeurosis at the upper tarsal border (2). It is important, as stated by Ellenbogen and Swara [26], to test the fixation by light caudal traction. If eyelashes evert after suturing, the stitches are replaced, taking a bite of the upper border of the tarsal plate. Additional stitches are placed to be approximately 3 mm apart. E. Excess preseptal orbicularis is removed. F. A running intradermal 6-0 Ethilon suture is used for skin closure.

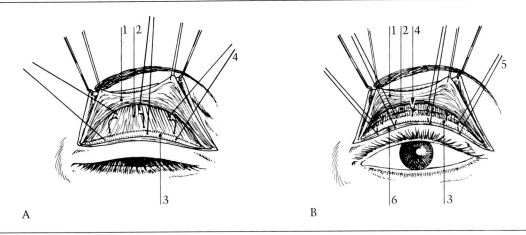

A                                    B

*Figure 20-12* *Technique of levator aponeurosis tucking and supratarsal fixation for treatment of the involutional eyelid with acquired ptosis. A. After skin excision and upward undermining of the preseptal orbicularis muscle (1), sectioned at the level of the lower skin incision, the septum is incised, the protruding fat removed, and the levator aponeurosis (2) identified. With disruptions, the edge is attached with a few Vicryl sutures to the upper border of the tarsal plate (3). With distentions, the width of aponeurosis to be shortened is determined by passing 5-0 Vicryl sutures (4) through the levator aponeurosis and the edge of the tarsal plate. By tightening with a single knot, the lid position is tested with regard to the limbus and to symmetry with the other side. In cases of excessive elevation, new sutures are placed and the situation of the lid margin tested again. B. The sutures are tightened (4) and a few more stitches placed to complete the tucking. For supratarsal fixation (5) 6-0 Vicryl stitches are placed between the anterior stitches, which unite the trimmed pretarsal orbicularis border (6) to the plicated levator aponeurosis edge. The excess of preseptal orbicularis muscle (1) is excised, and skin closure is completed with an intradermal running suture with 6-0 Ethilon.*

**8.** Pretarsal orbicularis border-levator aponeurosis fixation [26, 35, 78, 100, 101, 105] or fixation to the adventitia [111].

A dermal-levator aponeurosis fixation after clearance of the pretarsal space toward the lashline may evert the lashline, serving for treatment of entropion. On the other hand, if the pretarsal–orbicularis border fixation to the levator aponeurosis is performed at a somewhat higher level, the palpebral fissure may be widened [101].

I perform supratarsal fixation in patients with low or not well defined supratarsal folds, in those with asymmetries, and in the Asian "single" eyelid. Usually, fixation of the trimmed pretarsal orbicularis border to the levator aponeurosis at the tarsal edge or Flowers' "anchor blepharoplasty" with dermal fixation is used.

### Supratarsal Fixation and Levator Aponeurosis Tucking for Treatment of Acquired Ptosis

Surgery is performed under local anesthesia and moderate sedation to have the patient's cooperation for more precise determination of the level of the upper lid margin and for better achievement of symmetry. When the acquired ptosis is due to dehiscence, re-attachment of the levator aponeurosis is sufficient. With levator distentions, tucking su-tures of the aponeurosis to the tarsal plate are performed and combined with supratarsal fixation of the trimmed pretarsal orbicularis border to the levator aponeurosis edge (Figs. 20-12 and 20-13).

### Ptosis of the Lacrimal Gland

Ptosis of the lacrimal gland can be treated

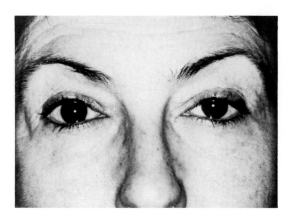
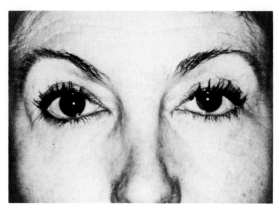

**Figure 20-13** *Supratarsal fixation with levator aponeurosis shortening in a patient with acquired ptosis of the left eye. A lower skin flap blepharoplasty was also performed. Preoperatively the patient tried to compensate the ptosis by elevating the eyebrow.*

(Figs. 20-14 and 20-15) by plication of the capsule of the orbital portion above the periosteal rim with a few 6-0 Vicryl sutures [29], by suspension under the orbital margin with a stitch given to the periosteum [64], or by using two or three mattress sutures through the body, tucking the gland posteriorly up under the rim [20, 107]. In very hypertrophic glands in patients with epiphora and without keratoconjunctivitis, the excess of the orbital portion may be grasped with forceps, ligated, and resected, with the ends of the ligatures sutured to the periosteum. The author has used the latter technique only twice, both times without complications.

BLEPHAROPLASTY ON
THE LOWER EYELID
*Skin-Orbicularis Excision
Lower Blepharoplasty*
During 1955 to 1965 in most patients and occasionally today, I perform a preplanned blepharoplasty by skin-orbicularis excision without skin flap undermining (Fig. 20-16) [39], a technique that, according to Rees [90], was first reported by Converse in 1964 [23] and is still used by Siegel [105]. The tech-

**Figure 20-14** *Dacryoadenopexy of the pars orbitalis of the lacrimal gland. After undermining the preseptal orbicularis muscle (2), the septum is incised and the ptotic lacrimal gland (1) identified by its different color from that of the protruding fat, which is removed. If the capsule has been opened, the firm lobulated consistency of the gland becomes visible. The lateral roof of the orbit (3) is visualized, the gland is reinserted, and with a few Vicryl sutures its capsule is united (4) to the periosteum. The excess preseptal orbicularis is then resected and skin closure performed.*

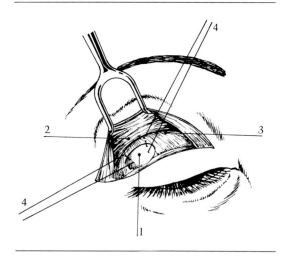

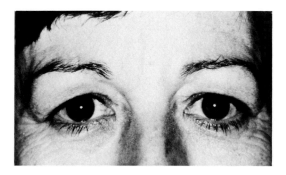

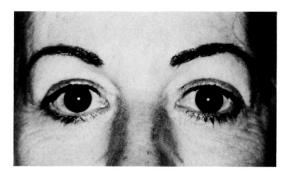

nique is indicated for patients with moderate upper skin excess and wrinkling or when blepharoplasty is combined with a facial rhytidectomy, just for removal of the upward shifted lower eyelid skin excess.

*Skin Flap Lower Blepharoplasty*
The skin flap blepharoplasty (Figs. 20-17 and 20-18) was the conventional technique used before popularization of the skin–muscle flap blepharoplasty. The technique is indicated in patients with large skin excess and wrinkling, moderate eyelid bags, and adequate tonus of the orbicularis muscle.

In patients with deep palpebromalar folds or "circles" between nose and eyelid, Regnault's technique [92] of suturing the medial edge of the orbicularis muscle to the tissue overlying the quadratus levator labii super-

**Figure 20-15** *Patient with hypertrophy of the right and ptosis of the left lacrimal glands. Lacrimal gland capsule suspension was performed and a partial excision of the orbital part of the lacrimal gland added on the right side. Lower eyelid skin flap blepharoplasty, supratarsal fixation, and browlift have also been performed.*

**Figure 20-16** *Skin–orbicularis excision blepharoplasty. A superficial layer of orbicularis muscle is removed together with the skin to avoid any thickening at the level of the suture line. Minimal undermining of the skin borders at the lateral canthus is occasionally necessary for better skin adaptation. Fat bags are removed through stab wounds. The technique requires exact preplanning of the excision.*

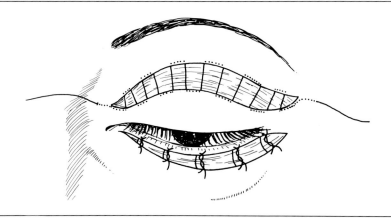

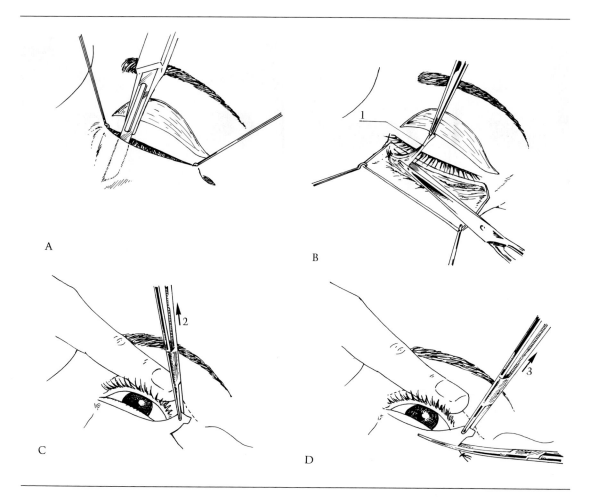

A

B

C

D

***Figure 20-17*** *Skin flap lower blepharoplasty. A. After incision, the skin is tensed upward with hooks and opposite traction on the cheeks and dissected downward with a scalpel beyond the lowest wrinkle. The depth of undermining is controlled from the surface, the blade showing through the skin. B. Hypertrophic fibers of the orbicularis, if present (1), are trimmed with scissors, and careful hemostasis is performed with delicate forceps and bipolar coagulation. Fat bags are removed at the site of protrusion after separating the orbicularis fibers with scissors and opening the septum. C. With moderate pressure on the eyeglobe, the skin medial to the canthus is displaced in an upward and medial direction (arrow 2), carefully redraped without "tenting." The excess is scratched with a scalpel and excised in a lateral to medial direction; two or three stitches are applied. D. The skin is then displaced upward (arrow 3) and redraped; the excess is then scratched with a scalpel, excised with scissors, and sutured with a few interrupted stitches. The lower skin border is thinned if necessary. Both upper and lower skin margins must be under similar longitudinal tension [88] to prevent a "round eye" due to scar retraction. Skin displacement—first in an upward medial direction and, after the first stitches have been applied laterally, in an upward lateral direction—corrects differences in length of the skin borders, keeping the incision, lateral to the canthus, short.*

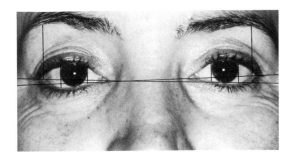 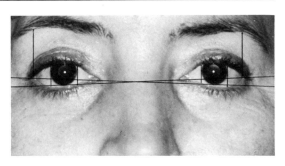

*Figure 20-20* Patient with large skin excess and major wrinkling. A skin flap–muscle flap technique was used.

With the skin–muscle flap blepharoplasty, the orbicularis muscle transection is performed 2 to 3 mm below the skin incision, between pretarsal and preseptal orbicularis to preserve function of the pretarsal orbicularis. This method is also recommended by Kostianovsky [55]. It avoids overlapping of the incision lines, and some pretarsal fullness is achieved as well, which according to Sheen [102] is, together with a well-defined palpebral furrow, a characteristic of the young eyelid. In the aged patient, flattening occurs caused by distention and descent of the pretarsal orbicularis. For its correction, Sheen advocated tarsal fixation of the orbicularis to the lower tarsal border with 7-0 silk sutures 4 mm apart and 6 mm from the skin edge.

*Skin Flap–Muscle Suspension Blepharoplasty*

The skin flap–muscle suspension blepharoplasty (Figs. 20-21 to 20–23) technique was first reported by the author in 1977 [46, 47, 49] for restoring the tension of the orbicularis muscle. This goal is achieved by upward and lateral displacement of the orbicularis muscle and its fixation, after resection of a superolateral wedge, to the raphe and periosteum.

The technique was also reported independently by Mladick [74] in 1979, who called it a "muscle suspension technique." Adamson et al. [1] suspended the lateral excess of orbicularis by passing it as a flap through a tunnel under the raphe toward the upper eyelid incision, performing fixation to the periosteum of the lateral orbital rim.

In 1978 Furnas [33] reported a technique based on a similar principle for treatment of festoons forming in the pretarsal, orbital, or jugal areas of the eyelids due to relaxation of the orbicularis muscle.

*Skin Flap-Muscle Suspension Technique with Wedge Excision of the Lower Tarsal Plate and Conjunctiva*

Wedge excision of the lower eyelid (rim, tarsus, conjunctiva, and orbicularis muscle) combined with a skin flap blepharoplasty (Fig. 20-24) is known as the modified Kuhnt-Szymanowsky procedure and has been recommended by Fomon [31], Castañares [15], and Rees [88, 90]. Fosatti [32] added suturing of the divergent fibers of the orbicularis muscle to the eyelid externally to the lateral canthus, using the technique for ocular branch palsy, senile relaxations, scar contractions, and maladaptations of eye prostheses. Leone [59, 60] suggested in 1970 that the tarsal excision be done at the lateral canthus, suturing the tarsal plate to the remnants of the lateral canthal tendon. In the author's modification, a step-like rim–tarsal plate excision is combined with a skin flap-muscle suspension blepharoplasty (Fig. 20-25).

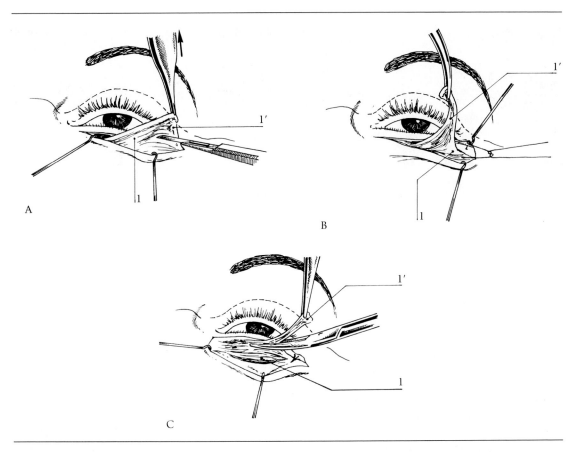

**Figure 20-21** Skin flap–muscle suspension lower blepharoplasty [46]. The skin is dissected with a scalpel at the lateral two-thirds of the lower eyelid down to the inferior eyelid wrinkles, toward the raphe, and at the crow's feet. The skin above the raphe is elevated with hooks and the orbicularis muscle horizontally incised immediately below the raphe down to the periosteum. The pretarsal orbicularis muscle is undermined and sectioned at the level of the skin incision. A hemostat is placed at the pretarsal connective tissue, and the orbicularis muscle is dissected downward beyond the palpebromalar sulcus. The septum is horizontally incised to remove the protruding fat. With smaller bags, restoration of the tension obtained with the technique adequately reinserts and retains the fat, without the need for removal. A. The orbicularis muscle (1) is displaced with moderate tension in an upward and medial direction, and the excess triangle surpassing the raphe is excised. B. The border sutured with 5-0 Vicryl to the raphe and the periosteum. C. An excess strip of the upper margin of the orbicularis is excised, mainly at the central one-third, so that the border contacts the preseptal orbicularis. The upper border must be at the level of the upper part of the tarsus to better adapt the eyelid to the eyeball. If the muscular border is below the tarsus, any excessive tension may tend to evert the rim. 6-0 Vicryl stitches may be used to join the muscular borders. The eyelid skin is redraped and the excess marked and excised as in the skin flap blepharoplasty technique.

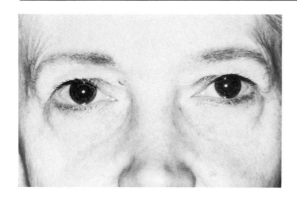

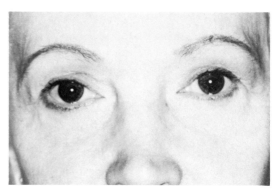

**Figure 20-22** *Skin flap–muscle flap suspension technique and rhytidectomy in a patient with major skin excess, decreased tonus of the orbicularis muscle, and large eyelid bags.*

In patients with involutional entropion, the author combines the preseptal muscular suspension and step-like tarsal excision. Vicryl tucking sutures are used to catch the aponeurosis of the capsulopalpebral head, the lower border of the tarsal plate, and the pretarsal orbicularis border. A strip is removed from the latter, with the purpose of increasing the horizontal tension at the level of the lower border of the tarsal plate and everting the rim.

Tucking sutures through the skin including the aponeurosis were first devised by Reh in 1972 to correct the distention or disruption of the aponeurosis from the tarsal plate [53]. These sutures permit inward rotation of the lower border of the thin tarsal plate toward the globe. A similar technique

has also been used by Morax [77]. Leber and Cramer [58] used an upward displaced orbicularis flap based on a technique previously published by Wheeler.

**Figure 20-23** *Patient with skin excess, wrinkles, wide palpebromalar folds, and severe decrease of the tonus of the orbicularis muscle. A skin flap–muscle suspension technique and browlift were performed. The tension of the orbicularis muscle improved considerably, and the lateral vertical apertures were augmented. Measurements confirmed that the skin flap–muscle suspension technique did not change the slant of the palpebral fissure (TALA unchanged).*

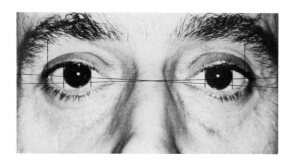

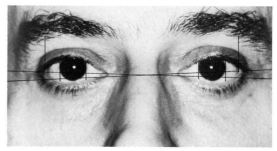

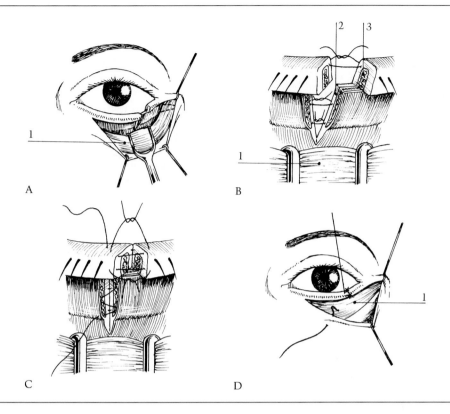

**Figure 20-24** Skin flap–muscle suspension lower blepharoplasty with step-like rim–tarsal plate excision (the author's modification of the Kuhnt-Syzmanowsky procedure). A. Skin flap dissection is performed. After incision immediately below the raphe, the pretarsal and preseptal orbicularis muscles (1) are undermined in a downward and lateral direction. B. The eyelid margin and tarsal plate are incised at the lateral one-third in a step-like fashion to prevent an indentation at the rim. For better appraisal of the width of the rim and tarsal plate to be excised, traction sutures may be passed a few millimeters from the canthus and at the midline. C. The eyelid margin is adapted and sutured with two 6-0 Ethilon stitches, the conjunctiva (2) with 6-0 catgut, and the edges of the tarsal plate (3) with a 6-0 Ethilon pull-out suture entering at the eyelid margin and emerging below through the orbicularis and the lower eyelid skin. D. The orbicularis muscle is displaced upward and laterally, the excess triangle excised, and the border sutured to the raphe and to the periosteum at the lateral canthal region (muscle suspension technique). The central border of the orbicularis is trimmed if necessary, the skin redraped, the excess removed, and the skin borders sutured as previously described.

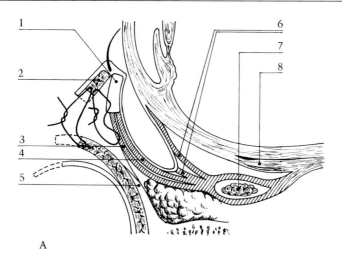

A

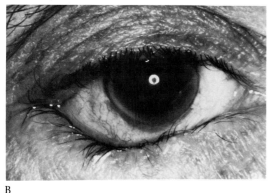

B

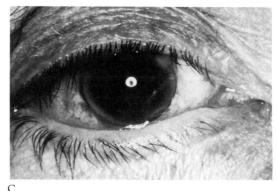

C

**Figure 20-25**  A. The author's technique for involutional entropion. After dissection of the skin, the orbicularis muscle is incised at the level of the lower border of the tarsal plate (1), the pretarsal orbicularis (2) is dissected in an upward direction, and the preseptal orbicularis muscle is dissected downward. Step-like rim–tarsal wedge excision is performed, and sutures are applied to restore the rim continuity. Tucking sutures of Vicryl are applied, catching the trimmed border of the pretarsal orbicularis muscle, the lower border of the tarsal plate, and the fascia of the capsulopalpebral head (3). The preseptal orbicularis muscle is tensed in an upward lateral direction, a triangular wedge at the lateral canthus is excised, and the free border is sutured to the raphe and periosteum with Vicryl sutures for muscular suspension. A few fine Vicryl stitches may be used to join the borders of the pretarsal and preseptal orbicularis muscle. Any skin excess is excised, and the skin is sutured independently. This technique achieves first reduction of a rim elongation, if present; second eversion of the rim is accomplished by increasing the horizontal tension at the level of the lower border of the tarsal plate with the muscular suspension technique and by attaching the border of the pretarsal orbicularis to the lower border of the tarsal plate and to the fascia of the capsulopalpebral head. 4 = inferior tarsalis muscle; 5 = septum; 6 = branches of the capsulopalpebral head of the inferior rectus muscle; 7 = inferior oblique muscle; 8 = inferior rectus muscle. Preoperative close-up view (B) result 1 year after surgery (C) of a 75-year-old patient with involutional entropion, rim elongation, and decreased tension of the orbicularis muscle operated with the technique shown in Fig. 20-25A.

PALPEBRAL FISSURE

*Blepharocanthoplasty with Browlift*

A lateral downward slant of the palpebral fissure confers a sad and aged appearance. In the involutional eyelid, the lateral canthal ligament, the orbicularis muscle, and the septum may distend, causing a reversed obliquity of the palpebral fissure. This problem may also be present constitutionally in the young person, may be a symptom of congenital malformations, or may be due to trauma. As has been proved by the author via quantitative evaluations, the slant of the palpebral fissure can be modified only by acting on the lateral supporting structures, i.e., the lateral canthal ligament.

The technique of blepharocanthoplasty with browlift (Figs. 20-26 to 20-28) was first described by the author in 1975 [44]. The technique was reviewed by Ortiz-Monasterio and Rodríguez in 1985 [81], who modified the approach to the lateral canthal ligament by vertically incising the periosteum of the lateral orbital rim and freeing the septum from the lateral and inferior orbital rim. These authors reported satisfactory results mainly for achieving an antimongoloid slant. Whitaker [120] dissected the lateral canthal soft tissue mass (periosteum, lateral canthal ligament, and raphe), which is subperiosteally freed from dermis to bone and from bone to conjunctiva to a point vertically below the pupil. After mobilization, the mass with the lateral canthus is fixed through two holes to the lateral orbital rim with wire or synthetic material.

With the author's technique, fixation of the lateral canthus was also first performed through holes in the lateral orbital rim, but this practice was discontinued as the periosteal fixation proved to be sufficiently stable. Elevation of the lateral canthus decreases its distance to the tail of the eyebrow. Therefore blepharocanthoplasty is always combined with a supraciliary or preferably forehead browlift. Thus the improvement obtained is not spoiled by the resulting shorter distance from the lateral canthus to the eyebrow.

*Medial Canthopexy*

Rarely, relaxation of the fibrous supporting structures of the eyelids affects the stronger medial canthal tendon, allowing the punctum to displace laterally and separate from the eyeball, thus interfering with normal tear transportation. A medial canthopexy is then indicated. The technique is as follows.

The incision of the lower eyelid is carried on medially beyond the punctum in a horizontal direction along the lower border of the medial canthal tendon while the eyelid is tensed laterally. The deep surface of the tendon is carefully freed from the connective tissue that surrounds the saccus lacrimalis up to its bony insertion. Usually, plication of the tendon is sufficient. However, an alternative method is to grasp the tendon with forceps close to the bony surface and sever the insertion. Tension applied to the medial end determines how much of the tendon should be removed. Reinsertion is performed with 4-0 unstained braided nylon, which is passed twice through the tendon and fastened to the remnants. If a large skin excess results from the canthal displacement, a small triangle of skin is also removed.

SOFT TISSUE FRAME OF THE EYELIDS

Ptosis of the soft tissues around the eyelid may preferentially involve the eyebrow and upper lateral eyelid, which can be corrected by a forehead–temporal lift of the lateral canthal region, or it may involve the complete periorbital region including the lower eyelid and cheek, in which case blepharoplasty is combined with a rhytidectomy of the upper two-thirds of the face, designated *blepharoperiorbitoplasty* by the author. In young patients, when only the lateral aspect of the eyebrow and the upper lateral eyelid are ptotic, in patients who reject the previously mentioned techniques, or in those in whom eyebrow asymmetries are present, a direct browlift by means of a supraciliary

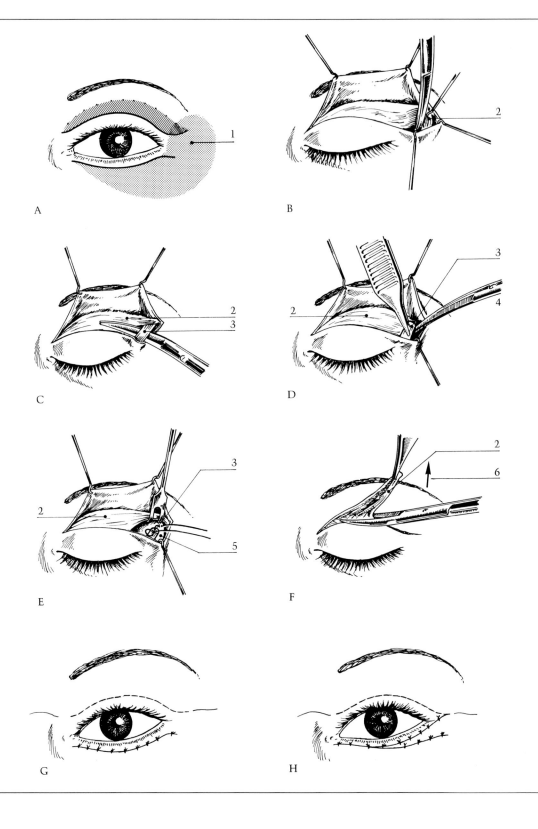

A

B

C

D

E

F

G

H

*Figure 20-26* *Blepharocanthoplasty with browlift [46]. A. Only the lower incision of the upper eyelid and the upper incision on the lower eyelid are performed. 1 = area of skin undermining. B. The orbicularis (2) above the raphe is split, and the lower orbicularis muscle is widely undermined (dotted line area). C. Scissors are inserted and turned at the lateral bony rim so that the tip goes around the lateral canthal ligament (3). D. The ligament is sectioned close to the bony rim. Some septal fibers close to the ligament must be sectioned with scissors (4) to obtain complete mobility of the lateral half of the eyelid. E. The ligament is sutured with two stiches of unstained braided nylon to the external periosteum (5) 4 to 8 mm above and lateral to its original insertion, depending on the slant to be obtained. F. The excess of upper preseptal orbicularis muscle and of skin are excised. A browlift (6) has to be added. Otherwise the distance lateral canthus–brow reduces without improvement of the sad and aged appearance. G. Skin sutures are completed as usual. H. In case of lack of skin at the external half of the lower eyelid, a Lewis Z-blepharoplasty [63] is added, bringing skin from the upper eyelid, based externally, to the lower eyelid.*

*Figure 20-27* *A, B. Patient aged 45 with skin excess, minor palpebral bags, and brow ptosis that is more marked on the right side. The vertical apertures are decreased owing to heavy upper eyelids. Blepharocanthoplasty with asymmetric supraciliary browlift was performed. The slant of the palpebral fissure improved (TALA +4 to +12 degrees), as did the vertical apertures. Symmetry of the eyebrow position was obtained, and the somewhat sad and asymmetric look was corrected. (From U. T. Hinderer. The aging palpebral and periorbital region. Transactions of the VII Congress of the IPRS, Rio de Janeiro, 1979).*

skin excision may be indicated in combination with the blepharoplasty.

*Supraciliary Browlift for Treatment of Ptosis of the Eyebrow and Hooding of the Upper Lateral Eyelid*

The supraciliary browlift, reported as early as 1930 by Passot and by Bames in 1958 [6], was popularized by Viñas [117] and Castañares [16]. Sokol and Sokol [109] and Smith and Newman [108] elevated the brow by means of a transblepharoplasty eyebrow suspension.

A supraciliary browlift is not performed in patients who have a tendency to keloid formation or hypertrophic scarring. When the technique is adequately performed, after 6 months to 1 year the scar is usually inconspicuous. However, the possibility of an unsightly scar must be discussed with the patient. During the first months when the scar is more visible because of its coloration, it can be covered by the bushy brow hair in men, or a brow pencil may be used by the female patient. As stated by Spira [110], the result is longer lasting than that of coronal browlifts.

The incision is performed obliquely to the skin surface, parallel to the hair shafts. The skin is carefully excised down to the orbicularis muscle. No undermining is required. Meticulous skin closure is performed using interrupted sutures of 6-0 Ethilon, and sur-

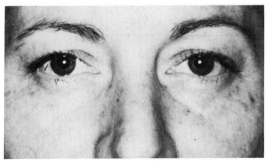

A

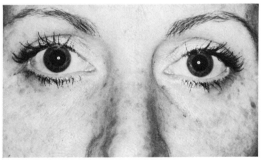

B

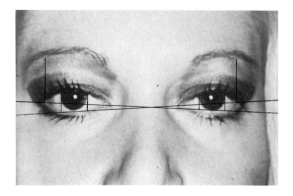
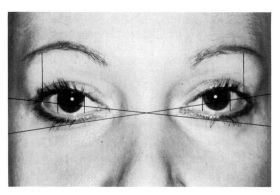

*face adaptation is carried out between the stitches using ⅛-inch adhesive paper tape strips. A subcuticular running suture is not used thereby avoiding constriction of hair follicles. Suturing starts at both ends to avoid any dog ear and to compensate for the differences in length of the wound margins. The stitches are removed on the third postoperative day.*

**Figure 20-28** *This patient, aged 28 with skin excess, minor bags, and moderate brow ptosis, requested a major slant of the palpebral fissure for achievement of almond-shaped eyes. A blepharocanthoplasty with browlift considerably increased the slant (TALA +6 to +15 degrees), also improving the vertical apertures and the distance from the lateral canthus to the brow. Despite the preoperative makeup, the postoperative photographs (without makeup) show the more youthful appearance of the ocular region. (From U. T. Hinderer. The aging palpebral and periorbital region.* Transactions of the VII Congress of the IPRS, *Rio de Janeiro, 1979).*

*Treatment of Ptosis of the Lateral Canthal Region Including "Crow's Feet"*
Correction of ptosis of the lateral soft tissues of the eye region is managed at the skin level. Upward and lateral displacement may be achieved by (1) joining the upper and lower blepharoplasty incision [36]; (2) rotating a flap from the upper to the lower eyelid [61]; (3) using a W-plasty or V-flaps, which permit a major skin excision and avoid scar webbing at the medial and lateral scar extensions [1, 24]; or (4) using a dermal flap for elevating the lateral lower eyelid [25]. With the last technique, however, epidermal cysts may occur [1]. In combination with a rhytidectomy, the orbicularis has been approached by Skoog [106], Aston [2], and Smith and Newman [108]. The orbicularis muscle is sharply dissected and its lateral segment spread and sutured under tension to the temporalis fascia in a cephaloposterior direction. According to Aston, the lateral di-

vision of the orbicularis muscle ring provides better improvement of folds and wrinkles, eliminating muscle function along the path of the transection. The technique also permits long-lasting elevation of the lateral brow.

*Treatment of Ptosis of the Periorbital Soft Tissues*
Whenever the eyebrow and the upper lateral palpebral and periorbital soft tissues are ptotic, I prefer to perform complete restoration of the tension. Such ptosis is present in most patients during the premenopausal decade.

In 1963 Marino [70–72] recommended an improvement of results of the forehead lift by performing deep dissection of the suprazygomatic superficial musculoaponeurotic system (SMAS) tissue, which he called the "meso temporalis," and detaching it from the orbital rim. In 1969 I reported the extended "blepharoplasty," a combination of a temporal lift with blepharoplasty [39]. Morales et al. [75, 76] in 1984 reported the temporal approach to a sub-SMAS elevation of the upper lateral periorbital tissues. Tessier in 1979 [114], followed by Psillakis in 1984 [85] and Mateo Santana, combined the forehead lift with a wide subperiosteal dissection, extended to the malar bone and maxilla to free the "facial mask" from the facial skeleton so it could be lifted independently from the skin. An additional vestibular approach, used by Tessier, completes the subperiosteal elevation from below—the so-called mask lift.

In 1985 and subsequently in 1986 and 1987 [48–51], the author reported the technique "blepharo-periorbitoplasty," based on a combined sub-SMAS-subperiosteal approach. Now, however, the subperiosteal dissection is limited exclusively to the site of the bony exit of the supraorbital bundle to make its dissection easier and safer (Figs. 20-29 to 20-33).

BLEPHARO-PERIORBITOPLASTY TECHNIQUE. With the blepharo-periorbitoplasty technique the following goals can be achieved.

1. Upward displacement of the forehead with correction of forehead and glabellar wrinkles. The forehead flap is dissected under the frontalis muscle and the galea and upper orbicularis toward the upper palpebral region. The frontalis muscle and galea, between 2.5 cm above the eyebrow and the hairline, are incised or removed (except at the pathway of the supraorbital nerves and vessels). The corrugators and the procerus muscle are dissected and partially removed (except immediately underneath the glabellar frowns). A downward slanting lateral orbital rim is corrected by ostectomy, if required.
2. Upward and moderately backward displacement of the temporal, periorbital, and maxillomalar soft tissues including the nasolabial fold. Thus also the upper orbicularis muscle, the raphe, and the

lower orbicularis muscle, except at its medial segment, are shifted upward. This maneuver is achieved through a connected deep superior dissection and a suborbicularis lower blepharoplasty approach.

An incision is made that follows the hairline at an 8-cm distance in a backward direction until reaching a vertical line above the ear. To prevent upward displacement of the sideburn and the preauricular skin immediately in front of the ear, the author's "hair-bearing rotation flap is used" [43]. This flap rotates backward while the facial skin in front of the flap is displaced upward and backward. The incision ends at the upper limit of the tragus. In case of a high forehead or temple recessions, a prehairline incision at the corresponding level is used.

From the temporal scalp incision, the pretemporal galea extension (fascia pretemporalis) is dissected on its deep surface along the temporal fascia at the anterior half of the zygomatic arch toward the orbital rim, the malar region, and the nasolabial fold. The tip of the scissors, directed toward the fascia, thus safely undermines the "meso temporalis," which contains the temporofrontal branch of the superficial temporal artery and the frontal, orbicular, and zygomatic rami of the facial nerve.

At the lower eyelid the fibers of the orbicularis muscle are split at the lateral third, and the lower orbicularis is deeply undermined toward the cheek and nasolabial fold and laterally until meeting the dissection from above. In case of major wrinkling and skin excess at the lower eyelid, a skin flap lower blepharoplasty is added.

Suturing the scalp and galea begins after adequate excision first at the midline of the forehead flap, then at the temporal flap, and finally at the intermediate segment. A soft suction drain toward the nasolabial fold is left in place for 12 hours, and the upper face is taped with 0.5-inch 3M strips.

The procedure can be combined with a lower face and neck rhytidectomy. Whenever indicated, malar augmentation is added,

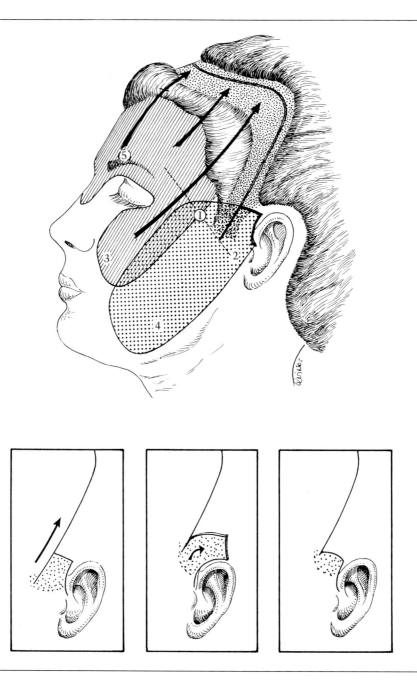

**Figure 20-29** *Blepharo-periorbitoplasty [48].*
*Top. The incision at the mid-forehead follows*
*the hairline for approximately 8 cm and then*
*proceeds backward to a level vertically above*
*the ear. Above the helix the author's*
*"preauricular hairbearing rotation flap" is*
*marked, which prevents excessive elevation of*
the sideburn. The incision ends above the
tragus. 1 = Markings for the pathway of the
frontal ramus of the facial nerve, at the
midpoint between helix and lateral canthus.
Posterior to this point the dissection should be
superficial and in front at a sub-SMAS level
along the temporal fascia. 2 = Pathway of the

**Figure 20-30** *Blepharo-periorbitoplasty (cadaver dissection). A. Cadaver dissection to show the safety of the scissors sub-SMAS dissection along the surface of the temporal aponeurosis with regard to the pathway of the frontal, orbicular, and zygomatic branches of the facial nerve. The pretemporal fascia has been sectioned between the radix helix and a point 2.5 cm above the tail of the eyebrow. After emerging from the superior pole of the parotid gland, 1.5 cm in front of the tragus, the frontozygomatic branches immediately enter the fat layer of the SMAS at the "meso temporalis" in which they are embedded. B. The facial nerve branches have been dissected from the SMAS. 1 = Pathway of the frontal branch. 2 = Area of the frontoorbiculozygomatic branches. 3 = Site of division of the frontal branch. 4 = Area of the rami of the frontal branch. 5 = Frontotemporal branch of the superficial temporal artery. 6 = Border of the divided pretemporal fascia. 7 = Border of the orbicularis muscle. 8 = Border of the frontalis muscle. 9 = Temporal fascia. 10 = Orbicular branches of the facial nerve. 11 = Zygomatic branches of the facial nerve. 12 = Lateral orbital rim; the periosteum is elevated.*

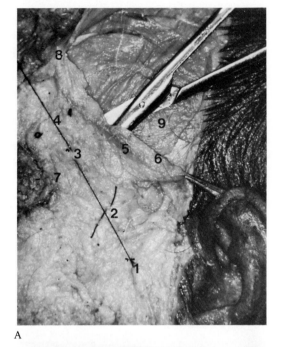

A

**Figure 20-29** *(continued) frontal ramus of the facial nerve (from 1.5 cm in front of the tragus, crossing point 1). 3 = Area of sub-SMAS dissection in front of point 1. Note that the deep dissection is carried out under the galea and frontalis muscle, the meso temporalis, the pars orbitalis of the orbicularis muscle at the upper palpebral region, at the raphe, and the lateral two-thirds of the preseptal and orbital part toward the cheek and nasolabial fold. 4 = Area of subcutaneous dissection. 5 = Only at the level of the supraorbital bundle, the dissection is made at the subperiosteal level, as it facilitates identification of the bundle. Bottom. Hairbearing preauricular rotation flap [43]. The facial tissues in front of the flap are displaced in an upward direction, and the flap rotates backward. This maneuver allows partial preservation of the sideburn except for the upper and posterior borders, which must be trimmed. The flap also allows a short scar, ending above the tragus, as the participation of the skin immediately in front of the ear on the upward lifting of the facial tissues is minimal.*

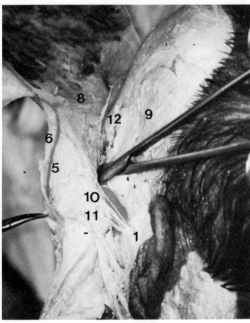

B

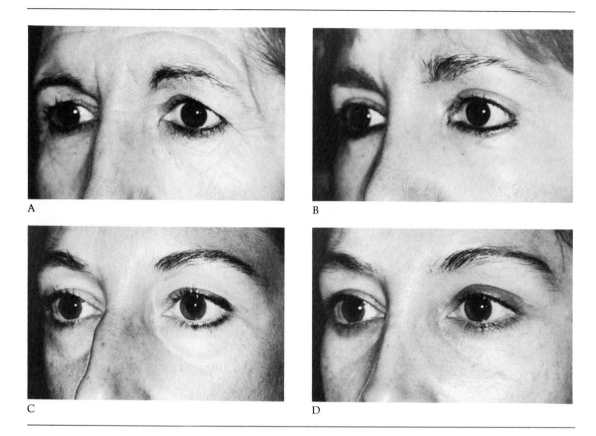

A   B   C   D

**Figure 20-31** A. Patient aged 49 with drooping of the eyebrow and upper palpebral region. B. One year after blepharo-periorbitoplasty. C. Patient aged 38 with drooping of the upper palpebral region, eyelid bags, deep palpebromalar sulcus, flat malar region, and hump nose. D. Five months after blepharo-periorbitoplasty, malar augmentation, and rhinoplasty.

**Figure 20-32** A, C. A 51-year-old patient with deep-set eyes, downward slanting of the upper lateral orbital rim, brow ptosis mainly of the medial half, decreased tonus of the orbicularis muscle and round-eye appearance, eyelid bags, deep palpebromalar sulcus, deep nasolabial folds, jowls, and turkey gobbler neck. B, D. Blepharo-periorbitoplasty with removal of eyelid bags, ostectomy of the downward slanting lateral supraorbital rim, and face and neck rhytidectomy achieved improvement of the ocular region and the ptotic periorbital soft tissues, conferring an almond-shaped appearance to the eyes.

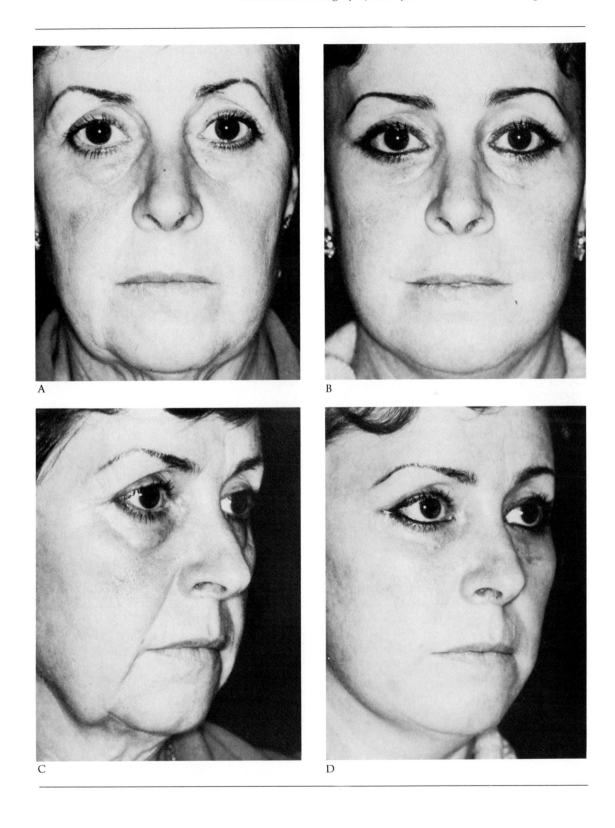

A

B

C

D

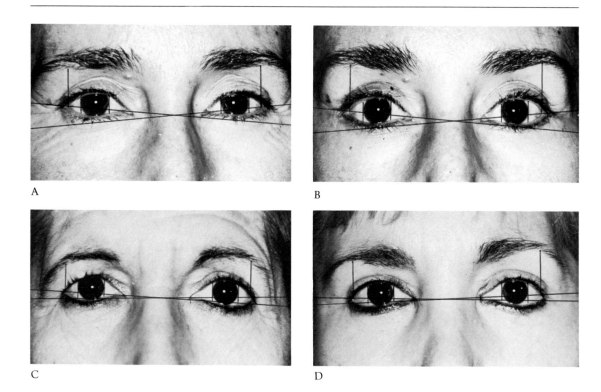

A

B

C

D

**Figure 20-33**  A. Patient aged 43 with drooping eyebrow and periorbital soft tissues and crow's feet. B. Six months after blepharo-periorbitoplasty. C, D. Front view of the patient corresponding to Fig. 20-31A, B. The preoperative (C) and postoperative (D) transverse axial line angles have not changed, indicating that although an improvement of the eye region is evident the slant of the eyelid remains unchanged. It can be modified only by a blepharocanthoplasty.

**Figure 20-34**  Patient aged 63 with a round-eye condition due to a previous blepharoplasty performed elsewhere. Lagophthalmos and the deep palpebromalar sulcus was improved by means of blepharo-periorbitoplasty. The upper eyelid has not been corrected. (The proposal for it to be added in a second stage under local anesthesia was refused.)

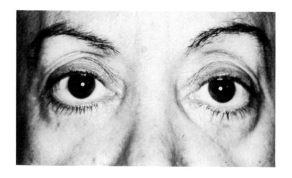

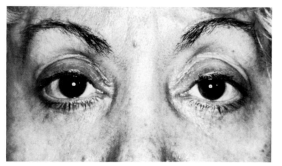

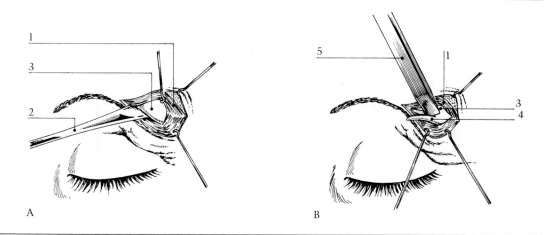

**Figure 20-35** *Correction of a low lateral orbital rim through the supraciliary approach (Lintilhac's technique). A. After suprabrow skin excision, the orbicularis muscle (1) is bluntly divided along its fibers for 1 to 2 cm, and the inferior border is retracted downward (2). A few millimeters above the supraorbital rim (3) the periosteum is horizontally incised and elevated caudally between the mid-pupillary line and the frontomalar suture and toward the orbital roof, taking care not to injure the supraorbital bundle. B. An osteotome (5) is used to reduce the downward convexity of the lateral supraorbital rim from the midline of the orbit toward the frontomalar suture (4) as well as of any forward protruding supraorbital ridges. Symmetry is checked by palpation. Any sharp edge of the orbital rim is smoothed. The periosteum, orbicularis muscle, and skin are sutured separately.*

as developed independently by Spadafora and by the author [40–42, 45].

Results show that all of the periorbital soft tissues, including the orbicularis muscle suprazygomatic soft tissues, and cheeks, are displaced in an upward direction (Fig. 20-34). The technique described is particularly useful for senile preectropion and postoperative "round eye" conditions with scleral show, as it elevates considerably the lateral lower eyelid and orbicularis muscle. It also achieves a pretarsal fullness, characteristic of the young eye. However, the inclination of the palpebral fissure itself is not changed, as it depends on the side of attachment and the ten-

sion of the lateral canthal ligament.

The result compensates for the somewhat longer recovery, which should be explained to the patient. The tonicity of the orbicularis muscle usually recovers with exercises of eyelid closure within two weeks. Occasionally a moderate edema at the malar area has been noticed but disappears within the first month.

### Correction of a Low Lateral Supraorbital Rim

So far as is known, Linthilhac [65] was the first to describe the reduction of prominent or low lateral supraorbital ridges through a supraciliary incision (Figs. 20-35 and 20-36). The blepharoplasty approach was reported by Lassus in 1979 [57]; Tessier [114] first recommended in 1979 removal through a coronal incision, and Flowers [30] reported a blepharoplasty approach.

### Correction of a Protruding Lower Orbital Rim

The correction of a protruding inferior orbital rim may contribute to the improvement of a depressed lower eyelid appearance, as was first reported by Rees in 1980 [90]. A skin–muscle flap blepharoplasty provides an easy approach to the lower orbital rim, which can be trimmed with an electric burr or an osteotome.

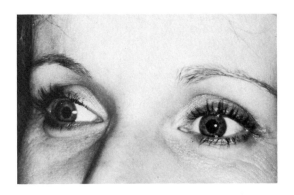

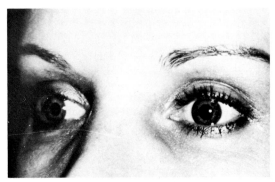

## Conclusions

Thorough preoperative qualitative and eventually quantitative evaluations of the various structures involved in the aging syndrome of the eyelids and periorbital region permit selection of the most suitable technique according to the patient's needs. Careful surgical performance is necessary to achieve a satisfactory aesthetic improvement, followed by a favorable psychic evolution—the ultimate goal of aesthetic operations. Whenever the periorbital frame of the eyelids is ptotic, tension has to be restored in addition to blepharosplasty.

**Figure 20-36** *This 37-year-old patient underwent rhinoplasty combined with supraciliary browlift of the tail of the eyebrow and ostectomy of a low lateral supraorbital rim. No blepharoplasty was needed to improve the somewhat sad appearance.*

## References

1. Adamson, J. E., McCraw, J. B., and Carraway, J. H. Use of a muscle flap in lower blepharoplasty. *Plast. Reconstr. Surg.* 63:359, 1979.
2. Aston, S. J. Orbicularis oculi muscle flaps: A technique to reduce crow's feet and lateral canthal skin folds. *Plast. Reconstr. Surg.* 65:206, 1980.
3. Aston, S. J. Skin–muscle flap lower lid blepharoplasty: An easier dissection. *Aesthetic Plast. Surg.* 6:217, 1982.
4. Aston, S. J. Panel discussion on lower lid blepharoplasty following presentations by the panel members. In S. J. Aston et al. (eds.), *Third International Symposium of Plastic and Reconstructive Surgery of the Eye and Adnexa.* Baltimore: Williams & Wilkins, 1982.
5. Baker, T. J., Gordon, H. L., and Mosienko, P. Upper lid blepharoplasty. *Plast. Reconstr. Surg.* 60:692, 1977.
6. Bames, H. O. Baggy eyelids. *Plast. Reconstr. Surg.* 22:264, 1958.
7. Beare, R. Surgical Treatment of Senile Changes in the Eyelids: The McIndoe–Beare technique. In B. Smith and J. M. Converse (eds.), *Proceedings Second International Symposium of Plastic and Reconstructive Surgery of the Eye and Adnexa.* St. Louis: Mosby, 1967.
8. Berry, E. P. Planning and evaluation blepharoplasty. *Plast. Reconstr. Surg.* 54:257, 1974.
9. Boo-Chai, K. Plastic construction of the superior palpebral fold. *Plast. Reconstr. Surg.* 31:74, 1963.
10. Boo-Chai, K. Surgery for Oriental eyelids: Some refinements in technique. *Aesthetic Plast. Surg.* 1:57, 1976.
11. Boo-Chai, K. Oriental Eyelid Surgery. In S. J. Aston et al. (eds.), *Third International Symposium of Plastic and Reconstructive Surgery of the Eye and Adnexa.* Baltimore: Williams & Wilkins, 1982.
12. Bourguet, J. La chirurgie esthetique de l'oeil et des paupiéres. *Monde Med.* 725, 1929.

13. Cardoso, A. D. Blepharoplasty by folding of the orbicularis muscle. In *Transactions of the VII Congress of the IPRS*, Rio de Janeiro, 1979.

14. Castañares, S. Blepharoplasty for herniated intraorbital fat. *Plast. Reconstr. Surg.* 8:46, 1951.

15. Castañares, S. Baggy eyelids: Physiological considerations and surgical techniques. *Excerpta Medica Int. Cong. Ser.* 66:499, 1963.

16. Castañares, S. Forehead wrinkles, glabellar frowns and ptosis of the eyebrows. *Plast. Reconstr. Surg.* 34:406, 1964.

17. Castañares, S. Blepharoplasty in exophthalmos. *Plast. Reconstr. Surg.* 47:215, 1971.

18. Castañares, S. Cosmetic Eyelid Plasty: Correction of Baggy Eyelids Deformity Produced by Herniation of Intraorbital Fat. In F. W. Masters and J. R. Lewis Jr. (eds.), *Symposium on Aesthetic Surgery of the Face, Eyelid and Breast* (Vol. 4). St. Louis: Mosby, 1972. P. 94.

19. Castañares, S. Classification of baggy eyelids deformity. *Plast. Reconstr. Surg.* 59:629, 1977.

20. Castañares, S. Colloquium. *Ann. Plast. Surg.* 1:69, 1978.

21. Castañares, S. Baggy Eyelids Deformity Classification. In S. J. Aston et al. (eds.), *Third International Symposium of Plastic and Reconstructive Surgery of the Eye and Adnexa.* Baltimore: Williams & Wilkins, 1982.

22. Connell, B. J. Eyebrow and Forehead Lifts. In E. Courtiss (ed.), *Male Aesthetic Surgery.* St. Louis: Mosby, 1982.

23. Converse, J. M. *Reconstructive Plastic Surgery.* Philadelphia: Saunders, 1964.

24. Courtiss, E. H., Webster, R. C., and White, M. F. Use of double W-plasty in upper blepharoplasty. *Plast. Reconstr. Surg.* 53:25, 1974.

25. Edgerton, M. T. Causes and prevention of lower lid ectropion following blepharoplasty. *Plast. Reconstr. Surg.*, 49:367, 1972.

26. Ellenbogen, R., and Swara, N. Correction of asymmetrical upper eyelids by measured levator adhesion technique. *Plast. Reconstr. Surg.* 69:433, 1982.

27. Fernandez, L. R. Double eyelid operation in the Oriental in Hawaii. *Plast. Reconstr. Surg.* 25:257, 1960.

28. Flowers, R. S. Colloquium. *Ann. Plast. Surg.* 1:66, 1978.

29. Flowers, R. S. Panel discussion following blepharoplasty. In S. J. Aston et al. (eds.), *Third International Symposium of Plastic and Reconstructive Surgery of the Eye and Adnexa.* Baltimore: Williams & Wilkins, 1982.

30. Flowers, R. S. Advanced Blepharoplasty: Principles of Precision. In M. Gonzalez Ulloa, et al. (eds.), *Aesthetic Plastic Surgery* (Vol. 2). Padua: Piccin Nuova Libraria, 1987. P. 115.

31. Fomon, S. *Cosmetic Surgery: Principles and Practice.* Philadelphia: Lippincott, 1960.

32. Fosatti, G. H. Tratamiento de la hipotonía del párpado inferior (a propósito de un nuevo procedimiento). *Rev. Cir. Plast. Urug.* 8(1):21, 1967.

33. Furnas, D. W. Festoons of orbicularis muscle as cause of baggy eyelids. *Plast. Reconstr. Surg.*, 61:540, 1978.

34. Furnas, D. W. Festoons of the Orbicularis Oculi: Correction and Precautions. In S. J. Aston et al. (eds.), *Third International Symposium of Plastic and Reconstructive Surgery of the Eye and Adnexa.* Baltimore: Williams & Wilkins, 1982.

35. Furukawa, M. Aesthetic surgery of Oriental eyelids. *Aesthetic Plast. Surg.* 1:139, 1977.

36. González-Ulloa, M., and Stevens, E. The treatment of palpebral bags. *Plast. Reconstr. Surg.*, 27:381, 1961.

37. Graham, W. P., Messner, K. H., and Miller, S. H. Keratoconjunctivitis sicca symptoms appearing after blepharoplasty: The "dry eye syndrome." *Plast. Reconstr. Surg.* 57:57, 1976.

38. Guy, G. C., Converse, J. M., and Morello, D. C. Aesthetic Surgery for the Aging Face. In J. M. Converse (ed.), *Reconstructive Plastic Surgery.* Philadelphia: Saunders, 1977.

39. Hinderer, U. T. Blefaroplástias simple y ampliada en el tratamiento de la blefarochalasis y las bolsas palpebrales. *Rev. Esp. Cir. Plast.* 2:229, 1969.

40. Hinderer, U. T. Profileplasty. *Int. Micr. J. Aesthetic Plast. Surg.* Card 1, No. 1, September 1971 (Profileplasty, 1972-A).

41. Hinderer, U. T. Profileplasty: Standard and new personal techniques. In *Transactions of the First International Congress ISAPS*, Rio de Janeiro, 1972. P. 52.

42. Hinderer, U. T. Treatment of the aging face. *Int. Micr. J. Aesthetic Plast. Surg.* (Facial Plasty 1974-B).

43. Hinderer, U. T. The Hairbearing Preauricular Rotation Flap and Additional Corrections in the Treatment of the Aging Face. In H. Höhler (ed.), *Plastische und Wiederherstellungschirurgie.* Stuttgart: Schattauer Verlag, 1975. P. 49.

44. Hinderer, U. T. Blepharocanthoplasty with eyebrow lift. *Plast. Reconstr. Surg.* 56:402, 1975.

45. Hinderer, U. T. Malar implants for improvement of the facial appearance. *Plast. Reconstr. Surg.* 56:157, 1975.

46. Hinderer, U. T. Additional procedures in aesthetic eyelid surgery. In *Transactions of the ISAPS IX Instruction Course,* Tokyo, 1977. P. 355.

47. Hinderer, U. T. The aging palpebral and periorbital region. In *Transactions of the VII Congress of IPRS.* Rio de Janeiro, 1979.

48. Hinderer, U. T. The blepharo-periorbitoplasty in rhytidectomy: anatomical basis. In *Transactions of the VIII ISAPS Congress,* Madrid, 1985.

49. Hinderer, U. Aging of the Palpebral and Periorbital Region. In M. Gonzalez-Ulloa et al. (eds.), *Aesthetic Plastic Surgery* (Vol. 2). Padua: Piccin Nuova Libraria, 1987. P. 1.

50. Hinderer, U. T., Urriolagoitia, F., and Vildosola, R. Nerven-Risikozonen bei der Rhytidektomie. *Handchirurgie* 18:370, 1986.

51. Hinderer, U. T., Urriolagoitia, F., and Vildosola, R. The blepharoperiorbitoplasty: Anatomical basis. *Ann. Plast. Surg.* 18:437, 1987.

52. Jones, L. T., and Wobig, J. L. *Surgery of the Eyelids and Lacrimal System.* Birmingham, AL: Aesculapius, 1974.

53. Jones, L. T., Reeh, M. J., and Wobig, J. L. Senile entropion: A new concept for correction. *Am. J. Ophthalmol.* 74:327, 1972.

54. Klatsky, S. A., and Manson, P. N. Separate skin and muscle flaps in lower-lid blepharoplasty. *Plast. Reconstr. Surg.* 67:151, 1981.

55. Kostianovsky, A. S. Modification of the cutaneous muscular flap approach for lower blepharoplasty. *Aesthetic Plast. Surg.* 3:153, 1979.

56. V. Lanz Wachsmuth. *Praktische Anatomie.* Erster Band, Erster Teil, Kopf, Teil B, Gehirnund Augenschädel, Springer-Verlag, 1979.

57. Lassus, C. Ostectomy of superior orbital rim in cosmetic blepharoplasty. *Plast. Reconstr. Surg.* 63:481, 1979.

58. Leber, D. C., and Cramer, L. M. Correction of entropion in the elderly: A muscle flap procedure. *Plast. Reconstr. Surg.* 60:704, 1977.

59. Leone, C. R. Repair of ectropion using the Bick procedure. *Am. J. Ophthalmol.* 70:233, 1970.

60. Leone, C. R. Repair of Senile Ectropion. In S. J. Aston et al. (eds.), *Third International Symposium of Plastic and Reconstructive Surgery of the Eye and Adnexa.* Baltimore: Williams & Wilkins, 1982.

61. Lewis, J. R., Jr. The Z-blepharoplasty. *Plast. Reconstr. Surg.* 44:331, 1969.

62. Lewis, J. R., Jr. A comparison of Blepharoplasty Techniques. In W. F. Masters and J. R. Lewis Jr. (eds.), *Symposium on Aesthetic Surgery of the Face, Eyelid and Breast* (Vol. 4). St. Louis: Mosby, 1972. P. 99.

63. Lewis, J. R., Jr. *Atlas of Aesthetic Plastic Surgery.* Boston: Little, Brown, 1973.

64. Lewis, J. R., Jr. Colloquium. *Ann. Plast. Surg.* 1:1, 1978.

65. Linthilhac, J. P. Reduction of the supraorbital ridges: A new cosmetic operation? *J. Int. Soc. Aesthetic Surg.* 1:61, 1981.

66. Loeb, R. La hipertrofia del músculo orbicular y su influencia en el relieve de las bolsas palpebrales. *Rev. Argent.* 1:7, 1966.

67. Loeb, R. Necessity for partial resection of the orbicularis oculi muscle in blepharoplasties in some young patients. *Plast. Reconstr. Surg.* 60:176, 1977.

68. Loeb, R. Improvements in blepharoplasty: Creating a flat surface for the lower lid. In *Transactions of the VII Congress of IPRS,* Rio de Janeiro, 1979.

69. Mahe, E., and Camblin, J. Blépharoplastie inférieure: la voie "transconjontivale." *Ann. Chir. Plast.* 23:171, 1978.

70. Marino, H. Frontal rhytidectomy. *Bol. Soc. Cir. B. Air.* 47:93, 1963.

71. Marino, H. The surgery of facial expression. *Transactions of the Fifth Congress of Plastic and Reconstructive Surgery.* London: Butterworths, 1971.

72. Marino, H. The forehead lift: Some hints to secure better results. *Aesthetic Plast. Surg.* 1:251, 1977.

73. Millard, D. R. Oriental peregrinations. *Plast. Reconstr. Surg.* 16:319, 1955.

74. Mladick, R. A. The muscle-suspension lower blepharoplasty. *Plast. Reconstr. Surg.* 64:171, 1979.

75. Morales, P. Fibro-muscular layer in the su-

prazygomatic rhytidectomy. In *Transactions of the Eighth Congress of Plastic and Reconstructive Surgery,* Montreal, 1983. P. 521.

76. Morales, P., et al. Suprazygomatic SMAS in rhytidectomy. *Aesthetic Plast. Surg.* 8:181, 1984.
77. Morax, S. Le viellissement des paupières. *Ann. Chir. Plast. Esthet.* 29:115, 1984.
78. Ohmori, S. Personal communication, 1977.
79. Ojeda, F. X., Rodrigues, A. G., and Espinoza, G. R. New dynamics in blepharoplasty. In *Transactions of the VII Congress of IPRS,* Rio de Janeiro, 1979.
80. Ortiz-Monasterio, F. X., and Krugman, M. Small incision blepharoplasty. *Aesthetic Plast. Surg.* 5:343, 1981.
81. Ortiz-Monasterio, F., and Rodríguez, A. Lateral canthoplasty to change the eye slant. *Plast. Reconstr. Surg.* 75:1, 1985.
82. Owsley, J. Q. Resection of the prominent lateral fat pad during upper lid blepharoplasty. *Plast. Reconstr. Surg.* 65:4, 1980.
83. Pearl, R. M. Acquired ptosis: A reexamination of etiology and treatment. *Plast. Reconstr. Surg.* 76:56, 1985.
84. Plaza de la, R., and Arroyo, J. M. A new technique for the treatment of inferior palpebral bags. In *Transactions of the VIII ISAPS Congress,* Madrid, 1985.
85. Psillakis, J. M. Empleo de técnicas de cirugía craneofacial en las ritidectomías del tercio superior de la cara. *Plast. Iberolatinoam.* 4:297, 1984.
86. Reeh, M. J. Pathophysiology and Surgery of Involutional Entropion. In S. J. Aston et al. (eds.), *Third International Symposium of Plastic and Reconstructive Surgery of the Eye and Adnexa.* Baltimore: Williams & Wilkins, 1982.
87. Rees, T. D. Technical aid in blepharoplasty: Ideas and innovations. *Plast. Reconstr. Surg.* 41:497, 1968.
88. Rees, T. D., and Wood-Smith, D. *Cosmetic Facial Surgery.* Philadelphia: Saunders, 1973.
89. Rees, T. D. The "dry eye" complication after a blepharoplasty. *Plast. Reconstr. Surg.* 56:375, 1975.
90. Rees, T. D. *Aesthetic Plastic Surgery.* Philadelphia: Saunders, 1980.
91. Rees, T. D., and Jelks, G. W. Blepharoplasty and the dry eye syndrome: Guidelines for surgery? *Plast. Reconstr. Surg.* 68:249, 1981.
92. Regnault, P. Correction of the infrapalpebral depression. *Aesthetic Plast. Surg.* 2:311, 1978.
93. Reidy, J. P. Swelling of eyelids. *Br. J. Plast. Surg.* 13:256, 1960.
94. Rogers, B. O. Cosmetic blepharoplasty using an electrocauterization technique. *Aesthetic Plast. Surg.* 1:263, 1977.
95. Rogers, B. O. History of Cosmetic Blepharoplasty. In S. J. Aston et al. (eds.), *Third International Symposium of Plastic and Reconstructive Surgery of the Eye and Adnexa.* Baltimore: Williams & Wilkins, 1982.
96. Sayoc, B. T. Plastic construction of the superior palpebral fold. *Am. J. Ophthalmol* 38:556, 1954.
97. Schaefer, A. J. Senile entropion. *Opthalmic Surg.* 5:33, 1974.
98. Schaefer, A. J. Statistical summary, senile entropion surgery. *Opthalmic Surg.* 8:125, 1977.
99. Schaefer, A. J. Lateral canthal tendon tuck. *Ophthalmology* 10:1879, 1979.
100. Sheen, J. H. Supratarsal fixation in upper blepharoplasty. *Plast. Reconstr. Surg.* 54:424, 1974.
101. Sheen, J. H. A change in the technique of supratarsal fixation on upper blepharoplasty. *Plast. Reconstr. Surg.* 59:831, 1977.
102. Sheen, J. H. Tarsal fixation in lower blepharoplasty. *Plast. Reconstr. Surg.* 62:24, 1978.
103. Shirakabe, T., Shirakabe, Y., and Shirakabe, T. Clinical results of Oriental double-eyelid operation: 4297 cases. In *Transactions of the VII Congress of IPRS,* Rio de Janeiro, 1979.
104. Shirakabe, Y. The double-eyelid operation in Japan: Its evolution as related to cultural changes. *Ann. Plast. Surg.* 15:3, 1985.
105. Siegel, R. J. Advanced blepharoplasty. In P. Regnault and R. K. Daniel (eds.), *Aesthetic Plastic Surgery.* Boston: Little, Brown, 1984.
106. Skoog, T. *Plastic Surgery.* Stuttgart: G. Thieme Verlag, 1974. P. 317.
107. Smith, B., and Lisman, R. D. Dacryoadenopexy as a recognized factor in upper lid blepharoplasty. *Plast. Reconstr. Surg.* 71:629, 1983.
108. Smith, J. W., and Newman, F. Blepharoplasty. In P. Regnault and R. K. Daniel (eds.), *Aesthetic Plastic Surgery.* Boston: Little, Brown, 1984.
109. Sokol, A. B., and Sokol, T. B. Transblepharoplasty brow suspension. *Plast. Reconstr. Surg.* 69:940, 1982.

110. Spira, M. Lower blepharoplasty—a clinical study. *Plast. Reconstr. Surg.* 59:35, 1977.

111. Spira, M. Blepharoplasty. In P. Regnault and R. K. Daniel (eds.), *Aesthetic Plastic Surgery.* Boston: Little, Brown, 1984.

112. Stasior, O. Repair of cicatricial Ectropion. In S. J. Aston et al. (eds.), *Third International Symposium of Plastic and Reconstructive Surgery of the Eye and Adnexa.* Baltimore: Williams & Wilkins, 1982.

113. Stephenson, K. L. The history of blepharoplasty to correct blepharochalasis. *Aesthetic Plast. Surg.* 1:177, 1977.

114. Tessier, P. Face lifting and frontal rhytidectomy. In *Transactions of the VII Congress of Plastic Reconstructive Surgery,* Brazil, 1979.

115. Tomlinson, F. B., and Hovey, L. M. Transconjunctival lower lid blepharoplasty for removal of fat. *Plast. Reconstr. Surg.* 56:314, 1975.

116. Uchida, J. A surgical procedure for blepharoptosis vera and for pseudoblepharoptosis orientalis. *Br. J. Plast. Surg.* 15:271, 1962.

117. Viñas, J. Ptosis de las cejas y arrugas paraoculares: Corrección quirúrgica simultánea. In *I Cong. Lat. Am. Cir. Plast. (Regional Sur),* Buenos Aires, 1962.

118. Wegener, E. H. Zur Frage der Stirnfaltenkorrektur. *Med. Kosmetik* 56:136, 1957.

119. Wesley, R. E., Pollard, Z. F., and McCord, C. D., Jr. Superior oblique paresis after blepharoplasty. *Plast. Reconstr. Surg.* 66:283, 1980.

120. Whitaker, L. A. Selective alteration of palpebral fissure form by lateral canthoplasty. *Plast. Reconstr. Surg.* 74:611, 1984.

121. Wilkins, R. B., and Patipa, M. The recognition of acquired ptosis in patients considered for upper-eyelid blepharoplasty. *Plast. Reconstr. Surg.* 70:431, 1982.

122. Wilkinson, T. S. Correction of the congenital short upper lip and heavy-lidded eyes. *Aesthetic Plast. Surg.* 4:73, 1980.

123. Zide, B. M. Anatomy of the eyelids. *Clin. Plast. Surg.* 8:623, 1981.

124. Zide, B. M., and Jelks, G. W. Surgical anatomy of the orbit. *Plast. Reconstr. Surg.* 74:301, 1984.

### Suggested Reading

Callahan, A. The correction of complications after levator resections for blepharoptosis. *Plast. Reconstr. Surg.* 52:616, 1973.

Castañares, S. Surgery of the Eyelids. In W. C. Grabb and J. W. Smith (eds.), *Plastic Surgery* (3rd ed.). Boston: Little Brown, 1979.

Connell, B. J. Brow Ptosis—Local Resections. In S. J. Aston et al. (eds.), *Third International Symposium of Plastic and Reconstructive Surgery of the Eye and Adnexa.* Baltimore: Williams & Wilkins, 1982.

DeMere, M., Wood, T., and Austrin, W. Eye complications with blepharoplasty or other eyelid surgery. *Plast Reconstr. Surg.* 53:634, 1974.

Herceg, S. J., and Harding, R. L. The trainor blepharoplasty for ptosis. *Plast. Reconstr. Surg.* 49:622, 1972.

Issakson, I. The surgical treatment of congenital genuine blepharoptosis. *Scand. J. Plast Reconstr. Surg.* 5:23, 1971.

Kaye, B. L. The forehead lift—a useful adjunct to facelift and blepharoplasty. *Plast Reconstr. Surg.* 60:161, 1977.

Kaye, B. L. Forehead and Brow. In T. Rees (ed.), *Aesthetic Plastic Surgery.* Philadelphia: Saunders, 1980. P. 731.

Klatsky, S. A., and Manson, P. N. Separate skin and muscle flaps in lower-lid blepharoplasty. *Plast. Reconstr. Surg.* 67:151, 1981.

Litton, C., and Trinidad, G. Chemosurgery of the Eyelids. In S. J. Aston et al. (eds.), *Third International Symposium of Plastic and Reconstructive Surgery of the Eye and Adnexa.* Baltimore: Williams & Wilkins, 1982.

Loeb, R. Aesthetic blepharoplasties based on the degree of wrinkling. *Plast. Reconstr. Surg.* 47:33, 1971.

Mustardé, J. C. Problems and pitfalls in blepharoplasty. *Aesthetic Plast. Surg.* 1:349, 1978.

Onizuka, T., and Iwanami, M. Blepharoplasty in Japan. *Aesthetic Plast. Surg.* 8:97, 1984.

Rees, T. D. Correction of ectropion resulting from blepharoplasty. *Plast Reconstr. Surg.* 50:1, 1972.

Stark, R. B. Blepharoplasty. *Ann. Plast. Surg.* 1:58, 1978.

Tenzel, R. R. Upper Lid Complications of Cosmetic Blepharoplasty. In S. J. Aston et al. (eds.), *Third International Symposium of Plastic and Reconstructive Surgery of the Eye and Adnexa.* Baltimore: Williams & Wilkins, 1982.

Tipton, J. B. Should incisions in the orbital septum be sutured in blepharoplasty? *Plast Reconstr. Surg.* 49:6131, 1972.

# 21

*Sherrell J. Aston*
*Charles H. M. Thorne*

# Aesthetic Surgery of the Aging Face

The history of facelifting has been comprehensively reviewed by Rogers [72] and Gonzalez-Ulloa [27]. Whether the first facelift was performed by Hollander [31, 32], Lexer [43], or Joseph [33] is not known for sure, but it is clear that by the early 1900s Bourget [13], Kolle [39], Lagarde [40], Morestin [53], Noel [55, 56], Passot [59–62], and Miller [49–51] had practices of aesthetic facial surgery. In 1920 Bettman [12] described the continuous facelift incision beginning in the temporal scalp and ending in the mastoid scalp, essentially the one used for rhytidectomy today. Bames [9], in 1927, contributed the concept of subcutaneous undermining (the earlier procedures had been limited to skin excision and closure without undermining).

The continuous incision described by Bettman and subcutaneous undermining recommended by Bames were the foundations of the classic facelift procedure that was performed without major modification for the succeeding four decades. The modern era of facelifting was inaugurated in 1974 when Skoog [75] described dissection of the superficial fascia of the face in continuity with the platysma muscle in the neck.

Because the aging process and the force of gravity affect not only the skin but also the structures deep to it, surgical modification of the deeper tissue layers are now an integral part of the facelift procedure. Mitz and Peyronie [52] wrote the classic paper in 1976 defining the anatomy of the superficial musculoaponeurotic system (SMAS). Several surgeons have reported modifications of the SMAS/platysma procedure to address specific problems [1, 6, 8, 17–19, 28–30, 35, 36, 42, 57, 58, 63, 64].

## Pathogenesis of Facial Aging

The process of facial aging represents a combination of atrophy, which is an intrinsic property of skin, and the effects of extrinsic factors, such as sun damage. At the histologic level, atrophy is manifested by flattening of the dermal–epidermal junction, a decrease in the number of melanocytes and Langerhans' cells, a reduction in the amount of glycosaminoglycan ground substance, progressive dropout of elastic fibers, and diminution in the total amount of collagen as well as the fraction of type III collagen (Table 21-1) [22, 24, 25, 81]. The histologic deterioration correlates with the clinical findings: thinning of the skin, decreased resistance to shearing forces, decreased elasticity, immunologic changes, and increased susceptibility to ultraviolet light and cutaneous malignancies.

Superimposed on the inevitable changes

**Table 21-1** *Histologic features of aging skin*

| Epidermis | Dermis | Appendages |
|---|---|---|
| Flat dermoepidermal junction | Atrophy (loss of dermal volume) | Graying of hair |
| Variable thickness | Fewer fibroblasts | Loss of hair |
| Variable cell size and shape | Fewer mast cells | Conversion of terminal to vellous hair |
| Occasional nuclear atypia | Shortened capillary loops | Abnormal nailplates |
| Loss of melanocytes | Abnormal nerve endings | Eccrine sweat gland—few and less responsive |
| Fewer Langerhans' cells | More hydroxyproline | Apocrine sweat glands—greater variation |
| | More insoluble collagen | Sebaceous glands—less sebum |
| | Less soluble collagen | |
| | More resistant collagen | |
| | Less extensible elastin | |
| | Less hexosamine and acid mucopolysaccharide | |

outlined above are the effects of sun damage, which result in epidermal dysplasia and dermal elastosis [38], and dramatically exacerbate the deterioration inherent in the aging process. As the skin becomes progressively atrophic, gravity causes it to hang from points of firmer, deep attachments. Structures deep to the skin, such as fat, muscle, and bone, also atrophy, accentuating the sagging of the altered cutaneous cover.

Clinically, the surface changes begin to appear at around age 30, when upper eyelid skin redundancy and crow's feet lines appear. At age 40 the nasolabial folds become more pronounced, and the glabella and forehead wrinkles are noticeable. Generally, by age 50 the neck is wrinkled, the jawline is less distinct, and the nasal tip may droop. At age 60 the progression of cutaneous and subcutaneous atrophy makes facial wrinkling and ptosis obvious in almost everyone.

## Unusual Skin Disorders

There are five rare skin conditions that may present as premature aging or skin laxity.

**1.** *Ehlers-Danlos syndrome.* The skin in this genetically transmitted disease is hyperextensible, and laxity occurs prematurely. Because of abnormal collagen maturation and tissue fragility, surgery in these patients has been associated with prolonged healing [70], hemorrhage [74], and darkly pigmented or telangiectactic hypertrophic scars [11]. Elective surgery is usually not advised in patients with this disease.

**2.** *Cutis laxa.* In this disorder there is a decrease in the number and size of the dermal elastin fibers, resulting in dramatic gravitational skin laxity. Repeated rhytidectomy can benefit these patients [20]. There is a subpopulation of patients, however, whose disease is not confined to the skin. These patients have generalized abnormalities such as pulmonary emphysema, heart disease, and aneurysms of the great vessels and are not likely to be candidates for facialplasty.

**3.** *Progeria.* Progeria is a systemic disease, inherited in an autosomal recessive pattern. It is characterized by growth retardation, atherosclerotic cardiovascular disease, and a shortened life-span. Although the facial appearance demonstrates premature aging, there is *no* role for aesthetic surgery in these patients.

**4.** *Werner's syndrome.* This rare disease is a systemic disorder characterized by autosomal recessive inheritance. The skin changes are similar to those of scleroderma. Elective surgery is contraindicated because of diabetic-like microangiopathy [23].

**5.** *Pseudoxanthoma elasticum.* This disorder has several forms with different inheritance patterns. With the recessive type II pattern the skin demonstrates degeneration of elastic fibers and premature skin laxity. Facialplasty can be beneficial.

## *Psychological Considerations*

As with any surgical procedure, the success of an aesthetic operation depends on the diagnostic and technical skill of the surgeon. In addition, however, psychological factors play a particularly important role [70]. One of the most difficult decisions for a plastic surgeon is deciding which patients are not candidates for elective, aesthetic surgery on an emotional or psychological basis.

Goin et al. [26] performed a prospective study on 50 facelift patients in which the patients stated both pre- and postoperatively their reasons for desiring surgery. Sixty percent of the patients provided a different reason postoperatively than preoperatively, suggesting that many patients harbor secret or unconscious motivations for undergoing facialplasty. Many patients who have realistic expectations preoperatively, such as wanting to look younger and perhaps to get a better job, state after the operation that they had hoped to avoid abandonment by husbands and friends or hoped the surgery would make them a "different person."

Patients who have difficulty delineating the anatomic alterations desired or in whom the degree of deformity does not correlate with the degree of personal inadequacy or misfortune ascribed to that deformity are not candidates for aesthetic surgery. Patients who are not considered good candidates for facelifting are given a thoughtful, but honest, explanation. The surgeon must not be persuaded to proceed with an operation when his or her instincts indicate that the patient is not an appropriate candidate.

## *Preoperative Evaluation*
### MEDICAL HISTORY

The same compulsive medical history that is indicated prior to any surgical procedure is required when evaluating a patient for aesthetic facial surgery. One must inquire specifically about and document any medications, allergies, medical problems, previous surgeries, and smoking and drinking habits. Because hematoma is the most common complication of facelifting, the history focuses on any factor that predisposes to postoperative hemorrhage, specifically hypertension and aspirin use. Surgery is postponed until blood pressure is under consistent control and until 2 weeks after any aspirin-containing medications are discontinued. Because of the risk of skin slough the smoking history is critical; if the patient smokes, the procedure is postponed until 2 weeks after smoking is discontinued. Aesthetic surgery is elective, and therefore whenever there is a question about a preoperative medical condition, the operation is postponed until appropriate consultations have been obtained and all issues settled.

### PHYSICAL EXAMINATION

Attention is first directed to the forehead, which is examined for transverse wrinkles, vertical glabella creases, transverse wrinkles at the root of the nose, and forehead/brow ptosis. These problems lend themselves to a forehead/brow lift. In many patients appropriate correction of brow ptosis is as important as blepharoplasty for deformities of the upper eyelid area.

The skin of the middle and lower thirds of the face is palpated for thickness, elasticity, and mobility. The malar area is observed for contour and symmetry. The contribution of the nasolabial folds to the patient's overall deformity is assessed, as nasolabial folds are not eliminated by facelifting. The jawline and jowl areas are examined for contour, fullness, and laxity. The lower jawline and neck are inspected for submental and submandibular fat deposits, submaxillary gland ptosis, mandibular contour, position of the hyoid bone, depth of the cervicomental angle, and platysma muscle anatomy. Voluntary platysma animation helps demonstrate the platysmal contribution to any folds that may be present in the submental region. The patient's hair is examined for thickness and hairline contour. Any incisions from previous surgery are noted.

PREOPERATIVE PHOTOGRAPHS

Preoperative photographs are essential and are ideally taken by a professional medical photographer. Photographs provide assistance in the preoperative planning and discussion with the patient, intraoperative decision-making, and postoperative counseling with patients who may not remember the exact preoperative appearance. Finally, photographs provide necessary medical-legal documentation.

LABORATORY EVALUATION

Preoperative laboratory evaluation must be individualized. It depends on the age and medical condition of the patient, the type of anesthesia, the particular requirements of the hospital, and the standard of care where one works.

PREOPERATIVE PATIENT COUNSELING

At the time of the preoperative consultation the patient is given written information concerning the planned procedure that reinforces the verbal information provided in the office. Patients are informed that aspirin-containing medications as well as cigarettes are forbidden during the 2 weeks prior to the procedure.

In addition to describing the anticipated results of the surgical procedure, it is necessary to point out the areas in which there can be little or no correction by the operation. Transverse forehead lines, deep glabellar creases, and transverse lines at the root of the nose can be improved with forehead/brow lifting, but the lines cannot be eliminated. Similarly, crow's feet lines can be improved to some degree but are never eliminated. Malar pouches that occur below the eyelid bags do not disappear after facelifting and frequently are accentuated during the immediate postoperative period. Nasolabial folds can be softened by skin undermining medial to the folds and accompanying suction lipectomy, but the folds are never eliminated. "Marionette lines" from the oral commissures down to the border of the mandible never disappear completely. A low hyoid bone position precludes an ideal cervicomental angle. Ptotic submandibular glands are difficult to improve. Finally, if the skin has numerous fine wrinkles they may need to be addressed with chemical peel after the patient has recovered from the facelift operation.

PREOPERATIVE ORDERS

Because of the proximity of the operative field to the oral cavity, it is difficult to perform a facelift under strictly sterile conditions. The patient must remove all makeup the night before surgery. A preoperative facial wash and shampoo with hexachlorophene (pHisoHex) or chlorhexidine (Hibiclens) is ordered for the night or morning before surgery. Because of potential contamination from the mouth and hair, a dose of prophylactic antibiotics is given intravenously prior to the initial skin incision.

Lorazepam (Ativan), 2 mg orally, is given the night before surgery to help calm the patient. It also contributes to the amnesia that is desirable if the procedure is performed under local anesthesia.

For procedures performed under general anesthesia an anesthesiologist evaluates the patient and selects the preanesthesia medications. For procedures performed under local anesthesia with intravenous sedation the premedications usually given are lorazepam (2 mg) orally 2 hours preoperatively followed by meperidine (Demerol; 75 to 100 mg), and hydroxyzine HCl (Vistaril; 75 to 100 mg) intramuscularly 1 hour preoperatively.

## Anesthesia

A facelift can be performed under either local anesthesia with intravenous sedation or general anesthesia with endotracheal intubation. If intravenous sedation is employed, diazepam (Valium) is the agent of choice. When sufficient diazepam has been administered to produce slurring of speech (5 to 20 mg), adequate sedation and amnesia are almost ensured without significantly compromising vital functions. Most patients require more than 10 mg of diazepam to produce amnesia, although an occasional patient demonstrates hemodynamic instability when that much is given. Therefore an initial dose of 1.0 to 2.5 mg is given to assess the responsiveness of the individual.

Regardless of the type of anesthesia (local or general), lidocaine (0.5%) with epinephrine (1:200,000) is used for local infiltration. The use of epinephrine allows a 50 percent increase in the tolerated dose of lidocaine (7 mg/kg) and prolongs the duration of local anesthesia. Approximately 60 ml of this solution is required for anesthetizing one side of the face and neck, and this dose provides a substantial margin of safety for the average-size patient. One-half the maximum dose of lidocaine can be safely infiltrated on the second side of the face when the first side is being closed. The onset of anesthesia with lidocaine is immediate, but the maximum vasoconstrictive effect of epinephrine is not evident for 8 to 10 minutes.

General anesthesia for facelifting requires an anesthesiologist who has experience with aesthetic surgery. If possible, the systolic blood pressure is maintained in the range of 100 to 120 mm Hg with the patient breathing spontaneously; hypotensive anesthesia is *not* desirable. Occasional assisted breaths are acceptable, but a mechanical ventilator is never used, as the positive pressure may cause unacceptable venous breathing.

Regardless of the anesthetic technique, full attention must be paid to the airway. A pulse oximeter is no substitute for attentiveness but is a helpful adjunct. When general anesthesia is employed, the endotracheal tube is frequently not taped to the face, thereby providing maximum exposure. Because the head is moved back and forth during the procedure, the tube may become disconnected or dislodged, and the pulse oximeter can help detect such potential catastrophes. The same is true under local anesthesia, where there is even less control of the airway; the pulse oximeter often provides the first indication that the airway is compromised. If any indication exists preoperatively that the patient is at high risk for anesthetic problems, the surgeon should obtain the assistance of an anesthesiologist rather than trying to perform both the surgery and the anesthesia.

## Surgical Techniques

### CLASSIC RHYTIDECTOMY

The classic facelift, which consists in subcutaneous undermining (with no alteration of the deeper structures), is indicated in an occasional patient who is young and has good bone structure, a thin neck, and a deep cervicomental angle. Although this technique is a good procedure for the ideal facelift patient, it does not address the effect of aging and the force of gravity on the tissues deep to the skin.

Prior to the administration of anesthesia, the planned incisions are marked. The facelift incision begins in the temporal scalp approximately 5 cm above the ear and 5 cm behind the hairline, curves down parallel to the hairline toward the superior root of the helix, and continues caudally in the natural preauricular skin crease (Fig. 21-1). The incision follows the crus of the helix into the incisura anterior, then curves slightly anterior to the tragus, continues inferiorly in the natural skin crease, and passes under the earlobe. Alternatively, the incision is made posterior to the tragus to eliminate the preauricular scar. The postauricular skin incision is outlined on the posterior surface of the concha 2 to 3 mm above the retroauric-

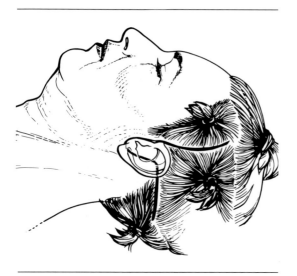

**Figure 21-1** *Facelift incision.*

ular sulcus so that the final scar lies in the concha–mastoid sulcus instead of on the exposed mastoid region. The superior extent of the posterior incision is high enough that the ear will cover the resulting scar. If the postauricular and mastoid incisions are too low, the scar may be conspicuous despite longer hairstyles. The length of the incision in the mastoid area is determined by the amount of excess neck skin. The incision must be long enough to accommodate redraping and excision of all excess skin without leaving a skin fold on the lateral neck and a "dog ear" in the scalp.

The hair is parted in the temporal and mastoid areas along the planned incisions and combed away without shaving. Antibiotic ointment may be combed into the hair to keep it flat. In addition, various other skin reference markings can be made to help ensure that the two sides of the face are dissected to the same extent and that the direction and amount of cephaloposterior advancement are the same on both sides.

One side of the face and neck is infiltrated with anesthetic/hemostatic solution (lidocaine 0.5% with epinephrine 1:200,000) before scrubbing for the surgical procedure.

During the 8 to 10 minutes required for the vasoconstrictive effect of epinephrine to develop, the patient is prepared and draped for surgery.

The previously outlined skin incision is made from the earlobe into the temporal region. In the temporal area the plane of dissection is deep to the superficial temporal fascia. This procedure helps minimize temporal alopecia by maintaining maximum blood flow to the hair follicles, is much faster than a subcutaneous dissection, and protects the frontal branch of the facial nerve. The transition to a subcutaneous plane of dissection is made at approximately the level of the lateral canthus (Fig. 21-2). The superficial temporal vessels are always cut when this transition is made.

After initiating the dissection with a scalpel, the remaining flap is elevated by scissor dissection, which is best performed under direct vision. When the mid-cheek is reached, a fiberoptic retractor is used to provide appropriate illumination for dissection and hemostasis. Care is taken to keep the dissection superficial at this point. It is easy to get too deep and risk damage to the buccal branches of the seventh cranial nerve (CN VII).

Subcutaneous undermining must extend beyond the area of redundancy. In general, dissection extends to within 1 cm of the lateral orbital rim, across the malar area, up to or medial to the nasolabial folds, to a point 1 cm lateral to the oral commissure, and inferiorly over the cervical area to the level of the thyroid cartilage (Fig. 21-3).

Major sensory nerves and all motor nerves are avoided using this approach. The great auricular nerve is just deep to the platysma, 6.5 cm below the external auditory meatus, and midway across the sternocleidomastoid muscle [48]. The trunk of the facial nerve is protected by its course within the parotid gland and by the SMAS/platysma layer beyond the parotid gland. Hemostasis is obtained by precise forceps electrocautery using long, insulated forceps. Blood vessels are

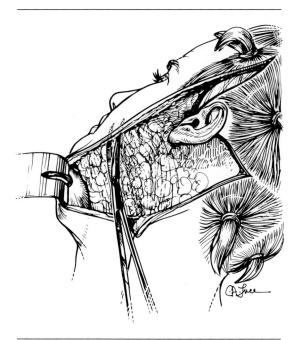

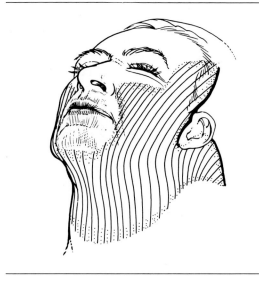

**Figure 21-3** *Extent of skin undermining.*

**Figure 21-2** *Subcutaneous undermining under direct vision using fiberoptic retractor. Transition from subcutaneous to deep dissection is seen in the temporal region.*

drawn slightly away from the skin flap and the deep tissues to avoid production of lumpy irregularities and burns on the skin flaps. This technique also reduces the chance of injury to the facial and sensory nerves.

The cervicofacial skin flap is advanced in a cephaloposterior direction, redraped over the underlying foundation, and fixed in its new position at two key points: one in the temporal scalp 1 cm above the ear, and the second at the apex of the postauricular incision. Excessive elevation of the temporal hairline is unnatural for both sexes and commits the patient to a camouflaging hairstyle. The sideburn is *never* rotated higher than the top of the ear. If placement of the sideburn at this level leaves residual skin laxity, a triangular skin excision below the sideburn is performed.

The overlapping skin in the temporal area is excised and the skin approximated with surgical staples in the hair-bearing area. In the mastoid area, the overlapping triangle of excess skin is excised in a straight line. A flat, closed-suction drain is brought out through a separate incision in the mastoid scalp. The mastoid incision and the postauricular skin incision are sutured with a running intracuticular 3-0 catgut. The overlapping skin in the preauricular area is excised to fit the skin incision without tension. If the original skin incision was made behind the tragus, it is of utmost importance to cut the flap so there is absolutely no tension on the retrotragal suture line. As the incision heals and the scar contracts, the tendency is to pull the tragus anteriorly resulting in an unnatural appearance.

Cephaloposterior flap advancement moves the flap under the earlobe, so conservative trimming in this area always yields a hidden scar underneath the earlobe and prevents earlobe distortion. Preauricular incisions are sutured with running 5-0 nylon.

SMAS/PLATYSMA FACIALPLASTY
Most patients requesting facialplasty have deformities that are more extensive than

simple skin laxity, such as: (1) submental and submandibular fat deposits; (2) platysma bands or other platysma deformities; (3) microgenia; (4) obtuse cervicomental angle; and (5) asymmetry. To correct such problems, the classic rhytidectomy procedure is not sufficient.

Selective alteration of the platysma in the neck and tightening of the SMAS in the cheeks benefits almost all patients. The nature of the platysma surgery is individualized, depending on a number of factors: the anatomy of the muscle, shape of the mandible, position of the hyoid bone, size of the thyroid cartilage, and amount of submental, submandibular, and subplatysma fat.

The platysma muscle is a thin, flat muscle that lies just underneath the skin of the anterior and lateral neck. Deep to the muscle lies the superficial layer of the deep cervical fascia. The plane between the platysma and the fascia is relatively avascular and easily dissected. Inferiorly, the platysma extends below the clavicles and attaches to the skin over the upper part of the pectoral and deltoid muscles. Superiorly, the platysma is continuous with the SMAS over the cheeks. The main body of the platysma is innervated by the cervical branch of CN VII. The upper medial portion of the platysma is innervated by small branches from the marginal mandibular nerve. At its anterosuperior margin, the platysma interdigitates with the depressor muscles of the lower lip and functions synchronously with the depressor labii inferioris and the depressor anguli oris muscles. Loss of function of the platysma muscle therefore may cause *transient* weakness of the depressor function of the lateral lower lip.

The right and left platysma muscles decussate in the submental region to a variable extent [15, 82]. When muscle fiber decussation is absent, the medial borders of each muscle may form bilateral vertical platysma bands, sometimes referred to as the *turkey gobbler deformity*. In some patients, medial platysma fibers decussate across the midline

above the hyoid bone, but platysma bands are nonetheless formed and lie lateral to the decussated fibers. In other words, the clinical presentation in these patients does not necessarily correlate with the actual platysma anatomy found during surgery.

The SMAS of the face [34, 52] is in continuity with the frontoparietal fascia superiorly and the platysma muscle inferiorly. The SMAS is attached to the dermis of the overlying skin by numerous fibrous septae, which separate the subcutaneous tissue into small fat lobules and establish multiple connections between the skin and the underlying SMAS. If correcting the patient's deformity has required extensive subcutaneous undermining, lifting the SMAS changes the underlying foundation over which the skin is redraped. If the patient's deformity is less severe and there is less skin undermining, lifting the SMAS helps lift the skin via the intact connection into the dermis.

Because the SMAS is continuous with the platysma, the two structures are dissected in continuity and advanced as a single flap. Rotation and advancement of this additional layer formed by the SMAS/platysma flap lifts and contours the cheeks, jawline, and neck.

Surgical alteration of the platysma muscle can be performed at its medial border, lateral border, or both. Medially, the surgeon may choose to employ submental defatting without altering the platysma muscle, midline plication of the platysma with wedge resection of the anterior borders, or vertical resection of platysma bands (Fig. 21-4). Laterally, the SMAS/platysma can be elevated and advanced without transecting the muscle, or, depending on the shape of the neck, partial-width or full-width platysma transection may be employed (Fig. 21-5).

Vertical platysma bands, one of the most frequent complaints of patients requesting cervicofacialplasty, frequently recur during the early postoperative period after conventional facelifting techniques. Midline plication of the platysma eliminates platysmal

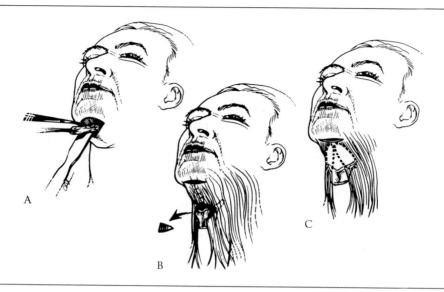

***Figure 21-4*** *Alternatives for medial platysma.*
*A. Submental defatting without platysma*
*modification. B. Midline platysma plication*
*with wedge resection. C. Vertical resection of*
*platysma bands.*

bands, deepens the cervicomental angle, and stabilizes the midline producing a secure sling effect when the lateral platysma flaps are advanced posteriorly.

After the SMAS/platysma has been elevated laterally, there are several alternatives. When the mandibular angles are prominent, the neck is thin, and the sternocleidomastoid muscles are well defined with a depression just anterior to them, even partial transection of the platysma may cause a depression that is too deep at the angles of the mandible. In this case, elevation and cephaloposterior advancement of the lateral platysma without transection eliminates the problem. If the posterior jawline and mandibular angles lack definition, however, partial-width platysma transection is the procedure of choice. The break in continuity of the lateral platysma, the cephaloposterior platysma/SMAS rotation, and the redraping of the platysma underneath the posterior mandible produces a relative concavity just anterior to the sternocleidomastoid muscle. It is critical that the lateral platysma

cut be made 6 cm below the mandibular border. Finally, in those patients with an obtuse cervicomental angle or a thick neck it may be desirable to perform full-width transection of the platysma. This procedure provides the maximum discrepancy between the mandible and the neck. Whereas conventional facelifting procedures are not beneficial for the patient with an obtuse cervicomental angle, full-width platysma transection may provide dramatic improvement.

SMAS/platysma surgery may be eliminated totally in favor of the classic rhytidectomy in patients with slight to moderate laxity. However, it is the opinion of the authors that SMAS/platysma tightening procedures decrease the incidence of recurrent laxity and provide a longer-lasting facelift result.

In patients who require submental lipectomy or surgery (or both) on the medial borders of the platysma muscle, the cervicofacialplasty is begun with a submental incision. In men the incision is placed directly in the submental crease where a hairless scar is least conspicuous. In women the incision is made slightly anterior to the crease to help offset, rather than deepen, the submental crease. The neck is hyperextended to

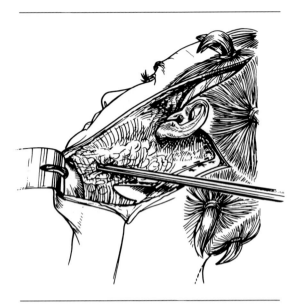

**Figure 21-8** *Final contouring of the neck after fixation of the SMAS/platysma. Care is taken not to defat immediately over the mandible.*

formed using either scissors or suction cannula under direct vision (Fig. 21-8). Care is taken not to defat immediately over the mandible to avoid adhesions between the dermis and the bone. The skin flaps are then rotated, advanced, and closed as described for the classic rhytidectomy.

### Dressing

At the conclusion of the procedure, a large-toothed comb is used to remove loose hair and dried blood. The face and hair are gently washed with saline. As many tangles and snarls as possible are removed from the hair. Flat cotton strips soaked in mineral oil are placed over the incisions and along the jawline. Gauze sponges are placed over the cheeks, and an elastic net dressing is passed over the head and opened anteriorly to expose the face and eyes. The dressing serves to cushion the skin flaps and helps eliminate deadspace underneath the flaps, absorbs drainage, and reminds the patient that he or she has had a surgical procedure. It is *not* a pressure dressing. Note that an excessively tight dressing is uncomfortable, does nothing to prevent hematoma, and can cause increased swelling by occluding venous and lymphatic outflow.

### Postoperative Management

To limit nausea, vomiting, and chewing, which can induce bleeding, the patient is started on a clear liquid diet and advanced to full liquids as tolerated. The day after surgery, a soft diet is provided and advanced to a regular diet by the second postoperative day.

For the first 24 hours after surgery the patient is encouraged to minimize head motion and maintain head elevation at approximately 30 degrees. Activity is limited as much as possible during the first 24 hours. The patient is instructed not to talk on the phone and to keep ambulation to a minimum. After 24 hours light activities may be resumed.

The patient may be discharged on the day of surgery if necessary and if appropriate care is available outside the hospital. It is the authors' preference, however, to keep the patient in the hospital for at least one night after surgery.

Shampooing is permitted and in fact is required on the third postoperative day. Hair washing is repeated at least every other day thereafter to keep the incisions clean. Men are permitted to shave on the third postoperative day. Because of skin numbness patients are encouraged to use an electric razor. Sun screens are advised for bright sunlight for 6 months.

The preauricular and submental sutures are removed on the fifth postoperative day. On postoperative day 9 or 10, all remaining postauricular and temporal sutures are removed, as are the staples in the hair. It is important to reassure the patient regarding the presence of edema, ecchymosis, and numbness. It is not uncommon for the patient to be mildly depressed during the early postoperative period. Reassurance and support are usually adequate to relieve this transient setback. In general, the patient feels self-confident enough to attend social functions after 3 weeks. It may take 2 to 3 months, however, for all the swelling and bruising to disappear. Patients return for follow-up at 6 weeks, 6 months, and 1 year, when the postoperative photographs are taken.

SECONDARY FACELIFTING
The goals of secondary facelifting are to (1) re-lift the face and neck; (2) remove the primary facelift scars; and (3) preserve maximum temporal and sideburn hair. The latter aim almost always requires a triangular excision of facial skin just below the sideburn, resulting in a transverse scar at the hairline. If this triangular excision is not performed, the temporal and sideburn hair is almost always rotated too far superiorly, yielding an unnatural, operated appearance.

Secondary flap dissection is usually easier than the primary dissection. Intraoperative bleeding and postoperative hematomas are also less frequent.

The amount of skin excised at a secondary lift is much less than at the primary procedure. For this reason preexcision of skin is never performed for a secondary facelift. In addition, care is taken to not promise the patient with preauricular scarring that all such scarring will be removed. As with primary facelifting, excessive tension is avoided, as it is predominantly rerotation of the flap, not tension, that provides the desired benefit.

Secondary SMAS/platysma surgery is performed as indicated by the patient's anatomy. It is somewhat hazardous, however, as tissue planes and possibly facial nerve branch location may be distorted by previous surgery.

MALE FACELIFTING
The social barriers against male facelifting have been broken. The main difference between male and female facelifting relates to shorter hairstyles and the denser connection between the skin and the underlying SMAS. Shorter hairstyles are not as forgiving as

some longer female ones, and therefore precise placement of the incisions is important. The triangular skin excision below the sideburn is almost always performed in the male patient. In addition, the fibrous connections between the SMAS and the skin are more tenacious in men, are more difficult to dissect, and result in more intraoperative bleeding than in women [2].

Studies indicate that the incidence of major hematomas is at least twice as high in men as in women. As discussed in the section on complications, Baker et al. [5], in a retrospective review of more than 7000 patients, reported an 8.7 percent incidence in men compared to 3.7 percent in the overall population. Pitanguy et al.'s series of male patients yielded similar results, with a 7.7 percent incidence of hematomas [67].

One must expect the procedure to require more surgical time in a male patient than in a female patient. This fact must be taken into consideration when scheduling the procedure.

## Complications
The complications that follow facelifting may be of minor significance (e.g., transient hair loss in the temporal area) or major significance (e.g., slough of a large area of preauricular skin). In addition, patients vary greatly in their ability to deal with complications. One patient may be frantic over a 1-cm postauricular skin slough, whereas another demonstrates only minimal anxiety while awaiting resolution of a margin mandibular nerve paresis. When complications appear, the surgeon must acknowledge what has occurred, take appropriate measures to remedy the problem, and be available to see the patient and discuss the situation as often as necessary.

HEMATOMA
Hematomas represent the most frequent complication following facialplasty and vary from large collections of blood that threaten

skin flap survival to small collections that are obvious only when facial edema has subsided. Most major hematomas occur during the first 10 to 12 hours postoperatively.

The most common presentation of a hematoma is an apprehensive, restless patient experiencing pain isolated to one side of the face or neck. Because pain is unusual following an uncomplicated facelift it must be regarded as a sign of hematoma until proved otherwise. Rather than provide analgesics for pain relief, the dressing is removed immediately to permit examination. In addition to causing skin flap ischemia, a large, expanding hematoma under tight skin flaps has the potential to cause respiratory compromise.

The treatment of expanding hematomas is always surgical. Sutures are removed to relieve tension on the skin flaps while making preparations for surgery. Usually the patient's anxiety and discomfort make general anesthesia preferable for hematoma evacuation. After preparing and draping the patient, the remaining sutures are removed, facial flaps are elevated for visualization, and the hematoma is completely evacuated. Rarely, a single bleeding vessel is detected.

The reported incidence of major hematomas requiring surgical evacuation ranges from 0.9 percent [83] to 8.0 percent [47]. Baker and colleagues [5] compiled statistics on 7700 facelift patients, 4 to 5 percent of whom were men, and found the average incidence of major hematomas to be 3.7 percent [2]. The incidence of hematomas in men is more than twice that in women. Pitanguy et al. reported a series specifically dealing with men and noted hematomas in 7.7 percent [67]. In the Baker et al. series there were 130 facelifts in men with a hematoma incidence of 8.7 percent.

The etiology of hematomas is multifactorial [47, 66, 68, 69, 77, 83] but correlates most closely with perioperative hypertension. Rees and coworkers, in a retrospective study of 23 hematomas in 26 rhytidectomy patients, noted an association with blood pressure elevation during the immediate postoperative period and development of hematomas at that time [69]. Straith and colleagues evaluated 500 consecutive facelift patients and found that blood pressures above 150/100 mm Hg on admission correlated with hematomas 2.6 times more frequently than normal blood pressures [80]. Because the ingestion of aspirin-containing medications is the other factor that correlates with postoperative hematomas, any such medications must be discontinued 2 weeks prior to the surgical procedure.

Small hematomas of 2 to 20 ml that are not apparent until edema begins to subside are a totally different entity and occur in 10 to 15 percent of patients. Initially, a small area of firmness is palpable followed by ecchymosis in the overlying skin, and depending on the amount of hematoma present, the skin surface may become irregular. Between the seventh and tenth days small hematomas liquefy, making it possible to express most of the blood by fingertip manipulation through a small stab incision.

A No. 11 blade placed tangentially through the skin gives access to the blood, and the scar heals well. Sometimes small hematomas can be aspirated using a 5-ml syringe and a 15-gauge needle. Either technique requires repetition on 2 to 4 successive days to remove as much blood as possible. Hematomas not detected and evacuated during the period of liquefaction result in skin firmness, irregularity, and discoloration that may persist for several weeks to months. Occasionally, hemosiderin deposits in the skin result in permanent discoloration. Patients who must return to the office frequently for aspiration of small hematomas require especially supportive care from the surgeon and the staff. Warm compresses and gentle daily massage may be helpful by making the patient an active participant in the healing process. Small intralesional injections of dilute steroids are occasionally helpful, but large doses produce subcutaneous fat atrophy and a depression when the hematoma has resolved.

## SKIN SLOUGH

Superficial sloughs of the epidermis usually heal with little or no residual scarring. Full-thickness skin sloughs always result in some degree of permanent scarring. The postauricular and mastoid areas are most frequently involved, presumably because the skin is thinnest in this area and is furthest from adequate circulation. Fortunately, small sloughs in this area are concealed by the ear and hair. A full-thickness slough in a visible area of the face and neck is a devastating complication. In most series, the incidence of skin slough after rhytidectomy is 1 to 3 percent [4, 47, 68]. It is not known why some patients develop skin sloughs, whereas most have no such problems. The most likely causes of skin slough are (1) undiagnosed hematomas; (2) a skin flap that is too thin or that is damaged during flap dissection; (3) excessive tension on wound closure; and (4) cigarette smoking.

There is no question that cigarette smoking increases the risk of skin slough. Rees and colleagues demonstrated a risk of skin slough 12 times greater in smokers than nonsmokers [71]. For this reason patients are required to abstain from smoking for 2 weeks preoperatively.

All facial skin sloughs, even when in a highly visible area, are treated by careful observation—*not* surgical intervention.

Areas of skin slough epithelialize and contract dramatically. The resulting scar is almost always better than would be anticipated from the initial wound appearance. Depending on the size of the sloughed area, it may be possible to excise the scar and readvance the facial skin, but it is generally years before sufficient skin laxity allows a secondary lift. One must be cognizant of the fact that during the secondary lift minimal excess skin is present, and it may not be possible to remove a scar that is more than 1 cm from the previous incision.

## NERVE INJURY

Transient numbness of the lower two-thirds of the ear, the preauricular area, and the cheeks for the first 2 to 6 weeks postoperatively occurs as a result of interrupting small sensory nerves during surgery and is unavoidable. The most common avoidable nerve injury during facialplasty is that of the great auricular nerve. This nerve is injured when dissection is too deep, piercing the fascia over the sternocleidomastoid muscle. McKinney and Katrana studied the course of the great auricular nerve and reported that, with the head turned 45 degrees toward the contralateral side, the nerve consistently crosses the midportion of the sternocleidomastoid muscle 6.5 cm below the caudal edge of the bony external auditory canal [48]. When injury to the great auricular nerve is recognized during surgery, an immediate, meticulous repair is performed.

Permanent injury of CN VII (facial nerve) is the most dreaded complication for any surgeon performing this operation. It is mandatory that the surgeon performing rhytidectomy be familiar with the anatomy and common variations of the facial nerve. Fortunately, permanent injury to the facial nerve branches is rare. Most patients regain full motor function after injury to a branch of the facial nerve within a few weeks to a year, although an occasional patient may take longer. Baker reviewed the literature and compiled statistics on 1500 patients and reported an incidence of facial nerve injury of 0.9 percent [4].

If transection of the facial nerve branch is detected during the procedure, immediate microsurgical repair must be performed. It is more likely, however, that nerve injury is not recognized during surgery, and the surgeon and patient are placed in the difficult position of waiting for return of function.

## ALOPECIA

Some degree of hair loss occurs after rhytidectomy. The incidence ranges from 1 percent [16] to 3 percent [41] of patients, depending on the report.

SCARRING

Facelift incisions generally heal with inconspicuous scars, accounting in a significant way for the popularity of the procedure. The most common causes of undesirable scarring after facialplasty are vascular compromise of the skin flaps (see Skin Slough, above) and excess tension on the closure. As discussed earlier, two points of maximum skin tension are established: in the temporal scalp just above the ear and at the apex of the postauricular incision. The remaining skin flaps are trimmed conservatively so there is minimal tension on the closure. This point is especially true in the preauricular area and around the earlobe, where the slightest tension widens the scar and distorts the earlobe.

Hypertrophic scarring is rare but does occur. The postauricular incision is the most frequent site of hypertrophic scars. Small-volume injections of dilute insoluble steroids often help flatten these scars.

Care is taken when placing the submental incision to minimize its length, so that when the skin flaps are advanced laterally the incision remains hidden underneath the mandible. Elliptical skin excision in the submental area tends to produce "dog ears" and is avoided if possible.

PIGMENTATION

Hyperpigmentation is caused by hemosiderin deposits in the dermis. Small, unevacuated hematomas that become apparent after edema subsides are frequent sites of hyperpigmentation. Such pigmentation is sometimes slow to resolve, occasionally taking 6 to 8 months; in rare circumstances the pigmentation is permanent.

## Ancillary Procedures

CHIN IMPLANTS

Microgenia is common in patients requesting facialplasty. A silicone chin implant can provide a dramatic improvement in facial harmony. Standard implants can be carved to the appropriate size and shape, and frequently a small implant is all that is required. A submental approach for placing a chin implant has the advantage that the implant can be sutured to the inferior border of the mandible, securing the implant position. Accurate, symmetric placement of the silicone chin implant is the most difficult part of the procedure.

MALAR IMPLANTS

Malar implants are beneficial in selected patients. They can be accomplished from an intraoral, subciliary, or facelift approach, but the intraoral approach is preferred. An incision is made in the gingivobuccal sulcus, and subperiosteal dissection is performed on the maxilla to gain access to the zygoma. Care is taken to not injure the infraorbital nerve. The difficulty with precise positioning during chin implant placement is even more significant with cheek implants.

BUCCAL FAT EXCISION

Buccal fat pad excision may further enhance the malar eminence and reduce the fullness of the cheeks. The fat pad can be removed through either an intraoral or a facelift approach. The intraoral incision begins at the first premolar and extends posteriorly for 2 cm. The fibers of the buccinator are separated bluntly, and the scissors are introduced in the direction of the temporomandibular joint to expose the well defined yellow buccal fat pad. Gentle traction with forceps draws the fat into the oral cavity, where it is excised and the base coagulated. The oral mucosa is approximated with absorbable sutures. Alternatively, the buccal fat pad is removed under direct vision from underneath the facial skin flap. After the SMAS dissection has been performed and the buccal branches of the facial nerve are visualized, blunt scissors are advanced into the fat pad anterior to the masseter muscle between the branches of the facial nerve. The yellow fat pad is seen and easily delivered.

## CHEMICAL PEEL

The primary indication for the use of chemical peel is the presence of fine wrinkles. Chemical peel may also be useful in the treatment of superficial keratoses and some areas of abnormal pigmentation. Deep surface irregularities, e.g., acne scarring, are better treated with dermabrasion. In general, chemical peel is not used for telangiectases, nevi, arteriovenous malformations, hemangiomas, or café au lait spots, and it has no place in the treatment of invasive malignancies.

The best candidates for chemical peel are patients with fair complexions. The more pigmented the skin, the greater is the line of demarcation between the treated and untreated areas.

The most commonly used agent for facial peeling is phenol. Several formulas have been proposed, but the one most commonly employed is the combination reported by Mosienko and Baker [54]. Their emulsion contains phenol 88% USP 3 ml, tap water 2 ml, liquid soap 8 drops, and croton oil 3 drops. The resultant concentration of phenol is approximately 50%, and the volume is sufficient for a full face treatment.

Litton and colleagues delineated the role of the various components of the mixture [44–46]. When topically administered, phenol causes denaturation and coagulation of the surface keratin. The role of croton oil is not known, but it is clear that its presence increases the effectiveness of the peel. It probably facilitates penetration of the phenol to the dermis. The liquid soap acts as an emulsifier and therefore aids in the penetration of the hydrophobic waxes and cholesterol esters on the skin surface. The tap water is used simply to dilute the concentration of phenol to the desired concentration (50%).

The effect of the phenolic peel is related to the depth of penetration. According to Spira and associates [76], the depth of penetration is proportional to the concentration of the phenol. This finding contradicts that of Rothman [73], who stated that the depth of penetration was inversely related to the phenol concentration. Rothman's explanation was that the higher the concentration of phenol the greater the coagulation of surface protein and the greater the *barrier* to further phenol penetration. For practical purposes, a 50% solution is as effective as more concentrated solutions without being associated with the additional risk of toxicity [76].

Although the therapeutic effect of chemical peel on skin exhibiting fine wrinkles is undeniable, the histologic changes accounting for this effect have been difficult to elucidate. Several investigators have observed a new zone of laminated collagen in the upper dermis of the peeled skin [3, 14, 40, 79]. Kligman and colleagues [37] studied the histologic changes in the excised skin from 11 women who had facelifts after previous chemical peels. The interval between the peel and the facelift varied from 18 months to 20 years. According to these authors, a band of new collagen 2 to 3 mm in width was formed in the upper dermis containing thin, compact, parallel collagen fibers arranged horizontally relative to the skin surface. Abundant, fine, elastic fibers were present as well. There was an abrupt demarcation between the orderly upper dermis and the underlying unpeeled dermis. In addition, the dysplastic changes prevalent in the unpeeled epidermis were absent in the peeled skin. Melanocyte populations were normal or increased in the previously peeled skin, but melanin production was decreased and more uniform, accounting for the bleaching effect characteristically seen after chemical peel. The authors emphasized that these changes were still present in the specimens obtained from patients who had been treated with chemical peel 20 years prior to their facelifts.

Chemical peel of the perioral region may be performed concomitantly with a facelift. Extensive chemical peeling of the face, however, is not performed at the same time as a facelift because of the possibility of hypertrophic scarring. Similarly, a lower eyelid peel is never performed at the same time as a lower eyelid blepharoplasty.

If chemical peel is to be performed for fine wrinkles around the mouth concomitantly with a facelift, no additional sedation or anesthesia is necessary. If the peel is being performed as a separate procedure, it is helpful to provide the patient with intravenous sedation. Infiltrating the area with local anesthetic is not necessary.

When performing the procedure, a cotton-tipped applicator is dipped in the freshly mixed solution, pressed on the edge of the container to near-dryness, and then gently rolled on the skin until there is a white, frosted appearance. Care is taken to leave the solution in the container on an adjacent table; the container is *not* held over the face of the patient where it might cause a disaster if spilled. Gentle stretching of the skin with the fingers of the other hand allows the fluid to coat the depths of the wrinkles. It is important to come right to the hairline and to the vermilion border of the lips to avoid a visible line of demarcation. On the lower lids the peel extends to within 2 mm of the ciliary margin. To deepen the penetration of the phenol, tape is applied to the treated area and left in place for 24 to 48 hours. Eyelids are not taped.

When the tape is removed, the treated area can be left to form a crust or can be dusted with thymol iodide to enhance crust formation. After approximately 10 days the crust separates, leaving behind pink skin. The pink color remains for 6 to 12 weeks. Patients must be careful to avoid direct sunlight during this period and even after 3 months are encouraged to make compulsive use of sun-blocking agents.

Complications of chemical peeling can be systemic or local. The most common systemic complication is the formation of cardiac arrhythmias, which can be avoided if the solution is applied slowly and in small amounts at one time. If a full face peel is performed, the face is divided into units and the treatment performed over a 60-minute period.

Local complications are most commonly changes in pigmentation. Hypopigmentation is the most common and produces a line of demarcation between the peeled and the unpeeled skin. Hyperpigmentation is generally caused by sun exposure to the peeled skin and is frequently blotchy. This nonuniform hyperpigmentation is more common in dark-skinned individuals. Scarring is unusual but has been seen in some patients who have undergone the deep peel (with tape) in combination with an extensive facelift. Scarring tends to occur more commonly on the neck, and therefore chemical peel is not used in this area. Telangiectasias are frequently made more prominent after peeling. Erythema is seen in all patients after chemical peel. Resolution is individual but usually occurs within 6 weeks, although, an occasional patient has prolonged erythema.

DERMABRASION

Dermabrasion is a useful technique in selected situations where surface irregularities exist from scarring, e.g., acne. The goal is to sand down the elevated areas so that the pits or depressions are less deep in comparison. Most, but not all, surgeons believe that chemical peel is superior to dermabrasion for fine wrinkles [7, 10, 37, 78, 79].

After dermabrasion the wound reepithelializes much as a skin graft donor site heals. The effect is permanent in that the thinned dermis never regains its original thickness. Care must be taken to preserve enough dermis for reepithelialization: the deeper the abrasion the slower the healing.

As with chemical peel, fair-skinned patients are the best candidates because healing is generally not accompanied by the pigmentation changes that are seen in darker-skinned individuals.

Several authors have compared the healing process following dermabrasion and chemical peel [7, 10, 78, 79]. There is some evidence that, except for thinning of the dermis, no histologic changes occur after dermabrasion, whereas chemical peel is followed by homogenization of the dermal collagen.

The technique of dermabrasion is well known. Local or general anesthesia is required. As the epidermis is abraded, the dermal papillae are noted as tiny sites of bleeding. Postoperatively, abraded areas can be treated with or without ointment.

Erythema can persist for several months or even longer after abrasion, and patients must be warned of this problem preoperatively. As with chemical peel, it is important to avoid sunlight several months after the procedure.

## Forehead/Brow Lift
### INDICATIONS
The primary indications for forehead/brow lifts are forehead/brow ptosis and lateral upper lid ptosis. However, a forehead/brow lift also helps correct transverse forehead lines and creases, glabellar creases, transverse folds at the root of the nose, upper nasal and medial eyelid fullness due to forehead/brow ptosis, and, to a lesser degree, nasal tip droop. many patients have upper lid fullness that *cannot* be corrected by blepharoplasty alone even with an extended incision.

In some patients correction of transverse forehead lines and/or glabellar creases, rather than brow ptosis, is the main indication for the procedure. In such patients, attention is directed toward interrupting the muscle activity rather than toward elevation of the forehead. Like any aesthetic procedure, it is tailored to suit the individual.

### PATIENT EVALUATION
The patient is examined while seated or standing, and attention is directed to the position of the upper eyelids and brow. The contribution of brow ptosis to upper lid fullness is determined by gently elevating the brow with the fingertips and observing the upper lid. Frequently the forehead/brow pto-

sis is the main component of upper lid fullness. If excess upper lid skin is still present with the brow elevated, upper lid blepharoplasty will be needed in addition to the forehead/brow lift and can be performed at the same time. The height of the forehead and the thickness of the hair must be evaluated to decide which incision is best for the individual patient.

Ellenbogen [21] delineated the criteria for the ideal eyebrow: (1) The brow begins medially at a vertical line drawn perpendicular through the alar base. (2) The brow terminates laterally at an oblique line drawn through the lateral canthus of the eye and the alar base. (3) The medial and lateral ends lie at approximately the same horizontal level. (4) The apex of the brow lies on the vertical line drawn directly through the lateral limbus of the eye. (5) The brow arches above the supraorbital rim in women and lies at approximately the level of the rim in men.

### FOREHEAD/BROW ANATOMY
The frontalis muscles are vertically oriented extensions of the galea that begin at the level of the anterior hairline and extend inferiorly to cover almost the entire forehead, inserting into the dermis of the forehead skin. The function of the frontalis is to elevate the eyebrows. Transverse forehead lines result from repeated frontalis contraction. The frontalis muscle is innervated by the frontal branch of the facial nerve. Loss of frontalis innervation always results in brow ptosis on the affected side.

In opposition to the brow-lifting activity of the frontalis muscles is the pull of the corrugator supercilii, procerus, and orbicularis oculi muscles. Contraction of these three muscles pulls the forehead and brow down.

The corrugator muscles arise from the periosteum along the superior medial orbital rim and insert into the dermis of the medial brow. Contraction pulls the brow medially and downward, producing a scowling appearance. Vertical glabellar creases develop as a result of repeated corrugator contrac-

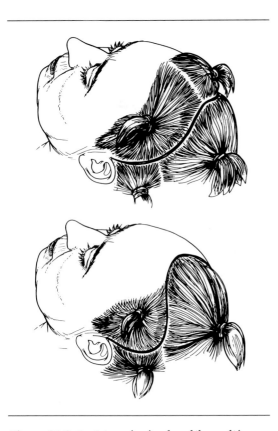

**Figure 21-9** *Incisions for forehead/brow lift.*

tion. The procerus muscles originate from the surface of the upper lateral cartilage and nasal bones and insert into the skin in the glabellar region. Contraction of the procerus muscle pulls the forehead down and the root of the nasal skin up, and causes transverse wrinkles at the root of the nose.

The frontal branch of the facial nerve emerges from underneath the parotid gland on a line extending from 0.5 cm below the tragus of the ear to a point 1.5 cm above the lateral brow, passing deep to the SMAS over the zygomatic arch [65]. The nerve enters the frontalis muscle on its deep surface.

TECHNIQUE

Either a bicoronal or a modified anterior hairline incision can be used for almost all patients requiring forehead/brow lift (Fig. 21-9). The bicoronal incision is the procedure of choice for patients with a normal

anterior hairline and normal hair growth. When the hairline is high, a modified anterior hairline incision is used that follows the frontal hair pattern in the middle portion of the forehead and then turns posteriorly for 7 to 9 cm before curving downward toward the top of the ear. If a facialplasty is being performed at the same time as the brow lift, the facelift is performed first, and the brow lift incision joins the temporal extension of the facelift incision.

Prior to induction of anesthesia or to administration of intravenous sedation, with the patient in the sitting position, vertical glabellar lines and transverse forehead lines are marked. The bicoronal incision is outlined in the scalp. The midpoint of the incision is marked 7 to 9 cm behind the anterior hairline so that, after scalp resection, at least 5 cm of hair-bearing scalp remains anterior to the incision in the midline. From the midline, the incision curves posterolaterally to join the temporal extension of the facelift incision. If a facelift is not being performed, the incision extends to the attachment of the ear, taking care to remain far enough behind the hairline so the resulting scar is at least 5 cm behind the hairline. The hair is parted along the planned incision. It is not necessary to shave hair.

Hemostatic/anesthetic solution (0.5% lidocaine with epinephrine 1:200,000) is infiltrated along the anticipated incision, across the supraorbital rim, and down the dorsum of the nose. After 8 to 10 minutes have elapsed, achieving the maximum vasoconstrictive effect, the incision is made. Protective plastic lenses are placed in the eye to protect the corneas from injuries when the forehead flap is turned down over the supraorbital rims. This step is particularly important when upper lid blepharoplasty has been performed, as the eyes are open and especially vulnerable to corneal abrasion.

The incision is beveled in the direction of the hair follicles, and the flap is elevated in the areolar plane between the galea and pericranium.

As the supraorbital rims are approached, care is taken to identify the supraorbital

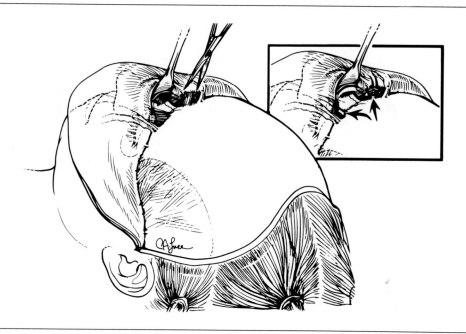

**Figure 21-10** *Exposure after subgaleal dissection of the forehead. The supraorbital nerves are easily seen, but the supratrochlear nerves are hidden by the corrugator muscles.*

neurovascular bundles. The supratrochlear nerves lie in the corrugator muscle and are not visualized until partial corrugator muscle resection has been accomplished (Fig. 21-10).

When the dissection reaches the supraorbital rims and the supraorbital nerves have been identified, the flap is released from the supraorbital rims. In the midline the dissection is extended onto the nasal process of the frontal bone. Large, blunt-tipped scissors are passed down the dorsum to the tip of the nose and spread to release soft tissue attachments on the upper one-half of the nose. Fine scissors are then used to spread the corrugator muscles to locate the branches of the supratrochlear nerves. Having identified the nerves, the corrugator muscles can then be resected, taking care to leave some corrugator muscle on the forehead flap to prevent a depression in this area.

Attention is then directed to the glabellar creases. Needles are passed through the flap from outside to inside at the upper and lower limits of the previously marked glabellar creases to locate them precisely on the inside of the flap (Fig. 21-11). A scalpel is used to incise the muscle on all four sides of each glabellar crease, forming an island of soft tissue under each crease that has been isolated from the surrounding muscle.

The course of the supraorbital nerves is then marked with ink to prepare for frontalis muscle resection. Needles are passed through the flap from outside to inside in order to outline the planned area of frontalis resection. The frontalis is resected as a rectangle from the hairline to a line 1 cm above the supraorbital rim and from supraorbital nerve to supraorbital nerve (Fig. 21-12). Another rectangle of frontalis can be removed lateral to each supraorbital nerve in the case of severe forehead wrinkles; however, in this case the rectangle of resected frontalis must not encroach as closely on the supraorbital rim, thereby preserving the frontal nerve.

The forehead/brow flap is then redraped in a posterior direction, overlapping the cut edge of the posterior scalp flap. Three key fixation points are established: the midline

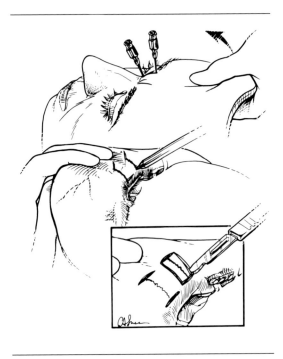

**Figure 21-11** *Treatment of glabellar creases.*

**Figure 21-12** *Resection of frontalis muscle, taking care not to injure the supraorbital neurovascular bundles.*

and bilaterally on lines extending vertically from the lateral limbus of the eye. Each of the three fixation points is secured with a surgical staple, and all overlapping excess flap is excised (Fig. 21-13). The fixation points are established with light tension, and the remainder of the flap is trimmed to have minimal tension on the flap closure.

Flap closure in the temporal area from the top of the ear to the top of the temporalis muscle is accomplished using a single layer of surgical staples. Across the top of the head where the flap is almost twice the thickness, the galea is closed with a running 4-0 vicryl suture, and the skin is approximated with surgical staples. Drains are not used. When wound closure is complete, the hair is combed over the incision to cover it and to remove any cut hair. A gauze bandage is placed over the incision and secured with a stockinette dressing, as described for the facelift.

Mild analgesics are prescribed for pain postoperatively. Patients generally complain of pressure and discomfort, but little pain. Any complaints of pain must be evaluated for possible hematoma, although it is a rare occurrence. The eyelids usually do not close

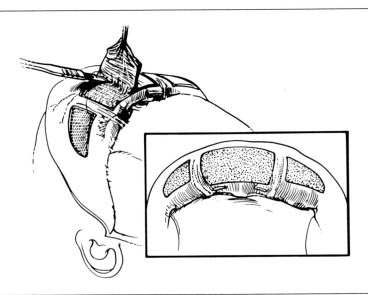

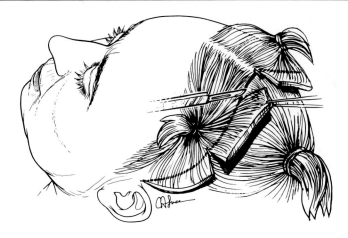

*Figure 21-13* *Redraping of the forehead/brow using three "key" fixation sutures.*

completely for the first 24 hours postoperatively, especially if an upper lid blepharoplasty has been performed concomitantly. Therefore generous application of ophthalmic lubricating ointment is necessary to prevent desiccation of the cornea. The dressing is removed on the first postoperative day if the forehead/brow lift is performed as an isolated procedure and on the second postoperative day if performed in conjunction with a facelift.

The patient is advised that swelling and periorbital ecchymosis are frequently worse on the second or third postoperative day. Hair can be washed on the second or third postoperative day and daily thereafter. All staples and sutures are removed between the eighth and tenth postoperative days.

COMPLICATIONS

Hematoma after forehead/brow lift is rare, occurring less frequently than after facelifting. A collection of blood under the flap, however, could conceivably lead to flap necrosis and alopecia, and therefore any complaints of pain must be carefully evaluated.

Significant alopecia is rare if the incision is closed without tension. Small areas of alopecia may occur at the three fixation points, where there is more tension and the suture cuts more deeply into the scalp. Patients with thin, fine hair, especially those who experience daily hair loss with routine brushing and combing, may have more hair loss during the first 3 to 6 weeks postoperatively.

Paralysis of the frontalis muscle is rare. Injury to the frontal branch of the facial nerve, however, can occur if flap dissection at the lateral orbital rim is too superficial. In the lateral orbital area the frontal branch of the facial nerve lies on the deep surface of the frontalis muscle and is frequently visualized when the flap is dissected. Resection of the frontalis muscle on the lateral portion of the flap, lateral to the supraorbital nerves, is kept at least 3 cm above the lateral orbital rim to avoid injuring the nerve.

When it does occur, frontalis paralysis is almost always transient. If any movement is present postoperatively, full return of function can be expected with time, but it may take 10 to 12 months.

Sensation of the forehead and anterior scalp is primarily by the supraorbital and supratrochlear nerves. The skin incision divides the sensory branches, and therefore numbness can be anticipated posterior to the incision. Patients may complain of itching or numbness of the forehead, which resolves over the course of 6 weeks to 6 months.

# References

1. Aston, S. J. Platysma muscle in rhytidoplasty. *Ann. Plast. Surg.* 3:529, 1979.
2. Aston, S. J. Male Cervicofacial Rhytidoplasty. In E. Courtiss (ed.), *Male Aesthetic Surgery.* St. Louis: Mosby, 1981.
3. Ayres, S. Superficial chemosurgery in treating aging skin. *Arch. Dermatol.* 85:385, 1962.
4. Baker, D. C. Complications of cervicofacial rhytidectomy. *Clin. Plast. Surg.* 10:543, 1983.
5. Baker, D. L., et al. The male rhytidectomy. *Plast. Reconstr. Surg.* 4:514, 1977.
6. Baker, T. J. Sectioning and plication of flaccid cervical bands. Presented at the 1st Congress of the Ibero-Latin American Federation of Plastic and Reconstructive Surgery, 1976.
7. Baker, T. J., and Gordon, H. L. Chemical face peeling and dermabrasion. *Surg. Clin. North Am.* 51:387, 1971.
8. Baker, T. J., Gordon, H. L., and Whitlow, D. R. Our present technique for rhytidectomy. *Plast. Reconstr. Surg.* 52:232, 1973.
9. Bames, H. O. Frown disfigurement and ptosis. *Plast. Reconstr. Surg.* 19:337, 1957.
10. Behiu, F., Feuerstein, S. S., and Markovitz, W. F. Comparative histologic study of mini pig skin after chemical peel and dermabrasion. *Arch. Otolaryngol.* 103:271, 1977.
11. Beighton, P., and Bull, J. C. Plastic surgery in the Ehlers-Danlos syndrome. *Plast. Reconstr. Surg.* 45:606, 1970.
12. Bettman, A. G. Plastic and cosmetic surgery of the face. *Northwest Med.* 19:205, 1920.
13. Bourget, J. Chirurgie esthétique de la face: Les nez concaves, les rides et les (poches) sous las-yeux. *Arch. Prov. Chir.* 28:293, 1925.
14. Brown, A. M., Kaplan, L. M., and Brown, M. D. Cutaneous alterations induced by phenol: A histologic bioessay. *J. Int. Coll. Surg.* 4:602, 1960.
15. Cardoso de Castro, C. The anatomy of the platysma muscle. *Plast. Reconstr. Surg.* 66:680, 1980.
16. Cohen, S. R., and Webster, R. C. Primary rhytidectomy—complications of the procedure and anesthetic. *Laryngoscope* 93:654, 1983.
17. Connell, B. F. Cervical lifts: The value of platysma muscle flaps. *Ann. Plast. Surg.* 1:34, 1978.
18. Connell, B. F. Cervical lift: Surgical correction of fat contour problems combined with full-width platysmal muscle flaps. *Aesthetic Plast. Surg.* 1:355, 1978.
19. Connell, B. F. Contouring the neck in rhytidectomy by lipectomy and a muscle sling. *Plast. Reconstr. Surg.* 61:376, 1978.
20. Dingman, R. O., Grabb, W. C., and Oneal, R. M. Cutis laxa congenita—generalized elastosis. *Plast. Reconstr. Surg.* 44:431, 1969.
21. Ellenbogen, R. Transcoronal eyebrow lift with concomitant upper blepharoplasty. *Plast. Reconstr. Surg.* 71:490, 1983.
22. Feuske, N. A., and Lober, C. W. Structural and functional changes of normal aging skin. *J. Am. Acad. Dermatol.* 15:571, 1986.
23. Fleischmajer, R., and Nedwich, A. Werner's syndrome. *Am. J. Med.* 54:111, 1973.
24. Freeman, R. G. Effects of Aging on the Skin. In E. B. Holwig and F. K. Mostofi (eds.), *The Skin.* Baltimore: Williams & Wilkins, 1971.
25. Gilchrest, B. A. Age-associated changes in the skin. *J. Am. Geriatr. Soc.* 30:139, 1982.
26. Goin, M. D., et al. A prospective psychological study of 50 female face-lift patients. *Plast. Reconstr. Surg.* 65:436, 1980.
27. Gonzalez-Ulloa, M. The history of rhytidectomy. *Aesthetic Plast. Surg.* 4:1, 1980.
28. Guerrero-Santos, J. The role of the platysma muscle in rhytidoplasty. *Clin. Plast. Surg.* 5:29, 1978.
29. Guerrero-Santos, J. Surgical correction of the fatty fallen neck. *Ann. Plast. Surg.* 2:389, 1979.
30. Guerrero-Santos, J., Espaillat, L., and Morales, F. Muscular lift in cervical rhytidoplasty. *Plast. Reconstr. Surg.* 54:127, 1974.
31. Hollander, E. Cosmetic Surgery. In M. Joseph (ed.), *Handbuch der Kosmetik.* Leipzig: Verlag von Veit, 1912.
32. Hollander, E. Plastiche (Kosmetische) Operation: Kritische Darstellung ihres gegenwärtigen Standes. In G. Klemperer and F. Klemperer (eds.), *Neue Deutsche Klinik* (Vol. 9). Berlin: Urban & Schwarzenberg, 1932.
33. Joseph, J. Hangewangenplastik (melomioplastik). *Dtsch. Med. Wochenschr.* 47:287, 1921.
34. Jost, G., and Levet, Y. Parotid fascia and face-lifting: A critical evaluation of the SMAS concept. *Plast. Reconstr. Surg.* 74:42, 1984.
35. Kaye, B. L. The extended neck lift: The "bottom line." *Plast. Reconstr. Surg.* 65:429, 1980.
36. Kaye, B. L. The extended facelift with ancillary procedures. *Ann. Plast. Surg.* 6:335, 1981.
37. Kligman, A. M., Baker, T. J., and Gordon, H. L. Long-term histologic follow-up of phenol face peels. *Plast. Reconstr. Surg.* 75:652, 1985.

38. Kligman, L. H. Photoaging, manifestations, prevention and treatment. *Dermatol. Clin.* 4:517, 1986.
39. Kolle, F. S. *Plastic and Cosmetic Surgery.* New York: Appleton, 1911. Pp. 116–117.
40. Lagarde, M. Nouvelles techniques pur le traitement des rides de la face et du cou. *Arch. Fr. Belge. Chir.* 31:154, 1928.
41. Leist, F., Masson, J., and Erich, J. B. A review of 324 rhytidectomies, emphasizing complications and patient dissatisfaction. *Plast. Reconstr. Surg.* 59:525, 1977.
42. Lemmon, M. L., and Hamra, S. T. Skoog rhytidectomy: A five-year experience with 577 patients. *Plast. Reconstr. Surg.* 65:283, 1980.
43. Lexer, E. *Die gesamte Wiederherstellungschirurgie* (Vol. 2). Leipzig: J. A. Barth, 1931, P. 548.
44. Litton, C. Chemical face lifting. *Plast. Reconstr. Surg.* 29:371, 1962.
45. Litton, C., Fournier, P., and Capinpin, A. A survey of chemical peeling of the face. *Plast. Reconstr. Surg.* 51:645, 1973.
46. Litton, C., Szachowicz, E. H., II, and Trinidad, G. P. Present day status of the chemical face peel. *Aesthetic Plast. Surg.* 10:1, 1986.
47. McDowell, A. J. Effective practical steps to avoid complications in face lifting. *Plast. Reconstr. Surg.* 50:563, 1972.
48. McKinney, P., and Katrana, D. J. Prevention of injury to the great auricular nerve during rhytidectomy. *Plast. Reconstr. Surg.* 66:675, 1980.
49. Miller, C. C. *The Correction of Featural Imperfections.* Chicago: Oak Printing Company, 1907.
50. Miller, C. C. *Cosmetic Surgery. The Correction of Featural Imperfections* (2nd ed.). Chicago: Oak Printing Company, 1908. Pp. 40–42.
51. Miller, C. C. *Cosmetic Surgery: The Correction of Featural Imperfections.* Philadelphia: Davis, 1925. Pp. 30–32.
52. Mitz, V., and Peyronie, M. The superficial musculoaponeurotic system (SMAS) in the parotid and cheek area. *Plast. Reconstr. Surg.* 58:80, 1976.
53. Morestin, H. La réduction graduelle des déformités tégumentaires Bull Méns. *Soc. Chir. Paris* 41:1233, 1915.
54. Mosienko, P., and Baker, T. J. Chemical peel. *Clin. Plast. Surg.* 5:79, 1978.
55. Noel, A. *La Chirurgie Esthetique. Son Role Social.* Paris: Masson et Cie, 1926. Pp. 62–66.
56. Noel, A. *La Chirurgie Esthetique.* Clermont (Oise): Thiron et Cie, 1928.
57. Owsley, J. Q., Jr. Platysma-fascial rhytidectomy. *Plast. Reconstr. Surg.* 60:843, 1977.
58. Owsley, J. Q., Jr. SMAS-platysma face lift. *Plast. Reconstr. Surg.* 71:573, 1983.
59. Passot, R. La chirurgie esthetique des rides du visage. *Presse Med.* 27:258, 1919.
60. Passot, R. L. *Chirurgie Esthetique Pure: Techniques et Resultats.* Paris: Doin et Cie, 1930.
61. Passot, R. *Chirurgie Esthetique Pure (Technique et Resultats).* Paris: Doin et Cie, 1931.
62. Passot, R. Quelques generalites sur l'operation correctif des rides du visage. *Rev. Chir. Plast.* 3:23, 1933.
63. Peterson, R. Cervical rhytidoplasty—a personal approach. Presented at the Annual Symposium on Aesthetic Plastic Surgery, Guadalajara, Mexico, October 1974.
64. Peterson, R. Cervical-rhytidoplasty. Presented at the Aesthetic Society Symposia on the Aging Face, 1976.
65. Pitanguy, I., and Silveira Ramos, A. The frontal branch of the facial nerve: The importance of its variations in face lifting. *Plast. Reconstr. Surg.* 38:352, 1966.
66. Pitanguy, I., Cansancao, A., and Daher, J. Resultados desfavoraveis em cirurgia plastica, hematomas pos ritidectomies. *Rev. Bras. Cir.* 61:155, 1971.
67. Pitanguy, I., et al. Ritodoplastia em homens. *Rev. Bras. Cir.* 63:209, 1973.
68. Rees, T. D., and Aston, S. J. Complications of rhytidectomy. *Clin. Plast. Surg.* 5:1, 1978.
69. Rees, T. D., Lee, Y. C., and Coburn, R. J. Expanding hematoma after rhytidectomy. *Plast. Reconstr. Surg.* 51:149, 1973.
70. Rees, T. D., Wood-Smith, D., and Converse, J. M. The Ehlers-Danlos syndrome. *Plast. Reconstr. Surg.* 32:39, 1963.
71. Rees, T. D., Liverett, D. M., and Guy, C. L. The effect of cigarette smoking on skin-flap survival in the face lift patient. *J. Plast. Reconstr. Surg.* 73:911, 1984.
72. Rogers, B. O. The development of aesthetic plastic surgery: A history. *Aesthetic Plast. Surg.* 1:3, 1976.
73. Rothman, S. The principles of percutaneous absorption. *J. Lab. Clin. Med.* 28:1305, 1943.
74. Rybka, E. J., and Ohara, E. T. Surgical significance of the Ehlers-Danlos Syndrome. *Am. J. Surg.* 113:431, 1967.

75. Skoog, T. *Plastic Surgery—New Methods and Refinements*. Philadelphia: Saunders, 1974.

76. Spira, M., et al. Chemosurgery—a histologic study. *Plast. Reconstr. Surg.* 45:247, 1970.

77. Stark, R. B. Follow-up clinic on deliberate hypotension for blepharoplasty and rhytidectomy. *Plast. Reconstr. Surg.* 49:453, 1972.

78. Stegman, S. J. A study of dermabrasion and chemical peels in an animal model. *J. Dermatol. Surg. Oncol.* 6:490, 1980.

79. Stegman, S. J. A comparative histologic study of the effects of three peeling agents and dermabrasion on normal and sun damaged skin. *Aesthetic Plast. Surg.* 6:123, 1982.

80. Straith, R. E., Raju, D., and Hipps, C. The study of hematomas in 500 consecutive face lifts. *Plast. Reconstr. Surg.* 59:694, 1977.

81. Uitto, J. Connective tissue biochemistry of the aging dermis: Age-related alterations in collagen and elastin. *Dermatol. Clin.* 4:433, 1986.

82. Vistnes, L. M., and Southern, S. G. The anatomical basis for common cosmetic anterior neck deformities. *Ann. Plast. Surg.* 2:381, 1979.

83. Webster, G. V. The ischemic face lift. *Plast. Reconstr. Surg.* 50:560, 1972.

# 22

*José Juri*

# Treatment of Baldness with the Use of Flaps

Hair loss, partial or complete interruption of the previous hair pattern, causes deep concern in men and women. Such concern is easy to understand because the loss of hair produces an aged and unaesthetic appearance.

The profuse vascularity of the scalp allows flaps to be designed in any way and direction. However, there are important vascular pedicles that must be considered to ensure the viability of the flaps, especially when the pedicles are long. It is also essential to follow the sagittal (anteroposterior) direction of the skull when designing flaps that are more than 2 cm wide. This design permits direct closure of the donor site with an advancement flap (see Fig. 22-13), thereby avoiding tension on the suture line or the need to apply skin grafts to the donor site. In addition, the appropriate flap for the specific alopecic area to be treated must be carefully selected, so the result gives a natural appearance.

These aims can be achieved using conventional or microvascular free flaps, or both. We have employed monopedicled flaps for the treatment of baldness and posttraumatic alopecia of different degrees. Basically, these flaps receive their blood supply through the temporal, retroauricular, and occipital pedicles, which, together with the frontal pedicles (supraorbital and supratrochlear), form the five major vascular pedicles that nourish the scalp.

## Classification

We have classified baldness into three degrees—I, II, and III (Fig. 22-1)—according to the area and topography of the glabrous region. Reconstruction employs one, two, or three flaps depending on the degree of baldness (Fig. 22-2), the possibilities offered by the donor site, and the patient's demands.

## Conventional Temporo-Parieto-Occipital Flap

### MARKING

The pulsating path of the superficial temporal artery, which will become the center of the flap base, is palpated. From this point, the desired length of the flap is measured on the glabrous frontal region. This length is taken to the donor site, where the flap is given its proper shape and design (Fig. 22-3). The width of the flap is 4 cm, and its average length is 23 cm.

### REPLACEMENT DELAY

It has been demonstrated that these flaps can be transferred without delay. However, because of their great length and the torsion

635

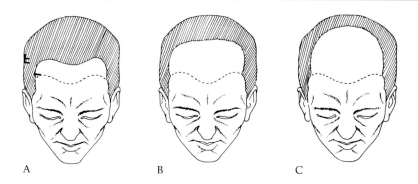

**Figure 22-1**  *Classification of baldness. A. Frontal baldness (degree I).
B. Frontoparietal baldness (degree II). C. Frontoparieto-occipital
baldness (degree III).*

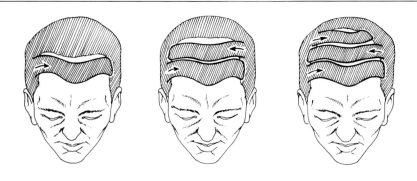

**Figure 22-2**  *Number and position of the flaps, according to the degree
of baldness.*

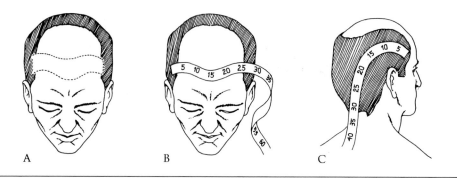

**Figure 22-3**  *Design (A) and measure (B & C) of the conventional
temporo-parieto-occipital flap.*

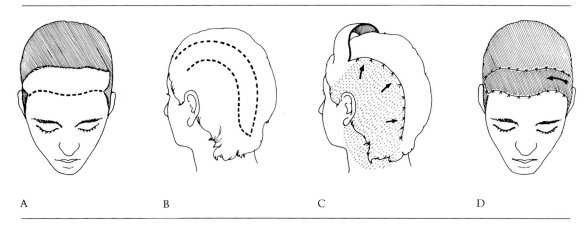

**Figure 22-4** *A. Design of the anterior frontal line. B. Design of the conventional temporo-parieto-occipital flap. C. Closure of the donor site allowed by wide undermining. D. Final suture of the flap.*

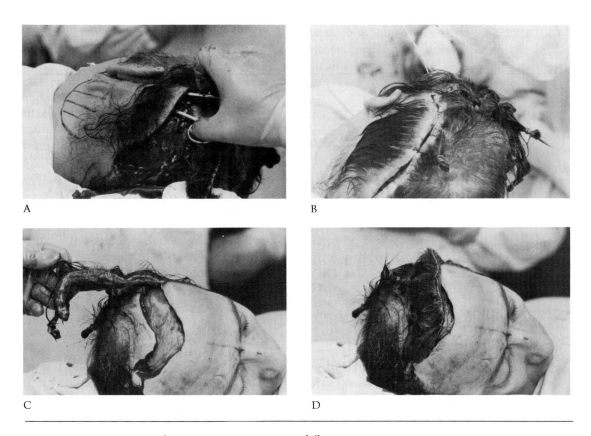

**Figure 22-5** *Conventional temporo-parieto-occipital flap: intraoperative views. A. Undermining of the retroauricular area and part of the neck. B. Suture of the donor site in two layers. C. Resection of the glabrous frontal region. D. Placement of the flap.*

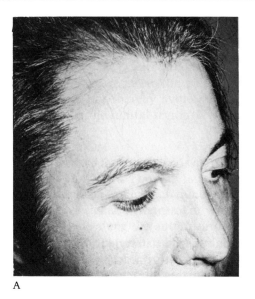
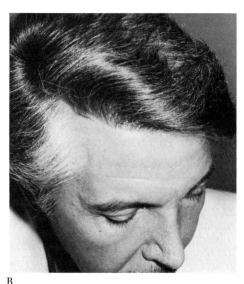

A

B

**Figure 22-8**  *Patient with degree I baldness treated with a temporo-parieto-occipital flap. A. Preoperative view. B. Postoperative view.*

**Figure 22-9**  *Patient with degree II baldness treated with two temporo-parieto-occipital flaps. A. Design of the lines for placement of the flaps. B. Immediate postoperative view. C. Long-term postoperative view (14 years later).*

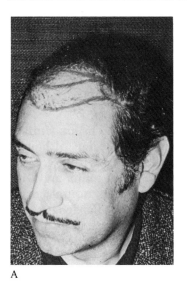
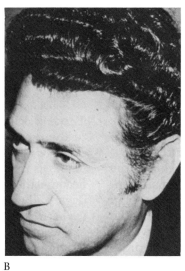
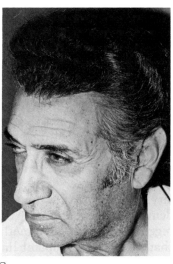

A

B

C

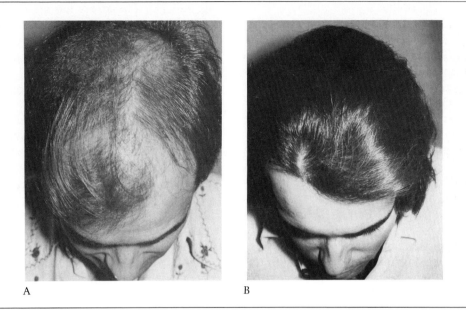

**Figure 22-10** *Patient with degree III baldness treated with two temporo-parieto-occipital flaps and a retroauricular flap. A. Preoperative view. B. Postoperative view.*

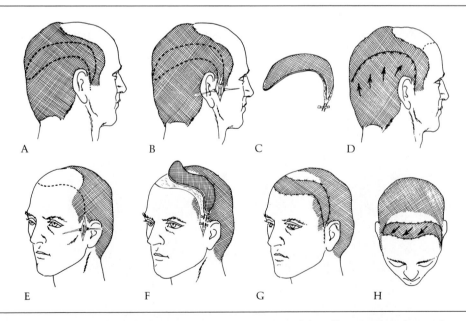

**Figure 22-11** *Surgical steps with the temporo-parieto-occipital free flap. A. Flap design (less curved than the conventional temporo-parieto-occipital flap). B. Exploring and dissecting the arteriovenous pedicle. C. View of the flap over the surgical table. D. Closure of the donor site with a retroauricular and cervical advancement and rotation flap. E. Exploring the contralateral vessels. F. Presentation of the flap and suture of the superficial temporal arteries and veins. G. Final suture after resection of the redundant glabrous surface. H. The arrows indicate the direction of the hair attained with this method.*

SURGICAL TECHNIQUE

The vessels of the flap pedicle are individualized (Fig. 22-11B). The flap pedicle is dissected, isolating the vessels of the neighboring tissue and the bed and ligating the corresponding collateral vessels (frontal, zygomatic, cutaneous, retroauricular). The flap is completely raised and separated from its bed (Fig. 22-11C), verifying the bleeding from the edges to the tip before clamping the vessels. A large area of aponeurotic fascia is preserved from the base to the tip of the flap to preserve the wide arteriovenous anastomotic network that nourishes it (see Fig. 22-12).

Closure of the donor site is performed before microanastomosis and placement of the flap in the frontal recipient site. To achieve this objective, wide undermining of the retroauricular and neck regions is required, as noted above. The only difference is that in this case forward rotation of the advancement flap is added (see Fig. 22-11D).

Individualization of the recipient vessels is necessary. The recipient superficial temporal artery and vein are microdissected (see Fig. 22-11E). The artery has an average caliber of 1.2 mm and the vein 1.5 mm (although sometimes we find arteries of wider caliber than veins). The selected suture site is at the level of the tragus (see Fig. 22-11F). (If the anastomosis can be performed at a higher level, the flap can be designed shorter.)

The flap is then transferred to the recipient site and fixed to the scalp with temporary stitches for immobilization. The arterial and venous anastomoses are then performed. When the clamps are released, flap bleeding is confirmed.

A previously designed incision in the anterior pilous implant line is then done, undermining the scalp in this region to place the flap, which is sutured along its anterior edge to the frontal skin (see Fig. 22-11F,G).

Finally, the alopecic region corresponding

**Figure 22-12** *Intraoperative views: details of the free temporo-parieto-occipital flap. A. The arrows indicate the aponeurotic fascia that ensures the integrity of the artery, the vein, and the anastomotic network that nourish the flap. B. The dissecting clamps spread the extensive aponeurotic fascia along the flap, ensuring the vascularization of supply and return.*

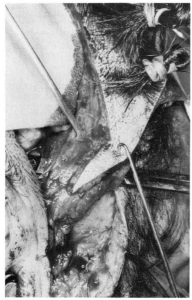

A

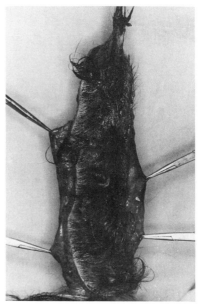

B

to the flap is resected, and the flap's posterior edge is sutured (see Fig. 22-11G). Two drains are placed: one in the retroauricular region and the other behind the flap. The operation is completed with an elastic padded dressing, leaving an opening to check the flap during the first 48 hours. The stitches are removed between the seventh and tenth postoperative days. The average total operative time is 5 hours.

**Figure 22-13** *Free temporo-parieto-occipital flap. A. Preoperative view. B. Anterior design. C. Postoperative view at 1 year.*

COMMENT

We believe that the free flap, because of its dimensions, its extraordinary blood supply, and the good caliber and similarity of its donor and recipient vessels, is an excellent technique (Figs. 22-13 to 22-15). It may be used for the treatment of hippocratic baldness and the alopecias of various etiologies, especially the partial alopecias that affect the scalp from the frontal to the occipital region, where hair grows in a forward direction. Finally, it is interesting to point out that at present we are performing these free

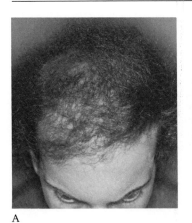 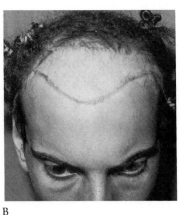 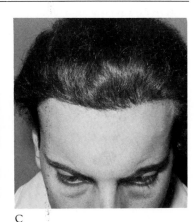

A   B   C

**Figure 22-14** *Free temporo-parieto-occipital flap. A. Preoperative view. B. Anterior design. C. Postoperative view at 1 year.*

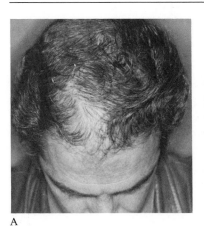 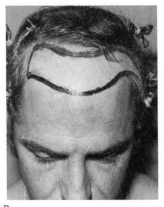 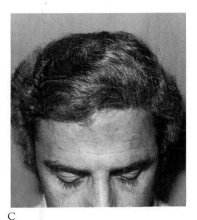

A   B   C

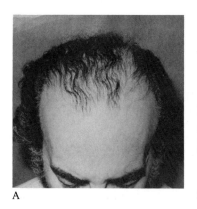
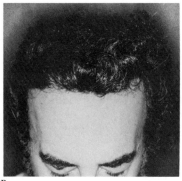
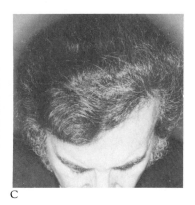

**Figure 22-15**  *Patient who underwent a surgical procedure with the free temporo-parieto-occipital flap. A. Preoperative view. B. Postoperative view at 6 months. C. Postoperative view at 3 years.*

**Figure 22-16**  *Intraoperative stages of the occipitoparietal flap (on an occipital pedicle). A. Flap design (on an occipital pedicle). B. Flap raising and transposition. C. Undermining (stripped area) for closure of the donor site. D. Closure of the donor site and undermining of the alopecic area. E. Suture of the flap in the anterior edge and resection of the glabrous region. F. Final suture. The arrows indicate the direction of the hair in the recipient site and in the flap.*

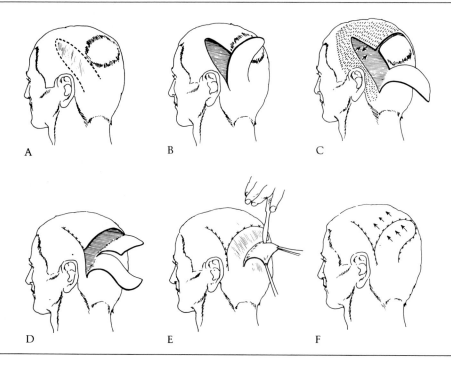

flap operations with local anesthesia, which avoids a lengthy anesthesia and its implied risks.

### *Occipital Baldness*

Occipital baldness usually occurs in isolation or as part of fronto-parieto-occipital

***Figure 22-17*** *Intraoperative stages of an occipitoparietal flap (on an occipital pedicle). A. Detachment of the flap and incision in the anterior line of the recipient site. B. Flap raised once the undermining has been completed. C. Closure of the donor site and final suture of the flap, after the alopecic region has been resected.*

baldness. The technique we use to solve this problem, which affects men as much as frontal baldness, is based on the use of a flap whose pedicle may be either retroauricular or occipital.

OCCIPITOPARIETAL FLAP
(ON AN OCCIPITAL PEDICLE) AND
PARIETOOCCIPITAL FLAP
(ON A RETROAURICULAR PEDICLE)
The selection of occipitoparietal and parietooccipital flaps is done according to the occipital region in which the bald area is located. If the occipital baldness is high, the flap pedicle chosen is occipital (Figs. 22-16 and 22-17) so the hair will grow in a forward

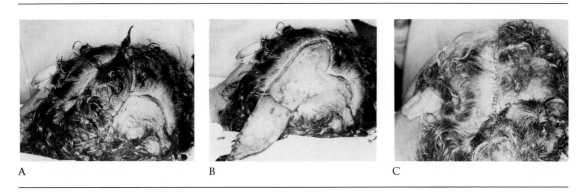

A        B        C

***Figure 22-18*** *Patient treated with an occipitoparietal flap (on an occipital pedicle). A. Preoperative view. B. Postoperative view.*

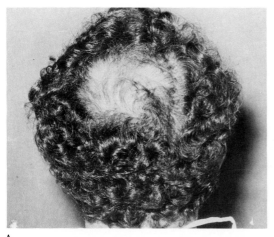
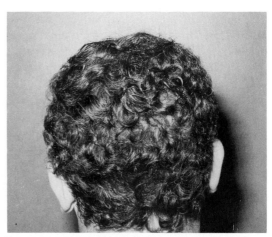

A                                                    B

direction (Fig. 22-18). If the occipital baldness is low, the flap pedicle chosen is retroauricular (Figs. 22-19 and 22-20), so the hair will grow backward (Fig. 22-21). In this manner, both variants of the occipital flap adapt to the normal hair growth in each of the regions. The design and surgical steps of both flaps are similar, and, in general, the tactics and techniques used in each case resemble those employed for the previously described temporo-parieto-occipital flap.

If the occipital alopecia occupies a larger area than the area that can be removed at the time of flap transfer, the redundant glabrous surface is removed 2 months later.

**Figure 22-19** *Intraoperative stages of the parietooccipital flap (on a retroauricular pedicle). A. The flap has been placed in the low occipital region, and the alopecic area is observed above the flap. B. Resection of the alopecic region. C. View of the final suture.*

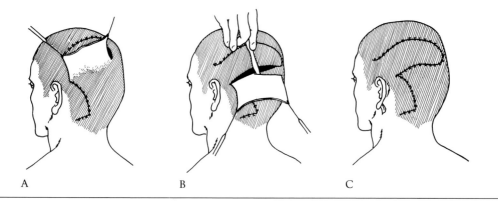

A    B    C

**Figure 22-20** *Intraoperative stages of a parietooccipital flap (on a retroauricular pedicle). A. Detachment of the flap from its bed and incision of the anterior recipient site. B. Wide undermining to achieve closure of the donor site without tension. C. Final suture.*

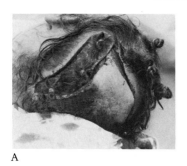
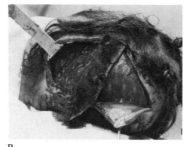
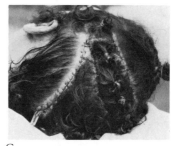

A    B    C

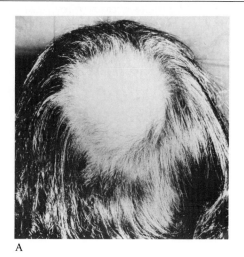

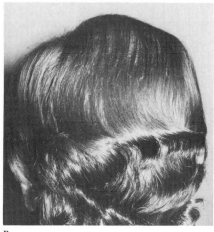

A                                                    B

**Figure 22-21** *Patient treated with a parietooccipital flap (on a retroauricular pedicle). A. Preoperative view. B. Postoperative view.*

## Final Comment

The use of monopedicled flaps, either conventional or free flaps, is the method of choice for treatment of the various types and degrees of baldness, as well as for treatment of the alopecias of various etiologies.

## Suggested Reading

Juri, J. Use of parieto-occipital flaps in the surgical treatment of baldness. *Plast. Reconstr. Surg.* 55:456, 1975.

Juri, J. Surgical Treatment of Baldness. In G. Sisson and M. Tardy (eds.), *Plastic and Reconstructive Surgery of the Head and Neck (Proceedings of the Second International Symposium).* New York: Grune & Stratton, 1977.

Juri, J. Use of Pedicled Flaps in the Surgical Treatment of Alopecias. In W. P. Unger (ed.), *Hair Transplantation.* New York: Marcel Dekker, 1979.

Juri, C., and Juri, J. Contribution to Plastic Surgery of the Scalp. In F. Ely (ed.), *Transactions of the Seventh International Congress of Plastic and Reconstructive Surgery.* São Paulo: Sociedade Brasileira de Cirugía Plástica (Cartgraf), 1979.

Juri, J., and Juri, C. Aesthetic aspects of reconstructive scalp surgery. *Clin. Plast. Surg.* 8:243, 1981.

Juri, J., and Juri, C. Two new methods for treating baldness: Temporo-parieto-occipito-parietal pedicled flap and temporo-parieto-occipital free flap. *Ann. Plast. Surg.* 6:38, 1981.

Juri, J., and Juri, C. Temporo-parieto-occipital flap for the treatment of baldness. *Clin. Plast. Surg.* 9:255, 1982.

Juri, J., and Juri, C. The Juri flap. *Facial Plast. Surg.* 2:269, 1985.

Juri, J., Juri, C., and Arufe, H. N. Tratamiento quirúrgico de la calvicie occipital. *Cir. Plast. Arg.* 1:32, 1977.

Juri, C., Juri, J., and Colnago, A. Monopedicled transposition flap for the treatment of scalp alopecias. *Ann. Plast. Surg.* 4:5, 1980.

Juri, J., Juri, C., and Colnago, A. Reconstruction of the scalp hemicircumference. *Ann. Plast. Surg.* 4:304, 1980.

Juri, J., Juri, C., and Colnago, A. The surgical treatment of temporal and side-burn alopecia. *Br. J. Plast. Surg.* 34:186, 1981.

Juri, J., Juri, C., and Ohmori, K. Colgajo libre témporo-parieto-occipital para la corrección de las alopecías postraumáticas de la región frontotemporal (técnica personal). *Cir. Plast. Ibero. Lat.* 8:179, 1982.

Juri, J., et al. Colgajo libre temporo-parieto-occipital para el tratamiento de la calvicie. *Cir. Plast. Arg.* 3:2, 1979.

Juri, J., et al. Nuevo concepto en el tratamiento de la calvicie occipital. *Cir. Plast. Arg.* 3:2, 1979.

Lamont, E. S. S. A plastic surgical transformation: Report of a case. *West. J. Surg.* 65:164, 1957.

Ohmori, K. Free flap surgery. *Ann. Plast. Surg.* 5:17, 1980.

Ohmori, K. Free scalp flap. *Plast. Reconstr. Surg.* 65:42, 1980.

Passot, R. *Chirurgie Esthetique Pure.* Paris: Doin & Cie, 1931.

# 23

# Primary and Secondary Aesthetic Rhinoplasty

## Primary Rhinoplasty

*Jack H. Sheen*
*Mark B. Constantian*

Rhinoplasty constitutes not primarily a challenge of technique but, rather, one of concept. Precision, versatility, and control in rhinoplasty depend most heavily on a working knowledge of the particularities of nasal functional anatomy and response to surgical alteration. Therefore we emphasize here the principles of nasal reconstruction that we consider essential and that cannot easily be found elsewhere. The authors' preferred techniques are described or referenced where applicable; countless variations and alternatives have been catalogued previously [7, 12, 13, 16, 21, 23–25].

### The Unique Nature of Rhinoplasty

Rhinoplasty is peculiar surgery. Traditionally conceived as a reduction operation by patients and physicians, the language, even the symbolism, of most patients seeking rhinoplasty describes excessive size. The "big nose," "bulbous tip," "wide bones," "bump"—all are requests for reduction; hence the evolution of a rhinoplasty model that prescribes "skeletal reduction, soft tissue contraction."

Consider, however, the uniqueness and inherent difficulty of this operative strategy: The surgeon is changing a structure whose final external appearance is critical if not paramount. This structure is configured as a skeleton with external and internal "cutaneous" coverings. The dynamics between (and within) skeletal and soft tissue layers are intricate (see below, Functional Anatomy), meaning that changes in one area affect function and appearance in the others. The considerable surgical goals are optimal function and aesthetics. Yet the usual surgical strategy prescribes reduction of the middle skeletal layer (often blindly) through the inner layer, expecting to precipitate uncontrollable contraction of the outer layer, whose detailed aesthetics constitute the critical surgical goal. Not that no similar strategy exists in other "reduction" operations, where the aesthetically paramount soft tissue surfaces are modified simultaneously.

Skeletal reduction followed by the inevitable soft tissue contraction is not always a benign phenomenon. On the contrary, this predictable biologic sequence directly causes the most common unfavorable sequelae of rhinoplasty (supratip deformity, middle vault collapse, columellar retraction, alar notching, and the like) [9, 10, 28].

The surgeon who intends to succeed in rhinoplasty must therefore develop a model of nasal behavior that integrates the particularities of nasal structure and function with the inherent limitations of the surgical approach. Every rhinoplasty is a compromise. Its goals are (1) improved function and (2) the closest possible illusion of the patient's preferred nasal configuration.

## The Model

### NASAL EQUILIBRIUM

Essential to the authors' rhinoplasty model is the concept that the nose represents not a static structure but, rather, a dynamic equilibrium, the sum of balanced, opposing forces [10].

Such equilibria occur commonly in nature. Stars, for example (including our sun), represent equilibria between gravitational collapse and the expansion generated by their central thermonuclear reactions; the processes are dynamic, but their configuration is stationary.

The preoperative nasal shape can be perceived as the same type of equilibrium between expansive and contractile forces. The nasal skeleton dynamically supports the skin, resisting the inwardly contracting skin sleeve and skeletal forces. Preoperatively, these forces are equilibrated. Skeletal reduction disrupts this equilibrium; the degree of disequilibrium at the end of the procedure determines the amount of redraping and contraction that will occur postoperatively and that can so defy and unsettle the recon-

structive surgeon. If the surgeon maintains nasal volume (and therefore nasal equilibrium) by skeletal "rearrangement," rather than "reduction," the surgeon immediately gains a powerful tool for (1) influencing postoperative nasal contour and (2) optimizing nasal function.

This tool works in two ways: by minimizing skin sleeve contraction and minimizing skeletal contraction. Unsupported soft tissues contract, and as they contract they thicken. The thickened skin sleeve effectively masks any skeletal contours the surgeon may have created. To the degree that the surgeon prohibits soft tissue contraction, thickening, and movement, there are increases in (1) the illusions of contour and refinement in the postoperative nose and (2) the predictability of the postoperative contour [9].

Skeletal contraction, though incompletely understood and infrequently discussed [10, 28], occurs as often as soft tissue contraction and can be equally disturbing to postoperative function and contour.* Consider, for example, the effect of middle vault collapse on airway size or of major alar cartilage resection on nostril support (see below, Functional Anatomy).

### SEQUELAE OF REDUCTION DISEQUILIBRIUM

The vectors of skin sleeve and skeletal contraction are predictable and are not always amenable to the desired aesthetic goal: caudally and medially over the bony and cartilaginous vaults, cephalad toward the caudal septum, posteriorly toward the maxilla, and posteriorly and concentrically around the tip. Unless resisted by proper and sufficient skeletal support, reduction disequilibrium proceeds toward a consistent endpoint that combines the most common features of the

---

*By the term *skeletal contraction* we connote movement resulting in volume reduction underneath the whole nasal skeleton, not "shrinkage" of individual osseous or cartilaginous parts.

overreduced postoperative nose: low dorsum, contracted middle vault, high supratip, round lobule, open nasolabial angle, retracted columella, retrusive upper lip, arching nostril rims, and flattened alar creases.

Whenever adjacent structural support is compromised but not rebalanced, and whenever soft tissue contraction is powerful enough to distort the underlying cartilages, skeletal and soft tissue collapse occurs. The surgeon must strive to reestablish the preoperative nasal equilibrium; the surgeon who controls the postsurgical equilibrium controls the postoperative result [10].

## *Functional Anatomy*
### NASAL LAYERS
Useful to the foregoing model is the concept of the nose as a system of two interrelated layers (Fig. 23-1A). The outer layer (Fig. 23-1B, left), like a knit elastic sleeve, slides over the inner, fixed, semirigid layer and contains the entire investing nasal skin plus the alar cartilages and their associated lining. The inner layer (Fig. 23-1B, right) contains everything else (bony and cartilaginous vaults, nasal septum, and associated linings) [10]. The "two-layer" concept of nasal architecture (1) associates the structures that behave together most clearly as a unit and (2) reminds the surgeon that changes in either the skeletal or skin layers have "global," not just regional, manifestations.

### STRUCTURAL INTERDEPENDENCE
The equilibrating forces discussed above operate in two ways: within each nasal layer and between the layers. Although the interrelations are numerous and often individualized, several are important to establish preoperatively: those within and between the bony and upper cartilaginous vaults, those within and between the middle and lower cartilaginous vaults, and those between the dorsum and tip (i.e., the "alar cap" [see below]).

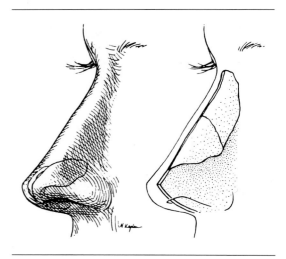

**Figure 23-1** *Nasal layers (see text).*

### *Bony and Upper Cartilaginous Vaults*
The width and stability of the upper cartilaginous vaults (the middle vault), a critical area of the nasal valve [16, 17], depend on the width of the bony vault as well as on the height and width of the roof of the middle vault. The upper lateral cartilages can be conceived as "braced" in their lateral positions by the width of the bony vault and (especially) the width of the middle vault roof. Resection of the roof (as during hump reduction) removes these outwardly distracting forces on the upper lateral cartilages, which, now medially unsupported, drift inward and can produce a characteristic "inverted V" deformity [30]. Osteotomy and in-fracture accentuate this inward drift, although the external discontinuity is often more visible if osteotomy has not been performed (Fig. 23-2). To avoid middle vault collapse and airway obstruction, the surgeon must plan to restore these distracting forces by dorsal grafts [28] or spreader grafts [30] whenever resection of the roof is intended.

### *Middle and Lower Cartilaginous Vaults*
The upper lateral cartilages are supported caudally by the alar cartilages, and radical

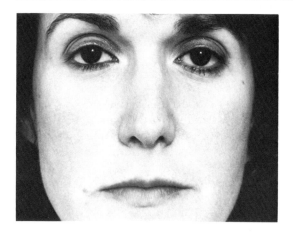 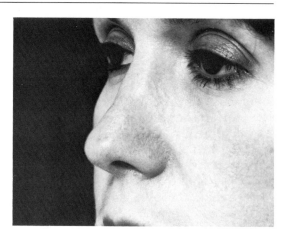

**Figure 23-2** *"Inverted V" deformity that occurs when the middle vault narrows after resection of the nasal roof.*

alar cartilage reduction can compromise middle vault support as well as tip and lateral alar wall support. In addition, the surgeon must note preoperatively the surface relations of the middle and lower cartilaginous vaults: Tip "projection" denotes the relative independence of the lower vault from the middle vault; the degree of tip projection must be a critical determinant of operative strategy.

*Dorsum and Tip*

Tip support and projection (i.e., the intrinsic ability of the tip to project anterior to the dorsum, especially the middle vault), depend in part on (1) alar cartilage shape, size, and substance, and to a lesser degree, (2) the relation of the bridge to the tip. Both factors are assessed preoperatively; the second is less often discussed. If the surgeon intends to reduce bridge height, the potential effect on tip support must be gauged.

The prior suggestion that the alar cartilages be considered part of the outer layer, external to the remaining nasal skeleton, emphasizes the broad impact of alar cartilage support on the nose. The tip, the lower nasal skin, and in fact nearly the entire lower half of the profile line depend on *suspension* of the skin sleeve by the alar cartilages, which, like a cap anterior to the rest

of the skeleton, maintain tension on the lower nose. It is this same lobular tension that drapes the skin to reveal the nasal planes and highlights [9]. The alar cartilages, or for that matter the grafted tip, carry a much larger responsibility for soft tissue support than is sometimes imagined [10].

## Preoperative Diagnosis

INTRANASAL EXAMINATION

Make a habit of examining the internal nose first, so that this most critical area is not forgotten during the discussion of the aesthetic details. Patients are always grateful to breathe well, even if an inadequate airway is not part of the preoperative complaint; more important, the surgeon must not decrease the airway by well intentioned aesthetic changes. Assess the septum for substance and deflection, mucosal cover (for signs of allergy, injury, atrophy, perforation), and (if needed) suitability for donor material. Specifically decide if a "high" (i.e., toward the dorsal border) septal deviation exists. Remember that hump removal unmasks the high septal curvature; you must be prepared to camouflage or correct the deflection so the nose does not appear newly crooked postoperatively. You may also consider performing no osteotomy; because the bones move inward unequally, fractures can make an apparently straight preoperative nose crooked postoperatively.

Assess turbinate size. At least 3 mm should exist between the inferior turbinate edges, the septum, and the nasal floor. Remember that the turbinates may be engorged during the initial examination; if so, assess them again prior to surgery. Finally, note the relation of nasal valves, septum, and turbinates. If the nasal roof is resected, the valve will narrow. The surgeon must plan to widen or reconstruct the valve postoperatively [30].

EXTERNAL EXAMINATION

The most prevalent misconceptions that patients hold about rhinoplasty follow the logic that the preoperative nose is a static structure in disequilibrium. Hence the argument follows that reduction can equilibrate the nasal skeleton and that the skin sleeve will contract uniformly and proportionately to reveal the attractive newer, "smaller," "thinner," "narrower" nose.

As has been discussed and is detailed further below (see Surgery), the evidence suggests otherwise. Equilibrium exists preoperatively; nasal shape is the result of a dynamic process in a stationary configuration. The skin contracts predictably but nonuniformly, the unrestricted endpoint of which is a thickened contour that does not provide a straight profile or normal nasal function [10, 28, 29] (Fig. 23-3).

The patient must therefore understand that every rhinoplasty is a compromise. The preoperative skeletal and skin volume, substance, and configuration have been predetermined; the goal is to produce the closest possible illusion of the patient's preferred configuration, consistent with optimal nasal function. Realistic aesthetics thus become not "narrower," "thinner," or "smaller" but, rather, "more balanced," "more proportionate," "more refined," "more functional." Re-

member that many of these "realistic" aesthetic goals may exist preoperatively; do not destroy them.

*Frontal View*

Examination of the nose on frontal view indicates the proportions between the widths of the upper and lower nose and the relative width of the middle vault. The desirable goals are that the lines from upper nose to base be gently divergent; the base should be wider than the bony vault. Specifically, the nose does not need to be "thin." If the middle vault is narrow preoperatively, remember that resection of the roof impairs support to the nasal valve and narrows the airway, even though the nose can appear wider postoperatively. Plan to restore lateral wall support to the middle vault [30].

*Oblique View*

Examination of the nose on oblique view indicates the relative confluence of the upper, middle, and lower nasal thirds; therefore this view also gives some evidence about tip projection. Remember that a discontinuity can be corrected by widening a narrow area as well as by narrowing a wide area. The more surgical options that are considered, the greater is the variety of nasal deformities that can be corrected.

Tip projection is assessed on lateral views as well. Guidelines for establishing adequate or inadequate projection, however, are difficult to provide; the extremes are easier to identify: An adequately projecting nasal tip lies anterior to the middle vault in oblique and lateral views; an inadequately projecting tip does not lie anterior in either. Between these extremes are tips that seem to project adequately on one view but not on another. Because tip position depends on the relative width of the middle vault and on relative dorsal height (see above, Structural Interdependence, Dorsum and Tip), these cases must be judged individually. Much depends on other parts of the surgical plan (e.g., the intended dorsal resection, treatment of the

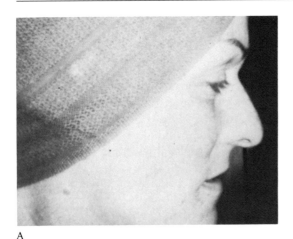

A

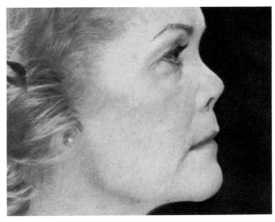

B

*Figure 23-3* *Unfavorable sequelae of reduction disequilibrium. A. Preoperative profile, showing low radix. B. After eight rhinoplasties. The first procedure created a large supratip deformity; the remaining surgeries aimed at reducing and thinning the nose further.*

middle vault, plans to reduce or augment the tip).

Second, comparison of both oblique views indicates the degree of preoperative symmetry. In well matched opposing oblique views, even subtle deviations of the bony or cartilaginous vaults become clearer; the most common combination is an apparent convexity in one dorsal line but a concavity in the other. Not only should the surgeon be aware of these irregularities but so must the patient. Finally, oblique views can indicate the relative masses between the upper and lower nose and therefore the disproportions that need correction by reduction or augmentation.

*Lateral View*
The lateral view is the profile about which patients are most explicit and have the strongest views, even though it is the angle from which they least often see themselves. Examination of the lateral view helps confirm the preoperative characteristics spotted on frontal and inferior views (relative upper and lower nasal masses, sectional discontinuities, tip projection). In addition, the lateral view provides some unique information: the relation between radix, dorsum, and tip. Of these structures, the radix is the least often

discussed. It is one of the most important points to be noted, however, because alteration of the radix provides the surgeon with a powerful tool for influencing overall postoperative nasal contour and balance.

In our culture, the ideal radix begins above the upper lid lash line; the dorsum is relatively straight, and the tip projects to, or slightly anterior to, the bridge line [28]. Note all deviations from this pattern and imagine the available strategic options. For example, in the patient with a low radix, slightly high dorsum, and inadequately projecting tip, it is often possible to achieve a straight dorsum by elevating the radix, reducing the bridge slightly (or not at all), and grafting the tip. Changes in all three areas need to be considered simultaneously; for example, elevating the radix decreases the nasofacial angle, whereas lowering the radix increases it. How does a proposed radix change, or change in tip projection, affect overall nasal balance and proportion? Which of the available options has the most predictable outcome? Over

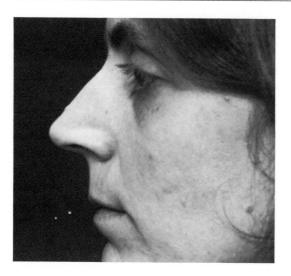 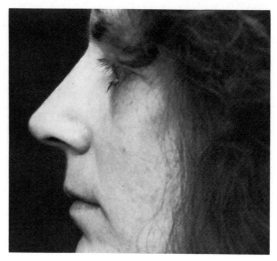

*Figure 23-4* Tip aesthetics. Preoperatively, this patient objected most to her projecting tip, yet when rebalancing her nose the tip was the structure least modified. Instead, the bridge and caudal septum were trimmed; radix grafting decreased the nasofacial angle and drew the skin sleeve cephalad to reveal more columella. Tip strategies must reflect the strategies for the entire nose.

which option does the surgeon have the greatest control? Most of all, what does the patient desire?

Some tip aesthetics are particularly important. The tip must be balanced, i.e., proportionate, both individually and as it relates to the remaining nose. With regard to individual balance, and despite the language of size used by many patients, the tip does not need to be "narrow." However, the supratip area should be flat, as should the superior lobule to the point of the tip. The mass of the tip should fall below the transverse light reflection that crosses the alar wall and runs toward the peaks of the domes of the alar cartilages [9]. The tip should be differentiated from the middle vault on all views [28]. At least portions of the lateral crura should be visible. Finally, the entire nasal base, including the lobule, should balance

the upper nose; this relation depends also, therefore, on the height of the bridge and the nasofacial angle [10] (Fig. 23-4).

Note also on lateral (and oblique) views the proportion of lobule to nostril length [28]. Remember that a small lobule/long nostril disproportion can be corrected by an increase in lobule size (as from tip grafting), a decrease in nostril size, or both. Finally, note the relation of columella to nostril rim and the nasolabial angle. Estimate preoperatively what corrections, if any, are needed; be cautious about straying from the plan during surgery because the latter areas are some of the most misleading to judge intraoperatively.

*Inferior View*

Examination of the nose on inferior view confirms nostril–lobule relations and can of course supply information about caudal septal deflections. Nostril asymmetries are especially common (see below).

ASYMMETRIES

All noses are asymmetric to varying degrees. Some patients are disgruntled to discover this fact; they must recognize instead how great the symmetries are despite independent development of the nasal halves [15]. The surgeon specifically points out all asymmetries preoperatively, both those that can be corrected and those that cannot. In this regard, the frontal, oblique, and inferior views are helpful.

PHOTOGRAPHS

Good quality photographs are taken to use at the preoperative visit and during surgery; it is dangerous to rely exclusively on intraoperative appearance and preoperative recollection. In addition, the photographs can help the surgeon explain the preoperative plan and the particular difficulties of the surgical challenge. At least one frontal view, both obliques, both laterals, and the inferior view are photographed; and the images are made large enough to allow recognition of minor asymmetries and skeletal features.

## Patient Preparation

INTERVIEW

The goals of the interview are to (1) find out what the patient wants specifically, and (2) explain what can be done specifically. Listen first to the patient's particular complaints ("I can't breathe;" "It's crooked," "I hate the bump") and then, letting the patient hold a mirror in one hand, inquire about each nasal area individually: the bony vault on frontal and lateral views, the dorsal shape, the tip on all views, nostrils, asymmetries, and so on. For the reasons discussed earlier, most patients describe their preferred configuration in terms of reduction: "thinner," "narrower," and especially "smaller." Unless you plan only to reduce the nose, you must help the patient understand the benefits of expansion (predictability, control, refinement, improved function). To this end, "balance" and "proportion" serve better than terms that signify only size.

Critical also are the details of the patient's preferred nasal configuration, particularly in regard to bridge contour, tip shape, and nasolabial angle. Both surgeon and patient must understand what is being asked, a goal

that is not as obvious as it sounds. For example, the patient who requests a "shorter" nose on profile (i.e., elevation of the tip) must appreciate and prefer the change that will also occur on frontal view.

Finally, reverse the nature of the questions and determine what nasal features the patient already likes. No step in rhinoplasty is mandatory. In fact, it is well to search as carefully for structures that ought to be preserved as for those that require change. Modest alterations that improve function and balance are always safer and easier for the patient to accept than are more comprehensive revisions.

SURGICAL PLAN

It is time to form a surgical plan and explain it to the patient. Both tasks tax the surgeon's skills. The data already collected describing the patient's goals, the present deformities, and the pecularities of nasal structure can usually be assembled around several surgical strategies; which one is picked depends on the specifics of the patient's desires, the individualities of this nose, and the surgeon's own experiences. Several iterations may be necessary before a plan can be devised that is comfortable. For example, with the nasal configuration described earlier (low radix, high dorsum, inadequately projecting tip), two obvious strategies are to (1) elevate the radix and tip, and lower the dorsum; or (2) lower the dorsum with minimal or no tip revision. Each "solution" yields a different nasal shape, balance, tip contour, and profile. Therefore you must prioritize. Does the patient believe that the tip projection is too great? Raise the radix. Is the tip lobule small in a relatively large nose? If so, graft the tip—and so on.

The patient must understand the plan *and prefer it to the other reasonable alternatives.* Be specific. Explain what is to be reduced. Explain what ought to remain unmodified—why nasal balance is already good in some areas or why it is not—why augmentation is necessary. The latter point may be the most difficult to make, especially because most patients think of rhinoplasty only as a reduction operation and therefore think of their preoperative deformity as always "too large." Secondary rhinoplasty patients, who have already seen the effects of reduction disequilibrium, are easier to convince.

Explain the choice of donor sites. We prefer nasal septum, if available; compared to conchal cartilage, it is faster to harvest, stiffer, usually flatter, easier to shape, and crushes well without shattering [28]. Concha serves if septum is missing or occasionally when a rounded contour is required.

Plan to bank any extra graft material underneath the retroauricular scalp [28] and obtain permission to do so preoperatively. Explain that the resected septal cartilage is not diseased, only crooked; that autogenous material is always superior to homografts or alloplastics; that, despite best efforts, soft tissue and skeletal contraction are not entirely controllable; and that therefore banked cartilage makes any secondary revision much simpler.

Finally, explain the sequelae and potential complications.

SEQUELAE
The surgeon requires much less antacid postoperatively if the patient has been acquainted with the sequelae of surgery, specifically packs, dressings, and especially "healing time." The latter topic is not intuitively obvious even to the most sophisticated patient. In a well judged rhinoplasty, in which equilibrium exists postoperatively and in which the soft tissues rest on the skeleton at the end of the operation, little change can occur. Nevertheless, things do happen. Contraction continues for a few weeks postoperatively, the amount of resulting visible change depending on the degree of adequate soft tissue support. The skin sleeve does not soften and become mobile for at least 3 months; some stiffness often lasts up to a year. Even if the skin cannot contract, it still "deskeletonizes": The tip rotates slightly caudad, the dorsal skin bet-

ter coapts the bony and cartilaginous vaults, the radix deepens. On frontal view, swelling over the bony vault can resolve slowly; because most patients are especially distressed by width in this area, they must be reassured. Finally, small skeletal irregularities can become palpable or even visible.

POSSIBILITY OF REVISION
Both patient and surgeon must remember together that revisions may be necessary and are almost predictable with some difficult configurations. Not only inexperience [24] but, more positively, a strong commitment to high surgical goals determines the percentage of revisions; in our practices, about 15 percent of primary rhinoplasties can benefit from some secondary modification. In many cases, these revisions are minor: modest contour changes or additional augmentation. Nevertheless, the patient must understand what cannot be predicted and therefore not mistake the uncontrollable for the uncontrolled.

POTENTIAL COMPLICATIONS
The topic of potential complications, formerly avoided by many patients, has moved up considerably on the list of items to discuss. If the patient avoids it, the surgeon must not. The patient who cannot be a dispassionate ally against complications at the preoperative consultation will not be one postoperatively.

*Hemorrhage* occurs rarely unless septal or turbinate surgery has been performed; in the latter groups the incidence is about 3 percent [14]. Reassure the patient that this sequela should not spoil the aesthetic result but may require extended packing or repacking.

*Infection* is rare following nasal surgery; the worst variant to be feared is spread to the cavernous sinus [8, 32], uncommon but reported. If prolonged packing (i.e., several days) is anticipated because of septal or turbinate surgery, perioperative antibiotics (maintained until the packs come out) may reduce the likelihood of suppurative sinusitis (a logical but unproved deduction). We use them.

*Asymmetry* may be viewed as a complication or a sequela; either way the patient should be willing to tolerate it, as sometimes it cannot be fixed. The key prognostic factor is the degree of preoperative asymmetry, including the less visible kinds, notably high septal deviation (see above, Intranasal Examination).

*Graft problems* are cited most often by surgeons who do not use grafts, as if complications from this technique distinguish nasal grafting from all other plastic surgical techniques. As the surgeon's mastery of grafting increases, the problems diminish in severity and number. Still, distortion, absorption, and visibility can occur. It is therefore imperative that surgeon and patient understand together the indications for grafting [27, 28], prefer the potential result to the alternative [11], and are prepared to correct or accept minor problems that arise.

## REFUSING TO OPERATE

By the time surgery is definitely planned, both patient and surgeon should understand each other. The surgeon must know the patient's goals in detail (and in order) and must believe them reasonable to achieve and reasonably motivated. The patient must understand enough of the surgeon's nasal model to appreciate the particulars of the surgical problem and the logic of the solution. Both must acknowledge and accept the potential sequelae and complications, and both must agree on the order of priorities: safety, function, and (lastly) aesthetics. Unless these criteria are comfortably met, the surgeon should not operate.

## Surgery

Intraoperative feedback during rhinoplasty is both difficult and unconventional. Unlike many operations, much more easily portrayed step by step in atlases, rhinoplasty differs because: (1) the surgeon does not eas-ily see the anatomy; (2) skin volume and texture produce constant variation among patients; (3) the strategies required for similar deformities may differ widely according to the particulars of the situation or the patient's desires; and (4) the outcome of the procedure does not appear immediately. The latter factor is widely acknowledged and troubles most surgeons, some concluding therefore that nasal surgery remains ungoverned by reliable biologic laws.

This inaccurate conclusion is avoidable if the surgeon remembers the equilibrium model and therefore learns to interpret the intraoperative nasal appearances as products of reduction, disequilibrium, expansion, and skin sleeve movement. We outline the cardinal points below. The authors' preferred techniques are detailed elsewhere [27, 28, 30]; refer to these sources for specific instructions.

## SKELETONIZATION

Remember that the alar cartilages are contained within the mobilized skin sleeve. Separation of the soft tissues from the skeleton thus rotate the tip cephalad and appear to demarcate it more sharply from the middle vault. By contrast, because the tip appears more projecting and because the outer sleeve has been loosened and rolled cephalad, the dorsum appears flatter, the radix more anterior, and the columella lower (Fig. 23-5A,B). The surgeon can thus be misled into reducing the dorsum less than planned and elevating the columella more than planned. Consult the preoperative photographs. "Deskeletonize" the nose with your fingers (i.e., push the skin sleeve gently caudad) and reassess before changing the preoperative plan.

If you plan to use spreader grafts (as part of the reconstruction), create the tunnels after dorsal resection. The intact mucosal attachment at the anterior edge of the septum prevents displacement of the spreader grafts.

Plan the septal resection after performing the dorsal resection. Remember that you must leave 1.5 cm dorsal and caudal septal strut supports. If you have made tunnels for the spreader grafts, which delineate the new dorsal edge, the tunnels also mark intranasally the upper edge of the new dorsum and can guide the septal resection safely.

## SEPTAL AND TURBINATE SURGERY

The surgeon who intends to control the postsurgical result must reestablish the preoperative nasal equilibrium and therefore depends heavily on appropriate graft material. The ability to remove usable septal cartilage safely depends on a careful, bloodless dissection. Make sure that the elevator is fully under the perichondrium; this plane dissects well once you find it. Elevation of perichondrium at the junction of septal cartilage and vomer is more difficult because of criss-crossing of the periosteal fibers; here, begin the dissection under the maxillary and vomerine mucoperiosteum and work cephalad [28]. It is usually possible to work well posteriorly onto the perpendicular plate of the ethmoid; as you remove cartilage or bone, check both airways to see that any airway obstruction is adequately corrected. Suture the flaps carefully and close any significant mucosal tears.

Inventory the cartilage after retrieving it. Assign priorities to the graft requirements and then make the best distribution possible of donor material to the task. Judge the grafts according to needed size, substance, and proposed location. If possible, use bony or irregular pieces where they cannot be seen (i.e., for spreader grafts or fill behind a cartilaginous tip graft). Crush or trim the grafts, as needed, smooth the edges carefully, and place them; if you are not satisfied *and improvement is still possible,* try again.

Partial inferior turbinectomy, especially a trim of the anterior edge (to obtain 3 mm clearance to septum or nasal floor) has value; like all nasal procedures, however, it has been overdone. Especially troublesome and as yet incompletely explained [2, 5, 6, 17, 34] is the poor correlation between patients' symptoms, subjective airway size, and objective findings. Certainly periodic and individual variations in turbinate size exist; try only to reduce the turbinates enough to achieve a satisfactory air space and to recreate the normal.

## DORSAL RESECTION

Producing a straight dorsum is not simply cutting along an imaginary line between the radix and the point of the tip. The nose is not a static structure. First, dorsal reduction often affects tip position. The nose can thus become longer or shorter after resection of the dorsum. Hump removal alters the dynamic anterior projection of the bony and upper cartilaginous vaults and therefore affects support to the dorsal nasal skin. Because of the global relations between the upper and lower nose, the tip can rotate. Whether this rotation is cephalad or caudad (i.e., whether the nose shortens or lengthens) depends on several factors, including preoperative tip position and projection, dorsal contour, skin sleeve size, skin character, and the location and amount of the dorsal resection.

Second, remember the interdependence of dorsum and tip (see above) and the relative preoperative position of each. Where is the radix (low, high, anterior, posterior, correct)? Where is the tip (i.e., is it projecting), and will the tip support itself after the dorsal resection? If not, a straight dorsum cannot be obtained until you augment tip projection.

Remember also that resection of a dorsal hump changes other relations: The middle vault contracts if the dorsal distracting forces of the roof have been removed [30] (Fig. 23-5D). Plan to reconstruct the roof by dorsal [28] or spreader [30] grafts if you resect it.

Dorsal resection throws the alar cartilages into greater relief, making them appear more prominent than they did preoperatively (Fig. 23-5C,D). Dorsal resection also widens the appearance of the bony vault on frontal view.

Hump removal can reveal a high septal deviation or can remove a prominent area of

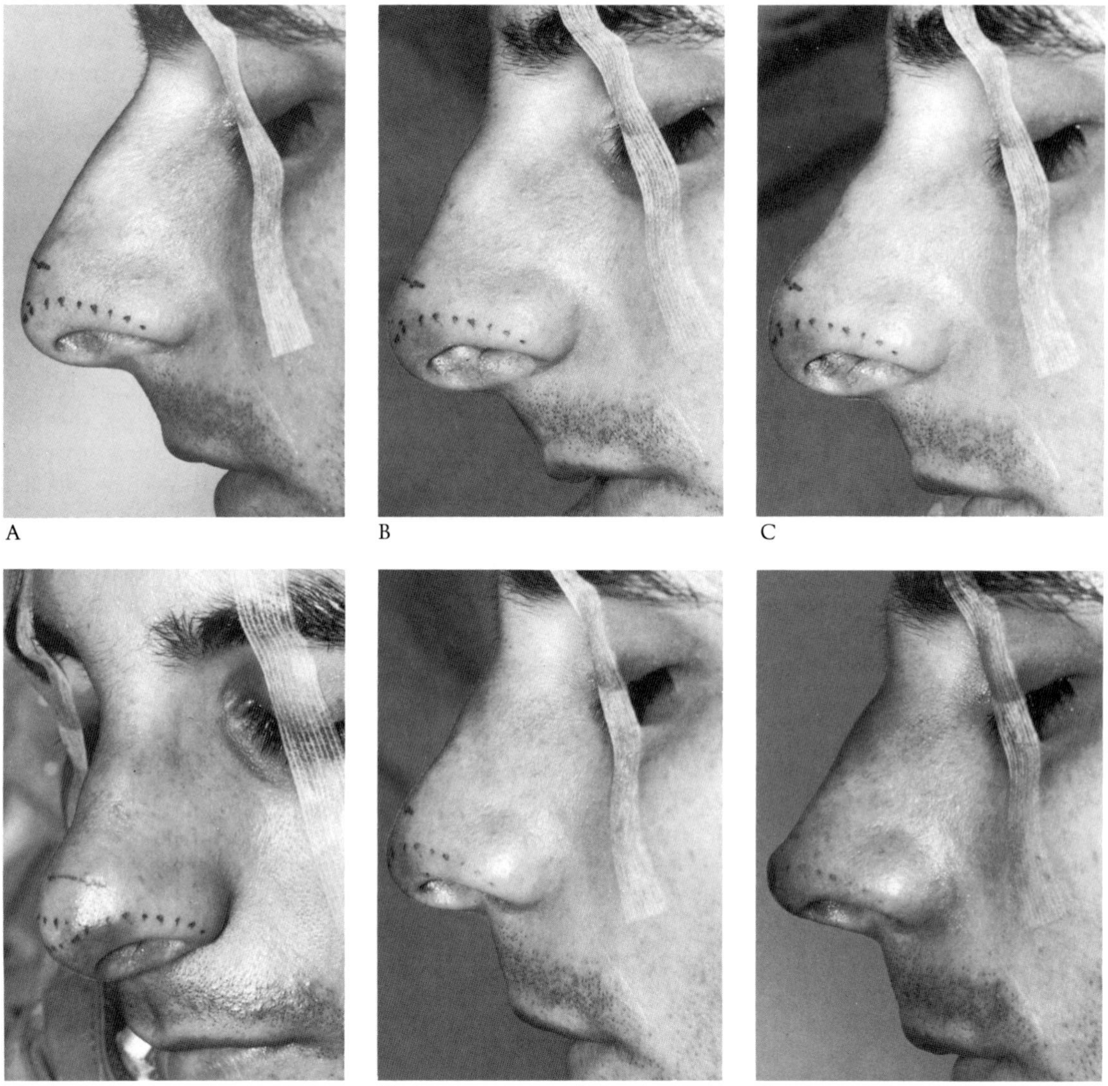

A

B

C

D

E

F

asymmetry in the crooked nose. In the former case, the nose suddenly looks newly deviated; in the latter situation, it appears newly straight. Look at the photographs.

## NASAL SPINE/CAUDAL SEPTUM

The area of the nasal spine/caudal septum, formerly considered intuitively obvious, defies complete description. One point to re-

*Figure 23-5* *A. Preoperative view. B. After skeletonization; note the positions of the radix, hump, tip, and columella. C. After dorsal resection; note the relative size and position of the tip. D. After dorsal resection; note the middle vault collapse. E. After alar cartilage reduction; compare to C. F. Immediate postoperative view after tip grafting.*

member is that resection of the caudal septum not only changes the relation of columella to nostril rim but also the sharpness of the subnasale and the carriage of the upper lip. Even without nasal spine reduction, caudal septal resection can produce lip retrusion. Be conservative. The end result of changes in the subnasale are not entirely obvious during surgery, often becoming more pronounced over the postoperative year. Finally, remember that both skeletonization and dorsal resection elevate the tip and alar rim and therefore make the caudal septum appear lower. Do not be misled into an unnecessary resection. Consult the preoperative photographs.

ALAR CARTILAGES
The alar cartilages, small structures, have received exhaustive attention in the literature [1, 4, 7, 11, 12, 13, 16, 18–28, 33, 35], and literally dozens of techniques have been proposed to enhance tip contour and projection. Remember that the alar "cap" supports a large area of lower nasal skin. If the tip is small, soft, round, or nonprojecting, reduction of alar cartilage volume cannot enlarge its supportive capacity. Alar cartilage resection is almost always overdone; "normal," attractive alar cartilages are 10 to 12 mm wide at the lateral crura [36], not 2 to 3 mm. Remember also that reduction of the alar cartilages, especially the domes, decreases tip projection (Fig. 23-5E). At this surgical stage the nasal contour can thus become convex again, misleading the surgeon into a deeper dorsal resection and compounding the problem. Using your fingers, position the tip where it should be before reducing the skeleton further.

OSTEOTOMY
Before performing an osteotomy, consider first that you may not need one; try to make this decision preoperatively. Patients are always delighted that fractures are not necessary. If the nasal base is already appropriately wider than the bony vault, narrowing the

upper nose further can make the base appear disproportionately large. If there is a high septal deviation, consider not performing osteotomy (see above, Intranasal Examination). If the nasal bones are short [28], if the patient is elderly and has brittle bones, or if he or she needs a wide bony base for eyeglasses, consider no osteotomy.

Osteotomy presumably achieves two goals: reduction of bony vault width and closure of the open nasal roof. Some aggressive maneuvers have been described to accomplish these modest objectives, including medial, superior, or percutaneous osteotomy, outfracture, or disarticulation. A single low-to-high osteotomy [28] is usually all that is needed; morbidity is always less with a lesser procedure.

UPPER LATERAL CARTILAGES
The caudal ends of the upper lateral cartilages may require trimming if the nose has been shortened; this maneuver is then the equivalent of shortening the inner nasal layer. The valve area is critical for unobstructed nasal airflow: Be conservative in the resection and recreate the normal anatomy [28].

ALAR WEDGE RESECTION
Like each preceding step except skeletonization (which itself can vary widely in degree), the alar wedge resection is an optional procedure, always best avoided if possible, as alar scars and nasal floor notching are horrible, common stigmata of rhinoplasty. Assess preoperatively the proportion of tip lobule to nostril and remember that tip grafting, if part of the plan, increases lobule size and may eliminate the need for nostril reduction. Because the alar rim has both external and vestibular surfaces, you must plan for each individually. Alar lobule size alone can be reduced without incising the vestibular surface. However, if nostril size must be reduced, preserve a medial flap at the sill to lessen the possibility of alar notching [28].

GRAFTS

The augmentation phase of the rhinoplasty is an opportunity to reestablish the preoperative nasal equilibrium. When electing, sizing, and executing the grafts, consider both the areas that needed augmentation preoperatively (e.g., radix, lateral walls, dorsum, tip) and those that may now need grafts because of the surgically created disequilibrium (most often the middle nasal vault or tip). If the goal is precision and control over the result, you must reestablish postoperative equilibrium and thereby prevent soft tissue and skeletal contraction [10]. Specifically, the skin should rest on the skeleton at the end of the procedure (Fig. 23-5F).

Each graft, especially the tip grafts, may require several sizings, removal, and replacement before it is just right. Insofar as possible, correct any palpable irregularities or asymmetries in the grafts or placement; they do not go away. Remember also that the grafts must be large enough to support the skin sleeve or skeleton and to resist the postoperative soft tissue contraction that always occurs. Although grafts do occasionally resorb, it is more common for postoperative contraction to obscure the grafts or blunt their effects. How much augmentation is necessary, desirable, or tolerable can be gauged only by experience. Be precise, document and photograph the results, and follow the patients.

## Postoperative Care

PACKING/SPLINTS

If septal or turbinate surgery has been performed, we use packs made of Adaptic Gauze (Johnson & Johnson Products, New Brunswick, N.J.) impregnated with bacitracin ointment (Pharmaderm, Hicksville, N.Y.) and layered over No. 18 French suction catheters placed in the floor of each nasal airway. The suction tubing extends to the posterior edge of the packing (about 4 cm).

Although complete patency does not usually last, the tubes help equalize middle ear pressure and allow enough nasal airflow to calm those patients anxious about their packing. The packs remain for 1 week.

In the absence of septal resection or turbinectomy, smaller packs can be used and need remain for only 24 to 48 hours. Patients mind packs least who have had the greatest airway obstruction preoperatively; some even remark that airflow is already better through the suction tubes than it was prior to surgery, a reassuring comment that calms the surgeon as much as the patient.

We prefer a tape and plaster nasal splint [28]; no alternative seems to coapt the reconstructed nose as precisely. Nasal splints, however, like extremity casts, can be placed too tightly; the nasal tip is at greatest risk. If tip reconstruction has been difficult, e.g., a small tip has been expanded with multiple grafts, check the patient conscientiously over the first postoperative week. At signs of reddening or prominent edema, be prepared to cut the tip sling, remove upper packs, and/or splint and restrict the patient's activity.

BLEEDING

The bleeding patient is usually terrified. He or she knows that no tourniquet can be applied, so before you arrive on the scene the patient normally constructs every imaginable outcome, from a dreadful aesthetic result to exsanguination. Your primary task, then, is to calm this anxious patient and elicit cooperation; as occurs in patients with upper gastrointestinal bleeding, calming alone often dramatically reduces the rate of bleeding. Frequently, removal of old packs, suctioning, identification of bleeding areas (usually the inferior turbinate), and reinsertion of a small pack of nonadherent gauze suffice. Occasionally, insertion of a posterior pack is necessary; familiarize yourself with this technique before you need it [16].

## INFECTION
Infection is a rare complication, although it is somewhat more common when conchal cartilage grafts have been used [31]. If fluctuant, drainage for culture and irrigation with the appropriate antibiotic has salvaged the graft; the technique is precise and must be accurately followed [31].

## POSTOPERATIVE RHINITIS
In patients without rhinitis preoperatively, persistent clear nasal discharge is often considered a common early sequela of rhinoplasty. In fact, rhinitis almost never occurs and, when it does, normally indicates excessive turbinectomy, a difficult problem for which there is currently no definitive solution.

## SEPTAL PERFORATIONS
Perforations occasionally occur after difficult septoplasties; they may or may not be symptomatic. Crusting, epistaxis, rhinitis, pain, or whistling can result. If you see a perforation, even if it is not symptomatic, tell the patient. Reassurance and treatment, if necessary [3, 12, 16, 24], satisfy most patients; the alternative is always surprise and anger when the same news comes from another physician.

## FOLLOW-UP AND REVISION
Patients should know beforehand that "healing" takes at least 1 year, and therefore follow-up must be at least that long. Much of rhinoplasty is "feel," which translates "experience." Experience and consequently surgical judgment derive only from a sufficiently complex nasal model. To a substantial degree each surgeon must develop his or her own model from repeated examinations, photographs, and hours with patients.

The decision to reoperate depends on the same factors involved in the primary rhinoplasty. The model and therefore the solution are usually clear and the goals reasonably motivated [28]. The surgery itself may be geometrically more difficult. Patient and surgeon must therefore understand each other explicitly. The elements of the decision and the surgery are found below, under Secondary Rhinoplasty.

# Secondary Rhinoplasty

*Jack H. Sheen*

It is better to consider secondary rhinoplasty in terms of rehabilitation rather than revision. Unsatisfactory primary rhinoplasty frequently causes functional and aesthetic impairment due to tissue deficit and damage. To say surgical revision or "redoing it" does not fully acknowledge the need to deal with a new set of problems, not just to find new or better ways to deal with the original problems.

Usually the major goals of a secondary procedure are to restore nasal function and nasal contour to a near-normal condition, i.e., to rehabilitate the nose. Scarring, tissue deficit, and decreased vascularity are factors that, if the surgeon fails to recognize their significance, may foil attempts at secondary correction.

Because secondary rhinoplasty requires the recognition and skillful treatment of special problems that worsen with each subsequent procedure (often causing irreversible tissue damage), it may be a disservice to patients to refer them back to the original surgeons who performed two or more unsuccessful operations. Patients must be spared the devastating effects of a series of untoward rhinoplasties.

## Ground Rules for Secondary Rhinoplasty

Because of the singularity and complexity of the problems associated with secondary rhinoplasty, there cannot be a standardized technique. However, there are ground rules that can be followed for a successful result.

*1.* Establish realistic patient expectations. A thorough, detailed discussion of expected results helps establish realistic patient expectations. The nose that is off midline is noted, and the patient is told that it will likely remain so. Crooked noses that are improved by camouflage techniques are always wider than they were before surgery, and the patients must accept this added width as a trade-off. Tip grafts may be asymmetric, but the slight asymmetry is a worthwhile trade-off for a more desirable position of the tip. Late adjustments can be made. Tip asymmetries are not the result of surgical error but are problems that can be anticipated from the formation of a new framework; they depend on the material used, the character of the patient's tissues, and the degree to which contour or position is changed.
*2.* Defer surgery until there is final resolution of tissues.
*3.* Limit the surgical dissection.
*4.* Use only autogenous graft material.
*5.* Have a well defined aesthetic goal.

### DEFER SURGERY
Minor surgical revision can be performed in 6 months; however, major reconstructions are deferred for at least 1 year. In some cases, 2 years or more are required for final resolution of tissues. The number and extent of prior procedures and the extent of the planned reconstruction are determinants for the timing of secondary rhinoplasty.

### LIMIT THE SURGICAL DISSECTION
The surgeon dissects only those areas that require surgical correction. A major difference between virgin and operated tissues is

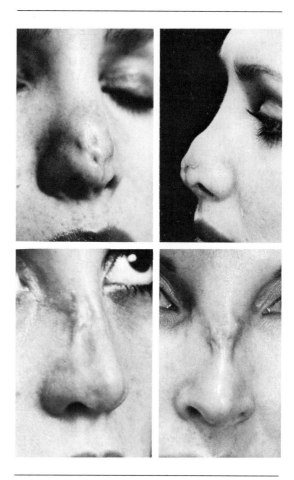

*Figure 23-6* *Patients after extrusion of alloplastic material with subsequent disfigurement.*

the decreased vascularity present in the latter. Injudicious undermining or incisions can further compromise vascularity, thereby sabotaging what might otherwise have been a good result.

### USE ONLY AUTOGENOUS GRAFT MATERIAL
The use of alloplastic material for secondary rhinoplasty is detrimental to the patient because of its poor long-term acceptance in the operated nose. The use of synthetic material is responsible for a high percentage of irreparably deformed noses, as the tissues re-

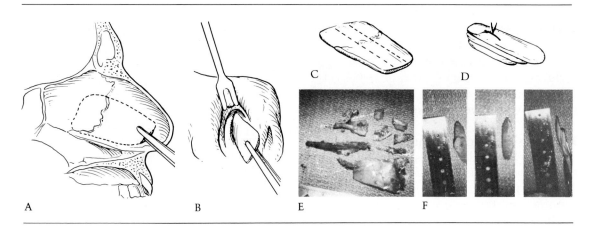

A    B    C    D    E    F

**Figure 23-7** *A–D. Available donor area and planned dorsal graft. E,F. Septal material obtained and dorsal graft ready for insertion.*

spond to infection and extrusion of the implants by disfiguring scarring (Fig. 23-6). Autographs of septal tissues, ear cartilage, rib bone or cartilage, and iliac bone are readily obtainable and provide the best chance for a permanent result.

## HAVE A WELL DEFINED AESTHETIC GOAL

A well defined aesthetic goal is not a vague generalization but, rather, a clearly defined set of relations that harmoniously integrate all of the anatomic parts of the nose.

## Graft Materials

With the above ground rules in mind, a discussion of the obtainment of graft material and its application to the most common problems in secondary rhinoplasty is in order.

## SEPTAL CARTILAGE

Whereas proficiency in the techniques of septal surgery is helpful for the plastic surgeon performing primary rhinoplasty, it is absolutely essential for the surgeon attempting to do secondary rhinoplasty because: (1) the patient requesting a secondary procedure

usually has nasal airway impairment; and (2) septal cartilage is the best material for nasal reconstruction. Improving the appearance of the nose using material removed to improve function is a winning combination. The surgeon's ability to extract the necessary material without jeopardizing the structure or function of the nose can make the difference between success and failure.

To harvest septal cartilage one must use an instrument that provides as much cartilage as possible in continuity with ethmoid to obtain optimal length of the graft. For this reason the use of a Ballenger knife is discouraged. In addition, the Ballenger knife cannot cross the osseochondral junction and is therefore useless for correction of functional problems involving the ethmoid or vomer. The Jackson nasal scissors is ideally suited to obtain excellent strips of donor cartilage with ethmoid attached; moreover, it can easily transsect irregular or distorted ethmoid and occasionally can be used to sever parts of the vomer.

Figure 23-7A illustrates the available donor area of the septum. Beveled septal cartilage can reduplicate the dorsum and has the effect of realigning the nasal contour by providing a straight, central framework for the soft tissues. The planning and preparation of a three-tiered graft for dorsal augmentation are shown in Figure 23-7C and D. Figure 23-

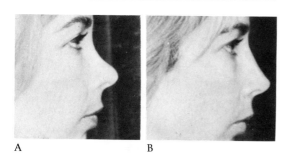

A                    B

**Figure 23-8** *A. Patient prior to insertion of graft (Fig. 23-7). B. After insertion of graft and chin augmentation.*

7E and F shows the material obtained and the prepared graft ready for insertion.

The patient on whom this graft was used is 23 years old, shown 10 years after a primary rhinoplasty (Fig. 23-8A). In Figure 23-8B the patient is shown after insertion of the above graft. Revision of the irregular tip cartilages and chin augmentation were also done.

## EAR CARTILAGE

Ear cartilage provides an abundant and readily available source of reconstructive material. The natural convolution of ear cartilage can make a superb dorsal graft. When obtaining ear cartilage, the anterior approach, as described by Brent [1] is the simplest, least deforming technique. It also produces the maximum amount of cartilage. Ear cartilage cannot be crushed or trimmed as satisfactorily as septal cartilage. However, it is more elastic and can be rolled into a usable graft and secured by nonabsorbable circumferential sutures.

Figure 23-9 illustrates a specimen obtained from the concha of an ear using the anterior approach. This maximal amount is resected only if it is needed. Because the structure of the ear is better if the concha cavum remains, just that amount necessary for a dorsal graft is removed.

The graft is designed so that the longest, most uniform part is obtained (Fig. 23-10). Most often the concha cavum is not used.

The completed graft (Fig. 23-11A,B), shown on dorsal and ventral views, demonstrates the use of circumferential nonabsorbable sutures to maintain form. The height and the

**Figure 23-9** *Conchal cartilage graft after removal from ear using the Brent anterior approach.*

**Figure 23-10** *Careful planning ensures the largest usable contour of the graft.*

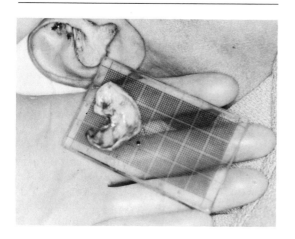

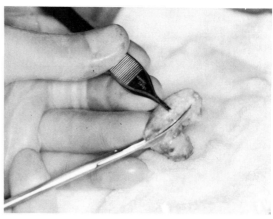

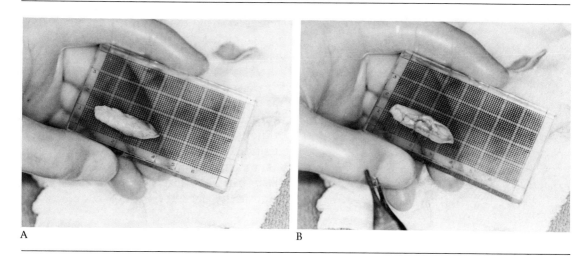

A    B

**Figure 23-11** *A. Dorsal view of prepared graft prior to insertion. B. Ventral view of graft.*

width of the graft can be controlled using this technique.

The patient shown in Figure 23-12A, C had undergone five prior surgeries, including

**Figure 23-12** *A,C. Patient after five procedures with no septal cartilage or bone available. B,D. After the sixth procedure using ear cartilage graft for reconstruction.*

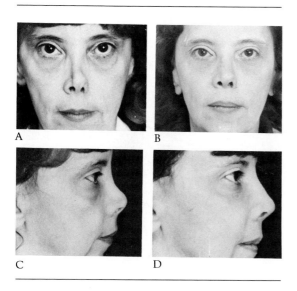

A    B

C    D

removal of most of the bony and cartilaginous septum. There was a 1.5-cm perforation at the angle of the septum. An alloplastic implant had been inserted through the tip, followed by infection and rejection, leaving a central scar and more distortion. The specimen shown in Figure 23-11A was used in the reconstruction of the dorsum. The effect of straightening the nose is apparent (Fig. 23-12B, D) with the new straight dorsal framework. In addition, the patient had bilateral flap rotations from the posterior membranous septum to close the septal perforation, a tip graft, lateral wall augmentation, and ethmoid bone grafts to the alar rims.

## Corrections
### FLAT TIP

A flattened, round, nonprojecting tip is a hallmark of the secondary rhinoplasty patient. A loss of tip definition usually is the result of surgical overtreatment of the lower lateral cartilages during primary rhinoplasty.

The use of supportive tip grafts of septal cartilage [2, 3] has proved to be a suitable method for achieving more projection of the nasal tip. Septal cartilage is my first choice for tip reconstruction, though ear cartilage

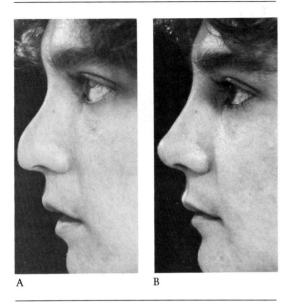

A                    B

*Figure 23-13* *A. Patient with flattened nasal tip after primary rhinoplasty. B. After secondary rhinoplasty, which included use of a septal cartilage tip graft.*

*Figure 23-14* *A,B. Frequently patients can have crooked appearing noses straightened by lateral onlay grafts of cartilage, which provide the illusion of straightness, as illustrated by this patient. C. Graft placement.*

has proved to survive better in those tips that are scarred with diminished blood supply. Though ear cartilage tip grafts seem to do better in low vascular areas, they do have a higher rate of irregularities and asymmetries than septal cartilage. Vomer or ethmoid has been used successfully in tip reconstruction as a barrier graft to support the position of the more caudally placed cartilage grafts. Figure 23-13A and B illustrates the dramatic effect of tip elevation on a secondary rhinoplasty patient whose flattened nasal tip was the primary cause of the unsatisfactory appearance of her nose.

CROOKED NOSE

Crookedness is frequently the result of asymmetry of the lateral contour rather than deviation of the central skeleton. Septal cartilage, intact or crushed, can be used to fill out lateral concavities to create the appearance of straightness.

The 44-year-old patient shown in Figure 23-14A had a crooked nose that was a consequence of asymmetric medial movement of nasal bones following osteotomy. The left nasal bone moved in too far because of the concavity of the septum on that side: The right nasal bone was held out laterally by the

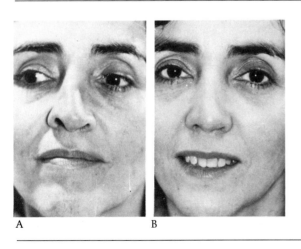

A                    B

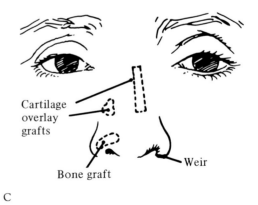

Cartilage overlay grafts

Bone graft

Weir

C

septal convexity on the right. After correction of the septal impaction against the right nasal bone, crushed cartilage was used to reform the contour of the nose, providing the illusion of straightness (Fig. 23-14B). No nasal bones were fractured.

Occasionally, a single dorsal graft can provide the illusion of straightness by creating a straight and uniform dorsal support. Often this procedure must be combined with lateral grafts, especially in patients who have thin tissues; otherwise the edges of dorsal graft become visible as the lateral walls sink.

The patient in Figure 23-15A had a low dorsum and a crooked-appearing nose after two previous rhinoplasties. A dorsal graft of ear cartilage provided a more symmetric nasal contour that showed less evidence of surgery.

## SUPRATIP DEFORMITY

The terms *supratip deformity, ram's head deformity,* and *parrot's beak* or *polybeak deformity* are used synonomously to describe a postsurgical fullness or convexity of the dorsal line, cephalad to the nasal tip. This problem is not the transient supratip swelling that frequently occurs during the immediate postoperative period; it is a supratip fullness that is definite and persistent. This unattractive hump of tissue is one of the most frequently found complications following primary rhinoplasty, and though it has been recognized and described, the problem and treatment have not been clearly understood.

In my opinion, the most frequent cause of supratip deformity is the reduction of dorsal skeleton to the point where the overlying soft tissue cannot drape over it. The thin tissue overlying the upper third of the nose tends to contract easily to the reduced dorsum, whereas the tissue overlying the caudal part of the nose does not. If this theory is correct, augmentation of the dorsal skeleton would correct the problem, and in my experience it has proved to be true.

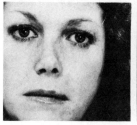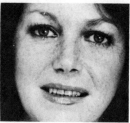

**Figure 23-15** *Straightening nasal contour using an ear cartilage graft, which provided a straight dorsal edge for tissues to drape over. Lateral grafts were also used.*

One hundred consecutive secondary rhinoplasty patients on whom I operated were analyzed as follows.

| | |
|---|---|
| Men | 23 |
| Women | 77 |
| Average age | 28.9 (youngest 16; oldest 67) |
| Average number of procedures | 2.7 (greatest number 8) |

The treatments employed were as follows.

| | |
|---|---|
| Dorsal augmentation | 82 (with or without tip graft) |
| Tip augmentation only | 8 |
| Reduction of dorsum | 8 |
| External excision | 7 (5 with dorsal augmentation) |
| Supratip thinning | 0 |

It is of significance that 82 percent of the patients in this series were treated by augmentation. Resection of scar tissue was not done in any of the cases.

The series of patients shown in Figure 23-16 have varying degrees of supratip fullness. Each patient was treated with dorsal augmentation without resection of any tissues to achieve the results presented.

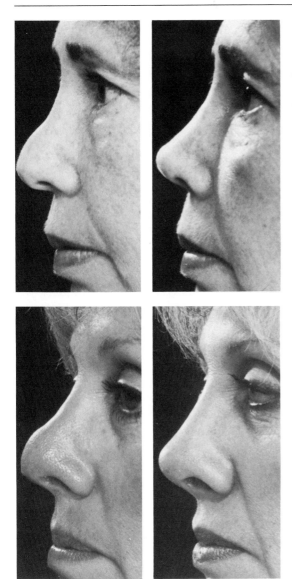
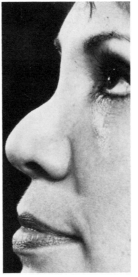
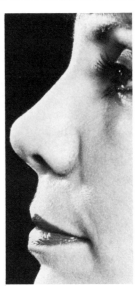

**Figure 23-16** *Patients with supratip deformity treated by augmentation. No dorsal tissues were resected from any of patients shown.*

## References

PRIMARY RHINOPLASTY

1. Beekhuis, G. T. Nasal tip projection. *Eye Ear Nose Throat Monthly* 51:92, 1972.
2. Beekhuis, G. T. Nasal obstruction after rhinoplasty: Etiology and techniques for correction. *Laryngoscope* 86:546, 1976.
3. Belmont, J. R. An approach to large nasoseptal perforations and attendant deformity. *Arch. Otolaryngol.* 111:450, 1985.
4. Bernstein, L. A basic technique for surgery of the nasal lobule. *Otolaryngol. Clin. North Am.* 8:599, 1975.
5. Berry, R. B. Nasal resistance before and after rhinoplasty. *Br. J. Plast. Surg.* 34:105, 1981.
6. Bridger, G. P. Physiology of the nasal valve. *Arch. Otolaryngol.* 92:543, 1970.
7. Brown, J. B., and McDowell, F. *Plastic Surgery of the Nose.* Springfield, IL: Thomas, 1965.
8. Casaubon, J., Dion, M. A., and Labrisseau, A. Septic cavernous sinus thrombosis after rhinoplasty. *Plast. Reconstr. Surg.* 59:119, 1977.

9. Constantian, M. B. Toward refinement in rhinoplasty. *Plast. Reconstr. Surg.* 74:19, 1984.

10. Constantian, M. B. A model for planning rhinoplasty. *Plast. Reconstr. Surg.* 79:472, 1987.

11. Constantian, M. B. Grafting the projecting nasal tip. *Ann. Plast. Surg.* 14:391, 1985.

12. Converse, J. M., et al. Deformities of the nose. In J. M. Converse (ed.), *Plastic and Reconstructive Surgery.* Philadelphia: Saunders, 1964. Pp. 869–948.

13. Deneke, H. J., and Meyer, R. *Plastic Surgery of the Head and Neck.* New York: Springer-Verlag, 1967.

14. Goldwyn, R. Unexpected bleeding after elective nasal surgery. *Ann. Plast. Surg.* 2:201, 1979.

15. Langman, J. *Medical Embryology.* Baltimore: Williams & Wilkins, 1963. P. 303.

16. Lore, J. M. *An Atlas of Head and Neck Surgery* (2nd ed.). Philadelphia: Saunders, 1973. Pp. 130–133, 162–191.

17. McCaffrey, T. V., and Kern, E. B. Clinical evaluation of nasal obstruction: A study of 1,000 patients. *Arch. Otolaryngol.* 105:542, 1979.

18. McCullough, E. G., and Mangot, D. Systematic approach to correction of the nasal tip in rhinoplasty. *Arch. Otolaryngol.* 107:12, 1981.

19. Ortiz-Monasterio, F., Olmedo, A., and Ortiz-Oscoy, L. The use of cartilage grafts in primary aesthetic rhinoplasty. *Plast. Reconstr. Surg.* 67:597, 1981.

20. Peck, G. The difficult nasal tip. *Clin. Plast. Surg.* 4:103, 1977.

21. Peck, G. Aesthetic Rhinoplasty. In W. B. Grabb and J. Smith (eds.), *Plastic Surgery.* Boston: Little, Brown, 1979. Pp. 424–433.

22. Peck, G. The onlay graft for nasal tip projection. *Plast. Reconstr. Surg.* 71:27, 1983.

23. Peck, G. *Techniques in Aesthetic Rhinoplasty.* New York: Thieme-Stratton, 1984.

24. Rees, T. D. *Aesthetic Plastic Surgery* (Vol. 1), Philadelphia: Saunders, 1980.

25. Rogers, B. O. Rhinoplasty. In R. M. Goldwyn (ed.), *The Unfavorable Result in Plastic Surgery.* Boston: Little, Brown, 1972.

26. Rubin, F. F. Controlled tip sculpturing with the morselizer. *Arch. Otolaryngol.* 109:160, 1983.

27. Sheen, J. H. Achieving more nasal tip projection by use of small autogenous vomer or septal cartilage grafts. *Plast. Reconstr. Surg.* 56:35, 1975.

28. Sheen, J. H. *Aesthetic Rhinoplasty.* St. Louis: Mosby, 1978.

29. Sheen, J. H. A new look at supratip deformity. *Ann. Plast. Surg.* 3:498, 1979.

30. Sheen, J. H. Spreader grafts: A method of reconstructing the roof of the middle nasal vault following rhinoplasty. *Plast. Reconstr. Surg.* 73:320, 1984.

31. Sheen, J. H., and Sheen, A. P. *Aesthetic Rhinoplasty* (2nd ed.). St. Louis: Mosby, 1987.

32. Slavin, S., et al. An investigation of bacteremia during rhinoplasty. *Plast. Reconstr. Surg.* 71:196, 1983.

33. Smith, T. Thoughtful nasal tip surgery. *Arch. Otolaryngol.* 109:160, 1983.

34. Stoksted, P., and Gutierrez, C. The nasal passage following rhinoplasty surgery. *J. Laryngol. Otol.* 97:49, 1983.

35. Webster, R. C., White, M. F., and Courtiss, E. H. Nasal tip correction in rhinoplasty. *Plast. Reconstr. Surg.* 51:385, 1974.

36. Zelnick, J., and Gingrass, R. Anatomy of the alar cartilage. *Plast. Reconstr. Surg.* 64:650, 1979.

SECONDARY RHINOPLASTY

1. Brent, B. Personal communication, 1977.

2. Brown, J. B. Secondary nasal operations. In *Plastic Surgery of the Nose* (2d ed.). Springfield, IL: Thomas, 1965.

3. Converse, J. M., et al. Rhinoplasty. In J. M. Converse (ed.), *Reconstructive Plastic Surgery.* Philadelphia: Saunders, 1964.

## Suggested Reading

Barton, F. E., Jr. Aesthetic aspects of partial nasal reconstruction. *Clin. Plast. Surg.* 8:77, 1981.

Beekhuis, G. J. Surgical correction of saddle nose deformity. *Trans. Am. Acad. Ophthalmol. Otolaryngol.* 80:596, 1975.

Berman, W. E. Secondary rhinoplasties and composite grafts. *Trans. Am. Acad. Ophthalmol. Otolaryngol.* 84:952, 1977.

Brown, J. B., and McDowell, F. *Plastic Surgery of the Nose.* St. Louis: Mosby, 1965.

Conley, J. Intranasal composite grafts for dorsal support. *Arch. Otolaryngol.* 111:241, 1985.

Converse, J. M. Corrective Rhinoplasty. In J. M. Converse (ed.), *Reconstructive Plastic Surgery* (Vol. 2). Philadelphia: Saunders, 1977. Pp. 1040–1163.

Converse, J. M. Deformities of the Nose. In J. M.

Converse (ed.), *Kazanjian & Converse Surgical Treatment of Facial Injuries*. Philadelphia: Saunders, 1974. Pp. 722–948.

Davis, P. K. B. The complications of Silastic implants: Experience with 137 consecutive cases. *Br. J. Plast. Surg.* 24:405, 1971.

Denecke, H. J., and Meyer, R. *Plastic Surgery of Head and Neck*. New York: Springer-Verlag, 1967

Elsahy, N. I. Prevention of parrot's beak deformity after reduction rhinoplasty. *Acta Chir. Plast. (Prague)* 19:63, 1977.

Fanous, N., and Webster, R. C. Revision rhinoplasty: A decision dilemma. *Arch. Otolaryngol.* 110:359, 1984.

Gerow, F. J., Stal, S., and Spira, M. The totem pole rib graft reconstruction of the nose. *Ann. Plast. Surg.* 11:273, 1983.

Goldwyn, R. M. *The Unfavorable Result in Plastic Surgery*. Boston: Little, Brown, 1972.

Jackson, I. T., Smith, J., and Mixter, R. C. Nasal bone grafting using split skull grafts. *Ann. Plast. Surg.* 11:533, 1983.

Juri, J., et al. Correction of the secondary nasal tip. *Ann. Plast. Surg.* 16:322, 1986.

Juri, J., et al. Neighboring flaps and cartilage grafts for correction of serious secondary nasal deformities. *Plast. Reconstr. Surg.* 76:876, 1985.

Kazanjian, V. H., and Converse, J. M. *The Surgical Treatment of Facial Injuries*. Baltimore: Williams & Wilkins, 1972.

McCabe, B. F. The problem of the collapsing upper lateral cartilage. *Ann. Otol. Rhinol. Laryngol.* 88:524, 1979.

Millard, D. R. Secondary corrective rhinoplasty. *Plast. Reconstr. Surg.* 15:404, 1955.

Millard, D. R., Jr. Reconstructive rhinoplasty for the lower two-thirds of the nose. *Plast. Reconstr. Surg.* 57:722, 1976.

Millard, D. R., Jr. (ed.). *Symposium on Corrective Rhinoplasty*. St. Louis: Mosby, 1976.

Millard, D. R. Jr. Secondary corrective rhinoplasty. *Plast. Reconstr. Surg.* 44:545, 1969.

Ortiz-Monasterio, F., and Olmedo, A. Reconstruction of major nasal defects. *Clin. Plast. Surg.* 8:535, 1981.

Peer, L. A. Fate of autogenous septal cartilage after transplantation in human tissue. *Arch. Otolaryngol.* 34:697, 1941.

Pitanguy, I., and Ceravolo, M. P. Secondary rhinoplasty. *Aesthetic Plast. Surg.* 6:47, 1982.

Pollet, J., and Weikel, A. M. Revision rhinoplasty. *Clin. Plast. Surg.* 4:47, 1977.

Rees, T., D., et al. Composite grafts. In *Third International Congress of Plastic Surgery*. Washington, DC: Excerpta Medica, 1963.

Rees, T. D., Krupp, S., and Wood-Smith, D. Secondary Rhinoplasty. *Plast. Reconstr. Surg.* 46:322, 1970.

Rees, T. D. *Aesthetic Plastic Surgery*. Philadelphia: Saunders, 1980.

Rees, T. D. An aid in the treatment of supratip swelling after rhinoplasty. *Laryngoscope* 81:308, 1971.

Regnault, P., and Daniel, R. K. *Aesthetic Plastic Surgery*. Boston: Little, Brown, 1984.

Rogers, B. O. The importance of delay in timing secondary and tertiary corrections of post-rhinoplastic deformities. In *Transactions of the Fourth International Congress of Plastic and Reconstructive Surgery*. Amsterdam: Excerpta Medica, 1967.

Rogers, B. O. Secondary and tertiary correction of postrhinoplastic deformities: Some dos and don'ts. In D. R. Millard (ed.), *Symposium on Corrective Rhinoplasty*. St. Louis: Mosby, 1976. P. 23.

Rogers, B. O. Secondary and tertiary rhinoplasty. In *Transactions of the 4th International Congress of Plastic and Reconstructive Surgery*. Amsterdam: Excerpta Medica, 1969. P. 1065.

Sheen, J. H. Achieving more nasal tip projection by the use of a small autogenous bone or cartilage graft. *Plast. Reconstr. Surg.* 56:35, 1975.

Sheen, J. H. Secondary rhinoplasty. *Plast. Reconstr. Surg.* 56:135, 1975.

Sheen, J. H. *Aesthetic Rhinoplasty*. St. Louis: Mosby, 1978.

Sheen, J. H. A new look at supratip deformity. *Ann. Plast. Surg.* 3:498, 1979.

Sheen, J. H. Aesthetic aspects of post-traumatic nasal reconstruction: A case study. *Clin. Plast. Surg.* 8:193, 1981.

Sheen, J. H., and Sheen, A. P. *Aesthetic Rhinoplasty* (2nd ed.). St. Louis: Mosby, 1987.

Sheen, J. H. Secondary rhinoplasty. *Plast. Reconstr. Surg.* 56:137, 1975.

Sheen, J. H. Secondary Rhinoplasty Surgery. In D. R. Millard (ed.), *Symposium on Corrective Rhinoplasty*. St. Louis: Mosby, 1976. P. 133.

Tobin, H. A., and Webster, R. C. The less-than-satisfactory rhinoplasty: Comparison of patient and surgeon satisfaction. *Otolaryngol. Head Neck Surg.* 94:86, 1986.

Webster, R. C. Revisional rhinoplasty. *Otolaryngol. Clin. North Am.* 8:753, 1975.

# III
# Skin and Adnexa

# 24

*Thermal and Electrical Injuries*

*Barry Press*

In the United States there are approximately 2 million thermal injuries every year, and 130,000 of them necessitate hospital admission. Approximately 10,000 to 12,000 of these individuals die as a direct result of the thermal injury annually [117]. Thermally injured patients spend 1.0 to 1.5 days per percent of total body surface area (TBSA) burned in the hospital. This number, however, represents only one-sixth of the total treatment, which includes intensive post-discharge reconstruction, rehabilitation, and readaptation to everyday life.

From 1961 to 1972 about 45,000 servicemen died in Vietnam and 300,000 were injured. During that same period 142,000 United States civilians died and 2.5 million were injured secondary to thermal injury [173]. It is apparent from the above figures that a severe burn is one of the most significant traumatic events a person can suffer and still survive. The prolonged morbidity of a burn injury is unsurpassed by that due to any other injury.

No one is immune from thermal injury, though demographic analysis shows four high risk groups that comprise the predominant victims of severe burn injuries: the young [154] (i.e., less than 2 years of age); the old (more than 65 years of age), the unlucky (National Burn Information Exchange [NBIE]

data indicate that 21 percent of burn victims are innocent bystanders to a fire [173]; and the careless. Again, NBIE data show that a full 75 percent of burn injuries result from the victim's own action [173], including such questionable practices as adding gasoline to an open pit fire to make it burn better or welding with an acetylene torch on an undrained automobile gasoline tank.

Many burns are caused by hot liquid scalds. Fifty percent of these burns occur in children [39]; the most common place for this injury to occur is the kitchen [174]. The most common kitchen scenario is a young child pulling on the cord or handle of a hot appliance, with the object falling onto the child from a countertop or range. The second most common place of occurrence in the home is the bathroom; most of these burns are caused by hot tap water. Table 24-1 shows the time to full-thickness burn at various water temperatures. Current recommendations for home hot water heaters call for a maximum temperature of 120°F. Most adult scald burns are caused by automobile radiator injuries.

Heating unit failure is the most common cause of residential fires [173]; failure of chimneys and vent flues account for 24 percent of such fires. Smoke detectors and home fire extinguishers can significantly in-

**Table 24-1** *Immersion time to produce full-thickness burns*

| Time | Temperature (°F) |
| --- | --- |
| 1 second | 158 |
| 2 seconds | 150 |
| 10 seconds | 140 |
| 30 seconds | 130 |
| 1 minute | 127 |
| 10 minutes | 120 |

Source: K. W. Feldman, R. T. Schaller, J. A. Feldman, et al. Tap water scald burns in children. *Pediatrics* 62:4, 1987.

crease warning time in residential fires and decrease the chance of death in the event of fire. They are mandatory for new construction in many areas of the United States.

Ignition of clothing is often a significant determinant of burn wound severity. When clothing ignites, the incidence of full-thickness burns increases six times and mortality approximately four times [190].

Cigarettes remain a common cause of fatal fires. In 1981 fires caused by cigarettes were the leading cause of residential fire deaths (27 percent) and accounted for 56 percent of deaths in hotel and motel room fires [191]. Many of these injuries and deaths are not to the smokers but, rather, to the nonsmokers in the area or adjoining rooms.

Historically, the tobacco industry has claimed that the technology does not exist to make fire-safe cigarettes. In 1984 tobacco manufacturers agreed to form a committee to direct, oversee, and review the work of a technical study group appointed to determine the technical and commercial feasibility, economic impact, and other consequences of developing fire-safe cigarettes [192]. The report of this committee, delivered in October 1987, suggested that with only minor modification a self-extinguishing cigarette could be produced. Prospects for eventual production of such a cigarette remain unclear at this time.

## Organization of Burn Care

The team approach to burn care has been validated in numerous settings. It works for both inpatients and outpatients. It is ideal for follow-up after discharge of the patient from the burn center. The team includes the director and resident physicians on the burn unit, nursing staff, nutritionist, physical and occupational therapists, psychologists, and social workers. We have found that weekly conferences are invaluable for assessing current patient care and developing care plans for subsequent therapy.

## Triage and Emergent Management

INITIAL TRIAGE AND MANAGEMENT
Thermally injured patients, like all other trauma victims, must be evaluated in a systematic fashion. No matter the extent of the patient's burns or other surface wounds, the first priorities are maintenance of a patent airway, effective ventilation, and support of the systemic circulation. Endotracheal intubation is performed liberally on patients who have suffered severe burns or when there is any question of an inhalation injury or a burn to the upper airway. An easy intubation on arrival in the emergency department may become impossible with the development of burn edema or the administration of large amounts of resuscitation fluid. In burn patients, orotracheal or nasotracheal intubation is preferable to tracheostomy, which is associated with a high complication rate [99, 137].

With the arrival of a "burn" patient to an emergency room from a house fire, automobile accident, or industrial accident, the major focus is often placed on expediting patient transfer to a burn care facility. Many of these patients have also suffered blunt or penetrating trauma, however, and all consequences of such trauma can be present in "burn" patients: closed head injury, pneumothorax and other thoracic trauma, spinal injuries, intraabdominal injuries (ruptured viscus, hemoperitoneum, or retroperitoneal hemorrhage), pelvic or long bone fractures, and significant blood loss. All of these injuries, although not obvious on external examination, can cause the patient's death more rapidly than does the burn wound itself. This fact underscores the importance of a systematic evaluation of the whole patient and, specifically, not attending to the burn wound to the exclusion of all else.

Patients with burns alone are often hypertensive. The appearance of early unexplainable hypotension or signs of systemic hypovolemia in a burn patient raises suspicions of another occult injury. Therefore after establishment of an airway, ventilation, and systemic perfusion, the next priority in evaluation of the burn patient is the diagnosis and treatment of other, concomitant life-threatening injuries. The history of the circumstances of the injury can be valuable in directing the search for associated trauma and indicating the possible presence of inhalation injury. Information about preexisting medical conditions, use of medications, and allergies is also helpful at the time of initial evaluation.

The patient is completely undressed, and all body surfaces are examined. Expeditious radiologic examination of the cervical spine, pelvis, and chest aids in the evaluation of possible blunt trauma.

After ruling out and treating other significant injuries, the burn wound can be evaluated. Regardless of the extent of the injury or if the patient is to be transferred to a specialized burn care facility, the two areas that need to be definitively managed prior to transfer are maintenance of adequate ventilation and, if indicated, release of constricting eschar.

## EMERGENT TREATMENT OF INHALATION INJURY

Inhalation injury is currently the major determinant of mortality due to burn injuries in the United States [83]. Treatment of these injuries is nonspecific and supportive only.

In the presence of a suspected inhalation injury, early endotracheal intubation is mandatory to prevent development of respiratory distress during transfer secondary to burn wound edema or the large amount of resuscitation fluid that is often needed [14]. The diagnosis of inhalation injury is often not clinically obvious, and one must maintain a high degree of suspicion of its presence. In addition, in the setting of a suspected inhalation injury, arterial blood gases including carboxyhemoglobin levels are measured; if the latter is elevated, 100% oxygen is administered [55]. Otherwise, adequate ventilation using normal ventilatory parameters is the goal.

## ESCHAROTOMY

Circumferential burns and the leathery eschar they produce can be a life- or limb-threatening problem in the chest and extremities. Circumferential eschar can cause sufficient decrease in chest wall excursion, resulting in respiratory embarrassment. Likewise, in the extremities constricting circumferential eschar can cause compartment syndromes or distal ischemia and necrosis [164]. The signs of impending circulatory or respiratory compromise from constricting eschar must be recognized and treated *prior* to transfer to a burn unit.

Limitation of chest wall excursion can be easily observed. If indicated, escharotomy is performed bilaterally in the anterior axillary lines, preferably using a cutting electrocautery current to incise the full length and depth of the eschar. With adequate incision of the eschar, obvious release of the underlying soft tissues is noted. Bleeding may be brisk but can generally be controlled with direct pressure. The application of topical hemostatic agents such as Avitene or Helistat may be necessary as well. Circumferential pressure dressings are obviously contraindicated. If chest excursion is still not adequate, incisions can be joined with a chevron-type incision over the costal margins. This maneuver allows sufficient release of the burned soft tissues of the chest wall to permit adequate ventilatory function.

In the extremities, pulses in the fingers and toes can be assessed using a Doppler apparatus. Several investigators have reported the utility of continuous pulse oximetry for such monitoring [13]. In the absence of these instruments, a large (16-gauge) needle can be used to prick the fingers and toes. Bright red capillary bleeding is a sign of adequate perfusion to the distal digit. Slow or no bleeding is indicative of diminished or absent arterial inflow, and rapid, dark bleeding is indicative of partial or complete venous occlusion. In either of the latter two circumstances, or if previously palpable or Doppler-detected pulses disappear, immediate escharotomy is performed on the affected extremity [165]. Bardakjian et al. have shown that oxygen saturation of less than 95 percent correlates well with the need for emergent escharotomy [13].

Extremity escharotomy is performed in the mid-lateral lines of the affected extremity, taking care in the arm to avoid the ulnar nerve posterior to the medial epicondyle, and in the lower extremity to avoid the common peroneal nerve posterior to the head of the fibula [163]. Again, it is essential that the escharotomy be performed through the entire *length* and *depth* of the eschar. Underlying soft tissue release indicates adequate incision. If the fingers are severely burned, digital escharotomy is performed along their mid-lateral lines, preferably on the ulnar aspects of the second, third, and fourth fingers and the radial aspect of the fifth. This method avoids painful scars on the primary working surfaces of the fingers [178]. Escharotomy of the thumb is best performed along the mid-lateral radial aspect. The thenar and hypothenar muscle compartments are often involved in severe burn injuries. Eschar over these compartments must be incised. If necessary, the fascia is opened as well [178]. For deep burns to the hand, dorsal escharotomy with interosseous compartment fasciotomy is also performed [164].

Interosseous compartment fasciotomy is performed through the dorsal escharotomy using a clamp spread longitudinally between the metacarpals. When incising a full-thickness burn eschar the procedure is rarely painful for the patient, but if the escharotomy is necessary for a combination of partial-thickness burn and edema secondary to fluid administration, pain may be significant. However, only rarely is this procedure required in the operating room, as intravenous analgesia and sedation carefully given and titrated to the patient's response is generally adequate.

For all extremities, sufficient release of eschar is performed until perfusion is restored to the distal limb. If perfusion is not restored after the performance of adequate escharotomy, inadequate fluid resuscitation must be suspected [178]. With deep thermal injury to the muscles or electrical injury, the escharotomy is combined with formal fasciotomy in affected muscle compartments [162]. For the severely burned limb, the decision to proceed with a formal fasciotomy is often difficult. However, the consequences of compartment syndrome are much more devastating to the patient's long-term rehabilitation than unnecessary fasciotomy. We therefore recommend liberal indications for fasciotomy in the presence of deep extremity thermal burns.

The size and extent of the burn wound is estimated at this time. The classic "rule of nines" has been shown to be inaccurate for establishing the extent of burn injury [69]. The Lund and Browder chart is easy to use, is more accurate, and provides a permanent medical record of the initial injury (Fig. 24-1). On initial evaluation, estimation of the burn depth is of less significance than its extent.

INDICATION FOR ADMISSION
The decision to admit a burn patient must be individualized. Generalized guidelines

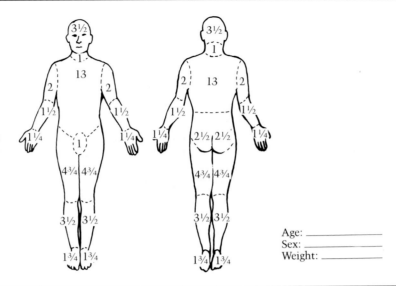

Age: _____
Sex: _____
Weight: _____

| Area | Birth–1 yr | 1–4 yr | 5–9 yr | 10–14 yr | 15 yr | Adult | Partial thickness 2° | Full thickness 3° | Total |
|---|---|---|---|---|---|---|---|---|---|
| Head | 19 | 17 | 13 | 11 | 9 | 7 | | | |
| Neck | 2 | 2 | 2 | 2 | 2 | 2 | | | |
| Anterior trunk | 13 | 13 | 13 | 13 | 13 | 13 | | | |
| Posterior trunk | 13 | 13 | 13 | 13 | 13 | 13 | | | |
| Right buttock | 2½ | 2½ | 2½ | 2½ | 2½ | 2½ | | | |
| Left buttock | 2½ | 2½ | 2½ | 2½ | 2½ | 2½ | | | |
| Genitalia | 1 | 1 | 1 | 1 | 1 | 1 | | | |
| Right upper arm | 4 | 4 | 4 | 4 | 4 | 4 | | | |
| Left upper arm | 4 | 4 | 4 | 4 | 4 | 4 | | | |
| Right lower arm | 3 | 3 | 3 | 3 | 3 | 3 | | | |
| Left lower arm | 3 | 3 | 3 | 3 | 3 | 3 | | | |
| Right hand | 2½ | 2½ | 2½ | 2½ | 2½ | 2½ | | | |
| Left hand | 2½ | 2½ | 2½ | 2½ | 2½ | 2½ | | | |
| Right thigh | 5½ | 6½ | 8 | 8½ | 9 | 9½ | | | |
| Left thigh | 5½ | 6½ | 8 | 8½ | 9 | 9½ | | | |
| Right leg | 5 | 5 | 5½ | 6 | 6½ | 7 | | | |
| Left leg | 5 | 5 | 5½ | 6 | 6½ | 8 | | | |
| Right foot | 3½ | 3½ | 3½ | 3½ | 3½ | 3½ | | | |
| Left foot | 3½ | 3½ | 3½ | 3½ | 3½ | 3½ | | | |
| | | | | | | Total | | | |

*Figure 24-1* Lund and Browder charts for establishing the extent of burn injury. These charts may be entered directly in the patient's record. (Reproduced by permission of Pediatrics 62:4, 1978.)

have been published [162] and include those patients with partial burns of 15 percent or more in adults, 10 percent or more in children, or any patient with a full-thickness burn of 10 percent or more. In addition, any patient with a burn to the face, hands, feet, or perineum, except burns of the most minor nature, must be admitted to the burn unit of a general hospital or be sent to a burn center, as is anyone with an electrical, chemical, frostbite, or inhalation injury. Even an individual with a minor burn in the context of associated major medical illness is seriously considered for burn center admission.

It is often advantageous, when minimizing patient pain and maximizing cooperation with wound care and rehabilitation, to admit patients with small burns to a burn unit for a period of 1 to 2 days to teach dressing changes and appropriate postinjury exercises. Again, considerations such as the patient's age, home situation, occupation, and level of cooperation enter into this decision.

INITIAL FLUID MANAGEMENT

Once the decision has been made to admit a patient, an intravenous line is established that can handle fluid resuscitation requirements (up to 2 liters per hour). Although it is preferable to establish vascular access through unburned skin, burned tissue is virtually sterile acutely. Intravenous cannulation can be performed through burned tissue if necessary for adequate volume delivery [162, 178]. Formulas for burn resuscitation are discussed in another section, but a rough estimate of the amount of fluid to be administered during the first hour after the burn can be obtained by the following formula: patient weight (kg) × % TBSA burned × 4/24 [162]. A Foley catheter is inserted, and urine output is measured hourly. Intravenous fluid (lactated Ringer's solution) is adjusted to maintain a urine output of 30 to 50 ml per hour in an adult and 0.5 to 1.0 ml/kg/hr in a child. Burns of over 20 to 25 percent TBSA are associated with a paralytic ileus.

A nasogastric tube is inserted and placed to suction to maintain gastric decompression. Analgesics and sedatives can be administered as needed but are given intravenously only; intramuscular absorption is erratic [162]. Small doses are used, titrated to the clinical response. The tetanus immunization of the burned patient is determined and brought up to date. The patient must be kept warm during transfer using warm intravenous fluids, warm gases if the patient is intubated, and adequate coverings; hypothermia is a frequent, often disastrous problem in these patients, and the patient's core temperature must be continually monitored.

Note that these measures are general guidelines only. The most optimal care of the seriously injured burned patient occurs only with coordination between the referring and accepting physicians regarding specific fluid management and monitoring of clinical status during transfer. These specifics must be agreed on prior to patient transfer.

## Treatment Principles for Outpatient Burn Management

A few basic principles ensure uncomplicated primary healing in most patients with minor burns. The magnitude of the patient's injury is determined with the patient completely undressed. Photographs are helpful to follow progress and for medicolegal purposes. The wounds are copiously lavaged with room-temperature saline solution and then gently washed using a mild soap and a wash cloth. Hexachlorophene is avoided, as large amounts of this drug can be absorbed systemically through burned tissue [162]. A substantial amount of pain relief can be obtained by applying cold towels to the burned area; these towels are left in place not longer than 15 to 20 minutes on large surface area burns, thereby preventing the development of hypothermia.

Treatment of blisters is controversial. Intact blisters with noncontaminated blister fluid provide a biologic dressing over a partial-thickness burn wound. There is some disputed evidence that the substances contained in the blister fluid promote healing [166]. It is the consensus that blisters that have ruptured or appear about to rupture must be débrided [162]. Moreover, any blister that interferes with function or movement (e.g., an eyelid blister that impairs vision) is débrided. The disadvantage of leaving blisters intact is that a less than cooperative outpatient may allow the blister fluid to become infected. Should infection occur, the partial-thickness injury under the blister may rapidly be converted to a full-thickness wound. Débriding *all* blisters prevents this possibility [178, 194].

With a noninfected partial-thickness burn wound, the use of topical or systemic antibiotics is controversial [194]. After blister débridement, the wound is covered with a moisture-retaining nonadherent dressing. Xeroform gauze is an excellent choice; bacitracin or Polysporin ointment can alternatively be used, especially on the face. Biobrane is a bilaminar synthetic biologic dressing that has shown great efficacy in the treatment of partial-thickness wounds [121]. When properly applied to a clean partial-thickness wound, Biobrane often adheres to the wound surface through the collagen impregnated on its inner surface. It remains adherent until healing occurs. Pain is minimal with this technique [121]. The initial cost of Biobrane is high, but as there is no need to change the dressing until the wound is healed, it can be effective and economical therapy for a clean partial-thickness burn.

If there is a question of contamination of the burn wound or of the presence of a devitalized eschar, a topical antibacterial such as silver sulfadiazine or mafenide can be used [127]. Mafenide is painful on application [127]; both of these agents tend to retard epithelialization [127]. For wound care, the patient or the family is instructed to remove the dressings once daily, wash the burn wound gently with a mild soap and warm water, and reapply the dressing after cleansing. If the patient or family is unwilling or unable to do it, often the hydrotherapy division of a hospital's outpatient therapy department can be utilized for dressing changes.

These patients are seen 24 to 48 hours after the first dressing change to rule out the presence of a streptococcal burn wound cellulitis. Should it occur in a small burn, it can usually be easily treated with a short course of oral penicillin. The patient is followed after the initial 48-hour evaluation at 2- to 3-day intervals until the burn wound heals. Wounds treated in this fashion should be totally reepithelialized within 2 to 3 weeks. If the wound does not epithelialize during this period, the original burn was probably deeper than thought on initial evaluation, and skin grafting is probably required to obtain the most durable and cosmetically acceptable skin cover [194].

Partial-thickness burns of any size are painful, and analgesia is prescribed for the patient for home use. Tylenol with codeine is usually satisfactory. Significant pain relief is also obtained by elevating the affected extremities, especially during the first 24 to 48 hours after injury. It may also be helpful to prescribe a mild sedative for the patient, e.g., oral diazepam, to be used with the analgesic medication 30 to 45 minutes prior to the daily wound care. This measure allows more vigorous washing and débridement of any adherent necrotic debris that may be present on the wound. The tetanus status of the patient must be ascertained and brought up to date.

Outpatients whose burns heal in an uncomplicated fashion are advised that it is probable no permanent scarring will occur, though pigment changes (hypo- or hyperpigmentation) are likely [194]. These changes fade with time, although there may be a permanent change in pigmentation from the surrounding nonburned skin. However, with healing in less than 3 weeks, true hypertrophic scarring is rare.

Burned skin, after healing, remains highly

sue. Several investigators have measured fluid loss into burn tissue and have found it to be in excess of what would be expected by an increase in vascular permeability alone [9, 68, 108].

Edema also occurs in unburned tissue. Demling et al. have calculated that 50 percent of the first 24-hour fluid requirement after a 50 percent burn in an experimental animal ends up as nonburned tissue edema if no colloid is used during the resuscitation [50]. Edema in nonburned tissue has classically been attributed to a generalized increase in microvascular permeability with a thermal injury in excess of 25 to 30 percent TBSA [17]. However, no increase in protein permeability has been shown in postburn lung [50, 72], and in fact there is no significant increase in lung water during resuscitation unless an inhalation injury is present [76, 189]. There is, however, still an increase in net transvascular fluid flux in soft tissue and lung after significant thermal injury.

This apparent paradox has been explained by Demling et al. to result from hypoproteinemia [49, 73]. It occurs because of protein loss from the capillary leak and accentuates edema in nonburned tissue by the following mechanisms. First, there is a decrease in the plasma/interstitial oncotic pressure that increases outward fluid flux. Second, Demling et al. and others believed there is a loosening of the intracellular matrix secondary to protein washout [102, 104]. Experimentally, they have shown that rapid colloid infusion can decrease edema in nonburned tissue by increasing the plasma/interstitial osmotic gradient [49]. There has been some concern by others that early administration of colloid during resuscitation increases the interstitial osmotic pressure as well and makes the resultant sequestered fluid in the interstitial compartment more difficult to remove during the diuretic phase of the resuscitation [62].

Postburn cell membrane alterations have been well documented. In burns of more than 30 percent TBSA, there is a generalized decrease in the cell transmembrane potential, especially in muscle [17]. Normal transmembrane potential is $-90$ mV. In burned tissue it is decreased to $-70$ to $-80$ mV, with cell death occurring at $-60$ mV. This change causes extracellular sodium to pass into cells, which in turn increases the cell water and intracellular edema. The decrease in cell membrane potential is attributed to a decrease in membrane-bound ATPase secondary to ischemia and may be influenced as well by the presence of free fatty acids produced by thermally injured tissue [48]. Restoration of membrane potential occurs 24 to 36 hours after injury depending on the adequacy of restoration of tissue perfusion. Therefore inadequate resuscitation results in a further decrease in membrane function and cell death.

## Clinical Response

The pathophysiologic changes outlined above result in a clinical response that is becoming increasingly well defined with the work of numerous investigators. Cardiovascular instability results from the microvascular and cell membrane changes described. The function of the cell membrane as a semipermeable barrier is lost in burned tissue, and therefore a functional plasma volume in burned tissue can be restored only with restoration of the extracellular space as well. Edema occurs later in nonburned tissue than in burned tissue because of hypoproteinemia. Protein loss peaks at 8 to 12 hours after the burn [48]. If adequate perfusion is maintained during resuscitation, plasma volume loss decreases substantially by 18 to 24 hours after injury [48].

Myocardial depression is a well described finding and is most evident in deep burns of more than 40 percent TBSA. A myocardial depressive factor has been postulated in the serum of burn patients but has never been identified. Cardiac output returns to near-normal levels before restoration of a normal plasma volume [17]. This situation leads to the existence in many severely burned patients of low central venous and pulmonary artery pressures in the face of adequate cardiac output and peripheral perfusion. Blood volume remains low for days in severely burned patients unless aggressively corrected. Red blood cell destruction in those with large burns may be up to 40 percent of the circulating volume. Eight to fifteen percent of the volume is thought to be destroyed initially by the thermal insult, with eventual loss of another 25 percent secondary to decreased survival time. Glucose intolerance may be seen during the early postburn period secondary to massive catecholamine release [200].

## Fluid Management for the First 24 Hours

The goal during the first 24 hours is to restore and maintain adequate tissue perfusion and oxygenation, avoid organ ischemia, and preserve heat-injured but viable soft tissue while minimizing any exogenous contribution to edema in nonburned tissue. Monitoring the burn patient is an important part of resuscitation, and no resuscitation formula is a "license" to put the patient on "autopilot." All formulas for resuscitation are *guidelines only.* Careful, precise monitoring of the patient's minute-to-minute status is much more important than the composition or amount of resuscitation fluid given. The release of catecholamines maintains blood pressure in the severely burned patient [200], which makes blood pressure a relatively insensitive monitor for adequacy of resuscitation. Pulse rate is a better indicator, with a rate of less than 120 per minute indicative of good fluid status in young patients. Older victims of burn injury may not be able to call on their cardiac reserve to increase the pulse rate in response to volume deficit. Pulse rate is thus regarded as a less reliable indicator of resuscitation in this older patient group.

Again, it is emphasized that the goal of initial resuscitation is to balance adequate perfusion with the detrimental effects of over-resuscitation. Microvascular instability in this group of patients is short term (24 to 36 hours). Satisfactory resuscitation carries the patient through this period with the least morbidity. Frequently seen is adequate perfusion and cardiac output in the presence of low filling pressures [17]. In those patients in whom invasive hemodynamic monitoring may be of benefit, e.g., the elderly patient with preexisting cardiac or respiratory disease or the massively burned patient with significant inhalation injury, Swan-Ganz monitoring of the pulmonary artery pressures and cardiac output is preferable to simple central venous pressure monitoring. Maintenance of an adequate cardiac output is better than a superadequate cardiac output. One must resist chasing a low central pressure or pulmonary artery pressure in the presence of clinical evidence of adequate resuscitation. The complications of central venous lines are increased in burn patients compared to those in other injured patients [54, 152]. Their use is reserved for the complicated or difficult resuscitations described above.

With the use of crystalloid resuscitation regimens such as the Parkland formula, urine output remains an excellent guideline for the adequacy of resuscitation [48]: 0.5 to 1.0 ml/kg/hr in the adult and 1 ml/kg/hr in the child are the target values. One may have to accept less urine output with severe inhalation injury [168], but some investigators have shown that under-resuscitation in the presence of inhalation injury is as detrimental as over-resuscitation [116]. To accurately reflect perfusion, the urine must be nonglycosuric and not produced by an osmotic load (e.g., dextran, hypertonic saline) [48]. Circulating levels of antidiuretic hormone are markedly elevated in severely burned patients for days and may contribute to sluggish urine output. The presence of persistent metabolic acidosis indicates inadequate perfusion and is an indication for increasing fluid administration [48], except in the setting of carbon monoxide poisoning [116] where the patient may be acidotic secondary to carbon monoxide inhalation. Acidosis, then, may not reflect true volume status. Inhalation injury may markedly increase fluid requirements because of the release of vasoactive mediators from the injured lung and an increase in surface area burned in significant lower respiratory tract inhalation injury [47]. Hematocrit determinations can also be indicative of the adequacy of resuscitation with initial hemoconcentration. A later decrease in hematocrit mainly reflects reexpansion of the intravascular compartment.

## Resuscitation Formulas

Many resuscitation formulas abound, and there are excellent summaries of their historical development [159]. All of the formulas serve as guides for fluid resuscitation only. Clinical monitoring of the response is more important; all authors acknowledge the existence of marked variability in individual patient response.

### ISOTONIC CRYSTALLOID

The Baxter [16–20, 22] or Parkland formula of crystalloid resuscitation during the first 24 hours followed by crystalloid and colloid during the second 24 hours is widely used in the United States. It has the significant advantages of a satisfactory response in most patients. It is simple, of low cost, and safe. It was developed from clinical and laboratory investigations that showed that colloid administered during the second 24 hours after burn was more effective than crystalloid for restoring plasma volume and maintaining cardiac output [17, 21]. This advantage was not seen with colloid during the first 24 hours. In addition to being more expensive, it is argued that extravasated colloid in the interstitial space obligates the formation of increased interstitial water and therefore may make later edema mobilization more

difficult [17]. However, evidence has shown that nonburned tissue and lung capillaries do continue to sieve protein with greater efficiency than was believed when the Parkland formula was developed [48]. The early addition of colloid to the resuscitation regimen may decrease the volumes given during the first 24 hours to the severely burned patient [48].

### HYPERTONIC SALINE

Hypertonic saline relies on the fact that inclusion of the sodium ion is the key element in crystalloid resuscitation [128]. It has been stated that any sodium-containing fluid can resuscitate the victim of a burn if given in adequate amounts [130, 149]. Hypertonic saline resuscitation regimens use intracellular water to fill the extracellular space deficit. Hypertonic saline has been reported to increase myocardial contractility and decrease systemic vascular resistance compared to isotonic regimens [193]. However, urine output is increased because of natriuresis and therefore is a less sensitive indicator of adequacy of resuscitation [48]. Soft tissue edema in nonburned tissue is unchanged with hypertonic saline compared to isotonic crystalloid.

How much hypertonic saline to use is controversial. Most regimens call for the serum sodium concentration to be kept under 160 mEq per liter [129, 136]. The rate of infusion is based on the same parameters as for isotonic saline. One-half of the first 24-hour total volume is given during the first 8 hours. Although the effects of this resuscitation regimen have not been totally worked out, it is clear that less fluid is required for initial resuscitation using this technique [48].

### PROTEIN

Protein infusions have been an important part of burn resuscitation for many years. They were significant components of early formulas for burn management, being included in varying degree in the Evans and

Brooke formula as well as Moore's Burn Budget. Plasma proteins generate an inward oncotic force that counteracts the outward hydrostatic force in the capillaries. Without proteins, massive interstitial edema occurs, such as that seen with the nephrotic syndrome.

The current argument about protein in burn resuscitation concerns the timing of its administration rather than whether to give it. Demling [48] categorized the three positions in this argument as follows.

**1.** Protein is not given during the first 24 hours for the reasons noted above.
**2.** Protein is given from the beginning of resuscitation preferably with crystalloid to maintain oncotic pressure.
**3.** Protein administration is started at 8 to 12 hours after injury using crystalloid or nonprotein colloid during the first 8 hours. The most massive fluid shifts occur during that period. There is, then, no indication for using the more expensive protein solutions initially.

For many of the reasons given above, it seems that the third position is the most logical. Several protein solutions are available. Heat-fixed proteins such as plasmanate have lost a portion of their oncotic activity because of agglutination and denaturation of protein. Albumin is the most oncotically active of the protein solutions and is associated with no disease transmission. Fresh frozen plasma contains the entire osmotic load of the plasma in addition to all of the clotting factors normally present; however, increased concern about disease transmission has made it a less attractive choice. It has also been shown that, in the absence of specific clotting defects, replacement of these factors is not necessary. As with many of the other resuscitative fluids, the precise amount needed is not defined. Infusion of protein at a constant rate seems preferable to pulsed administration: The requirements for protein are greater in patients with more than

50 percent burns, older patients, and those with significant inhalation injuries [48]. Protein experimentally in these situations is shown to decrease edema and increase hemodynamic stability [48]. It must be remembered that protein administration does not decrease edema in burned tissue but does attenuate nonburned tissue edema and maintains blood volume better than crystalloid alone.

NONPROTEIN COLLOID
Nonprotein colloid solutions have also been used for many years in Europe and the United States. Dextran is a colloid consisting of glucose molecules polymerized to form high-molecular-weight polysaccharides. They are classified on the basis of their molecular weights. Low-molecular-weight dextran (Rheomacrodex), with a molecular weight of 40,000, is the most widely used dextran in the United States. Combinations of crystalloid and dextran have been shown to decrease edema and improve survival compared to crystalloid alone [107]. One gram of dextran retains 20 to 30 ml of water compared to 13 ml of water for 1 gm of protein. Objections have been raised in the past regarding dextran because of allergic reactions and interference with blood typing. More recent data indicate that these problems occur much less frequently with the use of low-molecular-weight dextran than with dextran 70, which is primarily used in Europe [87, 118]. Demling et al. have found that the fluid requirement using a combination of dextran and crystalloid is one-half of that needed to keep vascular pressures at baseline during the first 24 hours after burn in an experimental animal compared to the use of crystalloid alone [50]. As with hypertonic saline, the use of dextran increases urine output owing to its osmotic effect, so that urine output cannot be used as well for judging the adequacy of resuscitation. Low-molecular-weight dextran is rapidly cleared from the plasma and must be infused to maintain a plasma level of 2 gm per deciliter

to maximize its volume properties [48]. It requires a rate of administration of 2 ml/kg/hr or more. As with all other nonprotein solutions, dextran does *not* attenuate burn tissue edema or hypoproteinemia. It does, however, attenuate edema in nonburned tissue.

Hetastarch is an alternative to dextran supplied in a 6% solution. This colloid has volume-expanding properties similar to those of a 6% protein solution, and its vascular retention is long [48]. We have used it successfully as the colloid administered during the second 24 hours of the Parkland regimen.

For the first 8 hours after a burn, four times as much crystalloid is required as a combination of dextran and crystalloid to maintain adequate perfusion in experimental animals [48]. Because of the rapid clearance of dextran it must be remembered that when changed to protein infusion after the first 8 hours volume requirements double to about 2 ml/kg/percent of burn. This effect is especially prominent with the use of low-molecular-weight dextran because of its rapid clearance.

## Choice of Fluids

The extensive amount of information above tends to obscure the fact that virtually all fluid resuscitation regimens are effective if monitored with care [48]. We attempt to individualize our resuscitation regimens based on the patient's age, general condition, other injuries, and preexisting medical considerations.

For young patients with burns of less than 50 percent TBSA without inhalation injury, the Parkland regimen is safe, effective, inexpensive, and satisfactory in most patients. For young, healthy patients with burns of more than 50 percent TBSA or in the presence of a significant inhalation injury, the use of hypertonic saline to minimize the total amount of fluid given is considered. In this group of patients, the elderly patient, or the patient admitted in frank shock at some

time after the burn injury, the use of low-molecular-weight dextran and crystalloid during the first 8 hours followed by protein and crystalloid may have salutary effects, as described above. Obviously, additional controlled clinical studies are indicated to delineate the potential benefits of these individualized resuscitation regimens.

## Inhalation Injury

With increased use of topical antimicrobials and early excision, the complications of surface thermal burns have become more defined and, in many cases, more controllable. In this setting, inhalation injury has become responsible for more deaths than surface burns [52]; 20 to 84 percent of burn mortality now results from pulmonary pathology, which is primarily due to inhalation of the products of combustion [84, 169, 172]. For any given patient, the presence or absence of inhalation injury may be a stronger determinant of mortality than the size of the burn wound [82]. It has been estimated that confirmed inhalation injury increases mortality by 30 to 40 percent [82].

PATHOGENESIS

The pathogenetic mechanisms of inhalation injury can be divided into three broad areas. Any one of these mechanisms may be present or absent in a given victim of inhalation injury, and all need to be searched for, diagnosed, and treated appropriately. These three major areas are (1) carbon monoxide inhalation, (2) direct thermal injury to the upper aerodigestive tract, and (3) effects of inhaling products of combustion.

Carbon monoxide is an odorless, tasteless gas that impairs tissue oxygenation by preferentially binding to hemoglobin and displacing oxygen from the hemoglobin molecule. Carbon monoxide's affinity for hemoglobin is 210 times that of oxygen [183]; the displacement of oxygen is its major pathogenetic effect [55, 67]. If carbon monoxide enters the cell's cytochrome system, it also impairs oxyen utilization. This mechanism is less important in the production of its deleterious effect, however.

Direct thermal injury to the lower airway is uncommon because of the great heat-dissipating capacity of the oro- and hypopharynx. An exception is inhalation of steam, which has 4000 times the heat-carrying capacity of air [82]. Superheated air can cause edema of the face and perioral tissues as well as the upper airway, which in turn causes increased work of breathing. The increase in visible edema parallels the generalized burn edema in any given patient, peaking at 18 to 24 hours after the burn and resolving over 4 to 5 days. Direct thermal injury of the upper airway mucosa is not necessary to cause respiratory embarrassment. Severe facial or neck burns may also lead to edema of the upper airway, thereby increasing the work of breathing. In addition to the direct effect of mucosal edema, mucosal swelling impairs clearance of secretions in the airway, which compounds the problem.

By far the most common and significant component of inhalation injury is the inhalation of products of combustion. Increased use of plastics and other synthetic materials in the everyday environment has caused the composition of smoke to become much more noxious to the respiratory system. Aldehydes, ketones, and organic acids are produced from combustion of these materials [38], and all cause significant chemical injury to the respiratory tract [38]. Although initial dramatic clinical response may be absent in these injuries, the result is similar to that seen with aspiration of acidic gastric contents.

Occasionally, moderate to severe bronchoconstriction and bronchorrhea cause an increase in $PCO_2$. Mucosal ciliary function may be markedly and almost instantaneously depressed, causing marked impairment of secretion clearance.

This chemical injury is the most significant in the lower respiratory tract. Severe cases may develop increased capillary permeability [188] and alveolar cell injury, which then lead to pulmonary edema and adult respiratory distress syndrome, which carries a mortality of 60 to 70 percent [2]. With severe damage to the airways and sloughing of the bronchial mucosa, plugging and secondary infection begin to supervene at 72 hours after the burn [169]. This situation predisposes the patient to the development of secondary pneumonia, with a poor prognosis. A deficiency of surfactant activity in the lung has also been documented in these cases, which appears to decrease lung compliance, thereby increasing the consequences of the injury [83].

DIAGNOSIS

Diagnosis has been classically based on clinical suspicion. The history of a burn occurring in a closed space has been highly correlated with the presence of significant inhalation injury, though approximately 12 percent of cases occur in open spaces. Singed nasal hairs, facial or oropharyngeal burns, and expectoration of carbonaceous sputum are occasionally seen but are nonspecific for the presence of inhalation injury. Signs of upper respiratory obstruction, e.g., crowing, stridor, or air hunger, usually signify a significant injury to the hypopharynx/larynx and mandate immediate intubation [196].

Often significant inhalation injury exists without immediate clinical findings; this situation can lead to a disastrous outcome if a patent airway is not ensured upon initial evaluation. All patients suspected of having inhalation injury must have assays for arterial blood gases, including determination of the carboxyhemoglobin level. Carboxyhemoglobin levels higher than 10 percent are probably significant and those over 50 percent are associated with death [116]. If the carboxyhemoglobin level is elevated, the patient is immediately administered 100% oxygen. This treatment decreases the washout time of the carbon monoxide from $T_{1/2}$ on room air = 250 minutes to $T_{1/2}$ with $FIO_2$ 1.0 = 40 to 50 minutes. Hyperbaric oxygen has not been shown to be of any more benefit than 100% oxygen in these patients [116]. Oxygen saturation may be misleading in this setting, as the saturation may be high but actual oxygen delivery to the tissues is low.

The mainstay of diagnosing inhalation injury to the oropharynx, hypopharynx, larynx, and upper airway has been fiberoptic bronchoscopy [135]. It is easy to perform during resuscitation of an unstable burn patient, as it can be done at the bedside with the patient intubated or prior to intubation if the airway is adequate. Significant findings in the hypopharynx and larynx include vocal cord edema and charring, sloughing, or edema of the hypopharyngeal and upper tracheal mucosa. An idea of lower respiratory tract inhalation injury can also be obtained using the fiberoptic bronchoscope to examine the primary, secondary, and in some cases tertiary bronchi, though the results have been reported to not correlate well with the extent or prognosis of the inhalation injury [25].

Xenon ventilation perfusion scanning has been advocated as a sensitive method for detecting inhalation injury to the lower respiratory tract [141]. Findings consistent with inhalation injury include air trapping behind edematous bronchioles for more than 120 seconds after injection. Such scanning allows localization of specifically injured areas of the lung, but it may be difficult to perform in the acute setting. Scans return to normal about 96 hours after the burn, yielding false-negative results [141]. Similarly, pulmonary function tests have been shown to be sensitive indicators of lower respiratory inhalation injury [198] but require more patient cooperation than is usually available in a significantly injured patient.

MANAGEMENT
The treatment of inhalation injury is supportive only, so that in a practical sense all that is needed to initiate treatment is an indication of the presence or absence of such an injury. The primary goal in the initial treatment of inhalation injury is airway maintenance. What may be an easy intubation at the initial evaluation in the emergency room may become an impossible situation later when resuscitation fluid and airway edema necessitate emergent tracheostomy. Therefore liberal use of endotracheal intubation is recommended in the setting of inhalation injury or its suspicion. If carbon monoxide poisoning is present, 100% oxygen is given. For the other two components of inhalation injury, treatment is ventilatory support until the mucosal barrier reforms (generally in 7 to 14 days). Chest radiographs are usually of little help [133, 134], as most of the damage is to the airways rather than to the lung parenchyma and chest radiographs are relatively insensitive to this level of injury. They do, however, assist in the diagnosis of secondary pneumonia and other pulmonary pathology, including pneumothorax and pleural effusion. The enthusiasm for corticosteroid administration for inhalation injury has waxed and waned [36] but data from well controlled prospective series indicate that these agents are in fact deleterious to survival, and their use is contraindicated [134].

Meticulous pulmonary toilet is helpful for clearing inspissated secretions and soft mucosal plugs. Repeat bronchoscopy, either fiberoptic or rigid, may be necessary to clear the airways. Adequate ventilatory support with the use of positive end-expiratory pressure (PEEP), if necessary, is mandatory to keep the systemic oxygenation in the normal range. The lowest delivered oxygen concentration ($FIO_2$) that accomplishes this goal is used.

Resuscitation volumes are carefully controlled. Over-resuscitation exacerbates the pulmonary injury, but it has been shown that attempts to under-resuscitate these patients are associated with disastrous clinical outcomes and a high incidence of invasive pulmonary sepsis [116]. The presence of an inhalation injury, especially in a patient with preexisting cardiac or respiratory disease, may be a strong indication for Swan-Ganz catheterization and monitoring of cardiac output (see Fluid Resuscitation and Monitoring, above).

There are conflicting data on the use of crystalloid versus colloid solutions in the presence of inhalation injury. There is evidence to show that protein restoration with the use of protein infusions may decrease the total fluid requirements during the initial resuscitation of a burned patient with an inhalation injury [48]. There is, however, no clear evidence that a carefully monitored crystalloid resuscitation is any more detrimental to pulmonary function in the presence of inhalation injury than the combination of crystalloid and colloid [63]. Further study is necessary to determine the optimal fluid regimen for these patients.

Documented infections must be treated aggressively with appropriate antibiotics. Empiric therapy early in the patient's course (3 to 10 days after the burn) must cover *Staphylococcus aureus* and gram-negative organisms [82]. Surveillance of lower respiratory tract flora is maintained to target potential invading organisms. Prophylactic systemic antibiotics are not indicated and can select resistant strains of colonizing organisms [133].

Should the patient survive the inhalation injury and burn, long-term sequelae are uncommon but will probably be seen with increasing frequency as more seriously injured patients survive their initial insult. These long-term sequelae include pulmonary fibrosis and tracheomalacia, and there is some evidence of growth disturbances in children [116].

## Wound Assessment and Care

Determination of burn depth is initially less important than the extent of the burn injury. Although superficial, partial-thickness, and full-thickness burns do have clinical characteristics that can be used for diagnosis and differentiation, they are frequently unreliable in the acute setting [80]. It is therefore wise to refrain from definitive pronouncements to the patient or the family about healing potential or the need for skin grafting or radical excision at the first burn examination.

The terms superficial, partial thickness, and full thickness are preferable to first, second, and third degree as confusion is sometimes engendered by the latter set, which have different meanings in Europe and the United States (Table 24-2). Superficial burns are usually easy to diagnose. The prototype is a sunburn with erythema and mild edema of the skin. The area involved is tender and warm, and there is rapid capillary refill after pressure is applied. All layers of the epidermis and dermis are intact, and so no topical antimicrobial is necessary. Uncomplicated healing is expected within 5 to 7 days.

Likewise, full-thickness burns have a relatively characteristic clinical appearance. With complete destruction of all epidermal and dermal elements, these areas are insensate and create little discomfort for the patient. The appearance may be of virtually any color because of breakdown of hemoglobin from vascular destruction. The appearance of the skin may be waxy and translucent. Visible thrombosed vessels underneath translucent skin are pathognomonic for full-thickness injury. If hair is still present on the skin it can easily be removed. The condition of the skin is often dry or waxy but may be leathery or frankly charred as well.

Partial-thickness burns encompass a wide spectrum of dermal injury and therefore initially may be difficult to diagnose with any degree of accuracy (Fig. 24-3). A partial-thickness burn involving the uppermost layers of the dermis is only slightly more serious than a superficial burn, whereas a deep partial-thickness burn may behave clinically like a full-thickness burn and be just as strong an indication for excision and grafting. The hallmark of the partial-thickness burn is blister formation. The presence of

*Table 24-2 Burn depth categories in the United States*

| Burn degree | Cause | Surface appearance | Color | Pain level |
|---|---|---|---|---|
| First (superficial) | Flash flame, ultraviolet (sunburn) | Dry, no blisters, no or minimal edema | Erythematous | Painful |
| Second (partial thickness) | Contact with hot liquids or solids, flash flame to clothing, direct flame, chemical, ultraviolet | Moist blebs, blisters | Mottled white to pink, cherry red | Very painful |
| Third (full thickness) | Contact with hot liquids or solids, flame, chemical, electrical | Dry with leathery eschar until débridement; charred vessels visible under eschar | Mixed white, waxy, pearly; dark, khaki, mahogany; charred | Little or no pain; hair pulls out easily |
| Fourth (involves underlying structure) | Prolonged contact with flame, electrical | Same as third degree, possibly with exposed bone, muscle, or tendon | Same as third degree | Same as third degree |

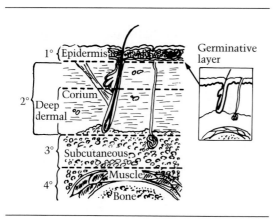

***Figure 24-3*** *Degree of burn in terms of depth. The inset emphasizes the manner in which partial-thickness burns heal from deep dermal structures of epithelial origin.*

blisters or bullae denotes at least some element of viable dermis underneath the blister fluid. Confusion may result, however, when partial-thickness burns are examined after blisters have been ruptured and uncovered. Classically, these burns are described as wet and exquisitely tender, though deep partial-thickness injuries may be relatively insensate. Blanching with pressure and capillary refill are other signs of dermal integrity but likewise may be virtually absent with deep partial-thickness injury. Hair is generally present in these burns, and its difficulty or ease of removal gives an idea of the depth of the dermal insult and injury to epithelial appendages. Often a red and white reticulated appearance is seen in these injuries after removal of the blister. This appearance is typical of what Heimbach and Engrav have coined the "indeterminate-thickness" burn [81]. It is so named because it correlates well with the inability of an experienced surgeon to predict spontaneous healing within less than 3 weeks. This concept is convenient for those oriented toward early excision and grafting; it removes the need to avoid excising any burn that may heal without skin grafts.

## Physical Wound Care: Initial Session

After establishment of adequate resuscitation infusions and ensurance of adequate ventilation, initial wound débridement and dressing is done in the burn center, in most cases in the hydrotherapy room. This room must be warm to minimize heat loss from the patient. Adequate analgesia, which is important for the procedure, can be easily achieved, even in the hemodynamically unstable patient, with small doses of intravenously administered morphine titrated to the patient's response. Obviously, constant monitoring of vital signs is mandatory. Admission photographs are taken at this time, providing a permanent visual record of the wounds as well as documentation for medicolegal purposes. Blisters and loose skin are débrided.

If indicated, this time is convenient for performing escharotomy. Cutting electrocautery is suitable and, if carefully performed, causes little or no pain to the patient. Fasciotomy can also be performed with cutting electrocautery. If care is taken only to divide the fascia, bleeding is minimal.

After débridement of loose skin and gentle washing of the wounds, the topical agent of choice is applied (see below). Dressing is completed expeditiously, monitoring patient core temperature throughout the procedure and using bulky absorbent dressings to control the massive amounts of exudate from these wounds. In some cases we have also found special beds such as the Clinitron air suspension bed or Flexicare bed helpful for treating burns of the back or other dependent areas [146]. It is of great importance to not apply dressings in a constricting fashion; distal extremities must be available for neurovascular monitoring. Loosely applied Flexinet effectively maintains the dressings in proper positions. Its use avoids the need for tape, which can be irritating to skin over a long period.

## Subsequent Wound Care Methods

The sessions of wound débridement and dressing change are often the most painful part of the day for the burn patient. Mechanical wound care is an important adjunct to application of topical antibiotics, and effective débridement is mandatory for removing nonadherent eschar, as it allows maximal penetration of topical agents to the wound surface. Effective débridement hastens healing of partial-thickness wounds and can make full-thickness wounds more quickly suitable for graft coverage. Adequate analgesia is essential and is most effective when given as short-term supplementation of routine analgesia and sedation. We have had success with one of two methods, depending on the patient's preinjury pain tolerance and mental state as well as the extent of the wounds. In patients who have adequate levels of narcotic analgesia (see Pain Control, below), effective wound débridement and dressing change can be performed with two Percocet tablets and 30 mg of oxazepam (Serax) orally 30 to 45 minutes prior to the dressing change. For those patients who are not able to tolerate dressing changes with this regimen, we have had successful results with small doses of intravenous fentanyl through a heparin lock totaling 50 to 300 μg in divided doses as needed over the course of a dressing change [177]. This narcotic agent has a rapid onset and short duration of action, thereby rendering the patient nearly pain-free for the dressing change but alert and awake almost immediately thereafter.

Classic burn wound care has been performed in a Hubbard tank or some other immersion facility. This apparatus creates a warm, pleasant, antigravity environment for the patient where range of motion can be performed in a relatively comfortable fashion by physical and occupational therapists. However, concern has been raised regarding potential cross-contamination of large wounds in the same patient with this type of aqueous immersion [140].

Therefore we have begun to shower the patients on a cart (Fig. 24-4) rather than immerse them, especially patients with large deep burn wounds. This method is somewhat more uncomfortable for the patient and must be done more quickly because of the greater tendency toward hypothermia even with a high ambient temperature in the tub room. There are advantages, however, in terms of infection control of the wound. Even intubated patients can be débrided and cleansed adequately in this fashion. Our therapists now generally use the dressing change period as one of assessment only to ascertain whether limitation of motion is caused by intrinsic wound or joint problems or by restrictive dressings.

Critically ill patients are still débrided and dressed in their beds, though it is done less frequently with increased use of the shower method. We still use tubbing for small wounds and when preparing patients to take care of their wounds before discharge. Dressings initially need to be bulky in the presence of eschar to absorb the substantial exudate created. After grafting, when the graft has revascularized, a properly applied dressing can protect the fragile grafts until they gain strength. Dressings, if too bulky, however, may decrease range of motion. Efforts are continually made to prevent this problem.

## Nutrition

With increasingly aggressive nutritional support, the benefits of adequate nutrition in severely burned patients have become apparent. The consequences of a major burn are so wide ranging that provision of adequate fuel for the reparative processes is absolutely essential if the patient is to have any chance of survival. The hypermetabolic state induced by a major burn is like that found with the stress response to trauma or sepsis but is much stronger and more long lasting [65, 113, 114, 155]. The hypermetabolic state in the patient with a major burn lasts until the wound is closed in some fashion [11]. A burn of more than 40 percent TBSA causes a

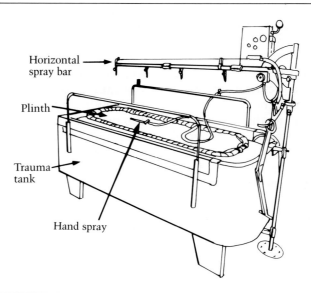

Horizontal spray bar

Plinth

Trauma tank

Hand spray

**Figure 24-4** *Horizontal spray system for avoidance of patient immersion.*

maximal metabolic effort greater than or equal to twice the basal energy expenditure [125, 202]. Although there is general agreement that this injury is the most stressful in terms of metabolic requirement and nutritional need, the reasons for the hypermetabolic burn state are not fully understood [202].

There is a consensus that the gastrointestinal tract of the burn patient is used for nutrition if it is available [144]. Fortunately, the combination of a major burn and other injury to the digestive system is rare, so the gastrointestinal tract is generally available for use. There is further agreement that adequate nutrition is an important factor in the complex of modalities necessary to maximize patient survival and minimize complications. Beyond this agreement there is a great deal of controversy on what and how much the burn patient should be fed [121]. As with methods of fluid resuscitation, formulas for determining caloric and protein requirements in burn patients abound [144]. There is a vast volume of data to support the various formulas. Analogous to resuscita-

tion methods, the response obtained by any given formula regimen is more important than the composition or amount of the formula given.

A time-honored formula in wide use today is that described by Curreri et al. [43], which describes the adult daily caloric requirements as 25 calories per kilogram plus 40 calories per percent of burn. For children, the formula is 60 calories per kilogram plus 35 calories per percent of burn. This formula appears to be accurate for assessing moderate-size burns in young, healthy patients. Several investigators have pointed out that caloric requirements are overestimated with this formula in large burns or in the elderly [125, 202]. All authors agree, however, that individual patient variability is considerable, and variations in utilization of nutrients with increasing magnitude of the primary injury is an important factor as well [121].

The Harris-Benedict equation is useful for predicting the basal energy expenditure (BEE) of a given patient [171]. Another method of computing calorie requirements in the burn patient is to simply double this BEE for a burn of more than 30 to 40 percent of the body surface area [125]. This method may well underestimate the caloric requirements of a given patient. Thus averaging the figures obtained from twice the Harris-Benedict equation and the Curreri formula may allow a reasonable starting target point for nutritional supplementation.

The protein content of the nutritional plan can be calculated using a calorie/nitrogen ratio of 100:1 to 150:1 with the higher nitrogen formulations reserved for the more highly stressed patients [161, 204]. By comparison, the normal diet has a calorie/nitrogen ratio of approximately 300:1. Delivery of adequate protein is usually more difficult than delivery of adequate calories. The average diet is comprised of 25 to 40 percent fat; essential free fatty acids must be supplied as well. Vitamin and mineral requirements are probably increased by the hypermetabolic state, though the exact quantities required for a given burn patient have not been determined [101]. Little is known about the utilization of these micronutrients in stress states, and stress may well be a limiting factor in the ability to deliver adequate nutrition to these patients. Vitamins C and A are necessary cofactors for wound healing and must be supplied in at least normal-diet amounts. Deficiencies of copper, zinc, and iron have been documented in burn patients, but requirements for their supplementation have not been defined.

A clinical dietitian is an essential member of the burn care team. Initial responsibility includes estimation of caloric needs with daily follow-up for calorie counts and a record of protein intake. Target values for calorie and protein intake must be determined early in the patient's course. If necessary to meet these goals, enteral feeding is started promptly. The dietitian is also instrumental in monitoring the response to nutritional replacement. It has been shown that significant systemic complications occur with a weight loss of more than 10 percent of the ideal lean body weight [43, 161, 201]. As a minimum goal, the patient's weight is not allowed to fall below this level during the hospitalization. Maintenance of the patient's weight at or above this baseline is one of the clinical indicators of adequate nutrient supplementation.

Some type of nutritional supplementation is required in most patients with burns of more than 20 percent TBSA. Oral intake is often limited by numerous factors, including compliance, palatability, and general energy level. It has been our practice to start aggressive nasogastric enteral feedings in such patients on postburn day 2 or 3, as soon as bowel sounds are present. Continuous feedings using an infusion pump are generally better tolerated than bolus feedings and avoid the problem of large residues in most patients. There are many small-bore, soft feeding tubes available that are easily passed and well tolerated for extended periods.

A detailed discussion of available formulas for tube feeding is beyond the scope of this chapter; references that allow selection of an appropriate formula are included at the end of this chapter [125, 126]. We, however, have had excellent results with a 1:1 mixture of Enrich and HCN Isocal given through a small (Keofeed) tube as a continuous infusion. The Enrich provides bulk, which has made diarrhea an infrequent problem in our patients [51]. When it occurs, it can usually be easily treated by slowing the infusion for a time, or, in extreme cases, adding an antidiarrheal medication to the tube feeding mixture. Separate supplementary protein packs can be added to this mixture to adjust the calorie/nitrogen ratio, which in most patients we prefer to be at 120:1 to 150:1. This regimen is started full strength at a slow rate and increased as tolerated to a target value calculated upon admission with the dietitians. It is important to check gastric residue frequently at the beginnings of feedings, but it has generally not been a problem. This mixture has worked so well that we use others only infrequently in our burn center. Again, monitoring the clinical response is more important than the formula used. We perform daily determinations of electrolytes, glucose, blood urea nitrogen (BUN), and creatinine until they are stable and weekly thereafter; weekly determinations of albumin, magnesium, phosphorus, and calcium are done as well.

Serum albumin has a long half-life and is therefore insensitive to acute changes in nutritional status. The mainstay of our clinical monitoring (though imperfect) is a weekly nitrogen balance study that is calculated from a 24-hour urine collection for urinary urea nitrogen in the standard fashion [201]. Our goal is a nitrogen balance of +4 to +6 gm or more per day in the acute patient. As the patient progresses through a course of operative procedures and wound closure, nutritional goals are constantly reevaluated and progress noted. Supplementation is adjusted accordingly.

Total parenteral nutrition is an option that must be used in some burned patients but is clearly a less preferable route than enteral feeding. There is little place for peripheral parenteral nutrition in these patients because of the usual paucity of peripheral venous cannulation sites and the inability to give adequate calorie and protein loads with this modality in severely burned patients [120]. If used, central venous catheters are changed every 72 hours.

The requirements for total parenteral nutrition are virtually the same as for enteral feedings. It is important to add fat emulsion to the feedings; 500 ml of a 10% solution two or three times a week provides adequate fat and fatty acids. Several investigators have calculated that the maximal acute glucose utilization rate in these patients in 5 mg/kg/min [34, 203, 205, 206]. Any excess is converted to fat with consequent increase in carbon dioxide production and deleterious effects on patients with pulmonary compromise or ventilator dependence.

The use of branched-chain amino-acid-enriched formulations in both the enteral and parenteral formulas has been advocated, and studies are currently in progress [57,

207]. As yet, there has been no clear advantage demonstrated with the use of these formulations in burned patients.

To summarize: adequate provision of nutrients is an essential part of the metabolic management of the burned patient. The goals are timely wound closure and prevention of loss of more than 10 percent of the preresuscitation body weight. Albumin is an unreliable monitor of the efficacy of nutritional therapy, especially in burn patients. There is a marked decrease in albumin with the burn, which is slow to change with even adequate nutritional supplementation.

Enteral feedings are used whenever possible. The easiest method for monitoring nutritional adequacy is a weekly nitrogen balance study. Much more work needs to be done in this important area, but the myriad variables induced by a severe burn injury and its sequelae make controlled studies to evaluate nutritional requirements and supplementation difficult.

### Prevention of Gastrointestinal Bleeding

Gastrointestinal bleeding, formerly a common complication in burned patients, is virtually nonexistent today [151]. Gastric and duodenal mucosal lesions have been shown to occur within 48 hours after the injury and have led to hemorrhage, ulceration, perforation, and death [180]. The use of effective antacid prophylaxis, however, has made this problem virtually unknown today [180]. We have found that in many cases prophylactic use of a histamine $H_2$ receptor blocker may make the administration of antacids less important. Our current preference is ranitidine or famotidine. The latter has the advantage of being able to be administered once a day through a feeding tube as an oral suspension. The pH is routinely checked every shift, but in most patients we have found that daily dosage with famotidine has resulted in the need for no additional antacid support to keep the gastric pH above 5.0 [148].

**Table 24-3** *Immunomodulating agents*

| Agent | Known or probable effects |
|---|---|
| Histamine-2 antagonists (e.g., cimetidine, ranitidine) | Cell-mediated immunity |
| Prostaglandin inhibitors (e.g., ibuprofen, indomethacin) | Cell-mediated immunity<br>Antibody response |
| Polymyxin B | Antibody response<br>Cell-mediated immunity |
| Ibuprofen, indomethacin | Cell-mediated immunity |
| Cyclophosphamide | Cell-mediated immunity |
| Cerium nitrate | Cell-mediated immunity |
| Thymosin | Cell-mediated immunity |
| Muramyl dipeptide | Cell-mediated immunity and monocyte stimulation |
| Vitamin A | Cell-mediated immunity |
| Vitamin E | Cell-mediated immunity |
| ARA-nucleotide | Cell-mediated immunity |
| *Corynebacterium parvum* vaccine | Nonspecific immunity; macrophage and neutrophil function; ? increase in colony-stimulating factor |
| Levamisole | Neutrophil functions |
| Fibronectin | Opsonic functions |
| Endotoxin (low dose) | Nonspecific immunity |
| Fresh frozen plasma | ? Replacement of complement, fibronectin, and other factors |
| Pyran | T-cell activation<br>Nonspecific immunity |
| CP-46, 665 | Improved phagocytosis |
| Pooled plasma and microorganism-specific antibody (i.e., passive immunization) | Phagocytosis and killing of microorganisms |
| Endotoxin-specific antibody | Inhibit endotoxin effects |
| Glucan | Reticuloendothelial system function; humoral and cellular immunity |
| Burn toxin-specific antibody | Inhibit various burn toxins |
| Microorganism-specific vaccine | Phagocytosis and killing of microorganisms |
| Thymopentin (TP5) | Neurophil and macrophage functions; antibody responses; cell-mediated immunity |
| Lymphokines, monokines (e.g., Il-1, Il-2) | Nonspecific and specific immune functions |
| Plasma exchange | Nonspecific and cell-mediated immunity |

[197]. The use of exogenous immunoglobulin preparations in burn patients has been advocated by many groups, but at this writing no clear clinical benefit has been demonstrated [71]. The use of lymphokines, especially interleukin 2, has produced experimental benefit and has theoretical significance [6, 123]. Interleukin 2 synthesized through recombinant DNA technology has only recently become available for human use, and clinical trials are now necessary to determine if it is of benefit.

## Topical Antibiotics

Prompt burn wound excision and closure is feasible only for patients with less than about 40 percent TBSA burn. For the remainder of patients, definitive wound closure may take a period of weeks even with the most aggressive operative approach. In these patients topical antibiotics are the single most important method of minimizing septic complications [127]. It is to be emphasized, however, that topical antibiotics are not a substitute for the supportive care for burn patients outlined in this chapter. They are only an adjunct to this care.

Theoretically, the basis for the use of topical antibiotics in burn patients is simple. Eschar forms on both partial-thickness and full-thickness burns. With increasingly thick eschar over deep burns, the distribution of systemically administered antibiotics to eschar cannot be relied on. Topical antibiotics are at greatest concentration on the wound surface, where the risk of exogenous contamination is the greatest.

With the untreated burn wound, cultures are negative during the first few hours. With deep wounds, the skin is effectively sterilized and can be contaminated early only by enteric or water contamination during transport. However, deep wounds become rapidly colonized within 24 hours by gram-positive cocci and within 3 to 7 days by gram-negative aerobes. Although this process is slower in less extensive burn wounds, the surface colonization eventually leads in the untreated wound to invasion of healthy tissue. It is therefore logical to institute topical antibiotic therapy as early as possible. The effective application of topical antibiotics reportedly decreases burn patient mortality by 50 percent.

No perfect topical antibiotics exist. The goals for therapy are to (1) delay colonization of the wound, (2) keep the wound bacterial density at lower levels than would otherwise occur, and (3) keep the wound flora more homogeneous and less diverse than would be present without therapy. The following sections summarize the topical agents in current use.

### SILVER SULFADIAZINE

Silver sulfadiazine is the most frequently used topical agent. It was introduced during the early 1970s after synthesis by Fox et al. [56]. It is supplied in a water-soluble base at a concentration of 1%, which is sufficient to inhibit growth of most sensitive microorganisms in vitro. It is generally applied every 12 to 24 hours and can be used with or without dressings. It is active in vitro against a number of gram-positive and gram-negative bacteria, *Candida albicans,* and perhaps herpes virus [127]. It is not entirely clear whether the antibacterial effect is from the parent compound, the silver ion, or the sulfadiazine moiety.

There is minimal pain associated with its application, and it is nonstaining. It does, however, form a thin pseudoeschar over the wound 2 to 3 days after its application, which may confuse the inexperienced examiner trying to determine wound depth. The pseudoeschar can generally be peeled off the wound with gentle débridement.

Wound penetration by silver sulfadiazine is intermediate between the rapidly absorbed mafenide and the poorly absorbed silver nitrate. Some systemic absorption does occur, but documented episodes of toxicity have been rare. Leukopenia is not infrequently seen after 2 to 3 days of treatment with this agent [127] and usually resolves without discontinuing the drug. Evidence suggests that this effect is not specific to silver sulfadiazine [187]. Leukopenia virtually never depresses the white blood cell (WBC) count to less than 2000 WBCs per cubic millimeter. There have been instances of induction of resistant organisms, mainly Enterobacteriaceae and *Pseudomonas aeruginosa* [28]. These reports have been sporadic, however, and there has not been a pattern of generally increasing resistance even with frequent use of this agent.

SILVER NITRATE (0.5% SOLUTION)

Silver nitrate solution is not toxic in a 0.5% concentration but has a significant antimicrobial effect. It was introduced in 1965 by Moyer et al. [132]. It is a broad-spectrum agent, and development of resistance to the silver ion is distinctly uncommon. There is minimal absorption from the burn wound, which makes toxicity virtually unknown. Because of its minimal absorption, it is an excellent prophylactic agent but is not indicated for established wound sepsis. The solubility properties of silver nitrate mandate preparation in distilled water; therefore a 0.5% solution is markedly hypotonic. Its use can lead to substantial leaching of sodium, potassium, and other plasma solutes from the burn wound. Careful monitoring of serum electrolytes is mandatory.

Occasionally some gram-positive and especially gram-negative organisms can reduce the nitrate from this compound to nitrite. Absorption of this nitrite may rarely lead to methemoglobinemia, occasionally necessitating treatment with intravenous methylene blue or other reducing agents [127]. Silver nitrate solution must be used by soaking bulky wet dressings. The dressings must be wetted every 2 hours to keep the concentration of the agent at less then 2%, at which point it becomes caustic and cytotoxic. Silver nitrate stains everything it touches brown or black. Removal of these stains from linen markedly shortens the life of the linen. It is not painful upon application.

MAFENIDE

Mafenide is usually applied every 12 hours without dressings. It has a broad antibacterial spectrum; its mechanism of action is unknown. It has the best penetration of eschar of any agent, and it penetrates cartilage well. This property makes it an excellent choice for use on burned ears and noses. With its active penetration, after 3 hours little agent is left on the wound surface, and so twice a day administration is necessary [127].

Mafenide is a strong carbonic anhydrase inhibitor, and its use results in an alkaline diuresis. It can lead to acid-base abnormalities when used on more than 20 percent of the body surface area. The polyuria induced by the agent can lead to a hyperchloremic metablic acidosis that, if compensated for by hyperventilation, may eventually lead to pulmonary failure in the compromised patient. This situation is a clear indication to discontinue the drug. With drug stoppage, this effect reverses in 24 to 36 hours. Significant pain results from the application of mafenide, probably due to its high osmolarity [127].

Mafenide is useful for control of established burn wound infection because of its excellent penetration but has largely been abandoned for routine use as a single agent. We have found that in high risk burn patients (e.g., those with burns of more than 40 percent TBSA or clinical sepsis) a regimen of dressing changes every 12 tours, alternating silver sulfadiazine and mafenide, is useful to minimize the complications from each agent and maximize their slightly different effects and spectrum [178]. Our practice for burns of less than 40 percent TBSA is dressing changes every 24 hours using silver sulfadiazine.

Mafenide inhibits reepithelialization, as does silver sulfadiazine. For this reason, we avoid use of these agents in the partial-thickness burn that is appearing to heal. A good choice for this type of wound is Xeroform-impregnated gauze. However, this agent occasionally excessively desiccates the wound. In this case, bacitracin ointment can be added to the Xeroform gauze. This method provides a bland, moist environment and does not inhibit reepithelialization.

MISCELLANEOUS AGENTS

Another topical agent that has been investigated is chlorhexidine gluconate, which has some promise for prophylaxis [12]. Second-line agents are nitrofurazone, neomycin, polymyxin B, bacitracin, and gentamicin. These agents are absorbed and have the potential for systemic toxicity, especially the aminoglycosides. They are thus used only for specific indications and are discontinued as soon as is practical.

## Recognition and Management of Infections

The burn patient without a significant inhalation injury is at the most danger of death from systemic sepsis [44]. There are a number of dose-related factors that make the burn patient highly susceptible to the development of invasive sepsis. First is the burn wound itself, which represents a major compromise in the body's defense mechanism. The burn wound, in addition to being locally susceptible to development of infection, is associated with dose-related immunosuppression of specific and nonspecific immune systems [138]. Furthermore, because these patients are often critically ill, they are subjected to a variety of invasive devices that bypass normal defense mechanisms including endotracheal tubes, bladder catheters, and arterial or venous intravascular catheters. Depending on other associated injuries, devices such as chest tubes, intracranial pressure monitors, and pulmonary artery catheters may be present for extended periods as well. Although the burn wound, especially when covered with necrotic eschar, is a common site of primary infection in the septic burn patient, other sites are common including the upper and lower respiratory tract, urinary tract, and less frequently infections from osteomyelitis or suppurative phlebitis. By far the most common four major categories of primary infection in burn patients, though, are the bloodstream, burn wound, lower respiratory tract, and urinary tract.

Because of the immunocompromised state of these patients as well as their intense and long-lasting hypermetabolism, usual clinical parameters of infection are lacking much as in other immunosuppressed patient populations (e.g., organ allograft recipients). Thus the burn surgeon must be constantly aware of the clinical status of the patient and be alert for any subtle changes, as they often are the first indicators of incipient sepsis.

The burn wound may change in appearance with the development of sepsis. A softening of the eschar or surrounding cellulitis may be seen, purulent material may begin to issue from the wound, or once-healthy granulation tissue may begin to deteriorate. Equally common, however, is no change in the wound appearance. Infection from the urinary tract or lower respiratory tract is infrequently accompanied by symptoms in these ill patients. Thus periodic culture surveillance is advisable to monitor the flora in these areas.

Careful serial clinical and laboratory monitoring of the patient is the most sensitive method of diagnosing sepsis before disastrous hemodynamic effects occur. We perform twice-weekly eschar biopsies [112, 150] for quantitative culture, though their value has been questioned [121]. Wound colonization with more than $10^5$ organisms per gram of tissue is an indication for us to perform expedient eschar excision, rather than start antibiotics.

Clinically, any change in the patient's general status leads to a high suspicion of sepsis. Such changes include unexplained hypotension, tachypnea, spiking fevers above the patient's daily baseline, tachycardia, new onset of ileus, altered mental status, decreased urine output, progressive leukocytosis with "left shift" including myelocytes and promyelocytes on the peripheral smear, thrombocytopenia, hyper- or hypoglycemia, hypoxia, or hypothermia. The development of hypothermia and leukopenia are particularly ominous signs in the patient who is clinically becoming septic and demands aggressive intervention.

Whereas the four anatomic areas mentioned above must be particularly considered, every potential site of infection must be examined, including donor sites, intravenous access sites, and skeletal pin insertion sites. Less commonly reported are meningitis, prostatitis, sinusitis, otitis, and endocarditis. These abnormalities must be ruled out in the patient with blood-borne sepsis of unknown origin. We have also treated an infant who became septic well into her hospital course because of an undiagnosed lung abscess and empyema [102].

A comprehensive discussion of organisms frequently encountered and appropriate antibiotics is beyond the scope of this chapter. There are many excellent summaries of approaches to this problem that are referenced at the end of this chapter [44, 163]. General principles follow.

*Pseudomonas aeruginosa* and *Staphylococcus aureus* are the dominant pathogens in burn centers. This statement is a general one only; it is more helpful for each burn center to know and monitor its own resident flora. *Candida* species are the most commonly isolated fungal organisms recovered from burn patients; other fungal infections are uncommon. Viral infections, particularly with cytomegalovirus, are being reported with increasing frequency, though their clinical impact is as yet undetermined [100].

Many of the adjunctive measures discussed elsewhere in this chapter are important in the prevention of infection and optimizing the patient's physiologic response mechanisms. Such measures include prompt excision, débridement and wound closure, adequate provision of nutrition, and immunization with tetanus toxoid.

There is little place for prophylactic antibiotic usage in burn patients [44]. Penicillin G used to be recommended for the first week to prevent group A beta-hemolytic streptococcal burn wound cellulitis. There is still arguably a place for this prophylaxis if topical antibiotics are not used, but several studies suggest that it is not necessary in addition to usual topical antibiotic treatment [53]. Although there are no studies to substantiate the efficacy of perioperative antibiotic prophylaxis for burn wound excision and grafting, it is reasonable to believe that a bacteremia does occur with manipulation of the burn wound. Prophylaxis during the perioperative period with a first-generation cephalosporin is practiced by a number of burn centers [44, 178]. There are no controlled studies that address the practice of continuous use of parenteral antibiotics. These agents are best reserved for use against documented infections with identified organisms [44].

## Wound Surveillance

There has been in the past a great deal of enthusiasm for monitoring the burn wound with quantitative eschar cultures. These tests, however, have been shown not to correlate well with healthy subeschar tissue invasion when more than $10^5$ organisms per gram of tissue are present [121]. They are expensive to perform but certainly give better information about the resident flora of a burn wound at any given time than does a surface swab culture [150]. Thus wound surveillance is a good means to monitor the wound's resident flora and to anticipate the potential offending organism(s) in invasive sepsis, but quantitative cultures may not be as useful as previously thought. The gold standard remains histologic examination of the subeschar tissue for visualization of invading microorganisms [121].

## Management of the Clinically Septic Patient

When sepsis is strongly suspected, support of the cardiopulmonary and gastrointestinal systems is of primary concern. Consideration is given to débridement on an urgent or emergent basis depending on the character of the burn eschar. Empiric antibiotic therapy is started after cultures are obtained [50].

Depending on the resident flora of a particular burn unit, some combination of agents to cover *Staphylococcus aureus* and gram-negative rods is given. A suitable combination is ampicillin or penicillin plus an aminoglycoside or a cephalosporin plus an aminoglycoside. Aminoglycoside dosage requirements are difficult to predict in burn patients, and individualized therapy is mandatory [167, 211, 212]. Drug level monitoring is advised as well for vancomycin, which is used increasingly as methicillin-resistant *S. aureus* becomes more of a problem [66]. It is important to obtain culture results as soon as possible including in vitro sensitivities, although the latter do not often correlate with in vivo behavior [44]. Antibiotic therapy is then targeted for the likely infecting organism(s). The use of new antibiotics or untested combination of antibiotics is recommended only as part of an investigational study or with the assistance of a physician fully versed in their usage and complications [44].

Fungal infections are an increasing problem. It is our current practice to treat burn patients systemically if fungus is found in two sites, i.e., sputum, intravenous catheter tip, urine, or wound. The most frequently seen organisms are *Candida* species, which appear 2 to 3 weeks after the burn [59]. We have aggressively treated these patients with systemic amphotericin B. This drug has a number of side effects but has clearly decreased the morbidity and mortality due to fungal infections [181].

Other adjunctive measures may be necessary in the patient with life-threatening infection. Adequate fluid must be given to maintain urine output in these patients, and invasive monitoring is added as the clinical situation demands. Steroids in pharmacologic doses have been suggested, but other evidence suggests that there is no beneficial effect. Often a change in topical antibiotic or increase in wound care frequency is added to the management of the burn patient with invasive infection. Certainly if one topical agent has been used for a long period, a change to another may be of benefit. In particular, mafenide has a much greater ability to penetrate the burn wound than other topical agents and is strongly considered in the presence of invasive burn wound infection, keeping in mind the complications of its use.

## Pain Control

Morphine given frequently in small intravenous doses titrated to the clinical response of the patient is an ideal method of pain control during the acute resuscitation period. We have found that for chronic pain control methadone, given every 8 hours (not as needed) in doses of 5 to 10 mg for adults, is excellent for most patients. Supplementation is generally needed for dressing changes, débridement, and some therapy manipulations, but the patients generally remain awake and alert. Power struggles for control of analgesic dosage between patient and nurse are usually avoided. Methadone takes 2 to 3 days to achieve a constant blood level with this regimen. This interval (at least) is allowed between dosage changes. The minimum dosage that causes the patient to be pain-free with minimal or no need of supplementary as-needed medication is utilized. Dependence on this drug does develop; therefore it is gradually tapered and discontinued 7 to 10 days prior to discharge. In the presence of severe pain even with methadone, often the addition of an antianxiety agent such as one of the benzodiazepines may be of help. Clinical psychologists can be of assistance in helping the patient to develop methods of nonpharmacologic pain control [182].

## Pulmonary Embolus

Questions often arise regarding the incidence of pulmonary embolus in burn patients, considering their prolonged immobilization and severe degree of injury. Little has been written on this subject, although Purdue and Hunt reviewed their experience with 2100 thermally injured patients [153], of whom 1439 were adults. There were no pulmonary emboli in children, and six adults (0.4 percent) sustained pulmonary emboli. There were no deaths among these six patients.

These authors concluded that although the risks of significant pulmonary emboli seem to be high in burn patients, clinical practice has not reflected it. This fact indicates that routine prophylactic heparinization is not justified in all burn patients. Certainly, preventive efforts must continue to be directed at those patients with classic risk factors for pulmonary emboli, including a history of thromboembolic disease, obesity, or burns of the lower extremities.

## Operative Therapy

Improvements in resuscitation have consistently presented the burn surgeon with patients who are stable 48 to 72 hours after the burn. These patients carry a variable load of dead tissue in immediate contact with healthy or injured but potentially salvageable tissue. Leaving this eschar in situ and waiting for separation due to autolysis to occur violates many surgical principles of débridement developed since the time of Paré. Although there were a few early reports of burn excision [96, 185, 186, 199], performance on a routine basis awaited development of critical care techniques, blood banking, anesthesia, and the ability to rapidly harvest and mesh skin to ensure graft survival on a less than perfect bed. Still, even with these improvements, one must agree with Jackson and colleagues that extensive excision "calls for greater experience and is considerably more trouble than delayed grafting in the third week" [96].

Additionally, development of powerful topical antibiotics during the mid-1960s caused most burn centers to lose interest in early excision and grafting. Especially with the use of silver sulfadiazine—with its pain-free

and consequent easy application and lack of metabolic problems compared to silver nitrate—primary excision and grafting may have become a thing of the past. During the early 1970s, however, overall mortality was noted not to have significantly changed even with the use of topical agents. Only through protracted follow-up was it realized that the epithelial coverage that forms over partial-thickness wounds, which take many weeks to heal, was unacceptable in terms of hypertrophic scar formation, lack of resistance to trauma, and pruritus. These points were reminders that topical chemotherapy was not the final solution to the burn wound [79].

In 1970 a Yugoslavian plastic surgeon, Janzekovic, published a short paper on the use of autografts to cover burn wounds [97]. Using the knowledge that deep donor sites could be overgrafted successfully with thin autografts, hastening donor site healing and improving its appearance, she applied this technique to dermal burns by repeatedly shaving layers of burned dermis until she reached a viable-appearing bed. She covered this bed with an immediate autograft. She reported that graft take was excellent and provided a clean, closed wound. Most of the burns she treated in this way were small, but, in her opinion, the hospital-stay-related pain and the need for reconstructive procedures decreased dramatically, and she reported that "esthetic disability" was also greatly reduced [97].

Burke and associates in Boston also developed an active program of early excision and grafting during the early 1970s. Long-term results were much better in their aggressively operated group of patients [29–32]. Controversy still surrounded the procedure during the late 1970s, however, and although there was general agreement that small full-thickness burns could be safely excised and grafted with good results, the issue of deep dermal burns had not been resolved. Clearly, a prospective randomized study was needed and was performed at the University of Washington [75]. Results clearly showed that the practice of early excision and grafting of indeterminate burns of less than 20 percent TBSA was superior to spontaneous healing. It decreased hospital stay and cost and lessened the need for secondary reconstruction. Moreover, these patients returned to work twice as fast as the nonoperated group [75].

Skeptics of this procedure have continued to point out that mortality is not improved in large burns treated in this way. As Heimbach explained [79], the reasons are threefold. First, as yet, no ideal skin substitute has been developed, which means that for large burns, although the eschar can be excised timely and rapidly, reliable wound closure can still not be performed simultaneously. The second reason is that burns of more than 70 percent TBSA or burns in the elderly are complex injuries with multifactorial deleterious effects on multiple organ systems that lead to morbidity or death. In this setting, reduction of the bacteriologic load from eschar excision may, in fact, not be enough to decrease overall mortality. Furthermore, the number of patients with this type of injury is small, and a great amount of time would be necessary to build a case load large enough to gather meaningful statistical data.

However, the value of this operative approach to burn wounds cannot be judged solely on survival statistics. Of the 2.0 million to 2.5 million burn injuries that occur every year, only about 30,000 are truly life-threatening. The others are problems of morbidity, i.e., cost, job time lost, pain, and chronic disability. It is here that early excision and grafting have made an obvious clinical difference in the experience of most who have tried it.

A detailed description of the techniques, patient selection, and operative and postoperative management involved in this approach to burns is beyond the scope of this chapter, but the reader is encouraged to study the excellent book by Heimbach and Engrav [81]. This volume sets out in great detail the procedures they follow.

For patient selection, Heimbach and Engrav made several excellent points. First,

small burns that will eventually heal can usually be excised with zero operative mortality. This fact implies that early excision requires an experienced surgeon. Inadequate excision and skin grafting lead to skin graft loss, thereby adding the size of the donor site to the total wound area and necessitating another operation. Second, non-life-threatening burns in patients with other medical problems must not be excised until the associated problems are under control so the operation is associated with no mortality and minimal morbidity. Third, hand and foot burns cause less time of disability if excision is performed shortly after admission. Fourth, large superficial burns with scattered small, deeper components are best treated nonoperatively until the shallow areas have healed. Fifth, significant problems with pain management may become indications for early excision [79].

## ORDER OF EXCISION IN MAJOR BURN INJURIES

In the absence of significant inhalation injury, it is rare for burns to cause significant infectious complications before the fifth to the tenth postburn day [81]. In the presence of a large burn the highest priority is to diminish the overall burn size and necrotic tissue load. Broad areas such as the trunk and lower extremities are given priority for excision [81]. Lower priority is given burns on the face and hands because they take more time to excise and cover with autograft. Goodwin et al. have shown that delayed excision on hands can result in acceptable function if accompanied by meticulous therapeutic assistance [63].

We agree with Heimbach that for a major burn the posterior trunk must be given high priority as the first area to be excised [81]. It is advantageous to do it early because the patient is relatively stable and tolerates the prone position better than later in the course. The posterior trunk and buttocks are frequent sites of burn wound infection and are difficult to inspect and keep well débrided; the flat, broad area lends itself well to quick excision and grafting. Complete full-thickness burns of the back are rare and in our experience often associated with non-survival. We therefore tangentially excise all but the most obvious full-thickness back burns.

TECHNIQUE OF TANGENTIAL EXCISION
Our preferred technique for tangential excision is with a Padgett electric dermatome set at 0.015 to 0.030 inch. Excision of full-thickness eschar is assisted by dressing the eschar 12 hours prior to excision with povidone-iodine foam, which dehydrates the eschar and makes it more physically amenable to tangential excision. A variety of hand dermatomes, e.g., the Goulian or Eschmann knives, may also be used. They are especially advantageous for small, irregular surfaces such as the hands and face, whereas the Padgett electric dermatome can be used to quickly remove uniform sheets of eschar from large surfaces. Excision is continued until punctate, uniform, brisk bleeding is obtained. If there is dermis left when this viable tissue level is reached, it is white and shiny. Gray, dull-appearing dermis is nonviable and does not, in our experience, support an immediately placed skin graft. If the dermis is burned through its full thickness, tangential excision is continued into the subcutaneous fat.

It is a common misconception that fat cannot support a skin graft. Certainly, nonviable fat does not support a skin graft, and any nonviable tissue is unsuitable for coverage in this manner. The scanty blood supply of fat relative to that of dermis and fascia makes differentiation of live and dead fat somewhat difficult. In general, any fat with hemorrhage or other discoloration (often brownish) must be excised. Healthy fat appears bright yellow and contains briskly bleeding vessels. We have found that with careful attention to detail and the application of relatively thin split-thickness skin grafts, 100 percent graft take can be achieved on fat excised in this manner.

We do not generally perform tangential excision under tourniquet control. The cadaveric appearance of the tissues distal to the inflated tourniquet makes differentiation of viable and nonviable tissues difficult even for the experienced observer [81]. The main danger is that one is tempted to take "just one more pass" to ensure a viable bed. Rosenburg and Zawacki described tangential excision and grafting in the extremities with tourniquet control. They reported reduced blood loss and acceptable graft take [158]. With the current rise in concern about blood transfusions, this technique may well increase in popularity. Tangential excisions are bloody procedures, and adequate blood must be available. We routinely type and crossmatch six units of packed red blood cells for major excisions of the trunk, four units for each lower extremity, and four units for each upper extremity including two units for hand excision alone. It has been our experience that the best method to limit blood loss is to work on only one area at a time and complete that area before proceeding. Extremities are excised working distal to proximal so that hemostatic compressive dressings applied after excision do not produce a tourniquet effect. Rapid, efficient eschar removal is the main technique for limiting hemorrhage in the absence of tourniquet control.

FASCIAL EXCISION
Fascial excision is the other method of immediate excision, and we reserve it for a few indications. Fascial excision offers the following advantages over tangential excision.

1. A viable bed for grafting is reliably provided.
2. Excision may be easily done on extremities under tourniquet control with decreased blood loss.
3. Less experience is required to obtain a good bed for grafting.

Fascial excision has a number of disadvantages, however. The excised fat does not regenerate, so permanent cosmetic deformity, which may be severe, is possible, especially in obese patients [98]. With circumferential excision, there is a risk of distal edema and an increased risk of damage to superficial nerves and tendons. There is a greater incidence of cutaneous denervation, and loss of sensation may be permanent. The fascia over joint surfaces such as the elbow, knee, and ankle is relative avascular. An ungraftable bed may result that requires eventual flap coverage.

We generally perform fascial excision using a cutting electrocautery or scalpel. We reserve this procedure for patients with deep burns with obvious extension well into the subcutaneous fat or large, life-threatening, full-thickness burns. In the elderly, fragile patient a small full-thickness burn may be much more suitable for fascial than tangential excision.

HEMOSTASIS

After completion of the excision, whether tangential or fascial, hemostasis must be attained. A number of methods have been advocated, including the use of microfibrillar collagen hemostat or topical thrombin. We have found disadvantages to the routine use of these agents because of cost and the clots that cover the wound surface. Such clots interfere with contact between the graft and graft bed, and often bleeding is restimulated when they are removed. Accordingly, we use application of sponges and laparotomy pads soaked in 1:200,000 epinephrine solution. The latter may be prepared in large quantities by adding 5 ml of 1:1000 epinephrine to 1 liter of normal saline. This solution is warmed and applied topically to the wound with the above-mentioned dressings. If the operative site is on an extremity, the epinephrine-soaked laparotomy pads are covered with a snug-fitting elastic wrap and the extremity elevated for 10 minutes. The dressings are then carefully removed, taking care not to traumatize the wound bed by

avulsing tiny clots. This sequence is repeated as often as necessary until hemostasis is obtained. Vessels that still have pulsatile flow after this sequence are precisely touched with the coagulating electrocautery. Substantial amounts of epinephrine are absorbed by the patient. The incidence of adverse effects is low, however [81], probably due to the large sustained endogenous catecholamine release in these patients.

Other modalities include topical thrombin in combination with topical epinephrine for tangential excisions of hand burns, which bleed freely. It is essential to remove all clots formed by the topical thrombin prior to application of skin grafts. Impressive blood loss is generated from tangential excision of the face and neck. To minimize it, we place the patient in a modified sitting position and perform the excision in a stage separate from the grafting, covering the face with either cadaver allograft or Biobrane between stages; the stages are generally separated by 24 to 72 hours. The face can be rendered more hemostatic by the application of sheets of Telfa soaked in epinephrine solution and sheets of Helistat, a topical collagen hemostat supplied in sheet form rather than powder form. This method has yielded excellent, rapid hemostasis for facial excisions.

AUTOGRAFT APPLICATION

In all areas but the face we proceed with immediate autografting if sufficient donor sites are available for allografting or coverage with Biobrane if autograft donor sites are not available. Whereas many recommend that sheet grafts be used whenever possible [81], skin meshed at 1.5:1.0 and minimally expanded can yield excellent cosmetic results that in many cases approach those obtained with sheet grafts. Meshed grafts, in addition, allow egress of subgraft fluid even with minimal expansion and can be used with excellent results in all areas except the face where the use of sheet grafts is mandatory.

We harvest most of our grafts using the Padgett electric dermatome, which is an unwieldy-appearing but superbly constructed instrument that allows even an inexperienced surgeon to obtain grafts that rival in quality the best of those taken by hand-drum-type dermatomes [81]. Most of our grafts are obtained at a thickness of 0.010 inch using the 3-inch (medium) guide for the Padgett dermatome. This method yields grafts that fit well on the Zimmer mesh grafter dermacarriers. The grafts are then meshed 1.5:1.0 and placed on the excised beds, securing them with stainless steel staples. We have found that wide staples can be placed just as precisely as the regular-width staples and are much easier for the patient to have removed 4 to 5 days after grafting. The exception is a graft on the face. We place these grafts in the aesthetic units of the face and fix them with fine interrupted and running sutures of 7-0 vicryl. These sutures do not need to be removed, and they yield precise approximation of the pieces of sheet graft.

Postoperative care of the grafts is an area in which there are many opinions but few facts. We have been impressed with the general use of wet dressings to maximize graft take and cause daily mild débridement of crust that forms on the graft during the first few days [178]. We wrap our grafts on extremities in five or six layers of fine mesh Kling roller gauze, which is soaked in a dilute antibiotic saline solution. Two ampules of GU irrigant are added to 1 liter of saline for this solution. The Kling is then rolled without tension directly onto the grafts, making sure that at least five layers of dressing cover the graft.

This dressing is then kept constantly moist by the nursing staff with identical solution and is changed once daily, taking care not to disrupt the grafts when removing the dressing. This care is continued until the interstices of the mesh are epithelialized. Alternative methods of graft coverage include Xeroform gauze and a bulky dressing or Biobrane, but we have found the best results for meshed grafts to come from the wet dressing technique.

Sheet grafts in the cooperative patient can be managed simply by leaving them open to air, which allows continuous inspection of the graft. The nursing staff continually rolls or aspirates small fluid collections that occur under the graft. This rolling must be done for 3 to 5 days after graft application. Obviously, immobilization of the graft on an affected part is crucial, as is elevation for grafts on extremities. When epithelialization is complete, we allow the reepithelialized graft to air-dry for 24 hours and then begin treatment with either Xeroform gauze or a moisturizing lotion. At this point, exposure of the grafts to air seems to cause them to become more durable rapidly.

## MANAGEMENT OF SPECIFIC AREAS
### Ears
The most important factor when treating ear burns is to prevent the development of suppurative chondritis. It can be exceedingly painful and difficult to eradicate, requiring filleting of the auricle and débridement of necrotic cartilage. The result is a shrunken, misshapen ear. Prevention involves topical antimicrobial therapy with mafenide because of its excellent cartilage penetration characteristics and avoidance of pressure. It is done by minimizing the dressing and not allowing the patient to use a pillow. Should suppurative chondritis supervene, débridement of cartilage is mandatory, as is treatment with an effective antipseudomonal antibiotic. *Pseudomonas* is the usual offending agent in this condition.

### Eyelids
Burns of the eyelids that require grafting usually require placement of grafts directly onto the orbicularis muscle [81, 90]. There is virtually no place for tarsorrhaphy in the management of the burned eyelid. A preferable strategy is continual regrafting of the eyelids as necessary to maintain eye closure [89]. Although multiple episodes of grafting may be necessary, the results are far superior to those achieved with tarsorrhaphy.

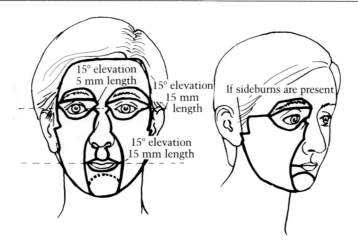

**Figure 24-6** *Aesthetic units of the face.*

## Nose

The nose is treated much like the ear. Sulfamylon is used because of its cartilage penetration; débridement is conservative. Flap reconstruction or composite graft reconstruction may be necessary but are best deferred until initial healing is complete [58].

## Face

Burns of the face are treated like any other burn in that wounds that appear not to be able to heal in 3 weeks are tangentially excised and grafted in aesthetic units. This undertaking is formidable in terms of time and blood loss. We perform a two-stage procedure with initial excision of the facial wounds to viable tissue and hemostasis followed by temporary closure with material such as cadaver allograft or Biobrane. Because of the disastrous cosmetic consequences with any graft loss in the face, we have also covered excised faces with antibiotic-soaked wet-to-wet gauze dressings changed every shift for 72 hours. When ready to graft the face, we have found that immobilization with a neurosurgical halo is an excellent means of protecting these large sheet grafts. This method was reported by Solem et al. [170], and we have had no com-

plications with it. Grafts are obtained at about 0.015 inch and applied to the aesthetic units of the face [60, 61] as much as possible without discarding large areas of normal skin. Precise fixation with fine sutures is performed as described above (Fig. 24-6).

Postoperative care is important. In an attempt to maximally immobilize these grafts, we use a neurosurgical halo in combination with a hyperextension mattress and occasionally a Steinman pin transversely through the mandible for postoperative neck hyperextension. Talking is not allowed for 5 days nor is chewing. The patient is tube-fed and sedated for comfort using regular doses of chlorpromazine 25 mg PO every 6 hours or a midazolam infusion. Grafts are exposed postoperatively and rolled as necessary by the nursing staff with aspiration of fluid collections as they occur. On the fourth or fifth postoperative day, a custom-fitted Uvex face mask mold is prepared from the patient, and when this appliance is available (generally in 24 hours), the halo is removed and the patient placed into the mask by the seventh postoperative day. We have had excellent results in several patients to whom this technique has been applied. Meticulous execution of this technique is mandatory, as is close observation to prevent respiratory compromise or aspiration.

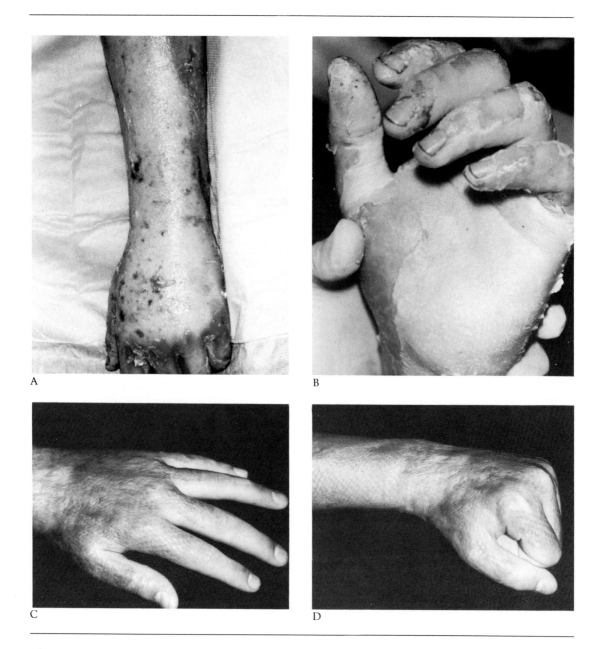

A

B

C

D

**Figure 24-7**  *A. A 15-year-old boy 4 days after thermal injury to the left forearm and hand. The burn is of indeterminate origin. B. Characteristic distribution of mild palmar injury with the most severe extent on the thenar eminence. Note edema and poor position of proximal interphalangeal joints in flexion and metacarpophalangeal joints in extension. The burn was tangentially excised and skin grafted on postinjury day 5. C,D. Healed skin graft and full active range of motion at 3 weeks after injury.*

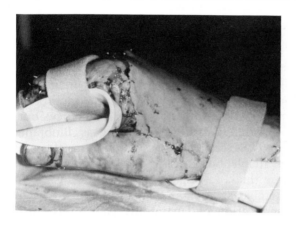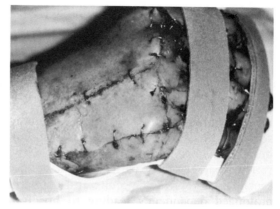

**Figure 24-8** *A 42-year-old man with an indeterminate burn of the right hand secondary to a water heater explosion. Tangential excision and sheet grafting were done on postburn day 6. Grafted hands are positioned in Orthoplast splints with care taken to avoid pressure over the fresh grafts. If meshed grafts are used, they are wrapped with moist gauze that incorporates the splints. Skeletal traction is rarely necessary.*

### Chest and Back

Back burns are excised conservatively, as there is virtually always some viable dermis. The area is then covered with allograft or Biobrane. We have allowed these patients to lie supine postoperatively in a Clinitron air-fluidized bed. Absorbent pads between patient and bed can be used if drying of the area is a problem. Healing often occurs in a surprisingly rapid fashion with this technique. Burns of the nipple and areola in the female breast are treated conservatively using secondary reconstruction of deep wounds.

### Hands

Hand burns are aggressively excised and grafted if they are of indeterminate or deep thickness. We agree with others that this method preserves the maximum function and causes the least time of disability with these wounds [63, 91, 94]. Burns of the palm (Fig. 24-7) rarely need grafting, as the protective fist-clenching reaction to injury pre-vents deep palmar burns in most adults. In fact, full-thickness palmar burns are often associated with burn wound mortality. We use sheet grafts or nonexpanded mesh grafts on the dorsum of the hand, as outlined by Heimbach and Engrav [81]. Meshed grafts are dressed with antibiotic-soaked gauze, which is wrapped over the grafts incorporating a previously made Orthoplast hand splint (Fig. 24-8). This method maintains the hand in a protected position of metacarpophalangeal joint flexion, interphalangeal joint extension, thumb abduction, and wrist extension during the healing period [23]. Skeletal traction is rarely necessary. Open interphalangeal joints are treated by careful débridement and percutaneous Kirshner wire pinning in 10 degrees of flexion. Often these open joints support thin skin grafts [23, 24], but one must be ready to perform flap closure if necessary. The problem of a major dorsal hand burn in combination with a major burn injury to the rest of the body is a difficult, often insoluble problem in burn surgery.

### Male Genitalia

The genitalia are treated conservatively. Burns of the penile shaft, unless extensive, almost never require skin grafting. The excess skin of the scrotum also precludes grafting; in

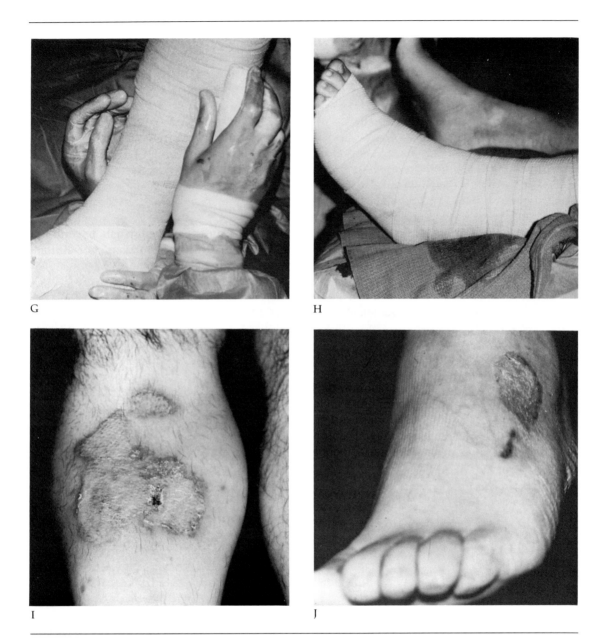

G

H

I

J

**Figure 24-9** (continued)
G. Unna boot dressing is applied over the N-terface from toes to knee
bilaterally. H. Dressing is completed with gauze roll and mildly compressive
Ace wrap over the Unna boot. The patient is discharged 24 hours
postoperatively and allowed to ambulate. I,J. Healed skin grafts 3 weeks
postoperatively.

aration and healing and is thus especially suited for donor sites where repeated harvesting is necessary.

Both Biobrane and N-terface are flexible but are porous enough to virtually never require aspiration of subdressing fluid collections, as is often the case with the polyurethane films (e.g., Op Site). In addition, use of polyurethane films requires normal skin to be present around the donor site for adherence of the edges of the film [81]. This situation is often not the case in a severely burned patient with limited donor sites that need to be harvested several times. Biobrane is also our donor site dressing of choice for small skin grafts taken for coverage of outpatient burns.

For small donor sites of less than 10 × 5 cm, we have found it advantageous to remove an ellipse of skin from the groin crease as a full-thickness graft. The linear wound, which is cosmetically acceptable, can then be closed in a standard fashion using intracuticular sutures and Steristrips. The full-thickness piece of skin thus harvested can be used either as a full-thickness graft or easily split using a Reese dermatome to yield a split-thickness graft of any thickness desired [23]. This method combines the versatility and excellent take of a split-thickness graft with the convenience and cosmetic superiority of a full-thickness donor site. We use this technique wherever possible.

In summary, an aggressive approach to burn wound excision by the experienced burn surgeon has many advantages and few disadvantages [64]. The disadvantages are increased operating time, blood loss, and episodes of anesthesia [81]. The advantages have been previously documented but also include greater acceptance on the part of the physicians, nurses, and patients involved in the treatment of these severe diseases. For this reason we believe that an aggressive approach to burn wound excision and grafting is the standard of care for most acute burn injuries.

## Electrical Injuries

Electrical injuries share many characteristics with thermal burns. There are differences, however, in the way that the passage of electrical current causes tissue injury [115]. Most tissue damage in electrical injury is due to heat generated by current flow [163]. It has classically been taught that different tissues of the body have varying electrical resistance, and that it is highest in bone [163], which results in bone acting like the heating element on an electric range. This theory is thought to explain the deep periosseous tissue damage that occurs in the relative absence of surface wounds. Subsequent data challenged this theory and stated that, in fact, the extremity may act as a unicompartmental model [109, 110]. Although the issue is unresolved, it is often found that deep tissue damage exceeds surface wounds observed after electrical (especially high voltage) injury.

An often observed phenomenon is an apparent progressive loss of viable tissue that occurs during the first few days after electrical injury [163]. Muscle tissue especially may appear viable and contractile shortly after injury but nonviable on subsequent exploration. The classic explanation for this difference is delayed thrombosis of microvasculature caused by the unique effect of electrical current [92]. It has been difficult, however, to demonstrate this progressive thrombosis experimentally, and the etiology of this delayed tissue loss thus remains unclear, though more recent evidence points to progressive tissue destruction caused by mediators released from injured cells [157].

Additional damage is caused during electrical injury by arc burn across flexion surfaces of the body [26]. It is most likely at the wrist, antecubital fossa, and popliteal fossa. Muscle contraction or tetany induced by electrical current results in an inability of the victim to release the current source, which may increase the magnitude of tissue destruction. Moreover, the victim's clothing

*Postgrad. Med.* 55:131, 1974.

23. Beasley, R. W. *Hand Injuries.* Philadelphia: Saunders, 1981.

24. Beasley, R. W. Secondary repair of burned hands. *Clin. Plast. Surg.* 8:141, 1981.

25. Bingham, H. D., Gallagher, T. J., Powell, M. D. Early bronchoscopy as a predictor of ventilatory support for burned patients. *J. Trauma* 27:1286, 1987.

26. Bingham, H. G. Electrical injuries to the upper extremity. *Burns* 7:155, 1981.

27. Boswick, J. A., Jr. Comprehensive rehabilitation after burn injury. *Surg. Clin. North Am.* 67:159, 1987.

28. Bridges, K., and Lowbury, E. J. L. Drug resistance in relation to use of silver sulphadiazine cream in a burn unit. *J. Clin. Pathol.* 30:160, 1977.

29. Burke, J. F., Bondoc, C. C., and Quinby, W. C. Primary burn excision and immediate grafting: A method for shortening illness. *J. Trauma* 14:389, 1974.

30. Burke, J. F., Bondoc, C. C., Quinby, W. C., et al. Primary surgical management of the deeply burned hand. *J. Trauma* 16:593, 1976.

31. Burke, J. F., May, J. W., Albright, N., et al. Temporary skin transplantation and immunosuppression for extensive burns. *N. Engl. J. Med.* 290:269, 1974.

32. Burke, J. F., Quinby, W. C., and Bondoc, C. C. Primary excision and prompt grafting as routine therapy for the treatment of thermal burns in children. *Surg. Clin. North Am.* 56:477, 1976.

33. Burke, J. F., Quinby, W. C., Bondoc, C. C., et al. Immunosuppression and temporary skin transplantation in the treatment of massive third degree burns. *Ann. Surg.* 182:183, 1975.

34. Burke, J. F., Wolfe, R. R., Mullany, C. J., et al. Glucose requirements following burn injury. *Ann. Surg.* 190:274, 1979.

35. Burke, J. F., Yannas, I. V., Quinby, W. C., et al. Successful use of a physiologically acceptable artificial skin in the treatment of extensive burn injury. *Ann. Surg.* 194:413, 1981.

36. Charnock, E. L., and Meehan, J. J. Postburn respiratory injuries in children. *Pediatr. Clin. North Am.* 27:661, 1980.

37. Cohen, M., Marshall, M. A., and Schafer, M. E. Tissue expansion for the reconstruction of burn defects. *J. Trauma* 28:158, 1988.

38. Cohen, M. A., and Guzzardi, L. J. Inhalation of products of combustion. *Ann. Emerg. Med.* 12:628, 1983.

39. Consumer Product Safety Commission: *Tap Water Scalds. Alert Sheet.* Washington, D.C.: Consumer Product Safety Commission, 1980.

40. Cotran, R. S. The delayed and prolonged vascular leakage in inflammation. II. An electron microscope study of the vascular response after thermal injury. *Am. J. Pathol.* 46:589, 1965.

41. Cuono, C. B., Langdon, R., Birchall, N., et al. Composite autologous-allogeneic skin replacement: Development and clinical application. *Plast. Reconstr. Surg.* 80:626, 1987.

42. Curreri, P. W., Luterman, A., Braun, D. W., et al. Burn injury: Analysis of survival and hospitalization time for 937 patients. *Ann. Surg.* 192:472, 1980.

43. Curreri, P. W., Richmond, D., Marvin, J., et al. Dietary requirements of patients with major burns. *J. Am. Diet. Assoc.* 65:415, 1974.

44. Dacso, C. C., Luterman, A., and Curreri, P. W. Systemic antibiotic treatment in burned patients. *Surg. Clin. North Am.* 67:57, 1987.

45. Deitch, E. A., Winterton, J., and Berg, R. Thermal injury promotes bacterial translocation from the gastrointestinal tract in mice with impaired T-cell-mediated immunity. *Arch. Surg.* 121:97, 1986.

46. Demling, R. H. Burn edema. I. Pathogenesis. *J. Burn Care Rehabil.* 3:138, 1982.

47. Demling, R. H. Early pulmonary abnormalities from smoke inhalation. *J.A.M.A.* 251:771, 1984.

48. Demling, R. H. Fluid replacement in burned patients. *Surg. Clin. North Am.* 67:15, 1987.

49. Demling, R. H., Kramer, G. C., and Harms, B. Role of thermal injury-induced hypoproteinemia on edema formation in burned and non-burned tissue. *Surgery* 95:136, 1984.

50. Demling, R. H., Kramer, G. C., Gunther, R., et al. Effect of non-protein colloid on post burn edema formation in soft tissues and lung. *Surgery* 95:593, 1984.

51. Denney, M. Personal communication, 1987.

52. DiVincenti, F. C., Pruitt, B. A., Jr., and Reckler, J. M. Inhalation injuries. *J. Trauma* 11:109, 1971.

53. Durtschi, M. B., Orgain, C., Counts, G. W., et al. A prospective study of prophylactic penicillin in acutely burned hospitalized pa-

tients. *J. Trauma* 22:11, 1982.

54. Ehrie, M., Morgan, A., Moore, F. D., et al. Endocarditis with the indwelling balloon tipped pulmonary artery catheter in burn patients. *J. Trauma* 18:664, 1978.

55. Fein, A., Leff, A., and Hopewell, P. C. Pathophysiology and management of the complications resulting from fire and the inhaled products of combustion: Review of the literature. *Crit. Care Med.* 8:94, 1980.

56. Fox, C. L., Monafo, W. W., Ayvazian, V. H., et al. Topical chemotherapy for burns using cerium salts and silver sulfadiazine. *Surg. Gynecol. Obstet.* 144:668, 1977.

57. Fratianne, R. B., Gerding, R. L., Zyga, M., et al. Branched chain amino acid enriched solutions in burn patients: A randomized prospective study. *Proc. Am. Burn Assoc.* 20:114, 1988 (abstract).

58. Furnas, D., Achauer, B. M., Bartlett, R. H., et al. Reconstruction of the burned nose. *J. Trauma* 20:25, 1980.

59. Gauto, A., Law, E. J., Holder, J. A., et al. Experience with amphotericin B in the treatment of systemic candidiasis in burn patients. *Am. J. Surg.* 133:174, 1977.

60. Gonzalez-Ulloa, M. Restoration of the face covering by means of selected skin of regional aesthetic units. *Br. J. Plast. Surg.* 9:212, 1956.

61. Gonzalez-Ulloa, M., Castillo, A., Stevens, E., et al. Preliminary study of the total restoration of the facial skin. *Plast. Reconstr. Surg.* 13:151, 1954.

62. Goodwin, C. W., Dorethy, J., Lam, V., et al. Randomized trial of efficacy of crystalloid and colloid resuscitation on hemodynamic response and lung water following thermal injury. *Ann. Surg.* 197:520, 1983.

63. Goodwin, C. W., Maguire, M. S., McManus, M. F., et al. Prospective study of burn wound excision of the hands. *J. Trauma* 23:510, 1983.

64. Gray, D. T., Pine, R. W., Harnar, T. J., et al. Early surgical excision versus conventional therapy in patients with 20 to 40 percent burns: A comparative study. *Am. J. Surg.* 144:76, 1982.

65. Gump, F. E., Price, J. B., and Kinney, J. M. Blood flow and oxygen consumption in patients with severe burns. *Surg. Gynecol. Obstet.* 130:23, 1970.

66. Haburchak, D. R., and Pruitt, B. A. Use of systemic antibiotics in the burned patient. *Surg. Clin. North Am.* 58:1119, 1978.

67. Halebian, P., Robinson, N., Barie, P., et al. Whole body oxygen utilization during carbon monoxide poisoning and isocapnic nitrogen hypoxia. *Proc. Am. Burn Assoc.* 17:5, 1985.

68. Ham, K. N., and Hurley, J. V. An electron microscope study of the vascular response to mild thermal injury in the rat. *J. Pathol. Bacteriol.* 95:175, 1968.

69. Hammond, J. S., and Ward, C. G. Transfer from emergency room to burn center: Errors in burn size estimate. *J. Trauma* 27:1161, 1987.

70. Hansbrough, J. F., Peterson, V., Kortz, E., et al. Postburn immunosuppression in an animal model: Monocyte dysfunction induced by burned tissue. *Surgery* 93:415, 1983.

71. Hansbrough, J. F., Zapata-Sirvent, R. L., and Peterson, V. M. Immunomodulation following burn injury. *Surg. Clin. North Am.* 67:69, 1987.

72. Harms, B. A., et al. Microvascular fluid and protein flux in pulmonary and systemic circulations after thermal injury. *Microvasc. Res.* 23:77, 1982.

73. Harms, B. A., Kramer, G. C., Bodai, B., et al. Effect of hypoproteinemia on pulmonary and soft tissue edema formation. *Crit. Care Med.* 9:503, 1981.

74. Harnar, T., Engrav, L. H., Marvin, J., et al. Dr. Paul Unna's boot and early ambulation after skin grafting the leg: A survey of burn centers and a report of 20 cases. *Plast. Reconstr. Surg.* 69:359, 1982.

75. Harnar, T. J., Heimbach, D. M., Engrav, L. H., et al. A randomized prospective study of early excision and grafting of indeterminant burns less than 20 percent TBSA. *J. Trauma* 23:1001, 1983.

76. Head, J. M. Inhalation injury in burns. *Am. J. Surg.* 139:508, 1980.

77. Heck, E. L., Bergstresser, P. R., and Baxter, C. R. Composite skin graft: Frozen dermal allografts support the engraftment and expansion of autologous epidermis. *J. Trauma* 25:106, 1985.

78. Heidman, M. Complement Activation by Thermal Injury and Its Possible Consequences for Immune Defense. In J. L. Ninnemann (ed.), *The Immune Consequences of Thermal Injury.* Baltimore: Williams & Wil-

kins, 1981. Pp. 127–133.

79. Heimbach, D. M. Early burn excision and grafting. *Surg. Clin. North Am.* 67:93, 1987.

80. Heimbach, D. M., Afromavitz, M. A., Engrav, L. H., et al. Burn depth estimation—man or machine? *J. Trauma* 24:373, 1984.

81. Heimbach, D. M., and Engrav, L. *Surgical Management of the Burn Wound.* New York: Raven, 1985.

82. Herndon, D. N., Langner, F., Thompson, P., et al. Pulmonary injury in burned patients. *Surg. Clin. North Am.* 67:31, 1987.

83. Herndon, D. N., Thompson, P. B., and Traber, D. L. Pulmonary injury in burned patients. *Crit. Care Clin.* 1:79, 1985.

84. Herndon, D. N., Traber, D. L., Niehaus, G. D., et al. The pathophysiology of smoke inhalation injury in a sheep model. *J. Trauma* 24:1043, 1984.

85. Herzog, S. R., Meyer, A., Woodley, D., et al. Wound coverage with cultured autologous keratinocytes: Use after burn wound excision, including biopsy follow up. *J. Trauma* 28:195, 1988.

86. High, R. M., Neale, H. W., Billmire, D. A., et al. Complications of controlled tissue expansion in pediatric burn patients. *Proc. Am. Burn Assoc.* 20:16, 1988 (abstract).

87. Hint, H. C. The relationship between the molecular weight of dextran and its effects: Rheomacrodex. In *Reports of Symposia at Cardiff, New Jersey.* Vol. 1. Piscataway, NJ: Pharmacia, 1964. Pp. 7–12.

88. Holliman, C. J., Saffle, J. R., Kravitz, M., et al. Early surgical decompression in the management of electrical injuries. *Am. J. Surg.* 144:733, 1982.

89. Hovey, L. Personal communication, 1988.

90. Huang, T. T., and Blackwell, S. J. Burn injuries of the eyelids. *Clin. Plast. Surg.* 5:571, 1978.

91. Hunt, J. L., and Sato, R. M. Early excision of full-thickness hand and digit burns; Factors affecting morbidity. *J. Trauma* 22:414, 1982.

92. Hunt, J. L., Mason, A. D., Masterson, T. S., et al. The pathophysiology of acute electric injuries. *J. Trauma* 16:335, 1976.

93. Hunt, J. L., Sato, R. M., and Baxter, C. R. Acute electric burns. *Arch. Surg.* 115:434, 1980.

94. Hunt, J. L., Sato, R., Baxter, C. R., et al. Early tangential excision and immediate mesh autografting of deep dermal hand burns. *Ann.*

Surg. 189:147, 1979.

95. Imbus, S. H., and Zawacki, B. E. Autonomy for burned patients when survival is unprecedented. *N. Engl. J. Med.* 297:308, 1977.

96. Jackson, D., Topley, E., Cason, J. S., et al. Primary excision and grafting of large burns. *Ann. Surg.* 152:167, 1960.

97. Janzekovic, Z. A new concept in the early excision and immediate grafting of burns. *J. Trauma* 10:1103, 1970.

98. Jones, T., McDonald, S., and Deitch, E. A. Effect of graft bed on long term functional results of extremity skin grafts. *J. Burn Care Rehabil.* 9:72, 1988.

99. Jones, W. G., Goodwin, C. W., Madden, M., et al. Tracheostomies in burned patients. *Proc. Am. Burn Assoc.* 20:82, 1988 (abstract).

100. Kealey, G. P., Bale, J., Jr., Strauss, R., et al. Reactivation of cytomegalovirus infections in burn patients. *Proc. Am. Burn Assoc.* 20:67, 1988 (abstract).

101. King, N., Goodwin, C. W., Jr. Use of vitamin supplements for burned patients: A national survey. *J. Am. Diet. Assoc.* 84:923, 1984.

102. Korman, J., and Press, B. Lung abscess and empyema complicating scald burns in an infant. Unpublished data, 1988.

103. Kramer, G. C., Harms, B. A., Bodai, B., et al. Mechanisms for redistribution of plasma protein following acute protein depletion. *Am. J. Physiol.* 243:803, 1982.

104. Kramer, G. C., Harms, B. A., Gunther, R., et al. The effects of hypoproteinemia on blood-to-lymph fluid transport on sheep lung. *Circ. Res.* 49:1173, 1981.

105. Krob, M. I., and Shelby, J. Enhanced allograft survival in H-2 compatible cyclosporine-treated mice. *J. Trauma* 28:225, 1988.

106. Kupper, T. S., Green, D. R., Chaudry, I. H., et al. A cyclophosphamide-sensitive T cell circuit induced by thermal injury. *Surgery* 95:699, 1984.

107. Lamki, L. O., and Liljedahl, S. O. Plasma volume changes after infusion of various plasma expanders. *Resuscitation* 5:93, 1976.

108. Leape, L. Tissue changes in burned and unburned skin of rhesus monkeys. *J. Trauma* 10:488, 1970.

109. Lee, R. C., and Kolodney, S. B. Electrical injury mechanisms: Dynamics of the thermal response. *Plast. Reconstr. Surg.* 80:663, 1987.

110. Lee, R. C., and Kolodney, S. B. Electrical in-

jury mechanisms: Electrical breakdown of cell membranes. *Plast. Reconstr. Surg.* 80: 672, 1987.

111. Levine, N. S., Atkins, H., McDeel, D. W. J., et al. Spinal cord injury following electrical accidents: Case reports. *J. Trauma* 15:459, 1975.

112. Loebl, E. C., Marvin, J. A., Heck, E. L., et al. The method of quantitative burn wound biopsy culture and its routine use in the care of the burned patient. *Am. J. Clin. Pathol.* 61:20, 1974.

113. Long, C. L. Energy and protein needs in the critically ill patient. *Contemp. Surg.* 16:29, 1980.

114. Long, C. L., Schaffel, N., Geiger, J. W., et al. Metabolic response to injury and illness: Estimation of energy and protein needs from an indirect calorimetry and nitrogen balance. *J. Parenter. Enteral Nutr.* 3:452, 1979.

115. Luce, E. A., and Gottlieb, S. E. "True" high tension electrical injuries. *Ann. Plast. Surg.* 12:321, 1984.

116. Madden, M. R., Finkelstein, J. L., and Goodwin, C. W. Respiratory care of the burn patient. *Clin. Plast. Surg.* 13:29, 1986.

117. Maley, M. P. Statistical data. In *Rekindle.* Ashland, MD: International Society of Fire Service Instructors, 1985.

118. Martez, A. T., and Zweifach, B. The high oncotic pressure effects of dextran. *Arch. Surg.* 101:421, 1970.

119. McBride, J. W., Labrosse, K. R., McCoy, H. G., et al. Is serum creatine kinase-MB in electrically injured patients predictive of myocardial injury? *J.A.M.A.* 255:764, 1986.

120. McDougal, W. S., Wilmore, D. W., and Pruit, B. A., Jr. Effect of intravenous near isosmotic nutrient infusions on nitrogen balance in critically injured patients. *Surg. Gynecol. Obstet.* 145:408, 1977.

121. McHugh, T. P., Robson, M. C., Heggers, J. P., et al. Therapeutic efficacy of Biobrane in partial and full-thickness thermal injury. *Surgery* 100:661, 1986.

122. McManus, A. T., Kim, S. H., Mason, A. D., Jr., et al. A comparison of quantitative microbiology and histopathology in divided burn wound biopsies. *Arch. Surg.* 122:74, 1987.

123. Meakins, J. L., Hohn, D. C., Hunt, T. K., et al. Host Defenses. In R. L. Simmons and R. J. Howard (eds.), *Surgical Infectious Dis-*

eases. East Norwalk, CT: Appleton-Century-Crofts, 1982. Pp. 235–284.

124. Miller, C. L., and Clandy, B. J. Suppressor T cell activity induced as a result of thermal injury. *Cell. Immunol.* 44:201, 1979.

125. Molnar, J. A., Bell, S. J., Goodenough, R. D., et al. Enteral Nutrition in Patients with Burns or Trauma. In J. L. Rombeau and M. D. Caldwell (eds.), *Enteral Nutrition.* Philadelphia: Saunders, 1984. Pp. 412–433.

126. Molnar, J. A., Wolfe, R. R., and Burke, J. F. Burns: Metabolism and Nutritional Therapy in Thermal Injury. In H. A. Schneider, C. E. Anderson, and D. B. Coursin (eds.), *Nutritional Support of Medical Practice.* (2nd ed.). Philadelphia: Lippincott, 1983. Pp. 260–281.

127. Monafo, W. W., and Freedman, B. Topical therapy for burns. *Surg. Clin. North Am.* 67:133–145, 1987.

128. Monafo, W. W., Chunktrasakul, C., and Ayvazian, V. H. Hypertonic sodium solutions in the treatment of burn shock. *Am. J. Surg.* 126:778, 1973.

129. Monafo, W. W., Halverson, J. D., and Schechtman, K. The role of concentrated sodium solutions in the resuscitation of patients with severe burns. *Surgery* 95:129, 1984.

130. Moncrief, J. A. Burn formulae. *J. Trauma.* 12:538, 1972 (editorial).

131. Moran, K., and Munster, A. M. Alterations of the host defense mechanisms in burned patients. *Surg. Clin. North Am.* 67:47, 1987.

132. Moyer, C. A., Brentano, L., Gravens, D. L., et al. Treatment of large human burns with 0.5 per cent silver nitrate solution. *Arch. Surg.* 90:812, 1965.

133. Moylan, J. A., and Alexander, G., Jr. Diagnosis and treatment of inhalation injury. *World J. Surg.* 2:185, 1978.

134. Moylan, J. A., and Chan, C. K. Inhalation injury—an increasing problem. *Surgery* 188: 34, 1978.

135. Moylan, J. A., Adib, K., and Birnbaum, M. Fiberoptic bronchoscopy following thermal injury. *Surg. Gynecol. Obstet.* 140:541, 1975.

136. Moylan, J. A., Reckler, J. M. C., and Mason, A. D. Resuscitation with hypertonic lactated saline in thermal injury. *Am. J. Surg.* 125: 580, 1973.

137. Moylan, J. A., West, J. T., Nash, G., et al. Tracheostomy in thermally injured patients: A review of five years experience. *Am. Surg.*

38:119, 1972.

138. Munster, A. M. Immunologic response of trauma and burns: An overview. *Am. J. Med.* 76:142, 1984.

139. Neligan, P. C., and Peters, W. J. The use of tissue expansion in burn scar reconstruction. *J. Burn Care Rehabil.* 8:107, 1987.

140. Newman, N. M. Nursing Procedures. In R. E. Salisbury, N. M. Newman, and G. P. Dingeldein Jr. (eds.), *Manual of Burn Therapeutics: An Interdisciplinary Approach.* Boston: Little, Brown, 1983. Pp. 137–140.

141. Nider, A. The effects of low levels of carbon monoxide on the fine structures of terminal airways. *Am. Rev. Respir. Dis.* 103:898, 1971.

142. Ohmori, K. Application of microvascular free flaps to burn deformities. *World J. Surg.* 2:193, 1978.

143. Parker, J., Rutan, R. L., Desai, M. H., et al. The scrotum as a donor site in burns greater than 80% total body surface area. *Proc. Am. Burn Assoc.* 20:129, 1988 (abstract).

144. Pasulka, P. S., and Wachtel, T. L. Nutritional considerations in the burned patient. *Surg. Clin. North Am.* 67:109, 1987.

145. Paul, W. E. (ed.). *Fundamental Immunology.* New York: Raven, 1984.

146. Peltier, G. L., Poppe, S. R., and Twomey, J. A. Controlled air suspension: An advantage in burn care. *J. Burn Care Rehabil.* 8:558, 1987.

147. Peterson, V., Hansbrough, J. F., Wang, X. W., et al. Topical cerium nitrate prevents postburn immunosuppression. *J. Trauma* 25:1039, 1985.

148. Press, B., and Dean, S. In press, 1990.

149. Pruitt, B. A., Jr. Fluid resuscitation for extensively burned patients. *J. Trauma* 21:690, 1981.

150. Pruitt, B. A., Jr., and Foley, F. D. The use of biopsies in burn patient care. *Surgery* 73:887, 1973.

151. Pruitt, B. A., Jr., and Goodwin, C. W. Stress ulcer disease in the burned patient. *World J. Surg.* 5:209, 1981.

152. Pruitt, B. A., Jr., McManus, W. F., Kim, S. H., et al. Diagnosis and treatment of cannula-related intravenous sepsis in burn patients. *Ann. Surg.* 181:546, 1980.

153. Purdue, G. F., and Hunt, J. L. Pulmonary emboli in burned patients. *J. Trauma* 28:218, 1988.

154. Purdue, G. F., Hunt, J. L., and Prescott, P. R. Child abuse by burning—an index of suspicion. *J. Trauma* 28:221, 1988.

155. Reiss, E., Pearson, E., Artz, C. P., et al. The metabolic response to burns. *J. Clin. Invest.* 35:62, 1956.

156. Rivers, E., Strate, R., and Solem, L. The transparent face mask. *Am. J. Occup. Ther.* 33:108, 1979.

157. Robson, M. C., Murphy, R. C., and Heggers, J. P. A new explanation for the progressive tissue loss in electrical injuries. *Plast. Reconstr. Surg.* 73:431, 1984.

158. Rosenburg, J. L., and Zawacki, B. E. Reduction of blood loss using tourniquets and "compression" dressings in excising limb burns. *J. Trauma* 26:47, 1986.

159. Rubin, W. D., Mani, M. M., and Hiebert, J. M. Fluid resuscitation of the thermally injured patient. *Clin. Past. Surg.* 13:9, 1986.

160. Rubli, E., Basard, S., Frei, E., et al. Plasma fibronectin and associated variables in surgical intensive care patients. *Ann. Surg.* 197:310, 1983.

161. Saffle, J. R., Medina, E., Raymond, J., et al. Use of indirect calorimetry in nutritional management of burned patients. *J. Trauma* 25:32, 1985.

162. Salisbury, R. E. Initial Management of Burns: Triage and Outpatient Care. In R. E. Salisbury, N. M. Newman, and G. P. Dingeldein, Jr. (eds.), *Manual of Burn Therapeutics: An Interdisciplinary Approach.* Boston: Little, Brown, 1983. Pp. 1–7.

163. Salisbury, R. E., and Dingeldein, G. P., Jr. Specific Burn Injuries. In R. E. Salisbury, N. M. Newman, and G. P. Dingeldein, Jr. (eds.), *Manual of Burn Therapeutics: An Interdisciplinary Approach.* Boston: Little, Brown, 1983.

164. Salisbury, R. E., McKeel, D. W., and Mason, A. D. Ischemic necrosis of the intrinsic muscles of the hand after thermal injury. *J. Bone Joint Surg. [Am.]* 56:1701, 1974.

165. Salisbury, R. E., Taylor, J. W., and Levine, N. S. Evaluation of digital escharotomy in burned hands. *Plast. Reconstr. Surg.* 58:440, 1976.

166. Saranto, J. R., Rubayi, S., and Zawacki, B. Blisters, cooling, antithromboxanes, and healing in experimental zone-of-stasis burns. *J. Trauma* 23:927, 1983.

167. Sawchuk, R. J., and Zaske, D. E. Pharmacokinetics of dosing regimens which utilize

multiple intravenous infusions: Gentamicin in burn patients. *J. Pharmacokinet. Biopharmacol.* 4:183, 1976.

168. Scheulen, J. J., and Munster, A. M. The Parkland formula in patients with burns and inhalation injury. *J. Trauma* 22:869, 1982.

169. Schlag, G., Redl, H., Traber, L., et al. Lung edema following smoke inhalation. *Eur. J. Surg. Res.* 16:106, 1984 (abstract).

170. Schubert, W., Kuehn, C., and Moudry, B. Halo immobilization in the treatment of burns to the head, face, and neck. *J. Burn Care Rehabil.* 9:187, 1988.

171. Silberman, H., and Eisenberg, D. *Parenteral and Enteral Nutrition for the Hospitalized Patient.* East Norwalk, CT: Appleton-Century-Crofts, 1982. Pp. 54–59.

172. Silverstein, P., and Dressler, D. P. Effect of current therapy on burn mortality. *Ann. Surg.* 171:124, 1970.

173. Silverstein, P., and Ladi, B. Fire prevention in the United States. *Surg. Clin. North Am.* 67:1, 1987.

174. Silverstein, P., and Wilson, R. Prevention of Pediatric Burn Injuries. In H. Carvajal (ed.), *Burns in Children.* Chicago: Year Book, 1988.

175. Slater, H., Newton, E. D., and Goldfarb, J. W. Free flaps in selected burn patients. *J. Burn Care Rehabil.* 7:385, 1986.

176. Smith, C. W., and Goldman, A. S. Selective effects of thermal injury on mouse peritoneal macrophages. *Infect. Immun.* 5:938, 1977.

177. Smith, L. Personal communication, 1987.

178. Solem, L. D. Personal communication, 1987.

179. Solem, L. D., Fischer, R. P., and Strate, R. G. The natural history of electrical injury. *J. Trauma* 17:487, 1977.

180. Solem, L. D., Strate, R. G., and Fischer, R. P. Antacid therapy and nutritional supplementation in the prevention of Curling's ulcer. *Surg. Gynecol. Obstet.* 148:367, 1979.

181. Spebar, M. J., and Pruitt, B. A. Candidiasis in the burned patient. *J. Trauma* 21:237, 1981.

182. Steinbach, R. A. Psychophysiology of pain. *Int. J. Psychiatry Med.* 6:63, 1975.

183. Stewart, R. D. The effect of carbon monoxide on humans. *Annu. Rev. Pharmacol.* 15:409, 1975.

184. Stratta, R. J., Saffle, J. R., Ninnemann, J. L., et al. The effect of surgical excision and grafting procedures on post-burn lymphocyte suppression. Presented at the 16th American Burn Association Meeting, San Francisco, 1984.

185. Switzer, W. E., Jones, J. W., and Moncrief, J. A. Evaluation of early excision of burns in children. *J. Trauma* 5:540, 1965.

186. Taylor, P. H., Moncrief, J. A., Augsley, L. Q., et al. The management of extensively burned patients by staged excision. *Surg. Gynecol. Obstet.* 115:347, 1962.

187. Thomson, P. D., Feller, I., Moore, N. P., et al. Evidence against leukopenia induced by silver sulfadiazine in acute burn injury. *Proc. Am. Burn Assoc.* 20:98, 1988 (abstract).

188. Tranbaugh, R. F., Elings, V. T., Christensen, J. M., et al. Effect of inhalation injury on lung water accumulation. *J. Trauma* 23:597, 1983.

189. Tranbaugh, R. F., Lewis, F. R., Christensen, J. M., et al. Lung water changes after thermal injury. *Ann. Surg.* 192:479, 1980.

190. U.S. Department of Health, Education and Welfare: *Studies on Death, Injuries and Economic Losses Resulting from Accidental Burning of Products, Fabrics or Related Materials.* Third Annual Report to the President of the United States and the Congress of the United States. Publication (FOA) 72-7013. Washington, D.C.: Government Printing Office, 1971. Pp. 36–37.

191. U.S. Fire Administration: *National Fire Incidence Reporting System and Federal Emergency Management Agency: Analysis of National Fire Protection Association Survey Data.* Washington, D.C.: Federal Emergency Management Agency, 1981.

192. U.S. House of Representatives, Dingell, J. D., Jr. *Committee on Energy and Commerce Report on House Bill 1880.* Washington, D.C.: Government Printing Office, 1984.

193. Velasco, I. T., Pontieri, V., Silva, R. E., et al. Hyperosmotic NaCl and severe hemorrhagic shock. *Am. J. Physiol.* 239:664, 1980.

194. Warden, G. D. Outpatient care of thermal injuries. *Surg. Clin. North Am.* 67:147, 1987.

195. Warden, G. D., Mason, A. D., Jr., and Pruitt, B. A., Jr. Evaluation of leukocyte chemotaxis in vitro in thermally injured patients. *J. Clin. Invest.* 54:1001, 1974.

196. Watanabe, K., and Makino, K. The role of carbon monoxide poisoning in the production of inhalation injury. *Ann. Plast. Surg.* 14:284, 1985.

197. Waymack, J. P., Miskell, P., Gonce, S. S., et al. Effect of ibuprofen on postburn metabolic and immunologic function. *Proc. Am. Burn Assoc.* 20:23, 1988 (abstract).

198. Whitener, D. R., Whitener, L. M., Robertson, K. J., et al. Pulmonary function measurements in patients with thermal injury and smoke inhalation. *Am. Rev. Respir. Dis.* 122:731, 1980.

199. Whittaker, A. H. Treatment of burns by excision and immediate skin grafting. *Am. J. Surg.* 85:411, 1953.

200. Wilmore, D. Metabolic Changes in Burns. In C. P. Artz, J. Moncrief, and B. A. Pruitt (eds.), *Burns: A Team Approach.* Philadelphia: Saunders, 1979. Pp. 120–131.

201. Wilmore, D. W. *The Metabolic Management of the Critically Ill.* New York: Plenum, 1977.

202. Wilmore, D. W., Long, J. M., Mason, A. D., et al. Catecholamines: Mediator of the hypermetabolic response to thermal injury. *Ann. Surg.* 180:653, 1974.

203. Wolfe, R. R., Durkot, M. J., Allsop, J. R., et al. Glucose metabolism in severely burned patients. *Metabolism* 28:1031, 1979.

204. Wolfe, R. R., Goodenough, R. D., Burke, J. F., et al. Response of protein and urea kinetics in burn patients to different levels of protein intake. *Ann. Surg.* 197:163, 1983.

205. Wolfe, R. R., Miller, H. I., Elahi, D., et al. Effect of burn injury on glucose turnover in guinea pigs. *Surg. Gynecol. Obstet.* 144:359, 1977.

206. Wolfe, R. R., O'Donnell, T. F., Stone, M. D., et al. Investigation of factors determining the optimal glucose infusion rate in total parenteral nutrition. *Metabolism* 29:892, 1980.

207. Yu, Y. M., Wagner, D. A., Walereswki, J. C., et al. A kinetic study of leucine metabolism in severely burned patients: Comparison between a conventional and branched chain amino acid enriched nutritional therapy. *Proc. Am. Burn Assoc.* 20:113, 1988 (abstract).

208. Zachary, L. S., Heggers, J. P., Robson, M. C., et al. Burns of the feet. *J. Burn Care Rehabil.* 8:192, 1987.

209. Zapata-Sirvent, R., Hansbrough, J. F., Carroll, W., et al. Comparison of Biobrane and scarlet red dressings for treatment of donor site wounds. *Arch. Surg.* 120:743, 1985.

210. Zapata-Sirvent, R., Hansbrough, J. F., Mansour, M. A., et al. Postburn immunosuppression in an animal model. IV. Immunomodulating drugs improve postburn resistance to sepsis. *Surgery* 99:53, 1986.

211. Zaske, D. E., Sawchuk, R. J., and Strate, R. G. The necessity of increased doses of amikacin in burn patients. *Surgery* 84:603, 1978.

212. Zaske, D. E., Sawchuk, R. J., Gerding, D. N., et al. Increased dosage requirements of gentamicin in burn patients. *J. Trauma* 16:824, 1976.

213. Zuker, R. M. The use of tissue expansion in pediatric scalp burn reconstruction. *J. Burn Care Rehabil.* 8:103, 1987.

# 25

*Melvin Spira*
*Samuel Stal*

# Basal and Squamous Cell Carcinoma of the Skin

## Embryology

The embryology of skin is worthy of discussion, as tumor genesis, treatment, and prognosis may be affected by the embryologic derivation of skin's components. The skin is derived from either ectoderm or mesoderm. Epithelial structures derived from the ectoderm include the epidermis, pilosebaceous and apocrine units, eccrine sweat glands, and nail units. Melanocytes, nerves, and specialized sensory preceptors arise from the neuroectoderm. Other elements within the skin, including macrophages and mast cells, Langerhans cells, Merkel cells, fibroblasts, blood vessels, lymph vessels, and fat cells, originate in the mesoderm (Fig. 25-1).

## Anatomy

The skin is composed of two layers, the epidermis and the dermis. The epidermis is the upper layer, ranging in thickness from 0.04 mm on the eyelids to 1.4 mm on the soles of the feet. The epithelium is stratified, squamous in nature, and cornified, with four cell types noted: keratinocytes, melanocytes, Langerhans cells, and Merkel cells, in decreasing numbers. The dermis consists primarily of a noncellular connective tissue composed of collagen, elastic fibers, and ground substance. Interspersed within are nerves, blood vessels, lymphatics, muscle units, pilosebaceous and apocrine units, and eccrine sweat units. The entire dermis, including papillary and reticular layers, is 15 to 40 times thicker than the epidermis. The dermis contains fibroblasts, mast cells, histiocytes, Langerhans cells, and lymphocytes and is generally divided into two layers, a thin upper zone underneath the epidermis, called the papillary dermis, and a thick lower zone, called the reticular layer, which is significantly larger and extends from the base of the papillary dermis to the subcutaneous fat. The reticular layer contains irregular, loosely arranged, coarse elastic fibers interspersed between thick collagen bundles with relatively few fibroblasts and blood vessels compared to the overlying papillary dermis [60, 62].

## Physiology

The skin is a multifunctional organ, providing the body an external cover to withstand minor trauma and invasion by microorganisms. With its underlying subcutaneous layer, it also protects against temperature extremes and water loss. It provides sensation, including point, temperature, pressure, and location discrimination. Skin regulates heat through the vasomotor activity of its blood vessels as well as through sweat gland activity [60, 62].

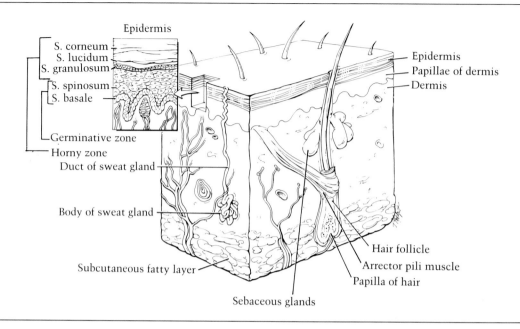

**Figure 25-1** *Cross-sectional view showing anatomic skin levels and associated pilosebaceous units.*

## Terminology

Many of the terms used in this chapter on basal and squamous cell carcinomas as well as commonly seen conditions of the skin are defined below (Fig. 25-2). An accurate description of these conditions is essential (Fig. 25-3).

Primary lesions can be described as skin abnormalities caused directly by disease processes with specific anatomic changes [60].

**Bulla.** A large blister (pemphigus, superficial burn).

**Cyst.** A tumor containing liquid or semi-solid material (epidermoid cyst).

**Macule.** A nonpalpable, circumscribed area usually demarcated by color change (freckle).

**Papule.** An elevated palpable lesion of varying size. A *papule* is less than 5 mm (wart), a *nodule* 5 mm to 5 cm (compound nevus), and a *tumor* more than 5 cm (squamous cell carcinoma, basal cell carcinoma).

**Patch.** A macule more than 5 cm in diameter (café au lait spot).

**Plaque.** A papule that is larger in surface area than in thickness, usually more than 2 cm in diameter, and usually flat (psoriasis).

**Pustule.** An elevated lesion containing pus (acne vulgaris).

**Vesicle.** Also called a blister; an elevated fluid-containing lesion usually less than 5 mm (herpes simplex, herpes zoster).

Secondary lesions are changes in the skin caused by excoriation, bleeding, atrophy, scarring, or infection in the area of primary pathology [60].

**Atrophy.** If epidermal, is associated with thinning of the epidermis, as seen in discoid lupus erythematosus; if dermal, is associated with a decrease in collagen ground substance and skin depression (steroid atrophy).

**Crust.** An accumulation of serum and cellular bacterial and squamous debris over damaged epidermis (impetigo, scab).

**Eczematoid lesion.** An inflamed lesion with

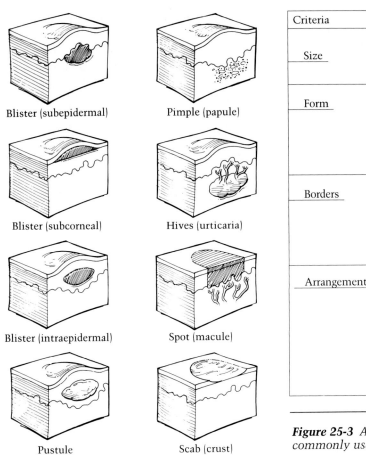

Figure 25-2 *Common primary skin lesions.*

| Criteria | Example | Description |
|---|---|---|
| Size | | 4 × 2 cm |
| Form | | Regular |
| | | Irregular |
| Borders | | Sharp |
| | | Diffuse |
| Arrangement | | Disseminated |
| | | Grouped |
| | | Confluent |

**Figure 25-3** *Accurate descriptive terms commonly used to denote skin lesions.*

scaling, crusting, and weeping (poison ivy, dermatitis).

**Erosion.** The loss of superficial epidermis: called *abrasion* when caused by trauma.

**Fissure.** A crack in the skin.

**Lichenification.** Areas of increased skin marking associated with thickening of the epidermis (neurodermatitis).

**Pedunculated lesion.** One on a stalk with a base smaller than the body.

**Sessile lesion.** Slopes into normal skin on a broad base.

**Telangiectasia.** The dilatation of superficial vessels, which sometimes become tortuous.

**Ulcer.** The loss of epidermis and all or part of the dermis; heals with scarring.

**Verruca.** A wart; the term verrucous or verrucoid means wart-like.

*Annular* denotes a ring-shaped lesion (ringworm). An *umbilicated* lesion has a central depression (moluscum contagiosum). *Confluent* lesions blend into each other. *Serpiginous* refers to an undulating, snake-shaped lesion whose border has formed several confluent lesions (hives, psoriasis).

Site is important, as certain precancerous lesions and cancers exhibit a distinct distribution pattern, occasionally allowing diagnosis by virture of tumor location [60].

## Etiology and Stimulators

The heading Etiology of Skin Cancer contains some broad categories. Certain skin carcinogens play an important part in the development of precancerous and cancerous growth. Exposure to ultraviolet radiation (UV) correlates directly with the development of skin cancer; the incidence of skin cancer is highest in sunny climates, in patients with light complexions, in people who work outdoors, and on areas of the body not covered by clothing. The photochemical effects of UV irradiation are due to electron excitation in the absorbing atoms and molecules, which induces damaging chemical reactions. Radiation-induced chemical damage in DNA may be responsible for cell death and neoplastic transformation. Normal DNA synthesis and cell mitosis are inhibited early in UV-exposed epidermis. The effect of a UV dose on the skin is reduced somewhat by the presence of hair, a thick stratum containing corneum, and melanin [2, 4, 18, 19, 22, 23, 31, 39].

Ionizing radiation has also been recognized as causing skin cancer and is widely used for the experimental induction of skin tumors. Physically, ionizing radiation includes electromagnetic radiations (x-rays and γ-rays) and particulate radiation (electrons, protons, neutrons, α-particles, and heavy nuclei). Both types of radiation elicit changes by ionizing important cell constituents. *An important feature of radiation-induced tumor is that a single radiation exposure may produce a tumor after a long latent period* [4, 19, 34].

Chemical carcinogenesis has been recognized for more than 200 years. In 1875 Potts blamed soot for the high incidence of scrotal cancer in chimney sweeps. The essential feature of the biochemical interaction of carcinogens in cells is the covalent bonding of carcinogen residues with cellular macromolecules, RNA, DNA, and protein. In mice, a single carcinogen application to the epidermis causes a mitotic block and prompt suppression of DNA synthesis. Repeated carcinogen applications associated with a sustained hyperplasia lead to superimposed transient periods of mitotic and DNA depression [2, 22].

During the past century viral carcinogens have been recognized, and numerous animal tumors are now known to be viral in origin, e.g., fowl sarcoma and mouse mammary tumors [2].

Relative to carcinogenesis, Albert summarized, "It is not clear whether there is a common pathway for cellular neoplastic transformation. It is possible that the carcinogenic process will prove to be similar to the process of the evolution of species and that random genetic damage of somatic cells produced by carcinogens is combined with selection of pressures to breed out a race of cells having growth advantages over their normal counterparts" [2].

A number of investigators have published accounts of families with a high incidence of cancer involving either a single organ or multiple anatomic sites. There are many factors involved that demonstrate the difficulty of human population studies of malignancy. Several skin cancers show mendelian inheritance. For example, in *xeroderma pigmentosum*, in which the tumors are multiple epitheliomas, the mode of inheritance is autosomal recessive; the mechanism is a defective DNA repair following UV irradiation [16, 18, 34, 47]. In *multiple nevoid basal cell carcinoma syndrome* the mode of inheritance is autosomal dominant, and the primary tumor is a basal cell carcinoma [5, 24, 41].

## Epidemiology of Premalignant and Malignant Epidermal Lesions

Epidemiology is an observational method of research concerned with the study of disease and disability in a human community rather than in a single individual. Many factors influence the incidence of skin cancer. The most important is excessive exposure to sunlight. There is a direct correlation between latitude and the incidence of skin cancer, given common pigmentation; the incidence is higher in those with lightly pigmented skin and in males rather than females. The lighter the skin pigmentation, the more likely it is that the cancer is a basal cell carcinoma. The darker the pigmentation, the more likely it is squamous cell carcinoma. The epidemiologist has information to offer relative to the causes of skin cancer. Population groups and their exposure to chemical carcinogens and UV light, skin pigmentation, the relation of skin cancer to anatomic areas exposed to sunlight, ancestral lines, a history of keratosis, outdoor occupation versus indoor occupation, the presence of scars and burns on the body, and radiation exposure history are important factors in the epidemiology of skin cancer [2, 4, 19, 22, 23, 31, 39].

There is agreement that squamous cell carcinomas arising in skin damaged by sunlight do not metastasize readily. Cancers that develop in scars or old burns or those that are produced by chemical carcinogens have a much higher rate of metastasis [6, 42]. A man who has had skin cancer has twice the probability of developing a second primary lesion compared to a woman. McDonald found that of every 100 people with a single primary lesion 12 annually developed a second primary cancer of the skin [34]. The incidence of second primary cancer of the skin is 140 times the incidence of the first primary [34].

In California (population 15 million) there are an estimated 6000 new cases of skin cancer each year, with almost 50 people dying annually as a result of such malignancies. More than half of these patients are 75 years or older. As a general rule the mortality rate is much less than 1 percent in the high-incidence areas [22].

## Premalignant Lesions
### ACTINIC KERATOSIS
Actinic keratosis is often referred to as "solar keratosis." It is the most common premalig-

nant lesion seen in older light-complexioned men. Actinic keratoses represent the cumulative effect of UV light exposure. These lesions are rare in blacks and other dark-skinned peoples [48, 49, 60].

Grossly, the lesions are discrete, well circumscribed, erythematous, and maculopapular; they are dry and scaly and vary in color from reddish to light brown. They appear primarily on sun-damaged or exposed skin and are frequently multiple (Fig. 25-4). Their roughness is due to adherent parakeratotic scales.

Microscopically, hyperkeratosis and parakeratosis, together with dyskeratosis and acanthosis, are prominent features in the epidermal layer. Within the dermis are distinct alterations, including an actinic elas-

***Figure 25-4*** *Actinic keratosis.*

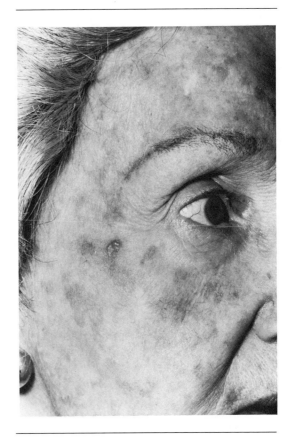

tosis, with these changes primarily in the upper dermis. The expression "basal degeneration of collagen" denotes an alteration or modification of collagen in the upper dermis. There is an associated inflammatory infiltrate consisting primarily of lymphocytes [14, 48, 49].

The differential diagnosis for actinic keratosis includes Bowen's disease and inflammatory lesions such as chronic eczematoid dermatitis, lichen simplex, and psoriasis. The distinguishing feature of the inflammatory lesions is their lack of cell-sharp border between normal and abnormal epithelium in contrast to actinic keratosis. Finally, benign nevi and other skin tumors on occasion are confusing. Most nevi and seborrheic keratoses are papillomas with a "stuck-on" appearance, whereas actinic keratoses are almost flat [14, 48, 49, 60].

The use of sunscreen, sun protective creams, lanolin, and vanishing cream to soften and protect the skin is included in the conservative care of the patient with actinic-damaged skin. Curettage and electrodesiccation form the foundation for treatment of most of these lesions [29, 33, 50]. Liquid nitrogen is also an effective modality [64]. More recently 5-fluorouracil (5-FU) in a 1 to 5% concentration (Efudex) has proved effective [17, 25, 26, 30, 54, 57]. Chemical peel and dermabrasion of the skin have also been effective but have largely been replaced by use of 5-FU [59].

The progression from actinic keratosis to invasive malignancy occurs by several routes, and *the resulting cancer is in almost all cases a squamous cell carcinoma* [48, 49]. The percentage of actinic keratoses that progress to invasive squamous cell carcinoma varies from 20 to 25 percent. These carcinomas that arise in actinically degenerated skin and in actinic keratoses rarely metastasize, suggesting that treatment should be conservative. *There is little place for "wide margins" in the surgical treatment of this lesion.*

## BOWEN'S DISEASE

Bowen's disease is seen in older patients in both sun-exposed and non-sun-exposed areas. It represents an intraepithelial squamous cell carcinoma (carcinoma in situ) and can involve the skin or mucous membranes, including mouth, anus, or genitalia. In most cases no specific etiologic factors can be determined. Most of the lesions are solitary, and men are afflicted more often than women. These lesions have a long clinical course, generally years [45, 49].

Clinically, the lesion appears as a solitary, rather sharply defined, erythematous, reddish, dull, scaly plaque (Fig. 25-5). Pruritus, superficial crusting, and oozing may be noted. Etiologic considerations include sunlight exposure, arsenic, viruses, chronic trauma, and heredity [45].

Microscopic examination reveals the stigmata of an intraepidermal squamous cell carcinoma with hyperkeratosis, parakeratosis, dyskeratosis, and acanthosis within the epithelial layers. Within the epithelium there is disorder. Cells are keratinized within the prickle cell layer, and hyperchromatic bizarre nuclei and increased cell mitosis are

*Figure 25-5 Bowen's disease of the forearm.*

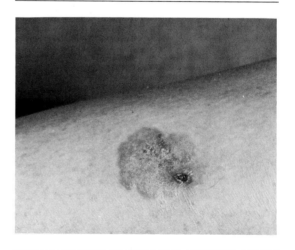

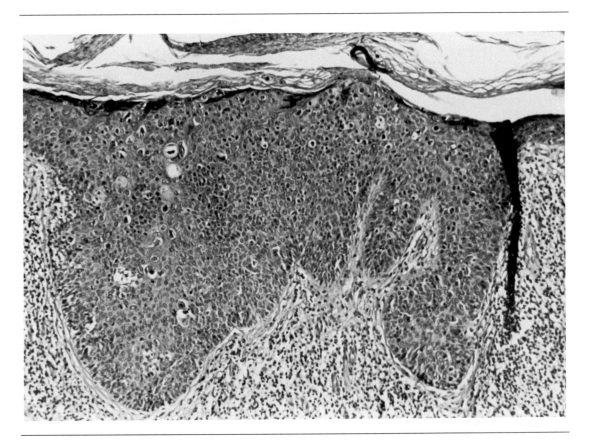

**Figure 25-6** *Bowen's disease (see text).*

observed. There is no dermal invasion, but a heavy inflammatory infiltrate is frequently noted in the papillar dermis with multinucleated giant cells [45] (Fig. 25-6).

The differential diagnosis includes superficial basal cell carcinoma, psoriasis, actinic keratosis, Paget's disease, and leukoplakia, as well as lichen sclerosus et atrophicus [49].

Straightforward surgical therapy includes either excision or a combination of curettage and electrodesiccation. Most surgeons favor the former and most dermatologists the latter. Adequate excision is indicated, as these lesions can subsequently become invasive squamous cell carcinomas and metastasize. When the lesion is seen on a mucosal surface, excision and primary closure or skin grafting may be required. Topical therapy, including 5-FU (in propylene glycol), is effective, particularly when multiple lesions are present [26, 30, 57]. The lesion responds poorly to x-irradiation [8, 45].

The prognosis is excellent with appropriate treatment. However, the prognosis is poor if a squamous cell carcinoma does develop; these lesions are much more aggressive than the squamous cell carcinomas that develop from actinic keratoses [48, 49]. There is also a relation between Bowen's disease and internal malignancies [8]. Knox and Joseph described a 7 percent incidence of cancer, including malignancies of the bladder, bronchus, breast, and esophagus, in patients with Bowen's disease [27].

## ERYTHROPLASIA OF QUEYRAT

Erythroplasia of Queyrat is often referred to as Bowen's disease of the mucous membranes. It most often affects the glans penis and is seen during the fifth and sixth decades of life, primarily in uncircumcised men [27, 43].

Grossly, erythroplasia consists of solitary or multiple erythematous lesions that are well circumscribed, moist, glistening, and velvety. Microscopically, the lesion resembles Bowen's disease. The differential diagnosis includes balanitis, lichen planus, and eczematoid eruptions [27]. The treatment is conservative surgery, employing curettage and desiccation. Topical 5-FU has been described as effective [27, 43]. Erythroplasia is much more likely than Bowen's disease to become malignant and carries with it an increased tendency to metastatic disease [27, 43].

## LEUKOPLAKIA

Leukoplakia, literally meaning "white patch," is seen primarily on oral, vulvar, or vaginal mucosa. Leukoplakia in the mouth is seen mostly in older men with a history of smoking. Ill-fitting dentures and teeth in poor repair often are associated with this condition [49].

Grossly, the lesions are elevated, sharply defined patchy areas of keratinization, generally lighter in color (white to gray) than the surrounding tissue, and of variable thickness (Fig. 25-7). When long-standing or chronic, the lesions may exhibit a verrucoid appearance [60].

Microscopically, we see the classic quartet of hyperkeratosis, parakeratosis, keratosis, and acanthosis. Within the epidermal layer, cellular atypia abounds, and within the dermis is seen an inflammatory infiltrate [22, 60]. The differential diagnosis includes lichen planus, kraurosis vulvae, erythroplasia, and frank squamous cell carcinoma.

The treatment, again, is generally conservative, with lip cream emollients or ointments. Smokers are advised to discontinue the habit. Poorly fitting dentures are refitted and operative dentistry carried out where indicated. Treatment thus includes prophylaxis with emollient sunscreens on the lips. The more florid lesions are generally biopsied. Toluidine blue is helpful in techniques that employ scraping, curettage, or electrodesiccation. Simple excision of the involved mucosa is generally employed. On the lips this procedure is called a lip shave or vermilionectomy and is an effective surgical technique for areas of leukoplakia *unresponsive* to conservative treatment [15].

As to prognosis for untreated lesions, 15 to 20 percent undergo malignant transformation. If there is evidence of ulceration or underlying induration, cancer is a real possibility [15]. The squamous cell carcinomas that develop from premalignant lesions on the mucous membranes are much more malignant than those associated with actinic keratoses.

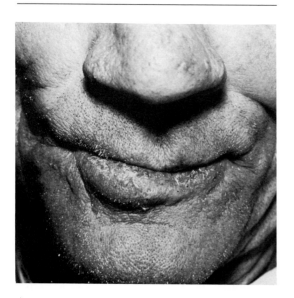

**Figure 25-7** *Leukoplakia of the lip of a 63-year-old chronic smoker.*

## KERATOACANTHOMA

*Keratoacanthoma* is the "self-healing" squamous cell carcinoma. Seen mostly on sun-exposed sites, it is usually solitary but can be multiple. Considerable difference of opinion exists as to whether the lesion is truly a low grade squamous cell carcinoma or it can be classified as a premalignant lesion [1, 7, 28, 49].

Grossly, the lesion is fleshy, elevated, and nodular, with a central hyperkeratotic core (Fig. 25-8). The most significant histologic factor is its rapid growth. Most lesions, when first seen, are weeks to several months old. Their short history and rapid increase in size suggests keratoacanthoma rather than squamous cell carcinoma [1, 60].

Microscopically, there is a keratin shell crater, with hyperplasia and dyskeratosis of the adjacent epithelium. Frequently, histologic differentiation is difficult but not impossible [1, 7, 28]. Differential diagnoses are basal cell carcinoma and squamous cell carcinoma [7, 60].

Treatment depends on surgical philosophy. In numerous published cases the lesion has involuted and disappeared without specific therapy. However, the malignant potential with subsequent ulceration and tissue destruction has been well described in other published series. Although the true incidence of keratoacanthoma is not known, in large clinics the ratio of keratoacanthoma to squamous cell carcinoma has been reported as 1:3 to 1.0:4.7. Thus although keratoacanthoma is classified as a benign and self-involuting neoplasm, most physicians seeing this problem advise early conservative excision of sufficient depth to eliminate the entire lesion. Rapid growth for a period of several weeks with spontaneous involution over a period of several months is supposedly a common occurrence but has never been witnessed by these authors [1, 7, 28, 49, 60].

### RADIATION DERMATITIS

The long-term sequelae of low-dose skin irradiation, a technique popular 50 years ago for the treatment of such conditions as chronic acne and fungal infections of the scalp, are familiar to surgeons today. An-

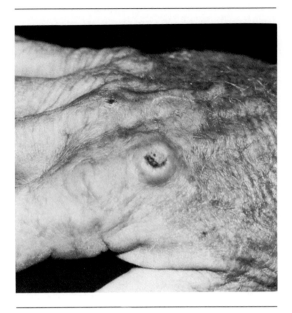

**Figure 25-8** *Keratoacanthoma of the dorsum of the hand.*

other form of chronic radiation exposure is found in the fingers and hands of dentists who hand-held intraoral x-ray film without protection during the long exposures required for obtaining dental radiographs. In either case, these patients may develop chronic radiation dermatitis, followed by the appearance of either basal cell or squamous cell carcinoma (Fig. 25-9). In the most severe conditions, even when malignancy cannot be proved, excision and resurfacing of the most involved areas is a consideration [8, 34, 49].

### PSEUDOEPITHELIOMATOUS HYPERPLASIA

Pseudoepitheliomatous hyperplasia is a condition seen in long-standing chronic ulcers, typically decubitus ulcers; it is evidenced as an epidermal thickening that can be mistaken for a neoplastic change or degeneration. Microscopically, there is a downward proliferation of epidermal cells associated with mild cellular atypia and an inflammatory infiltrate with microabscesses. This condition resembles squamous cell carci-

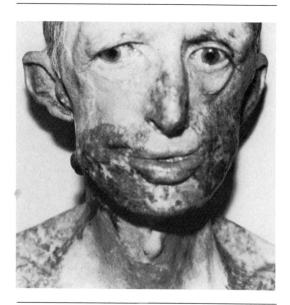

*Figure 25-9 A 69-year-old patient with multiple squamous cell carcinomas: status 30 years after irradiation for benign skin disease.*

noma at times and may be difficult to differentiate from malignancy. Generally, cell and nuclear changes are not as prominent in blood vessels, and nerve invasion is not seen. The condition responds to conservative treatment. In more long-standing cases, excision of the ulcer and grafting may be required [49, 60].

XERODERMA PIGMENTOSUM
Xeroderma pigmentosum is a relatively rare systemic disease transmitted through an incomplete sex-linked recessive gene. The disease, which has its onset during early childhood, is characterized by extreme sensitivity to sunlight. Initially, diffuse lentigos are noted with progressive drying and thinning of the skin. The primary deficiency is that of the enzyme endonuclease, which is needed to repair sunlight-damaged DNA. Malignant degeneration into basal cell or squamous cell carcinoma or melanoma is noted during early adult life, with death due to metastatic disease. Prolongation of life is possible by

absolute protection from sun exposure and continual aggressive treatment of all developing tumors. The prognosis is dismal [16, 47].

### Malignant Lesions
BASAL CELL CARCINOMA
Basal cell carcinoma is the most common malignancy of Caucasians, arising from cells of the basal layer of the epithelium or from the external root sheath of the hair follicle. It is directly related to sun exposure, the etiologic factor being UV radiation. Basal cell carcinomas occur most often at sites with the greatest concentration of pilosebaceous follicles. *Basal cell carcinoma differs from squamous cell carcinoma in that it does not arise from malignant changes occurring in preexisting mature epithelial structures; it requires stromal participation for survival. It does not possess the cellular anaplasia associated with true carcinoma, and it almost never metastasizes (Moxella and Hurley). It occurs with greatest frequency in individuals of northern European descent [2, 13, 22].* Grossly, several types are seen.

*1. Nodular ulcerative carcinoma.* These lesions are usually single, occur mostly on the face, and begin as small translucent papules that remain firm and exhibit telangiectasia. They grow slowly and tend to ulcerate, which can result in tissue destruction (Fig. 25-10). They are the most common by far of the basal cell carcinomas [13, 20, 38].
*2. Superficial basal cell carcinoma.* These lesions often occur multiply, usually on the trunk. They are lightly pigmented, erythematous, and patch-like. They may resemble eczema or psoriasis [13, 20].
*3. Sclerosing basal cell carcinoma.* Morphealike epitheliomas that are yellow-white with ill-defined borders, these lesions resemble small patches of scleroderma. This type of carcinoma is most frequently associated with recurrent disease. Characteristically, one sees peripheral growth, with central sclerosis and scarring [11, 20, 38, 55] (Fig. 25-11).

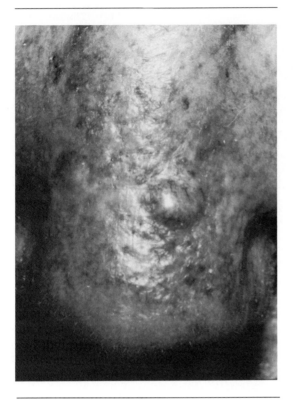

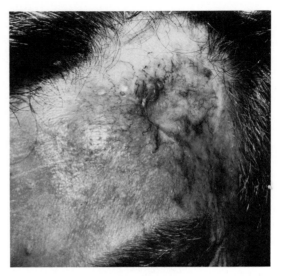

**Figure 25-11** *Sclerosing basal cell carcinoma. Note the morphea-like lesion with marked telangiectasia on the left forehead. Borders are ill-defined, which is commonly associated with recurrent disease.*

**Figure 25-10** *Nodular ulcerative basal cell carcinoma, presenting as a translucent papule, remaining firm and exhibiting telangiectasia.*

**Figure 25-12** *Pigmented basal cell carcinoma exhibiting the features of a nodular-ulcerative type with deep brownish-black pigmentation (must be differentiated from melanoma).*

**4.** *Pigmented basal cell carcinoma.* These lesions combine the features of the nodular ulcerative type with a deep brownish-black pigmentation [13] (Fig. 25-12).

**5.** *Basal cell nevus syndrome* (Fig. 25-13). Also known as Gorlin syndrome, this disorder is genetically determined, with childhood onset. Multiple basal cell carcinomas are associated with other anomalies, including skin pits on the palms of the hands and soles of the feet, epithelial jawline cysts, rib abnormalities such as splayed or bifid ribs, abnormal ectopic calcifications in the dura, and mental retardation. The disease is transmitted as an autosomal dominant with no sex linkage. Generally, the tumors have a benign clinical course until after puberty when malignant degeneration begins to take place.

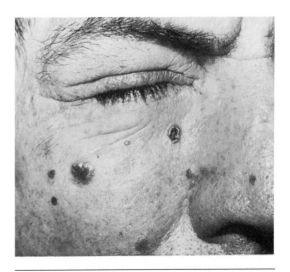

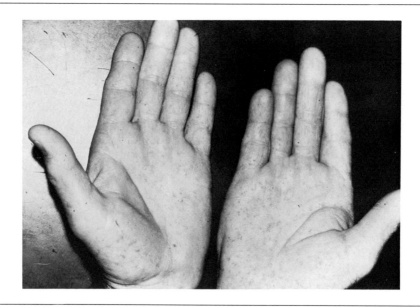

*Figure 25-13* *Multiple basal cells on the palms of the hand in a patient with basal cell nevus syndrome.*

The treatment consists in close observation with treatment of all malignancies by aggressive removal [5, 24, 39, 41].

6. *Trabecular (Merkel cell) carcinoma.* This relatively new entity resembles a basal cell carcinoma histologically and has been found to occur as a single tumor in older individuals. The tumor may be epidermal, dermal or even subcutaneous in origin, with a microscopic picture of irregularly anastomosing trabeculae and a rosette arrangement of deeply basophilic, uniform tumor cells. The name Merkel cell is derived from the fact that the tumor cells contain small granules identical to the neurosecretory granules of the epidermal Merkel cell. These tumors are aggressive and do metastasize, not only to local nodes but to viscera and bone. Treatment for cure is difficult [22, 39].

7. *Adnexal carcinoma.* These skin malignancies arise from sebaceous sweat glands. They are relatively uncommon and appear as solitary tumors in older patients. The tumors have no particular distinctive features, grow slowly, tend to recur locally after surgery, and metastasize regionally [39].

*Diagnosis*
Histopathologic confirmation is obtained with a biopsy. A variety of techniques is available. Their use depends on several factors, including size, location, clinical diagnosis, and the surgeon's preference.

1. *Curettage* is done under local anesthesia by scraping the tumor with a dermal curet. Tumor cell groups are soft and can often be curetted. Normal underlying dermis or scar tissue is hard and almost impossible to curet. When a basal cell carcinoma occurs in a scar or is morpheaform, it too is difficult to curet. The difference in ability to curet aids in differentiating normal tissue from some basal cell carcinomas [20, 28, 32, 50].

2. *Shave biopsy* of the upper half of the dermis is an excellent way to reveal a recurrent tumor, as a wide area can be sampled with minimal deformity. Rarely, a tumor is present so deeply that a shave biopsy

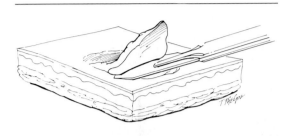

**Figure 25-14** *Technique of shave biopsy.*

does not reveal its presence. Also rarely, a basal cell carcinoma presents as a subcutaneous recurrence that would be missed by a shave biopsy; in this case, however, there is a *deep-seated nodule,* and the recurrence is easily recognized by tightly pulling normal or scarred overlying skin [9, 20] (Fig. 25-14).

3. *Punch biopsy,* 3 or 4 mm in diameter, while visualizing only a small area of the suspicious tissue, usually provides a specimen of sufficient size for diagnostic histologic evaluation. Some speculate that it might destroy the normal dermal barrier underlying a superficial tumor and possibly allow extension of the growth into deeper structures [20]. In our hands, to the best of our knowledge and after hundreds of punch biopsies, this possibility has not occurred.

4. *Excisional biopsy* is the treatment of choice when dealing with a primary basal cell carcinoma or a pigmented lesion. However, in the context of large tumors (as recurrences often are) and when location of the actual borders of the tumor are unknown, excision biopsy is impractical [13]. Deep wedge biopsy often gives valuable information regarding the depth below the dermis and breadth of infiltration of a *recurrent* basal cell carcinoma [20].

The microscopic pictures of the different basal cell carcinomas vary considerably. In all cases there is a proliferation of similar cells, oval in shape with deeply staining nuclei and scant cytoplasm. The tumors are composed of irregular masses of these basaloid cells in the dermis, with the outermost cells forming a palisading layer on the periphery. The surrounding stroma frequently exhibits a fibrous reaction. Microscopically, the nodular ulcerative type of basal cell tumor may show differentiation toward adnexal structures; there can be a solid, cystic, adenoid, or keratotic variety. The superficial basal cell carcinoma shows bands of basal cells in the dermis but maintains continuity with the overlying epidermis. This lesion is in contrast to the sclerosing basal cell carcinoma, which shows clusters and clumps of basal cells in the densely fibrotic stroma *without* continuity with the overlying epidermis, which in fact may be perfectly normal (Fig. 25-15). Severe actinic keratosis and squamous cell carcinoma may resemble basal cell carcinomas but are easily differentiated on biopsy. A deeply pigmented basal cell carcinoma may resemble a melanoma. Again, biopsy provides the diagnosis. A blue nevus can generally be differentiated from a deeply pigmented basal cell carcinoma by the character of the overlying epithelium (normal) and the duration of the tumor without growth [13, 22, 39].

It would be difficult to describe a form of treatment that has not been employed for basal cell carcinomas. Most are treated by curettage and desiccation or by simple excision as a fusiform ellipse and primary closure. Metastasis is rare. "Treatment planning assumes that the achievement of local control is synonymous with cure" [13]. Almost all of the techniques described and employed for the treatment of basal cell carcinomas have comparable cure rates if performed by experienced surgeons. Treatment depends on the age of the patient (older patients accept the scar and hypopigmentary changes associated with the prolonged healing after curettement and desiccation better than younger patients), site of disease (le-

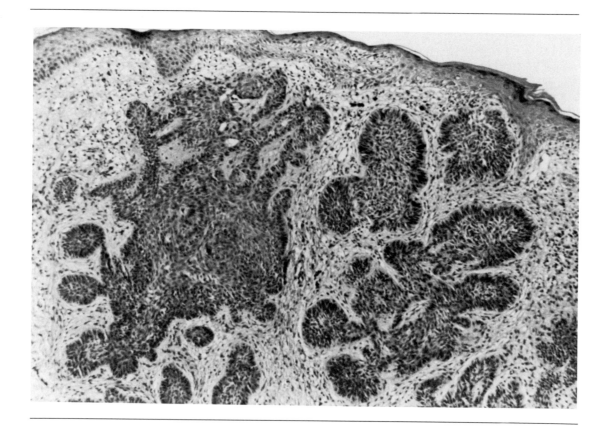

**Figure 25-15** *Basal cell carcinoma (see text).*

sions tend to recur in certain areas, e.g., the medial canthal area and the junction of cheek and nose, and may require more aggressive treatment [38], occupation (some patients' activities accept the delayed healing associated with curettement and desiccation better than others), and the type of carcinoma (nodular ulcerative carcinoma requires minimal margins and less aggressive treatment, being more exophytic than sclerosing; a sclerosing basal cell carcinoma may extend under normal epidermis [13]). In addition to curettage and desiccation, excision with margins and primary closure, closure with a skin graft, or closure with a local flap is most commonly employed [13, 20]. Other methods less widely used include cryotherapy, irradiation, and topical application or percutaneous injection of a chemical such as 5-FU.

Prognosis is excellent for this type of tumor. There are only about 150 cases of metastatic basal cell carcinoma documented in the literature [41]. If the treatment includes local eradication of the disease, the chance for cure is excellent. If submucosal extension is present as in lesions around the piriform aperture or orbit, there is less chance for a permanent cure [13, 38].

*Treatment Modalities*

CURETTAGE AND DESICCATION. Field block or infiltration anesthesia, using 1% lidocaine (Xylocaine) with epinephrine 1:200,000, is effective for most lesions. Curettage and desiccation are best suited to lesions less than 1 cm in diameter; however, surgeons experienced with the technique employ it in lesions up to 2 cm. The technique is best suited to lesions that are nodular, ulcerative, and exophytic in type [33, 50]. It is not suited to morphea-type basal cell carcinomas or to recurrent disease. Where a functional or anatomic deformity could result or where cartilage or bone are involved, other modalities are more effective. *The initial shaving preserves tissue for biopsy* [29, 33, 50]. The curet is used to remove the soft tumor down to firm dermis. Electrodesiccation follows, and curettage is repeated, with a second repeat of the sequence. The area is lightly dressed with an adhesive strip dressing, which is changed daily following a light wash. Separation of the eschar usually occurs within 2 to 3 weeks, and healing is complete shortly thereafter [20].

Other than delayed healing, hypopigmentation after healing, or the occasional pres-

ence of a hypertrophic scar, the aesthetic result is usually excellent [29, 33, 50]. As a general rule, the larger the lesion is, the greater the margin of normal tissue, with the small, nodular, ulcerative lesion requiring the least margin and the large, more extensive sclerosing basal cell lesion requiring the larger margin. The cure rate for primary treatment of basal cell carcinomas less than 2 cm in diameter by surgical excision is approximately 95 percent. For lesions 2 cm in diameter or larger, the rate falls to 90 percent [13].

SURGICAL EXCISION WITH MARGINS. Surgical excision provides an immediate pathologic inventory and an index of the adequacy of excision. The surgeon has a choice of closures—primary versus delayed primary versus secondary or delayed closure—depending on the pathology encountered and the availability of frozen section diagnosis. When frozen section diagnosis is not required, the lesion can be removed as a fusiform ellipse positioned along the lines of least skin tension. If the lesion is to be submitted for frozen section diagnosis, it is excised with a

**Figure 25-16** *Rotation-advancement flap used to close a defect of the nasal tip: status after excision of a recurrent basal cell carcinoma. A. Before treatment. B. After excision, with frozen section control. Note outline of the laterally based flap of the dorsal nasal skin. C. Six months after operation.*

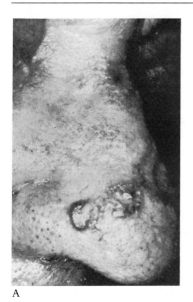
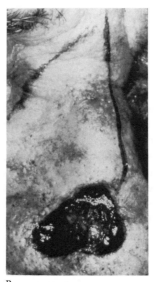
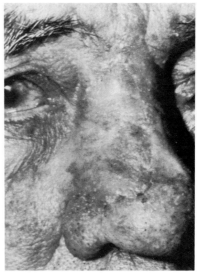

A                                  B                                  C

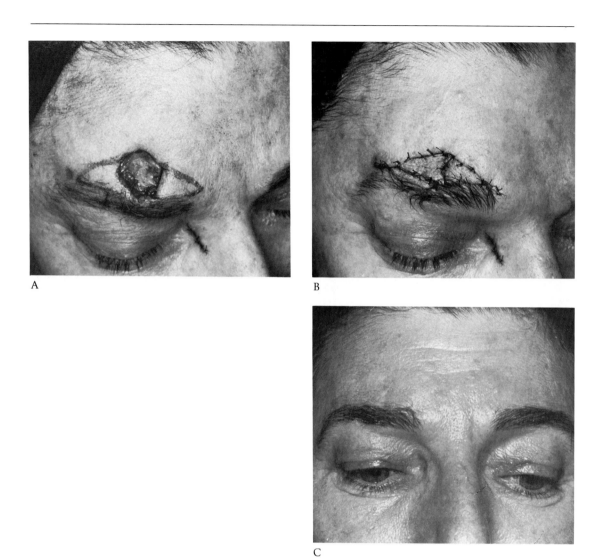

A

B

C

*Figure 25-19* *Closure of a 9 × 9 cm defect of the forehead with bilateral subcutaneous flaps. A. Immediately after excision with outline of the planned subcutaneous flaps. B. After mobilization of the flaps. C. One year after operation.*

able to any delay; Riefkohl and colleagues demonstrated a skin graft loss of 10 percent with delayed grafting [51]. A skin graft over a large area may be amenable to a tissue expansion technique several months later, allowing primary or staged excision of the graft and resurfacing with local tissue [20, 51]. In most instances the best donor sites for full-thickness skin grafts are the supraclavicular, infraclavicular, and postauricular regions. The skin grafts are thinned to remove all of the subcutaneous tissue and to

thin the dermis. The graft can be sutured in with 5-0 black silk tied over a stent dressing of fine gauze and moist cotton [20] (Fig. 25-20).

5-FLUOROURACIL. The topical use of 5-FU in concentrations higher than the 5% used

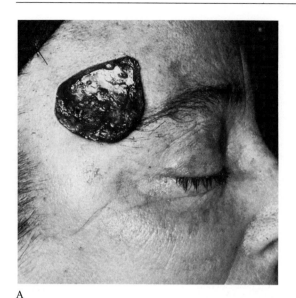
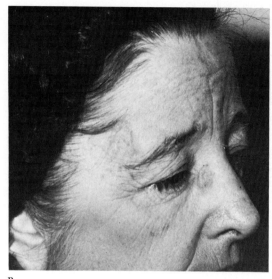

A                                    B

**Figure 25-20** *Full-thickness skin graft used to close a temple defect. A. Immediately after resection. B. One year after treatment with a thinned full-thickness skin graft from the postauricular region.*

for treating actinic keratosis has not been popular. Although Klein and others have used it in concentrations higher than 20%, it is better used as a treating and screening agent, particularly when actinic keratosis and basal cell or squamous cell carcinoma exist side by side [25]. Ryan et al. have used 5-FU in concentrations up to 20% as topical cytotoxic therapy with a degree of effectiveness [54] (Fig. 25-21). Methotrexate has also been injected into basal cell carcinoma lesions [39].

CRYOTHERAPY. For small lesions, liquid nitrogen applied with a cotton-tipped applicator or a spray that freezes the tumor and a 5-mm area of normal tissue for approximately 30 seconds has proved effective, particularly in the hands of experienced dermatologists. One sees immediate edema, exudation, subsequent necrosis, eschar formation, and healing.

Cryotherapy has, in recent years, been increasingly utilized in the management of skin tumors. It requires a degree of expertise generally not possessed by plastic surgeons, but when used appropriately it can result in high cure rates. It is associated with morbidity in terms of local tissue destruction and requires an incisional biopsy for tissue diagnosis prior to treatment [20, 64].

RADIATION THERAPY. In expert hands, low penetration x-irradiation to a tumor site in doses of 5000 R+ may be useful, particularly around orifices (eyelids, nares, and mouth) or where a scar resulting from surgical excision can be a difficult problem, as in the deltoid or sternal region. Remember that the scars from surgery generally improve with time, whereas those from radiation therapy worsen.

The late changes associated with any type of radiation treatment detract from its use in young and middle-age patients; however, it can be effective for treating an older individual with a large tumor in whom extensive resection is unacceptable or where the goal is palliation [8, 36, 45].

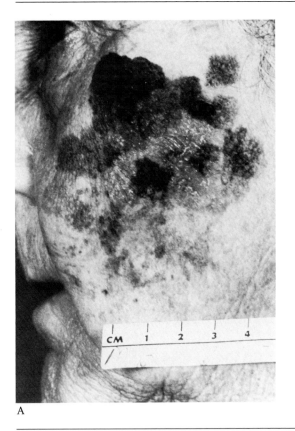

A

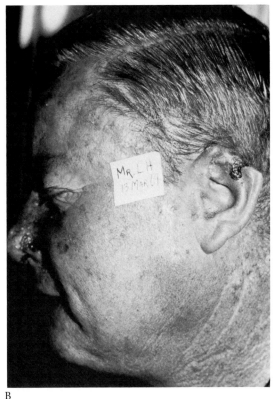

B

*Figure 25-21* Use of 5-FU to treat a large, diffuse lentigo maligna on the cheek. A. Before treatment. B. After treatment. (Courtesy of Dr. Robert F. Ryan, Tulane University.)

MOHS' FRESH FROZEN SECTION TECHNIQUE. In the original Mohs' technique (reported in 1941), zinc chloride paste was employed as a tissue fixative in situ [36, 37]. This technique now employs serial tangential excisions and is particularly useful for the treatment of sclerosing basal cell carcinomas, especially when dealing with a recurrent lesion [3, 10, 36, 37, 51–53, 65].

DERMABRASION AND CHEMICAL PEEL. Dermabrasion and chemical peel, which remove successive layers of skin, are useful for the treatment of premalignant lesions but have little use, if any, in the treatment of frank malignancies. Dermabrasion, when used over large segments of the face for multiple actinic keratoses or for the treatment of other benign tumors (trichoepithelioma, adenoides

cysticum), can be done under either local or general anesthesia. A diamond fraise wheel with a high-speed air-driven rotor gives the most satisfactory result. The error usually made in dermabrasion is not overtreatment but inadequacy of depth of abrasion. The abraded area is covered with a fine mesh gauze and then a wet dressing of fluffed gauze, which is removed within 24 to 48 hours, leaving the underlying gauze as a scaffolding for epithelialization. The crust and gauze usually come off within 7 to 8 days [58, 63].

## RECURRENT BASAL CELL CARCINOMA

Following extirpation, 5-year recurrence rates of 0 to 9 percent for primary tumors and of up to 47 percent for recurrent basal cell carcinoma have been reported in the literature [13, 20, 35]. Such rates depend on tumor size and location, sex and age of the patient, and previous therapy [13]. The clinical types of basal cell carcinoma most likely to recur after excision are the infiltrative nodular basal cell carcinoma with a poorly defined border (Fig. 25-10) and the sclerosing, morpheaform basal cell carcinoma [20] (Fig. 25-11). The outer borders of these tumors often cannot be accurately defined by clinical examination [20, 35].

Recurrent basal cell carcinoma poses a diagnostic problem because of the altered microscopic and clinical anatomy of the involved skin. These alterations are further complicated by fibrosis secondary to prior surgical procedures or radiation therapy. Recurrent tumor is a cancer that is diagnosed within the immediate area of a previously removed basal cell carcinoma up to 5 years after the initial removal. The recurrence must have the same histopathology as the original tumor. Recurrences can be classified into three categories [20].

1. Incomplete removal diagnosed during the immediate postoperative period after careful review of the histologic tissue margins
2. Continued growth of a tumor left in the immediate area becoming clinically manifest months or years after incomplete removal
3. New tumor formation in the immediate area of the previous tumor site that cannot be differentiated from the old lesion because of proximity to the scar

Definite clinical signs that alert the physician to the possible presence of a recurrent skin cancer are as follows [20].

1. Scarring with intermittent or nonhealing ulceration

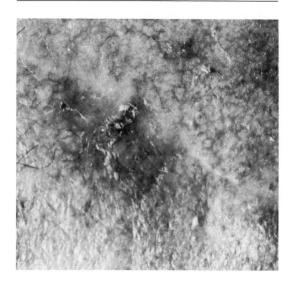

**Figure 25-22** *Recurrent basal cell lesion found in a scar that became red, scaly, and crusted 6 months after fusiform excision.*

2. A scar that becomes red, scaled, or crusted (Fig. 25-22)
3. An enlarging scar with increased telangiectasia in the adjacent area
4. Development of papule or nodule formation within the scar itself
5. Frank tissue destruction

When there is suspicion that a previously excised basal cell carcinoma has recurred, a biopsy is performed. Techniques that obtain sufficient tissue for pathologic examination and diagnosis are described above.

Surgical therapy by excision and microscopic control of tissue borders is the mainstay of treatment for recurrent basal cell carcinoma, but controversy remains. Surgical margins considered adequate for excision of a primary tumor are no longer satisfactory when dealing with recurrent cancers [12, 13, 20, 21, 46]. There is no consensus in the literature about adequacy of margins around a recurrent basal cell carcinoma. We believe that the safest method of ensuring complete excision is the individualization of each

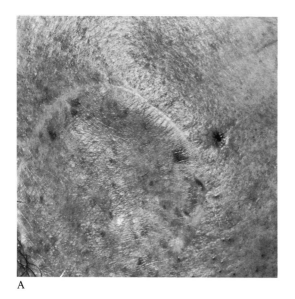

A

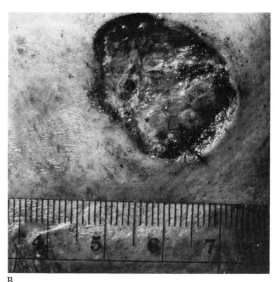

B

*Figure 25-23* *Excision with frozen section control. A. Basal cell carcinoma is adjacent to a previous full-thickness skin graft. B. Note the large excisional defect compared with the smaller defect, which appeared to be a small preoperative lesion.*

case, using microscopic examination of all borders of excised tissue to deep as well as lateral margins with meticulous frozen section control [3, 10, 13, 36, 37, 51–53, 65] (Fig. 25-23).

SQUAMOUS CELL CARCINOMA

Squamous cell carcinoma, originating from the keratinizing or malpighian (spindle) cell layer of the epithelium, is seen primarily in older patients, mostly men. Like basal cell carcinoma, its prime etiologic factor is solar radiation. In addition to radiation, however, chemicals, chronic ulcers including osteomyelitis, cytotoxic drugs, immunosuppressant drug treatment, chronic lesions, a wide variety of dermatoses, discoid lupus erythematosus, and hydradenitis suppurativa play a significant role in the development of the relatively small number of these skin cancers [44].

Hereditary factors are important, with blue-eyed, thin-skinned northern Europeans more likely to develop squamous cell carcinoma than darker, heavier-skinned individuals from southern Mediterranean areas.

Farmers, ranchers, sailors, and all those whose occupations require excessive sun exposure are predisposed to squamous cell carcinoma. Additional hereditary factors include xeroderma pigmentosum and albinism [2, 22, 23, 39].

Grossly, a solar-induced lesion (a squamous cell carcinoma) presents on a sun-exposed area. Inflammation and induration with thickening beyond the clinical lesion presages the malignant transformation of a precancerous lesion to a squamous cell carcinoma.

Two general types of squamous cell carcinoma are seen. The first is a *slow-growing* variety that is verrucous in nature and exophytic in appearance; although this type may be deeply locally invasive, it is less likely to metastasize. The second general type is more nodular and indurated, with *rapid growth* and early ulceration combined with local invasiveness (Fig. 25-24). With the histologic picture described below, the tendency to metastatic disease is greater [44].

Microscopically, masses of squamous epithelial cells invade the dermis with well differentiated keratinization. Keratin pearls surrounded by epithelial cells, as well as individual keratinizing cells, are noted (Fig. 25-25). With poorly differentiated lesions, keratinization may be minimal or absent, and there is decreased inflammatory response in the dermis (the more inflammation that is seen, the greater is the differentiation of the tumor). Intercellular bridges are absent. A poorly differentiated lesion may have a pseudoglandular appearance, and again the degree of differentiation is directly related to keratin pearl formation [39, 44].

Differential diagnosis includes actinic keratosis (induration and skin thickening would be absent), pseudoepitheliomatous hyperplasia (long history, chronic ulceration), basal cell carcinoma (biopsy and appearance), and keratoacanthoma (short history, characteristic central keratin plug, exophytic growth) [39, 44, 51].

Small, isolated skin ulcerations and lesions suspicious for carcinoma are treated conservatively for 2 to 3 weeks with a bland antibiotic ointment and a *continuous* light dressing. Any lesion that has not healed after 2 to 3 weeks of conservative treatment must be considered a skin cancer until proved otherwise. Treatment depends on the age of the patient and the size of the lesion. The various treatment techniques are covered in the section of this chapter concerning basal cell carcinoma. Older patients are treated conservatively. A lesion 1 cm or less in diameter may be treated by curettage and desiccation with histologic evaluation or simple fusiform elliptical excision. A lesion more than 1 cm in diameter may require a skin graft or flap. The location of the lesion is a factor when choosing the technique. Wound appearance may not matter so much to an older patient. A recurrent lesion is

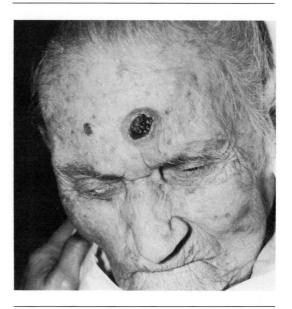

**Figure 25-24** *Nodular indurated squamous cell carcinoma.*

probably best treated by excision and skin grafting, rather than a skin flap. Dermatologists treat most squamous cell carcinomas by curettage and desiccation, whereas surgeons treat them with excision [19, 39, 44].

Microscopically controlled excision (modified Mohs' technique) is a good way to handle difficult and recurrent lesions, specifically in medial canthal and alar areas [36, 37, 53]. Radiation therapy can be effectively employed in patients over 55 years of age, particularly around the eyelids, nose, and lip [8, 43]. Radium implants have been largely replaced by irradiation employing supervoltage technique [8, 53]. Lymph node dissections are rarely performed electively, an exception being highly anaplastic tumors of more than 2 cm in patients under age 50 [44, 51].

Five to ten percent of these lesions metastasize. Those resulting from Marjolin's ulcer or xeroderma pigmentosum have a much greater tendency to metastasize than do those resulting from sun-induced skin changes [42]. The tendency for recurrence of squamous

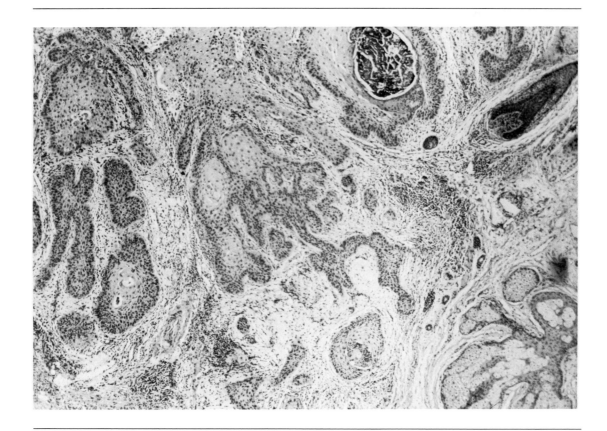

**Figure 25-25** *Squamous cell carcinoma (see text).*

cell carcinomas treated by any technique is approximately twice that for the best results treating basal cell carcinomas.

## Philosophical Approach to Treating Skin Cancers

TO BIOPSY OR NOT TO BIOPSY?
When teaching skin cancer surgery and in practice, the precept has been that excisional surgery can be based on the clinical presumptive diagnosis so long as a primary closure can be effected without resorting to other tissue rearrangement or skin grafting. Pigmented lesions are always submitted for biopsy. When a seborrheic keratosis or compound nevus is treated, the biopsy is always excisional. The office biopsy employs a 3-mm disposable punch, and the resulting wound requires no sutures.

WHEN ARE FROZEN SECTIONS NEEDED?
Most basal cell and squamous cell carcinomas can be treated without frozen section diagnosis. The treating surgeon must have sufficient diagnostic acumen to be able to differentiate between what is normal and what is disease and act accordingly. Frozen sections can be helpful when treating recurrent lesions or sclerosing basal cell carcinoma and in cases in which a lesion is in a site so critical that saving even a millimeter of tissue is important to the reconstructive effort. However, in this era of cost containment, the 20- to 30-minute wait in the operating room for the result of a frozen section may be a consideration.

HOW MUCH "MARGIN" IS NECESSARY?

The greater the exophytic character of the lesion, the less invasion there is and the less margin required. When the primary lesion is a nodule that extends into the dermis, a 2- to 3-mm margin of tissue is all that is required. It has been suggested that the margin of a morphea-type basal cell carcinoma be the first mesodermal barrier, followed by fascia, periosteum, perichondrium, and subcutaneous tissue [39]. To state categorically that the margin for basal cell carcinoma is 5 mm and for squamous cell carcinoma 10 mm, in the opinion of the authors, is an oversimplification and may actually represent a disservice to the patient. When determining margins, the type of tumor, its location, its size, whether it is recurrent, the age of the patient, and whether reconstruction is to be primary or delayed must all be considered.

INADEQUATE MARGINS: WHAT TO DO?
WHEN TO DO IT?

If there is gross tumor at the margins, it is the opinion of the authors that in most patients, particularly those under 50 years of age, reexcision is indicated. All plastic surgeons have anecdotes about tumors that were left in place with unquestionable residual disease but without clinical recurrence for years [12, 46, 51]. A problem arises when a pathologist reports that the tumor is "close" at the margins or "within one high power field of the border of the margin." In such instances it is the practice of the authors not to reexcise but to observe the patient closely, informing him or her of the potential problem. With a cooperative patient, reexcision is infrequent and close follow-up is adequate.

TO REPAIR OR NOT?

Factors that must be considered include the age and life expectancy of the patient, the presence of other disease, the histopathology of the neoplasm, the location of the lesion, the degree of disfigurement, the physical fit-

ness of the patient, the technical difficulties in repair, and the psychological fitness of the patient. Is the patient able to cope with the deformity? Covering residual disease with a local flap is a distressing situation experienced by many plastic surgeons [19]. A patient must be informed prior to surgery that the defect may be "left open to heal" or that the repair might be delayed until a later date, with reasons given for the occurrence of these two possibilities [40, 44]. Until 30 to 40 years ago, primary repair for extensive lesions was rarely considered, the idea being that a patient would live with his deformity for a year or two to be certain there was no recurrence, and repair would then be carried out. In addition to allowing time to observe for recurrent disease, this practice was intended to make the patient "appreciate the repair" that much more. It is the contention of the authors that most and possibly all skin cancers treated by a plastic surgeon can be repaired primarily, if not with a local flap then with a skin graft with consideration given to flap resurfacing at a later date for a more satisfactory cosmetic result. If repair of a facial defect is not undertaken because of any of the factors cited above, preparation must be made for construction of an adequate facial prosthesis before surgery.

SHOULD THE EXTENSIVE DEFECT
ASSOCIATED WITH A LARGER LESION
TREATED BY MOHS' FRESH TISSUE
TECHNIQUE BE SURGICALLY CLOSED?

Those experienced in Mohs' fresh tissue technique state that lesions under 2 cm heal within 3 to 4 weeks and generally are not a problem in terms of residual deformity or functional loss [40, 44].

WHAT IS THE SIGNIFICANCE
OF PERINEURAL AND
MUCOPERIOSTEAL INVASION?

Perineural, lymphatic, and mucoperiosteal invasion are usually indicative of advanced disease and worsen the prognosis for local cure and, in cases of squamous cell carcinoma, metastasis. In the opinion of the authors, the probability of cure when basal cell cancer has spread to the mucoperiosteum of the piriform aperture is remote. When such invasion is found, surgical treatment must be aggressive, with wide extirpation representing the patient's only hope for cure [39, 51].

## References

1. Ackerman, A. B. Histopathology of Keratoacanthoma. In R. Andrade, S. L. Gumport, G. L. Popkin, et al. (eds.), *Cancer of the Skin: Biology, Diagnosis, and Management.* Philadelphia: Saunders, 1976.

2. Albert, R. E. In R. Andrade, S. L. Gumport, G. L. Popkin, et al. (eds.), *Cancer of the Skin: Biology, Diagnosis, and Management.* Philadelphia: Saunders, 1976. Pp. 111–156.

3. Albright, S. D., III. Treatment of skin cancer using multiple modalities. *J. Am. Acad. Dermatol.* 7:143, 1982.

4. Allen, A. C. *The Skin: A Clinicopathologic Treatise* (2nd Ed.). Orlando: Grune & Stratton, 1967.

5. Anderson, D. E., Taylor, W. B., Falls, H. F., et al. The nevoid basal cell carcinoma syndrome. *Am. Hum. Genet.* 19:12, 1967.

6. Arons, M. S., Lynch, J. B., Lewis, S. R., et al. Scar tissue carcinoma. *Ann. Surg.* 161:170, 1965.

7. Baer, R. L., and Kopf, A. W. Keratoacanthoma. In *1962–63 Year Book of Dermatology.* Chicago: Year Book, 1963.

8. Bart, R. S., Kopf, A. W., and Petratos, M. A.: X-ray therapy of skin and cancer. In *Proceedings of the American Cancer Society.* Philadelphia: Lippincott, 1970.

9. Bart, R. S., Schrager, D., Kopf, A. W., et al. Scalpel excision of basal cell carcinomas. *Arch. Dermatol.* 114:739, 1978.

10. Barton, F. E., Jr., Cottel, W. I., and Walker, B. The principle of chemosurgery and delayed primary reconstruction in the management of difficult basal cell carcinomas. *Plast. Reconstr. Surg.* 68:746, 1981.

11. Bennett, J. P. From noli-me-tangere to rodent ulcer: The recognition of the basal cell carcinoma. *Br. J. Plast. Surg.* 28:144, 1974.

12. Burg, G., Hirsch, R. D., Konz, B., et al. Histographic surgery: Accuracy of visual assessment of the margins of basal cell epithelioma. *J. Dermatol. Surg. Oncol.* 1:21, 1975.

13. Casson, P. Basal cell carcinoma. *Clin. Plast. Surg.* 7:301, 1980.

14. Chernosky, M. E. Disseminated superficial actinic porokeratosis (DSAP). *Int. J. Dermatol.* 12:152, 1973.

15. Converse, J. M. *Symposium on Diagnosis and Treatment of Craniofacial Anomalies.* New York: NYU Medical Center, 1976. Pp. 2599–2600.

16. El-Hefnawi, H., El-Nabawi, M., and Rasheed, A. Xeroderma pigmentosum. I. *Br. J. Dermatol.* 74:214, 1962.

17. Epstein, E. Fluorouracil paste treatment of thin basal cell carcinomas. *Arch. Dermatol.* 121:207, 1985.

18. Epstein, W. L., Fukuyama, K., and Epstein, J. H. Early effects of ultraviolet light on DNA synthesis in human skin in vivo. *Arch. Dermatol.* 100:84, 1969.

19. Gibson, E. W., and Lopez-Garcia, J. Basal Cell and Squamous Cell Carcinoma of the Skin. In W. C. Grabb and J. W. Smith (eds.), *Plastic Surgery.* Boston: Little, Brown, 1979.

20. Goldberg, L., Stal, S., and Spira, M. Recognition and treatment of the recurrent basal cell carcinoma. *Ann. Plast. Surg.* 1983.

21. Gooding, C. A., White, G., and Yatuhashi, M. Significance of marginal extension in excised basal cell carcinoma. *N. Engl. J. Med.* 273:923, 1965.

22. Gordon, D., and Silverstone, H. *Cancer of the Skin: Biology, Diagnosis and Management.* Philadelphia: Saunders, 1976. Pp. 405–436.

23. Gordon, D., and Silverstone, H. Worldwide Epidemiology of Premalignant and Malignant Cutaneous Lesions. In R. Andrade, S. L. Gumport, G. L. Popkin, et al. (eds.), *Cancer of the Skin: Biology, Diagnosis, and Management.* Philadelphia: Saunders, 1976.

24. Howell, J. B., Anderson, D. E., and McClendon, J. L. The basal cell nevus syndrome. *J.A.M.A.* 190:274, 1964.

25. Klein, E., Stoll, H. L., Jr., Milgrom, H., et al. Tumors of the skin. XII. Topical 5-fluorouracil for epidermal neoplasma. *J. Surg. Oncol.* 3:331, 1971.

26. Klostermann, G. F. Effects of 5-fluorouracil (5-FU) ointment on normal and diseased skin: Histological findings and deep action. *Dermatologica* 140(suppl. 1):47, 1970.

27. Knox, J. M., and Joseph, L. M. Bowen's Disease and Erythroplasia. In R. Andrade, S. L. Gumport, G. L. Popkin, et al. (eds.), *Cancer of*

*the Skin: Biology, Diagnosis, and Management.* Philadelphia: Saunders, 1976.

28. Kopf, A. W. Keratoacanthoma—clinical aspects. In R. Andrade, S. L. Gumport, G. L. Popkin, et al. (eds.), *Cancer of the Skin: Biology, Diagnosis, and Management.* Philadelphia: Saunders, 1976.

29. Kopf, A. W., Bart, R. S., Schrager, D., et al. Curettage and electrodesiccation treatment of basal cell carcinoma. *Arch. Dermatol.* 113:439, 1977.

30. Litwin, M. S., et al. Topical chemotherapy of cutaneous malignancy of the head and neck. *South Med. J.* 62:556, 1969.

31. Lynch, H. T. Skin, heredity, and cancer. *Cancer* 24:277, 1969.

32. Martin, H., Strong, E., and Spiro, R. H. Radiation induced cancer of the head and neck. *Cancer* 25:61, 1970.

33. McDaniel, W. E. Surgical therapy for basal cell epitheliomas by curettage only. *Arch. Dermatol.* 114:1491, 1978.

34. McDonald. *J. Am. Womens Assoc.* 22:235, 1967.

35. Menn, H., Robin, P., Kopf, A. W., et al. The recurrent basal cell epitheliomas. *Arch. Dermatol.* 103:628, 1971.

36. Mohs, F. E. Chemosurgery: A microscopically controlled method of cancer excision. *Arch. Surg.* 42:279, 1941.

37. Mohs, F. E. Chemosurgery for skin cancer. *Arch. Dermatol.* 112:211, 1976.

38. Moore, J. R. Treatment of cicatrixing basal cell carcinomas. *Plast. Reconstr. Surg.* 47:371, 1971.

39. Moschella, S. L., and Hurley, H. J. Tumors of the Skin. In *Dermatology.* Vol. 2. Philadelphia: Saunders, 1985.

40. Moscona, R., Pnini, A., and Hirschowitz, B. In favor of healing by secondary intention after excision of medial canthal basal cell carcinoma. *Plast. Reconstr. Surg.* 2:189, 1983.

41. Murphy, K. J. Metastatic basal cell carcinoma with squamous appearance in the naevoid basal cell carcinoma syndrome. *Br. J. Plast. Surg.* 28:331, 1975.

42. Novick, M., Gard, D., Hardy, S. B., et al. Burn scar carcinoma: A review and analysis of 46 cases. *J. Trauma* Vol. 17, 1977.

43. Paletta, F. X. Erythroplasia of Queyrat. *Plast. Reconstr. Surg.* 23:195, 1959.

44. Paletta, F. X. Squamous cell carcinoma of the skin. *Clin. Plast. Surg.* 7:313, 1980.

45. Parker, R. G. Selective use of radiation therapy for neoplasms of the skin. *Clin. Plast. Surg.* 7:337, 1980.

46. Pascal, R. R., Hobby, L. W., Lattes, R., et al. Prognosis of "incompletely excised" versus "completely excised" basal cell carcinoma. *Plast. Reconstr. Surg.* 41:328, 1968.

47. Pickrell, K. Xeroderma pigmentosa. *Plast. Reconstr. Surg.* 49:83, 1972.

48. Pinkus, H. Actinic Keratosis—Actinic Skin. In R. Andrade, S. L. Gumport, G. L. Popkin, et al. (eds.), *Cancer of the Skin: Biology, Diagnosis, and Management.* Philadelphia: Saunders, 1976.

49. Pinkus, H., and Mehregan, A. H. Premalignant skin lesions. *Clin. Plast. Surg.* 7:289, 1980.

50. Reymann, F. Treatment of basal cell carcinoma of the skin with curettage.

51. Riefkohl, R., Pollack, S., and Georgiade, G. S. A rationale for the treatment of difficult basal cell and squamous cell carcinomas of the skin. *Ann. Plast. Surg.* 15(2):99, 1985.

52. Rigel, D. S., et al. Predicting recurrence of basal cell carcinoma treated by microscopically controlled excision: A recurrence index score. *J. Dermatol. Surg. Oncol.* 7:807, 1981.

53. Robins, P. Chemosurgery: My 15 years of experience. *J. Dermatol. Surg. Oncol.* 7:779, 1981.

54. Ryan, F. R., Litwin, M. S., Reed, R. S., et al. The use of 5-fluorouracil cream to define suitable areas. *Plast. Reconstr. Surg.* 46:433, 1970.

55. Salasche, S. J., and Amonette, R. A. Morphea form basal cell epitheliomas: A study of subclinical extensions in a series of 51 cases. *J. Dermatol. Surg. Oncol.* 7:387, 1981.

56. Shenaq, S. Personal communication.

57. Snyderman, R. K., and Starzynski, T. E. Clinical application of 5-fluorouracil in the treatment of skin lesions. *Plast. Reconstr. Surg.* 41:54, 1968.

58. Spira, M., and Stal, S. Dermabrasion, Chemical Peel, and Collagen Injection. In N. G. Georgiade (ed.), *Essentials of Plastic and Maxillofacial and Reconstructive Surgery.* Baltimore: William & Wilkins, 1986.

59. Spira, M., Freeman, B., Arfai, P., et al. Clinical comparison of chemical peeling dermabrasion and 5-FU for senile keratosis. *Plast. Reconstr. Surg.* 46:61, 1970.

60. Stal, S., and Spira, M. *Dermatology for Plastic Surgeons Handbook.* Presented at Annual

ASPRS Meeting, October 1984.

61. Stal, S., and Spira, M. Subcutaneous Pedicle Flap in Head and Neck Reconstruction. In P. Ward and W. Berman (eds.), *Plastic and Reconstructive Surgery of the Head and Neck: Proceedings of the Fourth International Symposium.* St. Louis: Mosby, 1985.

62. Stal, S., and Spira, M. In R. Stark (ed.), *Developmental Deformities of Skin.* New York: Churchill Livingstone, 1986.

63. Stal, S., and Spira, M. In R. Rudolph (ed.), *Dermabrasion and Chemical Peel. Biological Causes and Clinical Solutions.* St. Louis: Mosby, 1986.

64. Torre, E. Dermatological cryosurgery—a progress report. *Cutis* 11:782, 1973.

65. Tromovitch, T., and Stegman, S. Microscopic-controlled excision of cutaneous tumors. *Cancer* 41:653, 1978.

# 26

*Malignant Melanoma*

*Abdul-Ghani Kibbi*
*Arthur J. Sober*
*Martin C. Mihm, Jr.*

Interest in cutaneous malignant melanoma has increased greatly over the years. Such interest has resulted in early diagnosis, improved ability to assess the histologic and biologic attributes of this potentially lethal form of cutaneous cancer, and a reduction in the extent of surgical therapy needed.

Of great concern are the epidemiologic data, which have shown a continuous rise in the incidence of this neoplasm [41]. This increase is not confined to the United States but extends to many other countries where cancer registries have been kept [21, 53, 97]. About 28,000 people were estimated to develop malignant melanoma in 1989 and 6000 people to die of the disease [69, 91]. This number accounts for about three-fourths of all deaths from cutaneous cancers. In addition, data derived from the National Cancer Institute's Surveillance Epidemiology and End Result System indicated an 80 percent increase in the incidence of melanoma between 1973 and 1980 [88]. This rate of increase is second only to that of lung cancer in women over the same time period.

To reduce the mortality associated with this increasing incidence of melanoma, it is essential that new tumors be identified at an early phase in their natural history when prognosis for cure by surgical removal is excellent [51]. Indeed, a series of studies from various centers in which pigmented lesion clinics are established have shown that the clinical appearance of primary cutaneous melanoma is usually distinctive [12] and that at least 90 percent of the tumors can be diagnosed [40]. A high index of suspicion is essential to achieve this high frequency of diagnosis [26].

It is the aim of this chapter to present an approach to the management of cutaneous melanoma based on the clinical, histologic, and biologic features of this disease. Current precepts in the surgical management of this neoplasm are also discussed, based on the practice at this institution as well as a review of the literature.

## Clinical Diagnosis of Malignant Melanoma

The clinical diagnosis of primary cutaneous malignant melanoma rests on a careful history and physical examination [26]. Emphasis is placed on recognition of certain salient features in the early developmental phases of the tumor, at which point its surgical eradication is possible and cure is complete. An appreciation of the early gross characteristics of melanoma has resulted from a study of cases in the Pigmented Lesion Clinics in

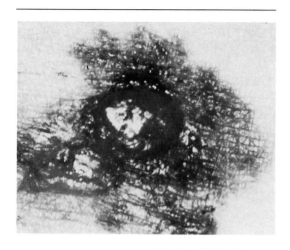

*Figure 26-1 A nodule within a superficial spreading malignant melanoma heralds the onset of deep invasion. The presence of white areas within a lesion that is otherwise composed of shades of brown, blue, or red is compatible with regression.*

## VARIEGATION OF COLORS AND PIGMENT PATTERN

Variegation of color is a frequent characteristic of malignant melanoma, especially of the superficial spreading type [67]. In one study [103] color change was observed in 55 percent of level II lesions. Colors heralding malignant transformation include shades of red, white, and blue in an otherwise brown or black lesion (Fig. 26-1). Red discoloration is often indicative of an inflammatory host response, sometimes associated with ongoing regression [65]. In certain instances the lesion is predominantly red-brown. White areas may be observed within the tumor that represent either an amelanotic component or partial or total regression of the lesion. The presence of gray-white in the center of a pigmented lesion always arouses strong suspicion [65]. Rarely, a halo of hypo- or depigmentation is noted around a pigmented lesion. If such a halo is asymmetric and the lesion is disposed asymmetrically therein, a malignant melanoma must be strongly suspected [65]. In some instances the lesion shows variegation in shades of brown and

many centers throughout the United States [67].

Based on clinical observation and photographic documentation of 150 patients seen at the Pigmented Lesion Clinic of the Massachusetts General Hospital from 1965 to 1973, Mihm et al. [67] described the clinical signs that facilitate diagnosis of early malignant melanoma. In order of importance, the positive signs that suggest malignant change include variegated color and pigment pattern, irregular border, and irregular surface. These signs have been confirmed by other investigators [95]. Additionally, several other criteria, such as lesion asymmetry [26], increase in size [71], increase in height, ulceration, tenderness [103], itching, and bleeding [70], have been documented in the literature. In our experience, ulceration and bleeding are telltale signs of advanced lesions and are consequently of little value for early recognition [103].

*Figure 26-2 This nodular malignant melanoma exhibits uniform discoloration, a glossy surface, and a faint rim of erythema around the border.*

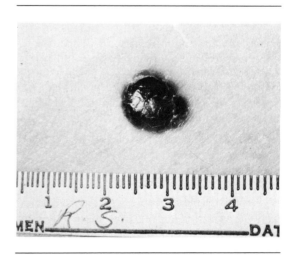

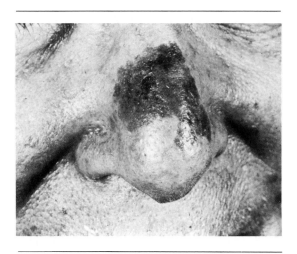

**Figure 26-3** *A tan, freckle-like lesion on an exposed surface of the body is exhibited in this precursor stage of lentigo maligna melanoma.*

tan, and other colors may be absent.

Although an irregular, haphazard array of colors is the hallmark sign of cutaneous melanoma, it is not observed in some tumors (Fig. 26-2), particularly those of the nodular type [38, 67]. These lesions are usually bluish-black, bluish-gray, or bluish-red. At times, nodular melanoma presents as an irregularly shaped blue-black plaque rather than a nodule [65]. This pattern of presentation is rare, and the clue to its diagnosis derives from other ancillary features such as surface and border characteristics. With regard to lentigo maligna (Fig. 26-3) and its invasive counterpart, lentigo maligna melanoma, variation in color occurs but is usually in shades of brown to dark brown except for the invasive component itself, which may be brown, black, blue-black, or rarely amelanotic [65]. Areas of regression may be noted as white, gray-white, or blue-gray spots within the lesion. As to acral lentiginous melanoma, the type occurring in the palms and soles, the haphazard array of color is characteristic [6]. These lesions often present as a tan or brown flat stain on the palm or sole (Fig. 26-4).

Subungual melanoma [76, 98], an infrequent type of acral lentiginous melanoma, prefers the great toe or thumb. This tumor often displays striking variegation in color. Streaks of brown, blue, white, and tan may be present under the nail. When these color changes are not obvious, the diagnosis of melanoma is more difficult. A high index of suspicion must be maintained when new pigmented lesions develop in the nail region; biopsy of the nail bed in the area of the nail fold and matrix is recommended.

IRREGULAR BORDER

An irregular border with pseudopods, a notch, or even a butterfly configuration is frequently noted in superficial spreading melanoma and lentigo maligna melanoma [67, 95]. This irregularity is more prominent as the lesion increases in size; it appears to result either from an uneven radial growth phase or from patchy spontaneous regression [66]. In contrast, nodular melanomas are often symmetric and display no border irregularity [65]. This uniform configuration may hamper the physician's ability to make the

**Figure 26-4** *Acral lentiginous melanoma exhibits a haphazard array of tan or brown color. The white areas within the lesion represent areas of regression.*

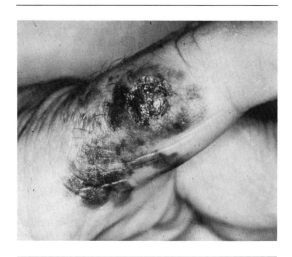

ritated seborrheic keratoses are clinically indistinguishable [92].

## HEMANGIOMA/PYOGENIC GRANULOMA

Amelanotic nodular melanoma can be confused with the vascular proliferations called hemangioma and pyogenic granuloma [65]. Pyogenic granuloma is a form of hemangioma that is characteristically dome-shaped and has a gray tinge with occasional blue-black or black flecks at its base. With its history of rapid growth and after careful inspection, the lesion can usually be differentiated from melanoma. With regard to the other types of hemangiomas, distinction is made on the basis of arrested growth, the reddish-brown or purple color, and the presence of profuse bleeding if traumatized [71].

## *Biopsy*

Acceptable methods for obtaining a biopsy specimen from a malignant melanoma have been the subject of great debate [52, 84]. It is imperative that all pigmented lesions with clinical features suspicious of melanoma be biopsied. The biopsy can be either excisional or incisional [47]. With either technique, the specimen must be full thickness, extending into the subcutaneous tissue to permit accurate microstaging of the lesion [17, 28]. Curet or shave biopsies are not recommended because such procedures often provide either inadequate amounts or poor quality of tissue, either of which conditions may reduce the accuracy of the histologic diagnosis [24, 48, 101]. Furthermore, such practices may preclude the determination of thickness should the diagnosis be melanoma. Because survival of patients with cutaneous melanoma has been shown to be inversely related to the thickness of the neoplasm [9], it is evident that a properly represented biopsy specimen is required for precise histopathologic assessment, without which further management maneuvers may be hampered.

## EXCISIONAL BIOPSY

An excisional biopsy is the procedure of choice [64]. This method is advocated by pathologists because it removes the tumor in toto and supplies the complete specimen for analysis. Unless the entire specimen is available, maximum tumor thickness cannot always be determined in a reliable fashion.

The excision outlines are usually marked so that a narrow margin (2 mm) of normal-appearing skin around the visible lesion is included [28]. The direction of the biopsy incision is selected so that primary closure is feasible and skin grafts are avoided at this primary stage of management. The physician performing the biopsy orients the specimen by placing a suture at a designated margin. This tactic is highly desirable because it allows the surgeon to determine if further ablative surgery is necessary in a given lesion.

## INCISIONAL BIOPSY

The incisional biopsy is an alternative if a lesion is large or anatomically located in a surgically sensitive area such as the nose or the periorbital or digital region [47]. In these cases an incisional biopsy specimen representative of the lesion is most desirable. Such a specimen can usually be obtained from either the most palpable portion of the tumor or the darkest part of the tumor in a flat lesion. The selected area must include tissue that is anticipated to contain the thickest portion of the tumor. However, whether the center or the edge is biopsied is determined on the basis of what the clinician considers to be the most representative portion of the tumor [48].

## EXCISIONAL VERSUS INCISIONAL BIOPSY FOR MELANOMA

Although an excisional biopsy is superior to an incisional one, evidence in the literature shows no statistically significant difference in survival rates based on biopsy type when data are analyzed by thickness categories [47]. One retrospective study, however, has demonstrated that an incisional biopsy has a deleterious effect on the patient's outcome [77]. The main argument against incisional biopsies stems from the concern that tumor cells may be dislodged into the surrounding skin structures. At the present time, the value of establishing an early diagnosis seems to outweigh the theoretical but unsubstantiated concern that incisional biopsy worsens prognosis.

The advantages of an excisional biopsy, as mentioned above, are the following: (1) It provides the pathologist with a complete specimen that permits microstaging the tumor. (2) If the lesion proves to be benign, the excision constitutes treatment.

## Histogenetic Types of Malignant Melanoma

During the late 1960s and early 1970s Clark et al. [13, 14] proposed that malignant melanoma can be divided into four or more distinct types, based on clinical and pathologic features. This concept has been challenged by Ackerman [1], who believed that all types of melanoma are basically the same lesion. Although it is true that we may be looking at different parts of a spectrum rather than at truly discrete subsets, this classification has stood the test of time, as it represents distinctive entities with different epidemiologic aspects, developmental biology, and behavioral characteristics [20]. Two principal phases of tumor development are recognized [13, 70]. The horizontal or so-called *radial growth phase* is characterized by proliferation of neoplastic melanocytes within the epidermis, with single cell invasion of the papillary dermis, that clinically forms a radially spreading patch. This phase is observed in superficial spreading melanoma, lentigo maligna melanoma, and acral lentiginous melanoma. The second phase, referred to as the *vertical growth phase,* exhibits proliferation of malignant melanocytes that take origin from the epidermis and expand the papillary dermis with invasion of the reticular

dermis and subcutaneous fat. The vertical growth phase presents usually as an expansile nodule [34]. Nodular melanoma is a prime example of such a growth pattern in which the vertical growth phase is observed without an associated radial growth phase. Subsequent discussion describes the clinical and histologic varieties of malignant melanoma as they relate to their patterns of growth.

### LENTIGO MALIGNA MELANOMA

Lentigo maligna melanoma (LMM) is a distinct entity and appears predominantly on the sun-exposed skin of older patients [59]. It accounts for about 5 to 12 percent of all melanomas [44]. Women are reportedly affected more frequently than men [57]; although a study by Koh et al. [39] has shown no sex predilection. The malar and temple regions of the face are the most common sites of LMM. On few occasions, it occurs in skin of other sites, e.g., the limbs, but usually only when there is significant solar damage [58]. The noninvasive phase of the tumor, called lentigo maligna, presents as an irregularly colored, tan-brown, freckle-like macule that in time undergoes changes in size and color. This lesion characteristically persists for a long period, even up to 30 or 40 years, before it acquires the capacity of invasion [70]. The appearance of raised, usually brown-black areas or even nodules heralds the onset of the invasion.

Histologically, in the noninvasive areas [58] of LMM and throughout lentigo maligna (LM), the lower portion of the epidermis shows proliferation of atypical melanocytes, as single cells and as nests (Fig. 26-7). The atypical melanocytes, unlike those of superficial spreading melanoma, arise in an atrophic epidermis, nearly always overlying a sun-damaged dermis, and frequently extend downward along hair follicles (Fig. 26-8). A distinctive feature of the LM–LMM process is the pleomorphism of melanocytes; bizarre, large, irregularly fusiform and dendritic melanocytes are often arranged adjacent to nor-

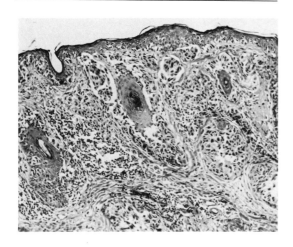

**Figure 26-7** *In this photomicrograph of lentigo maligna melanoma, nests and single cells of atypical pleomorphic melanocytes are confined to the dermoepidermal junction. The epidermis is atrophic.*

mal melanocytes. The vertical growth phase [37, 58] of LMM is often composed of spindle cells and is frequently accompanied by a desmoplastic response and invasion of neurovascular bundles (Fig. 26-8). This infiltration along neurovascular compartments is worthy of recognition, as it frequently leads to difficulty in histologic determination of the extent of certain lesions.

SUPERFICIAL SPREADING MELANOMA
Superficial spreading melanoma (SSM) is the most common type of melanoma in Caucasians and constitutes around 50 to 70 percent of all lesions in many published series [13, 14, 58, 65, 66]. These lesions occur anywhere on the skin surface but are commonly seen on the back and legs in women and on the trunk in men [94]. The mean age of affected patients is the early forties with no sex predilection in North American or Australian series. Their radial growth phase is shorter than that of LMM patients and is of the order of 6 months to 7 years [13, 51].

Early in its evolution, SSM is generally a flat to slightly raised, irregularly colored lesion [68]. It also exhibits border and surface irregularities. As the vertical growth phase begins, it gives rise to a prominent nodular component that may also be accompanied by surface ulceration [71].

Histologically, the radial growth phase [68] of this type of melanoma shows proliferation of rather uniformly atypical melanocytes singly and in nests at all levels of the epidermis (Fig. 26-9). Focal invasion by single cells or small nests in the papillary dermis may also be seen. The fully evolved malignant melanocytes are of the epithelioid cell type (Fig. 26-10), although the cytologic composition varies in certain instances. At times the epidermis is hyperplastic or papillomatous. A dense, superficial infiltrate of mature lymphocytes and papillary dermal fibrosis—possible evidence of regression—may accompany the radial growth phase.

Superficial spreading melanoma is often referred to as pagetoid melanoma [56] be-

**Figure 26-8** *Spindle cell-shaped malignant cells extend along the hair follicles in LM–LMM. A chronic inflammatory cell infiltrate is interspersed between invasive nests within the dermis.*

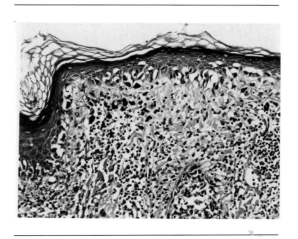

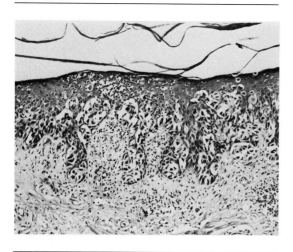

**Figure 26-9** *The radial growth phase of superficial spreading melanoma shows malignant epithelioid cells in the epidermis with characteristic pagetoid spread.*

cause of the tendency of the tumor cells to be disposed at all levels of the epidermis, a pattern reminiscent of Paget's disease. Indeed, when SSM occurs adjacent to the nipple or on the genitalia, differentiation between a malignant melanoma and Paget's disease can be a difficult task. The use of special stains for epithelial mucin is helpful for distinguishing between the two diseases [23].

With the onset of the vertical growth phase [68], malignant melanocytes fill the papillary dermis and extend downward to the reticular dermis and subcutaneous tissue. The cells of the invasive component may be similar to or different from those of the radial growth phase. Occasionally, small cell or nevocellular patterns of malignant melanocytes are observed and may be confused with a preexisting nevus. One helpful feature then is the tendency of nevi to show "maturation"; i.e., with increasing depth, cells in the deeper portion of a nevus are typically smaller and less pleomorphic in their cytologic appearance.

## NODULAR MELANOMA

Nodular melanoma is the second most common type of melanoma, comprising 10 to 20 percent of tumors [51]. In contrast to LMM and SSM, it is more aggressive and has a shorter clinical phase before deep invasion has occurred. This melanoma can affect any age group and is commonly seen on the trunk, head, or neck [71]. It is important to realize that not all melanomas with nodules on their surface are in fact nodular melanomas and that a nodule may develop on an SSM or an LMM. A distinct polypoid variant of nodular melanoma [55] is particularly aggressive and has a cauliflower appearance. This aggressiveness, however, has been primarily attributed to the greater thickness of these lesions rather than to their configuration [78].

Microscopically, nodular melanoma is a tumor in which no intraepidermal growth occurs without associated dermal invasion [58]. By convention, the epidermal melanocytic proliferation does not extend beyond

**Figure 26-10** *A large dyshesive nest of intraepidermal malignant epithelioid cells is seen. Note the single cell invasion of the papillary dermis, a feature associated with the onset of the vertical growth phase of malignant melanoma.*

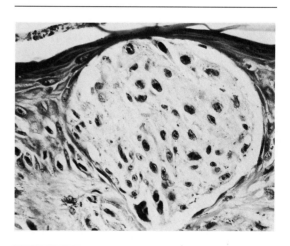

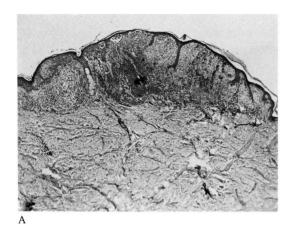

A

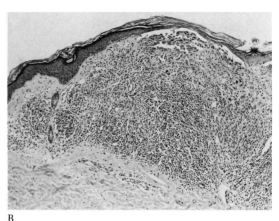

B

three rete ridges from the site of invasion (Fig. 26-11).

## ACRAL LENTIGINOUS MELANOMA

Acral lentiginous melanoma (ALM) occurs on the palms or soles [22, 43, 74], in mucosa or mucocutaneous junctions [86], or underneath the nail beds [22]. It accounts for 2 to 8 percent of all melanomas in Caucasians [50] and is reported in a substantially higher proportion (35 to 60 percent) of dark-skinned patients such as Blacks [79], American Indians [7], Orientals [87], and Hispanics. The evolution of this type of melanoma is unknown but appears to range from a few months to several years, with an average of 2.5 years according to Milton et al. [71]. Both radial and vertical growth phases are observed in ALM; however, unlike LMM and SSM, the vertical growth phase may follow the radial growth phase more rapidly in ALM [13]. Older individuals are frequently affected, with the tumor occurring, on average, during the sixties [71]. Although in some respects this tumor resembles LMM, its biologic behavior appears to be more aggressive, and it is more likely to metastasize [71].

Histologically, ALM in the radial growth

**Figure 26-11** *A. Proliferation of melanocytes in the dermis without significant radial spread beyond the invasive component typifies the growth pattern of nodular melanoma. B. Inflammatory cells interspersed between atypical melanocytes are seen in association with this tumor of nodular melanoma.*

phase [68] shows large, uniformly atypical melanocytes along the dermoepidermal junction within a hyperplastic epidermis (Fig. 26-12). This array of melanocytes is similar to that observed in lentigo maligna. Often these melanocytes have prominent dendrites that may extend even up to the granular cell layer of the epidermis. The dermal invasive component is typically composed of spindle cells (Fig. 26-13), but as is the case for all types of melanoma, the cytologic appearance of the tumor cells can be variable and this finding, in itself, is not diagnostic of any specific type. Like LMM, the vertical growth phase of ALM may show neuroidal fascicles or a desmoplastic response [37]. Indeed, desmoplasia in lesions occurring on the sole of the foot can be erroneously diagnosed as fibromatosis, and insinuation of tumor cells along neurovascular bundles must be care-

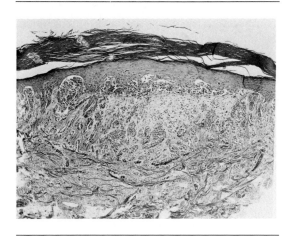

**Figure 26-12** *Arising in a hyperplastic epidermis and filling the papillary dermis are uniformly atypical melanocytes. These features are observed in acral lentiginous melanoma.*

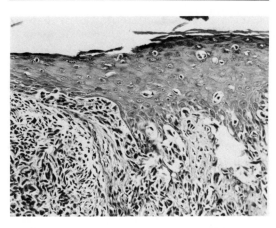

**Figure 26-13** *The invasive component of this acral lentiginous melanoma is made up of spindle-shaped cells. In the epidermis these atypical cells exhibit dendritic extensions.*

fully scrutinized to adequately evaluate margins of resection [37].

## Clinical and Pathologic Features as Prognostic Indicators

Multiple prognostic factors have been shown to predict the outcome of cutaneous melanoma. Accurate appreciation of these variables is a sine qua non for the choice of appropriate treatment procedures. With the use of multivariate models, it is now possible to identify with considerable accuracy the patients who are apt to do well and those who have lesions that are associated with low survival rates. Also, more advanced multivariable analysis techniques have enabled identification of the dominant prognostic variables while eliminating the factors that derive their significance by correlating with other dominant ones [5]. A review of the literature has shown that different lists of important prognostic factors have been generated from different centers studying melanoma. The

following is a summary of clinical and pathologic variables that influence prognosis.

CLINICAL VARIABLES
Clinical features of independent prognostic significance, in some studies, include the sex and age of the patient, site of the lesion, and evidence of a preexisting nevus.

*1. Sex of the patient.* Numerous studies have shown that female patients with melanomas have a better survival than men. In one study it was shown that there was little difference in survival of male and female patients for the first 2 years after diagnosis [54, 81, 89]. The survival curves for both sexes, however, diverged at this point, and 5-year survival for men was only 83 percent versus 90 percent for women [82]. One explanation for the better survival rates in women is that their melanomas occur more commonly on the extremities (a more favorable prognostic site) and are less commonly ulcerated [6].
*2. Age of the patient.* In most series pa-

tients younger than 50 years of age have a better prognosis than those older than 50 years of age [51, 54, 81]. The 5-year survival in the two groups is 90 and 84 percent, respectively. This difference in survival has been attributed to several factors, including lesion thickness [49] and hormone profiles [90]. Levine et al. [49] have demonstrated that older patients have thicker melanomas than do young ones. Thus the median thickness for melanoma patients in their third decade has been 1.1 mm, whereas it was 1.5 mm for those in the fifth decade and 2.8 mm for those in the seventh decade [6]. Furthermore, the changing hormonal milieu at menopause may account for the adverse effect of age on prognosis. Older individuals also have a higher percentage of acral lentiginous melanoma, which has on average a worse prognosis [22].

*3. Anatomic site of the lesion.* Several reports have demonstrated that patients with melanomas at certain anatomic sites have a worse prognosis than those with lesions at other sites. Scalp, hands, and feet appear to be areas of worse prognosis after correcting for thickness, and the remainder of the extremities appears to be a favorable location [18, 19]. Rogers and colleagues have shown that midline lesions as well as those in the acral areas on both the upper and lower extremities carry a poorer prognosis even after accounting for lesion thickness [83]. These investigators have divided body surface areas into high-, intermediate-, and low-risk sites, each of which is associated with a different 5-year survival. The biologic significance of this partition is as yet unknown and awaits further research work to validate its importance.

*4. Preexisting nevus.* It is well established that many cutaneous malignant melanomas arise in association with preexisting melanocytic nevi [16, 80]. In a study by Friedman and associates, approximately 20 percent of patients with malignant melanomas have had histologic evidence of a preexisting melanocytic nevus [27]. These melanomas have

been observed to have a better prognosis compared to those of similar thickness without an associated melanocytic nevus.

PATHOLOGIC VARIABLES
A plethora of pathologic variables that influence prognosis for malignant melanoma patients has been reported.

*1. Tumor thickness.* Tumor thickness is the dominant pathologic variable with significant prognostic implication [9, 10]. In fact, most other prognostic variables, e.g., level of invasion, derive their predictive ability from being highly correlated with tumor thickness [9, 48]. Thickness is measured vertically from the stratum granulosum to the deepest invasive part of the tumor using an ocular micrometer [9]. Such a measurement gives an inverse correlation between 5-year survival and tumor thickness. Breslow has suggested that lesions with a thickness of less than 0.76 mm have an excellent prognosis, whereas those with a thickness of more than 3 mm have a poor prognosis [10]. Other investigators have defined thickness subsets that better correlate with survival. The 5-year survival for thickness ranges of 0.85 mm or less, 0.86 to 1.69 mm, 1.70 to 3.64 mm, and 3.65 or more were 99, 94, 78, and 42 percent, respectively [93].

There are many important advantages of thickness microstaging that bear directly on the treatment approach. The risk of local recurrence, satellites, and in-transit metastases is directly correlated to thickness [6]. Hence tumor thickness can relatively accurately predict the risk of metastases and may then enable us to distinguish patient groups who may possibly benefit from elective lymph node dissection and adjuvant immunotherapy.

*2. Level of invasion.* Five levels of invasion have been described [14]: level I, melanoma cells are confined to the epidermis and its appendages; level II, melanoma cells extend into the papillary dermis; level III, melanoma cells fill the papillary dermis and impinge on the reticular dermis; level IV, melanoma cells invade the reticular dermis; and level V, melanoma cells invade the subcutaneous tissue. The 5-year survival in one study of 1130 patients with malignant melanoma has been reported to be 98, 96, 94, 78, and 44 percent for levels I, II, III, IV, and V, respectively [82].

**3.** *Ulceration.* The presence of ulceration in a lesion is regarded as a poor prognostic sign [63]. Measurement of the width of the ulceration with an ocular micrometer delineated two prognostic subgroups [6]. In one subgroup, ulcers less than 6 mm in width were associated with lesions thinner than those with ulcer widths of more than 6 mm; the 5-year survival rates for these two groups were 44 percent versus 5 percent. It is important to realize that ulcerated lesions tend to be thicker than nonulcerated ones; however, this factor remains significant even after lesion thickness has been taken into account [81].

**4.** *Growth pattern.* At present, all types of melanoma carry the same prognosis if compared thickness for thickness [6]. The observation that ALM patients have a lower survival rate is attributed to a delay in the diagnosis [22].

**5.** *Lymphocytic reaction.* The presence or absence of an inflammatory cell response around the tumor is, in most series [6, 58, 61], not regarded as being significant, although in one series the presence of a brisk lymphocytic response was associated with a decreased incidence of local recurrence [15].

**6.** *Mitotic activity.* Increased mitotic activity has been reported to add to thickness in determining prognosis [85]. In general, thick tumors have more mitoses than their thinner counterparts, and nodular melanomas have more mitotic activity than SSMs [60]. The mitotic rate must be recorded in the pathologist's report, as it may give some idea of the aggressiveness of the tumor.

**7.** *Other features.* Several other features are considered in some studies to have prognostic significance, including regression [99,

102], vascular invasion [45], cell type, pigmentation [62], and microscopic satellites [33]. Microscopic satellites in primary melanomas that are more than 1.50 mm thick are often associated with microscopic nodal metastasis in clinically negative nodes compared to those of similar thickness and without satellites [33].

## Management

### HISTORY AND PHYSICAL EXAMINATION

Once the diagnosis of cutaneous malignant melanoma is established, a plan of management is formulated with the hope of providing the best chance for cure [24, 38]. A complete history and physical examination are obtained. The history includes questions concerning lesion duration and history of change, the patient's history, the familial history of malignant melanoma and dysplastic nevi, and a review of any previous cutaneous surgery. The latter is particularly relevant in the evaluation of those 2 to 9 percent of patients with metastatic disease and an unknown primary site [11, 35]. Symptoms related to extracutaneous sites must be carefully assessed or elicited, as they may supply clues to the presence of widespread disease.

For the physical examination, the patient's skin must be examined completely. Careful inspection of the scalp, mucous membranes, and body folds is an important part of this examination. The skin is palpated for the presence of subcutaneous nodules. All potential lymph-node-bearing areas are carefully palpated. Any enlarged nodes, especially those with a firm consistency, must be strongly suspected of harboring metastatic disease. The specificity of this clinical assessment is approximately 70 percent; false positives result from nodal enlargement due to inflammation [4].

### LABORATORY INVESTIGATION

The routine preoperative laboratory investigation includes only the hospital requirements for surgery [24]. Abnormalities found on these examinations are further investigated by appropriate tests. Routine scans are not ordered unless suggested by an abnormality in the history and physical examination [24].

SURGERY
*Definitive Excision of the*
*Primary Tumor*
Wide surgical excision of the primary tumor is generally performed in all instances following the histopathologic diagnosis of melanoma. The purpose of a wide local excision is to remove any residual melanoma cells from the site and thus prevent local recurrence [48]. In the past, the recommended extent of the excision beyond the clinically visible perimeter of the lesion or beyond the scar from the site of the original biopsy has varied widely from 2 to 15 cm [17]. Currently, the resection margin we recommend is 1.0 cm for primary tumors less than 1.0 mm in thickness and 2.5 to 3.0 cm for all others [24, 38].

The depth of excision remains controversial. It is maintained that leaving the deep fascia intact improves survival and results in fewer subsequent metastases to the draining lymph nodes [36]. Proponents of such policy argue that the deep fascia acts as a barrier to continued lymphatic spread. In a study of 202 patients with stage I melanoma of the trunk and proximal limbs, there was no demonstrable statistical difference in the incidence of subsequent recurrence in 5-year survival time, whether the fascia was excised or left in situ [73]. It appears that removal of the fascia does not affect survival.

After local excision of the tumor with adequate margins, the wound is closed by direct apposition [64] if possible. If direct apposition is not feasible, a split-thickness skin graft, obtained from a donor site distant from the melanoma, or rotation flaps are used to cover the defect [28]. The results of studies comparing closure without grafting to closure with split-thickness skin grafts have shown no difference in incidence of local recurrence [3] or 5-year survival time [2].

*Elective Regional Lymph*
*Node Dissection*
Elective regional lymph node dissection (ERND) is one of the most controversial aspects of the surgical management of malignant melanoma [4, 64]. The debate centers around stage I melanoma patients in whom there is no clinical evidence of metastatic disease. In general, nonrandomized trials have demonstrated a benefit from ERND, whereas the randomized ones have failed to show benefit [64]. For those institutions that recommend ERND, the decision whether to embark on this elective procedure or to adopt a wait-and-see policy depends on several prognostic factors that can provide estimates of the risk for occult metastasis at regional nodes and distant sites. Once these prognostic variables are taken into consideration, clinical stage I melanoma patients can then be categorized according to their biologic risk for metastases and a rational surgical treatment strategy designed for each patient.

In our institution [24, 38], ERND is performed only after consideration of several factors: age, tumor type, location, tumor thickness, and patient preference. This procedure is not done in older patients and those in poor health. Individuals with tumors located in areas with potentially multiple lymph node drainage, especially on the torso, are not subject to lymphadenectomy. It is recommended that in these instances a technetium scan be performed, if lymph node dissection is contemplated, to delineate the basins of drainage. The presence of multiple drainage pathways would eliminate prophylactic dissection from consideration. Patients with lentigo maligna melanoma, regardless of tumor thickness and in the absence of clinically suspicious regional nodes, are exempt from ERND. Because the likelihood of microscopic tumor deposits in the regional nodes increases with increasing primary tumor thickness, we reserve ERND for a group of patients with tumor thickness of 1.7 mm to 2.0 mm. For tumors with thicknesses of more than 3.6 or 4.0 mm, the risk of metastasis is high, excluding any possible benefit from ERND. Finally, the patient's preference is considered in the decision in view of the controversial aspect of this procedure.

*Therapeutic Lymph Node Dissection*
A therapeutic lymphadenectomy is the universal treatment for patients with clinically suspicious lymph nodes [17, 32]. The number of lymph nodes with histopathologically detectable tumor is determined by the pathologist, as there is prevailing evidence to suggest that if one lymph node is involved with tumor the 8-year probability of survival is less than 40 percent, whereas when two or more lymph nodes are involved a lower survival rate is expected [4].

FOLLOW-UP
Once surgery is over, the need for periodic follow-up is emphasized [24, 38]. The risk of developing metastatic disease is likewise addressed. No patient with cutaneous melanoma can be assured of absolute cure, as even patients with thin primary melanomas occasionally develop metastases [75, 100, 104]. Patients are seen at 3- to 6-month intervals for 2 years, 6-month intervals for 3 subsequent years, and annually thereafter. All pigmented lesions are evaluated and if sufficiently atypical clinically are serially photographed to detect any changes that might herald a melanomatous transformation. Excessive sun exposure is discouraged. The use of sunscreens with a high sun protection factor (SPF) number is recommended. An annual chest radiograph is routinely advocated except for patients with tumors of less than 1 mm. The patient is advised to have his or her first-degree relatives examined, as the risk of melanoma developing in these kindreds is statistically significant [29, 31].

# References

1. Ackerman, A. B. Malignant melanoma: A unifying concept. *Hum. Pathol.* 11:591, 1980.
2. Aitken, D. R., Clausen, K., Klein, J. P., et al. The extent of primary melanoma excision: A reevaluation—how wide is wide? *Ann. Surg.* 198:634, 1983.
3. Bagley, F. H., Cady, B., Lee, A., et al. Changes in the clinical presentation and management of malignant melanoma. *Cancer* 47:2126, 1981.
4. Balch, C. M. Surgical management of regional lymph nodes in cutaneous melanoma. *J. Am. Acad. Dermatol.* 3:511, 1980.
5. Balch, C. M., Soong, S-J., Murad, T. M., et al. A multifactorial analysis of melanoma. II. Prognostic factors in patients with stage I (localized) melanoma. *Surgery* 86:3431, 1979.
6. Balch, C. M., Soong, S-J., Shaw, H. M., et al. An Analysis of Prognostic Factors in 4000 Patients with Cutaneous Melanoma. In C. M. Balch and G. W. Milton (eds.), *Cutaneous Melanoma: Clinical Management and Treatment Results Worldwide.* Philadelphia: Lippincott, 1985.
7. Black, W. C., and Wiggins, C. Melanoma among southwestern American Indians. *Cancer* 55:2899, 1985.
8. Bondi, E. E., Elder, D. E., Guerry, D., IV, et al. Skin markings in malignant melanoma. *J.A.M.A.* 250:503, 1983.
9. Breslow, A. Thickness, cross-sectional areas and depth of invasion in the prognosis of cutaneous melanoma. *Ann. Surg.* 172:902, 1970.
10. Breslow, A. Prognostic factors in the treatment of cutaneous malignant melanoma. *J. Cutan. Pathol.* 6:208, 1979.
11. Chang, P., and Knapper, W. H. Metastatic melanoma of unknown primary. *Cancer* 49:1106, 1982.
12. Clark, W. H., Jr. Clinical diagnosis of cutaneous malignant melanoma. *J.A.M.A.* 236:484, 1976.
13. Clark, W. H., Jr., Ainsworth, A. M., Bernardino, E. A., et al. The developmental biology of primary human malignant melanomas. *Semin. Oncol.* 2:83, 1975.
14. Clark, W. H., Jr., From, L., Bernardino, E. A., et al. The histogenesis and biologic behavior of primary human malignant melanomas of the skin. *Cancer Res.* 29:705, 1969.
15. Codman, A. J. Malignant melanoma: A re-

view of ten years' experience in Glasgow, Scotland. *Cancer* 23:1190, 1969.

16. Crucioli, V., and Stilwell, J. The histogenesis of malignant melanoma in relation to pre-existing pigmented lesions. *J. Cutan. Pathol.* 9:396, 1982.

17. Davis, N. C., Mcleod, G. R., Beardmore, G. L., et al. Primary cutaneous melanoma: A report from the Queensland Melanoma Project. *CA* 26:80, 1976.

18. Day, C. L., Sober, A. J., Kopf, A. W., et al. A prognostic model for clinical stage I melanoma of the lower extremity: Location on foot as independent risk factor for recurrent disease. *Surgery* 89:599, 1981.

19. Day, C. L., Sober, A. J., Kopf, A. W., et al. A prognostic model for clinical stage I melanoma of the upper extremity: The importance of anatomic subsites in predicting recurrent disease. *Ann. Surg.* 193:436, 1981.

20. Elder, D. E., Jucovy, P. M., and Clark, W. H., Jr. Melanoma classification: A testable hypothesis. *Am. J. Dermatopathol.* 4:443, 1982.

21. Elwood, J. M., and Lee, J. A. H. Recent data on the epidemiology of malignant melanoma. *Semin. Oncol.* 2:149, 1975.

22. Feibleman, C. E., Stoll, H., and Maize, J. C. Melanomas of the palm, sole, and nailbed. *Cancer* 46:2492, 1980.

23. Fisher, E. R., and Beyer, F., Jr. Differentiation of neoplastic lesions characterized by large vacuolated intraepidermal (pagetoid cells). *Arch. Pathol.* 67:140, 1959.

24. Fitzpatrick, T. B., and Sober, A. J. Primary Malignant Melanoma of the Skin. In T. T. Provost and E. R. Farmer (eds.), *Current Therapy in Dermatology*. Philadelphia: B. C. Decker, 1985.

25. Friedman, R. J., Heilman, E. R., Rigel, D. S., et al. The Dysplastic Nevus: Clinical and Pathologic Features. In D. S. Rigel and R. J. Friedman (eds.), *Dermatologic Clinics: Symposium on Melanoma and Pigmented Lesions*. Philadelphia: Saunders, 1985.

26. Friedman, R. J., Rigel, D. S., and Kopf, A. W. Early detection of malignant melanoma: The role of physical examination and self-examination of the skin. *CA* 35:130, 1985.

27. Friedman, R. J., Rigel, D. S., Kopf, A. W., et al. Favorable prognosis for malignant melanomas associated with acquired melanocytic nevi. *Arch. Dermatol.* 119:455, 1983.

28. Goldsmith, H. S. Melanoma: An overview. *CA* 29:194, 1979.

29. Greene, M. H. Dysplastic nevus syndrome. *Hosp. Pract.* 19:91, 1984.

30. Greene, M. H., Clark, W. H., Jr., Tucker, M. A., et al. Acquired precursors of cutaneous malignant melanoma. *N. Engl. J. Med.* 312:91, 1985.

31. Greene, M. H., Clark, W. H., Jr., Tucker, M. A., et al. High risk of malignant melanoma in melanoma-prone families with dysplastic nevi. *Ann. Intern. Med.* 102:458, 1985.

32. Guiliano, A. E., Mosely, H. S., and Morton, D. L. Clinical aspects of unknown primary melanoma. *Ann. Surg.* 191:98, 1980.

33. Harrist, T. J., Rigel, D. S., Day, C. L., Jr., et al. Microscopic satellites are more highly associated with regional lymph node metastases than is primary melanoma thickness. *Cancer* 53:2183, 1984.

34. Imber, M. J., and Mihm, M. C., Jr. Biological and Prognostic Significance of Vertical Growth Phase Characteristics in Malignant Melanoma. In Mihm, M. C. et al. (eds.), *Pathobiology and Recognition of Malignant Melanoma*. Baltimore: Williams & Wilkins, 1988. Pp. 19–34.

35. Ironside, P., Pitt, T. T. E., and Rank, B. K. Malignant melanoma: Some aspects of pathology and prognosis. *Aust. N.Z. J. Surg.* 47:70, 1977.

36. Kenady, D. E., Brown, B. W., and McBride, C. M. Excision of underlying fascia with a primary malignant melanoma: Effect on recurrence and survival rates. *Surgery* 92:615, 1982.

37. Kibbi, A., Bronstein, B. R., Sober, A. J., et al. The Vertical Growth Phase of Malignant Melanoma. In M. M. Wick (ed.), *Symposium on Brown Pigmentation*. Tokyo: University of Tokyo Press, 1986.

38. Kibbi, A., Sober, A. J., Fitzpatrick, T. B., et al. Diagnosis and management of malignant melanoma. *Compr. Ther.* 12:222, 1987.

39. Koh, H. K., Michalik, E., Sober, A. J., et al. Lentigo maligna melanoma has no better prognosis than other types of melanoma. *J. Clin. Oncol.* 2:994, 1984.

40. Kopf, A. W., Mintzis, M., and Bart, R. S. Diagnostic accuracy in malignant melanoma. *Arch. Dermatol.* 111:1291, 1975.

41. Kopf, A. W., Rigel, D. S., and Friedman, R. J.

The rising incidence and mortality rate of malignant melanoma. *J. Dermatol. Surg. Oncol.* 8:760, 1982.

42. Kraemer, K. H., and Greene, M. H. Dysplastic nevus syndrome: Familial and Sporadic Precursors of Cutaneous Melanoma. In D. S. Rigel and R. J. Friedman (eds.), *Dermatologic Clinics: Symposium on Melanoma and Pigmented Lesions.* Philadelphia: Saunders, 1985.

43. Krementz, E. T., Reed, R. J., Coleman, W. P., III, et al. Acral lentiginous melanoma: A clinicopathologic entity. *Ann. Surg.* 195:632, 1982.

44. Larsen, T. E., and Grude, T. H. A retrospective histological study of 669 cases of primary cutaneous malignant melanoma in clinical stage I. *Acta Pathol. Microbiol. Scand. [A]* 87:255, 1979.

45. Larsen, T. E., and Grude, T. H. A retrospective histological study of 669 cases of primary cutaneous malignant melanoma in clinical stage I. IV. The relation of cross-sectional profile, level of invasion, ulceration, and vascular invasion to tumor type and prognosis. *Acta Pathol. Microbiol. Immunol. Scand. [A]* 87:131, 1979.

46. Lederman, J. S., Fitzpatrick, T. B., and Sober, A. J. Skin markings in the diagnosis and prognosis of cutaneous melanoma. *Arch. Dermatol.* 120:1449, 1984.

47. Lederman, J. S., and Sober, A. J. Does biopsy type influence survival in clinical stage I cutaneous melanoma? *J. Am. Acad. Dermatol.* 13:983, 1985.

48. Lee, Y. N. Diagnosis, treatment, and prognosis of early melanoma: The importance of depth of microinvasion. *Ann. Surg.* 191:87, 1980.

49. Levine, J., Kopf, A. W., Rigel, D. S., et al. Correlation of thickness of superficial spreading malignant melanoma and ages of patients. *J. Dermatol. Surg. Oncol.* 7:311, 1981.

50. Lopansri, S., and Mihm, M. C., Jr. Clinical and pathological correlation of malignant melanoma. *J. Cutan. Pathol.* 6:180, 1979.

51. Mackie, R. M., and Young, D. Human malignant melanoma. *Int. J. Dermatol.* 23:433, 1984.

52. Macy-Roberts, E., and Ackerman, A. B. A critique of techniques for biopsy of clinically suspected malignant melanomas. *Am. J. Dermatopathol.* 4:391, 1982.

53. Magnus, K. Incidence of malignant melanoma of the skin in the five Nordic countries: Significance of solar radiation. *Int. J. Cancer* 20:477, 1977.

54. Magnus, K. Prognosis in malignant melanoma of the skin: Significance of stage of disease, anatomical site, sex, age and period of diagnosis. *Cancer* 40:389, 1977.

55. Manci, E. A., Balch, C. M., Murad, T. M., et al. Polypoid melanoma, a virulent variant of the nodular growth pattern. *Am. J. Clin. Pathol.* 75:810, 1981.

56. McGovern, V. J. The classification of melanoma and its relationship with prognosis. *Pathology* 2:85, 1970.

57. McGovern, V. J. The nature of melanoma: A critical review. *J. Cutan. Pathol.* 9:61, 1982.

58. McGovern, V. J., Mihm, M. C., Jr., Bailly, C., et al. The classification of malignant melanoma and its histologic reporting. *Cancer* 32:1446, 1973.

59. McGovern, V. J., Shaw, H. M., Milton, G. W., et al. Is malignant melanoma arising in Hutchinson's melanotic freckle a separate disease entity? *Histopathology* 4:235, 1980.

60. McGovern, V. J., Shaw, H. M., Milton, G. W., et al. Prognostic significance of the histological features of malignant melanoma. *Histopathology* 3:385, 1979.

61. McGovern, V. J., Shaw, H. M., Milton, G. W., et al. Lymphocytic Infiltration and Survival in Malignant Melanoma. In A. B. Ackerman (ed.), *Pathology of Malignant Melanoma.* New York: Masson, 1981.

62. McGovern, V. J., Shaw, H. M., Milton, G. W., et al. Cell Type and Pigment Content as Prognostic Indicators in Cutaneous Malignant Melanoma. In A. B. Ackerman (ed.), *Pathology of Malignant Melanoma.* New York: Masson, 1981.

63. McGovern, V. J., Shaw, H. M., Milton, G. W., et al. Ulceration and prognosis in cutaneous malignant melanoma. *Histopathology* 6:399, 1982.

64. Meyer, K. L., and Kenady, D. E. The surgical approach to primary malignant melanomas. *Surg. Gynecol. Obstet.* 160:379, 1985.

65. Mihm, M. C., Jr., Clark, W. H., Jr., and Reed, R. J. The clinical diagnosis of malignant melanoma. *Semin. Oncol.* 2:105, 1975.

66. Mihm, M. C., Jr., Clark, W. H., Jr., and From, L. The clinical diagnosis, classification and

histogenetic concepts of the early stages of cutaneous malignant melanoma. *N. Engl. J. Med.* 284:1078, 1971.

67. Mihm, M. C., Jr., Fitzpatrick, T. B., Lane Brown, M. M., et al. Early detection of primary cutaneous malignant melanoma: A color atlas. *N. Engl. J. Med.* 289:989, 1973.

68. Mihm, M. C., Jr., and Lopansri, S. A review of the classification of malignant melanoma. *J. Dermatol.* 6:131, 1979.

69. Mihm, M. C., Jr. Introduction. In M. C. Mihm Jr., et al. (eds.), *Pathobiology and Recognition of Malignant Melanoma.* Baltimore: Williams & Wilkins, 1988. Pp. 1–8.

70. Milton, G. W. Clinical diagnosis of malignant melanoma. *Br. J. Surg.* 55:755, 1968.

71. Milton, G. W., Balch, C. M., and Shaw, H. M. Clinical Characteristics. In C. M. Balch and G. W. Milton (eds.), *Cutaneous Melanoma: Clinical Management and Treatment Results Worldwide.* Philadelphia: Lippincott, 1985.

72. Nicholls, E. M. Development and elimination of pigmented moles, and the anatomical distribution of primary malignant melanoma. *Cancer* 32:191, 1973.

73. Olsen, G. Removal of fascia: Cause of more frequent metastases of malignant melanomas of the skin to regional lymph nodes? *Cancer* 17:1159, 1964.

74. Paladugu, R. R., Winberg, C. D., and Yonemoto, R. H. Acral lentiginous melanoma: A clinicopathologic study of 36 patients. *Cancer* 52:161, 1983.

75. Paladugu, R. R., and Yonemoto, R. H. Biologic behavior of thin malignant melanomas with regressive changes. *Arch. Surg.* 118:41, 1983.

76. Patterson, R. H., and Helwig, E. B. Subungual malignant melanoma: A clinicopathologic study. *Cancer* 55:2074, 1980.

77. Rampen, F. H. J., van Houten, W. A., and Hop, W. C. J. Incisional procedures and prognosis in malignant melanoma. *Clin. Exp. Dermatol.* 5:313, 1980.

78. Reed, K. M., Bronstein, B. R., Mihm, M. C., Jr., et al. Prognosis of polypoidal melanoma is determined by primary tumor thickness. *Cancer* 57:119, 1986.

79. Reintgen, D. S., McCarty, K. M., Jr., Cox, E., et al. Malignant melanoma in black American and white populations: A comparative review. *J.A.M.A.* 248:1856, 1982.

80. Rhodes, A. R., Harrist, T. J., Day, C. L., Jr., et al. Dysplastic melanocytic nevi in histologic association with 234 cutaneous melanomas. *J. Am. Acad. Dermatol.* 9:563, 1983.

81. Rigel, D. S., and Friedman, R. J. Malignant Melanoma. In J. Stone (ed.), *Dermatologic Allergy and Immunology.* St. Louis: Mosby, 1984.

82. Rigel, D. S., Rogers, G. S., and Friedman, R. J. Prognosis of Malignant Melanoma. In D. S. Rigel and R. J. Friedman (eds.), *Dermatologic Clinics: Symposium on Melanoma and Pigmented Lesions.* Philadelphia: Saunders, 1985.

83. Rogers, G. S., Kopf, A. W., Rigel, D. S., et al. Effect of anatomy location on prognosis in patients with clinical stage I melanoma. *Arch. Dermatol.* 119:644, 1983.

84. Roses, D. F. Proper biopsy of a lesion suspected of being a malignant melanoma. *Am. J. Dermatopathol.* 4:475, 1982.

85. Schmoekel, C., and Braun-Falco, O. Prognostic index in melanoma. *Arch. Dermatol.* 114:871, 1978.

86. Seiji, M., Mihm, M. C., Jr., Sober, A. J., et al. Malignant melanoma of the palmar-plantar-subungual-mucosal type: Clinical and histopathological features. *Pigment Cell.* 5:94, 1979.

87. Seiji, M., and Takahashi, M. Acral melanoma in Japan. *Hum. Pathol.* 13:607, 1982.

88. Shambaugh, E., Greene, M. H., and Young, J. Unpublished data, 1985.

89. Shaw, H. M., McGovern, V. J., Milton, G. W., et al. Histologic features of tumors and the female superiority in survival from malignant melanoma. *Cancer* 45:1604, 1980.

90. Shaw, H. M., Milton, G. W., Farago, G., et al. Endocrine influences on survival from malignant melanoma. *Cancer* 42:669, 1978.

91. Silverberg, E. Cancer statistics, 1989. *CA* 39:3, 1989.

92. Sober, A. J. Personal communication, 1986.

93. Sober, A. J., Day, C. L., Jr., Kohn, H. K., et al. Melanoma in the Northeastern United States: Experience of the Melanoma Clinical Cooperative Group. In C. M. Balch and G. W. Milton (eds.), *Cutaneous Melanoma: Clinical Management and Treatment Results Worldwide.* Philadelphia: Lippincott, 1985.

94. Sober, A. J., Fitzpatrick, T. B., and Mihm, M.

C., Jr. Primary melanoma of the skin: Recognition and management. *J. Am. Acad. Dermatol.* 2:179, 1980.

95. Sober, A. J., Fitzpatrick, T. B., Mihm, M. C., Jr., et al. Early recognition of cutaneous melanoma. *J.A.M.A.* 242:2795, 1979.

96. Subrt, P., Jorizzo, J. L., Apisarnthanarax, P., et al. Spreading pigmented actinic keratosis. *J. Am. Acad. Dermatol.* 8:63, 1983.

97. Swerdlow, A. J. Incidence of malignant melanoma of the skin in England and Wales and its relationship to sunshine. *Br. Med. J.* 2:1324, 1979.

98. Takematsu, H., Obata, M., Tomita, Y., et al. Subungual melanoma: A clinicopathologic study of 16 Japanese cases. *Cancer* 55:2725, 1985.

99. Trau, H., Kopf, A. W., Rigel, D. S., et al. Regression in malignant melanomas. *J. Am. Acad. Dermatol.* 8:363, 1983.

100. Trau, H., Rigel, D. S., Harris, M. N., et al. Metastases of thin melanomas. *Cancer* 51:553, 1983.

101. Wagner, D. E., and Cullen, R. A. Primary melanoma: Pitfalls in diagnostic biopsy techniques and interpretations. *Am. J. Surg.* 148:99, 1984.

102. Wanebo, H. J., Cooper, P. H., and Hagar, R. W. Thin (≤1 mm) melanomas of the extremities are biologically favorable lesions not influenced by regression. *Ann. Surg.* 201:499, 1985.

103. Wick, M. M., Sober, A. J., Fitzpatrick, T. B., et al. Clinical characteristics of early cutaneous melanoma. *Cancer* 45:2684, 1980.

104. Woods, J. E., Soule, E. H., and Creagan, E. T. Metastasis and death in patients with thin melanomas (less than 0.76 mm). *Ann. Surg.* 198:63, 1983.

# 27
# *Lasers*

## *Lasers in Surgery and Medicine*

*Ralph P. Pennino*

Laser is an acronym for *l*ight *a*mplification by the *s*timulated *e*mission of *r*adiation. A laser generates electromagnetic radiation at a particular wavelength and with unique properties. To use the laser effectively, efficiently, and safely, the surgeon must understand the basic principles of laser and apply them clinically. A working knowledge of these fundamentals is essential for technically proficient use of lasers and for comprehending and reproducing reported laser applications; it also enables one to help define the role of lasers in surgery.

The basic principles of the laser can be traced back to Albert Einstein who in 1917 postulated the process of stimulated emission of radiation [35]. This report laid the foundation for the work of Schawlow and Townes [84] and Vasov, who independently reported on the physical principles of the maser (*m*icrowave *a*mplification by the *s*timulated *e*mission of *r*adiation). Maiman [66] developed the first laser, a ruby laser, in 1960. It was followed by the development of the neodymium doped yttrium-aluminum-garnet (Nd:YAG) laser in the near-infrared region (1.06 μm) by Johnson in 1961, the argon laser at various wavelengths in the blue-green visible spectrum by Bennett et al. in 1962, and the carbon dioxide ($CO_2$) laser in the far-infrared spectrum (10.6 μm) in 1964 by Patel et al. Since that time we have seen an explosion in the use of lasers in the fields of voice and video communications, material processing, military applications, and more recently medicine and surgery.

### *Laser Physics*

What is electromagnetic radiation? The most familiar form is the visible light that surrounds us. However, it is just a small part of the electromagnetic spectrum. As shown in Figure 27-1, the electromagnetic spectrum starts with long wavelengths and short frequencies, and includes long radio waves, short radio waves, television, and so on. Moving up the scale toward shorter wavelengths and increasing frequencies, we enter the infrared region where there are two of the three most common lasers in use today, the carbon dioxide laser and the neodym-

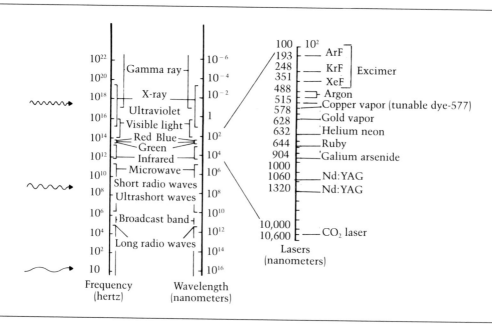

**Figure 27-1** *Electromagnetic spectrum.*

ium:YAG laser. This region is followed by the visible light region of the spectrum, which includes the argon laser. Moving further on there are still shorter wavelengths and higher frequencies, including the ultraviolet rays, x-rays, and gamma rays. The wavelength of the laser helps determine its biologic effect on tissue.

In its simplest form, an atom is composed of a nucleus with protons and neutrons surrounded by electrons (Fig. 27-2) [30, 41, 42, 78, 79]. The electrons can travel in designated energy levels or orbitals about the nucleus, as described by the laws of quantum mechanics. When all the electrons are in the lowest energy level, it is designated the *ground state.* To understand stimulated emission of radiation, let us use the hydrogen atom, which has one electron, as an example. When in its ground state this electron can absorb a photon, or radiant energy, and move to a higher energy level. This process is known as *absorption* and the atom is now in an "excited state." From its higher energy level the electron can return to a lower orbital or ground state and in the process

give off a photon of energy with a particular frequency and wavelength. This process is known as *spontaneous emission of radiation.* The frequency of this emission is related to the energy difference between the two orbitals. Frequency (v) and wavelength (λ) are inversely related according to: $c = \lambda v$ ($c$ = speed of light, $3 \times 10^{10}$ cm/sec). The excited state is analogous to a stretched, coiled spring. In a stretched state it is unstable and wishes to revert back to its resting state.

If an atom in an excited state is struck by a photon (whose energy is equal to the difference between two orbitals), it results in the electron returning to a lower orbital with the release of two photons of the same energy and wavelength and in phase with each other. This process is known as *stimulated emission of radiation* and serves as the basis for lasers.

The components of a laser (Fig. 27-3) include the laser medium, the power source known as the pumping system, the resonator or optical tube, and a delivery system [24,

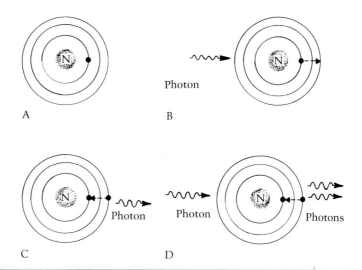

**Figure 27-2** *A. Composition of an atom.*
*B. Absorption. C. Spontaneous emission.*
*D. Stimulated emission. (N = nucleus.)*

30, 41, 78]. The laser medium is a source that generates a particular wavelength. The laser medium can be one of four types for clinical or experimental use: solid state, gas, dye, and semiconductor. A solid state laser consists of the laser medium in a solid matrix. These lasers include the ruby (694.3 nm) and Nd:YAG (1064 nm) lasers. A gas laser uses one gas or a gas mixture and includes the helium-neon (HeNe) (637.8 nm), $CO_2$ (10,600 nm), krypton, and argon (various wavelengths) lasers. A dye laser uses an organic dye that can be varied in type and concentration to provide different wavelengths in and around the visible spectrum. It is called a "tunable" dye laser. Semiconductor lasers, most recently introduced into medicine, are low-powered lasers that consist of two layers of semiconductor material sandwiched together. The gallium arsenide diode laser (830 and 904 nm) is an example of a semiconductor laser.

The laser medium is placed in a long optical cavity or resonator (see Fig. 27-3) that has parallel mirrors at either end. The rear mirror is 100 percent reflective, and the front mirror is partially transmitting. To produce stimulated emission the laser medium must be "pumped" into an excited state. When the number of atoms in the excited state is greater than the number of atoms in the ground state, a condition called *population inversion* occurs. Population inversion is necessary for a generation of stimulated emission. Various power sources are used to "pump" the laser medium into an excited state, including electrical sources (used for $CO_2$ lasers); optical sources (xenon or krypton flash lamps for the Nd:YAG laser); and even other lasers (the argon laser may be used as a power source for the pumped dye laser).

When population inversion occurs, various excited atoms undergo spontaneous emission of radiation and emit photons of a particular wavelength and frequency. Some strike other excited atoms and undergo stimulated emission of radiation and emit two photons. This process continues throughout the optical cavity. Those photons not parallel to the long axis of the optical cavity are lost as heat. The small percentage of photons that are given off parallel to the long axis form an energy wave, which strikes the mirrors and reflects back and forth, continuing the process of

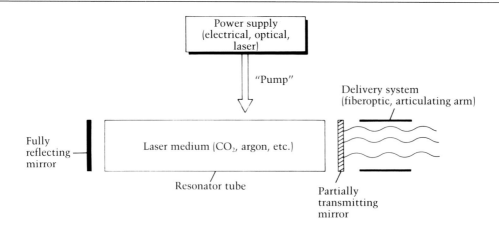

*Figure 27-3 Laser components.*

stimulated emission in the optical resonator. This energy can be released in a controlled fashion via the partially transmitting mirror and is then transmitted through a delivery system (i.e., fiberoptic, articulating arm with mirrors) to the target tissue. A lens or other focusing device (i.e., sapphire tips) may be incorporated at the end of the delivery system to focus the energy to a small spot size.

Laser emission has three properties (Fig. 27-4) that make it unique and valuable. First, it is monochromatic, or of one wavelength, determined by the laser medium. Second, all the electromagnetic radiation generated is spatially and temporally coherent, i.e., the energy waves are in phase with

*Figure 27-4 Properties of laser.*

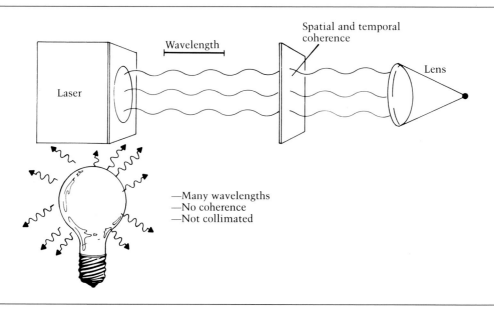

each other in both space and time. Third, the waves are collimated, which means they do not appreciably diverge from each other over distance (unlike a flashlight). This property allows the laser emission to be focused to a fine spot size. These three properties distinguish the laser from all other sources of electromagnetic radiation. Lasers are a source of intense energy that can be transmitted over distances with little loss of power and that can be focused to small spot sizes of tremendous power density.

## Power Density

The concept of power density, or irradiance, is one of the most important principles a surgeon must comprehend and apply when using the laser. *Power density* is the number of watts per unit area and is usually expressed as watts per square centimeter (Fig. 27-5). The area is defined as the area of the working spot generated at the laser–tissue interface. Therefore power density (PD) is equal to:

$$\frac{watts}{area} = \frac{watts}{\pi r^2}$$

where r = the radius of the spot size [9, 30, 38]. Watts is a unit of power.

*Energy fluence* is the total amount of energy (joules) directed to tissue during treatment [88]. It is a product of power density and time:

$$Fluence = PD \times t = joules/cm^2$$

The power density can be manipulated via changes in the numerator or denominator of this equation. Wattage is simply controlled by adjusting the output of the laser instrument. Increasing or decreasing the wattage increases or decreases power density. The area of the spot size can be controlled by a number of variables. When a focusing system is used at the end of a delivery system (i.e., $CO_2$ freehand laser surgery) to focus the

| • Power density = $\dfrac{Watts}{Area(A)} = \dfrac{Watts}{\pi R^2}$ | | | |
|---|---|---|---|
| Lens | 50 mm | 100 mm | 200 mm |
| Radius | R | 2R | 4R |
| Area | $\pi R^2 = A$ | 4A | 16A |
| Power density | PD | PD/4 | PD/16 |

**Figure 27-5** *Relation of power density, lens focal length, and spot size.*

beam, it determines the minimum spot size. The larger the lens, the larger the spot size. For example, a 50-mm lens of a $CO_2$ laser ($TEM_{00}$) generates a focused spot size of 0.09 mm. A 125-mm lens produces a spot size of 0.22 mm. Larger lenses result in longer focusing distances, which are needed in $CO_2$ laser endoscopic surgery where the beam is focused through rigid, hollow tubes (i.e., bronchoscope, sigmoidoscope) or for microscopic procedures with varying focal lengths. The trade-off for longer focal lengths is decreased power density. Increasing the focal length increases proportionately the radius or diameter of the spot size. However, the area is increased by a factor of the square of the radius (area = $\pi r^2$). Therefore doubling the focal length results in decreasing the power density to one-fourth of the original at the same wattage (see Fig. 27-5). Increasing the focal length by a factor of four results in $1/16$ of the original power density. If the surgeon wishes to maintain the same power density at this new larger spot size, he or she must compensate by increasing the wattage.

Another means of controlling the spot size is by a focus or defocus position of the delivery system. When the laser is used in focus (Fig. 27-6), the smallest possible spot size is generated and therefore maximum power density. However, it can be pulled back into a defocus position. The greater the defocus distance, the greater the spot size and subsequent reduction in power density. As is discussed later, this method is the one most

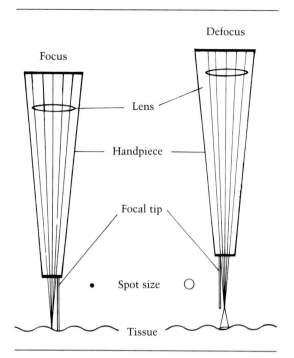

Focus

Defocus

Lens

Handpiece

Focal tip

Spot size

Tissue

**Figure 27-6** $CO_2$ handpiece of 125 mm. Left. In focus. Right. Defocused.

commonly employed to control power density during $CO_2$ laser freehand surgery.

## Laser–Tissue Interaction

The interaction of lasers with biologic tissue may be divided into thermal and nonthermal effects. Most nonophthalmologic surgical applications rely on the thermal effects to produce various desired results. Thermal effects consist of photocoagulation and photovaporization, which are temperature-dependent mechanisms [69]. Normal body temperature is 37°C. If tissue is transiently heated to less than 60°C, there is only a minimal effect, i.e., shrinkage, but no permanent damage. Above 60°C and below 100°C, coagulation of tissue occurs secondary to the denaturization of protein [88]. Macroscopically, it is seen as blanching of the irradiated tissue similar to the changes in egg white as it is heated. Collagen molecules lose their trihelical arrangement, shrink, and become randomized. This change is irreversible and results in cellular death, but it falls short of immediate tissue removal. Eventually this dead tissue sloughs.

At temperatures higher than 100°C, photovaporization of tissue occurs. Studies using the $CO_2$ laser show how the laser heats cellular water to boiling, resulting in a phase transition of water to steam. It is accompanied by a thousand-fold expansion and results in rupture of cellular membranes. Cellular fragments are blown up out of the wound and into the path of the laser, where they are heated to 300° to 400°C, resulting in carbonization, or to 500°C, resulting in combustion [48]. The temperature at the irradiated site is limited by the heat sink formed from the phase transition.

Photocoagulation and photovaporization depend on various parameters (Fig. 27-7), which include wavelength, power density, duration, spot size, and various tissue factors. When tissue is irradiated by a laser, the energy can be absorbed, reflected, scattered, or transmitted [44, 92]. The degree to which each of these events occurs depends on the wavelength of the laser and the physical and optical characteristics of the tissue. This point is best illustrated by comparing the three lasers most commonly used in clinical medicine and surgery today: the argon, Nd:YAG, and $CO_2$ lasers (Fig. 27-8).

At 10.6 µm the $CO_2$ is strongly absorbed by water or tissues containing water. Its absorption coefficient is 200 cm$^{-1}$, and its extinction length (distance traveled for 90 percent absorption of energy) is only 0.03 mm [44, 45, 79]. There is negligible or no backscatter, forward transmission, or lateral scattering. Because most biologic soft tissue is 70 to 90 percent water, the $CO_2$ laser can be used to cut or vaporize tissue with minimal tissue damage. Histologically, cellular damage can be divided into three zones. The first zone is the area of vaporization. The second zone consists of a rim of thermal necrosis less than 100 µm wide. The third zone consists of cellular edema. The total width of these three zones can range from 50 to 600

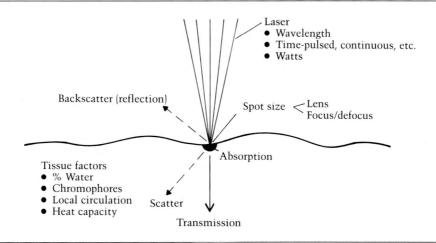

***Figure 27-7*** *Laser–tissue interaction.*

μm [8, 16, 19]. This cellular damage is secondary to heat transfer from the impact site [48]. Therefore thermal damage is time-related and increases with the length of time the tissue is exposed to the $CO_2$ laser.

***Figure 27-8*** *Comparison of $CO_2$, argon, and Nd:YAG lasers.*

The Nd:YAG at 1.06 nm has a small absorption coefficient of 0.1 $cm^{-1}$ and an extinction length of 90 mm in water [44, 79]. In biologic tissue its penetration is 3 to 5 mm, depending on the tissue irradiated. This factor is secondary to low tissue absorption plus high scattering (scattering coefficient =

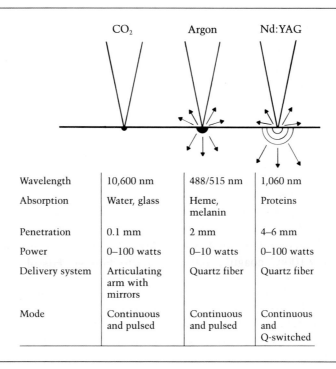

| | $CO_2$ | Argon | Nd:YAG |
|---|---|---|---|
| Wavelength | 10,600 nm | 488/515 nm | 1,060 nm |
| Absorption | Water, glass | Heme, melanin | Proteins |
| Penetration | 0.1 mm | 2 mm | 4–6 mm |
| Power | 0–100 watts | 0–10 watts | 0–100 watts |
| Delivery system | Articulating arm with mirrors | Quartz fiber | Quartz fiber |
| Mode | Continuous and pulsed | Continuous and pulsed | Continuous and Q-switched |

21; $CO_2 = 0$) and reflectance (backscatter), which lengthen its extinction length. It is this high scatter/absorption ratio that produces a beam profile that becomes wider with depth (see Fig. 27-8), resulting in a poor cutting device but an excellent tool to produce diffuse thermal coagulation [69]. Blood vessels 1 to 3 mm in size can be sealed, unlike with the $CO_2$ laser, which can seal vessels only up to 0.5 mm.

The argon laser produces energy at six wavelengths, 80 percent of which are at 488 nm and 514.5 nm in the blue-green visible spectrum [8, 42]. Its absorption coefficient is less than $0.001$ cm$^{-1}$ for water. However, argon laser energy is primarily absorbed by melanin, oxygenated hemoglobin (absorption coefficient in blood = 34 cm$^{-1}$), and chromophores in tissue; it is relatively poorly absorbed in nonpigmented tissue. Hemoglobin has absorption peaks at 418, 540, and 577 nm [92]. The argon laser has been used for the treatment of various pigmented vascular lesions, as its wavelength is close to the hemoglobin absorption peaks, and therefore a somewhat selective effect can be achieved [8]. The argon laser is used to penetrate the overlying epidermis and is absorbed by intravascular hemoglobin in the abnormal vessels. This light absorption is converted to heat, which results in coagulation of the abnormal vessel with relative sparing of deep epidermal appendages [3]. However, for superficial vascular lesions the argon laser may be replaced by a laser with a wavelength of 577 nm. Presently there are three lasers that generate the 577 nm wavelength: metal vapor laser, flush pumped dye laser, and tunable dye laser. They differ in spot size, power, and pulse duration. Melanin is a major light absorber in the epidermis, from the ultraviolet B spectrum through the visible to the near-infrared [8]. The longer the wavelength, the less melanin absorption and therefore greater transmission. Theoretically, a laser at 577 nm has an advantage over the argon laser because it would be transmitted through the epidermis with less

absorption and subsequent epidermal damage and have a more specific absorption for hemoglobin [46, 53]. Clinical trials using lasers at 577 nm for vascular lesions are currently under way [70, 98].

The next parameter that affects the laser–tissue interaction is the mode of delivery of laser energy. Until now continuous wave application has been discussed, i.e., continuous delivery of energy to the tissue. However, energy may also be delivered in pulses. The simplest form is achieved by gating a continuous-mode laser, which can produce pulse widths as small as 0.01 second. A superpulse mode has also been introduced to $CO_2$ lasers. It consists of a rapidly pulsed $CO_2$ laser with pulse widths from microseconds to milliseconds, 25 to 1000 pulses per second, peak powers of up to 500 watts, and average powers up to 35 watts at the tissue. The surgeon uses it like a continuous-wave laser. The theoretical advantage is less tissue damage. As previously noted, tissue damage is related to the length of time laser energy is in contact with tissue. The longer the time, the more thermal distribution of heat there is, resulting in a greater area of tissue damage. Less damage results from using high power over a short period of time than from using low power over a long period of time. Superpulse accomplishes this condition by breaking up the continuous laser into a series of short pulses each with a high power density. The only disadvantage is that with less thermal effect there is less hemostasis.

Even shorter pulse widths can be achieved by Q-switched lasers, which produce pulse widths of 10 to 20 nanoseconds and mode locked lasers producing a train of seven to ten pulses, each lasting 10 to 30 picoseconds. The last two processes are important for the generation of nonthermal effects and selective thermal effects. Thermal damage can be limited to small, more specific targets by varying the pulse duration and wavelength. For example, using a tunable dye laser at 577 nm, different effects on the skin can be produced by varying the pulse duration [2, 75, 92]. With a 1 μsec pulse the energy is absorbed by the hemoglobin in red blood cells within superficial vessels. However, because the thermal relaxation time of blood is greater than the pulse duration, there is no damage to the surrounding blood vessel. When the pulse duration is increased to 1 msec, the thermal relaxation time is exceeded and both the red blood cells and the blood vessel are damaged by thermal diffusion. Further increases damage the tissue around the blood vessel. This method may have potential future application for selective destruction of various tumors and disease processes.

Other factors affecting laser tissue interaction include the spot size of the laser. The spot size determines the power density and therefore various effects on tissue. In addition to chromophores, melanin, and hemoglobin, the local circulation of blood can provide a cooling effect on the tissue and alter the thermal effect of the laser.

Nonthermal or nonlinear effects of lasers comprise a relatively new area, and the terminology has not been consistent. Such actions include photochemical, photodisruptive (thermomechanical), and photoablative effects.

A photochemical effect is achieved by using a laser at a specific wavelength to activate a drug or chemical within a cell or tissue for a predetermined end effect [88]. It is best exemplified medically by the work with hematoporphyrin photoradiation therapy [31–33]. Simply explained, a photodynamic agent or exogenous chromophore such as a modified hematoporphyrin derivative is injected intravenously. It is subsequently distributed in body tissue and is then cleared from normal tissue but selectively retained by malignant tissue. This malignant tissue is then exposed to red light from a 630-nm laser, which activates the hematoporphyrin in the tumor, resulting in cellular death while preserving normal tissue. The exact mechanism of action is still debated. Other

uses of photochemical effects include laser-induced tissue fluorescence [80] and hematoporphyrin-derived fluorescence for the detection of various tumors [62].

Photodisruptive, or thermomechanical, laser effects use high peaked powers and short pulse intervals (Q-switched or mode locked) focused into small spot sizes (i.e., 50 μm) [65]. It results in an optical breakdown in tissue with momentary localized ionized plasma formation and a hydrodynamic shock wave that results in tissue disruption. It has been used in ophthalmology for noninvasive capsulotomy [96, 97].

Photoablative laser–tissue interaction is a process of nonthermal tissue destruction by excimer lasers, which produce wavelengths ranging from 193 (Ar F) to 351 (Xe F) in the ultraviolet region. An electric discharge is used to produce diatomic molecules (excited dimer-excimer) from the interaction of rare gases (zenon, krypton, argon) and halogen (fluorine or chlorine). When they return to the ground state, they release pulsed ultraviolet radiation. Tissue is destroyed as the ultraviolet light breaks the chemical bonds of the cell molecules. The major biologic target is protein. Early investigations have centered on corneal surgery (radial keratotomies) and ablation of atherosclerotic lesions. Pegman and Kuszak have found the photoablative action greater at short wavelengths. Experimental incisions have been made in excised guinea pig skin and human skin with 193-nm or 248-nm lasers. Electron microscopy shows a zone of injury confined to within 100 μm of the ablated area.

## Clinical Applications of the $CO_2$ Laser

The $CO_2$ laser may be used with four accessories that attach to the end of the articulating arm delivery system. First, the laser may be attached to a microslad unit, which is coupled to a microscope for various procedures. The $CO_2$ beam is reflected by a movable mirror controlled by a joystick. Spot

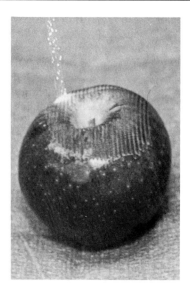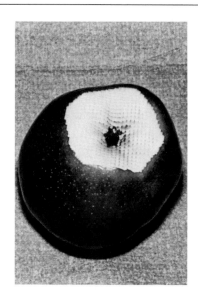

***Figure 27-9*** *Computerized scanner for $CO_2$ laser.*

size and focal length can be adjusted according to need. This technique has many applications in gynecology and otolaryngology.

Second, the laser may be attached to a rigid, hollow endoscope. The $CO_2$ laser cannot be transmitted by present day medical fiberoptics, which is a limiting factor. However, bronchoscopes, laparoscopes, and rectosigmoidoscopes have been developed and are in clinical use.

More recently, the laser has been coupled to a computerized scanner. The surgeon outlines the area to be ablated, sets the spot size, power, and speed, and the computer then vaporizes the tissue within the area outlined to the same depth throughout the lesion. This technique is illustrated on an apple in Figure 27-9. Presently, this device is more useful in the laboratory setting for controlled experiments but is slowly making its way into clinical use for dermabrasion and other applications.

The fourth and most common surgical use is $CO_2$ laser freehand surgery. The articulating arm is attached to a triple-jointed handpiece that has a focusing system. Of the above listed accessories, the technique of freehand laser surgery is the most difficult to learn. The surgeon must understand the principles of power density and how to apply them to achieve various effects on tissue.

## Technique of $CO_2$ Laser Freehand Surgery

With freehand $CO_2$ laser surgery the surgeon may use the laser to cut, vaporize, and sterilize surfaces and obtain hemostasis (Table 27-1) [76]. When using the laser as a scalpel, the handpiece must be in focus to generate the smallest spot size. Power density varies according to the tissue and the skill of the surgeon. Lower powers are used on the skin and are increased for subcutaneous tissue, muscle, and so on. The highest power densities are needed on parenchymous tissue such as the kidney to achieve better, though not complete, hemostasis. Overall, an experienced laser surgeon uses high power densities in the cutting mode to minimize thermal damage. When cutting, the tissue is

***Table 27-1*** *Technique of $CO_2$ laser freehand surgery*

| Technique | Spot size | Power density | Mode |
|---|---|---|---|
| Cut | Fine | Variable | Continuous |
| Vaporize | Large | High | Continuous/pulsed |
| "Sterilize" | Large | Low | Continuous |
| Hemostasis | Large | Low | Pulsed |

kept under constant tension and the laser moved at a slow, steady handspeed. The surgeon must think three-dimensionally and try to develop a "V-shaped" plane (Fig. 27-10). By keeping the tissue under tension and cutting at the apex of the V, a well defined incision or plane is developed. Remember that one is cutting with a spot size as small as 0.22 mm, and the novice laser surgeon can easily develop multiple planes resulting in ragged edges (Fig. 27-11).

The depth of an incision depends on various parameters, including handspeed, power, spot size, and percent water composition of the tissue. The greater the percentage of water in the tissue, the greater the efficiency of the $CO_2$ laser and therefore the deeper the incision when all other variables are held constant. Similarly, increasing power or using a small spot size maximizes the power density, resulting in a deeper incision. However, the most common method by which depth is controlled is the handspeed. The slower the handspeed, the deeper is the incision, and the faster the handspeed, the more shallow is the incision. $CO_2$ laser surgery must be performed with a slow, steady handspeed, as if painting. The surgeon must make an adjustment from the tactile sensation of conventional surgery to the hand-eye coordination of noncontact laser surgery. Proper technique is critical to achieve the desired result. $CO_2$ laser freehand surgery is user-dependent. What is one surgeon's reported result is another surgeon's disbelief when he or she cannot achieve similar results—which usually results from poor technique or improper settings (e.g., power, mode).

When the goal is to vaporize tissue, the spot size is increased, which is best accomplished by holding the handpiece in a defocus mode. The power must be increased to maintain a power density high enough to remove tissue quickly and efficiently.

The laser may be used to "sterilize" the surface of an infected lesion, such as a de-

***Figure 27-10*** *Cutting with the $CO_2$ laser. The surgeon develops a three-dimensional V-shaped plane.*

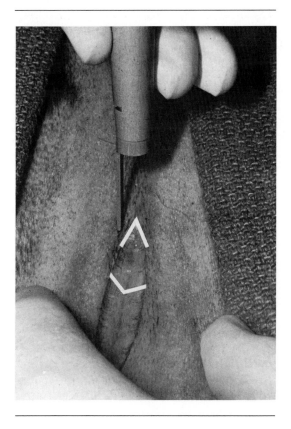

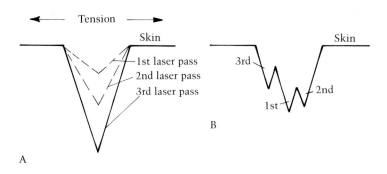

***Figure 27-11*** *A. When cutting with the $CO_2$ laser the surgeon keeps the wound under tension and develops a V-shaped plane cutting at the apex. B. Without tension, multiple planes can be developed because of the small cutting spot size.*

cubitus. It is accomplished with a large spot size via a defocused handpiece and low power density. Remember that only the surface is sterilized, not the entire lesion.

Finally, the $CO_2$ laser may be used for hemostasis by sealing vessels. The $CO_2$ laser is not the best hemostatic laser but can seal vessels up to 0.5 to 1.0 mm while cutting. There are two techniques that may be employed for vessels larger than 1 mm. First, when a vessel is seen in situ before it is cut, the laser may be put in a defocused mode via the handpiece. The amount of defocus depends on the wattage. One needs a low power density. Then, using short pulses of energy controlled with the foot pedal, the tissue alongside the vessel is irradiated, which results in the vessel shrinking in size as the surrounding tissue is desiccated. When the vessel is small enough, it may be irradiated directly, which seals it. The second method is for vessels that are clamped. Again, short bursts of defocused energy are used until the vessel is sealed (laser welding). Both of these techniques are difficult to learn, require practice, and are user-dependent. In most cases it is still best to use electrocautery and ligature where appropriate.

The main advantages of $CO_2$ laser surgery include noncontact surgery, sterility, decreased blood loss, reduced pain and edema, and a highly controllable effect on tissue [55, 57, 59, 64, 77]. Decreased blood loss results from the sealing of blood vessels up to 1 mm in diameter while cutting or vaporizing tis-

sue. The size of a vessel that can be sealed is increased to as much as 2 mm if local blood circulation is temporarily arrested via compression or tourniquet [48]. This effect has proved particularly beneficial for surgery on hemophiliacs [52], during extensive extirpative procedures where a significant blood loss may be anticipated [6, 56, 59, 89], and for surgery of highly vascular tumors [6, 55].

Carbon dioxide laser surgery destroys cells and their nuclei, including those of bacteria, by flash boiling of water and vaporization in the beam path. The $CO_2$ laser has been shown to reduce the bacterial population at the skin surface of previously inoculated pig skin by several orders of magnitude [72]. Similar results have been reported clinically during decubitus surgery [90, 91], including one series of more than 2000 decubitus operations performed with the $CO_2$ laser [43]. Bactericidal action and noncontact surgery make the $CO_2$ laser advantageous for surgery involving infected lesions or wounds [64]. One can cut without contaminating clean areas with dirty instruments. Note, however, that the reduction in bacteria is at the surface only.

Reduced pain with $CO_2$ laser surgery has been reported by various authors describing a wide range of procedures [6, 55, 60, 68]. However, this report is based on individual surgeons' personal observations, as no controlled studies have been performed to date. The etiology of this phenomenon has yet to be determined, but microscopic studies on cutaneous nerves cut with the laser showed the ends to be capped or welded. Nerves cut with a scalpel result in fraying of the nerve ending.

Finally, the $CO_2$ laser provides surgeons with a large amount of control for tissue ablation. By varying lenses, spot sizes, mode of operation (pulsed, continuous), power, and technique, the tissue can be cut and removed delicately, layer by layer, or rapidly in large amounts to suit the clinical situation. This ability is particularly advantageous for treatment of various dermatologic lesions and for oncologic surgery.

The main disadvantages of the $CO_2$ laser include the lack of mechanical contact with tissue, the need for specialized training, and the lack of maneuverability of equipment, which is limited to the configuration of the rigid delivery system. Surgeons depend on and are used to the tactile contact with tissue that is experienced with conventional surgery. The use of a nontouch instrument makes it necessary to switch to hand-eye coordination and the ability to translate surgery into a three-dimensional approach. It requires a certain learning period, which varies among surgeons. The laser is not an instrument that one can learn to use in the operating room without prior formalized training. The $CO_2$ laser handpiece is not as maneuverable as the cold knife despite various advances in the engineering features of the arm and handpieces.

Carbon dioxide laser surgery has been useful for treating a wide variety of skin and surface conditions. Both traumatic and professional tattoos have been treated with various lasers (ruby, argon, $CO_2$) when other modalities (e.g., dermabrasion, excision) were not appropriate [7, 15, 34, 37, 67, 82, 92]. Advantages of $CO_2$ laser removal of such lesions include accurate depth control, minimal thermal damage, and minimal blood loss. Using an airbrush technique, the epidermis and dermis are "planed away," layer by layer, until the pigment layer is reached. High levels of patient satisfaction has been reported despite a greater risk of hypertrophic scarring (7 to 40 percent) [29].

The argon and 577-μm lasers are those most commonly used for the treatment of port-wine stains. Bailin and others, however, reported that selected port-wine stains respond favorably to $CO_2$ laser therapy [28, 81]. The latter include port-wine stains that are light in color (pink versus purple), flat, and easily blanched with pressure. The $CO_2$ laser is used to vaporize the overlying epidermis to the level of the small superficial vessels, which are then vaporized or coagulated. The subsequent healing process is similar to that seen after argon laser therapy [21].

Good long-term results have been reported in the treatment of recurrent or therapy-resistant condylomata acuminatum [11, 13, 22, 61]. The $CO_2$ laser also allows easy treatment in such difficult areas as the nail bed (without removing the entire nail) and the urethra [83]. Proper technique is essential. Baggish demonstrated a significant increase in the primary cure rate (65.8 to 91.0 percent) when a "brush" technique is added to the therapy [12]. This technique is accomplished using spot sizes of 1.5 to 2.0 diameter and power settings of 2 to 5 watts. The laser is then moved rapidly over the tissue between the lesions, resulting in blanching, not blistering, of the skin. Histology shows destruction of the epidermis only. This added technique is intended to eliminate subclinical human papilloma virus within normal-appearing epithelium.

Rhinophyma can be treated with excellent cosmetic results [14, 36, 86]. Initially, the $CO_2$ laser is used to shave down the nose to the appropriate level. Then, with the laser handpiece defocused, final contouring is achieved by vaporization of selected areas.

Advantages include bloodless excision, minimal postoperative pain, and a better cosmetic result.

Other lesions treated with the $CO_2$ laser include congenital hemangioma [5], telangiectasia [58], blue rubber nevus [73], lymphangioma circumscriptum [17], facial angiofibromas of tuberous sclerosis [18, 93, 94], keloids [1, 4, 34, 54, 92], facial syringomas [95], warts [34, 68, 71], and other skin lesions [14].

The $CO_2$ laser has been used extensively for the management of oral cavity benign and malignant lesions in both adults and children. Crockett et al. reported on over 500 pediatric cases of benign lesions of the oral cavity and oropharynx exclusive of the larynx, including hemangioma, lymphangioma, and tongue lesions [27]. Advantages included decreased morbidity, shorter hospital stay, and decreased postoperative edema and bleeding. Ossoff reported that the $CO_2$ laser was beneficial for transoral resection of squamous cell carcinoma limited to superficial lesions up to 4 cm in diameter [74]. Benefits included precise dissection with microscopic control, decreased postoperative pain, decreased morbidity, and shortened hospital stay. Numerous other reports have concurred with these two studies and

have included treatment for sublingual keratosis [39, 40], leukoplakia [25], subglottic hemangioma [26, 49, 87], oral hemangioma, benign and malignant tongue lesions [20, 23, 50, 51], and turbinectomy [85].

The full potential of the $CO_2$ laser for plastic and dermatologic surgery has yet to be fully defined. The instrument has been used on an extended basis for about 10 years, although the earliest uses date to the 1970s. Presently, only 10 percent of plastic surgeons use the laser in their practice [63]. There has been both opposition and support of laser usage from inside and outside the medical profession. Although the $CO_2$ laser can be used to perform most surgical procedures, true indications must show a particular advantage over conventional methods for either the physician or the patient. These indications are still developing as new and better technology is introduced and as more surgeons report their experiences with the treatment of different disease processes. Unfortunately, in the present competitive medical market the laser has also become a victim of a marketing gimmick for those advertising certain questionable or misleading practices, e.g., laser facelift. Unfortunately, this problem has overshadowed the work of many serious investigators.

# Use of Argon and Carbon Dioxide Lasers in Clinical Plastic Surgery Practice

*David B. Apfelberg*
*Morton R. Maser*
*Harvey Lash*
*David N. White*

The use of lasers for plastic surgery has become well accepted as the standard treatment for many cutaneous disorders. The argon laser, which has the ability to selectively obliterate a wide variety of vascular and inflammatory lesions, was first employed during the early 1970s [1, 4, 5, 9, 10]. The carbon dioxide ($CO_2$) laser, which can accomplish a relatively bloodless incision or remove tissue by vaporization, has been used for surgical excision of vascular or contaminated lesions or vaporization of bulky masses since the mid-1960s [2, 3, 6–8]. This chapter describes the clinical use of both argon and $CO_2$ lasers and provides guidelines for the safe application of these five lasers in plastic surgery.

## Laser Physiology

All lasers produce intense light of high energy in the visible or invisible light spectrum. This energy can be focused by a series of optics to a point of maximum power density where the light can accomplish cutting, vaporization, cautery, and ablation. The high heat of the laser sterilizes bacterial and viral particles and malignant cells, thus rendering the laser valuable for treatment of inflammatory, infectious, or malignant diseases. Lasers also accomplish hemostasis during incision or ablation, thereby providing a relatively bloodless field of surgery. Precision as fine as destruction of individual 30-μm segments can be accomplished with microscopic control.

## Materials and Methods

The argon laser used by the authors produces intense blue-green light between 488 and 514 nm. This laser light is selectively absorbed by hemoglobin, which has a coefficient of light absorption at approximately 500 nm, or by pigment particles suspended in the upper dermis (decorative tattoo, melanin). The argon laser light is able to penetrate intact the overlying skin and is absorbed by hemoglobin-laden abnormal blood vessels or pigment particles. Light absorption is then converted to heat, which coagulates the abnormal vessels or vaporizes the pigment, sparing skin appendages such as sweat glands and pilosebaceous glands, which aid in rapid healing of the laser wound. Thus photocoagulation is the mechanism of action.

The $CO_2$ laser produces intense light in the invisible infrared spectrum (10,600 nm) that is capable of being absorbed by water. Because biologic tissues, especially vascular hemangiomas, contain 75 to 90 percent water, the laser acts by vaporizing tissue at its focal point, leaving adjacent tissue practically unaffected and thus enabling a fine hemostatic incision. The primary advantage of the $CO_2$ laser for hemangioma surgery is its ability to cut like a knife and seal small blood vessels at the same time. Postoperative scarring is similar to that seen with conventional techniques, and postoperative pain and edema are significantly reduced.

## Course of Treatment

The mechanism of action of the argon laser suggests its usage. This laser photocoagulates by the attraction of either hemoglobin, melanin, or suspended dermal pigment particles. The treatment is usually accomplished in an outpatient or office setting under local anesthesia. Epinephrine is not employed in the anesthetic to limit vasoconstriction, as maximum absorption of the light by hemoglobin-laden dermal lesions is expected to be achieved. After satisfactory local anesthesia and local skin antiseptic preparation, the laser instrument is set on the lowest power setting that can accomplish the desired clinical effect (blanching for a vascular lesion, vaporization for tattoos or melanotic lesions). A "test patch" always precedes treatment of a major area. The test patch accomplishes several things: It shows the patient the course of wound healing and the expected final result or blanching; it validates the machine settings; and it demonstrates the possible emergence of adverse healing problems. A major treatment may follow a test patch by 12 weeks or whenever clinical outcome can be confidently predicted.

The laser stylus is hand-held perpendicular to the skin surface at a distance of approximately 2 to 4 cm and slowly advanced across the skin according to the clinical effect (blanching for vascular lesions, vaporization for tattoos and solid lesions). A 1- to 2-mm spot size is most frequently used, and pulse duration may vary from 0.2 second to continuous exposure, depending on the experience of the operator. Practical treatment comprises a convenient treatment time of approximately 30 minutes and an adequate (but not toxic) amount of local anesthetic with a minimum of injections. Local nerve blocks (e.g., infraorbital, mental) may be employed with good patient comfort.

Follow-up care includes immediate application of ice compresses to limit edema and reduce burn injury. Most patients then treat their wounds as open partial-thickness losses, with topical antibiotics, daily cleansing, avoidance of contamination and sun exposure, and natural separation of eschars. The eschar that forms usually separates, and the wound is epithelialized within 10 to 14 days. Any unusual drainage, purulence, or fever is immediately treated with systemic and topical antibiotics (silver sulfadiazine, Silvadene). Although clinical blanching is usually immediately apparent, subsequent erythema in the area caused by inflammation may take a full 6 to 12 months to resolve.

The $CO_2$ laser may be utilized in a focused or defocused mode depending on the desired effect. $CO_2$ laser spot or aperture size varies between 0.2 and 1.0 mm, and power varies from 5 to 15 watts. For relatively bloodless incision, the laser beam is focused at the focal point (approximately 2 to 4 cm perpendicular to the skin) and moved slowly to make a fine incision. Blood vessels with lumen diameters of 0.5 mm and smaller are divided and sealed by the heat of the laser light, but larger vessels require clamping and ligation. Undermining of skin flaps and dissection of the margin or capsule of a lesion is accomplished by directing the laser in an oblique manner. Firm retraction aids in separation of the tissue layers. Cautery or vaporization may be accomplished by "defocusing" the laser beam, i.e., backing off from the focal distance about 4 to 8 cm. This modality results in ablation of bulky masses without significant bleeding. To accomplish $CO_2$ "laserbrasion" (laser dermabrasion), a defocused beam is rapidly "paint brushed" across the skin surface, producing selective superficial destruction of the uppermost layers of the epidermis and superficial dermis.

Laser incisional wounds are copiously irrigated to remove the charred debris before closure. Vaporization wounds are treated much like any superficial partial-thickness skin loss. The excellent hemostatic qualities of this laser make blood preparation and replacement seldom necessary. Postoperative pain, discomfort, and edema are usually minimal owing to the healing of small nerve endings and lymphatics. Sutures are left in the wounds slightly longer after laser incisions because of the initially lower tensile strength.

## Laser Safety

Laser safety factors must be understood and followed for the safety of the patient, the operator, and ancillary personnel. Major hazards are visual injury, inadvertent burns, and combustion. Ocular injury can be prevented by the wearing of laser safety glasses or goggles by the patient and all personnel. Alternatively, a moist gauze can be used to shield the patient's eyes. Bright or reflective instruments must be restricted. Restricted access to rooms where laser treatment is in progress also limits inadvertent eye exposure. The treatment area is shielded by moist gauze to prevent burns to adjacent areas. Aiming guides are employed prior to instituting treatment to be sure that the laser beam is properly aimed and aligned. Outright combustion and fires can be prevented by moistening the adjacent drapes and endotracheal tubes, using fire-retardant surgical drapes, and using safety shutters when the laser is not actually in use.

## Indications and Contraindications

Indications and contraindications for the use of both the argon and $CO_2$ lasers are demonstrated in Tables 27-2, 27-3, and 27-4. Suggestions for laser settings appear in Tables 27-5 and 27-6. Lesions amenable to the argon laser fall into four main categories. Vas-

**Table 27-2** *Treatment by classification: Argon laser*

Vascular disorders
    Port-wine hemangioma
    Capillary/cavernous hemangioma
    Strawberry mark (of infancy)
    Telangiectasia
    Acne rosacea
    Campbell-DeMorgan senile angiomas
    Venous lake
    Hereditary hemorrhagic telangiectasia
    Angioma serpiginosum
Miscellanous disorders
    Nevus of Ota
    Granuloma faciale

**Table 27-3** *Treatment by classification: $CO_2$ laser*

Vascular disorders
    Cavernous hemangioma
    Lymphangioma circumscripta
Pigmented lesions
    Nevus: epidermal, papillary, intradermal
      verrucous
    Seborrheic keratosis
    Café au lait spots
    Lentigo
Malignancies
    Superficial basal cell epithelioma, squamous
      cell carcinoma
    Bowen's disease
    Leukoplakia
Miscellaneous lesions
    Warts: plantar, hand, genital (condyloma
      acuminatum)
    Xanthelasma palpebrum
    Fungus nail: onychomycosis
    Nail matrixectomy: onychogryphosis,
      onychocryptosis
    Carnu cutaneum
    Porokeratosis
    Actinic keratosis
    Morton's neuroma
    Digital synovial (mucous) cyst

**Table 27-4** *Treatment by classification: Argon or $CO_2$ laser*

Vascular disorders
    Angiokeratoma
    Campbell-DeMorgan senile angioma
    Telangiectasia
Inflammatory disorders
    Pyogenic granuloma
    Rhinophyma
Decorative tattoo
Miscellaneous disorders
    Tuberous sclerosis (adenoma sebaceum)
    Trichoepithelioma
    Verrucae vulgaris: plantar, hand, genital
    Xanthelasma
    Granuloma faciale
    Kaposi's sarcoma
    Vitiligo
    Seborrheic hyperplasia (nevus sebaceum)
Not currently amenable to laser treatment
    Superficial varicosities of the lower
      extremity
    Hypertrophic scars and keloids

cular lesions include the hemangiomas and other superficial vascular lesions, e.g., telangiectasias and venous lakes (Figs. 27-12 and 27-13). Inflammatory lesions that contain numerous blood vessels, e.g., acne rosacea and granulomas, can also be treated. Moreover, miscellaneous superficial melanotic and pigmented lesions are amenable to treatment with the argon laser.

The $CO_2$ laser is indicated for excision of highly vascular lesions or situations where excessive bleeding may occur (patients with coagulapathies or highly vascular body areas) (Fig. 27-14). Contaminated or infected lesions are sterilized by the laser's heat (Fig. 27-15). Viral warts are particularly susceptible to this laser. Other superficial lesions are listed in Table 27-2.

The argon and $CO_2$ lasers can be used with equal effectiveness to treat decorative tattoos (Fig. 27-16), adenoma sebaceum or tuberous sclerosis, trichoepitheliomas, pyogenic granulomas (Fig. 27-17), and superficial vascular lesions such as angiokeratomas and capillary hemangiomas. Neither laser is effective for the treatment of hypertrophic or keloid scars or for the treatment of superficial telangiectasias or varicosities of the lower extremity.

**Table 27-5** *Treatment parameters for argon laser*

| Lesion | Spot size (mm) | Power (watts) | Pulse duration (sec) | Focus (F) Defocus (D) | Instructions |
|---|---|---|---|---|---|
| Port-wine hemangioma | 0.2–2.0 | 0.6–1.0 | 0.2–cont. | F | Minimal power to blanch |
| Capillary hemangioma | 0.2–2.0 | 0.8–1.2 | 0.2–cont. | F | Minimal power to blanch |
| Strawberry mark | 0.2–2.0 | 0.6–1.2 | 0.2–cont. | F | Minimal power to blanch |
| Telangiectasia | 0.2–1.0 | 0.6–1.2 | 0.2–cont. | F | Pinpoint blanch central vessel and radiating vessels |
| Acne rosacea | 0.2–1.0 | 0.6–1.2 | 0.2–cont. | F | Minimal power to blanch |
| Senile angioma | 0.2–1.0 | 1.0 | 0.2–cont. | F | Minimal power to blanch |
| Venous lake | 1.0–2.0 | 1.0 | 0.2–cont. | F | Minimal power to blanch |
| Granuloma faciale | 0.1–2.0 | 1.0–2.0 | 0.2–cont. | F | Blanch and shrink |
| Pyogenic granuloma | 0.2–2.0 | 1.0–2.5 | 0.2–cont. | F | Vaporize top, wipe, vaporize base vessel |
| Adenoma sebaceum | 0.2–1.0 | 1.0–1.5 | 0.2–cont. | F | Minimal power to blanch |
| Trichoepithelioma | 0.2–2.0 | 1.5–2.5 | 0.2–cont. | F | Blanch and shrink |
| Verruca (wart) | 0.2–2.0 | 1.5–2.5 | 0.2–cont. | F | Vaporize top, curet, vaporize basement membrane |
| Decorative tattoo | 0.2–2.0 | 1.0–2.5 | 0.2–cont. | F | Slow vaporization: top skin layers |

*Note:* The specific treatment parameters (power, spot size, pulse duration, focus) in this chart are to be considered *rough* guides only. Individual preference and operator experience may vary greatly. Also, the rapidity of advance of the laser stylus may markedly vary resulting in a vastly different power density for any given area. Similarly, laser manufacturers and optics are not necessarily similar for different lasers.

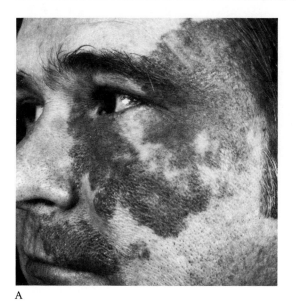

A

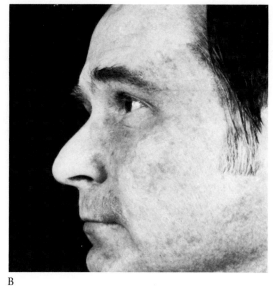

B

**Figure 27-12** ▲ *A. Port-wine hemangioma prior to treatment. B. Satisfactory blanching of port-wine hemangioma with smoothing of surface after argon laser treatment.*

**Figure 27-13** ▼ *A. Multiple facial telangiectasia. B. Elimination of facial veins following argon laser treatment.*

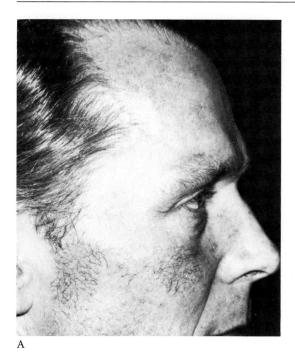

A

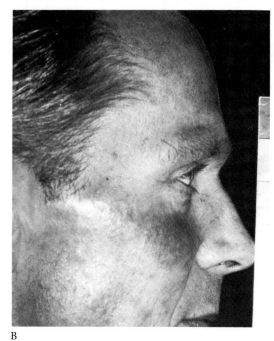

B

**Table 27-6** Treatment parameters for $CO_2$ laser

| Lesion | Spot size (mm) | Power (watts) | Pulse duration (sec) | Focus (F) Defocus (D) | Instructions |
|---|---|---|---|---|---|
| Excision hemangioma | 0.2–1.0 | 8–15 | Cont. | F/D | Focus to cut; defocus to cauterize |
| Malignancy | 0.2–1.0 | 8–15 | Cont. | F/D | Focus to cut; defocus to cauterize |
| Nevus | 1.0 | 5–10 | Cont. | D | Defocus to "laser-brade" to upper dermis |
| Keratosis | 1.0 | 5–10 | Cont. | D | Defocus to "laser-brade" to upper dermis |
| Lentigo | 1.0 | 5–10 | Cont. | D | Defocus to "laser-brade" to upper dermis |
| Leukoplakia | 1.0 | 5–10 | Cont. | D | Defocus to "laser-brade" to upper dermis |
| Adenoma sebaceum | 1.0 | 5–10 | Cont. | D | Defocus to "laser-brade" to upper dermis |
| Warts | 1.0 | 10/5 | Cont. | F/D | Focus to vaporize, curet, defocus to vaporize basement membrane |
| Xanthelasma | 0.2–1.0 | 5–8 | Cont. | D | Defocus to vaporize, curet, vaporize, etc. |
| Fungus nail | 1.0 | 10 | Cont. | D | Vaporize nail, remove, vaporize nailbed, curet |
| Matrixectomy | 0.2–1.0 | 10 | Cont. | F | Directly focus to destroy matrix |
| Telangiectasia | 0.2–1.0 | 5–8 | Cont. | F | Vaporize lightly |
| Pyogenic granuloma | 1.0 | 10/5 | Cont. | F/D | Focus to vaporize top, wipe, defocus to vaporize base vessel |
| Rhinophyma | 0.2–1.0 | 10/5 | Cont. | F/D | Focus to sculpt and cut; defocus to cauterize |
| Decorative tattoo | 1.0 | 10/5 | Cont. | F/D | Focus to vaporize epidermis, wipe, defocus, wipe, etc. (4–5 times) |
| Bowen's basal cell epithelioma | 1.0 | 10 | Cont. | F | Vaporize to upper dermis — secondary healing |
| Digital cyst | 1.0 | 10 | Cont. | F | Vaporize cyst, vaporize to base at joint |

*Note:* The specific treatment parameters (power, spot size, pulse duration, focus) in this chart are to be considered *rough* guides only. Individual preference and operator experience may vary greatly. Also, the rapidity of advance of the laser stylus may vary markedly, resulting in a vastly different power density for any given area. Similarly, laser manufacturers and optics are not necessarily similar for different lasers.

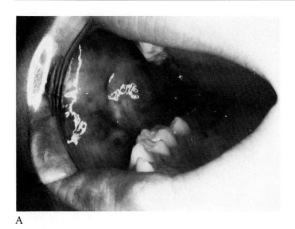

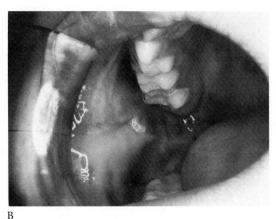

A                                    B

**Figure 27-14**  *A. Lymphangioma-hemangioma of buccal mucosa. B. Satisfactory excision of buccal hemangioma with $CO_2$ laser.*

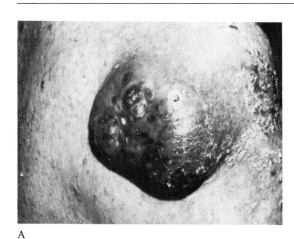

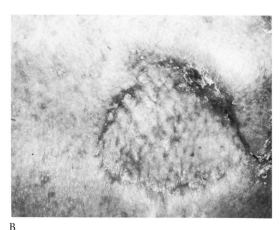

A                                    B

**Figure 27-15**  *A. Contaminated squamous cell carcinoma of right scapular area. B. Excision with the $CO_2$ laser followed by immediate split-thickness skin grafting.*

## Summary

Safe, effective treatment is outlined for the use of the argon and $CO_2$ lasers in plastic surgical practice. The argon laser is best used to photocoagulate superficial vascular or pigmented lesions. The $CO_2$ laser is effective as a hemostatic scalpel for more serious vascular situations or as a vaporizer of bulky, contaminated, infectious, or malignant lesions. Proper use of either laser depends on knowledge of laser pathophysiology, safety, and adherence to known indications and contraindications.

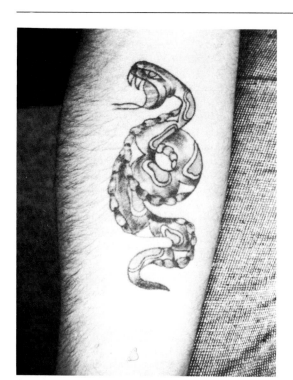

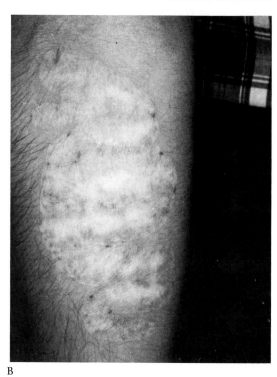

A

B

**Figure 27-16**  *A. Decorative tattoo.
B. Satisfactory resolution of tattoo pigment
after argon laser treatment.*

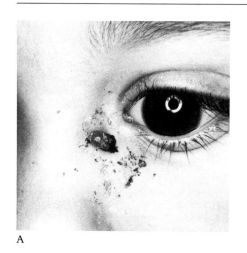

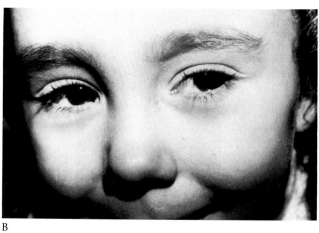

A

B

**Figure 27-17**  *A. Pyogenic granuloma of nasal
skin. B. Satisfactory resolution of pyogenic
granuloma without recurrence or scarring after
laser treatment.*

## References
### LASERS IN SURGERY AND MEDICINE

1. Abergel, R. P., et al. Laser treatment of keloids: A clinical trial and an in vitro study with Nd:YAG laser. *Lasers Surg. Med.* 4:291, 1984.

2. Anderson, R., and Parrish, J. Selective photothermolysis: Precise microsurgery by selective absorption of pulsed radiation. *Science* 220:524, 1983.

3. Apfelberg, D., et al. Histology of port wine stains. *Plast. Reconstr. Surg.* 32:232, 1979.

4. Apfelberg, D. B., et al. Preliminary report of argon and carbon dioxide laser treatment of keloid scars. *Lasers Surg. Med.* 4:283, 1984.

5. Apfelberg, D. B., et al. Review of usage of argon and carbon dioxide lasers for pediatric hemagiomas. *Ann. Plast. Surg.* 12:353, 1984.

6. Apfelberg, D. B., et al. Benefits of the $CO_2$ laser in oral hemangioma excision. *Plast. Reconstr. Surg.* 75:46, 1985.

7. Apfelberg, D. B., et al. Comparison of argon and carbon dioxide laser treatment of decorative tattoos: A preliminary report. *Ann. Plast. Surg.* 14:6, 1985.

8. Arndt, K., and Noe, J. Lasers in dermatology. *Arch. Dermatol.* 118:293, 1982.

9. Arndt, K. A., et al. Laser therapy: Basic concepts and nomenclature. *Am. Acad. Dermatol.* 5:649, 1981.

10. Ascher, P., et al. Ultrastructural Findings in CNS Tissue with $CO_2$ Laser. In I. Kaplan (ed.), *Laser Surgery II.* Jerusalem: Academic Press, 1976. Pp. 81–85.

11. Baggish, M. $CO_2$ laser treatment for condylomata acuminata venereal infections. *Obstet. Gynecol.* 55:711, 1980.

12. Baggish, M. S. Improved laser techniques for the elimination of genital and extragenital warts. *Am. J. Obstet. Gynecol.* 153:545, 1985.

13. Baggish, M. Treating venereal infections with the $CO_2$ laser. *J. Reprod. Mod.* 27:737, 1987.

14. Bailin, P., and Ratz, J. Use of the $CO_2$ Laser in Dermatologic Surgery. In J. Ratz (ed.), *Lasers in Cutaneous Medicine and Surgery.* Chicago: Year Book, 1986.

15. Bailin, P., et al. Removal of tattoos by $CO_2$ laser. *J. Dermatol. Surg. Oncol.* 6:977, 1980.

16. Bailin, P., et al. $CO_2$ laser modification of Moh's surgery. *J. Dermatol. Surg. Oncol.* 7:621, 1981.

17. Bailin, P. L., et al. Carbon dioxide laser vaporization of lymphangioma circumscriptum. *J. Am. Acad. Dermatol.* 14:257, 1986.

18. Bellack, G. S., and Shapshay, S. M. Management of facial angiofibromas in tuberous sclerosis: Use of the carbon dioxide laser. *Otolaryngol. Head Neck Surg.* 94:37, 1986.

19. Ben-Bassat, M., et al. A study of the ultrastructural features of the cut margin of skin and mucous membrane specimens excised by carbon dioxide laser. *J. Surg. Res.* 21:77, 1976.

20. Ben-Bassat, M., et al. The $CO_2$ laser in surgery of the tongue. *Br. J. Plast. Surg.* 31:155, 1978.

21. Buecker, J., et al. Histology of port-wine stains treated with carbon dioxide laser. *J. Am. Acad. Dermatol.* 10:1014, 1984.

22. Calkins, M. P., et al. Management of condylomata acuminata with the carbon dioxide laser. *Obstet. Gynecol.* 59:105, 1982.

23. Carruth, J. A. Resection of the tongue with the carbon dioxide laser: 100 cases. *J. Laryngol. Otol.* 99:887, 1985.

24. Carruth, J., and McKinzie, A. *Medical Lasers: Science and Clinical Practice.* Boston: Adam Hilger, 1986.

25. Chiesa, F., et al. Excision of oral leukoplakias by $CO_2$ laser on an out-patient basis: A useful procedure for prevention and early detection of oral carcinoma. *Tumori* 72:307, 1986.

26. Chora, D. I., et al. Subglottic hemangioma in children. *J. Laryngol. Otol.* 100:447, 1986.

27. Crockett, D. M., et al. Benign lesions of the nose, oral cavity and oropharynx in children: Excision by carbon dioxide laser. *Ann. Otol. Rhinol. Laryngol.* 94:489, 1985.

28. Dantow, J., et al. Treatment of port wine stains with the $CO_2$ laser. *J. Otolaryngol.* 15:35, 1986.

29. Dixon, J. A. Laser Treatment of Decorative Tattoos. In Arndt, Noe, and Rosen (eds.), *Cutaneous Laser Therapy, Principles and Methods.* New York: Wiley, 1983. Pp. 201–211.

30. Dixon, J. A. Lasers in surgery. *Curr. Probl. Surg.* 21:1, 1984.

31. Doiron, D., and Keller, G. Porphyrin photodynamic therapy: Principles and clinical applications. *Curr. Probl. Dermatol.* 15:85, 1986.

32. Dougherty, T. Hematoporphyrin as a photosensitizer of tumors. *Photochem. Photobiol.* 38:377, 1983.

33. Dougherty, T., et al. Photoradiation therapy for the treatment of malignant tumors. *Cancer Res.* 38:2628, 1978.

34. Eastern, J. Lasers in private dermatologic practice. *Cutis* 293, 1986.

35. Einstein, A. Zur Quantum Theori der Strahlung. *Phys. Z.* 18:121, 1917.

36. Eisen, R. F., et al. Surgical treatment of rhinophyma with the Shaw scalpel. *Arch. Dermatol.* 122:307, 1986.

37. Fankhauser, F., and Rol, P. Microsurgery with the Nd:YAG: An overview. *Int. Ophthalmol. Clin.* 25:55, 1985.

38. Fisher, J. D. The power density of a surgical laser beam: Its meaning and measurement. *Lasers Surg. Med.* 2:1, 1983.

39. Frame, J. W. Treatment of sublingual keratosis with $CO_2$ laser. *Br. Dermatol. J.* 156:243, 1984.

40. Frame, J. W. Removal of oral soft tissue pathology with the $CO_2$ laser. *J. Oral Maxillofac. Surg.* 43:850, 1985.

41. Fuller, T. Fundamentals of Lasers in Surgery and Medicine. In J. Dixon (ed.), *Surgical Applications of Lasers*. Chicago: Year Book, 1983.

42. Fuller, T. A. The physics of surgical lasers. *Lasers Surg. Med.* 1:5, 1980.

43. Glantz, G. Personal communication.

44. Glover, J. L., et al. The use of thermal knives in surgery: Electrosurgery lasers, plasma scalpel. *Curr. Probl. Surg.* 15:1, 1978.

45. Goldman, L., et al. *Lasers in Medicine.* New York: Gordon & Breach, 1971.

46. Greenwald, J., et al. Comparative histological studies of the tunable dye (at 577 nm) laser and argon laser: The specific vascular effects of the dye laser. *J. Invest. Dermatol.* 77:305, 1981.

47. Groot, D. W., and Johnston, P. A. Carbon dioxide treatment of porokeratosis of Mibelli. *Lasers Surg. Med.* 5:603, 1985.

48. Hall, R., et al. A carbon dioxide surgical laser. *Ann. R. Coll. Surg. Engl.* 48:181, 1971.

49. Healy, G., et al. Carbon dioxide laser in subglottic hemangioma: An update. *Ann. Otol. Rhinol. Laryngol.* 93:370, 1984.

50. Hirano, M., et al. $CO_2$ laser in treating carcinoma of the tongue. *Auris Nasus Larynx* 12:510, 1985.

51. Horch, H. H., et al. $CO_2$ laser surgery of oral premalignant lesions. *Int. J. Oral Maxillofac. Surg.* 15:19, 1986.

52. Hornblass, A., and Heischorn, B. J. $CO_2$ laser surgery in hemophilia. *Am. J. Ophthalmol.* 96:689, 1983.

53. Hulsberger-Henning, J. P., et al. Clinical and histological evaluation of port wine stains with a microsecond pulse dye laser at 577 nm. *Lasers Surg. Med.* 4:375, 1984.

54. Kanter, G. R., et al. Treatment of earlobe keloids with carbon dioxide laser excision: A report of 16 cases. *J. Dermatol. Surg. Oncol.* 11:1063, 1985.

55. Kaplan, I. Current $CO_2$ laser surgery. *Plast. Reconstr. Surg.* 69:552, 1982.

56. Kaplan, I., and Ger, R. Partial mastectomy and mammoplasty performed with $CO_2$ surgical laser: A comparative report. *Br. J. Plast. Surg.* 26:189, 1973.

57. Kaplan, I., and Giler, S. *$CO_2$ Laser Surgery.* Berlin: Springer-Verlag, 1984.

58. Kaplan, I., and Peled, I. The carbon dioxide laser in the treatment of superficial telangiectases. *Br. J. Plast. Surg.* 28:214, 1975.

59. Kaplan, I., and Sharon, U. Current laser surgery. *Ann. N.Y. Acad. Sci.* 267:247, 1976.

60. Klein, D. The use of the $CO_2$ laser in plastic surgery. *South. Med. J.* 70:429, 1977.

61. Krebs, H., and Wheelock, J. The $CO_2$ laser for recurrent and therapy-resistant condylomata acuminata. *J. Reprod. Med.* 30:489, 1985.

62. Lanzafame, R. J., et al. Hematoporphyrin derivative fluorescence: Photographic techniques for the localization of malignant tissue. *Lasers Med. Surg.* 6:328, 1986.

63. *Laser Med. Surg.* 4(6):15, 1986.

64. Levine, N., et al. Use of a carbon dioxide laser for the débridement of third degree burns. *Ann. Surg.* 179:246, 1974.

65. Loertscher, H., and Rol, P. Basic physics of Nd:YAG laser. *Int. Ophthalmol. Clin.* 25:1, 1985.

66. Maiman, T. Stimulated optical radiation in ruby lasers. *Nature* 187:493, 1960.

67. McBurney, E. $CO_2$ laser treatment of dermatologic lesions. *South Med. J.* 71:795, 1978.

68. McBurney, E. I., and Rosen, D. A. Carbon dioxide treatment of verruca vulgaris. *J. Dermatol. Surg. Oncol.* 10:45, 1984.

69. McKenzie, A. C., and Carruth, J. A. S. Lasers in surgery and medicine. *Phys. Med. Biol.* 29:619, 1984.

70. Morelli, J. G., et al. Tunable dye laser (577 nm) treatment of port wine stains. *Lasers Med. Surg.* 6:94, 1986.

71. Mueller, T. J., et al. The use of the $CO_2$ laser. *Am. J. Podiatry Assoc.* 70:136, 1980.

72. Mullarky, M. A., et al. The efficacy of the $CO_2$ laser in the sterilization of skin seeded with bacteria: Survival at the skin surface and in the plume emissions. *Laryngoscope* 95:186, 1985.

73. Olsen, T. G., et al. Laser surgery for blue rubber nevus. *Arch. Dermatol.* 115:81, 1979.

74. Ossoff, R. H. The use of modern technology in head and neck cancer. *Otolaryngol. Clin. North Am.* 18:515, 1985.

75. Parrish, J., et al. Selective thermal effects with pulsed irradiation from lasers: From organ to organelle. *J. Invest. Dermatol.* 80:075s, 1983.

76. Pennino, R., et al. Applications of the $CO_2$ laser in general surgery. *Cont. Surg.* 28:13, 1986.

77. Polanyi, T. Introduction. In A. Andrews and T. Polanyi (eds.), *Microscopic and Endoscopic Surgery with the $CO_2$ Laser.* Boston: John Wright, 1982.

78. Polanyi, T. Physics of Surgery with the $CO_2$ Laser. In A. Andrews and T. Polanyi (eds.), *Microscopic and Endoscopic Surgery with the $CO_2$ Laser.* Boston: John Wright, 1982.

79. Polanyi, T. G. Physics of surgery with lasers. *Clin. Chest Med.* 6:179, 1985.

80. Profio, E., et al. Laser-fluorescence bronchoscope for localization of occult lung tumors. *Med. Phys.* 6:523, 1979.

81. Ratz, J., et al. $CO_2$ laser treatment of portwine stains: A preliminary report. *J. Dermatol. Surg. Oncol.* 8:1039, 1982.

82. Reid, R., and Muller, S. Tattoo removal by $CO_2$ laser dermabrasion. *Plast. Reconstr. Surg.* 6:717, 1980.

83. Rosemberg, S. K., et al. Rapid superpulse carbon dioxide laser treatment of urethral condylomata. *Urology* 17:149, 1981.

84. Schawlow, A. L., and Townes, C. H. Infrared and optical masers. *Phys. Rev.* 112:1940, 1958.

85. Selkin, S. G. Laser turbinectomy as an adjunct to rhinoseptoplasty. *Arch. Otolaryngol.* 111:446, 1985.

86. Shapshay, S. M., et al. Removal of rhinophyma with $CO_2$ laser. *Arch. Otolaryngol.* 106:257, 1980.

87. Shikhani, A. H., et al. Infantile subglottic hemangiomas: An update. *Ann. Otol. Rhinol. Laryngol.* 95:336, 1986.

88. Sliney, D. Laser tissue interactions. *Clin. Chest Med.* 6:203, 1985.

89. Slutzki, S., et al. Use of the $CO_2$ laser for large excisions with minimal blood loss. *Plast. Reconstr. Surg.* 60:250, 1977.

90. Stellar, S. The $CO_2$ surgical lasers in neurological surgery, decubitus ulcers and burns. *Lasers Surg. Med.* 1:15, 1980.

91. Stellar, S., et al. $CO_2$ débridement of decubitus ulcers: Followed by immediate rotation flap or skin graft closure. *Ann. Surg.* 179:230, 1974.

92. Walsh, J., et al. Laser tissue interactions and their clinical applications. *Curr. Probl. Dermatol.* 115:94, 1986.

93. Weston, J., et al. Carbon dioxide laser brasion for treatment of adenoma sebaceum in tuberous sclerosis. *Ann. Plast. Surg.* 15:132, 1985.

94. Wheeland, R. G., et al. Treatment of adenoma sebaceum with carbon dioxide laser vaporization. *J. Dermatol. Surg. Oncol.* 11:861, 1985.

95. Wheeland, R. G., et al. Carbon dioxide ($CO_2$) laser vaporization of multiple facial syringomas. *J. Dermatol. Surg. Oncol.* 12:225, 1986.

96. Wilensky, J. The Use of Neodymium:YAG Lasers in the Treatment of Glaucoma. In J. Wilensky (ed.), *Laser Therapy in Glaucoma.* Norwalk, CT: Appleton-Century-Crofts, 1985.

97. Van der Zypen, E. The use of laser in eye surgery: Morphological principles. *Int. Ophthalmol. Clin.* 25:21, 1985.

98. Van Gemert, M., et al. Is there an optimal laser treatment for port wine stains? *Lasers Med. Surg.* 6:76, 1986.

## USE OF ARGON AND CARBON DIOXIDE LASERS IN CLINICAL PLASTIC SURGERY PRACTICE

1. Apfelberg, D. B., Maser, M. R., and Lash, H. Treatment of cutaneous vascular abnormalities with the argon laser—progress report. *Ann. Plast. Surg.* 1:14, 1978.

2. Apfelberg, D. B., Maser, M. R., and Lash, H. Review of usage of argon and carbon dioxide lasers for pediatric hemangiomas. *Ann. Plast. Surg.* 12:353, 1984.

3. Apfelberg, D. B., Maser, M. R., Lash, H., et al. $CO_2$ laser resection for giant perineal condyloma and verrucous carcinoma. *Plast. Surg.* 11:417, 1983.

4. Apfelberg, D. B., Maser, M. R., Lash, H., et al. Expanded role of the argon laser in plastic surgery. *J. Dermatol. Surg. Oncol.* 9:145, 1983.

5. Apfelberg, D. B., Lash, H., Maser, M. R., et al. A comparison of the argon and $CO_2$ lasers for the treatment of decorative tattoos—preliminary study. *Ann. Plast. Surg.* 14:6, 1985.

6. Apfelberg, D. B., Lash, H., Maser, M. R., et al. Benefits of the $CO_2$ laser for oral hemangioma excision. *Plast. Reconstr. Surg.* 75:46, 1985.

7. Brady, S. C., Blokmanis, A., and Jewett, L. Tattoo removal with the carbon dioxide laser. *Ann. Plast. Surg.* 2:482, 1979.

8. Fidler, J. F., Law, E., and Rockwell, R. J., Jr. Carbon dioxide laser excision of acute burns with immediate autografting. *J. Surg. Res.* 17:1, 1974.

9. Goldman, L., and Dreffer, R. Laser treatment of extended mixed cavernous and port wine stains. *Arch. Dermatol.* 113:504, 1977.

10. Noe, J. M., Barsky, S. H., Geer, D. E., et al. Port wine stains and the response to argon laser therapy: Successful treatment and the predictive role of color, age, and biopsy. *Plast. Reconstr. Surg.* 65:130, 1980.

# 28

*Gordon H. Sasaki*

# Hemangiomas, Arteriovenous Malformations, and Lymphangiomas

Hemangiomas and lymphangiomas remain the most common benign tumors the plastic surgeon sees in the skin and deeper tissues of the neonate. These angiomas represent sequestra of fetal tissue that consist primarily of endothelial cells. Such lesions may present at or before birth (congenital) or within the first 4 weeks of life (neonatal). Occasionally, acquired vascular malformations are reported during adulthood and are believed to be the result of trauma [27] or possibly hormonal influences [35]. Because each lesion has its own clinical course, management must be individually determined to meet the psychological and pathophysiologic consequences of each tumor.

Thomson [60] stated: "It is extremely important for the patient, the parents, and the physician to appreciate the natural history of each tumor in order to prepare the family unit for a specific treatment overview. In this regard, the most pivotal issue is the classification of a confusing nomenclature that can be of either a clinical or pathological nature."

A clinical classification of hemangiomas and lymphangiomas, as outlined by Thomson [60], is reproduced in Table 28-1.

## Significance

Most hemangiomas and lymphangiomas present as small, localized, superficial sequestra that are inconspicuously located on the body. A significant number undergo spontaneous regression or deflation and thus are considered transient cosmetic or functional deformities.

Whenever an elective aesthetic or functional reconstruction is required, however, it is best to have a patient who is old enough to cooperate during the surgical procedure and whose self image is developing. Elective surgical correction is recommended [20], in general, around ages 4 through 7, when the child becomes more aware of the deformity because of the development of body image at this age and the peer group's influence.

For problem lesions, the plastic surgeon is occasionally the primary physician who directs the overall management of the patient. Even in these cases, though, a multidisciplinary approach involving the pediatrician, geneticist, hematologist, oral surgeon, neurosurgeon, ophthalmologist, and social worker is required. Despite their benign histologic appearance, large and more critically located hemangiomas and lymphangiomas occasionally produce devastating physical deformities with associated psychological trauma. An example is the multiple disseminated hemangiomastosis of the newborn [6, 21], with diffuse involvement of the skin, liver, and intestinal tract. The mortality rate in these cases is significant despite aggressive medical and surgical management. Selection of the most appropriate emergent treatment for any of these problem lesions is varied and depends on the type, size, location, stage of development, clinical course, and degree of psychological impairment.

## Classification of Vascular Hamartomas

There is no uniformity in the classification of vascular hamartomas because of their great variation and overlap in clinical and histopathologic appearance. Attempts to classify these lesions, however, are important to reduce the confusion on diagnosis, management, and results.

Mulliken and Glowacki [43] and Pasyk et al. [49] proposed a classification based on the cellular dynamics of vascular hamartomas. Cellular dynamic lesions (hemangiomas, pyogenic granulomas, senile angiomas) possess definite *proliferative* and *regressive* phases, the proliferative phase being characterized by increased $^3$H-thymidine uptake, presence of tumor angiogenesis factors, mast cell activity, and syncytial cell formation. Cellular adynamic lesions (lymphangiomas, vascular ectasias, angiokeratomas, congenital arteriovenous malformations) have no *proliferation* or *regression* phase. The classification of Pasyk et al. is shown in Table 28-2.

The presence of steroid receptors (estradiol) within strawberry hemangiomas but not in cavernous hemangiomas, port-wine stain, or lymphangiomas may be another biologic indicator to aid in the classification, prognosis, and management of these common vascular lesions [54]. A more complete discussion of these findings is presented

**Table 28-1** *Classification of hemangiomas and lymphangiomas*

Capillary hemangioma
    Port-wine stain
    Strawberry
        Wild-fire
        Ulcerated
        Spontaneous regression
    Salmon patch
    Campbell de Morgan
    Telangiectasia
    Pyogenic granuloma
Capillary-cavernous hemangioma
Cavernous hemangioma
Other hemangiomas
    Verrucous
    Keratotic
    Venous
Lymphangioma
    Circumscripta
    Simplex
    Cavernous
    Cystic hygroma
Lymphangiohemangioma and
        hemangiolymphangioma
Arteriovenous malformation
Vascular gigantism

later under the management of strawberry hemangiomas.

In summary, the classification of vascular hamartomas is currently undergoing changes for the clinician. The term *hemangioma* (strawberry, cavernous, or mixed) may be best reserved to describe those lesions that cellularly and clinically undergo growth resolution. The term *vascular malformation* (port-wine stain and congenital or arteriovenous malformation) may accurately indicate those lesions that are cellularly adynamic and not responsive to change. Lymphangiomas are included within vascular malformations despite the fact that selected lesions do "regress." Regression, in most instances, however, represents deflation of lymph into a venous conduit.

***Table 28-2*** *Classification of vascular malformations*

| Cellularly dynamic lesions | Cellularly adynamic lesions |
| --- | --- |
| Hemangiomas<br>  Cellular<br>  Capillary<br>  Cavernous<br>  Mixed<br>  Verrucous<br>Pyogenic granuloma<br>Senile angioma | Vascular ectasias<br>  Salmon patches<br>  Nevus flammeus (port-wine stain)<br>  Nevus araneus<br>  Multiple telangiectasias<br>  Congenital phlebectasia<br>  Venous lake<br>Angiokeratomas<br>  Angiokeratoma Mibelli<br>  Angiokeratoma Fordyce<br>  Angiokeratoma circumscriptum<br>  Solitary and multiple angiokeratomas (imperial and Helwig type)<br>  Angiokeratoma corporis diffusum (Fabry's disease)<br>Congenital arteriovenous malformations* |

*Congenital arteriovenous malformations are *rheologically* dynamic but cellularly adynamic lesions.
*Source:* K. A. Pasyk, G. W. Cherry, W. C. Grabb, et al. Quantitative evaluation of mast cells in cellularly dynamic and adynamic vascular malformations. *Plast. Reconstr. Surg.* 73:69, 1984.

## Strawberry Hemangiomas (Newborn)

Strawberry hemangiomas are the most common birthmarks (4 to 5 percent incidence) [19] present at birth (70 percent) or within a few weeks during the neonatal period [24, 41]; the incidence is as high as 25 percent in premature infants. Females [24, 40, 41, 67] are more commonly affected than males, in a ratio of 2:1 to 3:1. Strawberry hemangiomas are relatively rare (0.1 percent) in blacks. More than one-half (56 percent) of all strawberry hemangiomas occur in the head and neck region; 23 percent occur in the trunk, 19 percent in the extremities, and 2 percent in the genitalia.

In general, strawberry hemangiomas grow rapidly in the first 5 to 8 months of life, reach a plateau between 6 and 12 months, and regress within 12 to 18 months. Regression follows a fairly consistent pattern for most uncomplicated superficial, mixed, and deep hemangiomas. Initially, there is cessation of growth in relation to the age of the child. The hemangioma becomes less tense to touch. Regression begins by the appearance of central blanching and coalescence of blue-gray areas of wrinkled skin that spread out peripherally over the lesion. Partial or complete regression and replacement fibrosis with fatty infiltration occurs later. Regression of the cavernous component is less obvious because it is less well delineated and the reduction of bulk is more gradual. Lister [36] reported the first statistical study of this phenomenon. Among 77 patients with 82 hemangiomas, 49 had disappeared completely, but 38 had demonstrated partial regression after 7 years of observation. Various authors have indicated the percentage of regression within 5 years: Wallace (97 percent) [64], Simpson (55 percent) [55], Bowers et al. (98 percent) [10], Walter (96 percent) [65], and Phelan and Grace (67 percent) [50]. In view of the high rate of spontaneous healing and small percentage of imperfect or unchanged lesions, it is particularly relevant to ask if any treatment is indicated. Over the years, the principle of *nil nocere* has been basically adhered to by most clinicians [1, 8, 29, 33, 40]. Such conservative theory has proved to be the safest, most efficacious management plan for most patients.

## INDICATIONS FOR EARLY MANAGEMENT

Complications are occasionally associated with the superficial and mixed (deep component) strawberry hemangiomas after rapid growth and spontaneous regression.

**1.** Severe progressive tissue destruction and distortion during the growth phase of the wildfire variant of strawberry hemangiomas may pursue a pseudomalignant course. Spontaneous hemorrhage can usually be controlled by firm pressure or surgical ligation. Ulceration can usually be managed by topical cleansing and ointment but is followed by a shiny, atrophic, contractured scar at the site of tissue breakdown. Infection occurs infrequently and is readily managed by local or systemic antibiotics.

**2.** Occasionally, strawberry hemangiomas grow by progressive degrees of tissue intrusion that obstructs small luminal structures such as the airways, introitus, and oral cavity [14]. In most cases these lesions involve the mucous membranes and are composed of the cavernous deeper vessels. These hemangiomas may persist into adult life.

**3.** Any obstruction of the visual axis is an indication for immediate treatment. Either transient amblyopia and astigmatism or permanent damage to the cortical visual center [52, 57, 60] can occur when there is total or partial visual obstruction for a short time during infancy.

**4.** With massive hemangiomas, disseminated intravascular coagulopathy may develop owing to thrombocytopenia [13, 18, 48]. The combination of bleeding and thrombocytopenia, described by Kasabach and Merritt [30], in large cavernous or mixed hemangiomas may be due to sequestration and platelet destruction. Straub et al. [58] suggested a localized intravascular consumption of fibrinogen, whereas others [9, 45] indicated a disseminated intravascular consumption coagulopathy and increased fibrinolysis.

## INDICATIONS FOR LATE MANAGEMENT

In occasional cases some form of late treatment may be indicated, often for reasons other than medical indications, such as emotional problems, parental concern, and the surgeon's anxiety. More often, delayed treatment may be indicated for those hemangiomas that have incompletely resolved. The remaining deformity may have produced contour or color discrepancies or may have distorted or destroyed facial features such as the nose, lips, and eyelids. Simpson and Lond [56] summed up a solution to this difficult problem: "If operation is deferred and performed only when natural resolution will clearly be unsatisfactory, simple excision of superfluous puckered skin may suffice and, at the worst, a more elaborate procedure can be undertaken with far less danger."

## MANAGEMENT ALTERNATIVES

In view of the wide range of opinions regarding management of the strawberry hemangioma or the mixed capillary-cavernous type, it is difficult to be dogmatic about which approach yields the optimal end result. Although the natural history of strawberry and mixed cavernous hemangiomas has been documented, a variety of opinions prevail regarding the behavior of these tumors. Reliance on the tendency to regress may be unwise for regression may not take place in selected lesions.

To establish a rational treatment plan, the first principle in the management of strawberry hemangiomas is to refrain from emergency therapy. There is time for consultation, proper diagnosis, and discussion of management alternatives. Continuous encouragement of the family unit is essential. The second principle is that, in the absence of factors that support active treatment, nothing is lost by attentive monitoring of the patient until at least 5 years of age. At that time, entry into a preschool, with its environmental influence, and the development of the patient's body image may produce psychological stress for the patient, family, and physician. A useful aid to improve parental apprehension is to have the family unit involved in group support sessions.

Grabb et al. [24] listed various treatments, in order of importance, as: (1) observation; (2) short course of alternate-day corticosteroid therapy; (3) compression; and (4) surgery. Other modalities include laser, radiation therapy, cryosurgery, and the use of sclerosing agents.

### Observation

During the period of attentive observation, 90 percent of these lesions either have involuted or are in the process of involution. An opaque cosmetic cream (e.g., Covermark; Lydia O'Leary, New York, N.Y.) that is tinted to match the patient's skin color is useful during this period.

### Corticosteroid Therapy

Systemic and local corticosteroids have been used to correct thrombocytopenia and prevent further bleeding diatheses in patients with giant hemangiomas (Kassabach-Meritt syndrome) [13, 48]. Although a few of these patients had regression of their hemangiomas, the steroid effects were unevaluable because combined forms of therapy were used, in particular surgery and irradiation. In 1967 Zarem and Edgerton [68] reported that seven patients with rapidly enlarging hemangiomas experienced premature involution after oral or locally injected steroids. Since then, three other clinical studies have confirmed their results and suggested modifications in the dosage and schedule of steroid treatment. In 1968 Fost and Easterly [20a] reported similar success in six patients. When therapy was begun, three patients were less than 6 months of age and the remaining three were 11, 13, and 16 months of age, respectively. Three patients, who relapsed after termination of therapy, were able to be controlled by a second course. In 1972 Brown et al. [12] presented a series of

nine patients with mixed capillary and cavernous hemangiomas. The enlarging lesions responded promptly after 20 to 40 mg of oral prednisone on alternate days for 1 to 3 months, with 4 to 6 weeks between succeeding courses. In 1972 Cohen and Wang [14] found steroid treatment effective in reducing the size of hemangiomas involving the airway, allowing early decannulation or eliminating the need for tracheostomy.

Sasaki et al. [54] reported that corticosteroid treatment of infant strawberry hemangiomas produced premature regression of growing lesions in patients, but not in those with cavernous or port-wine stain hemangiomas. Abnormally elevated serum estradiol-17β levels were found in strawberry hemangiomas: fourfold higher than in control, cavernous, or port-wine stain hemangiomas adjusted for age and sex of the patients.

Specific estradiol-17β receptor binding activity was studied in biopsy tissues obtained from normal prepubertal skin and skin from various kinds of hemangioma. Minimal specific estradiol-17β binding activity was detected in tissues of normal skin and involuting strawberry, cavernous, or port-wine hemangiomas. Abnormally high levels of specific estradiol-17β binding sites were demonstrated by receptor assays and in vitro tissue culture technique in nine tissue samples obtained from strawberry hemangiomas, seven of which responded definitely or probably to corticosteroid therapy. These data seem to suggest that there may be a causal relation between the presence of elevated serum estradiol and specific estradiol-17β receptors in the pathogenesis of strawberry hemangiomas and in response to corticosteroid treatment of the hormone-sensitive hemangiomas.

### Compression Therapy

Compression treatment of hemangiomas is believed to cause more rapid regression of selected hemangiomas. Case reports by Miller et al. [42] and Mangus [39] indicated that this therapy is safe, noninvasive, and efficacious.

The use of cosmetics (e.g., Covermark or Cover Girl), though not ideal, is still an acceptable form of management. These opaque cosmetic creams in combination with face powder can satisfactorily match the patient's skin tone and color.

Port-wine stains are resistant to the effects of steroids and radiation therapy. The adult vascular endothelium does not respond to irradiation, which may result in tissue hypoplasia, radiation dermatitis, and radiation carcinoma.

The argon laser has produced encouraging results [2, 16, 46] to modify significantly the color and presence of these lesions. With improvement in technique [22] and types of laser employed [63], residual scarring and irregularity of pigmentation are becoming less common. Scar incidence varies from 5 to 24 percent and is worse with lesions around the upper lips.

## Arteriovenous Malformations

The patient with true massive arteriovenous plexiform malformations has a potentially lethal problem causing extensive deformity and functional disturbance. Malan and Azzolini [38] emphasized that the physiologic significance of these lesions depended on the size of the arteriovenous shunt and its sequelae rather than the original morphologic type. Macroshunting may produce hypervolemia, cardiac hypertrophy, and congestive heart failure. Widespread involvement of the skin, subcutaneous tissue, muscle, and bone may lead to gigantism, tissue necrosis, and infection.

Clinical experience has demonstrated that surgical ligation of vessels may exacerbate the vascular hemodynamics of the lesion, opening previously collapsed vessels and thereby extending the distribution of the lesion. Treatment with sclerosing agents, radiation, steroids, and partial ligation has yielded poor results. For these reasons, intraarterial embolization with muscle fragments [5, 17, 34] and silicone spheres [37] has offered the surgeon a primary therapeutic alternative or a staged procedure prior to extirpation [32]. Control and regression of those difficult lesions by selective embolization alone has been encouraging [44, 51]. Provisions for extensive blood replacement and hypotensive anesthesia are made whenever wide resection is anticipated.

## Other Syndromes

Hemangiomatous syndromes are rare and may involve almost any area of the body. Williams [67] has written a concise review of the management of those complex problems.

The Sturge-Weber syndrome is a port-wine stain in the distribution of the ophthalmic and maxillary divisions of the trigeminal nerve of the face. However, the vascular lesion may also involve additional areas of the head, neck, and torso. There may be associated contralateral hemiplegia and focal, sometimes intractable, jacksonian epilepsy due to angioma of the leptomeninges. Calcification in a meningeal angioma may be seen in older children. Mental retardation is frequently observed. Various degrees of ophthalmic involvement include buphthalmos, megalocornea, hydrophthalmos, and glaucoma. Glaucoma is assumed to be present in more than 50 percent of patients who have a combination of trigeminal nerve distribution. If glaucoma is suspected and confirmed by tonometry and slit lamp analysis during the first 6 months of life, proper treatment by an ophthalmologist can prevent blindness.

The Klippel-Trenaunay-Weber syndrome (hemangiectatic hypertrophy and gigantism), which involves enlargement of an extremity due to capillary and cavernous hemangiomas, is associated with deeper venous varicosities, arteriovenous fistulas with micro-macroshunting, an increase in skin temperature, and perspiration of the affected extremity. Osteohypertrophy may result in a gross deformity of the extremity, associated with multiple complications, e.g., left ventricular hypertrophy or failure, ulceration and infection, diffuse consumption coagulopathy, and disuse due to gigantic tissue overgrowth [28, 31]. If the vascular involvement is large and life-threatening, amputation of the extremity may be required. For more localized forms of the disease to the digits or hand, soft tissue reduction, osteotomy, or epiphysiodesis may be indicated. Because delayed wound healing is common, such surgical interventions must be carefully considered.

Maffucci syndrome, or dyschondroplasia with cavernous hemangioma, demonstrates gross defects in ossification that lead to severe skeletal deformities. Chondrosarcoma and other neoplasia have been observed. Death is believed to occur because of multiple genetic defects [4].

The blue rubber bleb syndrome involves soft, compressible, deep cavernous hemangiomas found in the trunk, extremities, and submucosa of the gastrointestinal tract [4]. The number of lesions vary in size and location, and bleeding may be a significant problem for management.

CONCLUSION

The classification of hemangiomatous lesions is still undergoing revision to correlate more accurately their histopathologic characteristics with prognosis and treatment. Until the basic mechanisms of growth and regression are understood, the clinician must rely primarily on the growth characteristics of the lesion. Parental support and more sophisticated knowledge of these various lesions by the patient, family, and clinician are essential to proper management. The presence of steroid receptors has opened up new avenues for research and potential management of early lesions. Residual problem lesions may require a number of treatment modalities that must be based on solid rationale, safety, and efficacy.

## Lymphangioma

The lymphangioma represents a congenital and developmental lesion that continues to confuse clinicians by its imprecise etiology, natural maturation, and response to surgery [11, 53]. Lymphangiomas probably consist of an excess of lymphatic vasoformative tissue of fetal angiogenesis [59]. For purposes of discussion, lymphangiomas are classified as lymphangioma simplex, lymphangioma cavernous, and cystic hygroma.

Lymphangioma simplex is a rare, superficial lesion that may occur as a single nodule or may be arranged in groups. These capillary-sized lymphatic nodules have a grayish pink color and are most often seen on the genitalia, lips, and tongue.

Cavernous lymphangiomas may be small lesions or may involve an extensive area, causing, for example, macroglossia or macrochelia. The cavernous lesion usually involves deep structures with dilated lymphatic channels that are compressible.

Cystic hygromas represent a true congenital malformation of the lymphatics that most commonly arises in the neck, upper thorax, and groin. These lesions may be small and of only minor concern but occasionally involve large areas indifferent to normal fascial planes. Cystic hygromas may be unilocular or, more commonly, multilocular filled with clean fluid. The lesions may be present at birth and in 90 percent of cases become evident by the second year [26]. In general, the cystic hygroma is not compressible.

Lymphangiomas are often an admixture of capillary, cavernous, or cystic sinusoids. Frequently, large cystic spaces do not communicate with one another, so that decompression by aspiration technique requires entry into each cavity. On certain occasions, lymphangiomas present a diagnostic challenge to rule out similar lesions, such as lymphangiohemangioma. The presence of lymph fluid or erythrocytes within the endothelial channels may help to resolve the differential diagnosis [53]. Such differentiation can be facilitated by technetium isotope flow structure, which indicates the cystic hygroma to be a cold lesion.

There appears to be no hereditary predisposition to lymphangioma. Most large series report an equal ratio of males to females [53]. Gross and Goeringer [26] noted that 65 percent of 112 lymphangiomas were present at birth, 80 percent were noted by 1 year of life, and 90 percent by age 2. Bill and Sumner [7] found that only 4 percent of 61 lymphangiomas occurred after the third year. These authors found the neck most commonly involved, followed by the axillae and pectoral region. In the head area the tongue, cheek, and floor of the mouth were most commonly affected.

NATURAL HISTORY

Many clinicians believe that pure lymphangiomas tend to involute spontaneously or undergo partial regression. Others believe that there is no regression or deflation and therefore surgical intervention is indicated. Because the lesion has no regard to anatomic planes and involves tissue extensively, there may be increased morbidity due to transection of vital structures (muscle and nerves) during the surgical procedure.

Grabb et al. [24] reported complete involution or deflation in 41 percent and partial resolution in 29 percent by 5 years of age. Broomhead [11] first reported that 16 percent of cystic hygromas of the neck had complete resolution. The true incidence of involution is unknown, but Grabb et al. cited it as between 15 and 70 percent during the first 20 years of life.

Noninvoluting lymphangiomas may slowly enlarge at the same rate or faster than the growth of the child. Bill and Sumner [7] suggested that obstruction of lymph channels contributed to the growth phase of the lymphangioma. Often cystic hygromas enlarge during an upper respiratory infection over a period of hours and then return to their original size (deflation) over a period of a few days to months. There are no documented cases of carcinoma developing from a benign lymphangioma in the head and neck region [3].

MANAGEMENT

Because a significant number of lymphangiomas spontaneously resolve before 5 years of age, conservative treatment is recommended. Occasionally, a cystic hygroma impinges on the airway, and respiratory distress with the patient presenting with opisthotonos requires emergent decompression and tracheostomy.

Grabb et al. [24] outlined their approach to the general management of lymphangiomas and cystic hygromas as follows.

1. Expectant treatment is the rule.
2. Transient enlargement should not force a surgical intervention.
3. Staged partial excisions with preservation of vital structures may be considered for lymphangiomas that demonstrate no resolution by age 3 and provide significant functional and aesthetic considerations. With an extensive hygroma, it is well to limit one's sights to what can be accomplished at a single operation. One must never sacrifice important structures that are surrounded by the hygroma. Radical surgery is not necessary, as these lesions are not malignant. Several conservative debulking tailoring procedures are preferred to wide-scale dissection.
4. Surgical excision of small lesions may be indicated when the anticipated residual scar is acceptable.
5. Cysts that cannot be safely excised may be marsupialized, decompressed with multiple drains, or aspirated.
6. Radiation therapy, the injection of sclerosing agents, and steroid treatment have not produced satisfactory results.

SUMMARY

The diagnosis and treatment of lymphangiomas must be based on a combination of clinical pathologic findings. Conservative management is recommended for most lesions that may undergo resolution by deflation. The surgical approach must be individualized to preserve as many of the normal structures as possible and yet reduce the bulk of the problem lesions.

## References

1. Andrews, G. C., et al. Hemangiomas-treated and untreated. *J.A.M.A.* 165:1114, 1957.
2. Apfelberger, D. B., Maser, M. R., and Lash, H. Extended clinical use of the argon laser for cutaneous lesions. *Arch. Dermatol.* 115:719, 1979.
3. Batsakis, J. G. *Tumors of the Head and Neck: Clinical and Pathological Considerations* (2nd ed.). Baltimore: Williams & Wilkins, 1979.
4. Bean, W. B. *Vascular Spiders and Related Lesions of the Skin*. Springfield, IL: Thomas, 1958.
5. Bennett, J. E., and Zook, E. G. Treatment of arteriovenous fistulas in cavernous hemangiomas of the face by muscle embolization. *Plast. Reconstr. Surg.* 50:84, 1972.
6. Berman, B., and Wan-Peng, L. H. Concurrent cutaneous and hepatic hemangiomata in infancy: Report of a case and a review of the literature. *J. Dermatol. Surg. Oncol.* 4:869, 1978.
7. Bill, A. H., and Sumner, D. S. A unified concept of lymphangiomas and cystic hygromas. *Surg. Gynecol. Obstet.* 120:79, 1965.
8. Blackfield, H. M., Torrey, F. A., and Morris, W. J. The management of visible hemangioma. *Am. J. Surg.* 94:313, 1957.
9. Blix, S., and Aas, K. Giant hemangioma, thrombocytopenia, fibrinogenopenia, and fibrinolytic activity. *Acta Med. Scand.* 169:63, 1961.
10. Bowers, R. E., Graham, E. A., and Tomlinson, K. M. The natural history of the strawberry nevus. *Arch. Dermatol.* 82:59, 1960.
11. Broomhead, I. W. Cystic hygroma of the neck. *Br. J. Plast. Surg.* 17:225, 1964.
12. Brown, S. H., Neerhant, R. C., and Fonkalsrud, E. W. Prednisone therapy in the management of large hemangiomas in infants and children. *Surgery* 7:168, 1972.
13. Clemmensen, O. A case of multiple neonatal hemangiomatosis successfully treated with systemic corticosteroids. *Dermatologica* 159:495, 1979.
14. Cohen, S. R., and Wand, C. Steroid treatment of hemangioma of the head and neck in children. *Ann. Otol. Rhinol. Otolaryngol.* 81:584, 1972.
15. Conway, H., and Docktor, J. P. Neutralization of color in capillary hemangioma of the face by intradermal injection (tattooing) of permanent pigments. *Surg. Gynecol. Obstet.* 84:866, 1947.
16. Cosman, B. Experience in the argon laser therapy of portwine stains. *Plast. Reconstr. Surg.* 65:119, 1980.
17. Cunningham, D. S., and Palletta, F. Control of arteriovenous fistulae in massive facial hemangiomas by muscle emboli. *Plast. Reconstr. Surg.* 46:305, 1970.
18. Dargeon, H. W., Adio, A. C., and Pack, G. T. Hemangioma with thrombocytopenia. *J. Pediatr.* 54:285, 1959.
19. Edgerton, M. T., and Hiebert, J. M. Vascular and lymphatic tumors in infancy, childhood and adulthood: Challenge of diagnosis and treatment. *Curr. Probl. Cancer* 2(7):1, 1978.
20. Fisk, S. B., Pearl, R. M., Schulman, G. I., et al. Congenital facial anomalies among 4 through 7 year olds: Psychological efforts and surgical excisions. 14:37, 1985.
20a. Fost, N. C., and Easterly, N. B. Successful treatment of juvenile hemangiomas with prednisone. *J. Pediatr.* 2:351, 1968.
21. Fryns, J. P., Eggermont, E., and Eeckels, R. Multiple diffuse hemangiomatosis: Case report and review of the literature. *Z. Kinderheilkd.* 117:115, 1974.
22. Gilchrest, B. A., Rosen, S., and Noe, J. M. Chilling port wine stains improves the response to argon laser therapy. *Plast. Reconstr. Surg.* 69:278, 1982.
23. Goldwyn, R. M., and Rosoff, C. B. Cryosurgery for large hemangiomas in adults. *Plast. Reconstr. Surg.* 43:605, 1969.
24. Grabb, W. C., Dingman, R. O., Oneal, R. M., et al. Facial hamartomas in children: Neurofibroma, lymphangioma, and hemangioma. *Plast. Reconstr. Surg.* 66:509, 1980.
25. Grabb, W. C., MacCollum, M. S., and Tan, N. G. Results from tattooing port wine hemangioma. *Plast. Reconstr. Surg.* 59:667, 1977.
26. Gross, R. E., and Goeringer, C. F. Cystic hygromas of the neck. *Surg. Gynecol. Obstet.* 59:48, 1936.
27. Hall-Smith, S. P. Acquired haemangioma.

*Trans. St. Johns Hosp. Dermatol. Soc. Lond.* 48:190, 1962.

28. Herrington, J. L. Congenital angiomatous malformation involving the entire lower extremity: Report of hemipelvectomy in a 25 day old infant. *Surgery* 34:759, 1953.

29. Jacobs, A. H. Strawberry hemangiomas: The natural history of the untreated lesion. *Calif. Med.* 86:8, 1957.

30. Kasabach, H. H., and Merritt, K. K. Capillary hemangiomas with extensive purpura. *Am. J. Dis. Child.* 59:1063, 1940.

31. Khaw, J. H., and Datuk, O. Localized gigantism of the extremities. *Med. J. Malaysia* 27:292, 1973.

32. Kiehn, C. L., DesPrez, J. D., and Kaufman, B. Cavernous hemangiomas of the head and neck: Indications for arteriography and surgical treatment. *Plast. Reconstr. Surg.* 33:338, 1964.

33. Lampe, I., and Latourette, H. B. Management of hemangiomas in infants. *Pediatr. Clin. North Am.* 6:511, 1959.

34. Lang, E. R., and Bucy, P. C. Treatment of carotid-cavernous fistula by muscle embolization alone: The Brooks method. *J. Neurosurg.* 22:387, 1965.

35. Letterman, G., Schurter, M., Barter, R. H., et al. Hemangiomas of pregnancy. *South. Med. J.* 50:594, 1957.

36. Lister, W. A. The natural history of strawberry nevi. *Lancet* 1:1429, 1938.

37. Longacre, J. J., Benton, C., and Urterthiner, R. A. Treatment of facial hemangioma by intravascular embolization with silicone spheres. *Plast. Reconstr. Surg.* 50:618, 1972.

38. Malan, E., and Azzolini, A. Congenital arteriovenous malformation of the face and scalp. *J. Cardiovasc. Surg.* 9:109, 1968.

39. Mangus, D. J. Continuous compression treatment of hemangiomata: Evolution of two cases. *Plast. Reconstr. Surg.* 49:490, 1970.

40. Margileth, A. M., and Museles, M. Current concepts on diagnosis and management of congenital cutaneous hemangiomas. *Pediatrics* 36:410, 1965.

41. Matthews, D. N. Hemangiomata. *Plast. Reconstr. Surg.* 41:528, 1968.

42. Miller, S. H., Smith, R. L., and Schochat, S. J. Compression treatment of hemangiomas. *Plast. Surg.* 58:573, 1976.

43. Mulliken, J. B., and Glowacki, J. Hemangiomas and vascular malformations in infants and children: A classification based on endothelial characteristics. *Plast. Reconstr. Surg.* 69:412, 1982.

44. Natali, J., and Merland, J. J. Superselective arteriography and therapeutic embolization for vascular malformations (angiodysplasias). *J. Cardiovasc. Surg.* 17:465, 1976.

45. Neiderhart, J. A., and Rouch, R. W. Successful treatment of skeletal hemangioma and Kasabach-Merritt syndrome with aminocaproic acid. *Am. J. Med.* 73:434, 1982.

46. Noe, J. M., Barsky, S. H., Gear, D. E., et al. Portwine stains and the response to argon laser therapy: Successful treatment and the predictive role of color, age, and biopsy. *Plast. Reconstr. Surg.* 65:130, 1980.

47. Norberg, V. B., and Sunberg, J. Indications and methods for radiotherapy of cavernous hemangiomas. *Acta Radiol.* 1:257, 1963.

48. Paletta, F. X., Walker, J., and King, J. Hemangioma-thrombocytopenia syndrome. *Plast. Reconstr. Surg.* 23:615, 1959.

49. Pasyk, K. A., Cherry, G. W., Grabb, W. C., et al. Quantitative evaluation of mast cells in cellularly dynamic and adynamic vascular malformations. *Plast. Reconstr. Surg.* 73:69, 1984.

50. Phelan, J. T., and Grace, J. T. Conservative management of cutaneous capillary hemangioma. *J.A.M.A.* 185:100, 1963.

51. Riche, M. C., Hajean, E., Tran-Ba-Huy, P., et al. The treatment of capillary-venous malformations using a new fibrosing agent. *Plast. Reconstr. Surg.* 71:607, 1983.

52. Robb, R. M. Refractive errors associated with hemangiomas of the eyelids and orbits in infancy. *Am. J. Ophthalmol.* 83:52, 1977.

53. Saijo, M., Munro, I. R., and Mancer, K. Lymphangioma: A long-term follow-up study. *Plast. Reconstr. Surg.* 56:513, 1966.

54. Sasaki, G. H., Pang, C. Y., and Witliff, J. L. Pathogenesis and treatment of infant skin strawberry hemangiomas: Clinical and in vitro studies of hormonal effects. *Plast. Reconstr. Surg.* 73:359, 1984.

55. Simpson, J. R. Natural history of cavernous hemangiomata. *Lancet* 2:1057, 1959.

56. Simpson, J. R., and Lond, M. B. Natural history of cavernous hemangiomas. *Lancet* 2:1057, 1959.

57. Stigmar, G., et al. Ophthalmic sequelae of in-

fantile hemangiomas of the eyelid and orbit. *Am. J. Ophthalmol.* 85:806, 1978.

58. Straub, P. W., Kessler, S., Schreiber, A., et al. Chronic intravascular coagulation in Kasabach-Merritt syndrome. *Arch. Intern. Med.* 129:475, 1972.

59. Sulayman, R., and Cassels, D. E. Myocardial coronary hemangiomatous tumors in children. *Chest* 68:113, 1975.

60. Thomson, H. G. Hemangioma, Lymphangioma, and Arteriovenous Fistula. In W. C. Grabb and J. W. Smith (eds.), *Plastic Surgery.* Boston: Little, Brown, 1979. P. 518.

61. Thomson, H. G., and Lanigan, M. The cryanonose: A clinical review of hemangiomas of the nasal tip. *Plast. Reconstr. Surg.* 63:155, 1979.

62. Van Der Werf, E. Spontaneous disappearance of hemangiomata. *Nederl. Tijdschr. Geneesk.* 98:676, 1954.

63. Van Gemert, M. J. C., and Hulsbergen-Henning, J. P. A model approach to laser coagulation of dermal vascular lesions. *Arch. Dermatol. Res.* 270:429, 1981.

64. Wallace, H. J. The conservative treatment of hemangiomatous nevi. *Br. J. Plast. Surg.* 6:78, 1953.

65. Walter, J. On The treatment of cavernous hemangiomas with special reference to spontaneous regression. *J. Fac. Radiol.* 5:135, 1953.

66. Williams, H. B. Hemangiomas of the parotid gland in children. *Plast. Reconstr. Surg.* 56:29, 1975.

67. Williams, H. B. Vascular neoplasms. *Clin. Plast. Surg.* 7:397, 1980.

68. Zarem, H. A., and Edgerton, M. T. Induced resolution of cavernous hemangiomas following prednisolone therapy. *Plast. Reconstr. Surg.* 39:76, 1967.

# 29

Harvey A. Zarem
Nicholas J. Lowe

# Benign Growths and Generalized Skin Disorders

The purpose of this chapter is to review the subject of benign growths and generalized skin disorders. We have emphasized the clinical significance of the subjects in this area that present problems common to the dermatologist and plastic surgeon. Developments with regard to some relatively recently recognized entities, such as dysplastic nevi and the Kaposi sarcoma problem in acquired immunodeficiency syndrome, have been included. In addition, where relevant, advances in the therapy of skin diseases have been included.

## Benign Growths

Pigmented lesions present the physician with the dilemma of which are the potentially malignant or frankly malignant lesions and which lesions may be treated as benign. Clinically, the distinction between benign and malignant skin lesions is usually clear, but the physician must be cautious to remove those lesions that arouse suspicion of malignancy or that create anxiety in the patient. The characteristics of malignant melanoma have been defined in numerous articles, and most physicians are fully aware of the need to remove pigmented lesions that are enlarging, crusting, or bleeding or that show such activity as deepening pig-

mentation with surrounding inflammation. The real challenge is to understand the nature of the lesions that do not have obvious signs of malignancy but may create trouble in the future. Pathologists now agree that malignant melanoma may arise from a preexisting pigmented lesion or that it may arise de novo. Most malignant melanomas that arise from preexisting pigmented lesions do so from a melanotic freckle of Hutchinson [59]. Much less commonly, a junctional or compound nevus cell nevus, in particular a large nevus cell nevus that has been present since birth, can be the site of malignant melanoma. The ordinary nevus cell nevus—junctional, compound, or intradermal—is rarely complicated by the evolution of malignant melanoma [56].

The *junctional nevus* clinically is a smooth, flat, irregularly pigmented lesion. It may occur at any site on the body, but pigmented nevi on palmar or plantar skin or on transitional epithelium (e.g., glans penis, vulva, or vermilion border of the lip) are usually junctional nevi and remain so. Junctional nevi may appear at any age, but are most common during childhood, adolescence, and young adult life [48]. The junctional nevus seen during childhood is less common in adults, presumably because of the transformation of the junctional nevus to an intradermal compound nevus during adulthood.

Although it is uncommon for *malignant melanoma* to arise from an intradermal or a compound nevus, it may occur. However, it is generally agreed that unless such a lesion exhibits a notable change in size, crusting, surrounding inflammation, or increasing pigmentation, it need not be excised for fear of malignant degeneration.

### DYSPLASTIC NEVI

Dysplastic nevi are acquired pigmented lesions of the skin [49]. The precise definitions of dysplastic nevi have undergone reevaluation. Clinical features of dysplastic nevi are as follows: They often have a variable mixture of colors, their borders are irregular, and pigment may spread into the surrounding skin. They are usually more than 6 mm in diameter. Usually the person with dysplastic nevi has multiple nevi, often in excess of 100. Sun-exposed areas, especially the back, are the most common sites.

Dysplastic nevi may occur in families, or they may arise sporadically, without a family history. It is thought that with some familial dysplastic nevi inheritance is a dominant trait. One important aspect is that patients with dysplastic nevi have an approximately 5 to 10 percent risk of developing malignant melanoma compared to a risk of approximately 0.7 percent for the general population. For clinical purposes, these patients with dysplastic nevi require careful, continuous skin evaluation. Any suspicious lesions that clinically may have shown progression to melanoma must clearly be excised and subjected to careful histopathologic examination.

The *melanotic freckle of Hutchinson* (Fig. 29-1) early in its course resembles the junctional nevus but is characterized by continuing slow growth to form a path of irregular, polycyclic, variegated pigmentation usually larger than 1 cm. Although it characteristically occurs on the face, the melanotic freckle of Hutchinson may be seen on the neck, back, or anywhere else on the body. This lesion frequently precedes a superficial malignant melanoma, and its recognition is critical so that removal may be carried out before frank invasive melanoma develops. The excision of the melanotic freckle of Hutchinson need not be radical, but the entire lesion must be removed [59].

*Benign juvenile melanoma* has been clearly discussed in a comprehensive review article by Kopf and Andrade [28]. This lesion, despite some histologic characteristics that in the past led to confusion with malignant melanoma, is a variant of the nevus cell nevus and does not behave as a malignant lesion. These frequently nonpigmented, pale red, papular lesions usually occur before puberty and may even be present at birth. In 15 percent of cases, they are observed initially during adolescence or adulthood. The be-

*Figure 29-1* Melanotic freckle of Hutchinson showing irregular borders and variegated pigmentation. This lesion must be excised as there is a high incidence of progression to malignant melanoma.

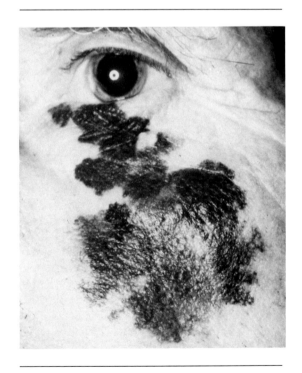

nign juvenile melanoma occurs most frequently on the face; only occasionally is it melanized. Although true malignant melanomas occur rarely in infants and children, it is important to recognize the more common benign juvenile melanoma to avoid unnecessary radical operative procedures necessary for the treatment of a malignant melanoma.

The *giant pigmented nevus* (Fig. 29-2) is a congenital lesion that sometimes demonstrates a tendency to occur in the distribution of dermatomes, or it may occur in a bathing trunk, vest, sleeve, or stocking pattern. It most commonly occurs on the head or pelvic area, appearing as a large, pigmented, hairy, soft verrucose lesion. The reported incidence of malignant melanoma arising in the giant pigmented nevus is variable—from less than 1 percent to as high as 10 to 25 percent [29, 44]. The issue of the malignant potential of congenital nevi is an important but confusing one. The "true incidence" of malignant degeneration in giant pigmented nevi is likely to be in the range of 1 to 2 percent, which was found in a 40-year follow-up in 110 defined cases of giant pigmented nevi: In that study, melanomas developed in two patients at ages 28 and 40 years, respectively, as cited by Dellon et al. [12] and Kaplan [24]. Kaplan reviewed the literature of 59 cases of malignant melanoma developing in giant pigmented nevi, adding seven other cases from their own institution, and demonstrated a peak incidence of malignant melanoma arising in the congenital giant pigmented nevi during the first 5 years of life.

It appears that those *lesions that exhibit verrucose characteristics* with deep pigmentation and thick skin are more likely to be complicated by malignant change and warrant operative removal. Most children or parents seek removal of these lesions because of aesthetic disfigurement [3]. The giant pigmented nevus creates a surgical challenge, especially about the face. Today it is generally agreed that such lesions on the

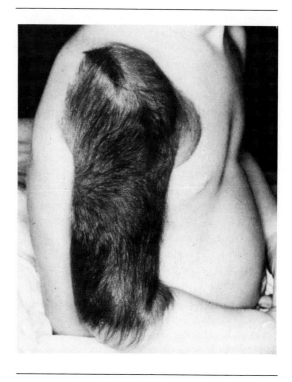

**Figure 29-2** *Giant hairy pigmented nevus.*

face are best removed and the face reconstructed with local skin flaps. Lesions on the trunk may be excised in stages with ultimate total removal. The extremity lesions are generally removed and resurfaced with free skin grafts. The melanocyte proliferative activity is frequently more extensive than is apparent from the margins of clinical pigmentation, so the appearance of pigmented cells in the scars or adjacent to the scars of previous excisions is not uncommon. For this reason it is important to remove some margin of seemingly normal skin beyond that indicated by the presence or absence of pigment. Neonatal dermabrasion has been used as an attempt to reduce the superficial pigmented cells present in giant nevi. Whether this procedure conducted early enough significantly reduces the risk of future malignancy is currently not known.

*Lentigo sinilis* is not a nevus cell lesion

but consists of a smooth, dark brown patch measuring up to 1.5 cm in diameter in which there are increased numbers of normal melanocytes. Lentigo senilis is frequently multiple in middle-aged or older people and appears especially in areas exposed to actinic rays, such as the dorsum of the hands, face, neck, and arms. Although lentigo senilis is on occasion difficult to differentiate clinically from freckles, junctional nevi, incipient seborrheic keratosis, and Hutchinson's melanotic freckle, it is rarely confused with malignant lesions. When the diagnosis of lentigo senilis is established, removal may be accomplished by operative excision when feasible or by proper cryotherapy.

A *freckle* (ephelis) represents a pigmented lesion with a normal number of melanocytes that produce an abnormally large number of melanin granules. The melanocytes in the freckle show no proliferative activity and as such do not exhibit any malignant potential.

The *blue nevus* is a firm, well defined small intradermal nodule composed of dermal melanocytes. Although malignant degeneration in blue nevi is a rarity, malignancy can occur in lesions that clinically resemble a blue nevus. Occasionally the differential diagnosis is difficult between blue nevus, metastasis of a malignant melanoma, and Kaposi sarcoma. A venous-like or other hemangioma may also present diagnostic confusion with the blue nevus, but usually compression of the lesion that is a hemangioma demonstrates some sponginess and blanching, which are not characteristic of the blue nevus.

The *nevus of Ota* is a blue-gray discoloration of the face in a pattern following the first and second branches of the fifth cranial nerve. The nevus of Ota most commonly involves the eye and the periorbital regions [64], and 60 percent are present at birth or within the first decade of life; 80 percent of the nevus of Ota lesions are seen in females. The lesion must be distinguished from a malignant melanoma, which it can closely resemble clinically.

EPIDERMAL LESIONS

*Nevus verrucosus* is a papillomatous yellowish tan keratotic plaque that appears at birth or during childhood. The lesion may be patchy or linear and often has the deceptive appearance of being limited to the superficial epidermis clinically. Superficial abrasion or electrodesiccation rarely removes the lesion permanently because there is an underlying dermal disturbance that induces the epidermal changes. Those lesions that create a significant diagnostic problem or cause a noticeable deformity can be excised with a full thickness of skin to ensure that they do not recur. Systemic agents currently being used in some patients with verrucous epidermal nevi are the synthetic retinoids. These agents are vitamin A analogs that may be used in appropriate patients to significantly reduce the degree of varicosity of these lesions. The two drugs used clinically are 13-*cis*-retinoic acid and the aromatic retinoid etretinate. These drugs are best managed by the dermatologist, as they have multiple mucocutaneous side effects as well as a significant potential for teratogenicity and skeletal hyperostosis. When the retinoids are discontinued, verrucous epidermal changes usually occur. These drugs are, however, valuable for selective patients with this condition.

*Keratosis follicularis* (Darier's disease) is a hereditary disorder of keratinization resulting in greasy, crusted, warty masses on the face, neck, chest, axilla, and inguinal areas. The unpleasant, malodorous masses have not responded to conservative treatment, and irradiation has been recommended in some dermatologic literature. One article has reported the successful treatment of these lesions by partial-thickness removal with split-thickness shaving or dermabrasion [11]. Again the synthetic retinoids have been used successfully to treat keratosis follicularis [51]. The guidelines for the use of these drugs must be followed carefully, and their use is best managed by a knowledgeable dermatologist.

*Hailey-Hailey disease,* a condition also known as chronic benign familial pemphigus, clinically affects the axillae and sub-mammary areas, although the groin may also be involved. It appears clinically as erosive exudative inflammatory areas of skin. It is histologically characterized by acantholysis. Treatment may be excision of the affected area with grafting. Dermatologic medical treatment involves the use of topical and systemic antibiotics as well as agents to reduce yeast colonization. It is often a difficult disease to manage.

*Tylosis* (keratosis palmaris et plantaris) is hereditary thickening of the palms and soles that becomes painful. Patients who are sufficiently symptomatic owing to the painful fissures may be treated with excision of the involved skin and resurfacing with split-thickness skin grafting [27]. There have been a small number of family members reported from England in whom tylosis was associated with the development of esophageal neoplasia. It occurs rarely, but a careful family history of this potential would be important for the management of such family members.

*Seborrheic keratosis* is a common lesion often seen in large numbers, especially on the trunk, face, and arms of middle-age and older individuals. The seborrheic keratosis is a sharply circumscribed, cauliflower-like, waxy papillomatous lesion with a friable hyperkeratotic surface. Most descriptively, it has a "stuck-on" appearance. Pigmentation of seborrheic keratosis is variable, from mild to deep black. The experienced physician can readily recognize seborrheic keratosis by its appearance and its characteristic superficiality, which allows the lesion to be readily scraped off level with surrounding skin, revealing a raw surface. Nevertheless, seborrheic keratosis is the most commonly encountered lesion in surgical pathology laboratories erroneously diagnosed by the clinician as malignant melanoma. Because many of these lesions are broad-based, excision is limited to those lesions for which there may be diagnostic uncertainty. Superficial examination of the histologic pattern of a seborrheic keratosis may create confusion with

squamous carcinoma in those inflamed lesions that have recently been subjected to trauma or irritation. The experienced pathologist is usually able to distinguish seborrheic keratosis from squamous cell carcinoma without hesitation. Adequate treatment of the seborrheic keratosis consists of curettage, superficial electrodesiccation, or freezing with liquid nitrogen, as this lesion does not undergo malignant degeneration.

The *actinic keratosis* (senile keratosis) must be distinguished from the seborrheic keratosis. The actinic keratosis is found primarily on exposed surfaces as discrete, flat, or slightly elevated lesions with hard, dry adherent hyperkeratosis and underlying erythema. Because these lesions are often numerous in elderly people with weather-beaten skin, it may be impractical to excise or biopsy all of them. The physician must select for excision those senile keratoses that occur in relatively young people, lesions that have become thickened or verrucose, and those that exhibit surrounding inflammation or crusting. Many dermatologists believe they are secure in removing lesions that do not have a suspicious characteristic using nonsurgical means such as liquid nitrogen or topical 5-fluorouracil. Histologically, the actinic keratosis may be similar to Bowen's disease. Except for the early superficial actinic keratosis lesions that are removed nonsurgically by the dermatologist, those lesions exhibiting the symptoms of activity with thickening skin, inflammation, and crusting must be adequately removed operatively and thoroughly examined histologically, as one may be dealing with a presquamous cancerous lesion. Patients are advised to use daily sunscreens to reduce further photodamage and perhaps avoid future actinic keratoses.

*Bowen's disease* (Fig. 29-3) presents as a persistent, red, rough, scaly patch that tends to spread slowly. When these lesions occur on the penis, they are referred to as erythroplasia of Queyrat. Bowen's disease is an intraepidermal squamous cell carcinoma in situ that can deteriorate to an invasive squamous

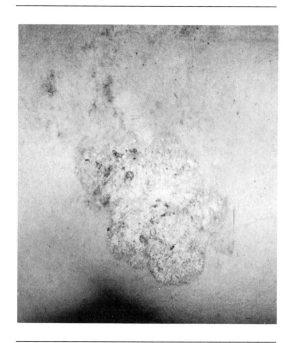

**Figure 29-3** *Bowen's disease on the leg, showing a rough, scaly patch with polycyclic borders.*

cell carcinoma if untreated. One-third of the Bowen's lesions occur secondary to chronic arsenic poisoning (e.g., from Fowler's solution), and they are associated with arsenical keratoses, leukomelanoderma, and a high incidence of visceral carcinoma, especially squamous cell carcinoma of the respiratory epithelium. The patient with multiple Bowen's lesions of the skin consistent with the arsenical-ingestion pattern deserves a visceral work-up, with repeated examinations [20].

*Keratoacanthoma* (Fig. 29-4) is a lesion that has been the subject of much discussion because of its unique qualities [9]. It is a rapidly growing papule that enlarges to 1 to 2 cm within a period of several weeks. It then undergoes spontaneous resolution within 6 months of its onset. The round, smooth, pink nodule encircles a massive keratinous plug. Histologically, the keratoacanthoma may be difficult to distinguish from a squa-

mous cell carcinoma, and frequently the diagnosis depends on the gross architecture of the lesion. Because the most critical diagnostic criterion of a keratoacanthoma may be spontaneous resolution, diagnosis with absolute certainty is often difficult. Incisional wedge biopsy is most important to determine the correct diagnosis of keratoacanthoma. The wedge of tissue must include a margin of normal skin, the raised shoulder of the keratoacanthoma, and some of the central crust. It must be deep enough to obtain tissue at the deep surface of the lesion to enable the pathologist to differentiate between keratoacanthoma and squamous cell carcinoma. If the lesion does not show a tendency to regress after several months, the physician must deal with the lesion as a squamous cell carcinoma. Rather than allow the lesion to declare itself as a benign keratoacanthoma, it is usually our preference to remove the tumor as if treating an early squamous cell carcinoma.

ADNEXAL TUMORS

In adnexal tumors the relations between epithelial and stromal components are maintained, even though distorted to varying degrees. Differentiation in the direction of hair follicles, sebaceous glands, apocrine or eccrine sweat glands, or various combinations of these cutaneous appendages occurs. Such tumors are classified according to their level of differentiation as well as their direction of differentiation, and a continuous spectrum ranging over all combinations of both parameters exists. Some general synonyms for adnexal tumors as a whole are organoid tumors, appendageal tumors, and hamartomas.

Where there is simply a localized excess of well differentiated, fully mature cutaneous appendageal structures with normal surrounding stroma, the lesions are called *nevi* of such appendages. The term *adenoma* is used when maturation of benign tumors is incomplete and their organization distorted, whereas the term *epithelioma* tends to be applied to poorly organized, immature tumors.

## TUMORS SHOWING HAIR FOLLICULAR DIFFERENTIATION

*Hair follicle nevus* (trichofolliculoma) presents on the face or scalp as a single, small, skin-colored papule, often with a highly characteristic central pore from which protrudes a wisp of white cottony hairs. Simple excisional biopsy suffices for diagnosis and treatment.

*Multiple trichoepithelioma* (epithelioma adenoides cysticum) is frequently a dominantly inherited disorder in which smooth, shiny, slightly translucent, firm, pale papules appear in increasing numbers during puberty or early adult life in somewhat symmetric distribution chiefly on the face, especially about the eyes but also on the scalp. Lesions may begin during early childhood, and they tend to be encountered more frequently in women. The lesions are benign and are best treated by electrodesiccation. Histologically, their differentiation from keratotic basal cell epithelioma may be difficult, whereas clinically they often resemble syringoma or the facial angiofibromas that characterize the tuberous sclerosis syndrome. So-called solitary trichoepithelioma is perhaps best included in the most highly differentiated end of the spectrum of keratotic basal cell epitheliomas.

*Pilomatricoma* (calcifying epithelioma of Malherbe) occurs as a single, hard, deeply seated, firm nodule covered by normal skin, usually 0.5 to 3.0 cm in size. It is found most commonly in children and young adults, especially on the face and arms. Clinically, it can be confused with a calcified epithelial cyst or even at times with carcinoma, when cutting into it, because of its solid, hard consistency. The lesion is benign and consists of an encapsulated mass of epidermoid cells with areas of small basophilic cells gradually merging into zones of pale eosinophilic "shadow" cells, among which there is usually calcium deposition. It is properly treated by simple excision.

*Tricholemmoma* shows downward proliferating buds of large, light-staining, glycogen-

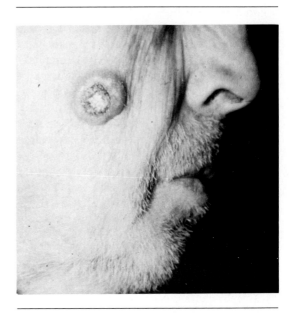

**Figure 29-4** *Keratoacanthoma on the cheek with a massive central keratotic core.*

rich, follicular sheath-type epithelial cells extending from the surface into the corium. The tumor buds are surrounded by a row of cells showing nuclear palisading to resemble the outer root sheath of hair follicles. This benign tumor usually occurs on the scalp and is amenable to simple excision.

## TUMORS SHOWING ECCRINE DIFFERENTIATION

*Syringomas* present occasionally as single, but more often as multiple, flesh-colored, pinkish or yellowish tan papules, usually 2 to 3 mm in diameter. They are often confused with trichoepithelioma, nevus, xanthelasma, or basal cell epithelioma. These lesions occur most often in adult women and usually involve the lower eyelids and upper cheeks, although they may also be found on the trunk, neck, and extremities. Removal for cosmetic purposes is best accomplished by electrodesiccation or cryotherapy with liquid nitrogen.

*Eccrine hidrocystoma* may resemble syringoma in distribution, but the lesions are translucent and appear as tense, slightly bluish, deep vesicles. These lesions are seen especially on the face of older women exposed to heat, which stimulates profuse perspiration. The lesions subside in a cool environment and represent passively dilated, obstructed sweat ducts. Avoidance of heat and simple puncturing of the lesions suffice for treatment.

*Eccrine poroma* usually occurs on plantar or palmar skin as a firm, sessile, reddish, papular or nodular tumor in a shallow cup-shaped depression surrounded by a narrow hyperkeratotic ridge. Clinically, it is easily confused with granuloma pyogenicum, amelanotic melanoma, or even Kaposi sarcoma. The lesions are benign and can be removed by simple excision biopsy for diagnosis followed by curettage and electrodesiccation.

*Eccrine spiradenoma* in 90 percent of cases is either painful, tender, or both. Paroxysms of severe pain triggered by manipulation may lead to clinical confusion with glomus tumor. The lesions are usually solitary, deep dermal or subcutaneous tumors about 1 cm in diameter, and they occur most often in young adults, frequently on the upper ventral body.

*Eccrine acrospiroma* (clear cell hidradenoma) may occur anywhere on the body, usually as a single, solid or cystic nodular, sometimes lobulated lesion that is flesh-colored or reddish and most often 1 to 2 cm in diameter. A few are tender on pressure, and a few show drainage or ulceration. Nodular hidradenoma is another term sometimes applied to this lesion as well as to other histologic variants of nodular, benign, solid, sweat gland tumors. All are easily treated by simple excision. Rarely, malignant clear cell hidradenoma and even malignant eccrine poroma have been noted and can usually be grouped under the general category of sweat gland carcinomas, which altogether are rare.

*Cylindroma* (turban tumor) (Fig. 29-5) occurs predominantly on the scalp or forehead as either solitary or multiple, firm, pink,

smooth nodules ranging in size up to several centimeters. They usually begin during adult life and are slow to grow. A dominantly inherited form, sometimes associated with multiple facial trichoepitheliomas, may form extensive grape-like clusters that cover the entire scalp like a turban. Simple excision suffices for treatment. In extensive cases, surgical removal of the most conspicuous tumors may be the most practical approach [19].

TUMORS SHOWING
APOCRINE DIFFERENTIATION
*Apocrine cystadenoma* is a small, benign, nevoid, dome-shaped, often translucent nodule, usually appearing on the face. It is frequently pigmented and on incision may contain brownish fluid. It may be clinically confused with pigmented or blue nevi and even with melanoma or pigmented basal cell epithelioma.

*Syringocystadenoma papilliferum* is usually a verrucose lesion that occurs most commonly on or near the scalp. It is a hamartomatous growth that frequently develops within an associated organoid nevus of the nevus sebaceous type. These lesions often

**Figure 29-5** *Cylindromas (turban tumors) of the scalp and forehead.*

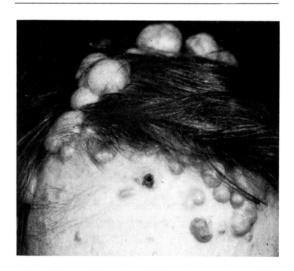

begin to develop during childhood and vary in size and appearance. They may be bulbous and exude fluid. Small lesions may be umbilicated and resemble molluscum contagiosum. Foci of basal cell epithelioma occur in about 10 percent of the lesions. Treatment consists in full-thickness excision of the lesion and any surrounding sebaceous nevus.

*Chondroid syringoma* (mixed tumor of skin, salivary gland type), like other mixed tumors, has both epithelial and mesenchymal tissue components, in this case sweat gland elements (syringoma) and cartilage-like chondroid. The lesions are stable, firm, asymptomatic, cutaneous nodules easily separated from the surrounding tissue and usually not connected to the normal overlying epidermis. The lesions are benign, and simple excision is needed only for cosmetic and diagnostic purposes.

## TUMORS SHOWING SEBACEOUS DIFFERENTIATION

*Nevus sebaceous (Jadassohn)*, also called organoid nevus, is a well circumscribed, verrucose or finely nodular, orange, raised, irregular, hairless plaque that occurs most frequently on the scalp and less often on the face and neck. It is present at birth and persists throughout life, being quiescent during childhood and tending to become verrucose and nodular during puberty. Clinically, it may resemble nevus verrucosus. In later stages of development, other tumors tend to arise in these lesions, with basal cell epithelioma arising in 15 to 20 percent. Syringocystadenoma papilliferum and other adenomatous appendageal tumors may also develop in them as well as keratoacanthoma. Rarely, even squamous cell carcinoma has been observed in the overlying epidermis. Because of the potential risk of aggressive tumor development in these lesions, their removal by simple excision during childhood or when first recognized is advisable.

*Senile sebaceous hyperplasia* occurs commonly on the face of middle-age or older persons, especially men with seborrheic complexions. The lesions usually present as multiple, soft, elevated, 2- to 3-mm papules with central umbilication and edges composed of confluent pinhead-sized yellowish white subunits. Fine superficial telangiectatic vessels may course over the edges of the papules. They often are easily mistaken for small basal cell epitheliomas. Treatment is usually not indicated, except for cosmetic purposes; they can be removed by simple electrodesiccation. Sebaceous adenomas, which are rare and benign, are solitary, smooth, firm tumors on the face of scalp, usually less than 1 cm in diameter.

*Sebaceous epithelioma* essentially looks and behaves clinically like basal cell epithelioma, except that the color is sometimes yellowish and there is a notable histologic tendency for their component cells to show sebaceous differentiation. These lesions are radiosensitive but are best treated by either excision or electrocoagulation and curettage, depending on their size and location. It may be necessary to differentiate this lesion from rare malignant sebaceous carcinoma, which usually develops in the tarsal region of the eyelids and may metastasize.

## SMOOTH MUSCLE TUMORS

Benign cutaneous tumors consisting of smooth muscle proliferation are called *leiomyomas.* Multiple cutaneous leiomyomas occur in widely varying numbers, sometimes diffusely scattered on the trunk, face, or extremities. They tend to increase gradually in number and are usually firm, pale, reddish brown, intradermal nodules less than 1 cm in size. Frequently they harden and become painful on pressure or application of cold. These multiple lesions are believed to arise from arrectores pilorum muscles. Solitary angioleiomyomas are usually small, encapsulated, subcutaneous nodules less than 2 cm in size, and they are seen mainly on the legs. They may be sensitive to pressure and cold and are believed to arise from venular smooth muscle. A third variety is the solitary genital lesion located in the subcutis on either the scrotum, labia majora, or nipple area. They may reach sizes of up to several centimeters. Solitary tender leiomyomas must be differentiated at times from glomus tumor and eccrine spiradenoma. Excision is the only suitable treatment for symptomatic leiomyomas. There is a fairly high tendency for recurrence.

EPITHELIAL CYSTS

Squamous epithelium-lined cysts of several types that contain lipid and keratinous material in the past have been encompassed under the general designation "sebaceous cysts." They are specifically classified as follows.

*Epidermoid cysts* are tense, somewhat fluctuant, smooth swellings to the dermis but freely movable over underlying tissues. They vary in size up to several centimeters in diameter and commonly occur on the face, neck, and trunk. Tending to enlarge slowly, they contain cheesy, lipid-rich material composed mainly of a lamellated, horny substance. Their squamous epithelial lining shows orderly keratinizing differentiation through a well developed granular layer. At times a central comedo-like point is present. These cysts may become infected, after which they are difficult to enucleate with the entire cyst wall because of adherence to surrounding tissues. There are no sebaceous glandular structures in the linings of these keratin cysts. Simple excision is the most suitable treatment for noninfected lesions. Small cyst linings can sometimes be teased out entirely through a small incision, which can heal with scarcely perceptible scarring. It is important to remove the lining sac completely; otherwise recurrence is likely. Mildly infected cysts with redness and tenderness can be treated with an oral antibiotic such as tetracycline for a few days until inflammation subsides, before excision is undertaken. Severely infected cysts may require incision, drainage, and curettage of the lining, followed by packing with iodoform gauze to allow healing from within.

*Pilar cysts* (also called wens or tricholemmal cysts) clinically resemble epidermoid cysts, except that they occur in 90 percent of cases on the scalp. They contain nonlamellous keratinous material that is not as cheesy as occurs in epidermoid cysts, and their lining shows pilar-type keratinization, with plump luminal cells without keratohyalin granules. They are managed similarly to epidermoid cysts. The dominant familial occurrence of large numbers of wens or epidermoid cysts alerts the clinician to look for the possible presence of Gardner's syndrome, with multiple polyposis of the colon and rectum. The high risk of early death from colon cancer in such patients makes early diagnosis and treatment by total colectomy imperative.

*Milia*, or whiteheads, are tiny 1- to 2-mm, superficially situated epidermal inclusion cysts that are miniature epidermoid cysts. They tend to occur most frequently about the eyes, where they are occasionally mistaken for xanthelasma, syringoma, or trichoepithelioma. They tend to develop at healing blister sites in some bullous diseases, e.g., epidermolysis bullosa, porphyria cutanea tarda, and pemphigus, and they may develop at dermabrasion sites. Treatment by simple needle teasing is effective, and the use of abrasive cleaners may also be helpful. Local electrocautery using a fine epilating needle is often useful for inducing clearance of multiple milia. This procedure is faster than attempting needle teasing if the patient has multiple lesions.

*Steatocystoma multiplex* is an autosomal dominantly inherited disorder in which numerous small (no larger than 1 cm) cystic intradermal nodules are found most commonly on the skin of the upper anterior midtrunk, axillae, scrotum, arms, and thighs. These small cysts contain an olive oil-like fluid, and sebaceous glandular elements are found in their thin squamous epithelial linings of two or three layers. Small lanugo hairs are also present in these cysts. Because of the large numbers of these harmless small lesions, their removal by excision is frequently impractical.

Dermoid cysts are congenital hamartomas, probably deriving from anomalous developmental inclusion of embryonic epidermis along embryonic cleft closure lines. Their most common sites are the lateral ends of the eyebrows and along the midline in the nasal root, neck, and sublingual, sternal, perineal, scrotal, and sacral areas. They are of variable size, at times as large as 10 cm. They are subcutaneous in location, resemble steatocystomas or epidermoid cysts, and usually have sebaceous glandular, rudimentary hair follicle, and sweat gland elements attached to their epithelial linings. At times, even cartilage and bone are present. Dermoid cysts must be completely excised.

## FIBROUS TUMORS

*Cutaneous tags and papillomas* occur in a variety of sizes and are soft and frequently pedunculated. They have been variously called cutaneous papilloma, fibroepithelial polyp, fibroma pendulum, acrochordon, soft fibroma (fibroma molle), and fibroma molluscum. They have a papillomatous, loose, finely fibrillar dermal core and often show epidermal changes resembling those in seborrheic keratoses. Occasionally, lesions on thin stalks become twisted, inflamed, and infarcted. The lesions are easily removed by clipping the stalks and lightly electrodesiccating the bases or by simple excision of the broad-based sessile lesions.

*Dermatofibroma, histiocytoma, nodular subepidermal fibrosis, fibroma simplex, sclerosing hemangioma, noduli cutanei,* and *fibroma durum* are various terms that have been applied to a common benign nonencapsulated, reactive, lenticular intradermal nodular lesion composed of proliferating fibrocytes, irregularly arranged bundles of fine collagen fibers, capillary blood vessels, histiocytes, and mononuclear inflammatory cells in varying proportions. At times the histiocytes in the lesions accumulate hemosiderin or become somewhat xanthomatized. The lesions are firm and range in color from pale skin hues through various shades of red, brown, and yellow. They occur most often on the lower extremities but also are seen on the arms and trunk in adults. They rarely exceed 1 to 2 cm in size. It is believed that some of these lesions develop at sites of minor trauma, e.g., mosquito bites. No treatment is usually needed unless excision becomes warranted for cosmetic or symptomatic reasons. Excision for histologic establishment of the diagnosis may be necessary. Incomplete removal tends to be followed by recurrence.

*Acquired digital fibrokeratoma* is a smooth, pinkish, hyperkeratotic, well demarcated, partly fleshy, horn-like projection emerging from a collarette of elevated skin on a finger. It may closely resemble a rudimentary supernumerary digit or small cutaneous horn. The core of the lesion contains thick collagen bundles. Excision at skin level with electrodesiccation of the base suitably removes this benign growth.

*Pseudosarcomatous lesions* are of interest because several clinically benign localized fibromatous proliferative lesions may show cellular changes and numerous mitoses that easily lead to a mistaken diagnosis of fibrosarcoma. Among such pseudosarcomatous lesions are the following: (1) Nodular pseudosarcomatous fasciitis (subcutaneous pseudosarcomatous fibromatosis) occurs most often on the upper extremities as a rapidly developing, slightly painful nodule, 1 to 3 cm in size, and attached to deep fascia. (2) Infantile digital fibromatosis is a rare pseudosarcomatosis characterized by asymptomatic, firm, red, smooth nodules up to 1 cm in size on the dorsal and lateral aspects of the distal phalanges of the toes and fingers during infancy and childhood. Surgical excision is the recommended treatment, but recurrences are reported to be frequent. (3) Atypical fibroxanthoma is a more common pseudosarcomatous lesion that appears on chronically sun-exposed parts of the head and neck, particularly in the preauricular area in older persons. The tumor is a small, firm nodule that may show some crusting and can resemble basal cell epithelioma. The bizarre, highly atypical spindle or histiocytoid cells and giant cells of the tumor, with abundant

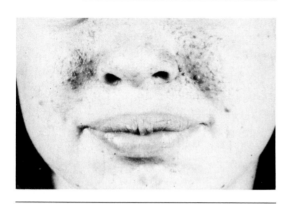

**Figure 29-6** *Multiple angiofibromas (adenoma sebaceum, Pringle type) associated with tuberous sclerosis.*

mitoses, are separated from the epidermis by a thin zone of collagen. Treatment is by simple excision.

*Dermatofibrosarcoma protuberans* usually presents as a slowly growing, hard, nodular protuberant mass arising in the dermis, mostly on the trunk and thighs. It may be erythematous or slightly dusky in color and is covered by smooth, shiny epithelium that gives a keloidal appearance. There may be complicating ulceration, infection, and scarring. As this local disorder becomes extensive, it may cause severe pain, contractures, and invalidism. Histologically, there is a characteristic "cartwheel" pattern of the hypercellular fibrous bundles in these nonencapsulated tumors that extend finger-like processes into adjacent subcutis and fascia. Mitotic figures may be numerous. Wide excision, including the deep fascia, is necessary to prevent recurrence. Long-standing, inadequately excised lesions have been known to metastasize [34].

*Angiofibroma* (Fig. 29-6) occurs on the lower central portions of the face and nose as firm, pale, sometimes telangiectatic fibrous or slightly erythematous papules 1 to 3 mm in size. Solitary lesions are inconsequential and can be removed for histologic diagnosis and cosmetic purposes by superficial biopsy and electrodesiccation. When multiple, these lesions had in times past been called adenoma sebaceum (Pringle type) and are associated with the tuberous sclerosis complex (Bourneville's disease). The fibrous papules of tuberous sclerosis that occur on the forehead, cheeks, chin, and nasolabial folds can be distressing to the patient. Dermabrasion and limited excision offer some improvement [37]. Characteristic periungual and subungual protruding digitate fibromas (Koenen's periungual tumors) also are often present in this syndrome.

*Myxoid cysts*, less appropriately called synovial cysts in the past, occur particularly on the dorsa of the distal phalanges of the fingers, just proximal to the nails. They are smooth, translucent nodules, usually less than 1 cm in size, that are filled with a crystal-clear mucin or jelly-like fluid. They are not truly cysts because they are not encapsulated by any lining. Their myxoid contents simply compress the adjacent superficial dermis. Removal can be achieved by excision or electrodesiccation and curettage.

*True myxomas* are rare tumors, resembling embryonal mesenchyme, that show infiltrating growth bryonal mesenchyme, and have uniform cellularity in contrast to the nonuniformity in mucinous cysts and mucinous degeneration. These tumors usually originate from deep fascia but in the skin may occur subungually. They require wide excision because of their high tendency to recur.

MISCELLANEOUS SKIN TUMORS

Xanthomas represent a variety of skin lesions characterized by focal accumulations of lipid-laden histiocytes and giant cells with foamy cytoplasm. Often these lesions are associated with a variety of hyperlipoproteinemias, and at times the morphologic type of xanthoma provides a clinical clue to the specific underlying lipidosis.

*Xanthelasma palpebarum*, the most common kind of xanthoma, occurs on the eyelids, usually near the inner canthi. It presents in the form of soft, thin, yellowish, slightly raised, elongated plaques, often symmetrically distributed. In a little more than one-half of individuals presenting with these lesions, there is associated hyperlipoproteinemia, a high risk of early atherosclerosis, and the accompanying cardiovascular complications. In many cases there is no apparent associated general disturbance of lipid metabolism, and xanthelasma is simply a local cosmetic problem. Extensive xanthelasma may also occur in biliary cirrhosis, with associated xanthomatosis, and in histiocytic disorders such as reticulohistiocytoma cutis, Hand-Schüller-Christian disease, and xanthoma disseminatum. Treatment of the cosmetic problem is relatively easy, as the lesions can be excised superficially, lightly electrodesiccated, or even treated topically with trichloracetic acid carefully applied with a flat toothpick applicator. A 20-year retrospective study on xanthelasma palpebarum reviewed 68 patients; 34 percent of the patients had an increased serum cholesterol level, but only 5 percent had a documented hyperlipemia [35]. Recurrence of the xanthelasma was noted in 40 percent of the patients who underwent excision of the xanthelasma; among the patients who had already had a recurrence of the xanthelasma after excision, a tertiary excision resulted in recurrence of the xanthelasma in 65 percent.

*Xanthoma planum* resembles xanthelasma but may involve extensive areas beyond the eyelids, especially the palmar creases, axillae, flexor areas of the extremities, neck, inner thighs, trunk, and shoulders.

*Glomus tumor* (glomangioma) is a benign vascular hamartomatous derivative of the glomus body—a normal intradermal arteriovenous anastomosis that arises from the normal neuromyoarterial glomus. It presents as a skin-colored or bluish, firm nodule a few millimeters to 1 to 2 cm in diameter. It is usually exceedingly sensitive, and paroxysms of severe radiating pain are often triggered by the slightest manipulation of the lesion. Nonpainful glomus tumors can

also occur. The lesions may be single or multiple and most characteristically occur on the hands and feet, especially subungually. Glomus tumors have also been reported on the face [7]. Treatment of symptomatic lesions requires complete excision, which dramatically relieves the severe episodes of pain. Subungual, highly sensitive lesions may be small and difficult to locate visibly. Hemangiopericytoma may resemble a painless glomus tumor and is rare and solitary; it may grow up to 10 cm in size. Rarely, hemangiopericytoma is malignant. Diagnosis requires histologic examination.

*Chondrodermatitis nodularis chronica helicis* is a fairly common chronic, inflammatory, painful, papular lesion on the upper rim of the ear that occurs with overwhelming preponderance in males. The lesions are tender and firmly attached to the cartilage, which histologically shows focal degenerative change and surrounding perichondritis. Overlying hyperkeratosis and acanthosis are present. Clinical differentiation from solar keratosis or incipient carcinoma may be difficult. Simple excision with removal of the focus of underlying degenerated cartilage suffices for treatment.

*Granular cell myoblastoma (Abrikossoff)* or *granular cell schwannoma* is a usually solitary, but occasionally multiple, hard, smooth, brownish red to flesh-colored intracutaneous nodular tumor, ranging up to 3 cm in size. Occasionally ulceration occurs, in which case it may clinically resemble squamous cell carcinoma. One-third of the lesions occur on the tongue. Some occur in internal organs, and rarely some behave in malignant fashion and metastasize. The lesions grow slowly and show characteristic, non-lipid-containing cells that resemble xanthoma cells, except that they have granular rather than foamy cytoplasm. Current opinion favors a relation of these cells to Schwann cells rather than muscle cells. The lesions are best removed by simple complete excision. Recurrence is likely if excision is incomplete.

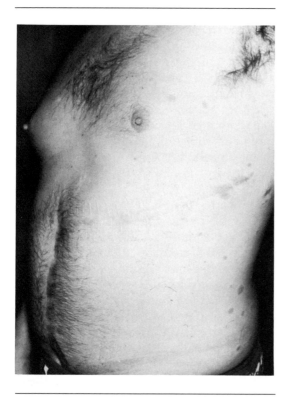

***Figure 29-7*** *Patient with psoriasis vulgaris. The psoriasis has occurred in a surgical scar: Köbner's phenomenon.*

## Generalized Disorders

It is important for the surgeon to be aware of the more common generalized skin disorders. With some of these conditions, surgery is ill-advised during certain phases of the disease. This point is true of, for example, psoriasis (Fig. 29-7), vitiligo (Fig. 29-8), and lichen planus. It is possible to induce Köbner's phenomenon, or the isomorphic response, if surgery is performed on the skin in patients where these diseases are active. The skin disease then occurs in the site of the surgical scar. With other dermatologic conditions, a plastic surgical procedure may be valuable after the disease has been controlled by dermatologic therapy. One example is the scarring that follows severe acne, which is often amenable to dermabrasion.

## PSORIASIS

Psoriasis is a benign, chronic, erythematous, scaling skin disease that occurs frequently. It has been variously estimated to affect between 1 and 3 percent of the population of the United States. The importance of recognizing psoriasis for the surgeon is that surgery must be avoided while the disease is actively worsening. In approximately one-third of patients at some stage during their disease there is the possibility of inducing Köbner's phenomenon, or the isomorphic response, wherein skin trauma results in new psoriatic lesions. In addition, psoriasis patients have a high skin colonization bacterial count, which may lead to an increased risk of postsurgical skin infections. Numerous treatments are available for psoriasis patients, ranging from topical therapy to phototherapy to various forms of systemic therapy [33]. It is recommended that these patients be treated by a dermatologist skilled in their care prior to any planned surgical procedure.

## DISCOID LUPUS ERYTHEMATOSUS

Discoid lupus erythematosus (DLE) is a chronic dermatitis (Fig. 29-9) that results in extensive atrophic scarring. The lesions of

***Figure 29-8*** *Patient with vitiligo of the dorsal hands, a frequently affected site. Vitiligo may also occur in surgical scars as Köbner's phenomenon.*

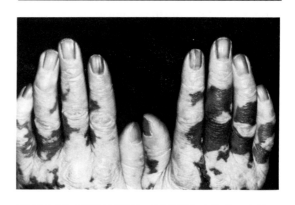

DLE may occur on the scalp, face, lips, and extensor surface of the arms and less often on the trunk. Although satisfactory treatment has been accomplished with topical steroid therapy and with antimalarial drugs such as chloroquine, there are many patients in whom DLE has caused persistent scarring and deformity of the nose and face, requiring the attention of the surgeon. The lesions are usually discrete, and surgical removal of the involved tissue permits successful reconstruction with the use of either free skin grafts of adjacent pedicle flaps after the activity of the lesions had been suppressed with the proper medical therapy. DLE treated in the past with radiation resulted in a significant incidence of squamous cell carcinoma over long periods of time. Mladick and colleagues [36] reported a case of squamous cell carcinoma developing on the face of a patient with DLE who had had no previous radiation therapy. Chronically active DLE lesions that result in severe atrophic scars complicated by secondary erosion and ulceration are excised after conservative measures have controlled the activity in the lesions because it is these long-standing chronically ulcerated scarred lesions that are particularly associated with the risk of carcinoma.

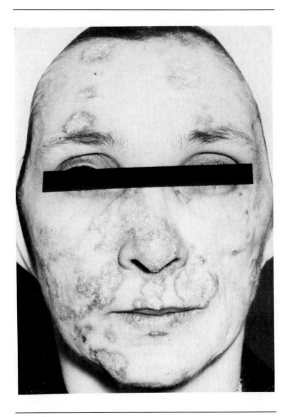

**Figure 29-9** *Chronic discoid lupus erythematosus.*

## SYSTEMIC LUPUS ERYTHEMATOSUS

Systemic lupus erythematosus (SLE) can vary from a mild to a severe and fatal disease. SLE activity is often reflected by leukopenia, anemia, increased erythrocyte sedimentation rate, positive antinuclear factor tests and lupus erythematosus preparations, and positive cutaneous immunofluorescence tests. Low serum complement levels are also present with active vasculitis.

After the systemic disease has been properly evaluated and controlled with appropriate therapy, the operative management of associated lesions has been safe. The use of skin grafts and flaps for reconstructive surgery in the patient with SLE has been successful in the presence of steroid therapy. It is clear that the benefits of steroid therapy for suppressing the vasculitis far exceed the drawbacks of delayed wound healing when undertaking an operative procedure in patients with this disease. Sjögren syndrome [6], consisting of xerostomia, keratoconjunctivitis sicca, and rheumatoid arthritis, has been associated in some instances with SLE. Occasional patients with Sjögren syndrome appear with a parotid mass secondary to parotitis that may be asymmetric or unilateral. Awareness of this entity often avoids a disastrous set of events due to the erroneous diagnosis of a parotid tumor without appreciation of systemic implications.

## SYSTEMIC SCLERODERMA

Systemic scleroderma is seen most frequently in the acrosclerotic form, especially in women

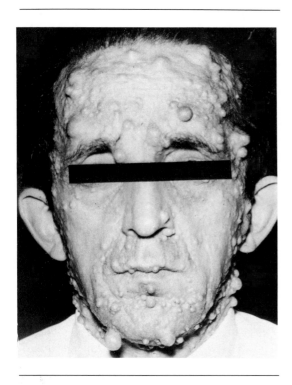

***Figure 29-10*** *Von Recklinghausen's neurofibromatosis.*

between the ages of 20 and 50 years. Because the initial process often begins in the distal extremities with such vasospastic changes as Raynaud's phenomenon and sclerodactyly, the surgeon is often consulted initially. Sclerodactyly designates the characteristic hand changes, consisting in hide-bound atrophic skin of the fingers held in partial flexion with limitation of motion in both flexion and extension. The cutaneous changes that lead to hide-bound atrophy and inelasticity of the skin, flexion deformities of the fingers, and ulcerations over joint and fingertip surfaces demand conservative treatment.

During the early stages of the disease, medical sympathetic block has been of some value in many people's mind. α-Methyldopa and guanethidine have been used as sympatholytic agents with some success in early scleroderma. Systemic steroid therapy has not helped in the course of this type of disease.

Operative intervention in scleroderma requires careful judgment, as the wound-healing characteristics of the tissues are tenuous. In the face of ulceration and gangrenous changes, the wound must be treated similarly to an ischemic ulcer, with careful débridement of the wound and resurfacing with split-thickness skin grafts when vascularity permits. Although operative procedures such as skin flaps and skin grafting have been successful in some patients [32], aggressive resection of tissue has been discouraging, as there may be progression of the necrosis following operative intervention. Although with the common acrosclerotic form of scleroderma steroid therapy has not been effective, there have been reports of cases of so-called mixed connective tissue disease that often present scleroderma-like features and do respond to steroid therapy [54].

SCLERODERMA CIRCUMSCRIPTUM
Morphea and band-like lesions characterize scleroderma circumscriptum. They often follow a dermatome pattern on the trunk or an extremity, or they appear in the paramedian region of the forehead, a condition referred to as scleroderma en coup de sabre. The latter disorder has been associated with progressive hemifacial atrophy in children. Severely deforming atrophy of skin, subcutaneous tissues, muscle, and bone may result from scleroderma. The eventual extent of the disease is unpredictable in its early stages, and spontaneous resolution occurs in some cases. The treatment must be conservative so long as there is active disease. When activity has ceased, the evidence suggests that operative intervention and correction of the deformity is safe and effective.

VON RECKLINGHAUSEN'S
NEUROFIBROMATOSIS
Known also as multiple neurofibromatosis (Fig. 29-10), von Recklinghausen's neurofibromatosis is a hereditary disorder manifested by numerous cutaneous neurofibromas and café au lait pigmentation, and

axillary freckling. It produces bone lesions and intracranial and gastrointestinal symptoms, and it is occasionally associated with mental retardation. The diagnosis is made on the basis of multiple neurofibromas, café au lait spots, and axillary freckling. Although the skin pigmentation may have been present since birth or early childhood, tumor formation is generally most aggressive at the time of puberty. The course of the disease is unpredictable. There is a rough correlation between the age of onset of the neurofibromas and the probable severity of the disease. Patients seen during their youth with disfiguring masses may go on to progressive difficulties, including palsies and pituitary hypofunction. To the surgeon, the most common presenting form of neurofibromatosis in the young patient is facial deformity with neurofibromatous masses, which are soft, flaccid subcutaneous tumors.

Treatment consists solely in excising the symptomatic lesions. Operative correction of these lesions is often only partial, as total excision of a large lesion in the facial region may create extensive deformity. The vascular pattern with large, thin-walled veins obscures the anatomy and makes hemostasis difficult. In the face, bony involvement results in facial deformity and asymmetry in addition to the soft tissue masses and thick, unsightly gingiva. Although malignant degeneration in multiple neurofibromatosis has been reported, it is not feasible to excise all the lesions in anticipation of malignant changes.

## XERODERMA PIGMENTOSUM

Xeroderma pigmentosum is an inherited disorder characterized by unusual sensitivity to actinic rays. Normally, there are special cellular enzyme systems that can remove and replace ultraviolet-damaged segments of DNA in which thymidine dimers have formed. In many cases of xeroderma pigmentosum, this DNA repair mechanism has been found deficient [8]. Theoretically, if the patient could be completely screened from actinic rays,

the skin would be protected and no lesions would occur. The patient develops keratoses and spotty pigmentation that ultimately involves all of the exposed surfaces of the body. Basal cell carcinomas, squamous cell carcinomas, and malignant melanomas occur. Patients with xeroderma pigmentosum may develop all of the cutaneous malignant neoplasms known. In the past most of these patients have succumbed to this disease by early adulthood. During the 1980s, however, careful protection from actinic rays, treating aggressive tumors with topical chemotherapeutic agents such as 5-fluorouracil, extensive dermabrasion, excision of malignant and premalignant lesions, and resurfacing with skin grafts significantly improved the outlook of these patients.

## DYSTROPHIC EPIDERMOLYSIS BULLOSA

Dystrophic epidermolysis bullosa is a hereditary disease of the skin and mucosa characterized by the formation of bullae after minor trauma that heal with scarring (Fig. 29-11). Excessive epidermal collagenase activity has been found in patients with this disorder [17, 40]. This enzyme is believed to attack the most superficially situated papillary dermal collagen fibers at a level where blister formation often begins. Although the entire skin and the mucosa of the hypopharynx and esophagus are subject to this breakdown, scarring secondary to the recurrent minor trauma is most obvious on exposed surfaces. The typical deformity is progressive encasement of the digits in a cocoon of atrophic scar, resulting in subsequent loss of the use of fingers and thumbs. There are varying degrees of clinical expression of this entity; some patients have a relatively normal life, but most suffer greatly and require careful attention from the family and the treating physician and surgeon.

To date, there is no basic therapy to remedy the defect that results in the formation of bullae. In some patients the vigorous use of topical steroid therapy has seemed to help reduce blistering and scar formation. Efforts

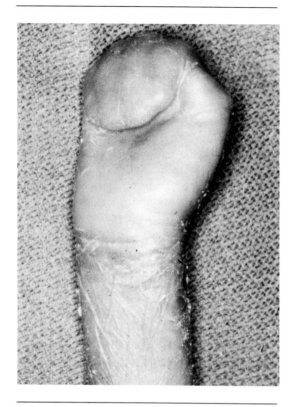

**Figure 29-11** *Dystrophic epidermolysis bullosa in a 6-year-old girl, showing entrapment of digits in a scar cocoon.*

to correct the severe hand deformities have been frustrating [23, 47]. Although the fingers are surprisingly mobile after being encased in the skin cocoon for many years, retention of the corrected position of the fingers after resection of the cocoon and resurfacing with skin grafts or flaps has been limited. Patients and their families have been enthused over the operative correction of the fingers and thumb deformities, but objectively there is loss of much of the correction with rescarring of the fingers. Our own experience with a modest number of patients has led us to correct the finger deformities repeatedly at intervals of several years because the patients believe that it improves their personal lives [65]. However, the patients must be realistically informed that the corrections are usually temporary.

## CUTIS LAXA

Cutis laxa is a rare skin disorder in which the skin hangs in loose folds owing to inadequacy of elastic fibers throughout the body, especially in the skin, lungs, and aorta [14, 45]. The defective elastic fibers in part account for the tendency to develop cardiorespiratory difficulties, which make the patient a significant operative risk. The systemic involvement in some patients contraindicates operative procedures. The primary presenting symptom is the extreme laxity of the skin, which causes the skin to hang in loose folds. The patient usually complains of appearing prematurely aged. Beighton and colleagues pointed out that the skin is not unduly fragile, wound healing is normal, and excessive bleeding is not a problem in these patients [4]. In the absence of cardiorespiratory difficulties, operative correction of the prematurely aged skin, excision of redundant tissues, and application of the standard rhytidectomy concepts have been gratifying.

## PSEUDOXANTHOMA ELASTICUM

Pseudoxanthoma elasticum is a heritable disorder in which the mechanically stressed skin (especially the base and sides of neck and axillae) takes on the texture of plucked chicken skin [25, 31]. The loose, inelastic skin has a yellowish, pebbled thickening. Widespread severe arteriosclerosis commonly develops as early as the third decade of life.

## CUTIS HYPERELASTICA

Known also as Ehlers-Danlos syndrome, cutis hyperelastica is a heritable disorder that must not be confused with cutis laxa [30]. Cutis hyperelastica is characterized by skin that is hyperextensible in a patient with extremely lax joints. These patients have a distinct fragility of the skin and blood vessels, and the patients report that their skin damages easily with frequent bruising and hematoma formation. In addition, these patients heal poorly, with gaping wounds that retract. The skin has a low tensile strength and does not hold suture material. The surgeon must clearly distinguish the patient with cutis hyperelastica from the patient with cutis laxa, as elective operative procedures on the former are fraught with disaster.

## VASCULITIS

Many disease processes have been termed some form of vasculitis, with the common denominator being an inflammation of blood vessels with subsequent thrombosis, ischemia, and necrosis of tissues. For clinical purposes, these diverse entities of necrotizing vasculitis can be classified according to the size of the vessels and the organ systems involved [61]. Pulmonary, renal, and gastrointestinal involvement may present severe problems in some forms. Large vessels are involved in periarteritis nodosa and temporal arteritis. Small vessel involvement occurs in such entities as Henoch-Schönlein purpura, Waterhouse-Friderichsen syndrome (where it is leukocytoclastic), and granulomatous forms of angiitis such as Wegener syndrome. The necrotic ulcers in various forms of necrotizing angiitis are ischemic lesions that are slow to débride and granulate. Recognition of the particular disease entity as a systemic necrotizing vasculitis and the initiation of systemic tumors, often with steroid or immunosuppressive agents, are of primary concern [13]. If the systemic disease can be brought under control, careful débridement and operative management require attention similar to that required for ischemic tissues [22]. Withdrawal of steroid therapy and activation of the vasculitis pose a serious threat to the successful management of necrotic lesions secondary to vasculitis.

Skin necrosis has occurred with many entities that result in increased coagulability or sludging of the blood. The Waterhouse-Friderichsen syndrome secondary to meningococcemia [53] and leg ulcers secondary to sickle cell anemia are well known entities to surgeons [62]. Cases of skin necrosis secondary to cryoglobulinemia and other paraproteinemias have been reported [52]. The presence of cryoglobulin in the blood has been associated with multiple myeloma, various

collagen diseases, and malignant lymphomas, and it has occurred idiopathically. Reports have documented the occurrence of skin necrosis following anticoagulant therapy, associated primarily with coumarin congeners [38, 42].

## NECROBIOSIS LIPOIDICA

Necrobiosis lipoidica is commonly associated with diabetes mellitus [5] (Fig. 29-12). Necrobiosis lipoidica may occur in patients without diabetes, and it may precede the clinical onset of diabetes mellitus. The lesion begins as a dusky red plaque that slowly progresses to atrophy of the skin; it may ulcerate in the center, secondary to minimal trauma. A distinct yellowish cast in the atrophic telangiectatic center of the lesion is characteristic. There seems to be a predilection for the pretibial area. The lesion is progressive, and control of diabetes and other medical modalities of tumors have not been effective. Some young women with necrobiosis lipoidica present with the primary complaint of disfigurement of the anterior

**Figure 29-12** *Necrobiosis lipoidica on the shins of a 32-year-old female diabetic.*

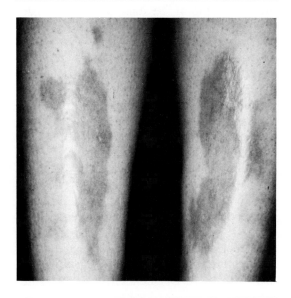

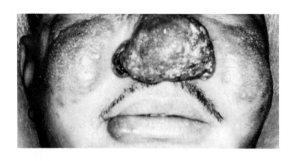

*Figure 29-13* Sarcoidosis with large nodular masses on the cheeks and nose.

lower legs. Although not widely recommended, operative resection of the involved area and resurfacing with split-thickness skin grafts have been successful [15].

### SARCOIDOSIS

The cutaneous manifestations of sarcoidosis (Fig. 29-13) may present initially as erythema nodosum, reddish tan, translucent, smooth papules on the eyelid and nasal margins or as a variety of deeper, indurated plaques and nodules. When the disease requires steroid therapy for control of systemic manifestations, the cutaneous lesions often respond in due time. Large, disfiguring, nodular masses may be excised after an adequate trial of medical therapy has failed to resolve the lesions [39].

### CUTANEOUS T CELL LYMPHOMAS

Cutaneous T cell lymphoma, or mycosis fungoides, is a cutaneous form of lymphoma that presents with pruritic erythematous scaly patches, infiltrated plaques, and irregular skin nodules and ulcers (Fig. 29-14). The diagnosis is established by histologic examination.

The usually extensive skin involvement precludes any definitive operative treatment except for purposes of diagnosis and for the management of ulcers. Topical nitrogen mustard or psoralen photochemotherapy utilizing the photoactive psoralen drugs followed by long-wavelength ultraviolet irradiation (UVA) may be utilized. Patients unresponsive to these treatments may be treated with electron beam therapy. If the ulcer is secondary to irradiation, the lesion must be managed conservatively or with appropriate débridement and resurfacing using split-thickness skin grafts or adjacent pedicle flaps when feasible. In most instances when irradiation ulcers have occurred, the extent of the disease and the extent of the previous electron beam therapy preclude the availability of adjacent tissues for pedicle flaps. Although mycosis fungoides is eventually a fatal disease, in some cases the course is prolonged. Hence extensive debridement and resurfacing of ulcerated areas with skin grafts or ped-

*Figure 29-14* Extensive mycosis fungoides in a 20-year-old woman.

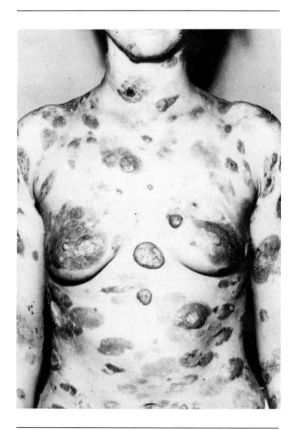

icle flaps are appropriate when the lesions create sufficient discomfort.

## KAPOSI SARCOMA

Kaposi sarcoma may be of two major types. The acquired immunodeficiency syndrome (AIDS) epidemic has resulted in a high number of Kaposi sarcoma cases. Kaposi sarcoma appears to arise with significant frequency in young patients with AIDS-related disease. In addition, there is the previously recognized form of Kaposi sarcoma that usually affects non-AIDS patients, usually the older or middle-aged man of Mediterranean racial origin. The importance of recognizing Kaposi sarcoma in AIDS patients has clear relevance for the surgeon and for the future management of that patient. Biopsy confirmation of the skin lesions is of clear importance; however, caution when handling such specimens is important in view of the potential for transmission of AIDS-related disease from blood products and biopsy tissue. The therapy of Kaposi sarcoma in AIDS patients is at an early stage of development [10]. Although further progress of tumors of these patients is important, it does not fall within the confines of this chapter.

Kaposi sarcoma in non-AIDS patients usually affects middle-age or older men with the highest frequency in people of Mediterranean origin, particularly Jews, Italians, and Greeks. The course of the disease in non-AIDS patients is slow, and frequently patients survive for more than 10 years after the onset of the disease. In some patients the disease remains localized to one body area, particularly the legs. This pattern is in contradistinction to that of AIDS-related Kaposi sarcoma, which can be rapidly fatal within 2 years from diagnosis.

The treatment of choice for non-AIDS-related Kaposi sarcoma has been predominantly radiotherapy. The surgeon may be asked to see the patient because of ulceration secondary to irradiation. There is little surgical reason to excise the Kaposi sarcoma lesion because the disease is multicentric

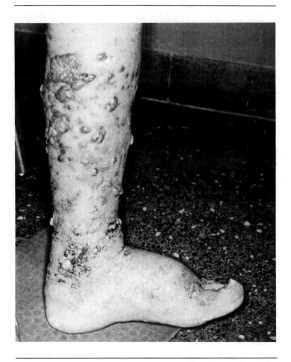

**Figure 29-15** *Kaposi sarcoma of 12 years' duration.*

and therefore recurs rapidly. One report also suggested that radiotherapy may be useful for controlling Kaposi sarcoma in some patients with AIDS-related disease.

It is a multicentric proliferative disorder of vasoformative tissue that ultimately follows a malignant neoplastic course (Fig. 29-15). In the early stages, lesions present as purplish pigmented patches of purpura, with hemosiderosis most often on the feet and lower legs. Later, indurated plaques and firm vascular polypoid excrescences appear. Chronic lymphedema also develops in affected areas.

Radiotherapy has been the treatment of choice. The surgeon is often asked to manage ulceration secondary to radiotherapy. The tissue diagnosis of the ulceration to distinguish irradiation necrosis from active tumor is mandatory to determine whether further radiotherapy or operative intervention is indicated. Surgical excision as the primary lesion in Kaposi sarcoma is futile, as the disease is multicentric. In the early stages of the disease, the surgeon must be aware of the possibility of this entity and its features so that the mistaken diagnosis of localized sarcoma is not made and inappropriate radical operative excision is not undertaken.

## ACNE VULGARIS

Acne vulgaris is a common skin disorder seen in adolescents and young adults. It consists of seborrhea, small comedones, and inflammatory papulopustules or cysts. In some instances the disease is severe, with deep cysts and burrowing sinus tracts that result in extensive scarring of the face, back, and anterior chest. The most severe form of cystic acne (acne conglobata) can be disabling, with undermining of the skin of the forehead, temporal regions, cheeks, and chin, as well as extensive pockets of a sanguinopurulent exudate. The usual pathogenic organisms are not found in these lesions.

Incision of the cystic lesions with a fine pointed blade or electric needle is used to drain the cysts and reduce the inflammation that produces the scarring. Dietary control, which in the past was an unpleasant ritual for patients with acne, is not thought to be important today. Topical medications with preparations containing sulfur, benzoyl peroxide, or vitamin A acid and careful skin hygiene, combined with long-term administration of systemic antibiotics such as tetracycline, have been helpful in controlling the disease. Ultraviolet rays are also beneficial. Although superficial x-ray therapy had been effective in controlling acne, the consequent atrophy of the skin and the increased risk of skin carcinomas have rendered this mode of therapy obsolete.

The synthetic retinoid derivative 13-cis-retinoic acid (Accutane) has revolutionized the therapy of severe acne. It has proved valuable in the therapy of severe nodulocystic acne [57]. It is taken orally usually in a dosage of 1 mg per kilogram body weight for an initial 4- to 5-month course of therapy. Many patients obtain long-term remission after discontinuation of the drug and at that stage are often amenable to further improvement with dermabrasion and the injection of collagen into depressed scars. Approximately 10 to 15 percent of patients require second courses of 13-cis-retinoic acid therapy. This drug is best prescribed by dermatologists because of mucocutaneous and other side effects. Women of childbearing potential must take adequate contraceptive precautions during and after therapy.

After the patient with acne has undertaken an optimal dermatologic regimen, dermabrasion in selected cases has been an effective tool for reducing the unsightliness of the acne scarring. Activity of the disease is not a contraindication to dermabrasion, and in some instances the dermabrasion seems to alleviate active pustules. Although frequently the objective improvement in the quality of the skin is not dramatic (perhaps 60 percent improvement), in most instances the results have yielded sufficient improvement in the appearance of the skin to gratify the patient. Shallow, sharply demarcated pits appear to benefit the most from dermabrasion. Dermabrasion essentially reduces the depth of the acne scar, and the resultant skin contracture further decreases the depth of the scar. Shadows are thereby minimized, and the patients are able to disguise the scarred acne skin effectively with appropriate cosmetics. Patients with olive or darker complexions are subject to depigmentation or hyperpigmentation after healing of the dermabrasion, so that the coloring of the skin may be blotchy. If the patient and the surgeon agree that the blotchy appearance presents less of a problem than the degree of pitting and scarring, dermabrasion may be undertaken, and judicious use of cosmetics yields a pleasant skin texture. Women are willing to use cosmetic makeup to disguise the blotchiness more often than men, who consider makeup inappropriate; this factor must be taken into consideration when selecting patients for dermabrasion. When the limitations of dermabrasion and the potential hazards of disturbed pigmentation are taken into consideration by the surgeon and patient, the procedure is a major means of alleviating the suffering of patients with acne vulgaris scarring.

Patients with severe cystic acne may develop extensive areas of undermining with epithelium-lined tunnels that harbor a sanguinopurulent material. These lesions do not heal and are a continuous source of purulent discharge that is unpleasant and embarrassing for the patient. Unroofing of the epithelium-lined tunnels helps to control the lesions and improves the gross appearance of the skin to the satisfaction of the patient.

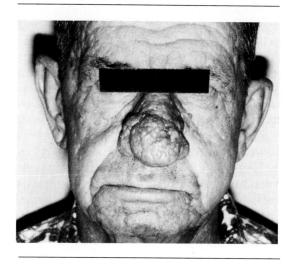

**Figure 29-16** *Rhinophyma.*

## ACNE ROSACEA AND RHINOPHYMA

Acne rosacea occurs primarily in middle-age individuals in the flush areas of the face. The nose, the medial aspects of the cheeks adjacent to the nose, and the chin exhibit patulous, dilated follicular openings with a lobulated dermal fibrosis that takes on a purplish hue with superficial large telangiectases. This disease has been associated with alcoholics because alcohol and spicy foods enhance the vasodilation of the central face in those patients prone to acne rosacea.

Rhinophyma (Fig. 29-16), or severe acne rosacea of the nose, carries the stigma of alcoholism as popularized in the literature. It is frequently rhinophyma that is the source of embarrassment for patients with acne rosacea, causing them to seek medical help. Understanding the disease and controlling the underlying process with an optimal dermatologic regimen are critical. Once rhinophyma is established, operative treatment with dermabrasion, surgical shaving of the thickened skin combined with dermabrasion, and total excision of the skin of the nose and resurfacing with skin grafts are effective treatments for this disease entity.

Although some surgeons have advocated excision of the diseased skin on the nose,

our preference in most cases is to shave the rhinophyma. The deep pores allow shaving of the thickened skin to a depth that leaves sufficient appendages for epithelialization. We have been unable to describe this level definitively, but in the thickened skin shaving may be carried to a depth beyond which one could ordinarily estimate without experience with this disease entity. Shaving is usually supplemented with dermabrasion to smooth the chiseled surface and to reduce the thickened skin on the medial cheeks adjacent to the nose.

After shaving and dermabrasion, hemostasis is aided by application of a gauze saturated with epinephrine 1:200,000 in saline. We have begun to apply a porcine graft dressing to the denuded nose rather than an antibiotic ointment and a greased gauze. Early experience suggests that the epithelialization under the porcine graft is comfortable and clean. After healing of the shaved nose, contracture of the newly epithelialized surface further enhances reduction of the bulbous nose.

When the surgeon chooses to excise the rhinophymatous skin, care must be taken to preserve the underlying perichondrium of the lateral cartilages for vascular support of a skin graft and to preserve the cartilage, which gives the natural contour of the nose. The alar rim is incised external to the nares to preserve the normal alar contour. Occasionally, excisions of the alar base are helpful for reducing the elongated nose. Resurfacing of the rhinophymatous nose after excision is best done with a full-thickness skin graft or thick split-thickness graft from a blush area when feasible. In some instances it is necessary to obtain a skin graft from a nonblush area, which is our primary objection to grafting in preference to shaving. The texture and color match of skin from the arm or trunk are rarely satisfactory compared with the natural blushed texture of the face, which is exaggerated in these patients.

ALOPECIA

The most common form of alopecia is early male-pattern baldness. Although surgeons have been correcting hair defects of the scalp for many years in patients with congenital absence of hair-bearing skin, burn scars, or traumatic scalp loss, current popularity of hair follicle transplants to correct male-pattern baldness has brought a rash of patients to the dermatologist and plastic surgeon seeking correction of baldness.

Topical minoxidil therapy has been approved for androgenetic alopecia. Minoxidil is a systemic antihypertensive drug that was found to have the side effect of producing unwanted hair growth. It may also be effective in some patients with alopecia areata.

Prior to undertaking any procedure, the differential diagnosis of alopecia must be considered. Alopecia areata consists in circumscribed patches of total baldness with otherwise normal scalp skin. Hair at the edges of active bald patches is easily extracted, and the root ends can be seen to taper to a point. Alopecia areata in children tends to be more extensive, and the return of hair is less likely. After puberty it is usually a self-limited disease, and regrowth of hair

in bald areas commonly occurs. The disease is not entirely predictable and may progress to permanent hair loss. Hair transplants in a patient with active alopecia areata would be injudicious. Cicatricial alopecias present as bald patches associated with areas of atrophic scarring. They occur after various disorders, including fungal and other infections, and with chronic discoid lupus erythematosus. After cicatricial alopecia has become inactive, it is appropriate in selected cases to undertake either excision of the scarred area or hair transplants if the vascularity of the tissue appears adequate to support such transplants.

Three operative procedures are available: insertion of plugs of scalp containing hair follicles, transplantation of strips of scalp hair, or transferral of local scalp flaps from the hair-bearing parietal region to the anterior scalp. The effectiveness of these procedures for satisfactorily correcting male-pattern baldness is an unanswered question in our minds. We have had sufficient experience to raise our skepticism over the ultimate success of these procedures. The plug technique consists in removing cylinders of hairless scalp with a sharp 4-mm round punch. Hemostasis is enhanced by cutting the cylinder with the punch and placing a cotton swab dipped in an epinephrine 1:200,000 solution into the defect while obtaining the hair-containing plugs. The plugs containing follicles are then obtained with a 5-mm punch from the lateral and posterior hair-bearing scalp. Instruments are available that facilitate taking plugs at an angle parallel to the hair follicle. On placing the plugs, the shafts of hair are oriented away from the direction in which the hair will lie in order to camouflage the scalp scar. Planning the area of implantation, including hair styling, allows some camouflage of the plugs with the existing hair. Strips of hair no wider than 1 cm can also be implanted in the hairless scalp to give a thick hairline. In the totally hairless area of the apex of the skull, it has been our experience that placement of plugs and strips has not given a natural appearance, and we have seen a significant number of patients who are dissatisfied. We have also not been able to offer these patients anything beyond further hair transplants to attempt to thicken the hair or cover up the spottiness of the transplants. Enthusiasm for this procedure on the part of other plastic surgeons and dermatologists implies that their experience has been more favorable than our own. We believe we are obligated to offer a word of caution that many men who have had hair follicle transplants by plugs and strips have been dissatisfied and have been dismayed to learn that there is no significant way of improving their situation once the procedures have been carried out. Our own position in this regard is one of extreme caution.

HYPERHIDROSIS

Some individuals are prone to hyperhidrosis—excessive sweating on the palms of the hands, the soles of the feet, and the axillae. Although these patients actually perspire more all over the body than the average person, areas just mentioned usually represent the focus of their complaint. Continued wetness of the hands, feet, and axillae is a source of great discomfort and extreme social embarrassment to the patient. Although these patients are somewhat improved in cool, dry climates, even under these conditions the perspiration is excessive, and there is literally a dripping of perspiration from the axillae. The condition may be improved with the usual antiperspirants, but the improvement is often insignificant. With excessive hyperhidrosis of the feet and hands, medical sympathetic block or surgical sympathectomy has been effective in carefully selected patients. Axillary hyperhidrosis has been treated effectively by wide elliptical excision of the apex of the axilla, including most of the eccrine sweat glands, which are concentrated in the axillary vault [50, 58].

The sweat glands extend in some areas below the dermis into the subcutaneous tissues, and for this reason some surgeons have advocated removing the subcutaneous tissues as well. It is more likely that any benefit from removing the subcutaneous tissue is derived from denervation of the remaining eccrine glands. On this basis we have chosen simply to do as wide an elliptical excision as feasible to permit primary closure and to undermine the adjacent tissues just below the dermis, thereby adequately denervating the remaining eccrine glands and facilitating skin closure.

EXCESSIVE HAIR

In young women excessive hair is of particular concern when present on the face, especially the upper lip or chin. The patient may require a medical work-up to rule out endocrine abnormalities. If there is no systemic basis for hirsutism, diathermy or electrolysis is a permanent means of hair removal, but these procedures do require the skill of an experienced operator to avoid scarring. Temporary removal of the hair is accomplished with the use of depilatories or epilating wax, which is acceptable in minor cases. Bleaching is also a means for reducing the conspicuousness of unwanted hair about the face. Shaving is an effective approach, despite the inaccurate belief that repeated shaving causes thickening of the hair.

HIDRADENITIS SUPPURATIVA

Hidradenitis suppurativa, an inflammatory disease of the apocrine glands, presents most frequently as deep recurrent abscesses in the axillae, which may result in scarred deep sinus tracts, fluctuant draining of abscesses, and excruciating pain with limitation of abduction of the shoulder. Although seen most commonly in young females in the axillae, it also occurs in the groin and perineum and in the areolae. Early acute cases may be treated with local therapy, such as incision and drainage of the abscess, followed by control with long-term antibiotic therapy. However, once the disease entity is established with deep scarring and sinus tracts, the only appropriate therapy is surgical excision of the

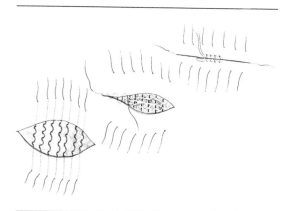

**Figure 29-17** *Excision and primary closure of axillary skin. Up to 8 × 15 cm (measured in contracted state) can be excised. Retention sutures of No. 1 nylon are placed about 4 cm from the wound edges, picking up the axillary fascia or two or three points (left). A 2-0 nylon subcuticular suture is then inserted (center), followed by interrupted 4-0 nylon vertical mattress sutures (right). (From W. J. Pollock, F. R. Virnelli, and R. F. Ryan. Axillary hidradenitis suppurativa: A simple and effective surgical technique.* Plast. Reconstr. Surg. 49:22, 1972.)

involved area. These patients are too frequently not offered the alternative of operative management of this disease until an unpleasant, prolonged course of conservative treatment for abscesses and pain has been undertaken. Rarely must patients be convinced of the need for operative interventions, as they have usually suffered extensively with the discomfort and unpleasantness of this disease. Culture of the purulent discharge and appropriate antibiotic therapy for a period of at least 10 days prior to operative intervention are important.

Excision of all of the involved tissue is the ultimate goal of the operative procedure. Primary closure can be accomplished with large defects, as pointed out by Pollock and colleagues [43], but the surgeon must not compromise the excision to accomplish primary closure. Large areas of involvement (8 × 15 cm) can be excised and closed primarily if the wound is closed with heavy retention sutures to approximate the axillary fascia

and subcutaneous tissues and if careful subcuticular skin closure is accomplished (Fig. 29-17). When primary closure is not feasible, split-thickness skin grafts and immobilization of the arm with Velpeau dressings comprise the next choice. We have not found it necessary to use any type of skin flap to accomplish skin coverage in the axillary vault after excision of hidradenitis suppurativa.

When the disease has extended beyond the axilla onto the chest wall or the upper arm, it is preferable to excise the involved areas entirely and apply split-thickness skin grafts. It has been our practice to undertake the excision and grafting on one axilla at a time so that the patient is not totally disabled during the healing period. When the surgeon can clearly excise and close the wounds primarily, it is feasible to undertake correction of the disease in both axillae with one operative procedure. Good healing and lack of wound infection are usual when all the diseased tissue is properly excised. If the scarred sinuses or involved glands are not completely excised, delayed wound healing and infection are common. Because these patients have had limited abduction of the shoulder for long periods prior to the operative intervention, the need for exercises to abduct the arm must be stressed and the patients followed until full abduction is accomplished.

DISSECTING CELLULITIS OF THE SCALP
Known also as perifolliculitis capitis abscedens et suffodiens, dissecting cellulitis of the scalp (Fig. 29-18) occurs most often in black men and is a disease of the scalp similar to hidradenitis suppurativa. The scalp is involved with a perifolliculitis that results in burrowing, encysted epithelium-lined tracts with associated chronic infection and granulation tissue. The conservative management of this extensive folliculitis has been discouraging. Once this disease entity is established, the only effective treatment is excision of the scarred, infected areas and re-

surfacing with split-thickness skin grafts or skin flaps from the adjacent scalp if the disease is limited.

PYODERMA GANGRENOSUM

Multiple skin abscesses with necrosis and undermining ulcerations occur in the necrotizing lesion of the skin called pyoderma gangrenosum. It is often associated with ulcerative colitis (50 percent of patients). It has also been reported to occur in association with other gastrointestinal disorders (diverticulosis, regional enteritis, peptic ulcer disease, hepatitis, and carcinoid tumor) as well as rheumatoid arthritis, pulmonary diseases, and hematologic disorders. No systemic disease is evident in 20 percent of the patients with pyoderma gangrenosum [26, 41, 63]. No specific organism or combination of organisms has been identified with this disease entity, although frequently *Proteus* and other gram-negative organisms and β-hemolytic streptococci have been cultured from these wounds. Systemic and topical antibiotic therapy has been of some use in controlling the active disease process. It appears today that the basic lesion is not a primary infection but may be a necrotizing cutaneous vasculitis with rapidly developing hemorrhagic liquefying tissue necrosis of the skin. It is characterized by ulceration surrounded by bluish hemorrhagic cribriform edges. The course is protracted and in some instances fulminant.

Careful control of pathogenic bacteria with culture and sensitivity tests preceding antibiotic therapy, associated with conservative débridement of the necrotic tissues, has been successful in many instances. It appears important to débride only the grossly necrotic tissue and not to incise the adjacent intact tissues, thereby avoiding extension of the disease beyond the operative débridement. Local and systemic steroid therapy immunosuppressives (e.g., azathioprine) and systemic sulfones have been helpful. Caution must be exercised when treating these patients with local injections because of the

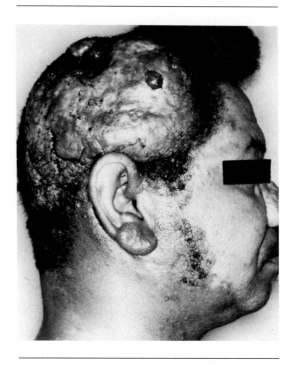

**Figure 29-18** *Dissecting cellulitis of the scalp.*

possibility of local skin trauma, which may induce new pyoderma gangrenosum lesions.

SKIN INFECTIONS
*Lupus Vulgaris*
Although once common, lupus vulgaris (Fig. 29-19) is now a rare form of cutaneous tuberculosis; it can produce slowly progressive destruction of soft tissues followed by atrophic scarring. Active areas of the disease are studded with superficial intradermal small reddish tan lupus nodules. Lupus vulgaris is a specific form of cutaneous tuberculosis that must be distinguished from scrofuloderma (cold abscess), either primary in the skin or extending to it secondarily from tuberculosis of bone or lymph nodes.

Lupus vulgaris is controlled with appropriate antituberculosis chemotherapy (long-term isoniazid administration). If resultant scarring is a problem, excision of the lesion, with prior antituberculosis therapy, is effec-

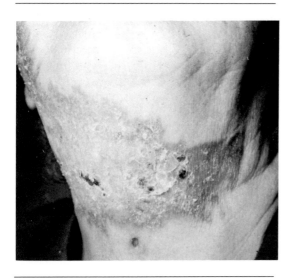

**Figure 29-19** *Lupus vulgaris of 20 years' duration, with atrophic scarring and active lupus nodules at the edges.*

tive and safe [2]. Treatment of lupus vulgaris with irradiation is now obsolete. In fact, it is appreciated that irradiation of lupus vulgaris contributed to the development of squamous cell carcinomas in these areas. Seventy-four percent of the patients seen by Griffith [21] with a carcinoma in the area of a lupus vulgaris lesion had had previous radiotherapy. In a group of patients with healed lupus vulgaris without previous radiotherapy, there was a 2 percent incidence of carcinoma. Rees [46] has demonstrated that there is an incidence of carcinoma in the unhealed lupus vulgaris lesion, even in the absence of irradiation.

### Leprosy

Leprosy affects primarily the skin and peripheral nerves, producing deformities that are of particular interest to the plastic surgeon. The classic picture of lepromatous leprosy incorporates the lepra facies, which has become a repulsive concept in our culture. Enna and Delgado [18] indicated three prerequisites before undertaking facial reconstruction for leprosy: (1) disease inactivity; (2) intact healthy skin; and (3) a stabilized deformity. The authors pointed out the common deformities that are typical of the face in leprosy: (1) megalolobule of the external ear; (2) loss of eyebrows; (3) nasal deformity; (4) sagging and wrinkled redundant facial skin; and (5) lagophthalmos. Correction of the nasal deformity associated with leprosy has been described in an experience with 86 patients, utilizing skin grafts to restore the nasal lining [1]. The problems encountered in leprosy subsequent to peripheral neuropathy have resulted in extensive literature on the management of hand deformities. The most commonly presenting dysfunction of the hand in the leprosy patient is ulnar nerve palsy, with the inability to fully extend the fingers for grasp, and median nerve palsy, with the inability of the thumb to oppose.

### Noma

Cancrum oris (noma) is a destructive infection of the face in African or Asian children under 5 years of age; the condition results in extensive unilateral loss of the lips, oral commissure, nose, cheek, and occasionally the lower eyelid. The bones of the maxilla, nose, zygoma, and mandible may be eroded, and masticatory muscle involvement often causes trismus [16].

### Fingernail Infections

Disturbances of the nail are frequent sources of concern for patients. Trauma, fungal infections, and psoriasis are the most common causes of nail deformities that lead patients to seek medical advice. Treatment of an acute paronychia consists in adequate drainage. The chronic paronychia presents a different problem. The surgeon must first look for a subungual abscess associated with a chronic paronychia. The small area of pus under the nail adjacent to the paronychia can be subtle and can result in a recurrent paronychia, requiring repeated operative drainage and search for an exotic causative organism. When the subungual abscess is recognized, unroofing the nail bed results in a certain solution to the problem. In the true chronic paronychia without a subungual component, candidiasis is the usual offender. The diabetic and patients whose hands are constantly wet—house cleaners, waitresses, bartenders, dentists—are susceptible to chronic paronychia associated with candidiasis.

Treatment of chronic paronychia associated with candidiasis is to remedy the wetness of the hands, apply nystatin locally, and flush the crevices and pockets under the nail with acetone to eliminate moisture. Congenital paronychia (Jadassohn-Lewandowsky syndrome) may require excision of the nail bed and nail plate, which can be resurfaced with split-thickness grafts [57].

*Wart Virus Infection*
Wart virus infections result in well circumscribed hyperkeratotic verrucose papules, nodules, spicules, or spiny clusters on the skin. On pressure-bearing plantar surfaces, large thick overlying callus accumulations can cause tenderness and pain on walking. In intertriginous and genital areas, such infections yield vegetating, gray or pinkish, cauliflower-like papillomatous soft excrescences and confluent masses called *condylomata acuminata*. These lesions are sometimes macerated, secondarily infected, and inflamed with malodorous purulent secretions developing in their crevices. Giant condylomata acuminata (Buschke-Lowenstein tumor) show pseudoepitheliomatous hyperplasia and may be clinically and histologically difficult to differentiate from epidermoid carcinoma. Plantar warts can be difficult to differentiate from corns and calluses. Black specks of degenerating hemorrhage and honeycomb patterning in the overlying hyperkeratosis are clinical signs that favor the diagnosis of wart. Tuberculosis verrucosa cutis (prospector's wart) may mimic the common wart but usually has some inflammatory reaction at its base and may show some exudation as well.

Common warts and especially plantar warts are not suitably treated by excision and suturing, as aggravated recurrences along the suture line from inoculated virus are common. Small lesions are best managed dermatologically with either curettage and electrodesiccation or liquid nitrogen. A host of other dermatologic approaches with such agents as caustics, vesicants, and formalin are available for the management of warts in addition to temporizing and suggestion that may result in suitable clearing. The surgeon is best advised to avoid futile attempts at clean excision. Massive condylomata acuminata at times require some surgical excision as part of the management program.

*Molluscum Contagiosum*
Molluscum contagiosum is a pox virus infection of the epidermis that results in the formation of translucent, umbilicated, smooth, pale semiglobular papules 1 to 3 mm in size. Rarely, such lesions become large (1 to 2 cm) and develop an inflammatory base, hyperkeratosis, and secondary infection; the lesions then resemble carcinoma or other skin tumors. Lesions in adults occur especially about the genital area and may be venereally transmitted. Giant molluscum contagiosum lesions have been reported to occur in AIDS patients. Clearly, the physician confronted with a large or unusual-appearing molluscum must take this possibility into account. There is a characteristic histologic picture in which infected cells develop huge cytoplasmic basophilic inclusions that compress the cell nucleus to a peripheral crescent. The lesions are best treated by curettage or light electrodesiccation and not by surgical excision.

## Laser Therapy
Argon and carbon dioxide lasers are now frequently used for therapy of various benign and malignant skin lesions. The argon laser and the flash pump dye laser seem to be particularly valuable for treating port-wine stains. The carbon dioxide laser may be used to

excise basal cell carcinoma, seborrheic keratoses, and verrucas, as well as other conditions such as hemangiomas and actinic cheilitis. Developments in laser technology that may have a place in dermatologic therapy include tunable dye lasers, where selections of ultraviolet wavelengths may create a more versatile apparatus.

## References

1. Antia, N. H., and Pandya, N. J. Surgical treatment of the nasal deformities of leprosy. *Plast. Reconstr. Surg.* 60:768, 1977.
2. Barker, L. P. Lupus vulgaris occurring in a skin graft. *Arch. Dermatol. Syph.* 54:758, 1946.
3. Bauer, B. S., and Vicasi, F. A. An approach to excision of congenital pigmented nevi in infancy and early childhood. *Plast. Reconstr. Surg.* 82:1012, 1988.
4. Beighton, P., Bull, J. C., and Edgerton, M. T. Plastic surgery in cutis laxa. *Br. J. Plast. Surg.* 23:285, 1970.
5. Binkley, G. W. Dermopathy in the diabetic syndrome. *Arch. Dermatol.* 92:625, 1965.
6. Block, J. J. Sjögren's syndrome: Clinical, pathological, and serological study of 62 cases. *Medicine (Baltimore)* 44:187, 1965.
7. Charles, N. Multiple glomus tumors of the face and eyelid. *Arch. Ophthalmol.* 94:1283, 1976.
8. Cleaver, J. E. DNA damage and repair in light sensitive human skin disease. *J. Invest. Dermatol.* 54:181, 1970.
9. Cohen, N., Plaschkes, Y., Pevzner, S., et al. Review of 57 cases of keratoacanthoma. *Plast. Reconstr. Surg.* 49:138, 1972.
10. Cooper, J. S., Fried, P. R., and Laubenstein, L. J. Initial observations on the effect of radiotherapy on epidemic Kaposi's sarcoma. *J.A.M.A.* 252:934, 1985.
11. Dellon, A. L., Chretien, P. B., and Peck, G. L. Successful treatment of Darier's disease by partial thickness removal of skin. *Plast. Reconstr. Surg.* 59:823, 1977.
12. Dellon, A. L., Edelson, R. L., and Chretien, P. B. Defining the malignant potential of the giant pigmented nevus. *Plast. Reconstr. Surg.* 57:611, 1976.
13. DePalma, R. G., Moskowitz, R. W., and Holden, W. D. Peripheral ischemia and collagen disease: Clinical manifestations, diagnosis, and treatment. *Arch. Surg.* 105:313, 1972.
14. Dingman, R. O., Grabb, W. C., and Oneal, R. M. Cutis laxa congenita—generalized elastosis. *Plast. Reconstr. Surg.* 44:431, 1969.
15. Dubin, B. J., and Kaplan, E. N. Surgical treatment of necrobiosis lipoidica, diabetocorum. *Plast. Reconstr. Surg.* 60:421, 1977.
16. Durrani, K. M. Surgical repair of defects from noma (cancrum oris). *Plast. Reconstr. Surg.* 52:629, 1973.
17. Eisen, A. Z. Human skin collagenase: Relationship to the pathogenesis of epidermolysis bullosa dystrophica. *J. Invest. Dermatol.* 52:449, 1969.
18. Enna, C. D., and Delgado, D. Surgical correction of common facial deformities due to leprosy. *Plast. Reconstr. Surg.* 42:422, 1968.
19. Given, K., Pickrell, K., and Smith, D. Dermal cylindroma (turban tumor). *Plast. Reconstr. Surg.* 59:582, 1977.
20. Graham, J. H., and Helwig, E. B. Bowen's disease and its relationship to systemic cancer. *Arch. Dermatol.* 80:133, 1959.
21. Griffith, B. H. The surgical treatment of lupus vulgaris and lupus carcinoma. *Plast. Reconstr. Surg.* 20:155, 1957.
22. Hill, E. J. Skin grafting in periarteritis nodosa. *Plast. Reconstr. Surg.* 15:186, 1955.
23. Horner, R. L., Wiedel, J. D., and Bralliar, F. Involvement of the hand in epidermolysis bullosa. *J. Bone Joint Surg. [Am.]* 53:1347, 1971.
24. Kaplan, E. N. The risk of malignancy in large congenital nevi. *Plast. Reconstr. Surg.* 53:186, 1976.
25. Kaplan, E. N., and Henjyoyi, E. Y. Pseudoxanthoma elasticum: A dermal elastosis with surgical implications. *Plast. Reconstr. Surg.* 58:595, 1976.
26. Kelley, M. L. Skin lesions associated with chronic ulcerative colitis. *Am. J. Dig. Dis.* 7:255, 1962.
27. Kisner, W. H., and Hendrix, J. H., Jr. Keratosis palmaris et plantaris. *Plast. Reconstr. Surg.* 51:424, 1973.
28. Kopf, A. W., and Andrade, R. Benign Juvenile Melanoma. In *Year Book of Dermatology* (1965–1966 series). Chicago: Year Book, 1966.
29. Lanier, V. C., Jr., Pickrell, K. L., and Georgiade, N. G. Congenital giant nevi: Clinical and pathological considerations. *Plast. Reconstr. Surg.* 58:48, 1976.

30. Lorincz, A. L. Ehlers-Danlos Syndrome (Cutis Hyperelastica). In D. J. Demis, R. G. Crounse, J. McGuire, et al. (eds.), *Clinical Dermatology* Vol. 1, Sect. 4, Unit 3. Hagerstown, MD: Harper & Row, 1972.

31. Lorincz, A. L. Pseudoxanthoma Elasticum. In D. J. Demis, R. G. Crounse, J. McGuire, et al. (eds.), *Clinical Dermatology.* Vol. 1, Sect. 4, Unit 2. Hagerstown, MD: Harper & Row, 1972.

32. Losken, H. W., Davies, D., and Gordon, W. Coverage of scalp and skull defect in a patient with the systemic form of scleroderma. *Plast. Reconstr. Surg.* 51:212, 1973.

33. Lowe, N. J. *Practical Psoriasis Therapy.* Chicago: Year Book, 1986.

34. McPeak, C. J., Cruz, T., and Nicastri, A. D. Dermatofibrosarcoma protuberans: An analysis of 86 cases—five with metastasis. *Ann. Surg.* 166:803, 1967.

35. Mendelson, B. C., and Masson, J. Xanthelasma: Follow-up on results after surgical excision. *Plast. Reconstr. Surg.* 58:535, 1976.

36. Mladick, R. A., Pickrell, K. L., Thorne, F. L., et al. Squamous cell cancer in discoid lupus erythematosus. *Plast. Reconstr. Surg.* 42:497, 1968.

37. Morgan, J. E., and Mulliken, J. B. Dermabrasion and limited excision of the fibrous papules of tuberous sclerosis. *Plast. Reconstr. Surg.* 59:124, 1977.

38. Nalbandian, R. M. *Skin necrosis induced by coumarin congeners. Excerpta Medica* 2:58, 1971.

39. O'Brien, P. Sarcoidosis of the nose. *Br. J. Plast. Surg.* 23:242, 1970.

40. Pearson, R. W. Mechano-Bullous Diseases (epidermolysis bullosa). In T. B. Fitzpatrick, K. A. Arndt, W. H. Clark, et al. (eds.), *Dermatology in General Medicine.* New York: McGraw-Hill, 1971.

41. Perry, H. O., and Brunsting, L. A. Pyoderma gangrenosum: Clinical study of 19 cases. *Arch. Dermatol.* 75:380, 1957.

42. Pierre, M., Jouglard, J. P., and Tramier, H. A case of skin necrosis following anticoagulant therapy. *Excerpta Medica* 2:109, 1971.

43. Pollock, W. J., Virnelli, F. R., and Ryan, R. F. Axillary hidradenitis suppurativa: A simple and effective surgical technique. *Plast. Reconstr. Surg.* 49:22, 1972.

44. Reed, W. B., Becker, S. W., Sr., Becker, S. W., Jr., et al. Giant pigmented nevi, melanoma, and leptomeningeal melanocytosis. *Arch. Dermatol.* 91:100, 1965.

45. Reed, W. B., Horowitz, R. E., and Beighton, P. Acquired cutis laxa. *Arch. Dermatol.* 103:661, 1971.

46. Rees, T. D. Surgical repair of lupus vulgaris. *Plast. Reconstr. Surg.* 20:147, 1957.

47. Rees, T. D., and Swinyard, C. A. Rehabilitative digital surgery in epidermolysis bullosa. *Plast. Reconstr. Surg.* 40:169, 1967.

48. Rhodes, A. R., and Melski, J. W. Small congenital nevocellular nevi and risk of cutaneous melanoma. *J. Pediatr.* 100:219, 1982.

49. Rigell, D. S., and Friedman, R. J. Clinical management of patients with dysplastic and congenital nevi. *Dermatol. Clin.* 3:251, 1985.

50. Rigg, B. M. Axillary hyperhidrosis. *Plast. Reconstr. Surg.* 59:334, 1977.

51. Risch, J., Ashton, R. E., Lowe, N. J., et al. 13-cis-Retinoic acid for dyskeratinizing diseases: Clinical pathological responses. *Clin. Exp. Dermatol.* 9:472, 1984.

52. Riu, R., Ruth, L. D., and Snyder, C. C. Skin necrosis secondary to cryoglobulinemia: Case report. *Plast. Reconstr. Surg.* 46:510, 1970.

53. Schultz, R. C. Skin sloughs in Waterhouse-Friderichsen syndrome. *Plast. Reconstr. Surg.* 42:598, 1968.

54. Sharpe, G. C., Irvin, W. S., Tan, E. M., et al. Mixed connective tissue disease—an apparently distinct rheumatic disease syndrome associated with a specific antibody to an extractable nuclear antigen (ENA). *Am. J. Med.* 52:148, 1972.

55. Stegmaier, O. C. Natural regression of the melanotic nevus. *J. Invest. Dermatol.* 32:413, 1959.

56. Stegmaier, O. C., and Montgomery, H. Histopathologic studies of pigmented nevi in children. *J. Invest. Dermatol.* 20:51, 1953.

57. Strauss, J. S., Rapini, R. P., Shalita, A., et al. Isotretinoin therapy for acne: Results of a multicentered dose response study. *J. Am. Acad. Dermatol.* 10:490, 1984.

58. Tipton, J. B. Axillary hyperhidrosis and its surgical treatment. *Plast. Reconstr. Surg.* 42:137, 1968.

59. Wayte, S. M., and Helwig, E. B. Melanotic freckle of Hutchinson. *Cancer* 21:893, 1968.

60. White, R. R., and Noone, R. B. Paronychia congenita (Jadassohn-Lewandowsky syndrome). *Plast. Reconstr. Surg.* 59:855, 1977.

61. Winkelmann, R. K., and Ditto, W. B. Cutaneous and visceral syndromes of necrotizing or "allergic" angiitis: A study of 38 cases. *Medicine (Baltimore)* 43:59, 1964.

62. Wolfort, F. G., and Krizek, T. J. Skin ulceration in sickle cell anemia. *Plast. Reconstr. Surg.* 43:71, 1969.

63. Wustrack, K., and Zarem, H. A. Pyoderma gangrenosum: Recognition and management. *Plast. Reconstr. Surg.* 62:423, 1978.

64. Yeschua, R., Wexler, M. R., and Neuman, Z. The nevus of Ota. *Plast. Reconstr. Surg.* 55:229, 1975.

65. Zarem, H. A., Pearson, R. W., and Leaf, N. Surgical management of hand deformities in recessive dystrophic epidermolysis bullosa. *Br. J. Plast. Surg.* 27:176, 1974.

## Suggested Reading

Arndt, K., Noe, J. M., and Rosen, S. *Cutaneous Laser Therapy: Principles and Methods.* New York: Wiley, 1983.

Braverman, I. M. *Skin Signs of Systemic Disease.* Philadelphia: Saunders, 1981.

Demis, D. J., Crounse, R. G., Dobson, R. L., et al. (eds.), *Clinical Dermatology.* Hagerstown, MD: Harper & Row, 1985.

Domonkos, A. N. *Andrews' Diseases of the Skin* (7th ed.). Philadelphia: Saunders, 1982.

Fitzpatrick, T. B., Eisen, A. Z., Wolff, K., et al. (eds.), *Dermatology in General Medicine* (3rd ed.). New York: McGraw-Hill, 1987.

Lever, W. F., and Schaumburg-Lever, G. *Histopathology of the Skin* (6th ed.). Philadelphia: Lippincott, 1983.

Rook, A., Wilkinson, D. S., Ebling, F. J. G., et al. *Textbook of Dermatology* (4th ed.). Oxford: Blackwell, 1986.

*Norman E. Hugo*

# Hypertrophic Scars and Keloids

Scar is the natural sequela of any wound and serves to impart strength through the elaboration and deposition of collagen. Scar knits the wound together, and much is made of the aesthetic appearance, the ultimate goal being an "invisible" scar. This goal, of course, is not attainable.

Medicolegal considerations of scars have become increasingly important as suits have been filed over the appearance of scars. It must be noted that the patient's contribution to scar formation is far more important than that of the surgeon. Wounds repaired meticulously by a surgeon can develop into hypertrophic/keloid scars. Not uncommonly, simultaneous wounds on a patient in the same area may heal in markedly different fashions, or different portions of the same scar may heal differently.

Certain regions of the body are especially prone to develop hypertrophic/keloid scars, including the back, shoulder, sternum, and earlobe. Although tension has been implicated in the formation of keloids, it is not a factor in the earlobe, and although inflammation is mentioned as a contributing factor, episiotomy wounds closed with chromic catgut rarely develop keloids, even in blacks. Thus there is no single unifying clinical reason for keloids to develop. Pigmented races, blacks and Asians, develop keloids more readily than whites.

## Collagen Structure

Because scar is basically collagen, it is imperative to understand the nature of collagen. Eleven types of collagen have been identified in vertebrate tissue [23]. They can be classified into groups characterized by chains of peptides with molecular weights equal to or greater than 95,000 and a continuous helical domain of approximately 300 nm (group 1: types I, II, III, V, K); helical domains separated by nonhelical segments (group 2: types IV, VI, VII, VIII); or a molecular weight less than 95,000 (group 3: types IX, X) [24]. Types I, II, and III are capable of forming fibers possibly by losing the major portions of their globular domains during extracellular processing [3].

## Scar Formation

The amount and type of collagen produced determines the type of scar. Collagen production by type is genetically determined, and their identification has been possible. The vertebrate fibrillar collagen genes evolved by duplication of a common multiexon structure that stemmed from a 54-basepair unit [28].

An abnormal scar results from the production of defective collagen or when collagen deposition or degradation is abnormal. An

*851*

example of abnormal collagen producing atrophic scars is the Ehlers-Danlos syndrome, which is a heterogeneous group of ten clinical types. Types I, II, III, and VIII are inherited as autosomal dominants, and type VI is inherited as an autosomal recessive. The biochemical disorder is unknown in types I, II, and III, but these types are characterized by large collagen fibrils many of which are irregular in shape. Type VI is caused by a lysyl hydroxylase deficiency and is characterized by small collagen bundles. The biochemical disorder in type VIII is also unknown [4].

Normal or aesthetically pleasing scars have an architecture approaching that of normal skin with well structured collagen bundles that course parallel with the epithelial surface. Hypertrophic scars, in contrast, have shorter, fragmented fibrils that are fewer and flatter. Keloid scars are characterized by disorganization [19]: Discrete bundle formation is absent, and whorls of collagen are present. It may be difficult to differentiate between hypertrophic scars and keloids on a morphologic basis [22], even though Cosman et al. established guidelines for such distinction [8].

An arrest in maturation also contributes to the unsightly scar. Collagen fibers measure 440 Å in granulation tissue, 600 Å in hypertrophic scars, 1000 Å in a mature scar, and 1050 Å in normal skin. Similarly, the shape of collagen fibrils is irregular and angular in granulation tissue, irregular to ovoid in hypertrophic scar, ovoid to round in mature scar, and round in normal skin [15].

Hypertrophic scars have an abundance of ground substance, suggesting a correlation with excessive mucopolysaccharides [5, 31]. Although there are close similarities with porcine xenografts in donor swine, keloid and hypertrophic scars are not found in experimental animals [32].

Initial observations suggested a correlation between hyperemia and hypertrophic scars [21]. Although hypertrophic and keloid scarring seem intimately linked with the state of their microvasculature, studies reveal that most of the microvessels are partially or completely occluded by endothelial proliferation and that hypoxia is the significant factor in producing hypertrophic and keloid scars [17, 18]. The abnormally high concentration of perivascular myofibroblasts may also contribute to the occlusion.

## Biochemical Differences Between Mature Scar and Hypertrophic/Keloid Scars

### COLLAGEN SYNTHESIS

There are excessive amounts of fibronectin in hypertrophic/keloid scars compared to that in mature scars [16, 27]. Whether this situation is cause or effect is conjectural.

Keloid scars produce significantly more collagen than hypertrophic scars, and both produce more collagen than mature scars or normal dermis [7]. Their fibroblasts are also stimulated to increase collagen production in the presence of histamine [6, 29]. Keloid fibroblasts synthesize collagen at a rate two to three times that of skin or mature scar [10].

Mature scars produce collagen at a relatively constant rate from 6 months to 20 years, whereas hypertrophic and keloid scars produce collagen at a level two times that for 2 to 3 years, then fall to a rate similar to that of mature scars. The collagen content in mature scars stays constant but increases for up to 4 years in hypertrophic and keloid scars [9].

### BIODEGRADATION

Collagen is in a state of constant turnover, and if synthesis exceeds degradation, an excess of collagen results. Although keloid/hypertrophic scars have a normal amount and type of collagenase [25], an activator of procollagenase is lacking [12]. Thus degradation of collagen is impaired.

## Treatment of Scars

### SURGERY

Scars that run perpendicular to the lines of minimal tension can be redirected by Z- or W-plasty. These procedures are especially effective on the face. Hypertrophic/keloid scars may be excised and followed by immediate injections of triamcinolone *(vide infra)*.

### PRESSURE

Use of pressure garments ameliorates hypertrophic/keloid scar formation by increasing the hypoxic condition, which results in focal degeneration of selective cells [17]. Physical flattening of collagen whorls also helps.

### DRUGS

Scar formation is inhibited by the incorporation of *cis*-hydroxyproline into the collagen molecule instead of proline [20]. Its toxicity is debated [2, 30]. β-Aminoproprionitrile (BAPN) prevents cross-linking in collagen and renders it susceptible to degradation [1]. Colchicine increases collagenase [26]. Intralesional injection of corticosteroids reduces hypertrophic/keloid scars owing to inhibition of inflammation and subsequent fibroplasia, if given early [11], or increased collagenolytic activity, if given late [14].

Interferon holds promise for the future. In experiments on cultured fibroblasts treated with interferon, a decrease in collagen production was accompanied by a decrease in type I collagen mRNA. This finding suggests that interferon decreases the rate at which the procollagen α1(I) gene is transcribed [13].

## References

1. Arem, A. J., Madden, J. W., Chrapil, M., et al. Effect of lysyloxidase inhibition on healing wounds. *Surg. Forum* 26:67, 1975.
2. Bora, F. W., Lane, J. M., and Prockop, D. J. Inhibition of collagen biosynthesis as a means of controlling scar formation in tendon injury. *J. Bone Joint Surg. [Am.]* 54:1501, 1972.
3. Burgerson, R. E., Morris, N. P., Murray, L. W., et al. The structure of type VII collagen. *Ann. N.Y. Acad. Sci.* 460:47, 1985.
4. Byers, B. H., and Holbrook, K. A. Molecular basis of clinical heterogeneity in the Ehlers-Danlos syndrome. *Ann. N.Y. Acad. Sci.* 460:298, 1985.
5. Chien, S. F., Shetlar, M. R., Shetlar, C. L., et al. The hypertrophic scar: Hexosamine containing components of burn scars. *Proc. Soc. Exp. Biol. Med.* 139:544, 1972.
6. Cohen, I. K., Beavan, M. A., Horakova, Q., et al. Histamine and collagen synthesis in keloid and hypertrophic scar. *Surg. Forum* 23:509, 1972.
7. Cohen, I. K., Keiser, H. R., and Sjoerdsma, A. Collagen synthesis in human keloid and hypertrophic scar. *Surg. Forum* 22:488, 1971.
8. Cosman, B., Crikelair, G. F., Ju, D. M. C., et al. The treatment of keloids. *Plast. Reconstr. Surg.* 27:335, 1961.
9. Craig, R. D. P., Schofield, J. D., and Jackson, D. S. Collagen biosynthesis in normal and hypertrophic scars and keloid as a function of the duration of the scar. *Br. J. Surg.* 62:741, 1975.
10. Diegelmann, R. F., Cohen, I. K., and McCoy, B. J. Growth kinetics and collagen synthesis of normal skin, normal scar, and keloid fibroblasts in vitro. *J. Coll. Physiol.* 98:341, 1979.
11. Griffith, B. H. Treatment of keloids with triamcinolone acetonide. *Plast. Reconstr. Surg.* 38:202, 1966.
12. Harper, E., and Gross, J. Collagenase and its Zymogen. In H. Peeters (ed.), *Protides of the Biological Fibrils, 21st Colloquium. Brugge, Belgium, 1973.* Oxford: Pergamon Press, 1974. Abstract 114.
13. Jimenez, S. A., and Rosenblum, J. Transcriptional control of human diploid fibroblast collagen synthesis by Y-interferon. *Ann. N.Y. Acad. Sci.* 460:453, 1985.
14. Ketchum, L. D., Smith, J., Robinson, D. W., et al. Treatment of hypertrophic scars, keloids and scar contracture by triamcinolone acetonide. *Plast. Reconstr. Surg.* 38:209, 1966.
15. Kischer, C. W. Collagen and dermal patterns in the hypertrophic scar. *Anat. Rec.* 179:137, 1974.
16. Kischer, C. W., and Hendrix, M. J. C. Fibronectin (FN) in hypertrophic scars and keloids. *Cell Tissue Res.* 231:29, 1983.
17. Kischer, C. W., and Shetlar, M. R. Microvasculature in hypertrophic scars and the effects of pressure. *J. Trauma* 19:757, 1979.

18. Kischer, C. W., Thies, A. C., and Chrapil, M. Perivascular myofibroblasts and microvascular occlusion in hypertrophic scars and keloids. *Hum. Pathol.* 13:819, 1982.

19. Knapp, T. R., Daniels, J. R., and Kaplan, E. N. Pathologic scar formation. *Ann. J. Pathol.* 86:47, 1977.

20. Lane, J. M., Bora, F. W., Prockop, D. J., et al. Inhibition of scar formation by the proline analog cis-hydroxyproline. *J. Surg. Res.* 3:135, 1972.

21. Larson, D. L., Abston, S., Evans, E. B., et al. Techniques for decreasing scar formation and contractures in the burned patient. *J. Trauma* 11:807, 1971.

22. Larson, D. L., Kischer, C. S., and Louis, S. R. Scanning and Transmission Electron Microscopic Studies of Hypertrophic Scar. In J. J. Longacre (ed.), *The Ultrastructure of Collagen.* Springfield, IL: Thomas, 1976. P. 263.

23. Miller, E. J. Recent Information on the Chemistry of the Collagens. In W. T. Butler. *The Chemistry and Biology of Mineralized Tissues.* Birmingham, AL: Ebasco Media, 1985. P. 80.

24. Miller, E. J. The structure of fibril-forming collagens. *Ann. N.Y. Acad. Sci.* 460:13, 1985.

25. Milson, J. P., and Craig, R. D. P. Collagen degradation in cultured keloid and hypertrophic scar tissue. *Br. J. Dermatol.* 89:635, 1973.

26. Morton, D., Steinbronn, K., Lato, M., et al. Effect of colchicine on wound healing in rats. *Surg. Forum* 25:47, 1974.

27. Nagata, H., Veki, H., and Moriguchi, T. Fibronectin. *Arch. Dermatol.* 121:997, 1985.

28. Ramirez, F., Bernard, M., Chu, M., et al. Isolation and characterization of the human fibrillar collagen genes. *Ann. N.Y. Acad. Sci.* 460:117, 1985.

29. Russell, J. D., Russell, S. D., and Tropin, I. K. M. The effect of histamine on the growth of cultured fibroblasts isolated from normal and keloid tissue. *J. Cell. Physiol.* 93:389, 1978.

30. Salvador, R. A., Tsai, I., Marcel, R. J., et al. The in vivo inhibition of collagen synthesis and the reduction of propyl hydroxylans activity by 3,4-dehydroxyproline. *Arch. Biochem. Biophys.* 174:381, 1976.

31. Shetlar, M. R., Doborkovsky, M., Linares, H., et al. The hypertrophic scar glycoprotein and collagen components of burn scars. *Proc. Soc. Exp. Biol. Med.* 138:298, 1971.

32. Silverstein, P., Goodwin, M. N., Raulston, G. L., et al. Hypertrophic Scar in the Experimental Animal. In J. J. Longacre (ed.), *The Ultrastructure of Collagen.* Springfield, IL: C. Thomas, 1976.

# IV
# Upper Extremity and Hand

# 31

Jeffrey P. Groner
Paul M. Weeks

# Skin and Soft Tissue Replacement in the Hand

When tissue loss in the hand prevents direct wound closure, adequate coverage usually requires either a skin graft or tissue flaps. Skin grafts can be partial or full thickness. Composite grafts contain the full thickness of skin and other tissues (e.g., nail bed). Flaps can be divided into two categories based on the preservation (pedicle flap) or interruption and surgical reestablishment of the blood supply (free flap). Pedicle flaps can be local (based in the same vicinity as the defect), regional (same extremity), or distant (elsewhere on the body).

## Skin Grafts

Skin grafts consist of the epidermis and varying amounts of dermis. Initially, fibrin adherence bonds the graft to the recipient site. At this stage the graft is nourished by plasmatic imbibition. Later, vascular buds from the recipient site connect to vessels at the undersurface of the graft (inosculation). The firm application of graft to recipient site is enhanced by using a stent. Graft nutrition is impaired by anything that is interposed between the recipient site and the skin graft, such as a hematoma or seroma. Bacteria that produce fibrinolytic enzymes or collagenase can loosen and destroy the graft. Shearing forces interfere with graft adherence [16].

Functional needs determine the use of either a full- or split-thickness graft. Split-thickness grafts (partial thickness) are revascularized more rapidly and have an easier "take" than full-thickness grafts. Full-thickness grafts provide more padding and less ultimate (secondary) wound contraction than split grafts. Thick split grafts combine the characteristics of both and are often used in the hand for this reason.

Skin grafts can be used to cover exposed subcutaneous tissues, periosteum, peritenon, and granulation tissue. Digital vessels and nerves are occasionally grafted as specific situations (such as replantation) dictate, but ordinarily greater padding and less tissue adherence and contraction than is provided by grafting are required. Circumstances may dictate the use of pedicle flaps to provide subcutaneous tissue or other specialized tissues (e.g., bone) in addition to skin. Treatment of hand burns demonstrates the utility of split-thickness grafting.

Full-thickness or deep-partial–thickness burns of the hand can benefit from prompt excision and grafting to reduce edema formation and permit early joint motion (Fig. 31-1). The hand is splinted with the metacarpophalangeal (MP) joints flexed and interphalangeal joints extended. The use of thick split grafts or full-thickness grafts will help

857

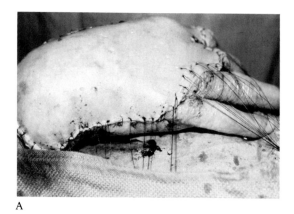

A

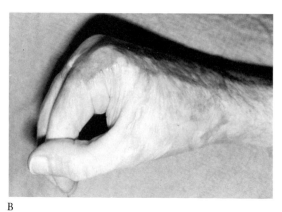

B

*Figure 31-1* *Skin graft coverage. A. Skin graft applied to burn site at dorsum of hand and. B. Final result.*

to minimize joint contracture. With aggressive management excellent hand function can be obtained.

Skin grafts can be taken from almost any area of the body. Split graft donor sites can demonstrate pigmentation changes and develop hypertrophic scarring. The lateral aspect of the thigh is a common donor site because large grafts can be obtained from a relatively concealed location. The lateral aspect of the buttock is more difficult to harvest but has the advantage of being hidden within the bikini area. Use of the ipsilateral forearm or arm for split grafts at best leaves a hypopigmented, obvious scar [128, 130]. Small split- or full-thickness grafts can be obtained from the hypothenar area [92]. Palmar areas in black individuals can be color-matched with plantar skin grafts [85].

Full thickness donor sites are usually closed leaving a linear scar. The graft is harvested in a fusiform shape along the lines of skin tension in areas with lax tissue. The donor site is often determined by the graft size requirement. Small grafts can be obtained from the ulnar side of the hypothenar eminence, the volar surface of the wrist, or the antecubital fossa. Larger grafts are obtained from the inner aspect of the arm or from the groin flexion crease. Patients frequently ob-

ject to use of the wrist crease, as the scar may imply a suicide attempt.

The ulnar side of the hypothenar eminence provides glabrous skin from a site that is readily available and can be closed primarily, resulting in an inconspicuous scar (Fig. 31-2). Excellent sensory function can be regained in these grafts [16, 85, 86].

## Pedicle Flaps

The blood supply to pedicle flaps is through an intact base, stalk, or pedicle. Pedicle flaps are either local, regional, or distant. Local flaps are obtained within the area of the defect and mobilized to fill the defect. Regional flaps are further removed from the defect but raised on the same extremity. Distant flaps are based elsewhere on the body. Donor sites are either closed primarily or skin grafted. Most regional and all distant pedicle flap coverage requires at least two stages. In the first stage the flap is inset at the recipient site. After the flap has established sufficient vascular connections with the recipient site, the second stage, pedicle transection and inset completion, is performed.

The more complete the inset at the primary stage, the more extensive the vascular ingrowth into the flap. The vascular supply of either a local or distant pedicle flap can be enhanced by the staged division of a portion of its vascular supply (delay maneuver), thereby encouraging a more efficient circulation. This permits use of a greater length-to-width ratio than would otherwise be possible.

Pedicle flaps can incorporate a variety of tissues, ranging from skin and subcutaneous fat to essentially a complete finger [15, 112]. The pedicle can be located in muscle, fascia, or skin or may be an arteriovenous stalk. Noncutaneous fascial and muscle flaps are skin grafted [84]. Pedicle flaps must be used to provide coverage in areas where tendon (denuded of epitenon), bone (denuded of periosteum), or joints are exposed. Areas that must support tendon grafting or transfers are best covered with a pedicle flap. Periosteal surfaces can be skin grafted, but flap coverage provides a more durable surface that is less prone to traumatic breakdown. Pedicle flaps can be used to provide sensation or specialized tissues.

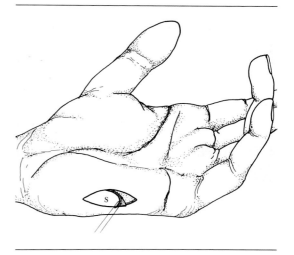

**Figure 31-2** *Hypothenar skin graft donor site. Position with skin graft (s) partially elevated.*

## CLASSIFICATION OF FLAPS ACCORDING TO BLOOD SUPPLY

Pedicle flaps can be classified by their blood supply as either random or axial pattern flaps. Random pattern flaps derive their blood supply from small unnamed vessels that are usually found in the dermal-subdermal plexus. The potential length varies with the robustness of the blood supply in the flap area.

Axial pattern flaps are nourished by a distinct artery that courses through the flap. This allows the design of a longer flap than would be possible with a random pattern flap based in the same area. The general outline of the flap is determined by the course of the direct artery included in the flap and its tributaries. Because the vascular supply is a discrete entity, a thin, flexible pedicle can be developed. Axial flaps have greater utility than random flaps.

Axial flaps have been further classified as either peninsular or island. Peninsular flaps maintain tissue continuity across the length of the flap to the donor area. Island flaps consist of an island of skin, muscle, fascia, or subcutaneous tissue maintained on a debulked or skeletonized pedicle [71].

## FLAP DYNAMICS

The transfer of a random regional or distant pedicle flap requires the maintenance of a donor site vascular supply until an adequate blood supply is established from the recipient site. Until that occurs, poor flap design, tension, edema, or inflammation can impair arterial inflow or venous return [108].

Proper flap design incorporates enough vessels within the pedicle to ensure adequate circulation. The permissible flap length is determined by the vascularity of the donor area. Flaps are often designed of greater dimension than initially estimated to avoid tension, since undue tension will initially impair venous return. Tension associated with a single suture can produce a white line across a flap, resulting in distal necrosis. Thick flaps are less pliable and compensations for their inelasticity must be made.

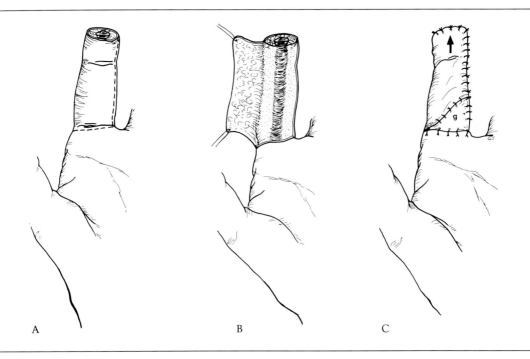

A                    B                    C

**Figure 31-3** *Hueston flap coverage of digital tip injury. A. Plan. B. Elevation, and C. Inset with full thickness graft (g) at donor site.*

Acute angulation or twisting can lead to venous congestion and edema. Edema magnifies the effects of tension and kinking, and when associated with inflammation, can further compromise circulation.

Pallor reflects inadequate arterial supply, while cyanosis indicates venous congestion. Mottling, cyanosis, and edema herald impending necrosis, and violet discoloration signals established tissue necrosis. Hematoma or seroma between the flap and recipient bed will impair healing and predispose to infection and flap necrosis. Hematoma formation can also reduce vascular flow through direct pressure effects [82].

CLASSIFICATION OF FLAPS
ACCORDING TO FUNCTION
Flaps may or may not contain a significant (constant, named) nerve branch in the pedicle. If not, innervation of the flap must be accomplished by ingrowth of neural elements from the recipient site.

INNERVATED PEDICLE FLAPS
Innervated flaps are used primarily to provide coverage of the working (opposable) surfaces of the hand. This includes the ulnovolar surface of the thumb pad and the radiovolar surfaces of the finger pads. These flaps can be developed from either local or regional tissues.

*Innervated Local Flaps*
HUESTON FLAPS. This axial flap incorporates an intact neurovascular bundle and provides excellent coverage of the fingertips with volar digital skin [46]. The flap is outlined proximally from the site of injury along the mid-lateral line of the digit until it reaches the second flexion line along its course (Fig. 31-3). The incision crosses the volar surface of the digit at this point. The flap is elevated superficial to the neurovascular bundle on

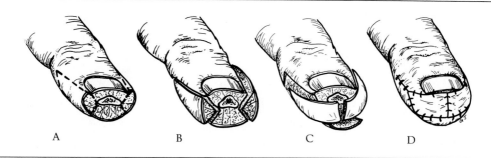

**Figure 31-4** *Kutler lateral advancement flap.*
*A. Injury and plan. B. Elevation.*
*C. Advancement. D. Inset.*

the same side as the mid-lateral incision; dissection is deep to the neurovascular bundle on the opposite side. With transposition, a significant kink ("dog-ear") occurs, which may require revision later. The donor area is covered with a full-thickness graft.

KUTLER LATERAL ADVANCEMENT FLAP. Two inverted triangular flaps are outlined, one on each side of the involved fingertip [30, 40, 60] (Fig. 31-4). The width of the flap is determined by the anteroposterior dimension of the wound. The apex of the triangle may extend proximal to the distal interphalangeal (DIP) joint flexion crease [7]. Osteocutaneous septa are divided, mobilizing the flaps from the bony phalanx while maintaining a subcutaneous pedicle that contains multiple, discrete neurovascular elements [105]. Adequate mobilization is required to avoid tension on closure; the bony phalanx is often rounded to help achieve this goal. The flaps are approximated over the fingertip and are sutured to the hyponychium or distal portion of the nail bed. The donor areas are closed directly in a V to Y pattern. If undue tension or blanching is encountered, the flap is mobilized further. Within 3 to 6 weeks, the finger pad will tolerate daily use. This flap best covers injuries with the same dorsal and volar levels (straight transection).

ATASOY-KLEINERT VOLAR ADVANCEMENT FLAP. A single triangular flap is mobilized from

the volar tissues of the fingertip in a similar manner as with the Kutler flap [3, 34] (Fig. 31-5). The base of the flap is the edge of the tissue defect and should be 2 to 3 mm wider than the distal edge of the nail matrix. The apex of the triangular flap may extend to the flexion crease of the DIP joint. The flap pedicle originates from the bony phalanx and digital sheath. The subcutaneous pedicle is freed from underlying osteocutaneous septa, which attach it to the skin surrounding the triangle. After division of the attachments at the apex of the triangle, the flap can be advanced more than a centimeter. The bony phalanx is contoured, and the nail bed is trimmed for direct suture of the flap to the hyponychium or nail bed. This flap best covers defects with a greater amount of volar tissue (oblique transection).

MOBERG VOLAR ADVANCEMENT FLAPS. The volar tissues along an entire digit or thumb are mobilized [1, 21, 53, 69, 95] (Fig. 31-6). Bilateral incisions are made in the mid-lateral lines. The neurovascular bundles are included in the volar flap. The flap is freed from the tendon sheath and advanced to cover the tip defect. The flap provides sensate coverage but the extensive mobilization required can devascularize dorsal skin. The incision of Burrow's triangles along the base of the flap may allow additional flap advancement.

LOCAL INNERVATED TRANSPOSITION FLAPS. A proximally based flap utilizing the digital neurovascular bundle as a pedicle can be

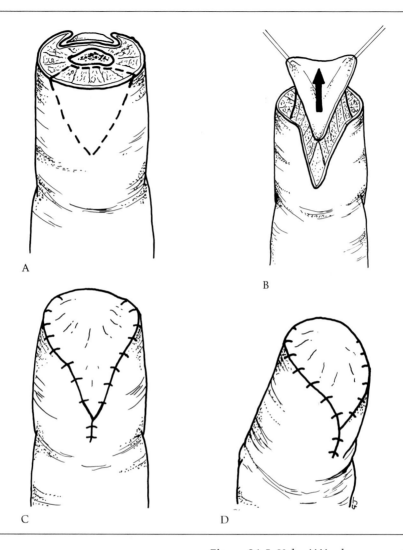

A

B

C

D

**Figure 31-5** *Volar V-Y advancement flap (Atasoy-Kleinert) coverage of distal digital injury. A. Plan. B. Advancement. C. Inset. D. Inset, oblique view.*

used to transfer dorsal skin to provide innervated coverage of a volar defect. Since the tissues distal to the flap tip will be denervated, this flap is most useful for coverage of amputation-type injuries with extensive volar soft-tissue loss or in the reconstruction of severely damaged distal tissues. A digital Allen's test is performed to determine the adequacy of blood supply to the digit. A template is made of the defect and transposed to the dorsal surface of the digit. The neurovascular bundle is isolated and the flap elevated, taking care to protect the dorsal

branches supplying the flap. The donor site is skin grafted.

A local neurovascular island flap has been described for soft-tissue coverage of the thumb pad [94]. Dorsoradial branches of the radial digital neurovascular bundle of the thumb are elevated along with overlying undamaged skin and transposed volarly to provide innervated coverage of small volar defects. The donor site is skin grafted.

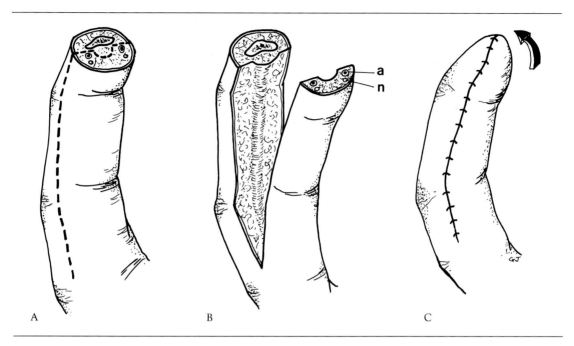

**Figure 31-6** *Moberg volar advancement flap.*
*A. Plan. B. Elevation. (a = digital artery;*
*n = nerve.) C. Advancement and inset.*

*Innervated Regional Flaps*
Littler perfected the island axial flap, which
incorporates a digital nerve into its pedicle.
Many modifications of the basic model have
been presented, including islands in continuity from two adjacent fingers and an island flap innervated by a dorsal sensory
branch of the radial nerve. One must carefully determine the adequacy of the blood
supply to each digit affected when a common digital artery is used as a pedicle.

LITTLER ISLAND TRANSFER ON A NEUROVAS-
CULAR BUNDLE. A pattern of the recipient
site is prepared and transferred to the ulnar
side of the ring or long finger [67] (Fig. 31-7).
The flap outline is modified to create a donor defect that will conform to favorable
flexion lines. The neurovascular bundle is
identified at the distal end of the island flap,
where it is divided and ligated. The flap is
elevated from the fibroosseous sheath and
the loose connective tissues over the extensor apparatus. The ulnar neurovascular bun-

dle is dissected proximally through a zigzag
skin incision to the superficial arch. At the
bifurcation of the common digital artery, the
digital artery to the adjacent finger is divided. The proper digital nerve contribution
to the common digital nerve is dissected
proximally to improve flap mobilization.
The flap and its pedicle are passed to the recipient site through a generous subcutaneous tunnel. Angulation and constriction
of the pedicle must be avoided. The pedicle
is inset and the donor area is covered with a
skin graft. The metacarpal artery can be used
as a vascular pedicle if the common digital
artery is absent [102].

Reports have been conflicting regarding
the usefulness of sensation that these flaps
provide. Criticisms center on the failure of
reorientation of sensation from the donor to
the recipient site and poor two-point discrimination [20, 59, 75, 83]. Reorientation of
sensation does occasionally occur, and some
authors report consistent attainment of two-
point discrimination less than 10 mm [41,
70]. Results are likely related, at least in
part, to technical factors [70, 91]. The flaps

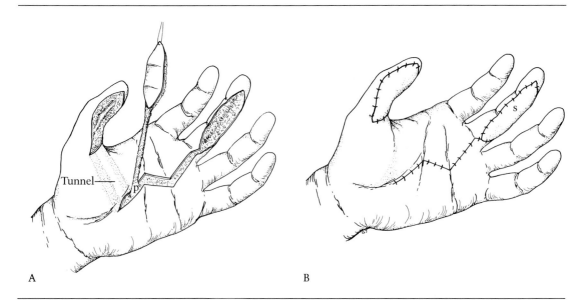

A                                    B

*Figure 31-7* Littler island transfer on a neurovascular pedicle. A. Elevation on neurovascular pedicle (p). Note tunneled area for passage of flap. B. Inset, donor site closure with full thickness skin graft (s).

are most often used to reconstruct a badly damaged thumb pad that is scarred, insensate, or ischemic. All three conditions are addressed by neurovascular island flaps [14, 113].

OMER MODIFICATION. Using the principles already described, a neurovascular pedicle flap can be developed in continuity from the radial and ulnar side of adjacent fingers to reconstruct a sensate first web space after median nerve injury [90, 91]. The cutaneous island is outlined along the ulnar aspect of the ring finger and the radial aspect of the little finger to include the skin of the web space. The vascular pedicle is the common digital artery. The donor site is grafted with the excised recipient site tissues.

HOLEVICH FLAP. Development of an island axial flap from the dorsum of the index finger that includes a branch of the superficial radial nerve can be used to reconstruct the thumb pulp [44]. As originally described this flap included only nerve, vessel, and subcutaneous tissue. Various modifications transfer a skin flap along with neurovascular tissues [9, 35, 61, 79, 96, 106, 115, 123]. Holevich also detailed a racquet-shaped skin flap based on the first dorsal metacarpal ar-

tery and associated veins (Fig. 31-8). The flap is transferred to the thumb through a dorsal incision on the thumb metacarpal extending to the volar defect.

NONINNERVATED PEDICLE FLAPS
Noninnervated flaps are used to cover defects of the forearm, hand, and fingers. These flaps are mobilized as local (from the dorsal or lateral surface of the involved digit), regional (adjacent finger, palm, thenar eminence), or distant flaps (chest, abdomen, or opposite arm) [23, 25, 45, 62, 73].

*Noninnervated Local Flaps*
LOCAL TRANSPOSITION FLAPS. Random flaps from the dorsal surface of the involved finger can be used to provide coverage of exposed denuded dorsal tendons, exposed joints, or volar defects [38, 50, 89]. Dorsal hand flaps can also be used in conjunction with Z-plasties or similar strategies to release scar contractures [25, 63, 99]. Careful planning is required to

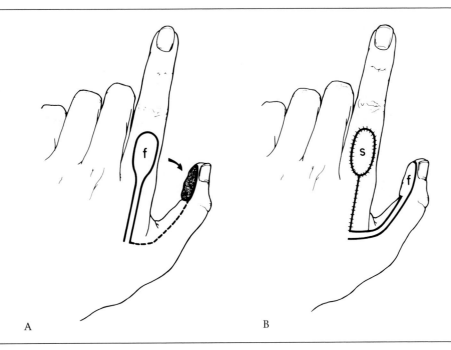

*Figure 31-8* Holevich flap. A. Plan with
proximally-based racquet-shaped skin flap (f).
B. Flap inset showing flap (f) and skin graft (s);
neurovascular elements (not shown) are
transferred along the axis of the flap.

ensure complete coverage of the recipient site. The pedicle can be based proximally, laterally, or distally. Digital flaps are elevated in the loose areolar tissue plane overlying the extensor apparatus. The peritenon should not be disturbed. A skin graft is used to cover the donor area. Use of volar skin to cover dorsal defects is rarely indicated.

LOCAL ISLAND AXIAL FLAP. When a local random flap is inadequate, a local axial island flap, based either proximally or distally as described by Weeks and Wray [125], can be used (Fig. 31-9). Adequacy of vascular flow to each side of the digit is confirmed. A pattern of the tissue defect is transposed to the side of a proximal phalanx. The radial side of the index and ulnar side of the little finger are avoided. The cutaneous island, centered over a digital artery, is elevated and the digital artery and nerve are identified. If

the flap is to be based distally, the artery is divided and ligated proximally; a proximally based flap will entail a distal pedicle division. Tissue along the artery is included in the pedicle to supply venous drainage. The flap is rotated and inset, and the donor site is skin grafted. If skin closure will compromise blood flow, the pedicle can be grafted or left exposed in the skin incision. This flap is particularly useful in the coverage of defects over the distal (DIP) or proximal interphalangeal (PIP) joints and the web space.

FLAG FLAPS. The flag flap described by Iselin [48] and by Vilain and Dupuis [122] has a long, narrow, proximally based dorsal pedicle supporting a broad distal flap component that includes the dorsal skin of the proximal or middle phalanx. The length of the pedicle allows transposition of the flap to the volar surface of the same digit, the dorsal surface of an adjacent digit, or the adjacent web space or palm.

Iselin [48] described homodigital (same finger) and heterodigital flag flaps. The homo-

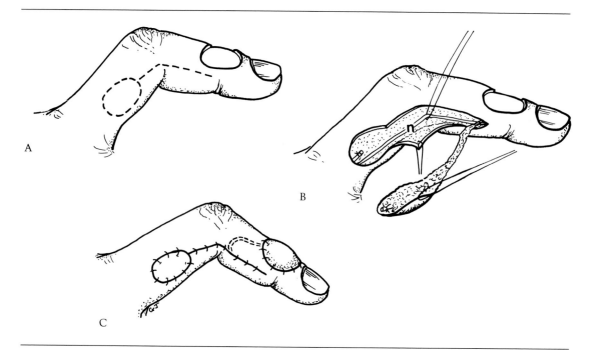

*Figure 31-9* *Distally-based local island axial (Weeks) flap. A. Plan. B. Elevation. Note preservation of digital nerve (n). C. Inset at distal dorsal defect.*

digital flap can cover volar defects, amputation stumps, and dorsal digital defects. The heterodigital flag flap can be used to cover the dorsum of an adjacent finger, to provide sensate skin for a thumb amputation stump (including radial nerve branches as in a "staged" Holevich flap), or to provide nonsensate coverage of a thumb amputation stump [123]. Flag flaps can be used in one or two stages.

The flap cannot be longer than the dorsal surface of the proximal or middle phalanx, and the width of the pedicle, which can be on either side of the phalanx, should be one-third to one-half the width of the dorsal surface of the phalanx. If the "flag" portion of the flap is over the dorsum of the proximal phalanx the pedicle is designed on the dorsum of the hand. The flap is elevated, preserving the peritenon. The blood supply is through the dermal-subdermal plexus, and as many longitudinal veins and cutaneous nerves as possible are included in the pedicle. The pedicle is divided in 15 to 21 days.

AXIAL FLAG FLAP. Lister [65] has described an axial flag flap that gains its blood supply

from either the dorsal metacarpal artery or a dorsal branch of the proper digital artery (Fig. 31-10). The artery is most reliably present in the second interspace and the index or long finger is most commonly used. The dorsal proximal phalangeal skin is mobilized on a narrow pedicle, which provides great utility for coverage of proximal, volar, or adjacent finger soft-tissue defects.

*Noninnervated Regional Flaps*
The surface of the palm or dorsal skin of an adjacent finger can provide a good tissue match. These flaps can be based laterally, distally, or proximally as need dictates [39, 45].

LATERALLY BASED CROSS-FINGER FLAP. This is the most commonly used form of the cross-finger flap and provides tissue for volar coverage [17, 28, 36, 51] (Fig. 31-11). A template of the defect is prepared and transposed to the dorsum of the adjacent finger. After a

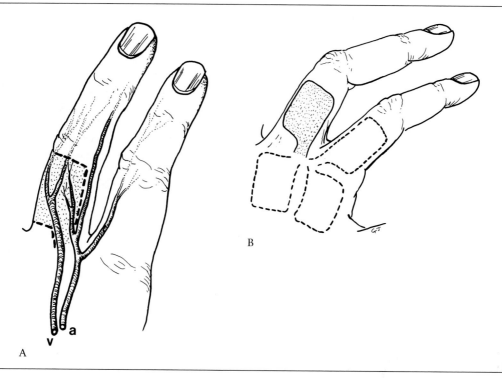

**Figure 31-10** *Axial flag flap (as described by G. Lister). A. Outline of flap: (a = artery; v = drainage by digital venous system.) B. Dorsal transposition options (flap may also be transposed volarly). (Adapted from G. D. Lister. Local flaps to the hand.* Hand Clin. *1:621,1985.)*

mid-lateral incision and two transverse incisions are made on the donor finger, the flap is reflected, much like turning the page of a book. The peritenon is left undisturbed over the extensor apparatus. The base of the flap is at the mid-lateral line opposite the injured digit. Incising Cleland's ligaments at the base of the pedicle significantly increases flap mobility. The fingers are positioned with the MP joints in maximal flexion, allowing the PIP joints to be slightly less flexed [56]. A full-thickness skin graft provides donor site coverage. The flap is detached at about 14 to 16 days after operation. Several series have demonstrated a return of useful sensation (as measured by two-point discrimination) when laterally based cross-

finger flaps are used for fingertip reconstruction [49, 57, 87, 107, 117].

REVERSED CROSS-FINGER FLAP. Dorsal defects of an adjacent finger can be covered with a laterally based flap of subcutaneous tissue [2]. A pattern is drawn on the donor digit. The skin is raised as a full-thickness graft hinged on the side away from the defect. The subcutaneous tissues are raised as a flap based on the mid-lateral axis adjacent to the injured digit. Care is taken not to disturb the paratenon while the flap is raised. The flap is inset and grafted and the donor site skin is returned to its original position as a full-thickness graft. The fingers can be sutured to each other to maintain positioning. Postoperative management is the same as for other cross-finger flaps.

PROXIMALLY OR DISTALLY BASED CROSS-FINGER FLAP. A pattern of the defect is transferred to the dorsum of an adjacent finger or occasionally to a distant finger (Fig. 31-12). The fingers are manipulated to determine

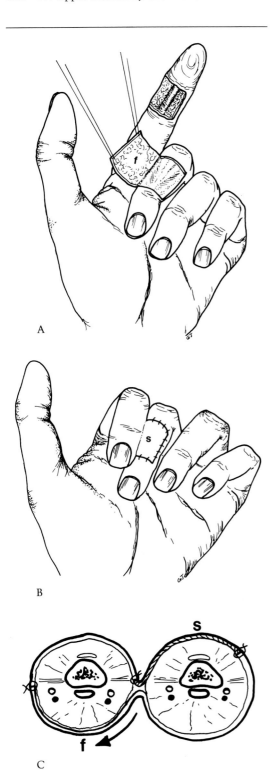

A

B

C

the most satisfactory position for joint immobilization. The flap is based to minimize tension; Kirschner's wires are occasionally used to maintain positioning. After 14 to 16 days, the flap is divided.

THENAR FLAPS. Coverage of the distal phalanx of the index or long finger can be provided by a flap from the thenar area (Fig. 31-13). A pattern of the tissue defect is outlined over the lateral aspect of the thenar eminence immediately proximal to the MP joint. The flap can be based either proximally or distally or a laterally based flap overlying the MP joint crease can be designed [5, 22, 78]. Though some authors claim that the PIP joint need be only slightly flexed, it is impossible to bring the finger tip to the palm without significant flexion at the PIP joint. A thick flap is raised in the subcutaneous tissue plane; near the MP crease the digital nerves are superficial and must be carefully avoided. The donor area is closed primarily or with a skin graft. The flap is inset and the finger immobilized with plaster, soft dressings, or a strip of tape extending from the dorsum of the hand around the dorsum of the finger to the volar surface of the thenar eminence and palm. The pedicle is transected at 14 days [77]. Mobilization of the joints is begun immediately.

The main disadvantages of this flap are the palmar donor site and flexed PIP joint position. The scar may be aesthetically unpleasing or tender. Designing the flap laterally (high) on the thenar eminence removes the donor site from the grip-pressure area of the palm. A PIP joint flexion contracture can occur, especially in older individu-

*Figure 31-11 Laterally-based cross-finger flap coverage of volar defect. A. Elevation with dorsal flap (f) raised on long finger. B. Inset with skin graft (s). C. Schematic cross section with dorsal flap (f) from donor digit, skin graft (s) at donor site. Note that actual plane of flap dissection will be deeper (at level of extensor paratenon).*

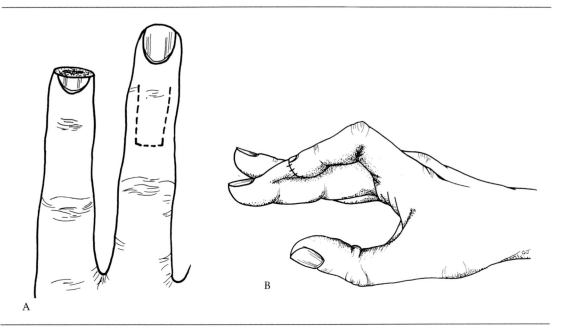

A

B

*Figure 31-12* Distally-based cross-finger flap coverage of index tip injury. A. Plan. B. Inset with index finger alongside long finger.

als. Some practitioners limit use of this flap to patients less than 30 to 35 years old.

PALMAR FLAPS. The palmar flap can provide coverage for small defects at the terminal phalanx of the thumb. The flap is based on the radial side of the palm between the first (MP) digital crease of the index finger and the proximal transverse palmar crease. The donor site is closed with a skin graft. The thumb is adducted for attachment of the flap into the recipient site without tension. After approximately 14 days the flap is divided. Disadvantages of this flap include the small amount of tissue available, the adducted positioning of the thumb, and the positioning of the donor site scar on a working surface.

FOREARM AXIAL FLAPS. The forearm can serve as a source of peninsular or island axial flaps for coverage of the hand. These reliable flaps are based on either the radial or ulnar arteries. The patency of both vessels must be determined preoperatively. Advantages include the use of a flap in the same opera-

tive field; skin of a similar texture, thickness, and color; predictable vascularity; and a straightforward dissection. Disadvantages are the sacrifice of a major artery and an aesthetically displeasing donor site scar. A forearm flap based on the posterior interosseous artery has also been described [6, 129].

The *radial forearm* flap is a fasciocuta-

*Figure 31-13* Distally-based thenar flap. Note position on thenar eminence, away from grip surface.

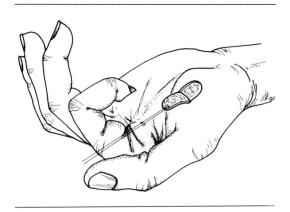

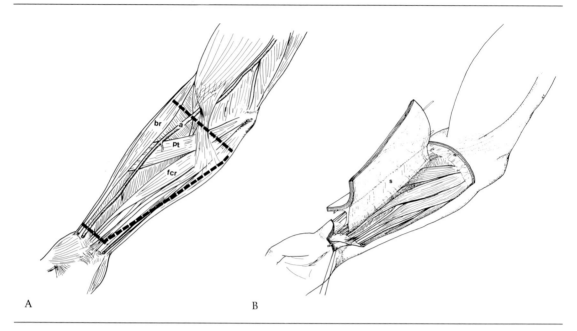

A                               B

*Figure 31-14* Radial forearm flap. A. Passage of radial artery beneath partial skin territory. (a = radial artery; br = brachioradialis muscle; pt = pronator teres muscle; fcr = flexor carpi radialis muscle.) B. Elevation of flap. Note radial artery and venae comitantes at base of fascial septa (s).

neous flap based on the radial artery and its venae comitantes, located in the lateral intermuscular septum [10, 32, 42, 81, 110, 111, 118] (Fig. 31-14). This septum lies between the flexor and extensor compartments of the forearm and is attached to the radius distal to the pronator teres insertion. The artery supplies most of the skin of the forearm, except the ulnar border, through several branches that pass through the deep fascia of the forearm forming a fascial plexus.

Usually, the flap is raised as a distally based island axial flap (Fig. 31-15). The course of the radial artery is marked on the forearm. The length of the vascular pedicle required is determined and the soft-tissue defect pattern is outlined on the volar surface of the proximal forearm. The radial artery is exposed, the skin flap raised, and the vascular pedicle mobilized. A cuff of soft tissue is maintained about the pedicle, which is important for maintenance of retrograde flow. The flap is inset and the donor site is closed either primarily or with a split graft

(Fig. 31-16). The flap can be distally based, as retrograde flow in the arterial and venous systems is usually excellent. Additional venous outflow must occasionally be supplied by microvascular anastomosis to recipient site veins [37].

The cephalic or saphenous veins can be used to reconstruct the radial artery. Approximately 60 percent of reconstructed radial or ulnar arteries remain patent [8]. This flap can be innervated by suturing a recipient site nerve to the lateral antebrachial cutaneous nerve, which can be incorporated into the flap.

A 10-cm bone segment up to 50 percent of the diameter of the radius can be elevated with the flap. The bone obtains its blood

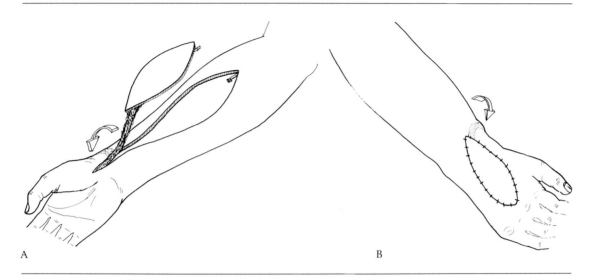

A

B

**Figure 31-15** *Reversed radial forearm flap coverage of dorsal hand defect. A. Elevation. B. Inset.*

**Figure 31-16** *Radial forearm flap coverage of exposed wrist prosthesis. A. Defect. B. Plan. C. Elevation (arrow at radial artery). D. Flap inset. (Courtesy L. Young, M.D.)*

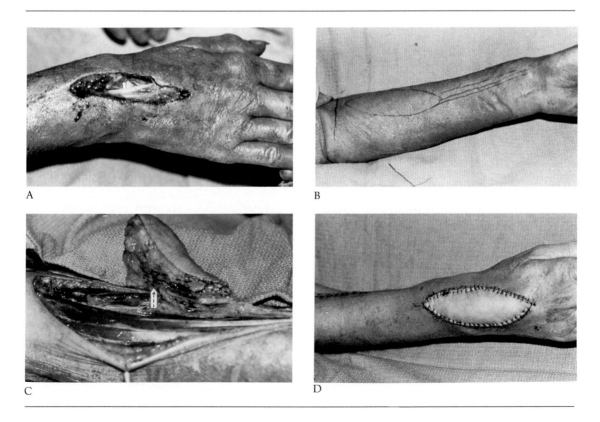

A

B

C

D

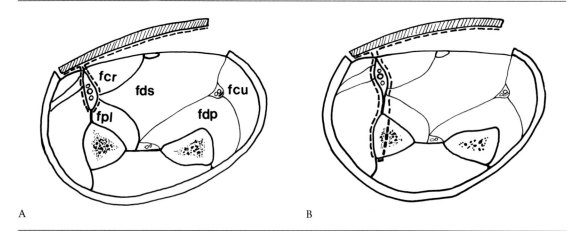

A                                        B

supply through the intermuscular septum distal to the insertion of the pronator teres [124] (Fig. 31-17). A cast is used to protect the radius for at least 3 weeks after operation.

A *fascial* flap incorporating the intermuscular septum and deep fascia of the forearm can be raised as an axial flap [98]. The fascia is covered with a skin graft. The advantages of using only fascia are its thinness and that its use avoids a skin graft on the forearm.

The *ulnar forearm* flap can be raised using the fasciocutaneous attachments of the ulnar artery to the deep fascia of the skin [26] (Fig. 31-18). In the proximal half of the forearm, the ulnar artery gives rise to approximately three vascular pedicles, which supply the deep fascia and forearm skin. These vessels pass between the flexor carpi ulnaris and flexor digitorum superficialis muscles and have a fairly reliable pattern. The most proximal pedicle is found 3 to 4 cm distal to the takeoff of the common interosseous artery, and the entire flap can be based on this pedicle. Venous drainage is provided by the venae comitantes of the ulnar artery or through the basilic vein. The pedicles supply the flexor carpi ulnaris and palmaris longus muscles, portions of which can be raised with the flap if bulk is needed. A segment of the ulna can be elevated with the flap; cast

*Figure 31-17* Radial forearm flap: cross-section of mid-third of forearm.
A. *Septofasciocutaneous flap. (fcr = flexor carpi radialis muscle; fds = flexor digitorum superficialis m.; fpl = flexor pollicis longus m.; fdp = flexor digitorum profundus m.; fcu = flexor carpi ulnaris m.)*
B. *Osteoseptofasciocutaneous flap.*

*Figure 31-18* Ulnar forearm flap: cross-section of mid-third of forearm. (fcr = flexor carpi radialis m.; fds = flexor digitorum superficialis m.; fdp = flexor digitorum profundus m.; fcu = flexor carpi ulnaris m.; ecu = extensor carpi ulnaris m.)

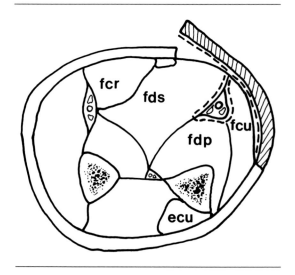

protection of the ulna is used [68]. Sensation to the flap can be gained by suturing the medial cutaneous nerve of the forearm to a recipient site nerve. The majority of the anterior surface and ulnar border of the forearm can be incorporated into this flap.

The flap is raised in the same fashion as the radial forearm flap. The course of the ulnar artery is marked, a template is made of the soft-tissue defect, and the length of the pedicle and size of the flap are planned. The flap is most frequently distally based, and retrograde flow of the arterial and venous systems is a sufficient vascular supply. If the donor site cannot be closed primarily, it is skin grafted. The ulnar artery is frequently the major vascular supply to the hand and a careful preoperative evaluation is essential. Vein graft reconstruction can be attempted.

DISTANT PEDICLE FLAPS

Distant flaps are not based on the involved extremity. They can be innervated only if a sensory nerve included in the flap is sutured to a nerve in the recipient site. Distant flaps are commonly based in the chest, abdomen, and groin areas [54]. Careful examination for previous surgical incisions is essential.

*Chest Flaps*

Anterior chest wall flaps can be taken from the contralateral or ipsilateral anterolateral chest wall or the infraclavicular region. The advantages of flaps from this area as compared to flaps from the lower abdomen include: thinner, more pliable skin and less subcutaneous fat; less dense hair growth; and the less dependent position of the hand. The main disadvantage is the poor donor site scar.

CONTRALATERAL ANTEROLATERAL CHEST-WALL FLAPS. The blood supply is derived from the intercostal vessels or the thoracoepigastric system [126] (Fig. 31-19). The vessels are oriented in a transverse to oblique direction toward the midline. Circulation across the midline is marginal and may not support an extension of a flap to the opposite side of the chest. Small donor areas can be closed directly; larger donor areas will require split grafts for closure. Skin grafts should be sutured to the underlying bed to minimize movement.

*Figure 31-19* Chest wall flap. A. Plan. B. Inset, with hand partially obscuring skin grafted donor site (crosshatched area).

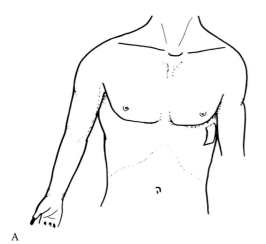

A

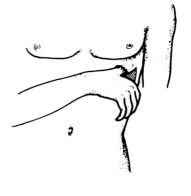

B

A transverse flap can be rotated 90 degrees cephalad or caudad. Rotation is facilitated by extending either the upper or lower limb of the incision for a distance equal to the width of the flap. Extension of the upper and lower limbs permits cephalad and caudad rotation, respectively.

Flaps raised above the umbilicus allow the forearm to rest comfortably across the lower chest with the elbow flexed. The patient can bend, stoop, walk or sit with ease. Care must be taken in positioning the arm to avoid tension or kinking of the flap. If the arm is placed too close to the flap area, the flap may be kinked on its base. If arm placement is not far enough across the chest, the flap may be under tension. To maintain proper positioning, the relative placement of the flexed elbow to the trunk is noted and maintained while a well-padded dressing is applied. The pedicle is transected at 14 to 21 days, depending on the degree of flap–recipient site inset, the healing of the flap edges to the recipient site, and the configuration and size of the flap.

IPSILATERAL CHEST-WALL FLAPS. Reliable immobilization of the arm after placement of an ipsilateral chest flap is difficult to achieve [126]. Consequently, these flaps are used more often for coverage of areas that lie against the ipsilateral side of the chest when the arm is rested on the chest or upper abdomen, for example, elbow, forearm, and wrist. These flaps can be based inferiorly, superiorly, or laterally. The donor site usually requires closure with a split graft.

INFRACLAVICULAR FLAPS. Available tissue is small and coverage is usually limited to digital defects. Tubed flaps developed immediately inferior to the clavicle are good for digital coverage, providing thin, well-vascularized skin. The donor site scars are severe and their location is even worse. This flap is used infrequently and rarely in women.

### Abdominal Flaps

Tissue coverage can be obtained from the abdomen above (epigastric) or below (abdominal) the umbilicus.

EPIGASTRIC FLAPS. These flaps are particularly useful when coverage of a large defect is required in the distal forearm or hand, or both. The flap base straddles the midline and obtains its blood supply from both sides [126] (Fig. 31-20). The dimensions available for development of the flap are determined by the curvature of the trunk and by the distance from the xiphoid to the umbilicus. The forearm is placed in a comfortable position across the lower chest and the flap is designed as needed. The donor area is covered by a split graft. Division and inset are similar to that of abdominal flaps.

ABDOMINAL-WALL SKIN FLAPS. Abdominal flaps are located below the umbilicus [126]. This skin is the least desirable for coverage of the digits or hand for the following reasons: (1) texture and color match to the recipient area is poor, (2) there is usually abundant subcutaneous fat, (3) it is hair-bearing skin, (4) weight gain will be reflected in the subcutaneous fat of the flap, (5) the skin is thick and inelastic, (6) flap sensation is poor, (7) the thick subcutaneous layer of the flap may prevent firm adhesion of the flap to bony areas and areas subjected to shear stresses, and (8) the flap dimensions are limited by the ratio of 1.0 : 1.5. The advantages are as follows: (1) donor area scarring is easily covered by clothing, (2) a large durable flap is available, and (3) the need for bulk to fill a depression can be readily met.

These are random pattern vascular flaps and attention must be paid to the length-to-width ratio and the anatomic positioning of the pedicle. Flap length should be restricted to 1.5 times the width. Unless both quadrants of the abdomen are raised as a flap, the flap should not extend across the midline of the abdomen. The width of the distal end of the flap can exceed the width of the base by 20 to 30 percent. A pattern of the tissue defect is prepared and placed over the donor area. Key points are marked on the recipient site and the flap to ensure accurate inset of the flap into the defect. Darts are of particular value when covering the thumb-index

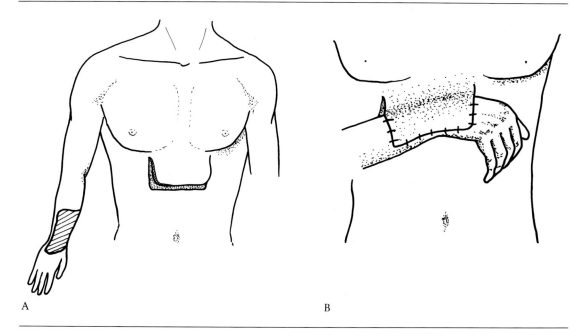

A                                                    B

**Figure 31-20** *Superiorly-based epigastric flap coverage. A. Elevation. B. Inset.*

web and the interdigital web spaces. As the flap is elevated, its subcutaneous tissues are trimmed until the transposed flap restores the normal contour of the recipient area [55].

A free skin graft is used to cover the donor site. Sutures are placed through the skin graft into the underlying bed for immobilization and protection of the graft from shear against the overlying extremity. A stent is not usually used. The flap is inset into as much of the recipient site as possible. When a large defect is being covered, the flap and recipient bed are coapted by occasional mattress sutures tied over a bolus or pledget. After 2 to 3 days of limited activity, the patient is allowed to ambulate. The dressing must be changed frequently to prevent maceration of the tissues. After 10 to 14 days, a light dressing is adequate for support. At 21 days the flap is detached. If there is any question about viability of the flap edges, completion of inset is delayed 3 to 5 days.

VARIATIONS OF THE ABDOMINAL FLAP. *Paired flaps* can be used to cover both the dorsal and volar surface of the hand [80]. An S-shaped incision is designed and drawn on the abdominal wall, creating adequate flaps for coverage of the defect (Fig. 31-21). The flaps are raised and rotated toward each other. The edges are joined with raw surface facing raw surface. A pocket is formed with a flap on each side, providing coverage for the volar and dorsal surface of the hand. This basically provides a mitten type of hand coverage that can subsequently be improved. Multiple soft-tissue defects can be covered by alternating sets of paired flaps [47].

*Louvre flaps* are multiple broad, thin flaps based mainly on subcutaneous pedicles that can be used for the resurfacing of multiple adjacent finger tissue defects [27] (Fig. 31-22). The lower abdomen is used as a donor site, taking advantage of the natural skin laxity. Though the flaps are nourished primarily from their subcutaneous connections, skin bridges are maintained to provide additional blood supply. The flaps can be raised at der-

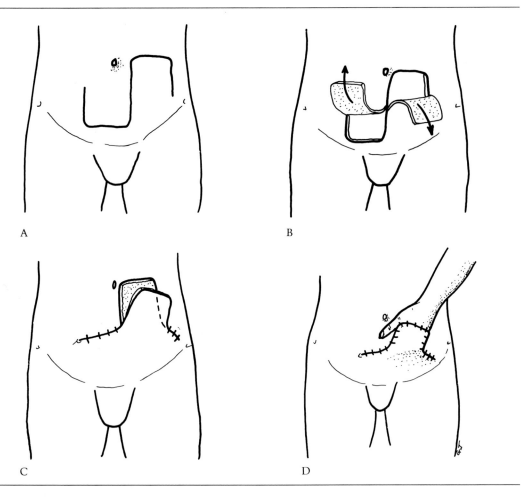

A

B

C

D

*Figure 31-21* *Paired abdominal flap. A. Plan. B. Elevation. C. Rotation. D. Inset.*

mal thickness in their distal half. Donor areas are covered with split grafts. The flaps are divided at 3 weeks.

A strip of abdominal skin can be elevated as a *bipedicled flap* for treatment of tissue loss along the dorsum of the hand or digits [120]. The bipedicled design allows the flap to be narrower than if it were supported by one pedicle. The area of tissue loss is covered by the flap; at 21 days the flap is divided or a delay procedure can be used. If multiple digits have been covered, they are separated at 10 to 14 days after flap division to ensure an adequate single digit vascular supply.

AXIAL PATTERN ABDOMINAL FLAPS. Shaw and Payne [104] described a one-stage, tubed abdominal pedicled flap that was based inferiorly on the superficial inferior epigastric artery and vein [43] (Fig. 31-23). The single pedicled flap varies in length from 5 to 18 cm, and in width from 2 to 7 cm. Superficial veins that are evident in the skin are used as a guide in outlining the flap. When veins are not visible, their approximate location over the femoral triangle is used. The flap is usually elevated just superficial to Scarpa's fascia. The base of the flap is undermined extensively to allow closure after tubing. By staggering the inferior ends of the incisions, the base of the tube can be rotated through

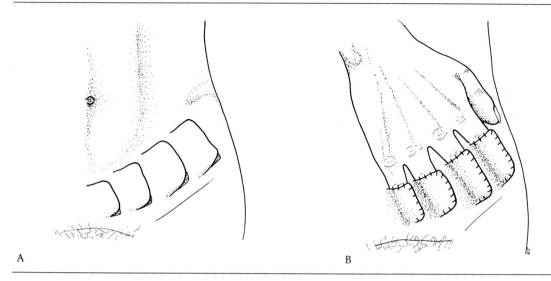

A           B

**Figure 31-22** *Abdominal louvre flap coverage of multiple dorsal digital injuries. A. Elevation. B. Inset.*

**Figure 31-23** *Superficial inferior epigastric artery-based flaps. A. As described by Shaw and Payne. B. Skin island modification for use as free flap. (siea = superficial inferior epigastric artery; scia = superficial circumflex iliac artery.)*

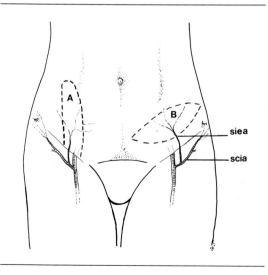

an arc of 180 degrees. If the medial incision is shorter, the tube will rotate laterally; if the lateral incision is shorter, the tube can be rotated medially. When the recipient area is completely covered at the time of pedicle development, the tube can be divided at 3 weeks. If, however, the tube itself is to be used to cover a portion of the defect, a delay procedure is required. A modification of the flap incorporating tissue across the midline can be used [114].

Barfred [4] made the following recommendations: Length should not exceed three times the width of the flap; the flap should be outlined parallel to the linea alba, but overlying the inferior superficial epigastric artery and vein; the distal pedicle is thinned for application to the recipient site and the proximal pedicle includes all tissues down to the level of the fascia; and direct closure of the donor area is usually possible. An advantage of this flap is the option it provides in positioning of the hand.

### Groin Flaps

The groin (or iliofemoral) flap, popularized by McGregor and Jackson [76], is based on the superficial circumflex iliac artery [66, 103]. Since this is an axial pattern flap, its

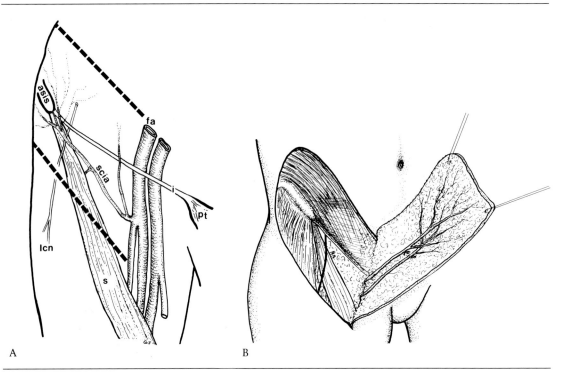

A                                    B

**Figure 31-24** *Groin (iliofemoral) flap.*
*A. passage of superficial circumflex iliac artery*
*(scia) beneath skin territory (dashed lines).*
*(i = inguinal ligament; scia = superficial*
*circumflex iliac artery; fa = femoral artery;*
*asis = anterosuperior iliac spine; pt = pubic*
*tubercle; lcn = lateral cutaneous nerve of the*
*thigh; s = sartorius muscle.) B. Elevation of*
*flap demonstrating plane of dissection.*

length-to-width ratio may far exceed that of
a random pattern flap. This flap is most useful for treatment of large soft-tissue defects
[33]. It can also be used as an osteocutaneous
flap [13, 29, 97].

The superficial circumflex iliac artery (SCIA)
usually arises from the femoral artery 2 to
3 cm below the midpoint of the inguinal ligament and courses laterally and parallel to
the inguinal ligament until it reaches the
medial border of the sartorius muscle [52,
109]. Here it divides into a deep branch and
a superficial branch, which passes upward,
entering into the soft tissues included in the
groin flap. It continues laterally parallel to
the inguinal ligament, dividing into an upper and lower branch just beyond the anterosuperior iliac spine. Lateral to this point on
the pelvis, it usually is no longer identifiable
as a discrete vessel.

The venous pattern in the groin is more
variable than the arterial pattern. These tributaries join the saphenous vein near its ori-

gin. This is very close to the origin of the
SCIA and thus any flap incorporating the artery will likely include the corresponding
venous system [93].

The flap is outlined as follows to ensure
inclusion of the SCIA and veins (Fig. 31-24).
A line is drawn from the anterosuperior iliac
spine to the pubic tubicle marking the
course of the inguinal ligament. The femoral
artery is palpated 2.5 cm below the ligament; this is the point of origin of the SCIA.
A line drawn laterally from this point and
parallel with the inguinal ligament will
mark the course of the superficial circum-

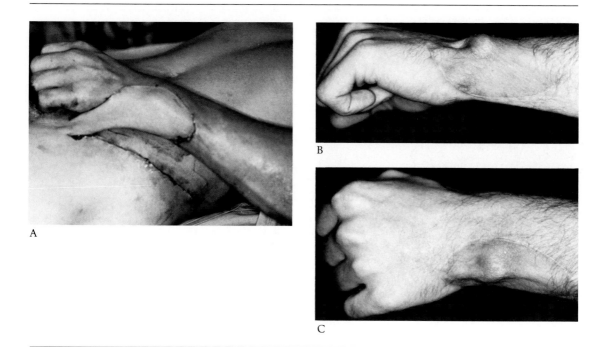

**Figure 31-25** *Groin flap coverage of ulnar wrist defect. A. Flap attached to defect. B,C. Final result. (Courtesy L. Young, M.D.)*

flex iliac artery. The flap is designed with the vessel running laterally along the mesial axis. In general, a flap that is 10 cm wide is recommended to allow tubing of the flap and to provide coverage. The length of the flap can be extended beyond the anterosuperior iliac spine by a distance equal to the breadth of the flap.

Dissection is begun laterally. The axial vessels are divided and dissection continued in the plane deep to these vessels. As dissection proceeds medially, the fascia over the lateral border of the sartorius is incised and reflected with the flap. The flap is elevated to the medial border of the sartorius. When coverage of small to moderate defects is required, the donor site can be closed in a transverse straight-line scar within the bikini area (Fig. 31-25). Larger donor areas are closed with split grafts.

McGregor and Jackson [76] noted from their experience with 50 cases that the responses of the groin flap to elevation are different from those of random pattern flaps. The differences included extreme pallor, absence of transient edema, and a prolonged time period required for necrosis to develop. The most common complication is partial flap necrosis due to ischemia, with an incidence in two series of approximately 20 percent [103, 127]. Postoperative management is similar to that for other pedicle flaps. If the defect has been entirely covered by the flap, the pedicle is divided at 3 weeks. Occasionally, it is not inset for an additional 5 to 7 days to prevent necrosis of the peripheral margin of the flap. If the defect has not been completely covered, the flap is delayed by division of the axial artery at 2 to 3 weeks, followed by complete division of the pedicle in 1 week. Intravenous fluorescein or laser Doppler can be used to determine revascularization of the flap [74].

## Free Flaps

Use of free flaps has become routine for covering defects [18, 64, 88]. They can provide well-tailored, high-quality, vascularized tissue to areas in which a local flap would not be possible or desirable. Bone or nerve can be incorporated, providing structural integrity and sensory potential [19]. Any axial flap can theoretically be used as a free flap.

### RADIAL AND ULNAR ARTERY FOREARM FLAPS

The radial and ulnar artery forearm free flaps have long, large-diameter vascular pedicles [42, 58, 68]. Retrograde vascular hook-up is usually tolerated but is occasionally problematic. The venae comitantes or cephalic (radial flap) or basilar (ulnar flap) veins can be used for venous outflow. The vascular component of the flap can be used as a graft to bridge an area in which the vascular continuity has been interrupted. Tendon, bone, or nerve can be incorporated within the flap.

The posterior interosseous artery has also been used as a pedicle for free tissue transfer [119].

The flaps are raised in a similar fashion as has been described. Again, it is extremely important that the vascular supply to the hand be ascertained with a preoperative Allen's test and intraoperatively by gentle occlusion of the flap arterial supply. Consideration may also be given to reconstruction of the arterial system to the hand.

*Figure 31-26* Lateral arm flap anatomy.
*A. Lateral view. (d = deltoid muscle;*
*bi = biceps m.; b = brachialis m.; t = lateral*
*head triceps m.; br = brachioradialis m.;*
*p = profunda brachii artery; rn = radial nerve;*
*prc = posterior radial collateral a.; dashed lines*
*= area of septal dissection.) B. Cross-section of*
*distal portion distal mid-arm level. (Shaded*
*area = septocutaneous flap; bi = biceps m.,*
*b = brachialis m.; t = lateral head triceps m.)*

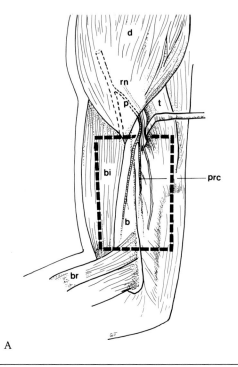

A

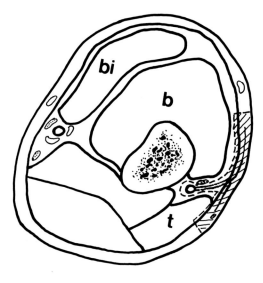

B

LATERAL ARM FLAP

The lateral arm flap, a fasciocutaneous flap raised on the lateral surface of the arm, is supplied by the posterior radial collateral artery, a branch of the profunda brachii artery [72] (Fig. 31-26). The artery penetrates the lateral intermuscular septum of the arm and gives off several septocutaneous branches, which supply the deep fascial plexus of the lateral arm skin. The lateral intermuscular septum lies in a line between the insertion of the deltoid and the lateral epicondyle of the humerus [100]. The skin and underlying soft tissues of the distal half of the lateral aspect of the arm and the proximal fifth of the forearm can be incorporated into this flap [101].

A template of the soft-tissue defect is transferred to the lateral aspect of the arm and centered over a line drawn from the deltoid insertion to the lateral epicondyle. The flap is raised to include the deep fascia and the dissection is carried to the lateral intermuscular septum. The posterior radial collateral artery enters the lateral intermuscular septum just distal to the deltoid insertion. Venous drainage is usually through venae comitantes though the superficial venous system can also be used. The flap can be innervated by utilizing the lateral cutaneous nerve of the arm. Donor defects up to 6 cm in width can be closed primarily; larger defects require skin grafting.

TEMPORPARIETAL FASCIA FREE FLAPS

This flap is obtained from the temporoparietal area of the skull [11, 121] (Fig. 31-27), located between the subcutaneous tissues and temporalis muscle fascia. The superficial temporal artery and vein provide the blood supply. Advantages of this flap are its thinness and well-hidden donor area. An excellent means of palmar reconstruction, it provides thin, well-vascularized coverage.

The hair over the temporoparietal area is shaved. A preauricular incision extending into the hair-bearing scalp skin is made. The superficial temporal artery and vein and the

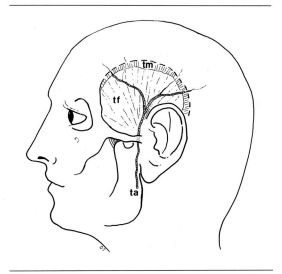

**Figure 31-27** *Temporoparietal fascia flap anatomy. (tm = temporalis muscle; tf = temporalis m. fascia; ta = superficial temporal artery.) Temporoparietal fascia not shown.*

auriculotemporal nerve are identified just anterior to the ear. The vessels always lie at a plane above or within the fascia and the branches of the seventh nerve lie below the fascia (Fig. 31-28). Dissection progresses in a cephalad direction and, if greater flap width is needed, in an occipital direction. Maximum dimensions of the flap usually do not exceed 13 by 9 cm. The skin flaps are closed primarily and the fascial flap, once inset, is skin grafted (Fig. 31-29).

OTHER FREE FLAPS

Free flaps for coverage of the hand can be based in other areas aside from those mentioned. A free groin flap based on the superficial circumflex iliac artery can be designed. By basing this free flap on the deep circumflex iliac artery a portion of the iliac crest can be included for bony reconstruction [116]. The dorsalis pedis flap is based on the dorsalis pedis artery, an extension of the anterior tibial artery [125]. The advantage of this flap is its thin, durable skin cover; the disadvantage is its poor-quality donor site.

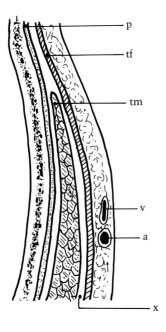

**Figure 31-28**  *Temporoparietal fascia flap, coronal section. (tm = temporalis muscle; p = periosteum; tf = temporoparietal fascia; x = plane of flap dissection; a,v = superficial temporal artery and vein. Temporalis m. fascia not shown. (Based on J. Upton, C. Rogers, G. Durham-Smith, et al. Clinical applications of free temporo parietal flaps in hand reconstruction. J. Hand Surg. 11A:475, 1986.)*

**Figure 31-29**  *Temporoparietal fascia flap. A. Flap. B. Defect. C. Skin graft coverage of fascial flap. D. Final result. (Courtesy J. Upton, M.D., and R. Khouri, M.D.)*

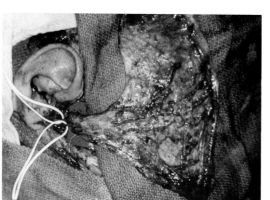

A

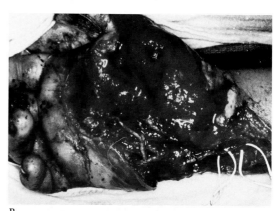

B

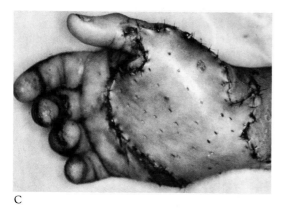

C

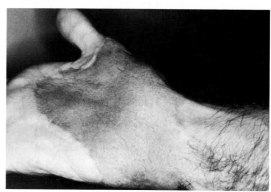

D

The scapular flap is based on the circumflex scapular artery, a branch of the scapular artery [24]. The artery passes through the triangular space and supplies the skin in a horizontal ellipse centered over the inferior angle of the scapula. A variation of this flap, the parascapular flap, uses a different cutaneous branch to provide a skin ellipse centered obliquely over the lateral border of the scapula [12]. The donor defect is most often closed directly and provides an acceptable linear scar. The vascular pedicle is reliable and the elevation of this flap is relatively straightforward. The skin is thin and of high quality and a fair amount can be obtained for free tissue transfer [31]. Disadvantages of this flap are a more difficult dissection in obese individuals, in whom the pedicle may be surrounded by fat, and the short pedicle length available with this flap.

Free flaps of muscle, which are then skin grafted, are useful in the coverage of large, hand and forearm soft-tissue defects. The latissimus dorsi muscle based on the thoracodorsal artery, the serratus anterior muscle based on the lateral thoracic artery, the rectus abdominis muscle based on the superior or inferior epigastric artery, the pectoralis minor muscle supplied by the pectoral branch of the thoracoacromial artery, and the tensor fascia lata muscle based on the terminal branch of the lateral circumflex femoral artery are possibilities [124].

Advanced microsurgical techniques have made possible the exacting reconstruction of structures in the hand using like structures obtained from other parts of the body. An example of this type of procedure is the reconstruction of a thumb using a wraparound flap from the big toe carried on a neurovascular pedicle (see Chaps. 41 and 42). Procedures such as this demand both skill and sophisticated operative resources but provide an option that must be weighed against the possible results obtainable with other avenues of reconstruction.

Many flaps and methods of coverage of soft-tissue defects of the hand have not been described in this chapter because of space limitations. The general goal of restoration of form and function within a reasonable period of time should be sought. The selection of a strategy for coverage of a particular soft-tissue defect may be influenced by the results obtained in published series. It should be kept in mind, however, that the results between different series vary widely, depending on the surgeon, country, and patient population. The functional use to which the patient will put the reconstructed extremity and the age of the patient are important factors in determining an appropriate surgical approach.

**ACKNOWLEDGMENT.** The authors thank Glyn Jones, M.D., for illustrating this chapter.

## References

1. Arons, M. S. Fingertip reconstruction with a palmar advancement flap and free dermal graft: A report of six cases. *J. Hand Surg.* 10A:230, 1985.
2. Atasoy, E. Reversed cross finger subcutaneous flap. *J. Hand Surg.* 7:481, 1982.
3. Atasoy, E., Ioakimidis, E., Kasdan, M. D., et al. Reconstruction of the amputated finger tip with a triangular volar flap; a new surgical procedure. *J. Bone Joint Surg.* 52A:921, 1970.
4. Barfred, T. The Shaw abdominal flap. *Scand. J. Plast. Surg.* 10:56, 1976.
5. Barton, N. J. A modified thenar flap. *Hand* 7:150, 1975.
6. Bayon, P., and Pho, R. W. H. Anatomical basis of dorsal forearm flap. *J. Hand Surg.* 13B:435, 1988.
7. Biddulph, S. L. The neurovascular flap in fingertip injuries. *Hand* 11:59, 1979.
8. Boorman, J. G., Brown, J. A., and Sykes, P. J. Morbidity in the forearm flap donor arm. *Br. J. Hand Surg.* 40:207, 1987.
9. Bralliar, F., and Horner, R. L. Sensory cross finger pedicle graft. *J. Bone Joint Surg.* 51A:1264, 1969.
10. Braun, F. M., Hoang, P., Merle, M., et al. Technique and indications of the forearm flap in hand surgery. *Ann. Chir. Main.* 4:85, 1985.
11. Brent, B., Upton, J., Acland, R. D., et al. Ex-

perience with the temporoparietal fascial free flap. *Plast. Reconstr. Surg.* 76:177, 1985.

12. Burns, J. T., and Schlafly, B. Use of the parascapular flap in hand reconstruction. *J. Hand Surg.* 11A:872, 1986.

13. Button, M., and Stone, E. J. Segmental bony reconstruction of the thumb by composite groin flap: A case report. *J. Hand Surg.* 5:488, 1980.

14. Campbell Reid, D. A. The neurovascular island flap in thumb reconstruction. *Br. J. Plast. Surg.* 19:234, 1966.

15. Chase, R. A. The damaged index digit: A source of components to restore the crippled hand. *J. Bone Joint Surg.* 50A:1152, 1968.

16. Chick, L. R. Brief history and biology of skin grafting. *Ann. Plast. Surg.* 21:358, 1988.

17. Cronin, T. D. The cross finger flap; a new method of repair. *Am. Surg.* 17:419, 1951.

18. Daniel, R. K., and Williams, H. B. The free transfer of skin flaps by microvascular anastomoses. *Plast. Reconstr. Surg.* 52:16, 1973.

19. Daniel, R. K., Terzis, J., and Schwarz, G. Neurovascular free flaps. *Plast. Reconstr. Surg.* 56:13, 1975.

20. Dellon, A. L. *Evaluation of Sensibility and Re-education of Sensation in the Hand.* Baltimore: Williams & Wilkins, 1981.

21. Dellon, A. L. The extended palmar advancement flap. *J. Hand Surg.* 8:190, 1983.

22. Dellon, A. L. The proximal inset thenar flap for fingertip reconstruction. *Plast. Reconstr. Surg.* 72:698, 1983.

23. Dickinson, J. C., and Roberts, A. H. N. Fasciocutaneous cross-arm flaps in hand reconstruction. *J. Hand Surg.* 11:394, 1986.

24. Dos Santos, L. F. The vascular anatomy and dissection of the free scapular flap. *Plast. Reconstr. Surg.* 73:599, 1984.

25. Earley, M. J. The first web hand flap. *J. Hand Surg.* 14B:65, 1989.

26. Elliot, D., and Bainbridge, L. C. Ulnar fasciocutaneous flap of the wrist. *J. Hand Surg.* 13B:311, 1988.

27. Emmett, A. J. J. Finger resurfacing by the multiple subcutaneous pedicle or louvre flaps. *Br. J. Plast. Surg.* 27:370, 1974.

28. Ersek, R. A., and Ersek, S. The sandwich switch flap. *J. Hand Surg.* 14A:746, 1989.

29. Finseth, F., May, J. W., and Smith, R. J. Composite groin flap with iliac-bone for primary thumb reconstruction. *J. Bone Joint Surg.* 58A:130, 1976.

30. Fisher, R. H. The Kutler method of repair of fingertip amputations. *J. Bone Joint Surg.* 49A:317, 1967.

31. Fissette, J., Lahaye, Th., and Colot, G. The use of the free parascapular flap in midpalmar soft tissue defect. *Ann. Plast. Surg.* 10:235, 1983.

32. Foucher, G., van Genechten, F., Merle, N., et al. A compound radial artery forearm flap in hand surgery: An original modification of the Chinese forearm flap. *Br. J. Plast. Surg.* 37:139, 1984.

33. Freedlander, E., Dickson, W. A., and McGrouther, D. A. The present role of the groin flap in hand trauma in the light of a long-term review. *J. Hand Surg.* 11B:187, 1986.

34. Furlow, L. T., Jr. V-Y "cup" flap for volar oblique amputation of fingers. *J. Hand Surg.* 9B:253, 1984.

35. Gaul, J. S. Radial-innervated cross finger flap from index to provide sensory pulp to injured thumb. *J. Bone Joint Surg.* 51A:1257, 1969.

36. Gault, D. T., and Quaba, A. A. The role of cross-finger flaps in the primary management of untidy flexor tendon injuries. *J. Hand Surg.* 13B:62, 1988.

37. Godfrey, A. M., Poole, M. D., Rowsell, A. R., et al. Local transposition of a distally-based island forearm flap to close a complicated excisional wrist defect in a nonagenarian: Some anatomical and clinical considerations. *Br. J. Plast. Surg.* 37:493, 1984.

38. Green, D. P., and Dominguez, O. J. A transpositional skin flap for release of volar contractures of a finger at the MP joint. *Plast. Reconstr. Surg.* 64:516, 1979.

39. Gurdin, M., and Pangman, W. J. The repair of surface defects of fingers by transdigital flaps. *Plast. Reconstr. Surg.* 5:368, 1950.

40. Haddad, R. J. The Kutler repair of fingertip amputation. *South Med. J.* 61:1264, 1968.

41. Henderson, H. P., and Reid, D. A. C. Long term follow-up of neurovascular island flaps. *Hand* 12:113, 1980.

42. Hentz, V. R., Pearl, R. M., Grossman, J. A. I., et al. The radial forearm flap: A versatile source of composite tissue. *Ann. Plast. Surg.* 19:485, 1987.

43. Hester, T. R., Nahai, F., Beegle, P. E., et al. Blood supply of the abdomen revisited, with

emphasis on the superficial inferior epigastric artery. *Plast. Reconstr. Surg.* 74:657, 1984.

44. Holevich, J. A new method of restoring sensibility to the thumb. *J. Bone Joint Surg.* 45A:496, 1963.

45. Horn, J. S. The use of full thickness hand skin flaps in the reconstruction of injured fingers. *Plast. Reconstr. Surg.* 7:463, 1951.

46. Hueston, J. Local flap repair of fingertip injuries. *Plast. Reconstr. Surg.* 38:349, 1966.

47. Hurtwitz, P. J. The many tailed flap for multiple finger injuries. *Br. J. Plast. Surg.* 33:230, 1980.

48. Iselin, F. The flag flap. *Plas. Reconstr. Surg.* 52:374, 1973.

49. Johnson, R. K., and Iverson, R. E. Cross finger pedicle flap in the hand. *J. Bone Joint Surg.* 53:913, 1971.

50. Joshi, B. B. Dorsolateral flap from same finger to relieve flexion contracture. *Plast. Reconstr. Surg.* 49:186, 1972.

51. Kappel, D. A., and Burech, J. G. The cross-finger flap: An established reconstructive procedure. *Hand Clin.* 1:677, 1985.

52. Katai, K., Kido, M., and Numaguchi, Y. Angiography of the iliofemoral arteriovenous system supplying free groin flaps and free hypogastric flaps. *Plast. Reconstr. Surg.* 63:671, 1979.

53. Keim, H. A., and Grantham, S. A. Volar flap advancement for thumb and fingertip injuries. *Clin. Orthop.* 66:109, 1961.

54. Kelleher, J. C., Sullivan, J. G., Baibak, G. J., et al. The distant pedicle flap in surgery of the hand. *Orthop. Clin. North Am.* 1:227, 1970.

55. Kelleher, J. C., Sullivan, J. G., Baibak, G. J., et al. Use of a tailored abdominal pedicle flap for surgical reconstruction of the hand. *J. Bone Joint Surg.* 52A:1552, 1970.

56. Kislov, R., and Kelly, A. P. Cross-finger flaps in digital injuries with notes on Kirschner wire fixation. *Plast. Reconstr. Surg.* 25:313, 1960.

57. Kleinert, H. E., McAlister, C. G., MacDonald, C. J., et al. A critical evaluation of cross finger flaps. *J. Trauma* 14:756, 1974.

58. Koshima, I., Iino, T., Fukuda, H., et al. The free ulnar forearm flap. *Ann. Plast. Surg.* 18:24, 1987.

59. Krag, C., and Rasmussen, K. B. The neurovascular island flap for defective sensibility of the thumb. *J. Bone Joint Surg.* 57B:495, 1974.

60. Kutler, W. A new method for fingertip amputation. *J.A.M.A.* 133:129, 1947.

61. Lesavoy, M. A. The dorsal index finger neurovascular island flap. *Orthop. Rev.* 9:91, 1980.

62. Leslie, B. M., and Ruby, L. K. Coverage of a carpal tunnel wound dehiscence with the abductor digiti minimi muscle flap. *J. Hand Surg.* 13A:36, 1988.

63. Lewis, R. C., Nordyke, M. D., and Duncan, K. H. Web space reconstruction with an M-V flap. *J. Hand Surg.* 13A:40, 1988.

64. Lister, G., and Scheker, L. Emergency free flaps to the upper extremity. *J. Hand Surg.* 13A:22, 1988.

65. Lister, G. D. Local flaps to the hand. *Hand Clin.* 1:621, 1985.

66. Lister, G. D., McGregor, I. A., and Jackson, I. T. The groin flap in hand injuries. *Injury* 4:229, 1973.

67. Littler, J. W. Principles of Reconstructive Surgery of the Hand. In J. W. Converse (ed.), *Reconstructive Plastic Surgery,* vol. 4. Philadelphia: Saunders, 1964.

68. Lovie, M. J., Duncan, G. M., and Glasson, D. W. The ulnar artery forearm free flap. *Br. J. Hand Surg.* 37:486, 1984.

69. Macht, S. D., and Watson, H. K. The Moberg volar advancement flap for digital reconstruction. *J. Hand Surg.* 5:372, 1980.

70. Markley, J. M. The preservation of close two-point discrimination in the interdigital transfer of neurovascular island flaps. *Plast. Reconstr. Surg.* 59:812, 1977.

71. Markley, J. M. Island flaps of the hand. *Hand Clin.* 1:689, 1985.

72. Matloub, H. S., Sanger, J. R., and Godina, M. The lateral arm neurosensory flap. *Transactions of the Eighth International Congress of Plastic Surgery and Reconstructive Surgery,* Montreal, 1983.

73. McCash, C. R. Cross-arm bridge flaps in the repair of flexion contractures of the fingers. *Br. J. Plast. Surg.* 9:25, 1956.

74. McGrath, M. H., Adelberg, D., and Finseth, F. The intravenous fluorescein test: Use in timing of groin flap division. *J. Hand Surg.* 4:19, 1979.

75. McGregor, I. A. Less satisfactory experiences

with neurovascular island flaps. *Hand* 1:21, 1969.

76. McGregor, I. A., and Jackson, I. T. The groin flap. *Br. J. Plast. Surg.* 25:3, 1972.

77. Melone, C. P., Beasley, R. W., and Carstens, J. H. The thenar flap: An analysis of its use in 150 cases. *J. Hand Surg.* 7:291, 1982.

78. Miller, A. J. Single finger tip injuries treated by thenar flap. *Hand* 6:311, 1974.

79. Miura, T. Thumb reconstruction using radial-innervated cross-finger pedicle graft. *J. Bone Joint Surg.* 55A:563, 1973.

80. Miura, T., and Nakamura, R. Use of paired flaps to simultaneously cover the dorsal and volar surfaces of a raw hand. *Plast. Reconstr. Surg.* 54:286, 1974.

81. Muhlbauer, W., Herndl, E., and Stock, W. The forearm flap. *Plast. Reconstr. Surg.* 70:336, 1982.

82. Mulliken, J. B., and Healey, N. A. Pathogenesis of skin flap necrosis from an underlying hematoma. *Plast. Reconstr. Surg.* 63:540, 1979.

83. Murray, J. F., Ord, J. V., and Gavelin, G. E. The neurovascular island pedicle flap: An assessment of late results in sixteen cases. *J. Bone Joint Surg.* 49A:1285, 1967.

84. Nahai, F., and Mathes, S. J. Musculocutaneous flap or muscle flap and skin graft. *Ann. Plast. Surg.* 12:199, 1984.

85. Nakamura, K., Namba, K., and Tsuchida, H. A retrospective study of thick split-thickness plantar skin grafts to resurface the palm. *Ann. Plast. Surg.* 12:508, 1984.

86. Napier, J. R. The return of pain sensibility in full thickness skin grafts. *Brain* 75:147, 1952.

87. Nicolai, J. P. A., and Hentenaar, G. Sensation in cross-finger flaps. *Hand* 13:12, 1981.

88. O'Brien, B. McC., Morrison, W. A., Ishida, H., et al. Free flap transfers with microvascular anastomoses. *Br. J. Plast. Surg.* 27:220, 1974.

89. Oguntro, O. Dorsal transposition flap for reconstruction of lateral or medial oblique amputations of the thumb with exposure of bone. *J. Hand Surg.* 9:894, 1983.

90. Omer, G. E., Jr. Evaluation and reconstruction of forearm and hand after acute traumatic peripheral nerve injuries. *J. Bone Joint Surg.* 50A:1454, 1968.

91. Omer, G. E., Jr., Day, D. J., Ratliff, H., et al.

Neurovascular cutaneous island pedicles for deficient median nerve sensibility. *J. Bone Joint Surg.* 52A:1181, 1970.

92. Patton, H. S. Split-skin grafts from hypothenar area for fingertip avulsions. *Plast. Reconstr. Surg.* 43:426, 1969.

93. Penteado, C. V. Venous drainage of the groin flap. *Plast. Reconstr. Surg.* 71:678, 1983.

94. Pho, R. W. H. Local composite neurovascular island flap for skin cover in pulp loss of the thumb. *J. Hand Surg.* 4:11, 1979.

95. Posner, M. A., and Smith, R. J. Advancement pedicle flap for thumb injuries. *J. Bone Joint Surg.* 53A:1618, 1971.

96. Rae, P. S., and Pho, R. W. H. The radial transposition flap: A useful composite flap. *Hand* 15:96, 1983.

97. Reinisch. J. F., Winters, R., and Puckett, C. L. The use of the osteocutaneous groin flap in gunshot wounds of the hand. *J. Hand Surg.* 9A:12, 1984.

98. Reyes, F. A., and Burkhalter, W. E. The fascial radial flap. *J. Hand Surg.* 13A:432, 1988.

99. Sandzen, S. C. Dorsal pedicle flap for resurfacing a moderate thumb-index web contracture release. *J. Hand Surg.* 7:21, 1982.

100. Scheker, L. R., Kleinert, H. E., and Hanel, D. P. Lateral arm composite tissue transfer to ipsilateral hand defects. *J. Hand Surg.* 12A:665, 1987.

101. Scheker, L. R., Lister, G. D., and Wolff, T. W. The lateral arm free flap in releasing severe contracture of the first web space. *J. Hand Surg.* 13B:146, 1988.

102. Schlenker, J. D. Transfer of a neurovascular island pedicle flap based upon the metacarpal artery: A case report. *J. Hand Surg.* 4:16, 1979.

103. Schlenker, J. D., and Averill, R. M. The iliofemoral (groin) flap for hand and forearm coverage. *Orthop. Rev.* 9:57, 1980.

104. Shaw, D. T., and Payne, R. L. One stage tubed abdominal flaps. *Surg. Gynecol. Obstet.* 83:205, 1946.

105. Shepard, G. H. The uses of lateral V-Y advancement flaps for fingertip reconstruction. *J. Hand Surg.* 8:254, 1983.

106. Small, J. O., and Brennen, M. D. The first dorsal metacarpal artery neurovascular island flap. *J. Hand Surg.* 13B:136, 1988.

107. Smith, J. R., and Boon, A. F. An evaluation of fingertip reconstruction by cross finger and

palmar pedicle flap. *Plast. Reconstr. Surg.* 35:409, 1965.

108. Smith, P. J. The importance of venous drainage in axial pattern flaps. *Br. J. Plast. Surg.* 31:233, 1978.

109. Smith, P. J., Foley, B., McGregor, I. A., et al. The anatomical basis of the groin flap. *Plast. Reconstr. Surg.* 49:41, 1972.

110. Song, R., et al. The forearm flap. *Clin. Plast. Surg.* 9:21, 1982.

111. Soutar, D. S., and Tanner, N. S. B. The radial forearm flap in the management of soft tissue injuries of the hand. *Br. J. Plast. Surg.* 37:18, 1984.

112. Stern, P. J., and Lister, G. D. Pollicization after traumatic amputation of the thumb. *Clin. Orthop. Rel. Res.* 155:85, 1981.

113. Stern, P. J., Kreilein, J. G., and Kleinert, H. E. Neurovascular cutaneous flaps for the management of radiation-induced fingertip dermal necrosis. *J. Hand Surg.* 8:88, 1983.

114. Stevenson, T. R., Hester, T. R., Duus, E. C., et al. The superficial inferior epigastric artery flap for coverage of hand and forearm defects. *Ann. Plast. Surg.* 12:333, 1984.

115. Sucur, D., and Radivojevic, M. Cross finger flap: A new technique. *J. Hand Surg.* 10B:425, 1985.

116. Swartz, W. M. Immediate reconstruction of the wrist and dorsum of the hand with a free osteocutaneous groin flap. *J. Hand Surg.* 9A:18, 1984.

117. Thomson, H. G., and Sorokolit, W. T. The cross finger flap in children; a follow-up study. *Plast. Reconstr. Surg.* 39:482, j967.

118. Timmons, M. J. The vascular basis of the radial forearm flap. *Plast. Reconstr. Surg.* 77:80, 1986.

119. Tonkin, M. A., and Stern H. The posterior interosseous artery free flap. *J. Hand Surg.* 14B:215, 1989.

120. Tsuge, K. *Comprehensive Atlas of Hand Surgery.* Chicago: Year Book, 1989.

121. Upton, J., Rogers, C., Durham-Smith, G., et al. Clinical applications of free temporoparietal flaps in hand reconstruction. *J. Hand Surg.* 11A:475, 1986.

122. Vilain, R., and Dupuis, J. F. Use of the flag flap for coverage of a small area on a finger or the palm: 20 years of experience. *Plast. Reconstr. Surg.* 51:397, 1973.

123. Walker, M. A., Hurley, C. B., and May, J. W. Radial nerve cross-finger flap differential nerve contribution in thumb reconstruction. *J. Hand Surg.* 11A:881, 1986.

124. Webster, M. H. C., and Soutar, D. S. *Practical Guide to Free Tissue Transfer.* London: Butterworth, 1986.

125. Weeks, P. M., and Wray, R. C. *Management of Acute Hand Injuries, A Biological Approach.* St. Louis: Mosby, 1973.

126. White, W. L. Flap grafts to the upper extremity. *Surg. Clin. North Am.* 40:389, 1960.

127. Wray, R. C., Wise, D. M., Young, V. L., et al. The groin flap in severe hand injuries. *Ann. Plast. Surg.* 9:459, 1982.

128. Xavier, T. S., and Lamb, D. W. The forearm as donor site for split skin grafts. *Hand* 6:243, 1974.

129. Zancolli, E. A., and Angrigiani, C. Posterior interosseous island forearm flap. *J. Hand Surg.* 13B:130, 1988.

130. Zoltie, N. Forearm split-skin donor sites: Are they cosmetically acceptable. *Ann. Plast. Surg.* 21:11, 1988.

# 32

## Sprains and Dislocations of the Fingers and Thumb

L. Andrew Koman
Ralph Coonrad
Gary G. Poehling

### General Principles

In order to treat appropriately an injured digit, it is crucial to establish a specific diagnosis and to understand the consequences of the injury on the delicate anatomic balance of the finger or thumb. The magnitude of ligamentous injury is often unappreciated except by an experienced observer. Objective tests such as roentgenograms seldom provide a definitive diagnosis or allow a true appreciation of the extent of the soft-tissue or ligamentous injury. A careful history and physical examination are therefore mandatory and are the only means by which the diagnosis can be made in the majority of digital sprains and dislocations.

The history must include the mechanism of injury, an estimate of the forces involved, and the effect of initial care on subsequent symptoms. The clinical examination should include careful inspection of the digit, localization of the site of maximal tenderness by palpation, an estimation of active and passive range of motion, and an evaluation of capsular and ligamentous stability. Estimation of joint stability often requires stress testing, both in extension and in flexion (Fig. 32-1), and, to be definitive, may require simultaneous roentgenographic or fluoroscopic assistance (stress testing). Plain roentgeno-grams (anteroposterior, lateral, and oblique) should be obtained before the stress testing. Arthrography, ultrasonography, computed tomography, magnetic resonance imaging, and arthroscopy may provide additional diagnostic information and allow confirmation of the suspected lesion.

Ligamentous injuries or sprains of digital joints can be classified into three groups according to the degree of injury. Grade I includes injuries with incomplete ligamentous and capsular tear or stretch and without any testable instability. Grade II is comprised of injuries of the joint with testable instability, but with incomplete ligamentous and capsular damage. Grade III includes injuries with total ligamentous disruption, capsular disruption, or both, with total instability of joint integrity by stress testing (Fig. 32-2).

Dislocations of digital joints may stretch the collateral ligaments without completely disrupting them, while still rupturing the volar capsule or volar plate. Dislocations are classified as simple or complex. Simple dislocations can be reduced by closed manipulation, whereas complex dislocations, often involving complete disruption or a herniation of the collateral ligaments, are usually irreducible except by open means. Complex

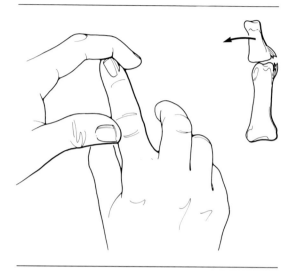

**Figure 32-1** *Stress testing is necessary to determine the degree of ligamentous injury and should be performed with the digit in full extension and 20 to 40 degrees of flexion.*

dislocations usually occur at the metacarpophalangeal (MP) joint as a result of "buttonholing" of the metacarpal head through the volar capsule and the subsequent interposition of the volar plate or other structures within the joint. Displacement of flexor tendons, cartilage flaps, periosteum, and extensor tendons can also impede closed manipulative reduction of both the proximal interphalangeal (PIP) and the MP joints.

## Carpometacarpal Joints
### DORSAL DISLOCATIONS (FINGERS)
Isolated ligamentous injury to the carpometacarpal (CMC) joints is rare, and most injuries in this area are dorsal fracture dislocations (Fig. 32-3). In the absence of fractures, the clinical suspicion of a dislocation is best confirmed by a 30-degree pronated view (Fisher [24, 25]) or computed tomography. Pure ligamentous injuries, produced by longitudinal compressive forces through the metacarpal head, are frequently associated with adjacent metacarpal fractures, dislocations, or fracture dislocations. Soft-tissue in-

juries of this magnitude may be sufficient to elevate pressure in the interosseous compartment. Dorsal dislocations are much more common than volar dislocations, and generally occur in the ulnar digits or thumb [33, 34].

*Pathologic Anatomy*
The relatively mobile fourth and fifth CMC joints are more susceptible to dislocation than the immobile second and third rays. The fifth CMC joint is most frequently injured. The volar plate and capsular ligaments and the collateral and intermetacarpal ligaments provide the most stability, and dorsal dislocation (often with small avulsion fractures) is the most frequent injury. During a dorsal dislocation, the convex bases of the fourth and fifth metacarpals, which provide inherent stability through their articulations with the carpal bones, are displaced dorsally, and extrinsic tendon power is unbalanced. This imbalance and subsequent overpull of the extensor carpi ulnaris in conjunction with interposition of capsular structures may prevent a stable reduction.

**Figure 32-2** *The spectrum of ligamentous injury. A. Incomplete ligamentous tear without joint subluxation. B. Incomplete ligamentous tear with joint instability. C. Complete ligament disruption and joint instability.*

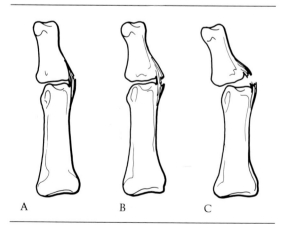

A         B         C

*Treatment*

Concentric and stable reduction of the fourth or fifth CMC joint is important for hand function. Uncomplicated and isolated dorsal dislocations can be managed by closed reduction and plaster immobilization or by percutaneous pinning. Excellent regional or general anesthesia is necessary because of the imbalance of the extrinsic motor groups. Capsular interposition or other soft-tissue blockage may prevent achievement of a stable concentric reduction and necessitate open reduction and internal fixation. Similarly, ligamentous injury in conjunction with extrinsic motor imbalance may make percutaneous pin fixation necessary.

Associated fractures or fracture dislocations of adjacent metacarpals and undiagnosed fracture dislocations generally require internal fixation. Open reduction through a dorsal incision is indicated if closed reduction is unsuccessful. It is important to monitor neurovascular compromise both preoperatively and postoperatively in order to detect the development of a compartment syndrome, which can be associated with these severe injuries, and to prevent ischemic contracture.

## LIGAMENTOUS INJURY (THUMB)
*Pathologic Anatomy and Diagnosis*

The concave saddle configuration of the first metacarpotrapezial joint provides enhanced stability, but the magnitude of forces across the joint necessitates ligamentous support for effective function. Pinch produces a dorsal subluxation force, which is magnified by hyperextension of the metacarpophalangeal joint. Subluxation or dislocation of the CMC joint will result in pain associated with activity and will diminish hand function. Injury to the palmar ligaments, if unrecognized and untreated, will result in instability of the basilar joint [14, 69].

The earliest recognized injury of this joint is a fracture dislocation (Bennett's fracture). The pure ligamentous injury is analogous to the fracture dislocation, but diagnosis is sig-

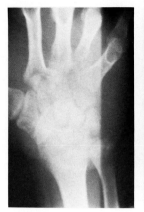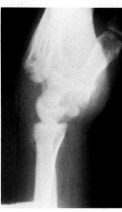

**Figure 32-3** *Anteroposterior and lateral roentgenograms of fracture dislocation of the fourth and dislocation of the fifth carpalmetacarpal joint.*

nificantly more difficult. The diagnosis of ligamentous injury should be suspected if acute clinical instability is detected; stress testing or arthrography may confirm the diagnosis. However, in the grade I or II sprain of the basilar joint, suspicion and careful clinical evaluation are important to avoid mismanagement and to prevent chronic ligamentous weakness.

*Treatment*

Partial tears of the first metacarpotrapezial joint (grade I and II sprains) with roentgenographic confirmation of concentric reduction should be protected with plaster immobilization of the metacarpal in extension and abduction for 4 to 6 weeks. Complete disruptions can be managed by plaster cast immobilization as well, but serial roentgenograms are necessary to confirm that subluxation does not occur during immobilization. Failure to maintain closed reduction or inability to obtain an anatomic reduction is an indication for open or closed reduction and internal fixation. If open reduction with internal fixation is undertaken, it may also be necessary to reinforce or reconstruct the

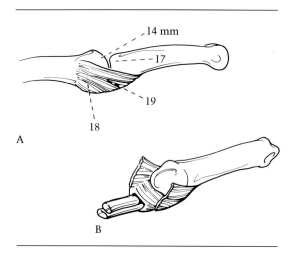

14 mm

17

19

18

A

B

**Figure 32-4** *A. Condyloid configuration of metacarpophalangeal joint and eccentric portion of collateral ligaments tighten collateral ligament during flexion and allow motion for abduction-adduction on full extension. B. Volar plate and collateral ligament support structure.*

palmar and dorsal ligaments at that time [21, 23].

## Metacarpophalangeal Joints (Fingers)

### DORSAL METACARPOPHALANGEAL DISLOCATIONS

#### Pathologic Anatomy and Diagnosis

The condyloid configuration of the MP joints in conjunction with their collateral ligaments and the support from surrounding structures provides significant protection from injury (see Fig. 32-3) and makes subluxation-dislocation a relatively infrequent occurrence. The volar plate, which blends into the deep transverse metacarpal ligament, provides additional support, as do the reflections of the intrinsic muscles and tendons. The dorsal capsular structures of the MP joint are the thinnest and weakest structures.

The volar plate and the MP joint are thick distally and thin proximally. The collateral ligaments and accessory collateral ligaments extend eccentrically from the metacarpal to the proximal phalanx and volar plate and provide lateral support (Fig. 32-4A). In flexion, collateral ligaments are tight and side support is maximal; the collateral ligaments are loose in extension to allow abduction-adduction (Fig. 32-4). Dislocations of the MP joint are generally caused by ulnar and dorsally directed forces (forced hyperextension) and involve the index finger most frequently [36]. Central digit dislocations without an associated injury to the adjacent index or little finger are rare [19].

The usual mechanism of injury is a fall on the outstretched hand, with the MP joint forced into hyperextension. As the proximal phalanx is displaced dorsally on the metacarpal, the volar plate is torn at its membranous attachment, usually at the base of the metacarpal. At this juncture, the extent of volar plate interposition and volar structure displacement determine whether the injury is simple or complex. The simple dislocation or subluxation can be reduced by closed manipulation, whereas the complex dislocations are irreducible by that means and require open reduction. Once reduced, both injuries are usually stable and will not dislocate spontaneously. However, there may be collateral ligament instability.

The diagnosis of dislocation of the MP joint is usually obvious, but roentgenograms should be obtained before reduction to rule out a concomitant fracture. In a simple dislocation, the proximal phalanx usually assumes a characteristic angulation of 60 to 80 degrees, with a dorsal displacement (Fig. 32-5A). The metacarpal head is prominent, and the prominence is easily visualized and palpable in the palm. In the complex dislocation, the proximal phalanx is less extended, the metacarpal head is prominent, and the pathognomonic sign of puckering of the skin over the area of the palmar crease may be present (Fig. 32-5B). Anteroposterior, lateral, and oblique roentgenograms should always be obtained to rule out fracture. In a complex dislocation, the widened joint space represents interposition of the volar plate, and the presence of a sesamoid within the

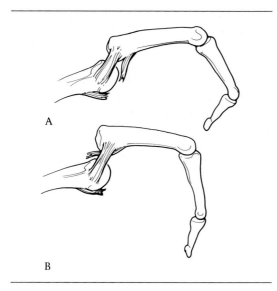

*Figure 32-5* *A. Simple dislocation of metacarpophalangeal joint. B. Complex dislocation of metacarpophalangeal joint.*

joint is pathognomonic of that type of dislocation. The importance of a sesamoid within the joint space is easily understood when it is remembered that the sesamoid lies in the lateral portion of the volar plate and therefore its presence in the joint space indicates the presence of the volar plate within the joint [2].

In a complex dislocation, the proximal phalanx is displaced dorsally, while the metacarpal head, because of the presence of the flexor tendons, is displaced radially and palmarly. As the proximal phalanx hyperextends, the volar plate and capsule rupture. Flexor tendons are displaced further ulnarly by the metacarpal head. With further hyperextension, the volar plate completely dislocates and comes to lie on the dorsum of the metacarpal head. The metacarpal head is then forced through the fibers of the palmar aponeurosis, leaving the transverse bands of the natatory ligament taut distally and the superficial transverse ligament taut proximally. Further radial deviation is prevented by the lumbrical. The metacarpal head lies fixed in this position, buttonholed through

these four structures and prevented from retraction by the volar plate [37, 39, 52] (Fig. 32-6). The finger assumes its characteristic attitude of ulnar deviation. Skin puckering is secondary to stretch of the longitudinal pretendinous band and transverse fibers of the palmar fascia, which are displaced. Neurovascular bundles lie taut lateral to the metacarpal head (Fig. 32-6D). In the thumb and fingers, the primary block to reduction is the volar plate.

### Treatment

SIMPLE DORSAL MP DISLOCATION. Care must be taken not to convert a simple dislocation into a complex one. Therefore, simultaneous hyperextension and longitudinal traction should be avoided during the reduction procedure. Excessive traction with additional hyperextension can cause further subluxation or complete tearing of the collateral lig-

*Figure 32-6* *Palmar visualization of complex MP dislocation. The volar plate is the primary block to reduction, which is further hindered by the natatory ligament (A), transverse palmar ligaments (B), flexor tendons (E), and palmar aponeurosis (C). Note the neurovascular bundle, which is stretched and immediately beneath the skin (D).*

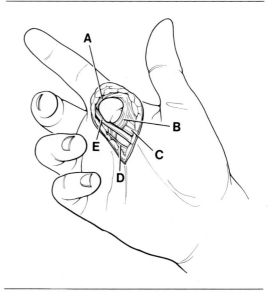

aments, allowing the volar plate to block reduction. Simple MP dislocations can be reduced by dorsal pressure on the proximal phalanx in conjunction with wrist flexion (see Fig. 32-5A). The finger should be stable after reduction but should be splinted for 3 to 4 weeks to prevent hyperextension. This is best achieved with a hand-based MP joint extension block splint.

COMPLEX DORSAL MP DISLOCATION. Attempts at closed reduction of complex dislocations are both futile and potentially damaging [5, 6]. If the diagnosis is in question, a single attempt at closed reduction is indicated under adequate anesthesia. Open reduction can be achieved through dorsal or palmar approaches. Regardless of the incision, reduction is achieved by proper repositioning of the volar plate. Palmar approaches are technically more demanding, since care must be taken to protect the neurovascular bundles, which may be tented just beneath the dermis. The palmar approach is advocated because it allows direct visualization of the volar plate, natatory ligament, superficial transverse ligaments, flexor tendons, and neurovascular bundles [19, 26, 32, 38, 53]. The dorsal approach is advocated because of its relative simplicity and because it avoids direct exposure of the more sensitive volar structures [19, 55, 65]. Arthroscopic visualization of complex MP dislocations has been achieved and allows the percutaneous insertion of instruments to reduce the volar plate. Regardless of the mechanisms of reduction, the joint is usually stable after reduction, and the reduction can be protected by extension block splinting for 3 to 5 weeks. During the early postreduction period, complete extension is blocked at 30 degrees of flexion, but full flexion is allowed. This block is decreased to neutral at weekly intervals.

PALMAR METACARPOPHALANGEAL DISLOCATIONS

Palmar dislocations of the MP joints are infrequent and irreducible (i.e., complex). Injuries with palmar displacement are rare.

Irreducible injuries are secondary to interposition of the dorsal capsule (detached from the metacarpal) or the volar plate (avulsed from its dorsal insertion) [8, 83]. In the uncomplicated injury, the dorsal capsule is torn and the collateral ligaments and volar plate remain in continuity, although they may be stretched. The diagnosis is easily made by clinical examination and routine roentgenograms. The uncomplicated injury is generally easily reduced and stable, although the integrity of the collateral ligament should be confirmed carefully after reduction. If closed reduction of complex injuries fails, open reduction through a dorsal incision is indicated.

COLLATERAL LIGAMENT INJURIES

Injuries of the collateral ligaments of the MP joint, except for those of the thumb, are rare. When one does occur, it is often a severe joint injury and is generally seen in conjunction with other injuries, such as fractures or lacerations, or both. The radial collateral ligament of the ulnar digits is the most likely to be injured. The mechanism of injury involves either abduction or adduction stress, and the symptoms are local pain, tenderness, and swelling in the area of the collateral ligament. After any dislocation, the collateral ligament must be stressed to ensure its integrity.

Treatment depends on the degree of ligamentous injury as well as the associated injuries. After stable concentric reduction of an isolated injury, protection with extension block splints modified to prevent radioulnar deviation for 3 weeks, followed by taping to the adjacent finger for an additional 2 to 3 weeks, is sufficient management [18, 19]. If concentric reduction is not possible, collateral ligament reconstruction is indicated.

## Metacarpophalangeal Joint (Thumb)

PATHOLOGIC ANATOMY

The condyloid configuration of the thumb MP joint and the fact that it is less spherical than digital MP joint heads provide variable flexion-extension as well as abduction-adduction of the thumb proximal phalanx. Stability is provided by true and accessory collateral ligaments, and by a thick volar plate strengthened by the sesamoids and reinforced by the intrinsic muscle insertions and the dynamic forces from intrinsic and extrinsic flexor and extensor tendons. However, the position of the thumb in an abducted position makes the MP joint susceptible to abduction and extension injuries [39].

### INJURIES OF THE DORSAL CAPSULE: DISLOCATIONS

Isolated injuries of the dorsal capsule of the thumb are frequent. They usually are seen after relatively minor trauma, with swelling and maximal tenderness over the dorsum of the MP joint [12, 15]. These injuries usually occur with a sudden flexion force while the extensor pollicis brevis tendon is actively contracting. The patient rarely sees a physician and believes that the thumb has been "sprained." Treatment is generally symptomatic, using splinting to achieve comfort and initiation of early range of motion.

Dorsal dislocation of the thumb MP joint occurs secondary to a hyperextensive force that ruptures the volar plate and capsule, and attenuates or disrupts the collateral ligaments. The volar plate generally tears proximally. Complex injuries with interposition of the volar plate, sesamoid, or both can occur. In simple injuries, the stability of the collateral ligaments after concentric reduction is the primary concern (see section on collateral ligament injuries). Complex injuries require open reduction. Incomplete ligamentous injuries can be managed by casting or splinting for 4 to 6 weeks (Fig. 32-7).

### VOLAR PLATE INJURIES

Isolated injuries of the volar plate (usually the ulnar aspect) of the thumb MP joint are uncommon and, when they occur, should be protected by splinting. It is important to look for an avulsion fracture at the insertion

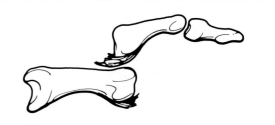

**Figure 32-7** *Dorsal dislocation of MP joint of the thumb. The volar plate is generally torn proximally. In the complex injury demonstrated, the volar plate is interposed between the metacarpal and proximal phalanx.*

of the volar plate at the base of the proximal phalanx [12, 28] and for intraarticular shearing fractures of the palmar metacarpal condyle [73–76]. Tenderness over the volar plate and pain on active or passive extension are indicative of volar plate injury. Extension block splinting for 2 to 3 weeks followed by protected range of motion is generally sufficient for mild to moderate injuries.

### COLLATERAL LIGAMENT INJURIES

Collateral ligament injuries of the thumb MP joint deserve special attention. Either the radial or the ulnar collateral ligament can be injured, with the latter injury being far more common. The term *gamekeeper's thumb* was coined by Campbell [13] in 1955 because of the damage sustained to the thumb ulnar collateral ligament by Scottish gamekeepers. This initial description was generally of a chronic stress of the ulnar collateral ligament. Currently, gamekeeper's thumb has come to designate any ulnar collateral ligament injury of the thumb, whether complete or incomplete, acute or chronic.

### Mechanism of Injury/Pathology

Any abduction force applied to the proximal phalanx of the thumb applies stress to the ulnar collateral ligament and can result in a partial or complete tear. The mechanism of injury is forced radial deviation (abduction stress), such as occurs with a ski pole. These abduction (valgus) stresses to the thumb MP joint can result in disruption of the volar plate, dorsal capsule, or dorsal aponeurosis, or all three, in conjunction with the ulnar collateral ligament. At the moment of injury, the true collateral ligament can be avulsed from its phalangeal attachment, or the entire ulnar complex, including the volar plate and dorsal capsule, can be disrupted. This disruption can include tearing of the adductor aponeurosis as well as the dorsal and volar capsule. The degree of injury depends on the force exerted, the position of the MP joint at the time of injury, and the rapidity of the loading. Stener [73] has postulated that the MP joint is in slight flexion at the time of abduction stress and the force is sufficient for complete disruption. The collateral ligament may be everted outside the adductor aponeurosis, which then slides forward and interposes itself between the torn ligament and its insertion, thereby creating the Stener lesion. As the MP joint then extends after the moment of injury, the aponeurosis slides proximally, trapping and everting the avulsed portion of the ligament. Recognition of this mechanism is important, because the presence of a Stener lesion will prevent the ligament from healing in an appropriate anatomic position.

*Diagnosis*
The diagnosis of collateral ligament injury of the thumb is based on the history and physical examination. The extent of injury, including the degree of ligamentous disruption and the amount of ligamentous displacement, may be difficult to evaluate using physical examination, plain roentgenograms, and stress roentgenograms. When an associated avulsion of the volar base of the proximal phalanx (distal insertion of the ulnar collateral ligament) occurs, the diagnosis is simplified by the degree of displacement recognizable on the roentgenograms [10, 12, 28–30, 80, 82]. Therefore, it is advisable to obtain plain roentgenograms before stress testing, because the diagnosis may be apparent and the displace-

ment of the collateral ligament is not placed at risk during stress testing. If the physical examination (exclusive of forced stress testing) is suggestive and roentgenograms fail to confirm an avulsion, the degree of collateral ligament injury is unknown. It is important, therefore, to ascertain the degree of ligament disruption and the degree of ligament displacement in order to choose the appropriate management. Additional information can be obtained by stress testing, arthrography [10, 64], or ultrasonography, or all three.

STRESS TESTING. The normal abduction-adduction laxity of the MP joint is 0 to 20 degrees (average, 10 degrees) and, while generally symmetric, can vary among individuals and with the degree of thumb flexion [15]. For this reason, asymmetry of the MP joint stress over 10 degrees is a relative indication of instability. The joint should be tested both in full extension and in 20 to 30 degrees of flexion. It is difficult to obtain a pure abduction force without rotation, even with proper anesthesia. During stress testing, laxity exceeding 30 degrees suggests a complete injury; an opening of greater than 45 degrees is believed to be pathognomonic of complete rupture of the ulnar collateral ligament [16, 18, 19, 73–76]. The potential dangers of stress testing are progression of an incomplete tear to a complete tear, the displacement of a nondisplaced injury (i.e., creation of a Stener lesion), and the inability to determine the presence of a Stener lesion despite documentation of a complete ligamentous disruption.

ARTHROGRAPHY-ULTRASONOGRAPHY. To improve diagnostic accuracy and prevent iatrogenic injury, arthrography was introduced and was shown to be a valuable diagnostic and prognostic tool [10, 64]. The technique is performed easily in an office or an emergency room setting. Fluoroscopy enhances arthrography, but it is not required. Local anesthetic (2.0 ml 1% lidocaine) is mixed with 2.0 ml diatrizoate meglumine–diatrizoate sodium (Renografin-60), and 0.5 to 1.0 ml of this mixture is injected into the MP joint

[10, 64]. The extent of capsular damage, the degree of collateral ligament disruption, and the extent of collateral ligament displacement can then be evaluated [10, 64]. Arthrography has helped to document injuries with complete collateral ligament tears and allows informed treatment decisions. Although the technique is not burdensome, painful, difficult to perform, or time consuming, it is seldom employed, despite the fact that operation shows collateral ligament displacement (Stener lesions) in only 30 to 60 percent of complete ligamentous injuries [16, 70, 73].

Real-time ultrasonography is capable of delineating the collateral ligament and aiding the diagnosis of complete versus partial injury. This noninvasive technique, which does not involve ionizing radiation or any known biologic hazard, should be beneficial in evaluating soft-tissue injuries of the hand and requires further evaluation to determine its role in the management of collateral ligament injuries of the thumb.

### Treatment

PARTIAL INJURIES. There is almost universal agreement that incomplete injuries (grade I and II sprains) of the ulnar or radial collateral ligament can be treated nonoperatively. Immobilization for 4 to 6 weeks followed by protected activity for 3 to 6 months allows the ligament, which is anatomically positioned, to recover sufficiently for excellent function. A thumb spica cast or rigid orthosis for 2 to 4 weeks is generally sufficient treatment. If a cast is chosen, it can be removed at 2 weeks and the joint reevaluated. If instability is present, additional casting is necessary. If instability is not demonstrated, an orthosis or bivalved cast can be used for the remainder of the treatment. The optimal position of immobilization is with the MP joint slightly flexed, the proximal phalanx ulnarly deviated, and the wrist in the functional position.

COMPLETE INJURIES. The management and evaluation of grade III collateral ligament injuries are controversial [35, 56]. Recent information suggests that surgical intervention does not improve the natural history of the injury [61]. Some experts recommend well-molded cast immobilization as an initial treatment for all such injuries [15, 54, 61]; others advocate surgical repair of all complete injuries [16, 19, 21, 23, 28, 30, 46, 49–51, 70, 73]. Some believe that the position of the ligament is important and that operation should be reserved for displaced ligamentous injuries. The rationale for surgery is that nonoperative treatment is unpredictable, anatomic restoration of the collateral ligament is essential, and the natural history of nonanatomic ligament alignment is chronic MP joint pain and disability. Recent prospective analysis of ulnar collateral ligament strain suggests that these tenets may be false [61] and that nonoperative management may provide equal or improved results. Unfortunately, no study addresses the crucial issue of degree of collateral ligament disruption and degree of displacement at the time of examination. In most studies, "complete" collateral ligament injuries are lumped with "partial" injuries and there is no distinction between displaced complete injuries versus nondisplaced complete injuries. Therefore, many of the conclusions drawn by these authors may not be valid.

Bowers and Hurst [10], on the basis of stress roentgenograms and arthrographic findings in 20 patients and a review of 197 previously reported cases, concluded that instability of the thumb MP joint (defined as greater than 30 degrees of abduction on stress roentgenograms), coupled with arthrographic evidence of a displaced or trapped ligament, was the only indication for operative repair. These data strongly suggest the importance of grouping complete injuries based on displacement and not on the degree of ligamentous disruption. Nonoperative management of complete lesions without displacement has not been demonstrated to be inferior to open management of the same lesion [15, 61]. Conversely, in spite of the work of Pichora and coworkers [61], it is difficult to justify not reapproximating a displaced ligament (Stener lesion). Furthermore, some data suggest that nonoperative management (cast duration, 4–6 weeks) followed by critical examination and open management of the 10 to 30 percent of thumbs with persistent instability, gives results comparable to those of early open procedures [15].

Many authors continue to ignore benign diagnostic techniques in favor of early surgical repair based on physical examination alone or physical examination combined with stress roentgenograms. They justify this approach by saying that greater than 95 percent of the patients were happy with the results and, if the lesion is overlooked, secondary reconstruction is not as successful. While this position can perhaps be rationalized in terms of expedience, it is difficult to justify. Displaced collateral ligaments, Stener lesions without bony attachments, or both are identifiable [10, 64], and the natural history of nonoperative lesions [61] suggests that this issue requires reappraisal. The following plan for the management of complete collateral ligament injuries is suggested.

A. For collateral ligament injuries with an avulsed bony fragment visualized roentgenographically and concentrically reduced MP joint:
1. If the fragment lies in continuity with the proximal phalanx, the joint should not be stressed and a thumb spica cast should be applied for 4 to 6 weeks. After this interval, the cast should be removed and the joint gently stressed. If it is unstable, operative repair should be considered. If it is stable at 6 weeks, active motion can be initiated, with protection for an additional 2 to 3 months.
2. If the avulsed fragment is displaced roentgenographically, operative intervention with anatomic restoration of the collateral ligament is indicated.

B. When no fragment is visualized on plain roentgenograms:
1. If the joint is stable (valgus stress ≤ 10 degrees different from the opposite thumb) and the joint concentrically reduced, the thumb can be casted, with reevaluation at 2 to 4 weeks and additional splinting or casting as necessary.
2. If the joint is unstable (completely disrupted), arthrography should be used to determine the degree of collateral ligament displacement or eversion. Anatomic restoration should then be obtained if the collateral ligament is everted or displaced (generally by surgical intervention). As an alternative to operation, plaster immobilization and retesting at 4 to 6 weeks can be offered the patient.
3. If arthrography confirms collateral ligament disruption (complete tear) but anatomic position of the collateral ligament, then closed treatment (cast immobilization with the MP joint in slight flexion) is the treatment of choice.

As for the technique of repair, the ulnar collateral ligament is best approached through an ulnar mid-lateral incision over the proximal phalanx that connects to an oblique dorsal incision extending proximally over the metacarpal (Fig. 32-8). The incision should allow access to the dorsal retinaculum, metacarpal head, proximal phalanx, and volar capsule. After the branches of the superficial radial nerve have been identified and protected, the adductor aponeurosis is identified. If a displaced collateral ligament is present, it is generally at the edge of the adductor aponeurosis, the smooth border of which it may partially obscure [18, 19]. If reduction of the collateral ligament is blocked by the adductor aponeurosis, the ligament should be dissected free, splitting the adductor aponeurosis longitudinally. If a Stener lesion is not present, the adductor aponeurosis is split to expose the ulnar and palmar aspects of the MP joint and to outline the po-

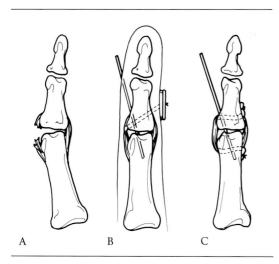

***Figure 32-8*** *Complete tears of collateral ligaments without joint subluxation (A) can be treated closed with modified extension block splinting. If the joint is unstable, open repair of the collateral ligament with a pullout button and joint stabilization can be performed (B), or reconstruction of the collateral ligament with a free tendon graft can be used if the ligament is not salvageable or with late repair (C).*

sition and continuity of the collateral ligament. The collateral ligament injury is then identified. If the ligament is avulsed from the proximal phalanx and has no bony attachment, it can be repaired directly, repositioned by a pullout technique (i.e., Bunell pullout wire or prolene suture over a button), or reinforced with local tissue (i.e., slip of the abductor pollicis longus) or a free tendon graft (i.e., palmaris longus) [4, 29, 54] (Fig. 32-8B, C). If there is a bony attachment, the type of repair depends on the size of the fragment. Small fragments are often reapproximated by pullout techniques, whereas large fragments can be fixed internally. If rupture occurs in the middle two-thirds of the tendon, it can be approximated with sutures. Proximal avulsions are rare and are managed in a similar manner as distal avulsions.

After reconstruction of the collateral ligament, the interface between the volar plate

and the collateral ligament must be reconstructed, and the dorsal capsule–collateral ligament juncture must be stabilized. Transarticular wire fixation depends on stability after ligamentous reconstruction and is often indicated. The MP joint should be immobilized in 20 degrees of flexion and deviated ulnarly. The adductor aponeurosis should be closed and the joint should be casted for 4 weeks and then splinted for an additional 2 to 3 weeks.

### CHRONIC ULNAR COLLATERAL LIGAMENT INJURIES

Chronic ulnar collateral ligament injuries can be managed by reconstruction of the ligament from local tissue and the scarred remnants of the collateral ligament [48, 50, 51], dynamic tendon transfers [39], stabilization by local static tendon transfers [29, 41, 42, 59, 66], free tissue transfers [29, 70], or MP fusion [28, 41, 42].

### RADIAL COLLATERAL LIGAMENT INJURIES

Although this entity is less frequent, its potential morbidity is equal to that of ulnar collateral ligament injuries, and the diagnosis and management are comparable.

## Interphalangeal Joints

### PROXIMAL INTERPHALANGEAL JOINT (FINGERS)

*Pathologic Anatomy*

The inherent stability of the PIP joint is produced by its articular configuration, intrinsic ligamentous and capsular integrity, and extrinsic flexor and extensor mechanisms [9, 11]. The lateral capsular collateral ligaments, accessory collateral ligaments, and volar plate provide intrinsic stability, and subluxation or dislocation cannot occur without injury to two or more components of the lateral volar complex.

Dorsal, lateral, or palmar dislocations can occur in the PIP joint. Dorsal injuries, in which the middle phalanx is displaced dor-

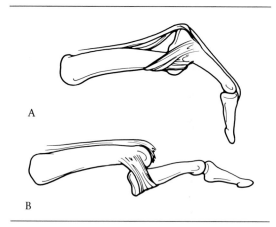

**Figure 32-9** *Dislocations of the proximal interphalangeal joint. A. Dorsal. B. Palmar.*

sally (Fig. 32-9A), are the most common and can involve avulsion of the volar plate from the middle phalanx and a split in the collateral ligaments, avulsion of the volar plate and a major split in the collateral ligaments, and fracture dislocation of the volar plate and a split in the collateral ligaments. The volar plate rarely ruptures proximally, but when it does, it can become interposed and prevent closed reduction (Table 32-1). Fracture dislocations are stable or unstable, generally depending on the percentage of intraarticular displacement. Lateral dislocations are secondary to abduction-adduction stress, generally associated with extension, and result in complete disruption of the collateral ligament and partial avulsion of the volar plate (Table 32-1). Palmar dislocations are rare and result from rotatory longitudinal compression on a semiflexed middle phalanx (Fig. 32-9B). Collateral ligament injury involves complete disruption of the collateral ligament, partial avulsion of the volar plate, and injury to the extensor mechanism [63].

## Classification

Subdivision of PIP injuries can be based on the direction of subluxation-dislocation and the potential for maintenance of concentric reduction with operative intervention or internal fixation (see Table 32-1). Unstable injuries are relatively rare without significant bony involvement [17, 19, 71].

For discussion purposes, injuries can be grouped according to the classification outlined in Table 32-1. Types I, II, and III are hyperextension injuries, and ligamentous or bony damage, or both, increase in the higher categories. The volar plate is always disrupted or avulsed and collateral ligaments are involved to varying degrees in all three injuries. Type IIA and IIIA injuries, in general, can be concentrically reduced and maintained in position by closed means. In type IIB, the volar plate is avulsed from the proximal phalanx and can be interposed, preventing reduction. In type IIIB injuries, the extent of the intraarticular fracture determines if the injury is unstable.

In type IV injuries, one collateral ligament is disrupted completely and the volar plate is partially injured. Type V injuries involve the extensor mechanism as well as the collateral ligament and the volar plate. In type VA injuries, the extensor mechanism is split between the central slip and lateral band; in type VB injuries, the central slip may be avulsed or torn.

## Evaluation

A careful physical examination, including palpation of the areas of maximal tenderness, estimation of lateral and posteroanterior stability, and appropriate roentgenograms (anteroposterior, lateral, oblique), are necessary for complete initial evaluation. Stability must be assessed during active and passive activity and, if doubt remains, fluoroscopic evaluation may be helpful; local anesthesia is often necessary for definitive evaluation. Complete injuries will demonstrate instability. Partial injuries will be stable, but point tenderness, pain with motion, and swelling will be elicited. Arthrography, plain roentgenograms, and fluoroscopy will be normal. Ultrasound or magnetic resonance imaging will demonstrate mid-substance lesions. The initial eval-

**Table 32-1** *Proximal interphalangeal injuries*

| Category | Mechanism | Pathology | |
|---|---|---|---|
| | | Volar plate | Collateral ligament |
| I. Dorsal subluxation | | | |
| Type I (subluxation) | Hyperextension | Middle phalanx avulsion | Split |
| II. Dorsal dislocation | | | |
| Type A (dorsal) | Hyperextension | Middle phalanx avulsion | Major split |
| Type B (complex) | Hyperextension | Proximal phalanx avulsion Interruption of volar plate | Major split |
| III. Fracture dislocation | | | |
| Type A | Compression-shear | Fracture dislocation of middle phalanx and volar plate Fracture fragment < 40% stable | Major split |
| Type B | Compression-shear | Fracture fragment > 40% unstable | |
| IV. Lateral dislocation | | | |
| Type A | Lateral force extension | Partial avulsion of middle phalanx | Complete rupture of at least one collateral ligament |
| Type B | Lateral force extension | Partial avulsion of middle phalanx | Complete rupture with interposition |
| V. Palmar dislocation | | | |
| Type A | Longitudinal compression, rotatory component, on semiflexed middle phalanx | Partial avulsion of middle phalanx | Complete rupture of at least one collateral ligament |
| Type B | Longitudinal compression, rotatory component, on semiflexed middle phalanx | Partial avulsion of middle phalanx | Extensor mechanism disruption |

uation should be repeated after reduction or manipulation to verify concentric reduction and the degree of relative stability.

*Treatment*
The treatment goal in PIP joint injuries should be to obtain a stable concentric reduction that will permit early range of motion. Decreased motion is the major unfavorable result in the management of PIP injuries and early active motion is important to prevent stiffness.

DORSAL PIP DISLOCATIONS (TYPES I–III, ACUTE). Dorsal dislocations, with the exception of type IIB (interposition of proximally avulsed volar plate), generally can be reduced easily with longitudinal radial and dorsal pressure on the middle phalanx. Types I, IIA, IIIA, and IVA injuries are relatively stable, and concentric reduction can be maintained during

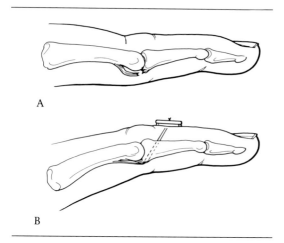

**Figure 32-10** *Reconstruction of torn volar plate (A) by pullout technique. Additional splinting (extension block type) is usually necessary.*

active and passive testing. Although traction devices have been recommended and are helpful in maintaining stability [3, 18, 19], these injuries, if stable, are best managed by extension block splinting [18, 19, 47] for 2 to 3 weeks. This technique allows active but restricted range of motion. Extension of the middle phalanx is blocked by a dorsal splint. The degree of flexion necessary to maintain concentric reduction is determined and the splint fabricated. Weekly, or more often as the injury stabilizes, the splint is extended. If the joint is unstable and concentric reduction is not maintained, open reduction with stability of the volar plate is indicated (Fig. 32-10).

Unstable injuries (IIB, IIIB) may require open reduction for concentric restoration of joint congruity or may be unstable unless range of motion is severely restricted. Rigid immobilization of the PIP, in general, results in a stiff, poorly functioning digit. Therefore, operative intervention to achieve stability sufficient to allow active or passive PIP range of motion is advocated by most authors [18, 20, 44, 45, 81]. In type IIIB injuries, large fragments can either be fixed internally by small wires or screws or be held in position by pullout sutures (Fig. 32-11). If the

fragments are too small or too severely comminuted for anatomic reduction, they can be resected and the volar plate advanced into the defect by a pullout technique [22]. Postoperative management is by extension block splinting for 2 to 4 weeks.

Complications of these techniques include failure to obtain and maintain concentric reduction, flexion contracture of the PIP joint, stiffness of the distal interphalangeal (DIP) joint if the extensor mechanism is tethered during open reduction or pullout techniques, and chronic volar plate laxity. Attention to detail will minimize failure to obtain and maintain concentric reduction and chronic volar plate laxity. Residual flexion deformity (5–10 degrees) is a common problem, and, in part, it is a reflection of the degree of soft-tissue damage and biologic response of the host. Flexion deformity can be minimized by careful observation and maximal maintenance of active and passive

**Figure 32-11** *Fracture dislocation, PIP joint (A). Management of avulsion of middle phalanx and volar plate by pullout technique (B) or screw (C).*

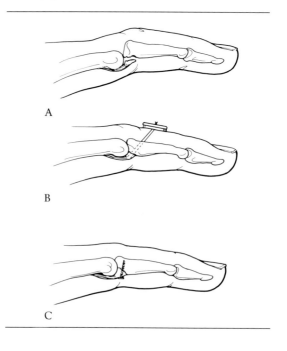

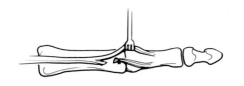

**Figure 32-12** *Chronic PIP hyperextension secondary to volar plate laxity can be reconstructed by using half of the flexor digitorum superficialis.*

range of motion within the restrictions of the magnitude of injury and trauma.

DORSAL PIP DISLOCATIONS (CHRONIC). Chronic volar plate laxity and hyperextension deformities are encountered, can be unstable, and can interfere with finger function or result in painful swan-neck deformities. The original deformity may be isolated to the volar plate or involve fragments from the middle phalanx. PIP hyperextension can result directly from volar plate laxity.

Treatment is surgical and involves advancement and reattachment of the volar plate [9, 11, 58, 62], plication of local tissue, use of a free tendon graft [1], reconstruction of collateral ligament–volar plate integrity [7], or superficialis tenodesis [43, 45, 58, 78] (Fig. 32-12).

LATERAL PIP DISLOCATIONS. When closed concentric reduction is successful, these injuries are best managed by extension block splinting modified to protect or prevent radial and ulnar forces on the PIP joint. Open reduction is necessary if stable concentric reduction is not possible.

PALMAR PIP DISLOCATIONS. These rare injuries are often incompletely appraised and the injury to the extensor mechanism is missed. Open reduction is indicated if extensor mechanism interposition prevents closed reduction (that is, management of boutonnière deformity). Reduction can be followed by gentle traction with MP and PIP flexion [79]. If the central slip is disrupted (as determined by operative inspection or clinical examination), postoperative management should

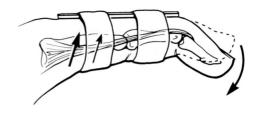

**Figure 32-13** *Management of buttonhole deformity by dorsal splinting of the proximal and middle phalanx and active range of motion of the DIP joint. Flexion of the DIP joint pulls the lateral band dorsally, preventing chronic deformity.*

be correction of the buttonhole deformity with dorsal splinting of the PIP joint, allowing active flexion of the DIP joint (Fig. 32-13).

## DISTAL INTERPHALANGEAL JOINT (FINGERS) AND INTERPHALANGEAL JOINT (THUMB)

Irreducible acute injuries can occur to the DIP joints of the digits or interphalangeal joint of the thumb, but they are infrequent

**Figure 32-14** *Traumatic mallet finger secondary to tear of extensor mechanism or avulsion of dorsal distal phalanx.*

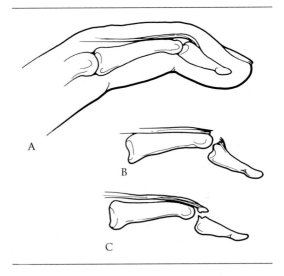

A

B

C

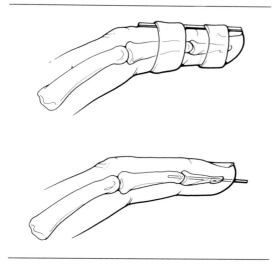

***Figure 32-15*** *Management of traumatic extensor mechanism disruption of DIP joint.*

[40, 57, 60, 67, 68, 77]. In general, these injuries are easily reduced and are relatively stable. Dorsal dislocations are most common and palmar subluxation with avulsion of the extensor mechanism from the distal phalanx (mallet finger) is frequent (Fig. 32-14). Reduction is obtained by gentle traction and can be maintained, and any associated mallet finger deformity managed, by dorsal splinting for 4 to 6 weeks [27, 31, 72] or by longitudinal pin fixation (Fig. 32-15).

# References

1. Adams, J. P. Correction of chronic dorsal subluxation of the proximal interphalangeal joint by means of a criss-cross volar graft. *J. Bone Joint Surg.* 41A:111, 1959.
2. Adler, G. A., and Light, T. R. Simultaneous complex dislocation of the metacarpophalangeal joints of the long and index fingers: A case report. *J. Bone Joint Surg.* 63A:1007, 1981.
3. Agee, J. M. Unstable fracture dislocations of the proximal interphalangeal joint of the fingers: A preliminary report of a new treatment technique. *J. Hand Surg.* 3:386, 1978.
4. Alldred, A. J. Rupture of the collateral ligament of the metacarpophalangeal joint of the thumb. *J. Bone Joint Surg.* 37B:443, 1955.
5. Barash, H. L. An unusual case of dorsal dislocation of the metacarpophalangeal joint of the index finger. *Clin. Orthop.* 83:121, 1972.
6. Barenfeld, P. A., and Weseley, M. S. Dorsal dislocation of the metacarpophalangeal joint of the index finger treated by late open reduction. *J. Bone Joint Surg.* 54A:1311, 1972.
7. Bate, J. T. An operation for the correction of locking of the proximal interphalangeal joint of the finger in hyperextension. *J. Bone Joint. Surg.* 27:142, 1945.
8. Betz, R. R., Browne, E. Z., Perry, G. B., et al. The complex volar metacarpophalangeal joint dislocation. A case report and review of the literature. *J. Bone Joint Surg.* 64A:1374, 1982.
9. Bowers, W. H. The proximal interphalangeal joint volar plate. II. A clinical study of hyperextension injury. *J. Hand Surg.* 6:77, 1981.
10. Bowers, W. H., and Hurst, L. C. Gamekeeper's thumb. Evaluation by arthrography and stress roentgenography. *J. Bone Joint Surg.* 59A:519, 1977.
11. Bowers, W. H., Wolf, J. W., Jr. Nehil, J., et al. The proximal interphalangeal joint volar plate. I. An anatomical and biomechanical study. *J. Hand Surg.* 5:79, 1980.
12. Browne, E., Dunn, H. K., and Snyder, C. C. Ski pole thumb injury. *Plast. Reconstr. Surg.* 58:19, 1976.
13. Campbell, C. S. Gamekeeper's thumb. *J. Bone Joint Surg.* 37B:148, 1955.
14. Chen, V. T. Dislocation of the carpometacarpal joint of the thumb. *J. Hand Surg.* 12B:246, 1987.
15. Coonrad, R. W., and Goldner, J. L. A study of the pathological findings and treatment in soft-tissue injury of the thumb metacarpophalangeal joint. *J. Bone Joint Surg.* 50A:439, 1968.
16. Derkash, R. S., et al. Acute surgical repair of the skier's thumb. *Clin. Orthop. Rel. Res.* 216:29, 1987.
17. Donaldson, W. R., and Millender, L. H. Chronic fracture-subluxation of the proximal interphalangeal joint. *J. Hand Surg.* 3:149, 1978.
18. Dray, G., Millender, L. H., and Nalebuff, E. A. Rupture of the radial collateral ligament of a metacarpophalangeal joint to one of the ulnar three fingers. *J. Hand Surg.* 4:346, 1979.
19. Dray, G. J., and Eaton, R. G. Dislocation and Ligament Injuries in the Digits. In D. P. Green (ed.), *Operative Hand Surgery.* New York:

Churchill Livingstone, 1988. Pp. 777–812.

20. Eaton, R. G. *Joint Injuries of the Hand.* Springfield, IL: Thomas, 1971. Pp. 51–66.

21. Eaton, R. G., and Littler, J. W. Ligament reconstruction for the painful thumb carpometacarpal joint. *J. Bone Joint Surg.* 55A:1655, 1973.

22. Eaton, R. G., and Malerich, M. M. Volar plate arthroplasty for the proximal interphalangeal joint: A ten year review. *J. Hand Surg.* 5:260, 1980.

23. Eaton, R. G., et al. Ligament reconstruction for the painful thumb carpometacarpal joints: A long-term assessment. *J. Hand Surg.* 9A:692, 1984.

24. Fisher, M. R., Rogers, L. F., and Hendrix, R. W. Systematic approach to identifying fourth and fifth carpometacarpal joint dislocations. *A.J.R.* 140:319, 1983.

25. Fisher, M. R., Rogers, L. F., Hendrix, R. W., et al. Carpometacarpal dislocations. *C.R.C. Crit. Rev. Diagn. Imaging* 22:95–126, 1984.

26. Flatt, A. E. Fracture-dislocation of an index metacarpophalangeal joint and ulnar deviating force in the flexor tendons. *J. Bone Joint Surg.* 48A:100, 1966.

27. Fowler, F. D. New splint for treatment of mallet finger. *J.A.M.A.* 170:945, 1959.

28. Frank, W. E., and Dobyns, J. H. Surgical pathology of collateral ligamentous injuries of the thumb. *Clin. Orthop.* 83:102, 1972.

29. Frykman, G., and Johansson, O. Surgical repair of rupture of the ulnar collateral ligament of the metacarpophalangeal joint of the thumb. *Acta Chir. Scand.* 112:58, 1956.

30. Gerber, C., Senn, E., and Matter, P. Skier's thumb. Surgical treatment of recent injuries to the ulnar collateral ligament of the thumb's metacarpophalangeal joint. *Am. J. Sports Med.* 9:171, 1981.

31. Gray, G. J., and Eaton, R. G. Dislocation and Ligament Injuries in the Digits. In D. P. Grem (ed.), *Operative Hand Surgery.* New York: Churchill Livingstone, 1988. Pp. 777–811.

32. Green, D. P., and Jerry, G. C. Complex dislocation of the metacarpophalangeal joint. *J. Bone Joint Surg.* 55A:1480, 1973.

33. Hartwig, R. H., and Louis, D. S. Multiple carpometacarpal dislocations. A review of four cases. *J. Bone Joint Surg.* 61A:906, 1979.

34. Hazlett, J. W. Carpometacarpal dislocations other than the thumb. A report of 11 cases. *Can. J. Surg.* 11:315, 1968.

35. Helm, R. H. Hand function after injuries to the collateral ligaments of the metacarpophalangeal joint of the thumb. *J. Hand Surg.* 12B:252, 1987.

36. Hunt, J. C., Watts, H. B., and Glasgow, J. D. Dorsal dislocation of the metacarpophalangeal joint of the index finger with particular reference to open dislocation. *J. Bone Joint Surg.* 49A:1572, 1967.

37. Johnson, F. G., and Greene, M. H. Another cause of irreducible dislocation of the proximal interphalangeal joint of a finger. *J. Bone Joint Surg.* 48A:542, 1966.

38. Kaplan, E. B. Dorsal dislocation of the metacarpophalangeal joint of the index finger. *J. Bone Joint Surg.* 39A:1081, 1957.

39. Kaplan, E. B. The pathology and treatment of radial subluxation of the thumb with ulnar displacement of the head of the first metacarpal. *J. Bone Joint Surg.* 43A:541, 1961.

40. Kitagawa, H., and Kashimoto, T. Locking of the thumb at the interphalangeal joint by one of the sesamoid bones. A case report. *J. Bone Joint Surg.* 66A:1300, 1984.

41. Lamb, D. W., and Angarita, G. Ulnar instability of the metacarpophalangeal joint of the thumb. *J. Hand Surg.* 10B:113, 1985.

42. Lamb, D. W., Abernathy, P. J., and Fragiadakis, E. Injuries of the metacarpophalangeal joint of the thumb. *Hand* 3:164, 1971.

43. Lane, C. S. Reconstruction of the unstable interphalangeal joint: The double superficialis tenodesis. *J. Hand Surg.* 3:368, 1978.

44. Lee, M. L. H. Intra-articular and peri-articular fractures of the phalanges. *J. Bone Joint Surg.* 45B:103, 1963.

45. McCue, F. C., Honner, R., Johnson, M. C. Jr., et al. Athletic injuries of the proximal interphalangeal joint requiring surgical treatment. *J. Bone Joint Surg.* 52A:937, 1970.

46. McCue, F. C., Hakala, M. W., Andrews, J. R., et al. Ulnar collateral ligament injuries of the thumb in athletes. *J. Sports Med.* 2:70, 1974.

47. McElfresh, E. C., Dobyns, J. H., and O'Brien, E. T. Management of fracture-dislocation of the proximal interphalangeal joints by extension-block splinting. *J. Bone Joint Surg.* 54A:1705, 1972.

48. Melone, C. P., Brodsky, J. W., and Hendrikson, R. P. Primary and secondary repair of thumb metacarpophalangeal joint collateral ligament injuries. *Orthop. Trans.* 8:382, 1984.

49. Milch, H. Recurrent dislocation of the thumb.

Capsulorrhaphy. *Am. J. Surg.* 6:327, 1929.

50. Moberg, E. Fractures and ligamentous injuries of the thumb and fingers. *Surg. Clin. North Am.* 40:297, 1960.

51. Moberg, E., and Stener, B. Injuries to the ligaments of the thumb and fingers. Diagnosis, treatment, and prognosis. *Acta Chir. Scand.* 106:166, 1953.

52. Moneim, M. S. Volar dislocation of the metacarpophalangeal joint: Pathological anatomy and report of two cases. *Clin. Orthop.* 176:186, 1983.

53. Murphy, A. F., and Stark, H. H. Closed dislocation of the metacarpophalangeal joint of the index finger. *J. Bone Joint Surg.* 49A:1579, 1967.

54. Neviaser, R. J., Wilson, J. N., and Lievano, A. Rupture of the ulnar collateral ligament of the thumb (gamekeeper's thumb). Correction by dynamic repair. *J. Bone Joint Surg.* 53A:1357, 1971.

55. Nutter, P. D. Interposition of sesamoids in metacarpophalangeal dislocations. *J. Bone Joint Surg.* 22:730, 1940.

56. Osterman, A. L., Hayken, G. D., and Bora, F. W. M. A quantitative evaluation of thumb function after ulnar collateral repair and reconstruction. *J. Trauma* 21:854, 1981.

57. Palmer, A. K., and Linscheid, R. L. Irreducible dorsal dislocation of the distal interphalangeal joint of the finger. *J. Hand Surg.* 2:406, 1977.

58. Palmer, A. K., and Linscheid, R. L. Chronic recurrent dislocation of the proximal interphalangeal joint of the finger. *J. Hand Surg.* 3:95, 1978.

59. Parikh, M., Nahigan, S., and Froimson, A. Gamekeeper's thumb. *Plast. Reconstr. Surg.* 58:24, 1976.

60. Phillips, J. H. Irreducible dislocation of a distal interphalangeal joint: Case report and review of literature. *Clin. Orthop.* 154:188, 1981.

61. Pichora, D. R., McMurtry, R. Y., and Bell, M. J. Gamekeeper's thumb: A prospective study of functional bracing. *J. Hand Surg.* 14A:567, 1989.

62. Portis, R. B. Hyperextensibility of the proximal interphalangeal joint of the finger following trauma. *J. Bone Joint Surg.* 36A:1141, 1954.

63. Redler, I., and Williams, J. T. Rupture of a collateral ligament of the proximal interphalangeal joints of the fingers. *J. Bone Joint Surg.* 49A:322, 1967.

64. Resnick, D., and Danzig, L. A. Arthrographic evaluation of injuries of the first metacarpophalangeal joint: Gamekeeper's thumb. *Am. J. R.* 126:1046, 1976.

65. Robbins, R. H. C. Injuries of the metacarpophalangeal joints. *Hand* 3:159, 1971.

66. Sakellarides, H. T., and DeWeese, J. W. Instability of the metacarpophalangeal joint of the thumb. Reconstruction of the collateral ligaments using the extensor pollicis brevis tendon. *J. Bone Joint Surg.* 58A:106, 1976.

67. Salamon, P. B., and Gelberman, R. H. Irreducible dislocation of the interphalangeal joint of the thumb. Report of 3 cases. *J. Bone Joint Surg.* 60A:400, 1978.

68. Selig, S., and Schein, A. Irreducible buttonhole dislocations of the fingers. *J. Bone Joint Surg.* 22A:436, 1940.

69. Shah, J., and Patel, M. Dislocation of the carpometacarpal joint of the thumb. A report of four cases. *Clin. Orthop.* 175:166, 1983.

70. Smith, R. J. Post-traumatic instability of the metacarpophalangeal joint of the thumb. *J. Bone Joint Surg.* 59A:14, 1977.

71. Spinner, M., and Choi, B. Y. Anterior dislocation of the proximal interphalangeal joint. *J. Bone Joint Surg.* 52A:1329, 1970.

72. Stark, H. H., Boyes, J. H., and Wilson, J. N. Mallet finger. *J. Bone Joint Surg.* 44A:1061, 1962.

73. Stener, B. Displacement of the ruptured ulnar collateral ligament of the metacarpophalangeal joint of the thumb. A clinical and anatomical study. *J. Bone Joint Surg.* 44B:869, 1962.

74. Stener, B. Hyperextension injuries to the metacarpophalangeal joint of the thumb—rupture of ligaments, fracture of sesamoid bones, rupture of the flexor pollicis brevis. An anatomical and clinical study. *Acta Chir. Scand.* 125:275, 1963.

75. Stener, B. Skeletal injuries associated with rupture of the ulnar collateral ligament of the metacarpophalangeal joint of the thumb. A clinical and anatomical study. *Acta Chir. Scand.* 125:583, 1963.

76. Stener, B., and Stener, I. Shearing fractures associated with rupture of the ulnar collateral ligament of the metacarpophalangeal joint of the thumb. *Injury* 1:12, 1969.

77. Stripling, W. D. Displaced intra-articular os-

teochondral fracture—cause for irreducible dislocation of the distal interphalangeal joint. *J. Hand Surg.* 7:77, 1982.

78. Swanson, A. B. Surgery of the hand in cerebral palsy and swan neck deformity. *J. Bone Joint Surg.* 42A:951, 1960.

79. Thompson, J. S., and Eaton, R. G. Volar dislocation of the proximal interphalangeal joint. *J. Hand Surg.* 2:232, 1977.

80. White, G. M. Ligamentous avulsion of the ulnar collateral ligament of the thumb in a child. *J. Hand Surg.* 11A:669, 1986.

81. Wiley, A. M. Instability of the proximal interphalangeal joint following dislocation and fracture dislocation: Surgical repair. *Hand* 2:185, 1970.

82. Winslet, M. C., et al. Breakdancer's thumb—partial rupture of the ulnar collateral ligament with fracture of the proximal phalanx of the thumb. *Injury* 17:201, 1986.

83. Wood, M. B., and Dobyns, J. H. Chronic complex volar dislocation of the metacarpophalangeal joint: Report of three cases. *J. Hand Surg.* 6:73, 1981.

# 33

*Harold M. Dick*
*Eric C. Carlson*

# Fractures of the Fingers and Thumb

The most common fractures in the skeleton occur in the small tubular bones of the hands and feet. Of these fractures the phalanges are the most frequently seen. In fact the distal phalanx has been estimated as representing the site of more than one-half of all hand fractures. The metacarpals and phalanges follow in the order of most frequently injured small tubular bones of the hand [6, 8].

All fractures of the hand can be, and often are, complicated by associated, multiple soft-tissue injuries, including crushing wounds, mangle, and partial amputations. The principles of fracture care are discussed in the individual sections dealing with specific tubular bones. Experiences during the recent wars have provided the basis for several specific principles [4]. First, skeletal injuries must be stabilized before one deals with the soft-tissue problems. Second, the early dressings should offer firm compression in the position of function or reduction to reduce edema. Third, and most important, early, active motion is the sine qua non for satisfactory small-joint motion after fracture. The compromise between stabilization for bone, nerve, and tendon healing versus early motion for small-joint recovery is the difficult dilemma all hand surgeons must solve on an individual patient basis [3, 8, 9].

## Roentgenographic Examination

X-ray examination is a prerequisite for all significant hand injuries. Children should always have both hands or digits x-rayed to help decide whether epiphyseal injuires are present. It is most helpful to x-ray the digit involved, not the entire hand, because of the problem of parallax. Three views are essential: anteroposterior, lateral, and 45-degree oblique. Articular fractures are often not seen without the oblique views. Small dental film has often been useful for better identification of small fragments. The metacarpals are best outlined in 10 degrees of supination (for the fourth and fifth metacarpals) or 10 degrees of pronation (for the second and third metacarpals) [8].

## Anesthesia

The majority of all hand injuries can be managed by regional anesthesia. General anesthesia becomes necessary only when concomitant injuries, or complex injuries in children under 7 years of age, are being treated. Axillary block is our procedure of choice although it has not been reliable in all circumstances. For brief procedures Bier's block using intravenous lidocaine and a double pneumatic tourniquet has been the most reliable and effective procedure. The combination of median and ulnar nerve blocks at the wrist level (with supplementary infiltration for the respective dorsal cutaneous branches) is advocated by Green and Rowland [6]. We deplore the use of digital blocks in the treatment of hand fractures or the use of any lidocaine with epinephrine. The possibility of digital circulation compromise in an already injured digit can produce ischemic necrosis. The techniques of regional blocks are well discussed in specific anesthesiology texts [6].

## Fracture of the Thumb Metacarpal

The thumb metacarpal base is frequently injured, largely due to a clenched fist receiving a direct blow to the metacarpal head. Three major fracture types can result: first, a transverse fracture through the shaft (Fig. 33-1); second, an intraarticular fracture of the base of the metacarpal with a web lateral fragment of varying size (Bennett's fracture, Fig. 33-2); and third, and most infrequently, a comminuted intraarticular fracture of the base of the metacarpal (Rolando's fracture; Fig. 33-3). The fresh, extraarticular fracture (type I) is usually reduced by a closed technique and held in a plaster thumb spica for 6 weeks. A percutaneous wire can be used if needed.

Since its first description in 1882, Bennett's fracture (type II) has been treated by more than a dozen different techniques. We believe that the *fresh* fracture deserves an open reduction and small, smooth K-wire fixation (0.045 inch), maintaining the metacarpal in 45 degrees of abduction and 45 degrees of opposition. The pins are placed percutaneously (one or two may be required). The thumb is then placed in a plaster spica for 6 weeks, and the pins are removed at 8 weeks. The goal of anatomic reduction of all intraarticular fractures seems the most rational, although the thumb carpometacarpal

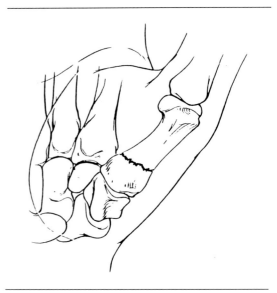

**Figure 33-1** *A 23-year-old man with transverse type I fracture shaft of the thumb metacarpal. The fracture was treated with splint protection for 4 weeks.*

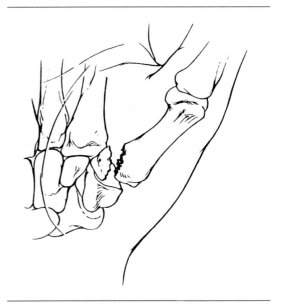

**Figure 33-2** *Type II, Bennett's fracture, an intraarticular fracture subluxation of the thumb metacarpocarpal joint.*

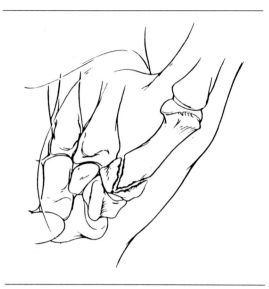

**Figure 33-3** *Type III, Rolando's fracture, a comminuted intraarticular fracture of the base of the metacarpocarpal joint.*

joint is very "forgiving" of joint incongruity. The size of the fracture fragment must be large enough to allow pin transfixion.

Rolando's fracture-dislocation is an even more challenging fracture to treat [8]. In the majority of cases, the comminution does not allow fragment pinning as described in Bennett's fracture. The two most helpful treatments are, first, a thumb spica cast in abduction and opposition of 45 degrees to relieve pain (10 to 12 days), followed by early active motion to remold the comminuted joint. The second choice of treatment is skeletal traction in 45 degrees of abduction and opposition with a K wire transversely through the proximal phalanx, held in a thumb spica cast with a rubber band outrigger for 6 to 8 weeks. The literature supports the principle that overzealous treatment is the cause of many poor results (especially open reduction in the face of severe comminution).

## Fracture of the Metacarpals

One of the most common sites of hand stiffness is the posttraumatic, or postimmobilization, stiff metacarpophalangeal joint. Most physicians believe that this is due to the common error of allowing the metacarpophalangeal joint to be immobilized in extension rather than flexion. The joint collateral ligaments are at maximum tightness in flexion. Thus, if they are allowed to remain in a cast in extension after adjacent injury and edema, the joint ligaments will contract and will be unable to easily renew good flexion motion because of the contracted collateral ligaments [2].

## Fracture of the Metacarpal Neck

Fractures of the metacarpal neck are the most common metacarpal fractures. They are seen most often in the fifth and fourth metacarpals, often after a direct blow by the closed fist. The angulation is always dorsal. There is approximately 15 degrees of anteroposterior motion of the fourth metacarpal and 25 degrees anteroposterior motion of the fifth metacarpal. The second and third metacarpals have negligible anteroposterior motion. This fact allows no angular deformity to be accepted by the index or third metacarpal or it will produce a painful prominence on grasping firm objects. The mobility of the fourth and fifth metacarpocarpal joints allows up to 25 degrees of angulation without grasp symptoms after healing. When there is a significant angulation (greater than 25 degrees) at the metacarpal neck site (Fig. 33-4), the fracture can be reduced closed, by placing the metacarpophalangeal joint in 90 degrees of flexion and pushing dorsally to reduce the fracture. The hazards of maintaining this position in plaster are too great, however; therefore, an intramedullary pin must be passed to hold the fracture. The fracture is held with a gutter splint for 3 weeks and the pin is removed at that time. The fracture is further protected

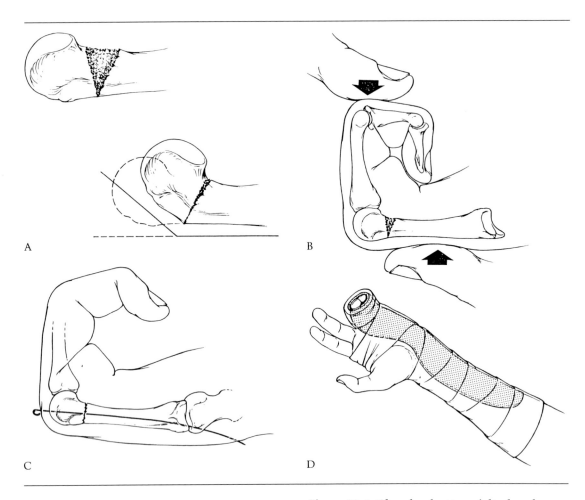

A

B

C

D

**Figure 33-4** *Closed reduction of displaced metacarpal neck fractures (especially the index and middle finger) with percutaneous pin fixation.*

for an additional 3 weeks by taping it to the adjacent finger [13].

The metacarpal shaft fracture falls into three categories: transverse fractures, short oblique fractures, and comminuted fractures. They usually have a dorsal angulation as a result of the pull of the interosseous muscles that arise from the shaft of the metacarpals. This deforming force exerts a greater force in flexion than the counterbalanced extrinsic extensor tendons resulting in the characteristic dorsal angulation of the metacarpal shafts.

The same principle applies for reduction of the metacarpal shaft as for metacarpal neck fractures. The fourth and fifth rays can accommodate angulations up to 10 and 25 degrees, respectively, without difficulty. Any angulation greater than this should be reduced. No angulation should be accepted in the third and second metacarpals. Once again the closed manipulation is not difficult, but most fractures require a percutaneous, smooth Kirschner's wire (0.045 inch) passed percutaneously down the medullary canal and out of the skin with the wrist flexed. The wires are removed at 3 weeks

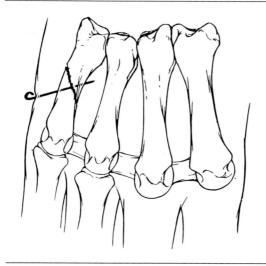

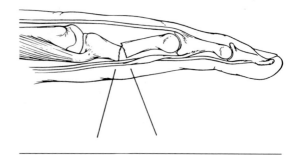

**Figure 33-6** *Displaced proximal phalanx fracture with volar angulation of the fracture site secondary to flexion of the proximal fragment by interossei and lumbricals. Extension of the distal fragment is caused by central slip and lateral bands.*

**Figure 33-5** *Percutaneous K-wire fixation of displaced oblique fracture of the fifth metacarpal shaft.*

and the fracture is protected in a plaster splint for 3 to 4 additional weeks.

Oblique fractures are best managed by passing Kirschner's wires at right angles to the shafts after reduction by traction and pinning them to the adjacent metacarpal tissue and below the fracture site (Fig. 33-5). The postreduction protocol remains the same [7].

Comminuted fractures of the shaft may require traction to maintain their length for 3 weeks' time. This is very hazardous because most traction wire usually passes through the proximal phalanx and the jeopardy to the extensor hood and intrinsic muscles is a real possibility. Fortunately, the indications are rarely encountered.

Bullet wounds commonly cause fractures of the metacarpal shaft. The bone-tissue loss in this circumstance may require a secondary bone graft. We generally prefer to maintain the metacarpal length with Kirschner's pins below the fracture site with the adjacent metacarpal, rather than face the hazards of traction. External fixators can be used alternatively.

## Fracture of the Proximal Phalanx

Fractures of the proximal phalanx are twice as common as fractures of the middle phalanx according to Belsky and associates [1]. The majority of fractures of the proximal phalanges are nondisplaced and only require taping to the adjacent normal finger for protection and assisted early active motion.

The fractures through the middle portion typically cause volar angulation of the fracture site. This is due to flexion of the proximal fragment by the transverse fibers of the interossei and lumbricals (Fig. 33-6). The angulation with the apex volar is produced by the distal fragment dorsiflexing because of the pull of the dorsal aponeurosis through the lateral bands and central slip of the extrinsic long extensor. With these forces in mind, in order to reduce the volar angulation it is necessary to flex the metacarpophalangeal joint to 60 or 70 degrees, with the proximal interphalangeal joint at no greater than 25 degrees of flexion (Fig. 33-7). Boyes [2a] recommends 50 to 70 degrees of flexion at the proximal interphalangeal joint. We believe that this may produce an uncommon amount of flexion contracture of the proximal interphalangeal joint. Much of the literature for maintaining these reductions

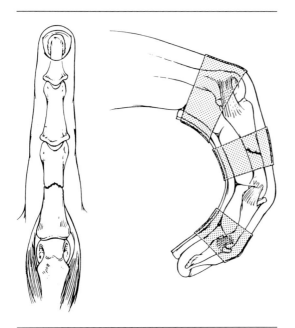

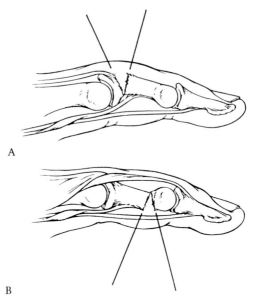

**Figure 33-7** *To reduce volar angulation relax interossei by flexing the metacarpophalangeal joint to 60 or 70 degrees.*

**Figure 33-8** *Middle phalanx fracture with volar or dorsal angulation depending on the fracture site and sublimus tendon insertion. When fracture is proximal to sublimus insertion, dorsal angulation results (A). When fracture is distal to sublimus insertion, volar angulation results (B).*

consists of elaborate and difficult traction apparatus [12].

For displaced or unstable fractures, we prefer closed reduction and percutaneous pinning of the fracture, followed by protective splinting and early motion. The traction techniques are reserved for the most difficult of the unstable fractures [1, 12].

### Fracture of the Middle Phalanx

The displaced fracture can have a volar or a dorsal angulation depending on the relationship of the fracture to the insertion of the sublimis tendon. When the fracture is proximal to the sublimis insertion, the extensor tendon central slip insertion extends the proximal phalanx and causes a dorsal angulation (Fig. 33-8A). When the fracture is distal to the sublimis insertion, the sublimis flexes the proximal fragment and causes volar angulation (Fig. 33-8B). Once again, in lieu of traction apparatus to maintain these

fractures, we have used percutaneous pins (Kirschner's wire, 0.045 inch) and early assisted active motion for these fractures [10].

The metacarpals, proximal phalanges, and middle phalanges must all be carefully evaluated after reduction for the proper rotational alignment. The proper alignment is confirmed by flexing the injured finger and moving its longitudinal axis, pointing to the tuberosity of the navicular. This should always be tested as a single finger, as multiple finger alignment prevents the adjacent fingers from pointing in the proper position [6, 8] (Fig. 33-9).

### Fracture of the Distal Phalanges

Fractures of the distal phalanges are probably the most frequent hand fractures (Fig. 33-10). They are rarely problems for healing

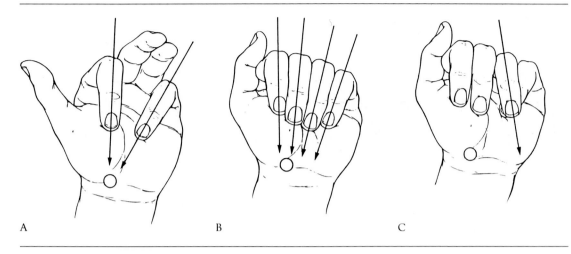

**Figure 33-9** *Rotational alignment is by individual digit alignment to point to the tuberosity of the navicular (A). If side by side (B) Malrotation will result (C).*

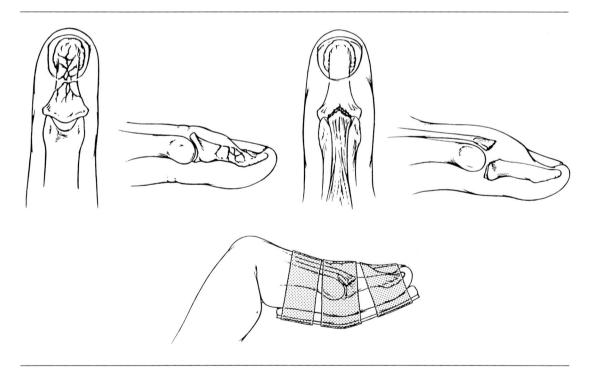

**Figure 33-10** *Comminuted distal phalanx fractures require no treatment other than symptomatic protection. The extensor tendons' fracture-avulsion can be treated open or closed.*

or deformity. The fresh injuries can be made less painful by releasing the subungual hematoma with a sterile no. 18 gauge needle. The only other treatment needed is for the purpose of protection from striking the painful tuft until healing has taken place in 10 to 14 days. We often use a bulky dressing for this reason. The hairpin splint described by Green and Rowland [6] is also helpful. It should be clear to the patient that any displaced intraarticular fracture involving more than 20 percent of the distal interphalangeal joints should be opened and reduced with Kirschner's wires or a pullout wire, as described by Wehbe and Schneider [11].

In summary, fractures of the small tubular bones of the hand are frequently overlooked and undertreated and often have poor results. We believe that a recognition of the dynamic anatomy, careful selection of the proper patient, and meticulous use of percutaneous pin insertion are the major techniques required to allow early motion and a satisfactory end result.

Unfortunately, intraarticular fractures of all the joints require open reductions and Kirschner's pin stabilization. This technique is very demanding even for the most expert surgeon, and the postoperative edema and scarring often produce as much stiffness as the intraarticular fracture. Rarely, extensive comminution may require skeletal traction in preference to open reduction.

# References

1. Belsky, M. R., Eaton, R. G., and Lane, L. B. Closed reduction and internal fixation of proximal phalangeal fractures. *J. Hand Surg.* 9A:725, 1984.
2. Belsole, R. Physiological fixation of displaced and unstable fractures of the hand. *Orthop. Clin. North Am.* 11:393, 1980.
2a. Boyes, J. H. *Bunnell's Surgery of the Hand,* (5th ed.). Philadelphia: Lippincott, 1970.
3. Breenwald, J. Bone healing in the hand. *Clin. Orthop.* 214:7, 1987.
4. Burkhalter, W. E., et al. Experiences with delayed primary closure of war wounds of the hand in Viet Nam. *J. Bone Joint Surg.* 50A:945, 1968.
5. Green, D. P., and O'Brien, E. T. Fractures of the thumb metacarpal. *South Med. J.* 65:807, 1972.
6. Green, D. P., and Rowland, S. A. Fractures and Dislocations in the Hand. In C. A. Rockwood and D. P. Green (eds.), *Fractures in Adults* (2nd ed.) Philadelphia: Lippincott, 1984.
7. Lamb, D. W., Abernathy, P. A., and Raine, P. A. M. Unstable fractures of the metacarpals: A new method of treatment by transverse wire fixation to intact metacarpals. *Hand* 5:43, 1973.
8. O'Brien, E. T. Fractures of the Metacarpals and Phalanges. In D. P. Green (ed.), *Operative Hand Surgery.* New York: Churchill Livingstone, 1988.
9. Packer, J. W., and Colditz, J. C. Bone injuries: Treatment and rehabilitation. *Hand Clin.* 2:81, 1986.
10. Schenck, R. R. Dynamic traction and early passive movement for fractures of the proximal interphalangeal joint. *J. Hand Surg.* 11A:850, 1986.
11. Wehbe, M. A., and Schneider, L. H. Mallet fractures. *J. Bone Joint Surg.* 66A:658, 1984.
12. Woods, G. L. Troublesome shaft fractures of the proximal phalanx. *Hand Clin.* 4:75, 1988.
13. Wright, T. A. Early mobilization in fractures of the metacarpals and phalanges. *Can. J. Surg.* 11:491, 1968.

H. Kirk Watson
M. Vincent Makhlouf

# 34
# Stiff Finger Joints

Joint stiffness is one of the more difficult problems in hand surgery. The ability to prevent contracture during the various phases of healing determines the ultimate success of treatment. Understanding how the anatomy influences contracture is paramount to dealing with it.

## Pathophysiology
### "NEGATIVE" HAND

The proximal and distal interphalangeal joints are different from the metacarpophalangeal joints. The initial response after trauma to a hand is an increase in tissue fluid—lymph, hemorrhage, or both, depending on the severity of the injury. Fluid increases in the tissues and in the joints. The fluid in the tissue of the capsule and collateral ligaments tends to produce effective shortening of these structures. The fluid inside the synovial space distends the capsule, and the joint assumes the position of maximum fluid capacity. The positional anatomic differences between flexion and extension are greatest in the metacarpophalangeal joints, and these joints are the key to the resultant negative hand. The *negative hand* is defined as the late fixed-hand deformity of finger interphalangeal flexion, meta-carpophalangeal extension, thumb adduction, and wrist flexion [2].

In a position just short of full extension, the metacarpophalangeal joint has maximum capsule laxity and maximum intracapsular fluid capacity. Abduction, adduction, and rotation are maximal, and the joint contact surface is small. When fully flexed, the intracapsular fluid capacity is minimal; the joint is stable, allowing little or no abduction, adduction, or rotation; and the collateral ligaments are tight with a broad, full-width joint contact surface.

After a crush, burn, or other injury, edema fluid hydraulically drives the metacarpophalangeal joints into extension. This position increases flexor tension and decreases extensor tension. The fingers flex at the proximal and distal interphalangeal joints. There is only minimal change in the fluid capacity of the flexed versus the extended interphalangeal joint and no hydraulic drive compared to the metacarpophalangeal joints. The positional changes in the interphalangeal joints are therefore secondary. The finger flexors tend to be central to the wrist motion axis because of their location in the carpal tunnel. However, their power is significant, and slight wrist flexion is usually present in a neglected, edematous hand (Fig. 34-1).

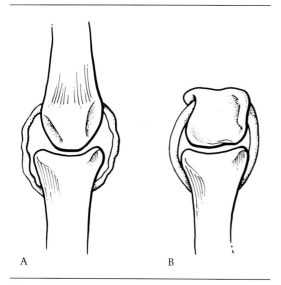

*Figure 34-1 The metacarpophalangeal joint in extension is different from the same joint in flexion. A. In full extension there is little contact area between the two articular surfaces. The capsule is lax, as are the collateral ligaments. Adduction-abduction and rotation are possible, and the joint has maximal fluid capacity. B. In flexion the contact area between the articular surfaces is large. The capsule is tight. The collateral ligaments are tight because of both cam action and their distention by the bony bulges of the volar metacarpal head. The joint is stable with nearly no abduction-adduction or rotation. There is minimal intrasynovial capacity. The joint easily returns to extension from this stable, tight, low tolerance state; this position, therefore, is ideal for immobilization.*

PATIENT EVALUATION

The most important part of dealing with stiffness or joint contracture is determining the etiology. One of the first principles is what we call the *seesaw effect*. This term simply means that a contractural structure spans two joints. If one joint is flexed, the other joint in the contractural system can then be extended. This seesaw effect is easily seen in a volar skin scar crossing the proximal and distal interphalangeal joints. The distal interphalangeal joint can be extended only if the proximal interphalangeal

joint is flexed and vice versa. This ability becomes less obvious, but no less important, when a tendinous structure crosses two joints.

A classic but slightly more complex instance is that of a tight oblique ligament of Landsmeer [7]. If fully contracted, the appearance is that of a boutonnière deformity. The seesaw band extends from the dorsal insertion of the extensor tendon at the distal phalanx to the volar bony ridge (assembly line) of the proximal phalanx [12] (Fig. 34-2). The band seesaws across two joints but is an extensor of the distal interphalangeal joint and a flexor of the proximal interphalangeal joint, which means that the distal joint may be flexed so long as the proximal interphalangeal joint is maintained in flexion. Passively extending the proximal interphalangeal joint brings the distal joint into full fixed extension. This particular example is called the *boutonnière test* and is positive in just this fashion with a boutonnière deformity.

Another example of this seesaw phenomena is the *Bunnell test* [3]. If the metacarpophalangeal joint is passively flexed in a patient with tight intrinsic muscles, the proximal and distal interphalangeal joints are easily flexed. If the metacarpophalangeal joint is extended, thereby tightening the already taut intrinsic mechanism, the middle and distal joints are forced into extension as the lateral band tightens over the dorsum of the proximal and distal interphalangeal joints. The inability to flex the proximal and distal interphalangeal joints with the metacarpophalangeal in zero flexion is indicative of tight intrinsic muscles as they affect more than one joint. Here the seesaw effect represents a positive Bunnell test [9].

FLEXION CONTRACTURES

Once stiffness and contracture have been limited to one joint, determining the offending structure becomes somewhat more difficult. A flexion contracture of the proximal interphalangeal joint, for instance, can be caused by any structure on the volar aspect of the proximal interphalangeal joint. Most volarly, Dupuytren's contracture can prevent extension. Deeper, an injured flexor sheath that has thickened and scarred may be producing flexion at the proximal interphalangeal joint. Either of the flexor tendons can be scarred down. Scar tissue itself can be preventing extension of the middle joint, and most commonly check reins are holding the volar plate fixed to the proximal phalanx. A bone block or articular damage represents the deepest cause of a flexed proximal interphalangeal joint [6].

Usually, an isolated problem in the extensor hood does not prevent passive extension. A useful tool is the "feel" of the joint as it is prevented from further extension. A more volar soft tissue structure can stop the joint with a gradually decreasing "rubbery" extensibility, whereas the check reins fixing the volar plate to the assembly line of the proximal phalanx stop extension in a sudden nonrubbery limit to extension. Much like the carriage of a typewriter at the end of its travel, there is an immediate, solid stop. Intraarticular deformity often produces rubbery, gradual prevention of further extension. Because the collaterals in the proximal and distal interphalangeal joints are generally tight in both flexion and extension, they are not usually a major etiologic factor in flexion or extension deformities of these two joints.

Prevention of flexion is occasionally secondary to a "jammed up" profundus tendon in an enclosed fibroosseous sheath. This problem can occur even if the tendon has been cut and scarred inside the sheath. The tendon fills and "jams" in the sheath, preventing the normal accordion collapse of the cruciform portions of the fibroosseous tunnel. The result is a slow, rubbery block to flexion.

EXTENSION CONTRACTURES
The extensor tendons are frequent causes of limitation to flexion of the proximal and dis-

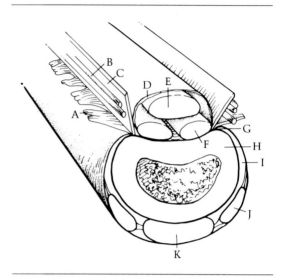

**Figure 34-2** *Section through the proximal aspect of the middle phalanx. (A = Cleland's ligament; B = neurovascular bundle; C = Grayson's ligament; D = flexor sheath; E = profundus tendon; F = sublimis tendon; G = "assembly line"; H = phalanx; I = transverse lamina of Landsmeer; J = lateral band; K = central slip.) The "assembly line" is the Sharpey fiber bone attachment area for the flexor sheath. All structures including Grayson's ligaments, Cleland's ligaments, transverse lamina of Landsmeer, and oblique ligament of Landsmeer. Dupuytren's and check reins attach to the "assembly line."*

tal interphalangeal joints. The hood commonly becomes bound to the bone proximal to the joint, which is usually a sudden, fixed stopping point to passive flexion.

Passive flexion prevented by a gentle, loose, rubbery stopping point that is extremely painful is most often a problem at the distal volar plate. The pain implies synovial involvement. The most common cause of a painful lack of passive flexion is a volar plate avulsion with or without a small fragment of bone torn from the base of the middle phalanx. We term this maneuver the *volar plate test*. A positive volar plate test after a minimum of 6 to 9 months postinjury usually warrants volar plate repair of the middle phalanx [1].

## TROPHIC CHANGE

Stiffness of a joint may be secondary to a panfibrosis as might be noted after reflex dystrophy or significant neurovascular injury. This overall stiffness and fibrosis is usually associated with trophic change. *Trophic change* is defined here as flattening of the cuticle base, increased nail curvature in both longitudinal and transverse planes, loss or decrease of bulk in the pulp of the finger, and flattening of the rugae pattern.

## *Distal Interphalangeal Joint Repair*

Stiffness in the distal joint is seldom a problem unless there is fixed flexion or hyperextension deformity. Stiffness with pain from arthritis is a joint problem, not a stiffness problem. Treatment of the underlying pathology resolves the stiffness of a swan neck or boutonnière deformity. A fixed extension deformity can often be treated by cutting the most dorsal and lateral fibers of the extensor tendon. Occasionally, complete transection of this tendon is indicated (severe burns and untreatable boutonnière deformity). Late untreated mallet deformities are seldom adequately salvaged by tendon work, and arthrodesis is frequently the procedure of choice.

## *Proximal Interphalangeal Joint Repair*

### NONOPERATIVE TREATMENT

*Splinting*

The conservative approach to interphalangeal contractures is basically the application of a nonelastic force in the direction of desired correction for long periods. Conservative treatment may be all that is necessary when minimal difficulties are anticipated, as in the prevention of contracture or during the postoperative period. A typical example is Dupuytren's contracture, where full simultaneous extension of all joints has been obtained at operation but the reaction in the

hand is expected to be significant. After the initial 3 days of total immobilization, a Joint-Spring (Joint Jack Company, East Hartford, CT) is used as a night splint. This same approach is usually beneficial after a trigger finger release. Its use at night for 1 to 2 weeks may be all the splinting that is necessary.

Ten days postoperatively or in circumstances of a more defined contracture of the proximal interphalangeal joint, stronger splinting measures are necessary. There are many splints available for this problem. We have found the Joint Jack to be the most powerful. The Joint Jack splint produces a vernier-controlled inelastic force. The splint is best applied 1 hour before bedtime, with the patient tightening the screw every 2 to 3 minutes to tolerance. At bedtime, the screw can be loosened a partial turn for comfort, and the patient sleeps with the splint in place with a piece of tape around the finger and the splint. The tape is necessary because the finger slowly and gradually straightens during the night, eventually causing the splint to drop off; thus the joint falls back into flexion if the splint is not secured. It is desirable to hold the extension for the maximum number of hours each night. If pain prevents sleep, the Joint Jack is applied in two 1-hour sessions each day. The screw is turned every 2 to 4 minutes initially and then less often as the rubbery phase, or "rapid gain phase," is overcome. Rapid correction occurs as fluid is driven from the tissues. The splint then works on the collagen. The rapid redeforming of the joint after splinting is indicative of the fluid return, and the patient must be made aware that the gains in collagen dissolution have not been in vain. Because of the "rapid gain phase" it is seldom beneficial to apply a Joint Jack for less than 30 to 40 minutes at a time. After surgery for severe joint damage or major joint trauma, it may be necessary to continue splinting for up to 1 year. One hour a day is usually sufficient. As weeks pass, the patient notes that less time and force are necessary to obtain full extension, and although the finger flexes after the splint is removed, it occurs more slowly and less severely as time goes on. Eventually the finger can be fully straightened in a minute or so, and finally active power alone can achieve full extension. At this stage, only the "rapid gain phase" itself exists, and the patient notes primarily morning stiffness (Fig. 34-3).

Splints such as the Wire-Foam spring finger extension splint are less powerful and less bulky and thus may be more acceptable for daytime use by the active or employed person. Single or multiple splints of this type can be worn either as the sole splint for proximal interphalangeal joint contractures or in conjunction with the Joint Jack, with the latter being used at night.

### Serial Casting

When dealing with resistant joint contractures, whether operated or nonoperated, the final nonoperative approach is serial casting. Usually, volar and dorsal splints are made from 2-inch plaster folded lengthwise to produce two 1-inch wide splints for the finger. They extend from the base of the palm to the tip of the finger and have one layer of cast padding. Three-point fixation is hand-held by the surgeon with significant force as the plaster dries. The volar distal pressure must be on the volar plate of the distal joint, not on the fingertip, and it must be at maximum patient tolerance. The splints are wrapped with gauze before drying and then taped when hard. The patient is instructed that burning pain over the contracted joint lasting for more than 2 hours must be relieved by cutting the tape or the gauze (or both) along the side of the finger [5]. Regardless of whether this step is necessary, the splint is taped increasingly tighter by the patient over a 1- to 3-day period. After approximately 3 days, a new splint is applied. In a difficult joint, the final straight splints are left in place for 1 to 2 weeks, at which time the Joint Jack program is started, often jack-

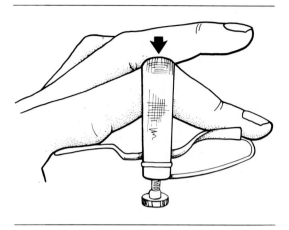

**Figure 34-3** *The Joint Jack places pressure on the volar plate of the distal joint, and the strap creates a volar moment on the proximal interphalangeal joint. The screw provides vernier control and significant drive to straighten the joint.*

ing the joint for most of the day initially and then progressing to the regular splinting program of 1 hour before bed and sleeping with the splint in place.

### OPERATIVE TREATMENT
### Flexion Deformity

The surgical approach to flexion contracture of the proximal interphalangeal joint begins with a zigzag incision volarly. These flaps can be advanced (YV) for skin length increase if necessary. Tight structures (Dupuytren's, sheath, tendons) are released or lysed as encountered. Check reins are the basic cause of flexion deformity [11] (Fig. 34-4). These two bands originate from thick, broad attachments along the proximal edge of the volar plate. They diverge proximally and insert separately along the volar lateral periosteum of the proximal phalanx along two bony ridges we call the "assembly line." Check reins are usually present as paired structures. The two digital arteries give off branches that run through the check reins to merge in the midline. These vessels feed the major vascular supply to the tendon vincular

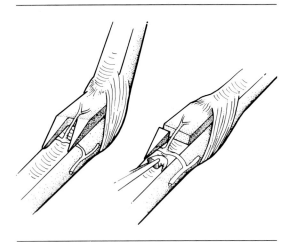

**Figure 34-4** *Check reins are responsible in almost all cases for contracture of the proximal interphalangeal joint. The volar plate is held to the "assembly line" by these two pyramidal collagenous structures. The vincular blood vessels are central and about 4 mm proximal to the volar plate. They arise from the transverse blood vessels that connect the two digital vascular bundles. They should be preserved during check rein release. Not shown here are dorsal portions of the check reins, which extend dorsal to the "assembly line" and can require release at the time of check rein excision. The release of the volar plate from the check reins does not violate the joint itself.*

system. It is essential that these vascular structures be preserved during check rein resection procedures. The proximal edge of the volar plate is identified, and the check reins are cut free from their broad triangular attachments to the proximal edge of the volar plate. This dissection must occasionally be carried laterally and dorsally along the side of the proximal phalanx in line with the proximal edge of the volar plate. The check rein is then elevated and removed, protecting the communicating nutrient vessel.

Because these structures lie well proximal to the most proximal edge of the volar plate, the joint is not violated by their resection. The collaterals have approximately the same tension in flexion as in extension, so it is almost never necessary to cut these ligaments. There is rarely a need to cut or remove the volar plate. This structure is essential to joint function. The check reins are the etiology of interphalangeal contracture, whether developmental (as in Dupuytren's) or traumatic (following crush injuries, fractures, and dislocations). A moderate amount of gentle, passive extension is often required to break up other small adhesions after check-rein resection, but full passive extension occurs every time if there is no bone block.

The joint is occasionally fixed in extension with a K-wire, but there are two problems that must be kept in mind with this technique: (1) The finger must be watched closely for neurovascular overstretch and embarrassment, particularly if it has been significantly flexed for a long period of time; and (2) cartilage necrosis can result if a cam action puts too much pressure on the fully extended joint surfaces. Rarely, at surgery the proximal interphalangeal joint "jumps" approaching full extension. This jump is a cam action, and the most dorsal fibers of both collaterals must be cut.

Postoperatively, the hand is immobilized in a bulky dressing and reinforced with a dorsal splint. After 3 to 7 days a light dressing is applied, and active movement of the joint is encouraged. A Joint Spring is applied at this stage. When the sutures are removed at approximately 14 days, a Joint Jack is applied in the standard fashion.

*Extension Deformity*
With pure joint extension contracture or when extension contracture develops associated with a nonjoint etiology, a dorsal capsulectomy is indicated [4, 8]. A dorsolateral approach exposes the hood. The transverse lamina of Landsmeer is cut, and the lateral band is elevated. The central slip must be preserved. The dorsal capsule is incised and the joint passively flexed. There usually are attachments of the extensor hood to the distal dorsal portion of the proximal phalanx. If

they are severe and the bed is poor, a small, thin Silastic sheet (0.005 inch or less) is placed underneath the hood over the scarred proximal phalanx. With severe articular fibrosis, it is occasionally necessary to cut the dorsalmost fibers of both collateral ligaments and free any volar plate pocket adhesions.

Unless the surgeon is absolutely sure that there are no other structures involved after release of an extension contracture of a finger joint, it is often wise to make a small incision in the volar wrist crease and demonstrate flexion of the finger by pulling on the profundus tendon (Fig. 34-5). Failure to produce good flexion by this maneuver indicates flexor tendon adherence.

**Figure 34-5** *Following capsulotomy or tenolysis, it is mandatory that the entire tendon system be checked for full and free excursion. It is usually accomplished through a small proximal incision.*

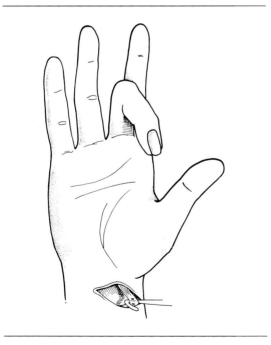

## Metacarpophalangeal Joint Repair

As noted earlier in the chapter, the metacarpophalangeal joint is actually two totally different joints. The anatomy of the extended metacarpophalangeal joint is different in the extreme from the anatomy of the flexed metacarpophalangeal joint. The loose collateral ligaments, free capsule, and small joint contact surface seen in the extended metacarpophalangeal joint produce a large intrasynovial capacity; the joint abducts and adducts easily and provides the only rotation in the entire digital ray. Any fibrosis of the collateral ligament or capsule with the joint in this position makes it difficult to achieve full flexion when the anatomy is at much closer tolerances. If the metacarpophalangeal joint is maintained in the flexed, tight-collateral position, it usually returns easily to extension. The anatomy of the volar plate is such that contractures seldom develop that can hold the metacarpophalangeal joint in the flexed position without external abnormalities, i.e., intrinsic and other nonjoint causes. The concept is so valid that Zancolli's volar plate capsulodesis into bone is probably contraindicated when the power of the extensor digitorum communis is normal. Even with such a surgically produced flexion contracture, the metacarpophalangeal joint gradually returns to full extension, stretching out the capsulodesis, and a claw deformity recurs. The fixed metacarpophalangeal flexion contracture is usually the result of dense postinjury fibrosis volar to the volar plate and involving the flexor sheath.

The problem then is to deal with extension contractures of the metacarpophalangeal joints. The initial conservative approach is usually a knuckle bender splint. Serial volar and dorsal plaster splints comprise the last-ditch conservative approach.

OPERATIVE TREATMENT
With a long-standing, severe contracture, the extended metacarpophalangeal joint is usually rigidly fixed by the collateral ligaments and dorsal capsule. These long-stand-

ing joint problems often require operative treatment. Through a dorsal zigzag incision, the dorsal neurovascular structures between the metacarpal heads are identified and carefully preserved in the areolar and fat tissue in which they lie. The sagittal band hood fibers are retracted distally or, if necessary, cut, usually on the ulnar side. These fibers of the sagittal band must be repaired during closure. The dorsal capsule is transected, and attempts at passive flexion are made. The collateral ligaments often cannot pass over the condyles, which are present on the volar aspect of the metacarpal head and support the proximal phalanx in full flexion. Under these circumstances, collateral ligament transection proximally at their attachments into the metacarpal head is indicated. Occasionally, cutting only the ulnar collateral ligament produces satisfactory flexion. However, both collateral ligaments usually must be cut because, although cutting one collateral allows the joint to be brought into flexion, careful observation demonstrates that the joint is springing open on the cut collateral side as flexion occurs. Under these circumstances, it is better to loosen the radial collateral as well, so that the proximal phalanx tracks normally over the head of the metacarpal. As with the extended interphalangeal joint, manipulation can probably free the volar plate; however, it is occasionally necessary to manually free volar plate adhesions. Postoperatively, these joints must be maintained in full flexion for the first week, and then active mobilization is allowed. Night splinting in full flexion may be necessary for several weeks.

## Congenital Disorders

A general approach for joint contractures present at birth is as follows: (1) Have the mother manipulate the joints into a corrected position several times a day. (2) Splinting is usually unsuccessful during the first 6 months of life because of the techni-cal limitations. (3) Volar skin tightness must be released and skin-grafted. Grafts must extend from midlateral to midlateral positions. (4) In general, surgical correction of a joint waits until the child is old enough to determine the presence of tendon control or that tendon control can be established around the time of surgical joint release.

A congenitally flexed thumb is usually due to one of three causes: (1) stenosing tenosynovitis; (2) spasticity; or (3) an inadequate extensor apparatus. Because the A-1 pulley is attached to the metacarpophalangeal joint volar plate, the stenosing tenosynovitis involves only the distal joint. Spasticity is easily distinguished from an inadequate extensor mechanism.

## Reflex Sympathetic Dystrophy

A patient with reflex dystrophy presents with an inability to flex or extend joints. It is then mandatory to make a distinction between the active dystrophy process and the ultimate fibrosis. Painful reflex sympathetic dystrophy is an active destructive process that requires immediate attention.

The "Dystrophile" tissue loading program is a successful approach with rapid results. This program consists in active traction and compression exercises that provide stress to the extremity without requiring joint motion that may aggravate the condition. Initially, increased pain and swelling may occur, but they generally subside within a few days as the neurovascular system begins to adapt [10].

The patient is instructed to use the Dystrophile in a "scrub the floor" pattern with the affected hand, applying increasing pressure as possible, as set on the Dystrophile three times a day for 3 to 7 minutes per session. The patient is also told to "carry" a weighted briefcase or purse in the affected hand throughout the day. The load is then increased as the patient's tolerance to the dystrophile program improves.

## Summary

With the exception of articular damage, almost all joint contractures can be eliminated or significantly improved. Approaching contracture with thorough analysis of the cause, applying a step-by-step program, and the patient "knowing" he or she will improve lead to confidence and satisfaction for both patient and surgeon.

## References

1. Bowers, W. H., Wolf, J. W., Nehil, J. L., et al. The proximal interphalangeal joint volar plate. I. An anatomical and biomechanical study. *J. Hand Surg.* 5:79, 1980.

2. Buch, V. I. Clinical and functional assessment of the hand after metacarpophalangeal capsulotomy. *Plast. Reconstr. Surg.* 53:452, 1974.

3. Bunnell, S., Doherty, E. W., and Curtis, R. M. Ischemic contracture, local, in the hand. *Plast. Reconstr. Surg.* 3:424, 1948.

4. Curtis, R. M. Stiff Finger Joints. In W. C. Grabb and J. W. Smith (eds.), *Plastic Surgery* (3rd ed.). Boston: Little, Brown, 1979. P. 598.

5. Field, P. L., and Heuston, J. T. Articular cartilage loss in long-standing immobilization of interphalangeal joints. *Br. J. Plast. Surg.* 23:186, 1970.

6. Kuczynski, K. The proximal interphalangeal joint: Anatomy and causes of stiffness in the fingers. *J. Bone Joint Surg.* [*Br.*] 50:656, 1968.

7. Landsmeer, J. M. F. The anatomy of the dorsal aponeurosis of the human finger and its functional significance. *Anat. Rec.* 104:31, 1949.

8. Rhode, C. M., and Jennings, W. D., Jr. Operative treatment of the stiff proximal interphalangeal joint. *Am. Surg.* 37:44, 1971.

9. Smith, R. J. Non-ischemic contractures of the intrinsic muscles of the hand. *J. Bone Joint Surg.* [*Am.*] 53:1313, 1971.

10. Watson, H. K., and Carlson, L. Treatment of reflex sympathetic dystrophy of the hand with an active "stress loading" program. *J. Hand Surg.* 12A:779, 1987.

11. Watson, H. K., and Turkeltaub, S. H. Stiff Joints. In D. P. Green (ed.), *Operative Hand Surgery* (2nd ed.). New York: Churchill Livingstone, 1988.

12. Watson, H. K., Light, T. R., and Johnson, T. R. Check rein resection for flexion contracture of the middle joint. *J. Hand Surg.* 4:67, 1979.

## Suggested Reading

Boyes, J. H. *Bunnell's Surgery of the Hand* (4th Ed.). Philadelphia: Lippincott, 1964.

Gigis, P. I., and Kuczynski, K. The distal interphalangeal joints of the human fingers. *J. Hand Surg.* 7:176, 1982.

Harrison, D. H. The stiff interphalangeal joint. *Hand* 9:102, 1977.

Jackson, I. T., and Brown, G. E. D. A method of treating chronic flexion contractures of the fingers. *Br. J. Plast. Surg.* 23:373, 1970.

Laseter, G. F. Management of the stiff hand: A practical approach. *Orthop. Clin. North Am.* 14:749, 1983.

Sprague, B. L. Proximal interphalangeal joint contractures and their treatment. *J. Trauma* 16:259, 1976.

Watson, H. K., Chicarilli, Z. H., Linberg, R., et al. Saddle deformity. *J. Hand Surg.* [*Am.*] 11:210, 1986.

*James W. Smith*

# 35

# Tendon Injuries in the Forearm and Hand

In 1918, Dr. Sterling Bunnell published his first medical treatise, "Repair of Tendons in the Fingers and Description of Two New Instruments" [8]. He reported many of his observations on this subject and concluded, "One of the most baffling problems in surgery is to restore normal function to a finger in which the tendons have been injured."

Since that time, our understanding of the anatomy and biology of tendons has increased considerably, as has our knowledge of wound repair in general and tendon healing in particular [2, 6, 15, 37, 49, 50, 57]. Important advancements have been made in the techniques of tendon repair, preservation and reconstruction of the flexor sheath, the late reconstruction of the flexor tendon system, and the postoperative rehabilitation of the hand and finger after tendon repair, grafting, or lysis [36, 43, 82].

With hand injuries, treatment must always be directed toward restoring the greatest possible function in the shortest time. In some cases, this goal can be accomplished by a single operative procedure, others will require multiple stages of reconstruction. When the injury is a complicated one, the repair of tendons is usually near the end of the list in nearly any plan of hand reconstruction. This is because so many prerequisites are required before one can expect a repaired tendon to have any chance of functioning normally again. The prerequisites include a blood supply that is adequate, satisfactory skin coverage, a well-aligned skeletal framework, good joint function, and the restoration of nerve continuity. The following discussion of tendon injuries and their treatment assumes that all these prerequisites can be or have been met. Extensor tendon injuries are considered first, followed by flexor tendon care.

## Extensor Tendon Injuries

We have divided injuries of the extensor tendons into five groups for the purpose of discussing their appearance and treatment (Fig. 35-1): (1) insertion injuries (mallet finger), (2) middle slip injuries (boutonnière deformity), (3) extensor hood injuries, (4) tendon injuries over the dorsum of the hand, and (5) tendon injuries at the wrist and in the forearm.

### MALLET FINGER

The mallet, or baseball, finger deformity [59, 70, 83] results from a disruption in the continuity of the extensor tendon at or near its site of insertion into the distal phalanx. This disruption can accompany an open laceration or be the result of a closed rupture or

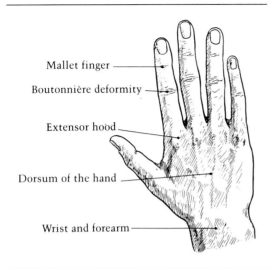

Figure 35-1 *Injuries to extensor tendons of the hand are here divided into groups for the purpose of describing their appearance and treatment.*

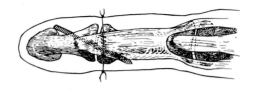

**Figure 35-2** *Mallet finger repair. An extensor tendon divided at or near its site of insertion can be repaired by approximating the two ends with a continuous nylon suture woven back and forth through the tendon. It is then brought out onto the skin on each side, where it can be fixed to the skin or tied to itself. After 3 weeks, the ends are cut and the suture is removed by gradual tension. Also shown is cross-pin fixation of the distal interphalangeal joint to maintain some degree of hyperextension. If the pin is placed longitudinally so that it protrudes through the tip of the finger, the patient experiences great discomfort with use.*

avulsion of the extensor tendon from its site of insertion. When an open wound is present and the extensor tendon has been cut by a sharp instrument, it can be repaired by carefully reapproximating its ends (Fig. 35-2). One technique is to anchor one end of a 4-0 nylon suture on the skin and then run it as a continuous suture, weaving it back and forth through the tendon ends from one side of the finger to the other. With closed injuries, when a rupture results, extensive fraying of the tendon ends usually occurs at the point of separation. This makes any surgical repair more difficult and gives results that are less satisfactory than those that can be obtained by splinting alone. The exception to this statement occurs when a chip of bone adjacent to the site of tendon insertion is avulsed from the distal phalanx along with the tendon. A preoperative x-ray film will help to identify the type of injury that should be repaired surgically by reattaching the bony fragment to its former site [9, 31, 70]. Some surgeons believe that if the bony fragment represents less than 30 percent of

the total articular surface of the distal interphalangeal joint, the injury should not be treated by the open technique.

When injuries are treated closed, the residual disability at most will be some slight swelling of the dorsum of the joint and perhaps a 10-degree defect in extension. In most cases of uncomplicated tendon disruption, it is best to immobilize the finger in either a plastic or metal splint. It should hold the distal joint in nearly full hyperextension and the proximal interphalangeal joint in moderate flexion [83]. This relaxes the lateral bands of the extensor mechanism and permits scar tissue to bridge the gap for the restoration of extensor tendon continuity. Splinting should be continuous for 6 weeks (Table 35-1).

Another technique that has been useful is fixation of the distal interphalangeal joint in extension with a Kirschner's pin [59]. The proximal interphalangeal joint can be held in moderate flexion with a splint or with the same pin. However, unless the operator is experienced with the placement of these pins through both joints, he or she should not do so because the possible complications

**Table 35-1** *Routine periods of immobilization**

| Site | Tendon injury | Time (weeks) |
|------|---------------|--------------|
| Finger | Flexor tendons | 3 |
| | Extensor tendons | 4 |
| Forearm | Wrist flexors and extensors (larger tendons) | 5 |
| Others | Mallet finger | 6 |
| | Boutonnière | 6 |

*It is easier to remember the periods of immobilization by thinking of them as the "3,4,5,6" rule; an additional week of guarded motion should be added to each period before normal activity is resumed.

of further tendon damage, loss of soft tissue, and joint contracture may outweigh the possible advantages.

## BOUTONNIÈRE DEFORMITY

The boutonnière deformity [14, 46, 83] results from a disruption in the continuity of the central (middle) tendon slip at the level of the proximal interphalangeal joint (Fig. 35-3). Here, the extensor mechanism is made up of two lateral bands and a central slip, which, because of its dorsal location, is frequently damaged. When it is divided, the proximal interphalangeal joint may at first be capable of weak finger extension because the lateral bands, if not displaced, can still aid in finger extension at this joint. With continued use, however, the lateral bands slip volarward on either side of the joint and become less effective as extensors. When their displacement becomes extreme and they lie below the axis of joint rotation, they can act like joint flexors and produce a flexion deformity. In such a circumstance, the angle of approach of these lateral slips to the distal interphalangeal joint is altered and can cause its hyperextension.

Verdan suggests that, in the long-standing injury, the middle slip of the extensor tendon should be shortened over the middle third of the proximal phalanx [83]. With the finger in full extension, enough of the scar is resected to permit an end-to-end suture of the central slip. The lateral bands are then replaced in their physiologic positions and held there by a few fine catgut sutures. The

6-week period of splinting is as necessary as before.

Many other methods have been described for treating long-standing, proximal, interphalangeal tendon injuries. Most have provided less than a satisfactory result (Fig. 35-4).

For long-standing cases of boutonnière deformity complicated with marked hyperextension of the distal phalanx, Dolphin [14] has suggested transecting the central part of

**Figure 35-3** *In the boutonnière deformity, lacerations at the level of the proximal interphalangeal joint frequently divide the middle slip of the extensor tendon mechanism. Unless these injuries are wide and deep, the lateral bands will frequently be spared. The potential gravity of the problem may not be appreciated if some extension remains at this joint. Finally, the lateral bands slip volarward to a point where they lie below the axis of rotation and begin to act as joint flexors. They then begin to aid the development of a typical boutonnière deformity. Note that the distal interphalangeal joint falls into hyperextension with this deformity.*

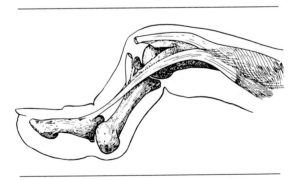

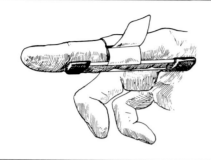

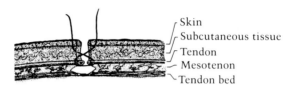

**Figure 35-4** *Any extension splint can be used that holds the metacarpophalangeal and proximal interphalangeal joints in hyperextension during the 6-week period of treatment. Flexion of the distal joint should be encouraged during this time.*

**Figure 35-5** *Figure-of-eight suture. Suture is begun by passing one end through each side of the tendon, then crisscrossing the ends and bringing them out through the subcutaneous tissue and skin. Closing the wound by tying sutures also approximates the ends of the tendon. Later, the sutures can be removed so that no buried suture material is left in the tendon.*

the extensor tendon apparatus over the middle phalanx. This transection permits the patient to regain flexion of the distal phalanx and often improves extension of the proximal interphalangeal joint.

EXTENSOR HOOD INJURIES
Injuries at the metacarpophalangeal joint level [15, 57, 83] frequently damage the extensor tendon mechanism and expose the underlying joint. In these cases, it is important to close the synovial lining of the joint before repairing the tendon. This double closure restores the architecture of the joint and provides a soft-tissue bed on which the tendon can glide. Continuity of the extensor mechanism is restored by weaving a suture of 4-0 nylon back and forth between the two cut edges of the tendon. Each end of the suture is passed through the skin beyond the site of repair and tied to itself. This, along with 4 weeks of splinting the parts in extension, helps to maintain the proper tension necessary to hold the tendon ends together. The suture can be removed by cutting the knots and pulling on one end until the suture comes out.

EXTENSOR TENDON INJURIES ON THE
DORSUM OF THE HAND
Over the dorsum of the hand, the simple figure-of-eight suture, as suggested by Bunnell

[9], provides a good means for either primary or secondary approximation of divided extensor tendons (Fig. 35-5). This suture, however, has no holding power, and splinting is necessary for 4 weeks as an aid to immobilization and proper tendon healing (Fig. 35-6). This suture can also be used effectively for reapproximating divided extensor tendons in the forearm. When the point of suture is expected to pass beneath the dorsal carpal ligament once healing is complete and motion restored, it may be necessary to sacrifice part or all of this ligament to prevent it from limiting tendon amplitude.

EXTENSOR TENDON INJURIES IN
THE FOREARM
Tendons in the forearm can be injured either at their musculotendinous junction or within the substance of the muscle. Primary care should always include restoration of musculotendinous continuity when feasible. Failure to approximate tendon ends or restore muscle continuity can result in a gap that becomes filled with scar tissue. It is difficult later to excise the scar and bridge the gap. Even where the gap between the tendon end and its muscle is not too great, the interposition of scar tissue with healing prevents tendon motion more distally. Therefore, before a secondary musculotendinous repair is performed in these cases, all scar tissue

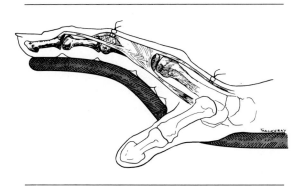

*Figure 35-6 Figure-of-eight sutures and splinting for the repair of an extensor tendon injury. If division of the middle slip is recognized at the time of injury, it can be repaired by several simple figure-of-eight sutures as shown here, or by weaving a suture transversely back and forth between the two ends of the tendon. It is important to the final healing that the wrist and fingers be placed in extension postoperatively for 6 weeks. Any division of extensor tendons proximal to the metacarpophalangeal joint can be repaired in a similar fashion. These tendon repairs should be splinted for 4 weeks in complete extension before a final week of guarded motion is begun.*

must be removed completely. Sometimes it is possible to fill the gap and restore musculotendinous continuity by advancing the tendon on the muscles at their juncture. Finally, it is important to close the fascia over the muscle junction and make a satisfactory soft-tissue bed in which the repaired muscles or musculotendinous units can glide.

## Flexor Tendon Injuries

With the development of better techniques for the atraumatic repair of flexor tendons, the recommended treatment of flexor tendon injuries has changed significantly. The primary repair of flexor tendons has almost universally replaced the "no-man's-land" concept, which favored secondary grafting [3, 10, 19, 36]. The advantages of primary tendon repair include restoration of the tendon to its normal length, reduction of the period of disability created by wound healing

and late grafting, a lessening of the tendency for joint stiffening, and better results of secondary tenolysis, when the procedure is necessary.

The belief that flexor tendon repair should be treated as a surgical emergency has been altered significantly by several reports suggesting that equal or better results can be achieved from delayed primary flexor tendon suture [24, 67]. In some patients, a delayed repair was possible after an interval of a month after injury when the end of the proximal flexor tendon had been held in the flexor sheath by an intact vinculum.

It has been demonstrated that, in most instances, it is better in "no-man's-land" to repair both the flexor digitorum profundus and superficialis tendons rather than the profundus alone, as was thought to be the wiser choice at one time [36]. Repair of both tendons appears to have the advantage of preserving the vincular blood supply to the profundus tendon, retaining the independent finger motion with stronger flexor power and providing a smooth bed for gliding of the profundus tendon. Combined repair also lessens the possibility of hyperextension deformities of the proximal interphalangeal joint and can reduce the incidence of rupture while providing a better functional recovery than single-tendon suture.

It is important to appreciate the fact that severed flexor tendon ends will usually retract well away from the digital laceration site. Particularly when the digit is in flexion at the time of injury, the distal stumps of the severed tendons will come to lie a centimeter or more distal to the level of sheath disruption when the digit is in full extension. For that reason, it is mandatory to extend the wound of injury in both the proximal and distal directions to provide wide visibility of the area of an injury.

On occasion, it may be possible to identify and retrieve the retracted tendon ends by passing small forceps into the flexor tendon sheath, grasping the tendon and gently returning it to the area of injury [65]. One should not, however, engage in indiscriminate, repetitive attempts. A good working rule should be that when the severed flexor tendon ends are not visible in the proximal tendon sheath when the wrist and metacarpophalangeal joint are flexed, it is probably better to extend the proximal incision or to make a separate incision in the palm to gain access to the flexor tendons and to delicately pass them back through the sheath to the level of repair.

SUTURE MATERIAL AND TECHNIQUES

Although there is wide variation in the selection of suture material for flexion tendon repairs, most surgeons now prefer braided synthetic polyester material (Ethibond), usually of a 4-0 caliber [43, 49], although monofilament sutures are used by some. The specific techniques for tendon sutures have changed considerably from those used in the past. Bunnell's pullout or crisscross suture has lost its popularity in favor of simpler or stronger repairs.

Urbaniak [78], in an excellent study of the tensile strength of different tendon junctures, indicated the superiority of the Kessler repair for the type of end-to-end suture that is required for the severed flexor tendon. The Kessler "grasping" stitch [28] or similar "core" suture methods have emerged as the most popular types of flexor tendon repair. The Tajima modification [77], in which the suture knots are tied within the repair site, is particularly convenient because the suture can be placed in the tendon ends as soon as they are identified and the ends can then be used to pass the tendon through the flexor tendon sheath and into position for repair without the need to further damage the tendon by instrumentation.

The repair is usually completed by the use of a running suture utilizing 6-0 nonabsorbable monofilament material in an effort to "tidy up" the repair site and invert the tendon [40, 48]. Lister has emphasized that the epitendinous suture should be shallow and inverting to diminish the tendon bulk at the site of repair [42].

Kleinert classified flexor tendon injuries into separate surgical topographic zones (Fig. 35-7) to facilitate discussions of their treatment and prognosis [31, 33, 34, 35]. This helps us to give attention to the technical consideration of each area and to emphasize the differences in their treatment, postoperative care, and prognosis.

ZONE 1

Zone 1 represents that part of the fibroosseous canal between the insertion of the superficialis and the insertion of the flexor profundus tendon. When the flexor profundus tendon is divided at this level, there is a loss of active flexion of the distal phalanx, as well as a hyperextension instability of the distal interphalangeal joint. This can result in a great deal of disability, particularly when these injuries are in the index and middle finger, because, with an unstable pinch, patients tend to drop things easily. With zone 1 profundus tendon injuries, function of the proximal interphalangeal joint can be altered, too. If the proximal end of the flexor profundus becomes caught at the level of the sublimis chiasm, it can markedly affect the range of active movement at the proximal interphalangeal joint.

With these injuries, the location of the proximal tendon stump is an important factor [38]. If the proximal end of the tendon has retracted into the palm, it is difficult to reattach the stump if the injury is beyond 10 days old.

If the tendon has been caught at the level of the chiasm of the superficialis tendon, the delay time is up to 3 weeks. If it is near the distal end, the repair can be performed at a significantly delayed period of time if necessary.

For tendon lacerations within 1.5 cm of the insertion, the profundus tendon can be advanced and attached to the distal phalanx. For clean, fresh, sharp lacerations more than 1.5 cm away from the insertion, primary tenorrhaphy is the treatment of choice. In the past, these tendon junctures have not in-

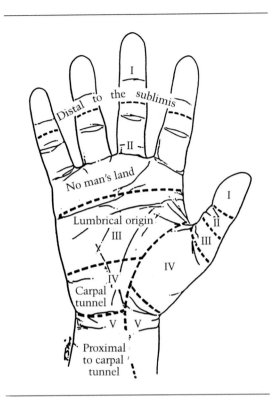

**Figure 35-7** *Flexor tendon zones in the hand and zones of the flexor pollicis longus. (From H. E. Kleinert et al. Primary repair of flexor tendons. Orthop. Clin. North Am. 4:866, 1973; and J. R. Urbaniak. Repair of the flexor pollicis longus. Hand Clin. 1:69, 1985.)*

frequently adhered to the underlying bed at the point of repair. More exacting tendon repairs have lessened this frequency of adherence. Delayed repair and secondary tenorrhaphy, tendon grafting, and other joint stabilization procedures all should be considered in the management of zone 1 tendon lacerations.

## ZONE 2: NO-MAN'S-LAND (CRITICAL ZONE)

Tendons are frequently injured within an anatomic area that, in the past, was labeled "the critical zone" or "no-man's-land." This is the area where both flexor tendons run together in the flexor sheath beginning at the A1 pulley and ending at the superficialis in-

sertion. Since the repair of tendons lacerated in this region was often followed by their adherence to the adjacent fixed structures, most textbooks in the past recommended as the best primary treatment suture of the skin only and an attempt to restore active flexion at a later date by tendon grafting [9, 46].

More recently, Kleinert and Verdan reporting for the Committee on Tendon Injuries, recommended the repair of both the profundus and superficialis tendons [16, 33, 36, 43, 83]. Resection of the flexor superficialis insertion was believed to adversely affect the blood supply of the profundus tendon through the connecting vincula, thus worsening the conditions for healing of the profundus. Superficialis excision is a consideration only when tendon repair requires the sacrifice of critical pulleys or when both tendons are lacerated and need to be immobilized at the same level. Most surgeons now recommend repair of the superficialis whenever possible because this appears to improve functional results.

The significance of the tendon sheath synovium on nutrition, healing, and the subsequent function of tendons has received increasing attention [27, 56] (Fig. 35-8). In the past, excising a portion of the flexor tendon sheath through which the tendon repair would travel was recommended, while maintaining adequate pulleys to prevent bowstringing. At present, many authorities suggest closing the tendon sheath after tendon repair. Clinical studies support the belief that sheath closure can be beneficial when it is relatively easy and convenient. In certain specific circumstances closure can help to eliminate any mechanical impingement on the tendon repair.

For exposing the injured profundus and superficialis tendons, either a midaxial finger incision or Brunner's zigzag incision should be used to extend the original laceration. Then the tendon sheath should be elevated for the repair, taking care to preserve and not damage the essential pulleys. After the re-

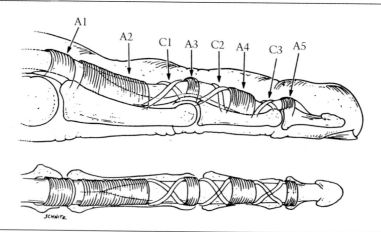

**Figure 35-8** *The flexor retinaculum in the fingers, showing five annular and three cruciform pulleys. The sturdy pulleys are important biomechanically in guaranteeing efficient digital motion by keeping the tendon closely applied to the phalanges. The thin, pliable cruciate pulleys permit the flexor sheath to be flexible while maintaining its integrity. (From Idler, R.S. Anatomy and biomechanics of the digital flexor tendons. Hand Clinics. 1:3, 1985.)*

pair, the flap of tendon sheath should be closed by suture and carefully preserved [42]. It is believed that closing the sheath can reduce adhesions. Furthermore, the site of the repair and the tendon juncture are less likely to catch on the edge of the sheath window with the start of finger mobilization.

The proximal end of the lacerated tendon has usually retracted proximally and can be retrieved by flexing all of the joints and "milking" the tendon back from the palm. Extending the incision proximally in order to find the tendon end is sometimes necessary.

Once retrieved, the two ends are abutted by flexing all joints. The proximal tendon is transfixed about 2 cm from its cut end by passing a straight needle (No. 25) through the skin and tendon sheath of the finger from one side to the other, being careful to avoid the neurovascular structures. The cut edges of the tendon should be small and regular. If they are not, or if a part of the tendon is frayed, these fragments should be removed to square off the tendon.

Suturing is performed without tension; exacting approximation of the tendon ends is essential if fine sutures are to be used. The accordionlike effect that Bunnell shows in all of his drawings must be avoided when the tendon suture is tied, in order to minimize the intratendinous damage (Fig. 35-9). The Kessler modification of the Mason-Allen suture is preferred by some because it reduces longitudinal compression and, at the same time, increases longitudinal alignment [27, 28]. It is thought that this should help to deter separation of the tendon ends (Fig. 35-10).

Either a coated or uncoated, braided, synthetic polyester suture (4-0) is used, depending on the size of the tendon. Handling the outer surface of the tendon with instruments is likely to cause additional adhesions. Instead, the cut end of the tendon should be grasped with a fine-tooth dissecting forceps. The suture can be passed through the tendon with greater ease and more control if the tendon is pressed against the adjacent soft tissues while the suture is inserted.

After the Kessler suture has been tied, the margins of the tendon juncture are more accurately approximated with a running suture of 6-0 or 7-0 monofilament nylon (Fig.

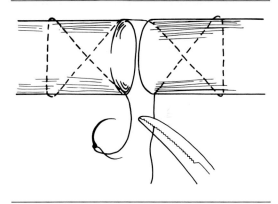

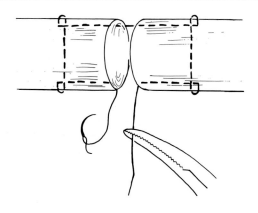

**Figure 35-9** *Modified Bunnell suture. When tying the suture, one should approximate the ends without producing an accordion effect or undue tension.*

**Figure 35-10** *The modified Kessler–Mason-Allen suture.*

35-11). To prevent adhesions, which might limit tendon movement within the tendon sheath later in healing, each part of the suture should help to enclose any exposed area of raw tendon.

When both the profundus and superficialis tendons have been divided, Lister and Kleinert [43] believe that they both should be repaired. If both slips of the superficialis tendon have been divided, they should be repaired separately with inverted "figure of eight" sutures. Once suturing is completed, most surgeons close the fibrous sheath loosely using a 6-0 nonabsorbable synthetic suture. Recent evidence suggests that preserving the sheath reduces the subsequent formation of adhesions.

At the end of the operation, the extremity is elevated and gentle pressure is placed over the area of repair while the tourniquet is released. A bipolar coagulator is used to help gain exacting hemostasis after the hyperemia has subsided. The wound is irrigated with Ringer's lactate solution to ensure that all blood clots have been removed. The wound is closed with 6-0 monofilament nylon. The straight needle that was placed in the tendon earlier can be removed at this point.

Dressings are applied and a dorsal plaster

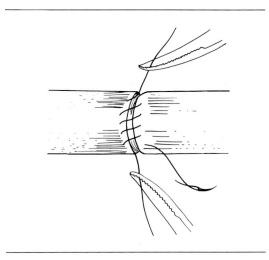

**Figure 35-11** *The tenorrhaphy is completed by placing a running suture of fine material around the periphery of the tendon. One should try to approximate the margins, eliminate raw surfaces, and invaginate any protruding tendon fibers.*

splint is positioned to extend from the upper forearm to reach just beyond the tips of the fingers. The plaster holds the wrist in approximately 60 to 70 degrees of flexion, which represents a position about 20 degrees less than full flexion. The metacarpophalangeal joints are flexed 20 degrees and the interphalangeal joints about 10 degrees. The cast is molded to prevent finger extension. Since controlled mobilization of repaired tendons is begun immediately, rubber bands are attached to the nails of the fingers with transfixing sutures or by fastening a seamstress's hook and eye to the nail of the finger with cryanoacrylate adhesive.

Once the cast is hardened, the rubber bands are attached to the nails and the other end is fastened to the dressing at the wrist level with a safety pin. This sort of attachment should hold the fingers at rest but with slight positive flexion toward the forearm. The rubber bands should be of a strength that will allow the patient to extend the fingers against resistance as far as the dorsal guard. The patient is encouraged to do this as often as possible during the 3 weeks until the splint is removed. After the splint has been removed, the rubber bands from the injured finger are attached to an Ace bandage at the wrist for an additional 2 weeks. Kleinert and colleagues [33] have shown that this method of controlled mobilization is effective in part because the contraction of one group of muscles against resistance results in a synergistic relaxation of antagonist muscles. Thus, during sustained extension there is no activity in the flexor digitorum profundus or flexor digitorum superficialis tendons. As the fingers are relaxed and returned to full flexion, some power of contraction returns to the flexor units, but little force can be generated because of the position of the tendon.

### THE THUMB
Most tendon injuries in the thumb occur at the level of the interphalangeal crease, which is near the point of the flexor profundus insertion. So long as the wound is clean, the flexor profundus tendon can be repaired either primarily or secondarily. At the time of tendon surgery, the flexor tendon sheath must be resected widely so that the edge of the resected sheath lies about 1 cm beyond the excursion of the thickened area of sutured tendon.

Tendon injuries that lie more proximal, at the level of the sesamoids and the metacarpal pulley, should be evaluated carefully before a primary repair is undertaken. Secondary repair might be preferable unless circumstances are ideal for primary repair. In either case the metacarpal pulley is widely excised.

Over the thenar eminence, injuries to the flexor pollicis longus tendon are likely to occur in conjunction with injuries to the thenar muscles and the recurrent branch of the median nerve. Because all these structures lie so close together, each of these possibilities should be considered in examining injuries to this location. Flexor pollicis longus repairs can be performed in this area either primarily or secondarily.

### THE PALM
Tendons are damaged less frequently with injuries in the palm, because of the protection of the palmar fascia and the fact that the tendons lie farther away from the surface. When only the superficialis tendon is divided in the midpalmar area, its repair is unnecessary. When both tendons are divided in ideal circumstances, and when the juncture does not appear to pass beneath the carpal ligament with full flexion, both of the tendons can be repaired with a fairly good chance that some independence of action can be achieved. In less tidy circumstances, perhaps only the profundus should be repaired and the adjacent parts of the superficialis resected. Because the mesenterylike arrangement that carries their segmental blood supply to them lies between the two tendons, it is best not to do any more separation than necessary in preparation for their repair.

It is much more useful merely to place sutures through the tendon ends and bring them into proper approximation.

### THE WRIST
Restoration of good hand function may prove difficult after tendon lacerations at the wrist

for two reasons: (1) More than one tendon is divided, and (2) the proximity of their junctures after repair results in cross-adherence between them. In cases in which the junctures of sutured tendons will, with finger movement, pass beneath the transverse carpal ligament, a reapproximation of the profundus tendons alone may be advantageous. Since tendon junctures nearly always have a greater circumstance than a normal tendon, multiple junctures may produce an increased volume for the limited space of the carpal ligament.

THE FOREARM
When flexor tendons and their muscles are injured proximal to the carpal ligament, primary repair is preferred. Delayed repair beyond 4 weeks can cause such shortening of the muscle that tendon grafting is needed for correction. In these cases, grafting decreases muscle-tendon excursion and incomplete finger flexion is not uncommon. Both superficialis and profundus tendons should be repaired. Tendon gliding is not as much of a problem as one would expect.

More proximal injuries in the forearm can include divided muscles. They should be repaired primarily, if at all possible, before muscle contractures create a gap and make later approximation more difficult. The fascia that covers each muscle should be carefully sutured after hemostasis has been achieved. Draining the wound helps to decrease skin tension. Surprisingly good results can be gained in these cases. A division of the median and ulnar nerves frequently accompanies tendon lacerations in the forearm and wrist.

Regardless of the technique chosen, some means of nerve approximation should be employed to prevent the retraction of their ends. Failure in this regard makes any secondary suture a great deal more difficult and nerve grafts may be required. Postoperatively, splinting of the wrist in the position of flexion should be continued for 4 to 5 weeks after tendon repairs in the wrist and forearm level.

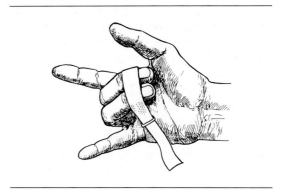

**Figure 35-12** *Web strap and buckle worn nearly all the time during the preparation for tendon grafting. It is necessary to have the joints of the injured finger as supple as those in adjacent normal fingers.*

FLEXOR TENDON GRAFTS
The primary suturing of divided flexor tendons within the digital sheath has eliminated the need for tendon grafting for the less complicated cases. However, there is still a great need for tendon grafting in the treatment of more severely injured fingers.

Factors important to the success of tendon grafting are complete wound healing, an absence of edema and induration, satisfactory skeletal alignment, and a full range of passive motion in the joints (Fig. 35-12). The ease with which this passive joint motion can be accomplished should be comparable to that in a normal finger.

TECHNIQUE OF FLEXOR
TENDON GRAFTING
A midaxial incision [9] or the zigzag volar-digital incision, described by Bruner [7], provides good exposure for the surgical procedure of tendon grafting. The exact site for placing the midaxial incision can be determined by flexing the finger and identifying the point at each joint where the flexion crease ends (Fig. 35-13). If the points are connected, they will create a line that passes through the axis of rotation of each joint (midaxial line), and therefore the line remains the same length whether the finger is

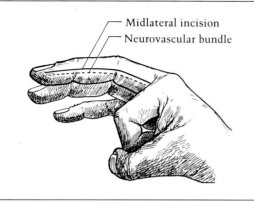

**Figure 35-13** *The midlateral line or midaxial line passes through the axis of rotation of each joint.*

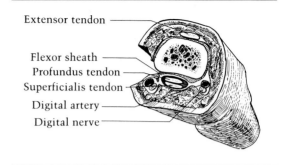

**Figure 35-14** *Cross-sectional view of approach to the flexor tendon sheath. Note that the digital nerve and artery in the volar flap are preserved by this method.*

flexed or extended. After the skin has been incised along this line, it is best to continue to gain exposure in the central portion of any one finger segment. Here, the fat is more plentiful than it is over the joint, which thus allows a greater margin of safety. As deeper dissection is begun, the first structure encountered will be Cleland's ligament [46]. This contains fingers that run almost in a volar-dorsal direction and connect the thinner fascial layers surrounding the digital nerve and artery with the skin.

The digital nerve and artery lie approximately 2 mm volar to the margin of the incision, so it is best to preserve the thickness of fat on the volar flap (Fig. 35-14). Cleland's ligament can be isolated from the adjacent fat at the level of the proximal interphalangeal joint to a degree sufficient that it can be identified later and resutured. Such resuturing appears to prevent hyperextension deformities at the proximal interphalangeal joint after tendon grafting.

Once Cleland's ligament has been divided, deeper dissection will expose the side of the phalanx, with the margin of the flexor sheath extending forward along the volar surface much like the vista dome on the roof of a sightseeing bus. The tendon sheath can be identified more easily in an area away

from the site of previous injury, where the scar tissue will be minimal, and here it can be readily separated away from the fat.

As the dissection is continued near the tip of the finger, it is important that the skin incision lie adjacent to the side of the fingernail and that most of the fat be left on the flap, because beyond the distal interphalangeal joint, the digital nerve divides and some branches lie on the side of the finger very close to the nail. It is easy to cut them at this location if the surgeon is not careful.

Once the "vista dome" of the flexor tendon sheath has been identified in the midphalangeal portion of each segment, the dissected segments can be connected over the areas of the joints. It is best to preserve all the pulleys possible in the finger, as well as the sheath when feasible. The natural location of the pulleys can be confirmed by determining the points where the flexor tendon sheath is thickest. They are usually located in the proximal one-third of the middle phalanx and in the midportion of the proximal phalanx (Fig. 35-15). Such pulleys, when left, prevent "spanning" of the tendon graft. If a tendon injury has damaged the sheath at these levels, it is worthwhile to try to preserve them and to relocate one more proximal or more distal, depending on the location of the scar, so that a suitable pulley

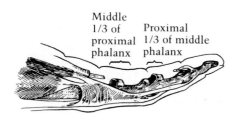

**Figure 35-15** *Location of pulleys that are essential to minimize or prevent the "spanning" of the tendon grafts and to make them work more efficiently. When it is possible, try to preserve the entire A1 pulley, located over the proximal one-third of the middle phalanx, and the A2 pulley, located at the middle portion of the proximal phalanx.*

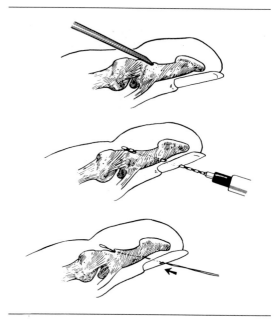

**Figure 35-16** *Technique for elevating a bone flap in preparation for distal fixation of the tendon graft. Some surgeons try to drill in a reverse direction to minimize the chance of damaging the fingernail bed. Others prefer to suture the graft to the remnant of the profundus tendon.*

will remain. All other remnants of the flexor tendon sheath can be opened so the profundus remnants can be resected, but the sheath should be preserved wherever possible for later closure. Effort should be made to create a good bed through which a tendon graft can glide. In the joint areas, the vincula of the superficialis and profundus tendons are preserved because this lessens tissue reactions during the time of tendon healing.

Distally, preparation must be made either for fixing the tendon graft to the remnant of the profundus tendon or for inserting it beneath a bone flap in the distal phalanx. Bone flaps [5, 9] are developed with a chisel at the usual site of the profundus tendon insertion (Fig. 35-16). The chisel perforates the volar surface of the cortical bone and a little trap door of bone is elevated. A small drill bit is used to establish a tunnel between the bone flap and the overlying nail, with care taken not to damage the nail bed. A wire is threaded through this tunnel and used as an aid for later placement of the tendon graft beneath the bone flap.

In the palm, a separate incision is used to identify and elevate a window of the palmar fascia so that the more proximal segments of the divided tendons can be freed. In identifying the superficialis and profundus ten-

dons, it should be remembered that the superficialis is more volar. The attachment of lumbrical muscle to the profundus tendon helps to identify it and usually prevents its proximal end from slipping back beyond this point.

When both tendons have been divided in a finger injury, the thin filmy covering (paratenon) overlying the tendons proximal to the metacarpophalangeal joint usually thickens during the several weeks that elapse between injury and repair. This thickened paratenon should be incised and a large amount removed so that the superficialis tendon can be identified and separated from the profundus tendon. Straight clamps are placed on each proximal tendon end, and the superficialis is identified so that if the wrist incision is performed later to obtain the palmaris tendon for a graft, the superficialis can be removed back to this level. The proximal tendon juncture is made by suturing the graft to the profundus tendon at the level of the lumbrical muscle or just distal to it. Parkes [45a] as well as Littler [46] have emphasized the disastrous role the lumbrical can play; if it becomes shortened, it can exert a force on the finger in the wrong direction through the extensor tendon mechanism. For this reason, it may be better to resect the lumbrical if it appears damaged. Finally, before taking the graft, it is worthwhile to thread a suture or a pediatric feeding catheter through the pulleys and into the palm in preparation for sliding the tendon graft through the finger and into place.

The palmaris longus tendon is available for use as a graft in 85 percent of cases [86]. Its presence should be determined before operation, if possible, so that the leg can be prepared if it is absent. The palmaris longus tendon can be removed through several small parallel incisions in the forearm. The procedure is as follows: The distal end of the palmaris longus tendon is identified at the wrist through a transverse incision. Tension is placed on its course to identify the point of its muscle juncture. A second transverse incision is made at this level and the skin and subcutaneous tissue are separated until the tendon can be identified in the filmy tissue beneath. The distal end of the tendon should be isolated at the point of its attachment to the palmar fascia at the wrist level, and a double right-angle suture or some similar suture should be inserted through it for the purpose of handling and later transfer. In the proximal end of the tendon, another double right-angle suture is placed. Then the tendon is carefully separated from its paratenon and mesotendon so that it is free and no attachments remain. To accomplish this, it may be necessary to make a third small transverse incision. If any residual fibers of paratenon are intact, they will prevent mobilization of the tendon. With sutures in

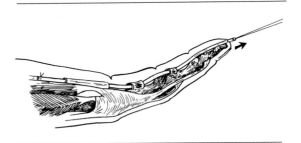

*Figure 35-17* *End-to-end suture of the tendon graft to the motor unit at the base of the palm after tendon graft has been placed in tendon bed.*

each end, the tendon graft is free so that it can be transferred to the finger (Fig. 35-17).

The distal end of the tendon graft is placed under tension to aid in its identification at the wrist level. Through the wrist incision, a clamp is placed beneath the superficialis tendon and the tendon is withdrawn back at this level. As it is pulled out at the wrist level, the suture previously placed beneath the pulleys comes out with it. Some surgeons believe it is advantageous to slide the tendon graft from the forearm to the finger through the existing incisions, without actually removing it from the body. This decreases the possibility of injury to the surface of the tendon and keeps it from drying out. If this seems to be an acceptable option, the end of the tendon graft with the double right-angle suture in it is attached to the proximal end of the catheter. As it is pulled distally, the tendon graft will slide through the profundus tunnel and into the digit until its proximal end is in juxtaposition to the distal end of the profundus tendon and ready for an end-to-end suture of the modified Bunnell or Kessler type.

With a No. 11 knife blade, a small stab wound is made in the tip of the finger just beneath the nail (Fig. 35-18). A mosquito clamp or tendon passer is used to establish a

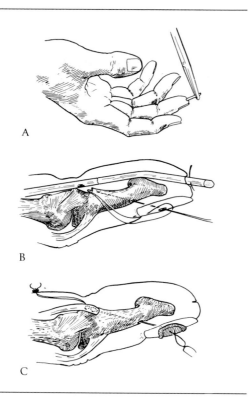

*Figure 35-18* Insertion of tendon graft. A. The tendon graft is pulled through a stab wound in the fingertip to determine the point where it will be under the desired degree of tension. B. A small curved needle is placed through the tendon to keep it from retracting into the finger as tension is evaluated. Once the proper tension is achieved and the length of the graft is known, the point where the graft lies adjacent to the bone flap can be marked on the tendon. C. The distal end of the tendon is fixed beneath the bone flap and tied over a button at the end of the finger.

channel from this point to the site of profundus insertion, and the distal end of the tendon graft is pulled back through to the tip of the finger to determine the point at which it will be under the desired degree of tension. A small, curved, empty needle can be placed through the tendon to keep it from retracting into the finger, and the needle is repositioned until the proper tension in the graft appears to correspond to that of tendons in the adjacent fingers. Through the midlateral incision the point is noted at which the tendon graft under proper tension approximates to the profundus remnant or the bone-flap window. The point is marked on the tendon graft and the distal suture is placed. The monofilament nylon suture placed in it and passed beneath the bone flap and through the nail bed to the nail level is held in its position beneath the volar bone flap by tying the ends of the tendon suture over a button on top of the fingernail. No pullout wire is necessary because at 3 to 4 weeks, the monofilament nylon can be cut and removed at the nail level with gentle tension.

When the palmaris tendon is absent, the superficialis, the plantaris tendon, or an extensor digitorum longus tendon will prove a satisfactory substitute. If the latter is selected, it must be removed from the second, third, or fourth toe and not from the great toe or little toe. Removal of the long extensor from the great toe jeopardizes too important a function. In the little toe, there is no short extensor to substitute for the function of the long extensor if it is removed.

When the time between injury and tendon grafting is long, as a general rule the tendon graft should be a little shorter so that the finger will be under slightly greater flexor tension than an adjacent normal finger. Some surgeons have suggested that the tendon be interwoven in the palm to decrease the chances of its becoming fixed at the point of juncture [61]. This could be detrimental if the bulkiness of a tendon juncture prevents it from sliding beneath the carpal tunnel, limiting the degree of flexion. In many cases it may be preferable to perform an end-to-end suture of the tendons (see Fig. 35-17).

It is important to release the tourniquet before the wounds are closed in order to establish good hemostasis. If the tendon graft were not vascularized because of a hematoma, a portion might undergo necrosis and become adherent to the scar. The hand is usually elevated for 10 minutes after release of the tourniquet to allow the hyperemia to subside before an attempt is made to establish hemostasis.

After hemostasis has been achieved, the arm is again elevated for a minute's time to allow venous blood to drain from the arm. Then the tourniquet is reinflated to avoid the accumulation of additional blood in the wound while it is being sutured. The small forearm incisions can be closed by a running suture, but perhaps it is better to put interrupted sutures in the fingers and palm to permit any serum or blood that might accumulate to leak out through the suture line during the early postoperative period.

The wrist is immobilized with a plaster splint in a position of 10 to 15 degrees less than maximum flexion; the fingers are allowed to fall into some degree of extension to compensate for the wrist flexion (Fig. 35-19). This type of immobilization is maintained for 3 weeks after operation. Active but guarded motion can be started during the fourth postoperative week, with the splint reapplied between exercise periods. No passive motion should be carried out before the end of the fourth week.

During the period of mobilization it is important to concentrate initially on gaining full flexion rather than extension. The patient should be encouraged to flex the proximal and distal interphalangeal joints, and the metacarpophalangeal joints can be positioned in extension with a small exercise block placed in the palm. In this way the tendon graft must produce the finger movement, rather than having the metacarpophalangeal joint flex through the action of the lumbricals and interossei without necessitating movement of the tendon graft. The patient should be warned that 2 or 3 months may be required to achieve full flexion. At the same time all attempts to extend the fingers by strong passive force should be discouraged, because the result can be an overstretching of the tendon juncture; if this juncture becomes too long, full flexion will never be possible.

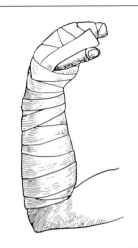

**Figure 35-19** *A plaster splint is used to immobilize the hand with the wrist in some degree of flexion for 3 weeks. In the fourth week, guarded active motion is suggested before the cast is discarded. It is important not to place a bolus dressing in the palm at the time of wound closure, since this will not permit the tendon graft to move with the finger in case any unexpected muscle contraction occurs during the healing period.*

SILASTIC RODS

Nonreactive Silastic rods, popularized by Hunter and Salisbury [20], can sometimes serve as a valuable aid in tendon surgery. The term *space maintainer* seems to best describe their potential function. Sometimes, when both tendons have been divided in no man's land, tendon grafting can be performed as a delayed procedure, 7 to 10 days later. Before the overlying skin is closed, a small segment of Silastic rod is inserted into the tendon sheath so that it will span across the site of the injury to prevent the collapse of this structure. Then, at the time of the grafting, it is removed.

These rods are also helpful in severely scarred finger with stiff joints and no flexor tendon function. After all possible scarring is removed from the finger, a Silastic rod is inserted beneath old pulleys and anchored distally to the stump of the profundus tendon at the terminal phalanx. Proximally, it can extend into the palm or to the wrist. After 3 or more months, when the tissue reaction has subsided and joint mobility has reached a maximum, the rod is replaced with a tendon graft.

## References

1. Allen, B. N., et al. Ruptured flexor tendon tenorrhaphies in zone II: Repair and rehabilitation. *J. Hand Surg. [Am.]* 12:18, 1987.
2. Amadio, P. C., et al. The effect of vincular injury on the results of flexor tendon surgery in zone 2. *J. Hand Surg. [Am.]* 10:626, 1985.
3. Bieskar, A. Flexor tendon repair in no man's land. *Scand. J. Plast. Reconstr. Surg.* 14:279, 1980.
4. Boyes, J. H. Evaluation of results of digital flexor tendon grafts. *Am. J. Surg.* 89:1116, 1955.
5. Boyes, J. H., and Stark, H. H. Flexor-tendon grafts in the fingers and thumb. *J. Bone Joint Surg. [Am.]* 53:1332, 1971.
6. Brand, P. W. *Clinical Mechanics of the Hand.* St. Louis: Mosby, 1985.
7. Bruner, J. M. The zig-zag volar digital incision for flexor-tendon surgery. *Plast. Reconstr. Surg.* 40:571, 1967.
8. Bunnell, S. Repair of tendons in the fingers and description of two new instruments. *Surg. Gynecol. Obstet.* 26:103, 1918.
9. Bunnell, S. Tendon Injuries. In J. H. Boyes (ed.), *Surgery of the Hand* (5th ed.). Philadelphia: Lippincott, 1970.
10. Burton, R. I. Severed Tendons and Nerves Distal to Metacarpophalangeal Joint. In J. W. Littler, L. M. Cramer, and J. W. Smith (eds.), *Symposium on Reconstructive Hand Surgery.* St. Louis: Mosby, 1974. Pp. 117–128.
11. Chow, J. A., Thomes, L. J., Dovelle, S. W., et al. A combined regimen of controlled motion following flexor tendon repair in "no man's land." *Plast. Reconstr. Surg.* 79:447, 1987.
12. Citron, N. D., and Forster, A. Dynamic splinting following flexor tendon repair. *J. Hand Surg. [Br.]* 12:96, 1987.
13. Cohen, M. J., and Kaplan, L. Histology and ultrastructure of the human flexor tendon sheath. *J. Hand Surg. [Am.]* 12:25, 1987.
14. Dolphin, J. A. Extensor tenotomy for bouton-

nière deformity of the finger. Presented at the 18th Annual Meeting of the American Society for Surgery of the Hand, Jan. 18, 1963.
15. Doyle, J. R., and Blythe, W. F. Anatomy of the flexor tendon sheath and pulleys of the thumb. *J. Hand Surg.* 2:149, 1977.
16. Duran, R. J. Controlled Passive Motion Following Flexor Tendon Repair in Zones Two and Three. In *AAOS Symposium on Tendon Surgery in the Hand.* St. Louis: Mosby, 1975.
17. Eiken, O., Lundborg, G., and Rank, F. The role of the digital synovial sheath in tendon grafting. *Scand. J. Plast. Reconstr. Surg.* 9:182, 1975.
18. Furlow, L. T. The role of tendon tissues in tendon healing. *Plast. Reconstr. Surg.* 57:39, 1976.
19. Green, W. L., and Niebauer, J. J. Results of primary and secondary flexor-tendon repairs in no man's land. *J. Bone Joint Surg.* 56:1216, 1974.
20. Hunter, J. M., and Salisbury, R. E. Flexor-tendon reconstruction in severely damaged hands. *J. Bone Joint Surg. [Am.]* 53:829, 1971.
21. Hunter, J. M., et al: The pseudosynovial sheath—its characteristics in a primate model. *J. Hand Surg.* 8:461, 1983.
22. Hurst, L. N., McCain, W. G., and Lindsay, W. K. Results of tenolysis. *Plast. Reconstr. Surg.* 52:171, 1973.
23. Idler, R. S. Anatomy and biomechanics of the digital flexor tendons. *Hand Clin.* 1:3, 1985.
24. Iselin, F. Early Management of Fresh Hand Wounds with Specific Reference to Delayed Repair. In *AAOS Symposium on Tendon Surgery in the Hand.* St. Louis: Mosby, 1975. Pp. 88–90.
25. Kaplan, E. B. *Functional and Surgical Anatomy of the Hand.* Philadelphia: Lippincott, 1953.
26. Katsumi, M., and Tajima, T. Experimental investigation of healing process of tendons with or without synovial coverage in or outside of the synovial cavity. *J. Nigata Med. Assoc.* 95:532, 1981.
27. Kessler, F. B., et al. Fascia patch graft for a digital flexor sheath defect over primary tendon repair in the chicken. *J. Hand Surg. [Am.]* 11:241, 1986.
28. Kessler, I. The grasping technique for tendon repair. *Hand* 5:253, 1973.
29. Ketchum, L. D. Primary tendon healing: A re-

view. *J. Hand Surg.* 2:428, 1977.

30. Ketchum, L. D., Martin, N., and Kappel, D. Factors affecting tendon gap and tendon strength at the site of tendon repair. *Plast. Reconstr. Surg.* 59:708, 1977.

31. Kleinert, H. E., and Bahn, L. The current state of flexor tendon surgery. *Ann Chir. Main* 3:7, 1984.

32. Kleinert, H. E., Kutz, J. E., Ashbell, T. S., et al. Primary repair of flexor tendons in "no man's land." *J. Bone Joint Surg. [Am.]* 49:577, 1969.

33. Kleinert, H. E., Kutz, J. E., Atasoy, E., et al. Primary repair of flexor tendons. *Orthop. Clin. North Am.* 4:865, 1973.

34. Kleinert, H. E., Schepels, S., and Gill, T. Flexor tendon injuries. *Surg. Clin. North Am.* 61:267, 1981.

35. Kleinert, H. E., and Smith, D. J., Jr. Primary and Secondary Repairs of Flexor and Extensor Tendon Injuries. In J. E. Flynn (ed.), *Hand Surgery* (3rd ed.). Baltimore: Williams & Wilkins, 1982. Pp. 220–231.

36. Kleinert, H. E., and Verdan, C. Report of the Committee on Tendon Injuries. *J. Hand Surg.* 8:794, 1983.

37. Landsmeer, J. M. F. A report on the coordination of the interphalangeal joints of the human finger and its disturbances. *Acta Morphol. Neerl. Scand.* 2:59, 1959.

38. Leddy, J. P., and Packer, J. W. Avulsion of the profundus tendon insertion in athletes. *J. Hand Surg.* 2:66, 1977.

39. Leffert, R. D., Weiss, C., and Athanasoulis, C. A. The vincula. *J. Bone Joint Surg. [Am.]* 56:1191, 1974.

40. Lin, G. T., An, K. N., Amadio, P. C., et al. Biomechanical studies of running suture for flexor tendon repair in dogs. *J. Hand Surg. [Am.]* 13:553, 1988.

41. Lindsay, W. K., and Thomson, H. G. Digital flexor tendons: An experimental study. Part 1. The significance of each component of the flexor mechanism in tendon healing. *Br. J. Plast. Surg.* 12:289, 1960.

42. Lister, G. Pitfalls and complications of flexor tendon surgery. *Hand Clin.* 1:140, 1985.

43. Lister, G. D., Kleinert, H. E., Kutz, J. E., et al. Primary flexor tendon repair followed by immediate controlled mobilization. *J. Hand Surg.* 2:441, 1977.

44. Littler, J. W. Free tendon grafts in secondary tendon repair. *Am. J. Surg.* 74:315, 1947.

45. Littler, J. W. The severed flexor tendon. *Surg. Clin. North Am.* 39:435, 1959.

45a. Parkes, A. The "lumbricalis plus" finger. *J. Bone Joint Surg.* 53:236, 1971.

46. Littler, J. W. Principles of Reconstructive Surgery of the Hand. In J. M. Converse (ed.), *Reconstructive Plastic Surgery* (2nd ed.). Philadelphia: Saunders, 1977.

47. Lundborg, G., Myrhage, R., and Rydevik, B. The vascularization of human flexor tendons within the digital synovial sheath region—structural and functional aspects. *J. Hand Surg.* 2:417, 1977.

48. Manske, P. R. Review article: Flexor tendon healing. *J. Hand Surg. [Br.]* 13:237, 1988.

49. Manske, P. R., et al: Intrinsic flexor-tendon repair. A morphological study in vitro. *J. Bone Joint Surg. [Am.]* 66:385, 1984.

50. Manske, P. R., and Lesker, P. A. Nutrient pathways of flexor tendons in primates. *J. Hand Surg.* 7:436, 1982.

51. Mason, M. L., and Allen, H. S. The rate of healing of tendons: An experimental study of tensile strength. *Ann. Surg.* 113:424, 1941.

52. Matthews, P., and Richards, H. The repair potential of digital flexor tendons. *J. Bone Joint Surg. [Br.]* 56:618, 1974.

53. Matthews, P., and Richards, H. Factors in the adherence of flexor tendon after repair. *J. Bone Joint Surg. [Br.]* 58:230, 1976.

54. Peacock, E. E., Jr. A study of circulation in normal tendons and healing grafts. *Ann. Surg.* 149:415, 1959.

55. Peacock, E. E., Jr. Biological principles in the healing of long tendons. *Surg. Clin. North Am.* 45:461, 1965.

56. Peterson, W. W., Manske, P. R., and Lesker, P. A. The effect of flexor sheath integrity on nutrient uptake by primate flexor tendons. *J. Hand Surg. [Am.]* 11:413, 1986.

57. Protenza, A. D. The healing of autogenous tendon grafts within the flexor digital sheath in dogs. *J. Bone Joint Surg. [Am.]* 46:1462, 1964.

58. Potenza, A. D. Philosophy of flexor tendon surgery. *Orthop. Clin. North Am.* 17:349, 1986.

59. Pratt, D. R. Internal splint for closed and open treatment of injuries of the extensor tendon. *J. Bone Joint Surg. [Am.]* 34:785, 1952.

60. Pulvertaft, R. G. Tendon grafts for flexor tendon injuries in the fingers and thumb. *J. Bone*

*Joint Surg.* [*Br.*] 38:175, 1956.

61. Pulvertaft, R. G. Suture materials and tendon junctures. *Am. J. Surg.* 109:346, 1965.

62. Pulvertaft, R. G. Tendon grafting for the isolated injury of the flexor digitorum profundus. *Bull. Hosp. Jt. Dis. Orthop. Inst.* 44:424, 1984.

63. Schlenker, J. D., Lister, G. D., and Kleinert, H. E. Three complications of untreated partial laceration of flexor tendon-entrapment, rupture, and triggering. *J. Hand Surg.* 6:392, 1981.

64. Schneider, L. H., et al. Delayed flexor tendon repair in no man's land. *J. Hand Surg.* 2:452, 1977.

65. Schneider, L. H. *Flexor Tendon Injuries.* Boston: Little Brown, 1985.

66. Schneider, L. H. Staged tendon reconstruction. *Hand Clin.* 1:109, 1985.

67. Schneider, L. H., Hunter, J. M., Norris, T. R., et al. Delayed flexor tendon repair in "no-man's land." *J. Hand Surg.* 2:252, 1977.

68. Smith, J. W. Blood supply of tendons. *Am. J. Surg.* 109:272, 1965.

69. Sourmelis, S. G., and McGrouther, D. A. Retrieval of the retracted flexor tendon. *J. Hand Surg.* [*Br.*] 12:109, 1987.

70. Stark, H. H., Boyes, J. H., and Wilson, J. N. Mallet finger. *J. Bone Joint Surg.* [*Am.*] 44:1062, 1962.

71. Stark, H. H., Zemel, N. P., Boyes, J. H., et al. Flexor tendon graft through intact superficialis tendon. *J. Hand Surg.* 2:456, 1977.

72. Strickland, J. W. The management of acute flexor tendon injuries. *Orthop. Clin. North Am.* 14:827, 1983.

73. Strickland, J. W. Flexor tendon repair. *Hand Clin.* 1(1):55, 1985.

74. Strickland, J. W. Results of flexor tendon surgery in zone II. *Hand Clin.* 1:167, 1985.

75. Strickland, J. W. Flexor tendon injuries. Part 3. Free tendon grafts. *Orthop. Rev.* 16:18, 1987.

76. Strickland, J. W., and Glogovac, S. V. Digital function following flexor tendon repair in zone II: A comparison of immobilization and controlled passive motion technique. *J. Hand Surg.* 5:537, 1980.

77. Strickland, J. W. Management of acute flexor tendon injuries. *Orthop. Clin. North Am.* 14:837, 1983.

78. Urbaniak, J. R., Cahill, J. D., Jr., and Mortenson, R. A. Tendon suturing methods: Analysis of tensile strengths. In *AAOS Symposium on Tendon Surgery in the Hand.* St. Louis: Mosby, 1975. Pp. 70–80.

79. Urbaniak, J. R. Repair of the flexor pollicis longus. *Hand Clin.* 1:69, 1985.

80. Urbaniak, J. Flexor tendon injuries. *Orthop. Rev.* 15: 1986.

81. Verdan, C. Primary repair of flexor tendons (with discussion by Mason, Littler, and Boyes). *J. Bone Joint Surg.* [*Am.*] 42:647, 1960.

82. Verdan, C. E. Half a century of flexor-tendon surgery. *J. Bone Joint Surg.* [*Am.*] 54:472, 1972.

83. Verdan, C. E. Primary and Secondary Repair of Flexor and Extensor Tendon Injuries. In J. E. Flynn (ed.), *Hand Surgery (2nd ed.).* Baltimore: Williams & Wilkins, 1975.

84. Wade, P. J. F., Muir, I. F. K., and Hutcheon, L. L. Primary flexor tendon repair: The mechanical limitations of the modified Kessler technique. *J. Hand Surg.* [*Br.*] 11:71, 1986.

85. Weeks, P. M., and Wray, R. C. Rate and extent of functional recovery after flexor tendon grafting with and without silicone rod preparation. *J. Hand Surg.* 1:174, 1976.

86. White, W. L. The unique, accessible, and useful plantaris tendon. *Plast. Reconstr. Surg.* 25:133, 1960.

87. Wilson, R. L. Flexor Tendon Grafting. In *Flexor Tendon Surgery, Hand Clinics.* Philadelphia: Saunders, 1985.

88. Wilson, R. L., Carter, M. S., Holdeman, V. A., et al. Flexor profundus injuries treated with delayed two-staged tendon grafting. *J. Hand Surg.* 5:74, 1980.

# 36

*F. William Bora, Jr.*
*Mark A. Urban*

# Nerve Injury and Treatment

Trauma to peripheral nerves, resulting in partial or complete nerve section, is frequent in both civilian and military populations. After continuity of a nerve is interrupted, the axons and myelin sheaths degenerate distal to the laceration (wallerian degeneration). Within 2 days of section, axonal disruptions can be discerned by electron microscopy. Later, axonal fragmentation can be visualized by light microscopy of silver-stained sections; myelin sheaths retract and form into globules of fat, and phagocytosis of myelin and axonal fragments occurs. In addition to paralysis and anesthesia in the territory innervated by the severed nerve, the trophic influences of the nerve on muscle, joints, nails, and skin are lost, which results in progressive atrophy of muscle, bone, and skin, as well as degenerative changes in the joints.

To restore normal neurologic function, axons in the proximal stump of the interrupted nerve must sprout, migrate through the scar between proximal and distal stumps, and reach end-organs. Proteins required for the formation of these regenerating axons must be synthesized, chiefly in the nerve cell bodies in the anterior horn of the spinal cord and dorsal root ganglia, and be transported peripherally to the axon tips. Most such proteins are transported through the axons from the nerve cell bodies at a rate of 2 to 5 mm per day in mammals, a rate comparable to the observed rate of axonal regeneration [17]. The specific protein constituting the bulk of this flow is neurotubular monomer, a 60,000-dalton (molecular weight) globular protein [9].

Ideally, after nerve section, axonal outgrowth and remyelination occur promptly and in an orderly fashion before end-muscle deterioration can occur, and full neurologic function is restored. In practice, unfortunately, nerve regeneration is often prolonged, misdirected, and incomplete, and full sensory and motor trophic functions of nerve are not achieved. Several factors are responsible for this incomplete recovery:

**1.** Axons may penetrate the scar promptly but grow into the incorrect fascicle in the distal nerve stump so that they never reach the appropriate end-organs. This problem can be reduced by careful matching of nerve fascicles in the proximal and distal stumps at the time of surgical repair of a severed nerve [4]. It might be further reduced by control of scar formation at the site of laceration of the nerve.

**2.** Axons may fail to penetrate the scar, so that a neuroma forms at the site of section. The neuroma consists of whorls and tangled

**Table 36-1** *Comparison of compliance and cross-sectional areas of nonoperated normal and operated rat nerves*[a]

| Nerve | Compliance (sq mm/gm $\times$ 10$^{-3}$) | Cross-sectional area (sq mm) |
|---|---|---|
| Nonoperated normal | 1.101 ± 0.074 | 1.010 ± 0.027 |
| Cut and repair | 1.162 ± 0.180 | 1.141 ± 0.115 |
| Block excised | | |
| 2 mm | 1.427 ± 0.233[b] | 1.105 ± 0.059 |
| 5 mm | 1.369 ± 0.204[b] | 1.132 ± 0.145 |
| 5 mm (neuroma not included) | 1.154 ± 0.170 | 1.025 ± 0.090 |

[a]All data presented as the mean ± 95% confidence interval.
[b]$p<0.05$ from other groups.
Source: F. W. Bora, Jr., S. Richardson, and J. Black. The biomechanical responses to tension in a peripheral nerve. *J. Hand Surg.* 5:21, 1980.

block excised), and the 5-mm block-excised group with the neuroma excluded from the test specimen—were also so similar that all three are represented by a single curve.

The results (Table 36-1) show that the compliance and cross-sectional areas of the 2- and 5-mm block-excised groups of nerves were statistically similar to each other and statistically different ($p < 0.05$) from the unoperated controls, the cut and repaired nerves, and the 5-mm block-excised nerves without neuroma.

A histologic comparison between the normal unoperated nerve and an operated nerve with a 5-mm gap-excised and sutured that was studied 7 weeks after surgery showed the following changes in the operated nerve:

an increase in epineurium and endoneurium, unchanged perineurium, and an increase in Schwann cell proliferation within the fascicular area. The axons in the operated nerves were decreased in number and size, and their myelin wraps were less elaborate than one would expect for the diameter of the axon with which they were associated (Fig. 36-3).

**Figure 36-3** *Histologic comparison of the normal unoperated nerve on the left and a section of an operated nerve (5-mm block-excised group) on the right from the same level, 5 mm proximal to the neuroma. (From F. W. Bora, Jr., S. Richardson, and J. Black. The biomechanical responses to tension in a peripheral nerve. J. Hand Surg. 5:21, 1980.)*

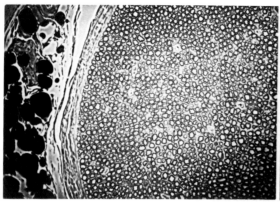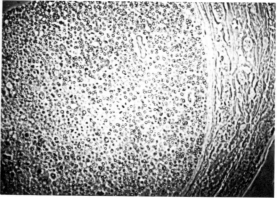

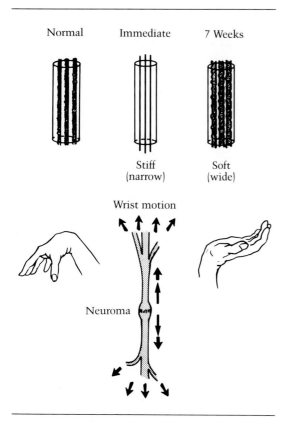

**Figure 36-4** *The three figures at the top compare normal nerve to the immediate adjustments a nerve makes to tension and to the changes found 7 weeks after surgery. Cross-sectional narrowing and an increase in compliance are the initial changes, but at 7 weeks after surgery the nerve tissue hypertrophies and increases its cross-sectional area as well as its compliance. These biomechanical changes show how nerve tissue adapts to tension during a 7-week period after nerve suture. These nerve adaptions permit the nerve extensibility necessary for joint mobilization during the extremity rehabilitation period, as shown at the bottom. (From F. W. Bora, Jr., S. Richardson, and J. Black. The biomechanical responses to tension in a peripheral nerve. J. Hand Surg. 5:21, 1980.)*

Data from these experiments show an initial stiffening response of the peripheral nerve to tension, but when tested 7 weeks after surgery, the surgically manipulated nerve with the neuroma in the test specimen had a softer curve than the normal curve. These biomechanical adjustments assist nerve extensibility and joint extension when extremity rehabilitation is begun 7 weeks after suture (Fig. 36-4).

### Epineurial Versus Perineurial Suture

Most nerve lacerations are clean and proximal to their terminal fascicular division. Two of the most important decisions to be made by the surgeon treating acute nerve lacerations are how and when to suture these multifascicular injuries. Authors have reported that epineurial suture is unreliable for restoring accurate fascicular anatomy after nerve laceration and that perineurial sutures give more satisfactory results in both clinical and experimental situations [4]. Because the use of perineurial suture is more difficult technically, is more time-consuming, and if not properly executed creates more intraneurial scar, which is more directly obstructive to axon regrowth than in epineurial suture, accurate reproducible methods of study are needed to compare the return of nerve function after nerve repair by the two techniques. Exact biochemical methods were used in a study [5] to compare the extent to nerve regeneration after epineurial, perineurial, and a combination of the two suture repairs in rabbits in early and late situations.

Sixty adult male Dutch-belted rabbits were anesthetized with spinal anesthesia. One sciatic nerve was transected midway between the sciatic notch and the knee in each rabbit. The 60 rabbits were divided into six groups of ten rabbits per group, and the lacerated nerve was repaired by placement of two 7-0 silk sutures and studied at the following two locations: (1) the sciatic nerve neuroma immediately distal to the suture (Fig. 36-5); and (2) the myelin content in the posterior tibial nerve (Fig. 36-6). These specimens were studied by the following methods to evaluate the amount of scar caused by

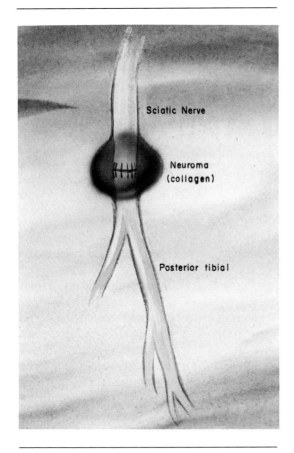

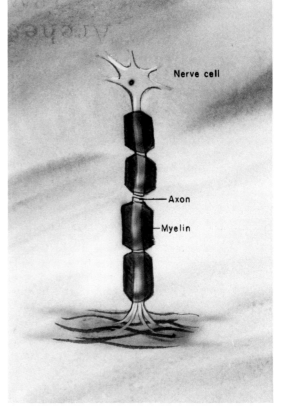

*Figure 36-5* Sciatic nerve neuroma. (From F. W. Bora, Jr., D. E. Pleasure, and N. A. Didizian. A study of nerve regeneration and neuroma formation after nerve suture by various techniques. J. Hand Surg. 1:138, 1976.)

*Figure 36-6* Nerve with myelin cover. (From F. W. Bora, Jr., D. E. Pleasure, and N. A. Didizian. A study of nerve regeneration and neuroma formation after nerve suture by various techniques. J. Hand Surg. 1:138, 1976.)

each technique as well as the return of nerve function after the various suture methods used in this study: (1) collagen in the sciatic neuroma immediately distal to the suture (by hydroxyproline assay) [18]; (2) collagen in the posterior tibial nerve (by hydroxyproline assay); and (3) biochemical assay of myelin content of the posterior tibial nerve (myelin was isolated by sucrose density gradient ultracentrifugation [14] and quantitated by sterol [19], phospholipid [11], sulfatide [12], and protein [13] assays).

No functional return of muscle strength was observed below the knee on the oper-

ated side in the various groups. Biochemical data in Tables 36-2 and 36-3 compare the percent of collagen in total protein [23] found in the sciatic nerve neuroma immediately distal to the suture and in the posterior tibial nerve.

Myelin production is an index of axon growth and maturation and was used in this study to determine nerve regeneration at sacrifice of the animal at 10 weeks. The biochemical data in Table 36-4 compare the percent of normal myelin in the operated nerve in the various suture technique groups studied. Myelin content was estimated as the

**Table 36-2** *Collagen: Percent of total protein in sciatic nerve immediately distal to suture*

| Technique | Operated sciatic nerve (%) | Unoperated sciatic nerve (%) |
|---|---|---|
| Epineurial immediate | 59.1 | 45.4 |
| Perineurial immediate | 44.4 | 48.6 |
| Epineurial and perineurial immediate | 50.1 | 47.1 |
| Epineurial delayed | 69.1 | 46.8 |
| Perineurial delayed | 61.2 | 44.7 |
| Epineurial and perineurial delayed | 55.2 | 48.5 |

Source: F. W. Bora, Jr., D. E. Pleasure, and N. A. Didizian. A study of nerve regeneration and neuroma formation after nerve suture by various techniques. *J. Hand Surg.* 1:138, 1976.

sum of cholesterol, phospholipid, sulfatide, and protein. Cerebroside was not assayed.

The myelin content of injured nerves increases as axons penetrate the distal segment and mature [16, 21]. A sensitive, quantitative method for determining the extent of nerve regeneration after laceration and suture is to assay myelin in the distal segment. The most significant finding in this study was that 60 percent of normal myelin production was found in the posterior tibial nerve after nerve lacerations repaired by immediate epineurial suture, compared to 23.8 percent in the immediate perineurial suture group and less in the delayed groups. This finding suggests to the operating surgeon that immediate epineurial repair is the best treatment for the clean, multifascicular laceration in clinical practice.

Most of the collagen in peripheral nerves is in the epineurium, separated from the myelinated and unmyelinated axons by the perineurium, a multilamellar sheath of mesothelial cells [22]. The well defined normal fascicular pattern is lost at the site of nerve transection; during nerve regeneration, multiple slender "pseudofascicles" form in the anastomotic zone, each surrounded by a slender perineurial layer, all within a much thickened epineurium [3]. Collagen content of the anastomotic zone, as judged by hydroxyproline assay, increases progressively after nerve section and repair and may reach more than 60 percent of total protein, particularly when epineurial suturing techniques are used [16, 24]. It is likely that the scar induced by epineurial suture is predominantly in the periphery of the nerve and not so

**Table 36-3** *Collagen: Percent of total protein in posterior tibial nerve*

| Technique | Operated posterior tibial nerve (%) | Unoperated posterior tibial nerve (%) |
|---|---|---|
| Epineurial immediate | 31 | 41 |
| Perineurial immediate | 34 | 35 |
| Epineurial and perineurial immediate | 35 | 31 |
| Epineurial delayed | 30 | 29 |
| Perineurial delayed | 31 | 34 |
| Epineurial and perineurial | 32 | 35 |

Source: F. W. Bora, Jr., D. E. Pleasure, and N. A. Didizian. A study of nerve regeneration and neuroma formation after nerve suture by various techniques. *J. Hand Surg.* 1:138, 1976.

*Table 36-4* Normal myelin: Percent in
operated posterior tibial nerve

| Technique | % |
| --- | --- |
| Epineurial immediate | 60 |
| Perineurial immediate | 24 |
| Epineurial and perineurial immediate | 10 |
| Epineurial delayed | 9 |
| Perineurial delayed | 14 |
| Epineurial and perineurial delayed | 7 |

Source: F. W. Bora, Jr., D. E. Pleasure, and N. A. Didizian. A study of nerve regeneration and neuroma formation after nerve suture by various techniques. *J. Hand Surg.* 1:138, 1976.

much an impediment to penetration of axonal sprouts as the perineurial scar induced by fascicular suturing. It is probably for this reason that the rate of nerve regeneration in rabbits after immediate epineurial repair of a sectioned sciatic nerve is greater than that with immediate perineurial repair.

Morphologic observations by Holmes, Saunders, and Young [10, 20] suggested that, after nerve transection, the endoneurial Schwann cell tubes in the distal nerve segment become progressively constricted by deposition of endoneurial collagen, and that this endoneurial fibrosis results in a permanent reduction in the diameter attained by regenerating axons. Abercrombie and Johnson [1, 2] found that the collagen content of the distal nerve segment of a transected rabbit sciatic nerve increases linearly for more than a year after the injury and concluded that the entire distal segment was involved. This study confirmed that collagen scar formation does occur in the distal stump of transected nerves, regardless of whether the nerves are repaired, but that the scar is confined to the initial few millimeters below the injury and does not extend into the remainder of the distal nerve segment. It has been suggested that one of the reasons for failure to recover full muscle power after nerve transection and regeneration is progressive fibrosis of denervated muscle so that the mechanical properties of the muscle

are impaired permanently despite reinnervation. Histologic observations of denervated muscle confirmed that the proportion of the muscle cross section taken up by fibrous tissue increased, but this study found that the total collagen content in triceps surae muscle after sciatic nerve transection in rats did not increase even a year after denervation. Rather, collagen content remained constant while the muscle fibers atrophied (Pleasure and Bora, unpublished data). These observations indicated that collagen scar formation after nerve transection was confined to the immediate region of the traumatic zone and suggested that measures limiting scar in this region might be successful in improving the prognosis of patients with nerve injuries.

In clinical practice, immediate repair of the nerve injury often is not possible owing to contamination of the wound and associated injuries of other tissues. Delayed suture must be done then and is best accomplished by specialized personnel with microsurgical instrumentation. At this time, better functional results are found most consistently after epineurial suture is used to repair clean multifascicular nerve injuries.

Epineurial sutures (Fig. 36-7) are used for most nerve lacerations, but the fascicular technique (Fig. 36-8) is used when the nerve is cut where it divides into its terminal fascicular branches. Fascicular suture is used when the median nerve is cut at the level of the carpal canal, where several (four to seven) fascicles must be sutured back to the stem median nerve. In such cases, the epineurium is removed proximally and the fascicles identified so that specific fascicles are sutured individually. The ulnar nerve, when cut 2 inches proximal to the wrist or where it branches in Guyon's canal, is repaired by a perineurial stitch. Lacerated radial nerves at the elbow and lacerations of the common digital nerve where it divides into its proper branches at the base of the finger are also sutured by the fascicular method. Sutured main trunk lacerations are immobilized for

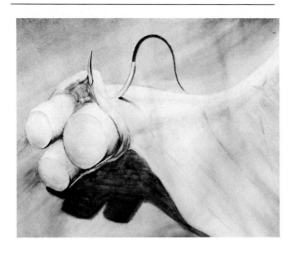

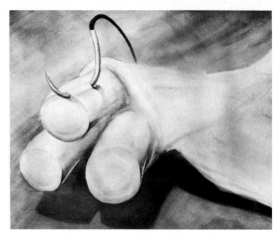

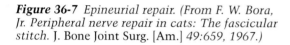

**Figure 36-7** *Epineurial repair. (From F. W. Bora, Jr. Peripheral nerve repair in cats: The fascicular stitch.* J. Bone Joint Surg. [Am.] *49:659, 1967.)*

**Figure 36-8** *Perineurial repair.*

6 weeks, and cut digital nerves with little tension are held for 3 weeks.

## Recommended Treatment for Nerve Suture

### JUDGMENT

Factors to be considered when deciding whether to repair a nerve laceration primarily or secondarily are (1) the circumstances of the injury (a knife wound in a kitchen favors primary repair, a wound in a machine shop favors secondary repair); (2) the time elapsed between the injury and treatment (1 hour favors primary suture, 24 hours favors secondary repair); (3) the character of the wound (a clean wound favors primary repair, a dirty wound favors secondary repair); (4) the presence of other injuries (a cut involving skin, nerve, and one or two tendons favors primary suture; multiple injuries, e.g., head or abdomen or multiple tendon lacerations, favor secondary nerve repair); and (5) the status of the surgeon (a well rested operator performs a more exact suture, and the ultimate functional result of a nerve repair reflects the technical exactness of the

method of suture). The examples cited above are obviously at the extremes of the scale of each consideration; when they approach the middle of the scale, as they frequently do, each factor must be evaluated not only by itself but in relation to all other factors presented. In general, open nerve lacerations are repaired primarily. Closed nerve injuries are generally kept under observation until it has been determined that a period has elapsed in which one would expect end-organ reinnervation; if recovery has not taken place as expected, secondary surgery is then performed.

### TIMING

Suturing a nerve primarily subjects the patient to only one operation and one hospitalization. Primary nerve suture lessens the reinnervation time of muscle and sensory receptor end-organs. If the acute injury is complicated by multiple injuries or possible infection of the wound, secondary repair is the treatment of choice. Factors favoring secondary suture are as follows: (1) The epineurium is thicker, enabling the surgeon to place sutures more accurately, and the thicker epineurium holds the suture more firmly, making tying easier. (2) The interneurial fibrosis that occurs at the cut ends after nerve laceration can be more easily assessed at secondary suturing, making trimming of the nerve ends easier. Based on observations made when evaluating the functional results in clinical cases as well as on data from experimental situations, it is clear that the prime objective of a surgeon treating a nerve laceration is to suture the cut as soon as it is conveniently possible.

TECHNIQUE

Acute skin lacerations can usually be incorporated into physiologic incisions that make nerve exposure suitable for mobilization and suture. After skin and subcutaneous dissection, normal nerve is identified proximal and distal to the neuroma, after which the neuroma, including some of the surrounding scar tissue, is isolated by sharp dissection. With this technique, intact fascicles may be preserved, and only the injured fascicles within the neuroma are isolated and sutured. Acute lacerations have a blood clot in various degrees of maturation between the cut ends rather than the tough fibrous tissue that is present in late nerve repair situations. After the neuroma or injured nerve ends are isolated, a No. 11 scalpel blade is used to trim the nerve to normal fascicular tissue. A moistened tongue blade is placed behind the nerve to protect other structures and to provide cutting resistance as the nerve ends are freshened. Magnification is helpful when aligning rotation, matching fascicles, and placing and tying sutures. The microscope is used for most upper extremity repairs; however, loupes are used for epineurial repairs of large proximal nerves, e.g., the sciatic and the brachial plexus.

The use of 10-0 monofilament nylon is recommended for nerve suture, but a larger suture size may be utilized if more strength is needed to bring nerve ends together. Many cases require two to three 6-0 or 7-0 nylon sutures to hold the nerve ends together; then, after tension is overcome, smaller 10-0 sutures are used to approximate the lac-erated epineurial edges. Fine jeweler's forceps, a nonlocking eye needle holder, and sharp nerve scissors are especially helpful for this delicate surgery.

Anatomy that assists the surgeon in fascicular orientation are vascular markings on the outside of the nerve and the size of the fascicles on the proximal and distal faces of the lacerated nerve edges, especially if the cut ends have not been trimmed. If an acute laceration is clean, one can remove the blood clots between the fascicles and the epineurium, thereby eliminating all trimming. This technique increases the chance of good fascicular matching because axons do change places within the peripheral nerve as they run from the shoulder to the fingertip, and trimming changes the fascicular patterns at the cut ends. Nerve mobilization and joint positioning is helpful for overcoming moderate gaps so that nerve suture holds the nerve ends together with minimal tension and buckling. Fibrous tissue is provoked by each nerve suture, obstructing axonal sprouting and maturation; therefore a minimum number of stitches is recommended for nerve and repairs. Fascicular sutures require at least one suture per fascicle and, in some cases, two or three. Judgment regarding the number of sutures depends on how each fascicle lies after the placement of each suture.

Nerve function is compromised by injuries other than transection. Bullet wounds, needle injections, and localized pressure on the skin produce hemorrhage and ultimate scarring in and around the nerve in the area of injury. Patients with such injuries who have altered nerve function are followed carefully by repeated clinical examination and electrical diagnostic testing; if the nerve function deteriorates or does not return to an acceptable level within a reasonable period of time, these patients are candidates for surgical release. Neurolysis, using magnification and microsurgical techniques, may be helpful in such cases.

After nerve laceration and suture, the

regular evaluation of cutaneous sensibility helps to define the surgical result and establish a functional treatment program for the patient. Sensation is evaluated at 6-week intervals by the following modalities:

*1.* The Tinel sign (cutaneous percussion of the injured nerve) is used to define the level to which axons have regenerated after nerve injury and its treatment. The patient determines the point of maximum sensitivity to the stimulus and realizes paresthesias in the area of innervation by the nerve, distal to the injury. After axons have penetrated the neuroma, a Tinel sign advances along the course of the nerve at a rate of about 1 mm per day or 1 inch per month.

*2.* Measurements of the size of the anesthetic and dysesthetic zone are determined by the patient's subjective description of the quality of the sensibility. From this information, a sensory mapping is obtained that is used as a baseline to which future mappings are compared.

*3.* Sensory localization is determined using a moving-touch stimulus as a constant-touch stimulus. This method of testing evaluates the quickly and slowly adapting capacities of the group A-beta fibers, which control the perception of touch [7]. This modality measures a pattern of sensory recovery in which moving touch is perceived and localized prior to constant touch. This sensory evaluation aids in determining the appropriate time to institute a program of sensory reeducation. Tests for the appreciation of light touch to deep pressure, through the process of localization, are made using Von Frey hairs or Weinstein-Seinones pressure aesthesiometer filaments. These filaments quantitatively measure light touch and deep pressure sensation. The fibers of varying diameters are placed against the skin. Pressure is exerted until the fiber bends as filaments of various diameters are used until a sensory response is elicited. This quantitative examination is measured in milligrams and is a study of the patient's sensibility, the variable being the

diameter of the fiber [25]. The test provides an opportunity for charting the patient's recognition of touch. These examinations can be compared as the patient is tested at subsequent visits. Two-point discrimination tests use a two-point aesthesiometer calibrated in millimeters for each zone of the hand. The patient discriminates between one and two points of stimulation, which are applied longitudinally within each zone. After the discriminatory abilities are determined, they are related to functional use by comparing the results to the test that measures the tactile manipulation of objects, i.e., Moberg pickup.

Although sensory evaluation is important for determining the results of a nerve injury, other rehabilitative programs are also important. Sensory reeducation teaches the patient to maximize sensibility and improve hand function. This exercise programs the patient to relearn altered sensory impulses. Various stimuli (moving touch, constant touch, and objects of varying size and shapes) are placed in contact with impaired sensory areas, and the patient is taught to reassociate the new sensation with an old activity. Sensory relearning by active motion is another modality that helps patients improve their impaired sensibility. This program uses active manipulation of blocks of various shapes and textures, as well as objects used in everyday life, to improve the appreciation of touch localization [8, 26].

Although sensory evaluation and sensory reeducation programs are useful for the nerve injury patient, it is also important to prevent deformity and to strengthen weak muscles. Dynamic and functional splints prevent joint contracture and keep joints in their functional positions while muscles are reinervated. This program maximizes hand function when muscles start to recover because the joints are mobile and the muscle action is delivered to the joint in its most functional position. Patients are further instructed about passive exercises to increase joint motion.

Postoperative treatment also includes various methods to increase muscle strength by employing therapeutic putty, as well as resistive muscle exercises during the performance of functional activities. Grip strength is measured periodically with the Jamar dynamometer. Lateral and palmar pinch exercises to individual fingers are encouraged and their strengths recorded.

Periodic electromyographic testing can be helpful for determining the reinnervation of paralyzed muscles by defining functioning motor unit potentials. Biofeedback techniques may be used on surface muscles, in some cases as a strengthening modality.

## References

1. Abercrombie, M., and Johnson, M. Collagen content of rabbit sciatic nerve during Wallerial degeneration. *J. Neurol. Neurosurg. Psychiatry* 9:113, 1946.
2. Abercrombie, M., and Johnson, M. The effect of reinnervation on collagen formation in generating sciatic nerves of rabbits. *J. Neurol. Neurosurg. Psychiatry* 10:89, 1947.
3. Ballantyne, J. P., Jr., and Campbell, M. Electrophysiological study after surgical repair of sectioned human peripheral nerves. *J. Neurol. Neurosurg. Psychiatry* 36:797, 1973.
4. Bora, F. W. Peripheral nerve repair in cats: The fascicular stitch. *J. Bone Joint Surg. [Am.]* 49:659, 1967.
5. Bora, F. W., Jr., Pleasure, D. E., and Didizian, N. A. A study of nerve regeneration and neuroma formation after nerve suture by various techniques. *J. Hand Surg.* 1:138, 1976.
6. Bora, F. W., Jr., Richardson, S., and Black, J. The biomechanical responses to tension in a peripheral nerve. *J. Hand Surg.* 5:21, 1980.
7. Dellon, A. L., Curtis, R. M., and Edgerton, M. T. Evaluating recovery of sensation of the hand following nerve injury. *Johns Hopkins Med. J.* 139:235, 1972.
8. Dellon, A. L., Curtis, R. M., and Edgerton, M. T. Re-education of sensation in the hand after nerve injury and repair. *Plast. Reconstr. Surg.* 53:297, 1974.
9. Grafstein, B., McEwen, B. S., and Shelandski, M. L. Axonal transport of neurotubule protein. *Nature* 227:289, 1970.
10. Holmes, W., and Young, Y. Nerve regeneration after immediate and delayed suture. *J. Anat.* 77:63, 1942.
11. Kates, M. *Techniques of Lipidology*. Amsterdam: Elsevier 1972. Pp. 424–425.
12. Kean, E. Rapid, sensitive spectrophotometric method for quantitative determination of sulfatides. *J. Lipid Res.* 9:319, 1968.
13. Lowry, O., Rosenbrough, N., Farr, A., et al. Protein measurement with the Folin phenol reagent. *J. Biol. Chem.* 193:265, 1951.
14. Norton, W. Isolation of myelin from nerve tissue. *Methods Enzymol.* 31A:435, 1974.
15. Pleasure, D. E., and Towfighi, J. Onion bulb neuropathies. *Arch. Neurol.* 26:289, 1972.
16. Pleasure, D., Bora, F. W., Jr., Lane, J., et al. Regeneration after nerve transection: Effect of inhibition of collagen synthesis. *Exp. Neurol.* 45:72, 1974.
17. Pleasure, D. E., Mishler, K., and Engle, W. K. Axoplasmic transport of proteins in experimental neuropathies. *Science* 166:524, 1969.
18. Prockop, D., and Undenfriend, S. A specified method for the analysis of hydroxyproline in tissues and urine. *Anal. Biochem.* 1:228, 1960.
19. Rudel, L., and Morris, M. Determination of cholesterol using ophthaldehyde. *J. Lipid Res.* 14:354, 1973.
20. Saunders, F., and Young, Y. The role of the peripheral stump in the control of fiber diameter in regenerating nerves. *J. Physiol. (Lond.)* 103:119, 1944.
21. Schroder, J. Altered ratio between axon diameter and myelin sheath thickness in regenerating nerves. *Brain Res.* 45:49, 1972.
22. Shantaveerappa, T., and Bourne, G. Perineurial epithelium: A new concept of its role in the integrity of the peripheral nervous system. *Science* 154:1464, 1966.
23. Spies, J. Colorimetric procedures for amino acids. *Methods Enzymol.* 3:467, 1957.
24. Sunderland, S. *Nerves and Nerve Injuries*, Baltimore: Williams & Wilkins, 1968.
25. Werner, J. L., and Omer, G. E. Evaluating cutaneous pressure sensation of the hand. *Am. J. Occup. Ther.* 24:347, 1970.
26. Wynn-Parry, C. B., and Salter, M. Sensory reeducation after median nerve lesions. *Hand* 8:250, 1976.

# 37

*Mark R. Belsky*
*Richard G. Eaton*

# Degenerative and Posttraumatic Arthritis of the Hand

Osteoarthritis, the most common form of arthritis, frequently involves the hand. Radiographic evidence of hand involvement increases with age: Less than 3 percent of all persons in the 18 to 24 age group have some evidence, whereas almost 80 percent of men and 90 percent of women have evidence of involvement after age 75 [12]. The economic impact of arthritis in the United States has been estimated to be a staggering 13 billion dollars [12]. Thus, the significance of osteoarthritic involvement must not be underestimated. *Osteoarthritis, degenerative arthritis, degenerative joint disease,* and *posttraumatic arthritis* are terms used to describe a similar process that may be variable in its presentation and, except for a specific traumatic event, usually obscure in its cause.

The cardinal symptom of osteoarthritis is pain, which occurs with activity and is relieved with rest. The pain is aching in character and usually poorly localized. Stiffness and eventually weakness follow closely behind. The source of the pain is unclear since cartilage has no apparent nerve supply, but it may arise from the noncartilaginous intraarticular and periarticular structures. Synovitis secondary to cartilaginous debris may be the cause. Ther stiffness is a result of the degenerative process, with new bone formation and loss of the "elasticity" of the capsular and ligamentous structures. The weakness results from pain and disuse.

Although usually insidious and dry, osteoarthritis can be associated with an acute inflammation. Erosive osteoarthritis can present this way and can cause severe destruction [15]. Clinically and histologically, its similarities to rheumatoid arthritis are striking.

The most common involvements of osteoarthritis in the hand will be described with regard to clinical presentation and treatment. Distal interphalangeal involvement, seen chiefly in women, usually has initial symptoms of stiffness and dorsal bony protuberances, referred to as Heberden's nodes [12, 13]. These changes can develop insidiously and progress unnoticed for years without pain or can present as short, intermittent periods of pain associated with inflammation and aching particularly after activity. Involvement is usually asymmetrical. There is believed to be a genetic predisposition, being autosomal dominant in women and recessive in men [12, 13].

The pathology is primary degeneration of the articular cartilage with narrowing of the joint space. The nodes represent hypertrophic bone formation of the condyles of the middle phalanx and adjacent base of the distal phalanx. There may be an associated lateral angulation as the joint destruction is followed by erosion. These changes can be best demonstrated on anteroposterior and true lateral x-ray films.

The nodes are easily palpable and visible. Often, patients complain more of the cosmetic appearance than the actual pain. Otherwise pain and stiffness of these joints are the major complaints. Symptomatic treatment is usually helpful. Mild, nonsteroidal antiinflammatory (NSAID) medications, such as aspirin, ibuprofen, and indomethacin, have been used with considerable early success.

For those with persistent symptoms, a small dorsal splint can be applied to prevent motion at the distal interphalangeal joint to relieve pain. The patient can apply the splint as needed. On occasion a Band-Aid is all that is needed to alleviate mild discomfort.

For unrelenting pain and marked deformity, the most predictable surgical treatment is arthrodesis. The functional loss is minimal if stiffness is already present and the cosmetic appearance improves with removal of the hypertrophic bone.

Occasionally, osteophytectomy without arthrodesis, with preservation of an adequate joint surface, has been performed to improve appearance, but pain relief is less predictable. Zimmerman and associates [20] reported the use of silicone interpositional arthroplasty in the distal interphalangeal joint. Despite an extensor lag that averaged 12 degrees, they were able to retain 33 degrees of stable motion.

A mucous cyst can occur over the dorsolateral aspect of the distal interphalangeal joint and is thought to be a manifestation of degenerative arthritis of that joint [8] (Fig. 37-1). This is a small gelatinous cyst, often covered by a delicate thinned skin, that appears proximal to the nail plate.

Often, the nail plate is grooved longitudinally due to pressure by the cyst on the germinal matrix. These cysts can rupture or, through well-intended aspirations, become infected. Treatment of the cyst is surgical [8]. The cyst wall can be separated from the overlying skin and the ever-present dorsal osteophyte, underlying the cyst, should be

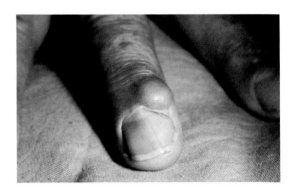

**Figure 37-1** *A small gelatinous cyst is noted in the eponychium with an associated longitudinal groove of the nail plate.*

excised. Recurrence after this form of treatment is extremely rare.

The second most frequent location for degenerative arthritis in the hand is the basal joint of the thumb [2, 12, 13]. This key articulation between the trapezium and the first metacarpal is prone to degeneration because of its unique mobility. This reciprocally biconcave saddle joint allows flexion, extension, abduction, and adduction of the thumb ray [6, 7]. The scaphotrapezial joint, another key linkage in the thumb-wrist compression axis, is also prone to degenerative change. As in the distal interphalangeal joint, the involvement is more common in women, especially after age 40. When it occurs in men, there is often a history of previous injury. Basal joint degenerative arthritis is often seen after recognized Bennett's or other occult fractures.

Patients with osteoarthritis of the hand often have a history of crocheting or needlepointing that has been curtailed because of pain. The patient complains of pain and weakness of the hand that is aggravated with activity and relieved with rest. Often it is difficult for patients to localize the pain to the base of the thumb and they may complain of diffuse wrist or hand pain.

It has been instructive to classify the degree of joint deterioration into four recogniz-

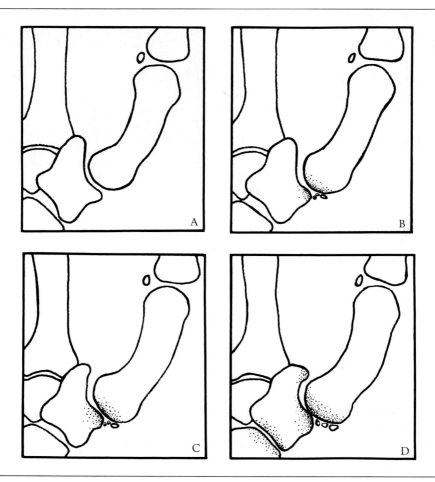

**Figure 37-2**  *A. As represented in this drawing of the lateral radiograph of the thumb ray, stage I involvement includes less than one-third subluxation of the trapezial–first metacarpal joint and normal articular contours. B. Stage II includes early evidence of degenerative changes, such as small bony fragments at the joint margins and early erosion of the dorsoradial facet of the trapezium. C. Marked joint space narrowing, larger debris (>2 mm), and sclerosis along the joint margins characterize stage III disease. D. Stage IV disease involves advanced degenerative changes of the trapeziometacarpal joint as well as the scaphotrapezial joint.*

able radiographic stages [3]. The symptoms, clinical and radiographic findings, and treatment vary with each stage.

Proper radiographic evaluation is manda-

tory to permit accurate evaluation of the extent of involvement. Staging is based on the lateral radiograph. In addition a true posteroanterior stress radiographic view, made while firmly pressing the radial border of the distal phalanx of each thumb together, demonstrates capsular laxity as well as visualization of all four trapezial articulations.

Stage I involvement of the basal joint begins with the insidious onset of pain and of the basal joint but usually no grinding or crepitus. Motion is full but often painful. Roentgenography may show slight widening of the joint space, less than one-third subluxation in any projection, and normal articular contours (Fig. 37-2A).

During acute flares, molded splints and antiinflammatory medication such as salicylates or one of the nonsteroidal antiinflammatories are helpful in reducing the symptoms. If instability can be demonstrated, reconstruction of the volar ligament restores stability and alleviates pain and further degeneration [6, 7].

Stage II disease includes significant capsular laxity and more than one-third subluxation of the joint. Small bony or calcific fragments along the joint margins of less than 2 mm in size are noted dorsally or volarly (Fig. 37-2B). Early erosion of the dorsoradial facet of the trapezium is seen. Clinically, this stage is distinguishable only by degree of pain from stage I and its treatment should not vary.

By stage III stiffness and deformity have developed. Radiographs show joint space narrowing and evidence of further degeneration. Larger debris with fragments greater than 2 mm in size are seen dorsally and volarly (see Fig. 37-2C). Some sclerosis may be seen along the joint margin as well but all involvement noted on the radiograph is confined to the trapezial first and second metacarpal joints. Crepitus may be noted, with twisting of the basal joint. Significant joint subluxation with palpable flexion deformity of the basal joint may be present.

Depending on the duration of the disease, associated changes may be seen. Adduction deformity of the thumb metacarpal, reciprocal hyperextension of the metacarpophalangeal joint, instability of the metacarpophalangeal joint, and thenar atrophy can occur (Fig. 37-3). Three-point check pinch and key pinch strength are diminished.

If symptoms are present medical management similar to that for stage I disease relieves some of these patients. Intraarticular injection of cortisone has been reported to relieve symptoms in some individuals.

With failure of conservative management, our preference for surgical reconstruction is a partial trapezial resection (that part of the trapezium articulating with the first and second metacarpals) and interposition arthroplasty [9, 14]. This procedure includes a

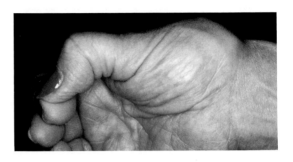

**Figure 37-3** *Adduction deformity of the thumb metacarpal and reciprocal hyperextension of the metacarpophalangeal joint are noted in this patient with stage III disease.*

ligament reconstruction of the essential volar ligament after interposition of a folded segment of flexor carpi radialis into the defect created. If there is associated hyperextension of the metacarpophalangeal joint or excessive laxity of the ulnar collateral ligament, a stabilization procedure is performed at this level.

Stage IV is reached when advanced degenerative changes are present in the basal joint and degenerative changes are also noted in the scaphotrapezial joint. This is a modification of the original classification. Severe joint space destruction is associated with cystic and sclerotic subchondral bone changes (see Fig. 37-2D). Significant erosion of the dorsal facet of the trapezium is present.

Clinically, these patients have deformities similar to those of patients with stage III disease except that the deformities may be more marked. Treatment is surgical and total trapezial excision and arthroplasty are recommended because of the pantrapezial involvement.

Reconstruction at this advanced stage includes trapezial resection, arthroplasty, and implant arthroplasty. The two most popular procedures are resection arthroplasty followed by implantation with either a folded fascial implant or a silicone implant [3, 9, 14]. Although these operations have undergone considerable evolution since their design, essentially the procedure removes the trapezium and its articulations and replaces them with a spacer. The spacer is constructed from rolled-up tendon [14], folded fascia [9], or a silicone implant [1, 3, 18, 20]. The important principles include maintaining length and stability while restoring motion.

A successful basal joint arthroplasty requires a stable, adjacent metacarpophalangeal joint. If it is hyperextensible, ligament stabilization, a capsulodesis, or arthrodesis is recommended [5].

Another modification of the resection arthroplasty is the suspension arthroplasty described by Thompson [19] in his excellent review of trapeziometacarpal arthrosis. In arthroplasties this procedure obviates the need for any interposition.

Since the development of interposition arthroplasty for stage III disease and implant arthroplasty for stage IV disease, basal joint arthrodesis is rarely indicated. In some cases, arthrodesis of the basal joint has predisposed to eventual degeneration of the adjacent metacarpophalangeal joint.

The next most commonly involved joints in the hand are the proximal interphalangeal joints and the metacarpophalangeal joints. The degenerative process in the proximal interphalangeal joints is likened to that of the distal interphalangeal joints. Nodes similar to Heberden's nodes are seen and are called Bouchard's nodes [13]. Clinically, these patients have pain, stiffness, and deformity. Joint space narrowing and abundant osteophyte formation are seen. Irregular erosion of the joint can occur, leading to angular deformities.

If medical management of the symptoms fails, several surgical alternatives are available. Early in the disease if a reasonable joint space persists, joint margin débridement with osteophytectomy and resection of tight collateral ligaments may improve motion and relieve pain.

With more severe joint destruction and loss of motion, arthroplasty may be required to relieve pain and restore motion. Implant arthroplasties of the Swanson design have been performed in selected cases, with successful relief of pain and only limited improvement in range of motion [16, 17]. The indications for proximal interphalangeal implant arthroplasty must include a significant loss of motion. The preoperative motion should be less than 60 degrees since the anticipated postoperative range of motion is 60 to 70 degrees in most cases.

For posttraumatic arthritis our preference has been the volar plate arthroplasty [4]. Pain and stiffness are frequent sequellae of dorsal fracture dislocation of the proximal interphalangeal joint, particularly when greater than 40 percent of the volar articular surface of the middle phalanx is disrupted (Fig. 37-4A). The mechanism of injury includes a longitudinal compression force across the proximal interphalangeal joint, driving the middle phalanx dorsally and impacting its volar articular surface. Volar plate arthroplasty provides a resurfacing of the defect in the middle phalanx and a volar restraint to maintain a congruous reduction (Fig. 37-4B). Similarly, there is relief of pain, but improvement in range of motion has been more significant. Regardless of the choice of arthroplasty used, the result of the proximal interphalangeal joint in osteoarthritis has been less than satisfactory.

Another treatment alternative is arthrodesis of the proximal interphalangeal joint in a functional position. This may be the preferred treatment in the flanking index and fifth fingers; however, since these joints contribute 100 degrees to the total active motion (TAM = 240–260 degrees) of the ray, its loss of motion may be a significant hardship. This treatment is less commonly indicated than arthroplasty but can predictably relieve pain.

Primary osteoarthritis of the metacarpophalangeal (MP) joints of the fingers is not common. It usually follows trauma or infection. The initial treatment is symptomatic and buddy taping may be very helpful in ad-

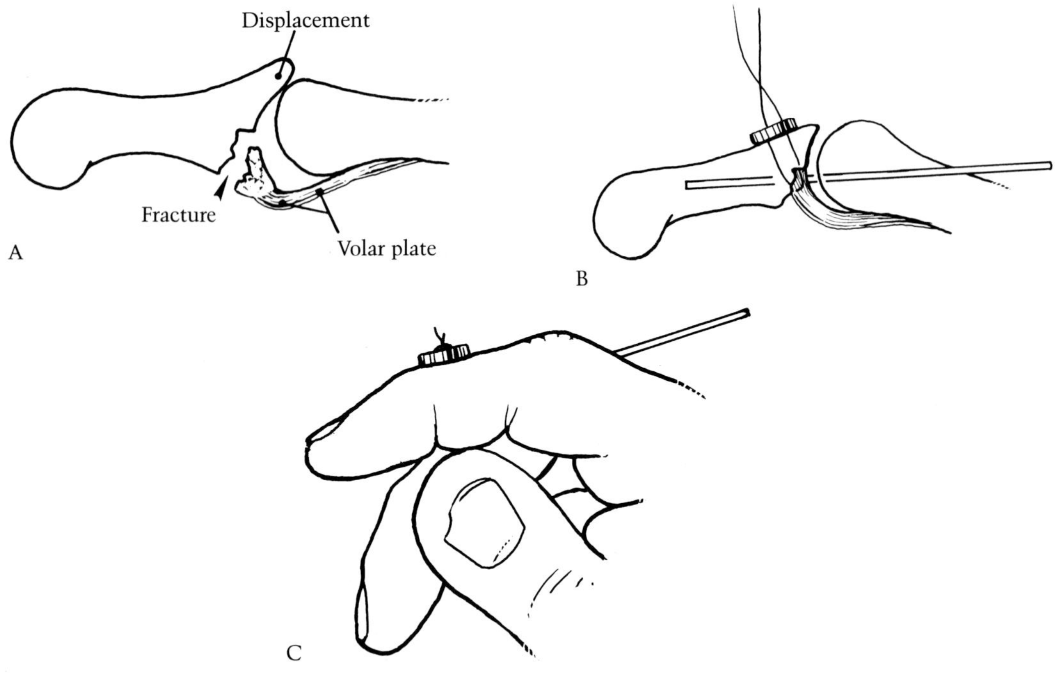

**Figure 37-4** *A. Dorsal dislocation associated with a large articular fracture of the base of the middle phalanx. Some of the articular cartilage is compressed into the defect. B. Resurfacing of the defect with advancement of the volar plate.*

dition to NSAIDs.

Surgical treatment varies, depending on adjacent joint involvement and the particular digit in need of repair. The thumb MP joint and occasionally the index MP joint are best arthrodesed. The thumb MP is arthrodesed in neutral or slight flexion with 10 degrees of pronation; the index MP is fused in 25 degrees of flexion [11].

Implant arthroplasty as described by Swanson [18] is still the most popular arthroplasty of the MP joint. It relieves pain and provides reasonable motion even in a high-demand individual. The technique is well described [1, 17, 18].

One subtle cause of arthritic pain in the thumb MP joint is sesamoiditis [15]. Although it is usually due to injury, degenerative radiographic changes can be seen, with joint space narrowing and osteophyte formation. The patient complains of pain around the MP joint; it is more commonly on the radial side at the radial sesamoid-metacarpal artic-

ulation, where the pain and tenderness are maximal. Steroid injection and occasionally excision may be necessary to relieve the pain. This can also be a cause for persistent pain after MP arthrodesis.

## References

1. Beckenbaugh, R. D. Arthroplasty in the Hand and Wrist. In D. P. Green (ed.), *Operative Hand Surgery* (2nd ed.). New York: Churchill Livingstone, 1988.
2. Burton, R. I. Basal joint arthrosis of the thumb. *Orthop. Clin. North Am.* 4:331, 1973.
3. Eaton, R. G. Replacement of the trapezium for arthritis of the basal articulations. *J. Bone Joint Surg.* 61A:76–82, 1979.
4. Eaton, R. G. Volar plate arthroplasty of the

proximal interphalangeal joint: A review of ten years' experience. *J. Hand Surg.* 5:260–268, 1980.

5. Eaton, R. G., and Floyd, W. E., III. Thumb metacarpophalangeal capsulodesis: An adjunct to basal joint arthroplasty for collapse deformity of the first ray. *J. Hand Surg.* 13A:449–453, 1988.

6. Eaton, R. G., and Littler, J. W. A study of the basal joint of the thumb. *J. Bone Joint Surg.* 51A:661–668, 1969.

7. Eaton, R. G., and Littler, J. W. Ligament reconstruction for the painful thumb carpometacarpal joint. *J. Bone Joint Surg.* 55A:1655–1666, 1973.

8. Eaton, R. G., Dobranski, J. W., and Littler, J. W. Marginal osteophyte excision in treatment of mucous cysts. *J. Bone Joint Surg.* 55A:550–574, 1973.

9. Eaton, R. G., Glickel, S. Z., and Littler, J. W. Tendon interposition for degenerative arthritis of the trapeziometacarpal joint of the thumbs. *J. Hand Surg.* 10A:645, 1985.

10. Eaton, R. G., Lane, L. B., and Littler, J. W. Ligament reconstruction for the painful thumb carpometacarpal joint: A long-term assessment. *J. Hand Surg.* 9A:692, 1984.

11. Feldon, P., and Belsky, M. R. Degenerative diseases of the metacarpophalangeal joints. *Hand Clin.* 3:429–445, 1987.

12. Kelsey, J. L., et al. *Upper Extremity Disorders.* St. Louis: Mosby, 1980. Pp. 19–22.

13. Moskowitz, R. W. Clinical and Laboratory Findings in Osteoarthritis. In D. J. McCarty (ed.), *Arthritis and Allied Conditions.* Philadelphia: Lea & Febiger, 1979.

14. Pelligrini, V. D., and Burton, R. J. Surgical management of basal joint arthritis of the thumb (Parts I and II). *J. Hand Surg.* 11:309–332, 1986.

15. Peter, J. B., Pearson, C. M., and Marmor, L. Erosive osteoarthritis of the hands. *Arthritis Rheum.* 9:365–368, 1966.

16. Ruby, L. K. Arthroplasty of the proximal interphalangeal joint. *Orthop. Rev.* 10:111–114, 1981.

17. Swanson, A. B. Flexible implant arthroplasty for arthritic finger joints. *J. Bone Joint Surg.* 54A:435, 1972.

18. Swanson, A. B. Osteoarthritis in the hand. *J. Hand Surg.* 8:669–674, 1983.

19. Thompson, J. S. Treatment of trapeziometacarpal arthrosis. *Adv. Orthop. Surg.* 105–120, 1986.

20. Zimmerman, N. B., et al. Silicone interpositional arthroplasty of the distal interphalangeal joint. *J. Hand Surg.* 14A:116–214, 1989.

# 38

H. Kirk Watson
Deborah Ekstrom

# Dupuytren's Contracture

Dupuytren's disease is characterized by contraction of the palmar fascia, forming nodules and cords primarily superficial to the neurovascular and tendinous structures of the palm. Extension of the contracting fascia into the digits can cause significant disability due to flexion contracture at the metacarpophalangeal, proximal interphalangeal, and occasionally distal interphalangeal joints.

Anatomic distortion of the digital nerves and vessels by contracting fascial tissue bands make this entity one of the most challenging technical procedures confronting the hand surgeon. Therefore, thorough knowledge of hand anatomy and close acquaintance with the predictable changes caused by the contracting fascial bands are the key to a successful outcome of surgical therapy.

## Pathophysiology

Both conjecture and scientific investigation have, as yet, failed to reveal the exact etiology of Dupuytren's contracture, although the myofibroblast has been implicated in the physiology of the disease [1, 7, 14, 17, 23, 29]. Increased amounts of type III collagen [2, 3, 8, 19], hexosamine, and hydroxylysine [3], compared to their levels in undiseased adult fascia, have also been found; and manipulation of the contractile mechanism of

myofibroblasts cultured from Dupuytren's tissue has shown responses to prostaglandins [12]. Investigation has failed to find any specific hormone receptors for estrogens or progesterone in the diseased palmar fascia [10], and no clear HLA patterns are yet discernible [26]. Perhaps additional investigation together with current data will clarify the precise etiology and pathogenesis of Dupuytren's contracture.

## Incidence

Dupuytren's disease is a heritable condition common among northern European stock, particularly those of Celtic origin, whereas its occurrence among the Chinese and pure black African races is rare [4, 18, 22]. Classically, Dupuytren's disease has been linked to epilepsy, alcoholism, diabetes, and tuberculosis. Men are affected more frequently than women and are more likely to come to surgery, suffering perhaps more severe manifestations of the disease. A small percentage of patients may also demonstrate plantar (Lederhosen's disease) or penile involvement (Peyronie's disease) or have associated knuckle pads on the proximal interphalangeal (PIP) and metacarpophalangeal (MP) joints dorsally. Interestingly, the knuckle pads seem to be a precursor of contractibility and often

967

disappear as the palmar fascia hypertrophies. Acute trauma may accelerate the condition [27]; however, the opposite result has also been reported [9, 20]. The ring finger is most commonly involved, followed in frequency by the little, middle, and index fingers. Disease is sometimes found in the thumb but is unusual [5].

## Dupuytren's Diathesis

Dupuytren's diathesis refers to the constitutional predisposition for developing this disease, inferring a more rapidly aggressive course and the expectation for early recurrence. Occurrence in a younger age group and the presence of a strong family history, knuckle pads, or plantar involvement may herald the presence of a Dupuytren's diathesis.

## Anatomy

Anatomically, the palmar aponeurosis may be completely involved in the disease process usually with sparing of the superficial transverse ligament of the palm. The pretendinous fascia as well as Grayson's ligament, the lateral digital sheet, and natatory ligament may contract, forming the spiral band displacing the neurovascular bundle medially and superficially (Fig. 38-1). Involvement of the fascia deep to the digital neurovascular structures called retrovascular fascia, if not recognized, may be a cause of recurrent disease. Disease in the thumb and first web is uncommon and not usually a cause of disability. The only cause of contracture at the MP joint is the pretendinous band. Contracture of the PIP joint is affected by contracture of the natatory ligament as well as the digital fascia. Although less commonly involved than the two more proximal joints, the distal interphalangeal (DIP) joint is also sometimes affected.

## Surgical Indications

Correction of deformity and restoration of hand function are the goals of surgical ther-

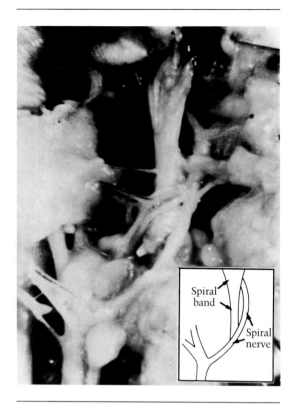

*Figure 38-1* The nerve and artery progress from the lower left of the photograph around the spiral band lying subcutaneously. They progress deep distally to their normal position alongside the fibroosseous tunnel. The nerve and artery are particularly at risk when they lie immediately subcutaneously volar to the spiral band.

apy for Dupuytren's disease. It follows, then, that functional disability is the major indication for surgical intervention.

The mere presence of a palmar nodule is otherwise not an indication for surgery. There are three indications for noncontractile fasciectomy: (1) unremitting tenosynovitis caused by a palmar nodule overlying the A-1 pulley or by constricting vertical septae at that location; (2) common digital nerve involvement in the palm producing burning pain in the finger (rare); and (3) the occasional patient who emotionally cannot accept nodular palmar Dupuytren's under any circumstances and who may fall victim to less skilled practitioners. Although MP joint contracture may cause disability, it can be corrected at any time as the flexed position protects that joint's function. Surgery is indicated for MP joint contracture alone, however, primarily as functional deficit occurs. Contraction of the DIP joint of only 15 to 20 degrees, in contrast, demands rapid surgical intervention to ensure the outcome. Long-standing PIP joint contractures develop articular cartilage changes, loss of subchondral bone, and dorsal adhesion of the extensor mechanism [6]. Almost any degree of contracture of the PIP joint is an indication for surgery. An uncommon indication for surgery for Dupuytren's contracture is neurovascular compromise with involvement of median, ulnar, and digital nerves reported [11, 21, 24]. In rare instances, joint replacement, arthrodesis, or even amputation of the digit may be indicated for severe disease. There are differing views as to whether incidental palmar fascia should be removed when operating in the area for another condition, e.g., stenosing tenosynovitis or carpal tunnel syndrome. In our experience, the Dupuytren's contracture reacts and hypertrophies rapidly if fasciectomy is not performed simultaneously.

## Operative Technique

Whereas transverse incisions have been advocated by some, longitudinal zigzag incisions from the palm extending into the digits have many advantages [13]. Exposure is excellent, and there is continuity of the dissection with skin bridges. The flaps may be advanced (Y-V) providing significant skin gain into the digits (Fig. 38-2). Parallel longitudinal zigzag incisions in the palm do well, and scarring is minimal. Full-thickness skin grafts are rarely needed. It is preferable to close all wounds because of the highly specialized nature of the palmar structures; however, it is worth noting that under difficult circumstances portions of the wound

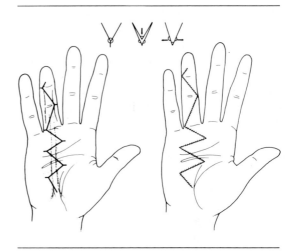

**Figure 38-2** *When the entire incision is necessary, there are approximately four flaps in the palm with approximately 90 degrees or slightly less angular measurement at the apex. The length of the backcut is shorter on the most proximal flap, and the longest backcut is on the flap that encompasses the proximal finger crease. The average length of the backcuts is about one-third the side of a flap. The degree of movement of the V-flap into the Y-cut varies with the need for skin length gain. This same incision feeds skin into the finger of camptodactyly and other surgical conditions. Inset. Skin length gain is achieved through a wedge effect. As the V moves into the Y, it drives the skin of the Y apart, effectively gaining length. It is usually necessary to have a minimum of two flaps, as the base of a single flap would limit the distal advance of the skin.*

may be left open [16]. They close well within about 2 to 3 weeks.

A basic technical principle in Dupuytren's surgery is dissection around, but never within, the diseased fascia. We prefer excision of all diseased fascia in the involved area. Under tourniquet control, the skin flaps are raised and dissection begins in the mid to proximal palm. The palmar fascia is transected here where it can be easily raised off the tendons and the neurovascular structures. Subsequent dissection proceeds proximally, removing that entire portion of the proximal palmar fascia. The distal segment is then removed by elevating the fascia and cutting the vertical septae that extend dorsally along the sides of the tendons. Heavy vertical septae are often found on each side of the A-1 pulley and must be excised similarly. In this manner, the palmar disease can be rapidly excised.

In the digit, the skin flaps are raised and the diseased fascia exposed. Care must be taken to watch for a soft, pulpy skin prominence at the base of the digit proximal to the proximal finger skin crease. This finding warns of spiral band formation with displacement of the neurovascular bundle medially and superficially [25]. In the finger, the central fascial band usually splits just over the PIP joint. These bands course deep to the neurovascular bundles. Distally they attach to the "assembly line" on the middle phalanx. After complete excision the PIP joint must be checked for full extension, and check rein ligament release is performed if necessary.

Check reins are the basic cause of flexion deformity. They diverge proximally from the volar plate and insert separately along the volar lateral periosteum of the proximal phalanx along two bony ridges that we call the "assembly line." Check reins are usually present as paired structures. The two digital arteries give off branches that pass through the check reins to merge in the midline. These vessels feed the major vascular supply to the tendon vincular system [29] and must be preserved during check rein resection procedures (Fig. 38-3).

The release is done by identifying the proximal edge of the volar plate and cutting the check reins free from their broad triangular attachments to the proximal edge of the volar plate. This dissection must occasionally be carried laterally and dorsally along the side of the proximal phalanx in line with the proximal edge of the volar plate. The check rein is then elevated and removed, protecting the communicating nutrient vessel. The joint is straightened.

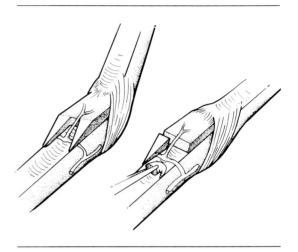

*Figure 38-3* *The check reins exist as thickened, triangular, abnormal scar tissue from the proximal edge of the volar plate to the "assembly line." They often extend somewhat dorsally (not shown here). With incision or excision of the check reins, the joint can be brought to full 180-degree extension. Preservation of the communicating vessels is important as the main vincular blood supply passes volarly to the tendons just proximal to the volar plate.*

After excision of all accessible diseased fascia and check rein release, the wound is closed. Backcuts can be made at the apex of the incisions, allowing advancement of additional skin into the finger. This maneuver facilitates tension-free closure and primary healing, avoiding open wounds, skin grafts, and Z-plasties. Before releasing the tourniquet, a compressive dressing and plaster splint are applied. The anteroposterior diameter of the dressing must just exceed the lateral dressing diameter, producing palmar pressure. No pressure should be present on the sides of the index and little finger metacarpals. Some surgeons prefer to release the tourniquet and seek control of any hemorrhage prior to skin closure.

Excision of all accessible diseased fascia (limited radical fasciectomy) is the procedure now most commonly done for Dupuytren's disease. Occasionally, a patient of advanced age with limited life expectancy can most appropriately be treated with fasciotomy alone.

## Postoperative Management

Postoperatively, mobilization is begun in light dressing at 48 hours. A Joint Spring (Joint Jack Co., Glastonbury, CT) splint is applied to involved fingers at the time of initial dressing change. By 10 days, Joint Jack (Joint Jack Co.) splints may be used on the PIP joints.

## Complications

Early complications include hematoma, infection, and skin slough, with scarring and recurrence common late complications. A frequent complication of Dupuytren's surgery is the excessive tissue reaction typical of this disease. Although relatively few Dupuytren's patients progress to a full reflex sympathetic dystrophy, many reach the "at risk" level, demonstrating excessive pain and swelling that leads to stiffness.

The tissue "dystrophile" loading program is a successful approach to both the "at risk" patient and the "full blown" dystrophy patient. This program consists in active traction and compression exercises that provide stress to the extremity without requiring joint motion that may aggravate the condition. Initially, increased pain and swelling may occur, but they subside within a few days as the neurovascular system begins to adapt.

The patient is instructed in the use of the dystrophile [28], applying as much pressure as possible three times a day for 3 to 7 minutes per session. The patient is also told to "carry" a weighted briefcase or purse in the affected hand throughout the day. The load is increased as the patient's tolerance improves.

A not uncommon complication is the contracted PIP of the little finger after two or more operations. Commonly, there is trophic change in the digit. Compromise of both the nerve and the vascular system is

**Figure 38-4** *The severely flexed trophic multiinsult finger can be functionally preserved by approaching the finger dorsally and achieving sufficient extension by shortening the bone at the middle phalanx. It is important to maintain the cancellous metaphyseal bone of the base of the middle phalanx so that one is not dealing with two cortical midshaft bones when the shortening has been completed. The distance A to A¹ is the same preoperatively as postoperatively, emphasizing that the length of neurovascular damage and scar tissue has not been changed.*

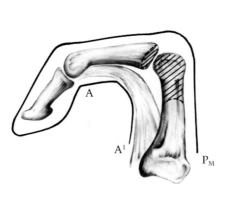
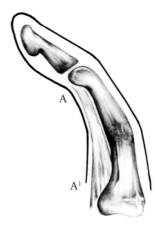

common. Further volar release is nearly impossible, and amputation is frequently recommended. These digits are functionally and cosmetically preserved via a dorsal approach, shortening to correct the flexion, and arthrodesis of the PIP joint (Fig. 38-4).

## Summary

Dupuytren's disease is a tenacious hereditary recurrent problem. Early surgery (once contractures develop) produces improved results. Palmar localized radical fasciectomy seems to preclude recurrence and leaves later finger Dupuytren's devoid of proximal attachments. Close attention during the postoperative period is important.

## References

1. Badalamente, M. A., Stern, L., and Hurst, L. C. The pathogenesis of Dupuytren's contracture: Contractile mechanisms of the myofibroblasts. *J. Hand Surg.* 8:235, 1983.
2. Bailey, A., Sims, T., Gabbiani, G., et al. Collagen of Dupuytren's disease. *Clin. Sci.* 53:499, 1977.
3. Brickley-Parsons, D., Glimcher, M., Smith, R., et al. Biochemical changes in the collagen of the palmar fascia in patients with Dupuytren's disease. *J. Bone Joint Surg. [Am.]* 63:787, 1981.
4. Chow, S. P., Luk, K. D., and Kung, T. M. Dupuytren's contracture in Chinese: A report of three cases. *J. R. Coll. Surg. Edinb.* 29:49, 1984.
5. Cleland, H., and Morrison, W. A. Dupuytren's disease in the thumb: Two cases of a central cord. *Hand Surg. [Br.]* 11:68, 1986.
6. Field, P. L., and Hueston, J. T. Articular cartilage loss in long-standing flexion deformity of the proximal interphalangeal joints. *Aust. N.Z. J. Surg.* 40:70, 1980.
7. Gabbiani, G., and Majno, G. Dupuytren's contracture: Fibroblast contraction? An ultrastructural study. *Am. J. Pathol.* 66:131, 1972.
8. Gelberman, R., Amiel, D., Rudolph, R., and Vance, R. Dupuytren's contracture: Electron microscopic, biochemical and clinical correlative study. *J. Bone Joint Surg. [Am.]* 62:425, 1980.
9. Grace, D. L., McGrouther, D. A., and Phillips,

10. Hankin, F. M., Eckenrode, J., and Louis, D. S. Oestrogen and progesterone hormone receptors in Dupuytren's disease. *J. Hand Surg. [Br.]* 11:463, 1986.
11. Hueston, J. T. Digital Wolfe grafts in recurrent Dupuytren's contracture. *Plast. Reconstr. Surg.* 29:342, 1962.
12. Hurst, L. C., Badalamente, M. A., and Makowski, J. The pathobiology of Dupuytren's contracture: Effects of prostaglandins on myofibroblasts. *J. Hand Surg.* 11:18, 1986.
13. King E., Bass, D., and Watson, H. K. Treatment of Dupuytren's contracture by extensive fasciectomy through multiple Y-V plasty incisions: Short-term evaluation of 170 consecutive operations. *J. Hand Surg.* 4:234, 1979.
14. Majno, G., Gabbiani, G., Hirschel, B. J., et al. Contraction of granulation tissue in vitro: Similarity to smooth muscle. *Science* 173:548, 1971.
15. McCash, C. R. Open palm technique in Dupuytren's contracture. *Br. J. Plast. Surg.* 17:271, 1964.
16. McFarlane, R., and Chiu, H. Pathogenesis of Dupuytren's contracture: A correlative clinical-pathological study. *J. Hand Surg.* 3:1, 1978.
17. Mennen, U. Dupuytren's contracture in the Negro. *J. Hand Surg. [Br.]* 11:61, 1986.
18. Menzel, E., Piza, H., Zielinski, C., et al. Collagen types and anticollagen-antibodies in Dupuytren's disease. *Hand* 11:243, 1979.
19. Milner, R. H., and Reid, C. A. Dupuytren's contracture which resolved following a traumatic incident. *J. Hand Surg. [Br.]* 10:277, 1985 (letter).
20. Nissenbaum, M., and Keinert, H. E. Treatment considerations in carpal tunnel syndrome with coexistent Dupuytren's disease. *J. Hand Surg.* 5:544, 1980.
21. Rosenfeld, N., Mavor, E., and Wise, L. Dupuytren's contracture in a black female child. *Hand* 15:82, 1983.
22. Salamon, A., and Hamori, J. Possible role of myofibroblasts in the pathogenesis of Dupuytren's contracture. *Acta Morphol. Acad. Sci. Hung.* 28:71, 1980.
23. Salzberg, C. A., and Weinberg, H. Dupuytren's disease as a cause of ulnar tunnel syndrome. *J. Hand Surg.* 12:91, 1987.
24. Short, W. H., and Watson, H. K. Prediction of

H. Traumatic correction of Dupuytren's contracture. *J. Hand Surg.* 9:59, 1984.

the spiral nerve in Dupuytren's contracture. *J. Hand Surg* 7:84, 1982.

25. Spencer, J. D., and Walsh, K. I. Histocompatibility antigen patterns in Dupuytren's contracture. *J. Hand Surg. [Br.]* 9:276, 1984.

26. Stewart, H. D., Innes, A. R., and Burke, F. D. The hand complications of Colles' fractures. *J. Hand Surg. [Br.]* 10:103, 1985.

27. Tomasek, J. J., Schultz, R. J., Episalla, C. W., and Newman, S. A. The cytoskeleton and extracellular matrix of the Dupuytren's disease "myofibroblast": An immunofluorescence study of a nonmuscle cell type. *J. Hand Surg.* 11:365, 1986.

28. Watson, H. K., and Carlson, L. Treatment of reflex sympathetic dystrophy of the hand with an active "stress loading" program. *J. Hand Surg.* 12A:779, 1987.

29. Watson, H. K., Light, T., and Johnson, T. Checkrein resection for flexion contracture of the middle joint. *J. Hand Surg.* 4:67, 1979.

## Suggested Reading

Barton, N. J. Dupuytren's disease arising from the abductor digiti minimi. *J. Hand Surg. [Br.]* 9:265–270, 1984.

Burgess, R. D., and Watson, H. K. Stenosing tenosynovitis in Dupuytren's contracture. *J. Hand Surg.* 12:89–90, 1987.

Dupuytren, G. *Leçons Orales de Clinique Chirurgicale.* Vol. 1. Paris: G. Baillière, 1832.

Evans, R. A. The aetiology of Dupuytren's disease. *Br. J. Hosp. Med.* 36:198–199, 1986.

Gonzalez, R. I. The use of skin grafts in the treatment of Dupuytren's contracture. *Hand Clin.* 1:641–647, 1985.

Hill, N. A. Dupuytren's contracture. *J. Bone Joint Surg. [Am.]* 67:1439–1443, 1985.

Hueston, J. T. Current state of treatment of Dupuytren's disease. *Ann. Chir. Main* 3:81–92, 1984.

Hueston, J. T. The extensor apparatus in Dupuytren's disease. *Ann. Chir. Main* 4:7–10, 1985.

James, W. D., and Odom, R. B. The role of the myofibroblast in Dupuytren's contracture. *Arch. Dermatol.* 116:807–811, 1980.

Kischer, C. W., and Speer, D. P. Microvascular changes in Dupuytren's contracture. *J. Hand Surg.* 9A:58–62, 1984.

Larkin, J. G., and Frier, B. M. Limited joint mobility and Dupuytren's contracture in diabetic, hypertensive, and normal populations. *Br. Med. J. [Clin. Res.]* 7:292(6534):1494, 1986.

Lease, J. W. Dupuytren's disease. *Surg. Annu.* 17:355–368, 1985.

Lubahn, J. D., Lister, G. D., and Wolfe, T. Fasciectomy and Dupuytren's disease: A comparison between the open-palm technique and wound closure. *J. Hand Surg.* 9A:53–58, 1984.

McFarlane, R. M. The current status of Dupuytren's disease. *J. Hand Surg.* 8:703–708, 1983.

McFarlane, R. M. The anatomy of Dupuytren's disease. *Bull. Hosp. Jt. Dis. Orthop. Inst.* 44:318–337, 1984.

McGrouther, D. A. The microanatomy of Dupuytren's contracture. *Hand* 14:215–236, 1982.

Nagay, B. Dupuytren's contracture—contemporary views on the etiopathogenesis and clinic of the disease. *Mater Med. Pol.* 17:251–256, 1985.

Noble, J., Heathcote, J. G., and Cohen, H. Diabetes mellitus in the aetiology of Dupuytren's disease. *J. Bone Joint Surg. [Br.]* 66:322–325, 1984.

Pereira, R. S., Black, C. M., Turner, S. M., et al. Antibodies to collagen types I–VI in Dupuytren's contracture. *J. Hand Surg. [Br.]* 11:58–60, 1986.

Schneider, L. H., Hankin, F. M., and Eisenberg, T. Surgery of Dupuytren's disease: A review of the open palm method. *J. Hand Surg.* 11:23–27, 1986.

Short, W., and Watson, H. K. Predication of the spiral nerve in Dupuytren's contracture. *J. Hand Surg.* 7:84–86, 1982.

Skoag, T. Dupuytren's contracture: Pathogenesis and surgical treatment. *Surg. Clin. North Am.* 47:433, 1967.

Tonkin, M. A., and Lennon, W. P. Dermofasciectomy and proximal interphalangeal joint replacement in Dupuytren's disease. *J. Hand Surg. [Br.]* 10:351–352, 1985.

Tonkin, M. A., Burke, F. D., and Varian, J. P. Dupuytren's contracture: A comparative study of fasciectomy and dermofasciectomy in one hundred patients. *J. Hand Surg. [Br.]* 9:156–162, 1984.

Tonkin, M. A., Burke, F. D., and Varian, J. P. The proximal interphalangeal joint in Dupuytren's disease. *J. Hand Surg. [Br.]* 10:358–364, 1985.

Tubiana, R. Evaluation of deformities in Dupuytren's disease. *Ann. Chir. Main* 5:5–11, 1986.

Tubiana, R., Fahrer, M., and McCullough, C. J. Recurrence and other complications in surgery of Dupuytren's contracture. *Clin. Plast. Surg.* 8:45–50, 1981.

# 39

*Earl J. Fleegler*

# Tumors of the Upper Extremity

Masses may arise from any of the tissues of the upper extremity. Therefore, this tumor group is a broad collection that challenges the diagnostic acumen of any physician willing to take on the responsibility of its treatment. Although frequently benign, these lesions may produce unsightly contour changes, cause difficulty putting on rings, gloves, or other items of clothing, and produce an alteration in finger range of motion. They may interfere with nerve, muscle, tendon, or joint function, and some produce pain. Those tumors that are more aggressive may recur locally, be destructive to surrounding tissues, and even metastasize, ultimately leading to the death of the patient. In such cases the approach to these "lumps" may be more difficult than is initially apparent. Principles involved in their diagnosis and management require an understanding of the staging of neoplasms, appropriate methods of biopsy, and principles of treatment [58]. The best treatment modalities for some of these tumors are still not established.

## Benign Tumors
### GANGLIA
Ganglia are probably the most common masses encountered in the hand. They are frequently firm, often located in the dorsum of the wrist, and when in this location be-come more prominent on wrist flexion. They are usually attached to the underlying joint capsule. These cysts may also be attached to tendon sheaths and less frequently involve the tendons or even bony structures.

Patients are frequently bothered by deformity produced by ganglia, although additional complaints include weakness, numbness, and pain. Other than those lesions associated with a clear history of trauma or with underlying bony abnormalities, it is often difficult to explain their etiology.

The clinical course of ganglia varies. Some regress spontaneously, whereas others continue to become more prominent. Recurrence is common even with surgical treatment. However, methods that do not completely remove the ganglion, although they may have their indications, are more frequently associated with recurrence of complaints.

At surgery these white to gray cysts are filled with a viscid, clear, muscin-containing fluid [1]. Common sites for ganglia include the dorsoradial aspect of the wrist followed by the palmar aspect of the base of fingers, and the palmar-radial aspect of the wrist. A similar lesion is found in the area of the distal phalanx of the dorsum of the finger, and in this location it is frequently associated with an underlying osteoarthritic spur [19].

Treatment includes a variety of approaches, including many means of disrupting the ganglion while leaving them in situ, aspiration with or without injection of corticosteroids, and surgical excision with some form of splinting. "Second hand" experience with the first-mentioned modality has not revealed significant long-term freedom from these cysts treated by smashing them. Because of a similar experience with the aspiration and injection technique, this possibility is discussed with the patient but is reserved for recurrent cysts unless specifically requested by the patient. Surgical excision of the cyst is undertaken after complete discussion of differential diagnosis, alternatives of treatment, and all the considerations usually reviewed with patients presenting with masses. Such surgery is carried out in the regular operating suite under pneumatic tourniquet control and appropriate anesthesia, usually an axillary block. Incisions, usually transverse for dorsal wrist lesions, must give adequate exposure. Important structures include underlying sensory nerve branches, which if injured may lead to long-term disability, are carefully protected. The cysts are followed to their origin, magnification is used, and the ganglion is completely excised. Postoperative splinting is routine.

Such splinting is carried out with a wrist "cock-up" splint keeping the wrist in the neutral position. If, as occasionally is seen, the cyst involves more superficial structures such as the extensor retinaculum and synovial tissues surrounding the extensor tendons, splinting is discontinued after about a week and a half when sutures are removed. However, concern for ligamentous stability has led to 3 weeks of splinting for many of the patients whose ganglion extends down to the dorsal wrist ligaments. With this approach, hand therapy is usually required, and some limitation of range of motion, which is discussed with the patients, is possible.

## EPIDERMAL AND SEBACEOUS (TRICHILEMMAL) CYSTS
More confusion in the differential diagnosis of tumors of the hand may be created by other types of cyst, e.g., the epidermal inclusion cyst and sebaceous or trichilemmal cyst. Inclusion cysts have been thought to result from epidermal tissue displaced into the deeper tissues secondary to trauma. However, our experience with this relatively common mass is that patients frequently do not recall a specific traumatic episode in the area of the mass.

The presenting complaint is usually that of a firm mass not previously noted; discomfort occasionally brings these lesions to the patient's awareness. On examination inclusion cysts are frequently firm, smooth, and of varying fixation, from freely movable to slightly fixed. They may also be found within bone, in which case radiographic examination reveals "solitary, unmineralized, radiolucent lesions in distal phalanges" [32]. This site is a rare one for primary bone tumors. Usually the bony defect has a sharply defined margin with a thin layer of sclerotic bone [32]. Treatment of these cysts is complete excision and primary reconstruction of the area, which also provides a specimen for histologic evaluation.

Sebaceous cysts are confined to the hair-bearing skin areas [54] and are frequently attached to an overlying small dimpled area. Infection may be a presenting complaint.

If it is not clinically infected, treatment is surgical removal that includes an ellipse of the attached skin. Infection may require incision and drainage first, then antibiotics and local care with warm compresses, after which the cyst may be excised.

## VERRUCAE (WARTS)
Warts are raised, hard lesions with irregular surfaces (Fig. 39-1). They may be seen in a variety of areas including the palmar and dorsal skin of the hand and the nail bed area. These warts are caused by the human papilloma virus, which is a DNA-containing tumor-producing virus [33]. Warts about the fingernail area can be especially difficult to treat because of deformity produced in the nail folds and nail bed area. Persistent or recurrent "warts" in this area often require

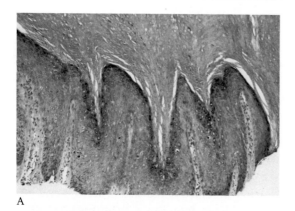

A

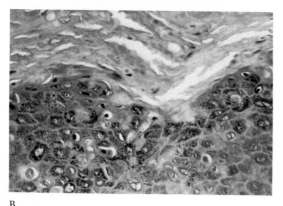

B

*Figure 39-1* A. *Irregular papillary surface is seen in a wart of the nail bed. B. Note the vacuolated cells, retention of nuclei into the keratinized layer (parakeratosis), and prominent keratohyalin granules, which are all typical of verruca vulgaris (wart).*

biopsy because of the difficult differential diagnosis between them and nail area squamous cell carcinoma (see discussion later in this chapter).

Treatment of these warts may include use of agents that are locally destructive [54, 76]. Recurrent lesions, once biopsied and proved to be benign verrucae, may be treated with bleomycin by those experienced with this mode of therapy [75]. Dermatologic colleagues also utilize cryotherapy for certain warts. Although these virus-produced skin tumors may resolve spontaneously or with one of the modalities of treatment described above, recurrence is sometimes a difficult problem. Occasional excision followed by local tissue reconstruction or skin graft may be utilized depending on the judgment of the surgeon [43].

KERATOSES

Seborrheic keratosis, characterized by a relatively flat to slightly elevated, waxy or greasy looking lesion, may vary in color from light tan to yellow to brown. Malignant change in such lesions is not common.

Once histologic diagnosis is obtained a variety of destructive therapeutic modalities seem reasonable, including various types of excision, electrodestruction, cryotherapy, or even 5-fluorouracil cream [26, 76]. My preference is excision followed by local reconstruction. This method usually results in early healing and yields excellent tissue samples for careful histologic evaluation.

Actinic (senile or solar) keratoses are premalignant tumors. It may be difficult to distinguish them from a seborrheic keratosis, and biopsy is recommended. In their premalignant condition these tumors are usually cured by excision and primary reconstruction.

Arsenical keratoses are commonly located on the palmar aspect of the hand (as well as plantar aspects of the feet) (Fig. 39-2). These tumors are firm, irregular, and rough feeling; they are multiple and vary somewhat from having almost a normal skin color to an erythematous, scaly, wart-like appearance.

After histologic diagnosis, treatment may vary from excision with primary closure or skin grafting for lesions that are either bothering the patient, ulcerating, or showing evidence of malignancy, to wide excisions of groups of lesions followed by skin grafting. Control of the extensive involvement by these tumors may be difficult.

Radiation dermatitis and cutaneous horn are premalignant conditions. They require regular follow-up reevaluation after ablative treatment (Fig. 39-3).

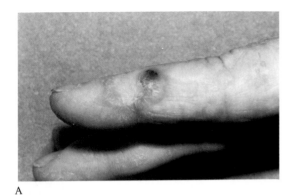

A

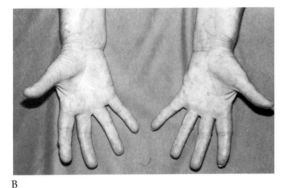

B

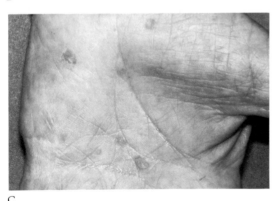

C

**Figure 39-2** *A. A 66-year-old woman had been treated during childhood with an arsenic compound for acne. She presented here with an ulcerated lesion with a hyperkeratotic edge that had previously undergone biopsy, revealing areas of carcinoma in situ. B, C. Palmar views demonstrate the hyperkeratotic lesions that were slightly elevated. The skin is pink and rough in texture.*

## NEVI

Pigmented tumors of the upper extremity may cause even more confusion than is encountered in the differential diagnosis of the masses already mentioned. Malignant variations of pigmented tumors are becoming more common on sun-exposed areas of the upper extremity.

Diagnosis requires that one is alert to these dangerous tumors and carries out appropriate biopsy. It is our responsibility, when pigmented lesions are called to our attention, to clarify their exact nature and potential. The pigment-containing cell, the melanocyte, is situated in the basal layer of the epidermis and is capable of manufacturing melanin. If a collection of these cells are present in the dermis itself, they are referred to as *nevus cells.* Tumors composed of collections of such cells may be divided into those present at birth (congenital) and those that were acquired later in life. The patient pictured in Figure 39-4 is an elderly woman who presented with a brown macule on the dorsum of her hand in a sun-exposed area. Such lesions are characteristically flat and on histologic examination are characterized by increased numbers of normal melanocytes above the basement membrane [54]. This benign, senile lentigo needs no further treatment unless other changes develop. The debate as to whether benign moles or nevi can become malignancies is still not settled. Benign, acquired, melanocytic nevi are generally smaller, perhaps not more than 6 mm in diameter, although larger ones are encountered; these nevi usually have regular or uniform color patterns [71]. In addition, the overlying skin markings are intact or normal (which is best observed with the assistance of magnification). Nevi usually occur after birth and continue to appear as the individual matures, goes through puberty, and experiences pregnancy [34]. In later life moles may actually become less conspicuous—at least they do not increase in size and new ones do not develop in middle life.

Among the types of benign nevi junctional

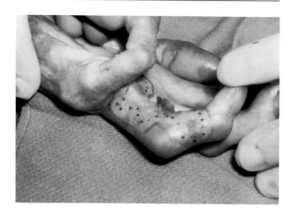

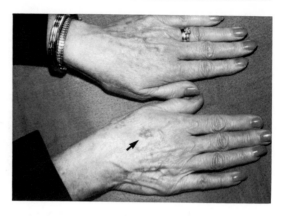

**Figure 39-3** *Note the cutaneous horn surrounded by atrophic skin containing multiple keratoses in a previously irradiated patient.*

**Figure 39-4** *Senile or solar lentigo. These lesions are common on the dorsum of the hands in older patients [54].*

nevi are those that are clinically flat and may have dark brownish pigmentation (Fig. 39-5). Histologically, their melanocytes are noted within the epidermis; they do not appear to reach up into the upper portions of the epidermis; and their nests of cells are located above the basement membrane [54].

Compound nevi have their melanocytes located in both the dermis and the epidermis [54] (Fig. 39-5B). Clinically, they are well circumscribed, frequently dark brown, and evenly pigmented with intact overlying skin markings.

When benign melanocytic cells come to lie completely within the dermis, the nevus is then termed *intradermal melanocytic nevus* [54] (Fig. 39-5C). Clinically, this lesion appears raised above the skin surface, has a uniform color (which may vary from skin-color tan to brown), and has a well defined, regular border. Histologically, the nuclei become smaller with progressively deeper movement of the lesion into the dermis. This development of the nuclei is considered to be a sign of maturation [71]. Contrast this benign cell maturation process with subsequent patient examples showing malignant melanoma. Blue nevi are benign lesions

whose blue color derives from melanocytes that contain a considerable amount of pigment located within the dermis.

Treatment of the patient complaining of a pigmented skin tumor requires a careful history and physical examination. The differentiation just reviewed of commonly encountered lesions may be helpful in arriving at a diagnosis. However, in each case it must be understood that the ultimate information is derived from histologic evaluation of an appropriate specimen, which requires at least excision of the lesion for pathologic evaluation in the case of small lesions or incisional biopsy including the junction of the lesion with normal skin for large ones. Incisional biopsies must include both the area of junction of the lesion with normal-looking skin and that portion of the pigmented lesion that might exhibit the most advanced stage of the tumor, such as a nodular area in an otherwise flat lesion. When the pathology report defines a malignant pigmented tumor, review of the specimen with the pathologist can help provide additional information that has implications concerning malignant potential and even surgical planning. Combining the classification of Clark et al. and

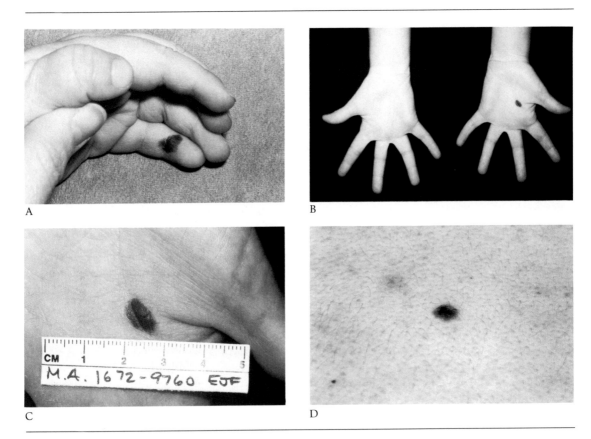

A

B

C

D

Breslow can help the surgeon understand a particular tumor's potential [8, 15, 16]. (See the later section in this chapter dealing with malignant tumors.)

TUMORS OF VASCULAR TISSUE

This section discusses masses composed of various types of blood and lymph vessels. Although some of these tumors come to the physician's attention when the patient is older, they are commonly seen during childhood and are usually congenital in origin. They are often among the more difficult lesions to understand and treat.

Capillary hemangiomas are areas of red to purple discoloration seen through the skin. In the capillary-strawberry type hemangioma there is usually a history of the patient being born with a small, "pale pink-white

*Figure 39-5* A. A 3-year-old male child presented with a congenital, flat, somewhat irregularly marginated, uniformly pigmented dark brown lesion on the palmar-radial aspect of the left little finger. Excisional biopsy revealed that it was a junctional nevus. B. This hand belongs to a 5-year-old girl with a regularly marginated, slightly raised, uniformly dark brown tumor that had increased slightly in size. Biopsy revealed that it was a compound congenital nevus. C. A closer view of the compound nevus described above reveals intact skin markings with a smooth, nonulcerated surface. D. Note the somewhat lighter brown, elevated pigmented tumor that had a regular margin. At biopsy it was determined to be an intradermal nevus.

patch" [50]. The lesion usually enlarges to form a spongy red mass—a strawberry hemangioma. So long as no other associated pathology, such as discrepancy in limb growth or evidence of arteriovenous fistula, is found on examination, the compression method of nonsurgical treatment is usually recommended [50]. Regression of such lesions can be achieved by the therapy described. However, I prefer not to make any promises with regard to the extent of such improvement. Syndromes that must be ruled out include the Maffucci syndrome, which includes multiple mixed capillary-cavernous hemangiomas associated with osteochondromas. Jaffe indicated that chondrosarcoma may occur in more than 50% of patients with the Maffucci syndrome [48, 84]. Multiple hemangiomas may be associated with gastrointestinal hemangiomas and bleeding and are also sought during the general evaluation of the patient [50].

Cavernous hemangiomas contain larger vessels (frequently of mixed venous and arterial components); the lesions can grow to a large size, are often poorly marginated, and are frequently deep-seated. They do not appear to regress [50]. One approach to their treatment is the utilization of carefully applied and monitored, gentle pressure gradient garments (Jobst Co., Toledo, Ohio). Such treatment is an effort to obtain some improvement with regard to overall size and rate of growth. However, the results are variable. The literature also describes utilization of systemic steroid treatment. Such workers have employed a trial course of systemic steroids when lesions were extensive, enlarging, and "nonamenable to surgical excision" [86]. This approach was utilized for young children. The interested physician may carefully review the report in our reference section as well as the precautions. On occasion these lesions, which may enlarge and produce discomfort including a heavy sensation, are found to be localized enough to permit surgical treatment in the upper extremity. Preoperatively, careful evaluation includes angiography to ascertain the extent of the tumor and its relation to important vessels and to help decide if vascular reconstruction will be required [69] (Fig. 39-6).

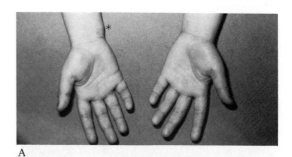

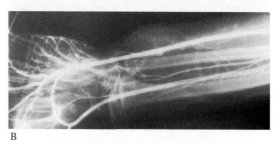

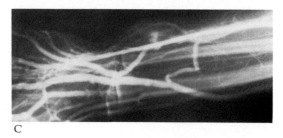

**Figure 39-6** *A. A 6-year-old girl has a mass (\*) that was soft on palpation involving the ulnar border of her right distal forearm. It was first noted about a year before the photograph was taken, after a fall during which the patient struck her ulnar forearm against a stone. When held in the dependent position, the mass measured approximately 3 × 3 cm and decreased to about 1.5 × 1.5 cm when the arm was elevated above the heart level. The mass was nontender; by history it had an occasionally bluish discoloration, and it enlarged to involve the dorsum of the hand on occasion. The child complained of discomfort in the area of the mass when her hand was held in the dependent position. No bruit could be heard on auscultation of the mass, and no thrill could be palpated. After the evaluation and routine radiographic studies, an arteriogram (B) revealed a 3 × 2 cm hemangioma fed by arterial branches of the ulnar artery (C) with some venous displacement seen around the mass.*

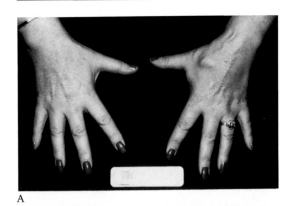

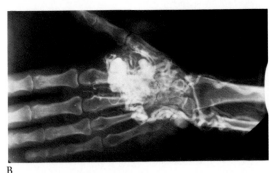

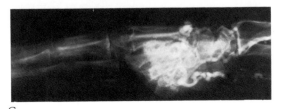

*Figure 39-7* A. Hands of a 46-year-old woman who had complained of some pinprick sensation in the palm of her nondominant left hand for approximately 8 years. During that time she had noted a prominent venous pattern in the thumb and thumb web area. She was sent for evaluation because of vague discomfort in the area (which was subsequently considered to be related to basal joint arthritic changes in the thumb) and recommendation by at least one physician that the mass be surgically removed. A bruit could be heard over the mass, and a thrill could be palpated.
*B, C.* Angiographic extent of this large A-V malformation. Follow-up over the next 8 years, as well as evaluation by numerous other physicians, led to the recommendation of no surgical treatment for this patient's lesion.

During the history and physical examination of these patients we must keep in mind the potential problems related to syndromes associated with hemangiomas, including intravascular coagulation problems with sequestration of platelets within the tumors: the Kasabach-Merritt syndrome [9].

Congenital arteriovenous (A-V) fistulas were well reviewed by Griffin and colleagues [42]. Symptoms such as unrelenting pain and ulceration, in addition to the A-V malformation, occasionally forces the issue and requires a surgical procedure. However, whether this form of therapy or a lesser intervention is undertaken, the patient and physician are embarking on a course that may result in a spectrum of problems from worsening pain, to enlargement of the mass, to loss of the extremity (Fig. 39-7).

Angiography evaluation is required to appreciate the extent of these communications. Gelberman and Goldner further defined indications and contraindications utilizing radiography, xerography, and angiography to detect the absence or presence of interosseous extension. They urged the use of all available diagnostic facilities to define the extent of these tumors and to determine alterations that may come about in blood flow in relation to extirpation [39]. Radiotherapy for this benign disorder is fraught with not only the benign changes that follow such treatment but the later development of malignant neoplasms [64].

GIANT CELL TUMORS (XANTHOMAS)
Xanthomas are common hand tumors that are most often seen during middle age. Complaints include those of a slowly growing mass that may interfere with placing the hands in gloves or putting on rings when the tumor reaches relatively large size; otherwise they frequently cause few other complaints. They are often found in the vicinity of joints.

Although referred to as giant cell tumors of the tendon sheath, it is difficult to specify from which structure they arise. Radio-

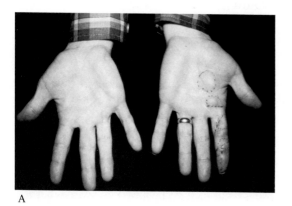

A

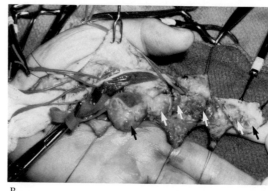

B

**Figure 39-8** *A. A 36-year-old woman was seen after three recurrences of biopsy-proved benign giant cell tumor of the tendon sheath. The dotted lines outline the extent of the tumor on clinical examination. B. Surgical exploration confirmed this recurrence of the yellow-tan to brown tumor. Giant cell tumor extended into the interphalangeal joints around digital vascular structures; it was intimately adherent to the flexor tendons. This massive involvement required ray amputation for treatment. The patient has done well over the next 5 years of follow-up, with no evidence of local recurrence.*

graphic evaluation may produce confusion with more "worrisome" lesions because of erosion of bone produced by pressure. Giant cell tumors are frequently multilobular and moderately firm. As they enlarge they may produce mechanical interference with finger function; they can surround digital nerves, producing numbness or discomfort; and ultimately they can become large, filling joint spaces and tendon sheaths (Fig. 39-8).

Because of their ability to enlarge, after evaluation of the patient exploration is recommended with a bloodless field. However, as with tumors involved in the differential diagnosis of more aggressive neoplasms, it is believed that exsanguination of the limb with an Esmarch tourniquet is contraindicated. Therefore the hand is elevated to allow venous drainage prior to inflation of the pneumatic tourniquet at the arm level. After important anatomic structures are appropri-

ately exposed, these tumors must be carefully followed. Frequently the yellow-tan, multilobulated small bits of tumor can be detected with the aid of magnification extending into joints and around important structures. In an effort to prevent recurrence, which is not uncommon, careful extirpation of these tumors is necessary.

LIPOMAS

Tumors of fat are often soft but can present difficulty in differential diagnosis when encapsulated or surrounded by other anatomic structures that limit them and produce a firm feel on palpation (Fig. 39-9). As can be seen in Figure 39-9, when strategically located lipomas may produce a significant problem: Not only deformity but compression of important nerves may produce functional deficits.

Magnetic resonance imaging (MRI) can be helpful for identifying lipomas. When clinically indicated, exploration with careful excision is the treatment of choice.

TUMORS OF FIBROUS TISSUE
*Fibromas*

Although considered rare, fibromas, which consist of dense fibrous tissue associated with benign-appearing fibroblasts, can be a significant nuisance in the upper extremity (Fig. 39-10). They must be distinguished

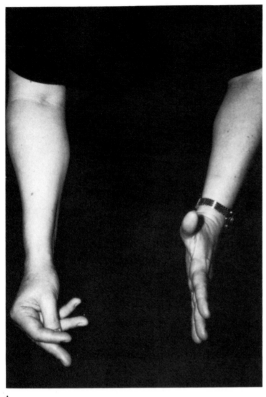

A

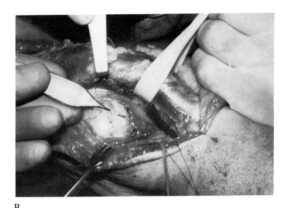

B

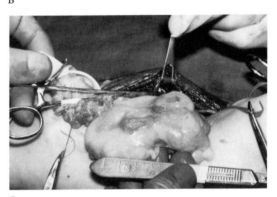

C

from more serious lesions in the clinical differential diagnosis. As illustrated, they can grow to a significant size and even produce a functional disability in the hand [14, 31, 41, 47, 66].

Clinical presentation is usually as a small, asymptomatic palmar or digital mass that may be fixed to deeper structures and may produce vague discomfort. However, more extensive involvement, as illustrated in Figure 39-10, does occur. Exploration may reveal a moderately firm, cream-colored mass that may have an almost mucoid appearance.

After establishing the diagnosis, treatment is complete excision. In our limited experience with this tumor, such therapy has not usually been associated with recurrent tumor.

*Figure 39-9* A. This 49-year-old woman had a 13-year history of a slowly enlarging mass that involved the right proximal forearm. She developed an inability to extend her thumb and fingers. B. Surgical exploration revealed a large lipoma with a markedly thinned posterior interosseous nerve stretched over it (nerve demonstrated over the forceps). C. Completed extirpation of the lipoma. Because of chronic pressure damage to the posterior interosseous nerve, subsequent tendon transfers were required.

### Dermatofibromas

Dermatofibroma becomes important from the standpoint of differentiating it from more serious conditions. It is usually a single lesion, although it may be multiple. When pigmented it can lead to some confusion in terms of its differentiation from serious pigmented tumors. Dermatofibromas

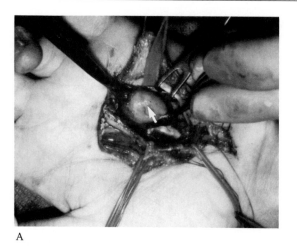

A

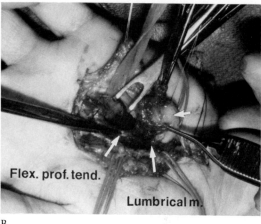

B

**Figure 39-10** *A. This mass was found at exploration in the palm of a 30-year-old right-handed woman who presented with a 1½- to 2-year history of palmar tenderness and, subsequently, a mass. Exposure at surgery (arrow) revealed that this tumor was larger than could be appreciated clinically. B. It was firm and adherent to adjacent lumbrical muscle. In order not to open other planes at the initial stage of dissection an incisional biopsy was carried out, and a benign fibroma of tendon sheath was found. Complex excision of the lesion was carried out. No evidence of recurrent mass has been found during her 5-year follow-up.*

are fibrous tissue tumors that involve the skin and must be differentiated from dermatofibrosarcoma protuberans, fibrosarcoma, and malignant fibrous histiocytoma [54].

Treatment for the benign dermatofibroma is usually concluded with the excisional biopsy. However, and despite histologic appearance, we have encountered some difficulties with these lesions, including recurrence and interference with finger motion [36].

## Fibromatosis: Palmar Fasciitis (Dupuytren's Disease or Contracture)

Although the etiology and pathogenesis of the disease is still uncertain, palmar fasciitis produces significant hand deformities. Thick-

ened cords, skin damage, and contractures may require extensive surgical procedures and, even so, sometimes results in recurrence and increasing deformity.

Treatment is removal of the offending abnormal fascia and appropriate additional procedures to release contractures (e.g., joint capsulotomy) and prevent their recurrence (Z-plasty, skin replacement by skin grafts, or both when there is significant skin involvement).

## TUMORS OF PERIPHERAL NERVE

Depending on the recognition and appropriate treatment of peripheral nerve tumors (a relatively uncommon group) a spectrum of problems from sensory or motor deficit, chronic pain, local recurrence, or even a threat to life may result. This area is a difficult one in which to develop one's knowledge because of the exceedingly rare nature of some of these tumors, especially the malignant forms [45].

## Neurilemmoma (Schwannoma)

Neurilemmomas are the most common benign peripheral nerve tumors encountered [79]. They arise from peripheral nerve Schwann cells [56]. The tumors are not common in the hand but may be seen as a painful forearm mass involving one of the major peripheral nerves. Percussion over them may produce a "pins and needles" or "electric shock" dysesthesia.

These patients are treated by "shelling out" the tumor from the peripheral nerve while preserving the nerve after incision in the epineurium. However, difficult removal with damage to the nerve is also possible.

### Neurofibromas

Neurofibromas are tumors that consist of both nerve and fibrous tissue. They are often seen in patients who have von Recklinghausen's disease (neurofibromatosis). In addition to presenting with single or multiple masses, these patients may have problems of digital overgrowth related to their syndrome. Although an isolated neurofibroma has a low incidence of malignant change, there is a significant incidence of malignant degeneration into neurosarcomas in patients with von Recklinghausen's disease [76].

Treatment includes excisional biopsy followed by appropriate additional treatment for neurofibromas that become painful or enlarge.

### Tumors of Nonneural Origin Involving Peripheral Nerves

Both lipomas and hemangiomas have been encountered in association with nerve compression symptoms. Treatment, other than nerve decompression with extirpation of the compressing lipoma, remains in some question. Intraneural lesions can be difficult to remove and, despite our best efforts, are still associated with pain and increasing neurologic deficit [57].

### GLOMUS TUMOR

Glomus tumors are small masses that contain glomus cells and pericytes associated with smooth muscle. The actual glomus is a type of arteriovenous communication (Fig. 39-11). Although pain can be a prominent symptom of those lesions that are frequently subungual in location, they are occasionally

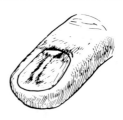

**Figure 39-11** *Glomus tumor. A bluish, or cyanotic, streak underneath the fingernail, accompanied by pain, suggests the presence of a glomus tumor. These tumors are also sensitive to changes in temperature.*

asymptomatic and are also found in the area surrounding the nail and in the pulp [40].

When in the subungual location they may produce elevation or a ridge-type deformity to the nail plate. Discoloration places them in the differential diagnosis for other important subungual tumors such as melanoma [40, 82].

Treatment of these tumors requires adequate exposure, which can be difficult under the nail plate and requires partial or complete nail plate removal. The important anatomy of this area, including the nail matrix-extensor tendon and joint relations, must be preserved when possible for the treatment of this tumor [37]. After removal of these pink to violaceous masses and histologic confirmation, the repaired nail matrix and bed requires protection and separation from the overlying nail fold (e.g., by replacement of the cleaned nail plate or substitute material).

### ANEURYSMS

Although rare, aneurysms in the hand enter into the differential diagnosis of tumors. Figure 39-12 shows a 19-year-old man who underwent incision and drainage of what was thought to be an infection in the ulnar aspect of his palm. The procedure's results led to a rapid consultation request. Such "false aneurysms" of the palmar arteries are often associated with a history of trauma

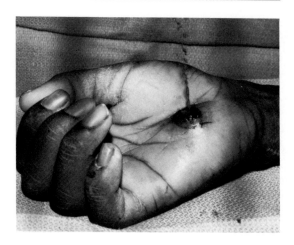

**Figure 39-12** *A 19-year-old man presented with a warm, ulnar palmar mass that was diagnosed as an abscess in the emergency room. One month prior he had undergone suturing of a laceration that occurred when he fell onto glass. The immediate results of incision and drainage of his ulnar artery aneurysm are apparent.*

[40]. False aneurysms are distinguished from true aneurysms by their lack of all the anatomic layers in their arterial walls. The area of injury is replaced by fibrous tissue. Another relatively common history is that of blunt trauma, often repetitive, to an area of the hand, especially the ulnar aspect. Such was the case with the 32-year-old patient shown in Figure 39-13. He had associated decreased light touch sensation in the ring and little fingers. After resection of the aneurysm and replacement with a reversed vein graft (Fig. 39-13B) the patient noted improved sensibility. Although the success of long-term patentcy of such grafts is not as good as would be hoped, this patient's Allen test revealed good flow through the vascular reconstruction 16 months postoperatively.

Some rare aneurysms are caused by "fibromuscular dysplasia." When such a diagnosis is made, the patient must be evaluated for the possibility of multiple aneurysms.

Atherosclerotic aneurysm, as demonstrated in the 65-year-old woman in Figure 39-14, is

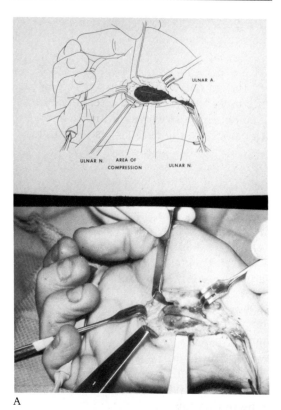

A

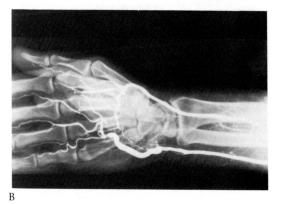

B

**Figure 39-13** *A. Exploration of a 32-year-old man's ulnar artery aneurysm that resulted from blunt trauma. Note the ulnar nerve being compressed by the underlying aneurysm. B. Angiogram obtained approximately 10 months after resection and reverse vein graft reconstruction. The appearance of this interposed vein graft was considered normal.*

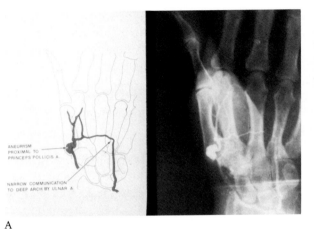

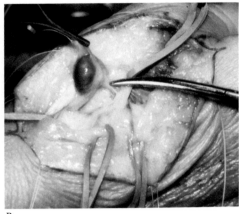

A                                                                                                    B

*Figure 39-14* A. Angiogram and drawing depicting a radial artery aneurysm that occurred spontaneously in a 65-year-old woman in the dorsum of her dominant right hand. Initial evaluation considered that it might be a ganglion. In addition, the patient subsequently developed color change (white discoloration) in the index finger when exposed to cold. The importance of correct diagnosis and treatment were stressed in this patient because of a tenuous communication between the radial and ulnar sides of her vascular arch. Pulse volume recordings and vascular evaluation confirmed the need to reconstruct her radial blood supply after aneurysm resection. B. Surgical dissection reveals that the aneurysm involves the radial artery on the dorsum of the hand as it continues between the thumb and index metacarpals.

a true aneurysm. They may be located in such a way that they require resection and reconstruction. Although the vicinity of the hamate bone is a common site for development of aneurysms, the above examples emphasize the varied nature of these lesions and multiple anatomic sites for their development.

Symptoms and signs range from an asymptomatic mass to a feeling of warmth, soreness, and tenderness. Pulsations may be palpated for but can be misleading. They may or may not be easily discerned depending on obliteration of the aneurysm by clot. Confusion may be produced by transmitted pulsation through adjacent masses, e.g., cysts. Even arteriography may yield inaccurate conclusions. Neurologic deficits that may be related to pressure may therefore respond to resection of the aneurysm. Raynaud's phenomenon, as seen in the 65-year-old woman in Figure 39-14 with the atherosclerotic aneurysm, may occur in a limited anatomic area, rather than involving the entire hand. It occurs when there is an underlying source of emboli.

Treatment requires a thorough understanding of the anatomy of the blood supply [17, 78]. Incisions are designed with respect to the usual considerations in hand surgery, in-

cluding the avoidance of right angle incisions across skin creases while planning for the ability to extend incisions for anatomic exposure. Although there is debate as to whether simple ligation and excision or vascular reconstruction is required, one must consider climate, e.g., individuals who work in cold climates. Anatomic variations (e.g., lack of complete arterial arches such as in the 65-year-old patient described) and multiple other factors go into assessing injured, elderly, and ill patients [52].

## TUMORS OF CARTILAGE AND BONE

During the development of the human skeleton two basic types of bone formation occur: (1) intramembranous ossification and (2) enchondral ossification [61]. Intramembranous ossification is that method by which large areas of the body skeleton are formed, including the compact bone of the shafts of long bones. These bones utilize formation of osteoid without requiring a cartilaginous scaffold. However, enchondral ossification (e.g., seen in finger bones) utilizes the formation of a cartilaginous scaffold on which ossification occurs. In this second category, a line of chondrocytes is first established, and maturing cartilage found in the epiphyseal area of tubular bones follows. Maturation develops through four zones: resting, proliferating, and zones resulting in progressive cell maturation and death followed by absorption of dead cells and calcification [61].

Osteochondroma is considered to be a common bone tumor [21] (Fig. 39-15). However, in the hand these lesions are less frequently encountered than enchondromas [63]. In contradistinction to enchondroma, osteochondroma is a subperiosteal proliferation of a bony mass capped by cartilage that grows perpendicular to the orientation of the growth plate.

Among the more common complaints are limitation of function as well as deformity and growth alteration. Discomfort may occur as well.

Radiography may reveal osteochondroma bone connecting with the cortex of the underlying bone. There may be some irregular calcification in the cartilaginous cap. However, extensive calcification with irregularities in the cap raise the question of the development of a chondrosarcoma [21].

These tumors are common in children and adolescents as well as in young adults [63]. At surgery the bony lesion capped with glistening, perhaps blue-white or pale cartilage is seen. Huvos pointed out that finding a cartilaginous cap exceeding 1 cm in thickness raises the question of chondrosarcoma [46].

Treatment is recommended for symptomatic lesions and those showing change in size or the above radiographic findings. If these tumors occur after growth has been completed, one must be especially suspicious. Excision includes resection of the mass including its periosteum [46, 61].

## ENCHONDROMAS

Enchondromas may be solitary or multiple tumors that, like osteochondromas, may originate in the epiphyseal area but are within the shaft of the bone. They are thought to be of congenital origin [12]. Enchondromas are frequently located in the metaphyseal area. They are believed to arise from cartilaginous rests. Presenting complaints frequently include alteration in form (secondary to an enlargement or expansion of the bone) and pain (fractures are not unusual through these thin bones) (Fig. 39-16).

Many people are not even aware they have these tumors. They are frequently encountered as incidental findings on radiographic evaluation. The radiographs show an irregular, stippled calcification in an otherwise lytic area. The cortex of the bone is frequently intact but expanded. Differential diagnosis of these cystic lesions includes simple bone cyst (Fig. 39-17) and giant cell tumor of bone (Fig. 39-18). At surgery gross pathologic evaluation reveals thinned or expanding cortical bone. Subjacent to this area is a gelatinous, often pale blue to white material.

Treatment carried out when the diagnosis is histologically established includes curettage of the tumor and packing the cavity with cancellous bone chips. If possible, in patients who have sustained a pathologic fracture, it is best to obtain fracture healing and bony alignment before carrying out the surgery described. Although the outlook is usually good for these patients, though rare for the single lesion, possible development of chondrosarcoma from enchondromas is now recognized [20, 49, 85].

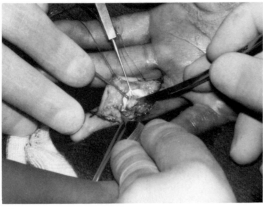

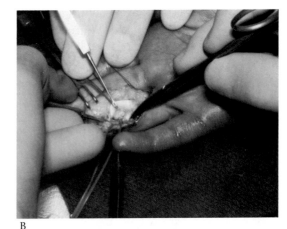

A

B

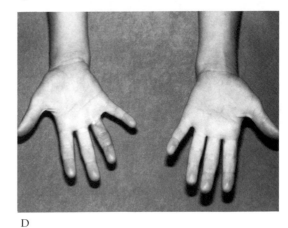

C

D

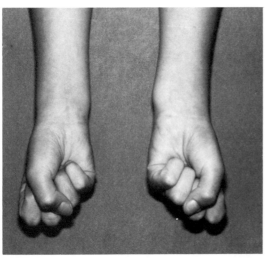

E

**Figure 39-15** *A. A 9-year-old girl presented with a previously operated osteochondroma of the right ring finger middle phalanx (dotted line outlines the previous surgical site and tumor). Her writing in school was noted to have become progressively less legible in association with pain in the area of the mass. A palpable mass was present in the area described in association with some radial deviation of the finger. B–E. After evaluation, including radiographic study (which revealed closure of the epiphysis in this area) exploration (B) with excision of the mass (C, osteotomy carried out to remove the osteochondroma) was followed by (D,E) good healing and satisfactory range of motion. By 4 months after operation she had regained full range of motion, could write better, and was more comfortable.*

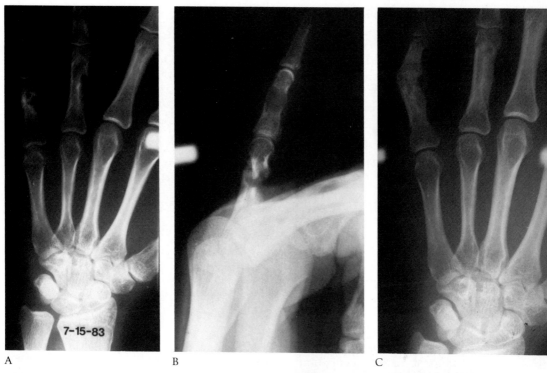

A                                    B                                    C

**Figure 39-16**  A. Dominant right hand ring and
little finger involvement by lytic lesions
involving the proximal and middle phalanges.
A displaced fracture had occurred through the
proximal phalanx of the right little finger.
Expansion of the bone with actual bulging of
the cortices is also noted. B. Note the fracture
through the enchondroma of the right little
finger. C. Appearance after curettage and bone
grafting of the involved sites. D, E. Patient
could flex and extend her fingers after this
relatively significant involvement by
enchondromas necessitating the treatment
described. Note that a bone scan had been
obtained preoperatively in an effort to rule out
other sites of involvement and help confirm the
differential diagnosis.

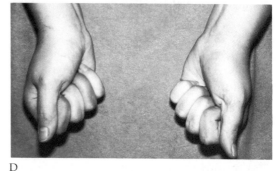

D

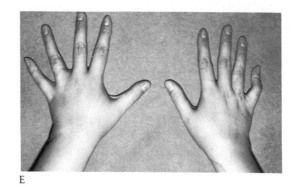

E

If there is rapid enlargement of the lesion with disruption of the cortex without trauma and increasing pain, physicians must be alert to the possibility of multiple enchondromas, Ollier's disease, multiple enchondromas associated with cavernous hemangiomas, or Maffucci's syndrome, which are well documented in the literature [22, 25, 40, 46].

Both syndromes remind us to evaluate the patient's skeletal system completely in the search for multiple lesions.

## OSTEOID OSTEOMAS

Osteoid osteomas are rare, in my experience, with regard to hand tumors. These patients are frequently young, 15 to 30 years of age. Localized pain and swelling with a radiographic picture showing a small nidus of increased density alert the physician to this possibility. Patients often obtain relief of their complaints after pathologic diagnosis, complete removal of the lesion, and appropriate bone replacement (usually cancellous bone chips) [70].

## GIANT CELL TUMORS

Giant cell tumors of bone must be distinguished from other primary bone tumors, including osteogenic sarcoma and fibrosarcoma. These lesions can even produce metastasis, and local recurrence is common. Such local recurrence (Fig. 39-18) is especially prevalent after limited treatment modalities, such as curettage and bone grafting [70]. Especially when applied at an early age, radiation, which has not been shown to be curative for these tumors, has the potential to produce malignant tumors [21, 70, 73].

These patients may present with areas of nodularity, enlargement, and deformity. Fracture may occur through the lesion, producing pain. Their differentiation into low or high grade lesions or even benign or malignant forms of giant cell tumor must not be utilized to justify inadequate forms of therapy.

Age distribution is in the young adult range. Radiographic examination reveals a

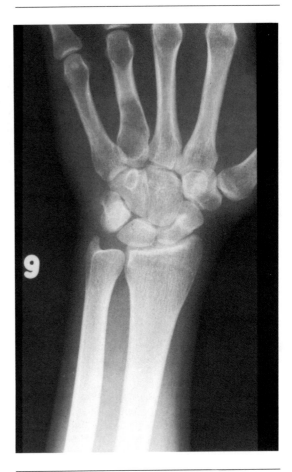

*Figure 39-17* Radiograph of a 20-year-old woman who was found incidentally to have an expanding lesion of the base of the right ring finger metacarpal during examination to follow a healing navicular fracture. Because of the enlargement, surgical exploration was carried out after the patient was fully evaluated. Curettage and cancellous bone chip packing were considered adequate treatment for what was determined to be a cyst.

lytic lesion frequently in the epiphyseal area. It is not unusual to see expansion of the cortex of the bone with a fracture [2]. Multicentric tumors must be sought. Therefore, in addition to routine radiographic evaluation, a skeletal work-up, including bone scan and computed tomography (CT) of the lungs, are important.

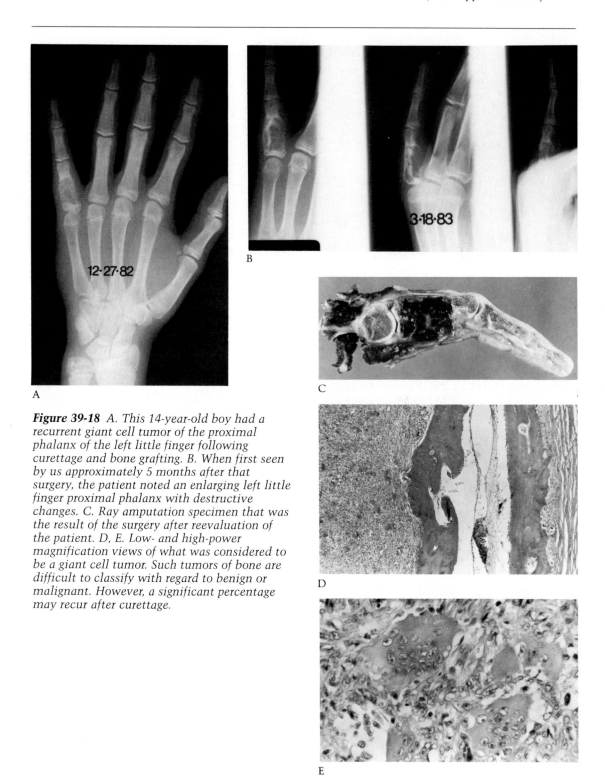

**Figure 39-18** *A. This 14-year-old boy had a recurrent giant cell tumor of the proximal phalanx of the left little finger following curettage and bone grafting. B. When first seen by us approximately 5 months after that surgery, the patient noted an enlarging left little finger proximal phalanx with destructive changes. C. Ray amputation specimen that was the result of the surgery after reevaluation of the patient. D, E. Low- and high-power magnification views of what was considered to be a giant cell tumor. Such tumors of bone are difficult to classify with regard to benign or malignant. However, a significant percentage may recur after curettage.*

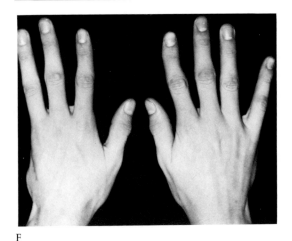

F

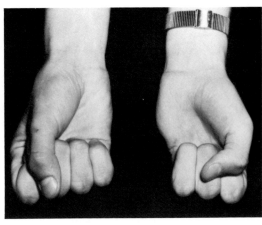

G

*Figure 39-18* *(continued) F, G. After ray amputation the patient had good range of motion. He remained free of tumor by clinical reevaluation and radiographic reevaluation at an almost 4-year postoperative follow-up.*

Treatment of giant cell tumors of bone must consider the high incidence of their local recurrence with incomplete removal [11]. Therefore our approach to the 14-year-old boy shown in Figure 39-18 (who already had a recurrent lesion of his nondominant little finger after curettage and bone graft that had "broken through" the bony cortex) included a ray amputation. Soft tissues about the tumor site were kept with the specimen [5, 44, 74, 77].

One must keep in mind that certain patients with giant cell tumors of bone are at risk to develop pulmonary metastases.

## Malignant Tumors

During the evaluation of patients presenting with tumors, a careful history with regard to initial discovery of the mass and evolution of the lesion must be obtained. Changes in size, color, surface characteristics, discomfort, and alterations in hand function suggest the need for a biopsy. Historical information concerning exposure to possible inciting agents, e.g., sun, radiation, chemicals, or the presence of a chronic wound, is important. Family history may link a person's complaint to malignancies with a genetic pattern [27, 58]. The social history may help the examiner differentiate a common paronychial infection from the manifestation of a Kaposi sarcoma that might be related to acquired immunodeficiency syndrome (AIDS) [51].

Physical examination of such patients requires not only measuring and recording size and other characteristics of the neoplasm but also careful assessment of the regional lymphatic pathways and distant potential sites for metastatic deposit. Laboratory studies that evaluate the patient's general health as well as giving possible indications of potential metastatic disease must be considered.

Screening radiographic procedures include chest x-ray films as well as radiographic views of the area of the tumor. Soft tissue lesions might be better evaluated by a xerogram. MRI or CT scans may give additional information concerning the nature of the lesion as well as its anatomic extent. Vascular studies may be useful for evaluating the mass as well as for the surgical dissection.

Consultation with the appropriate pathologist prior to carrying out a biopsy is frequently helpful. Biopsy techniques require planning for adequate tissue samples while creating the least tumor manipulation. Incision planning requires consideration of future tumor surgery. Whereas small lesions can be excised completely with a margin of normal tissue, large ones may be better handled with an appropriate incisional biopsy. The pathologist's findings help determine the excision necessary to encompass the site of surgical manipulation as well as to provide adequate surrounding tissue to serve as a barrier between the tumor and its extension. Once the preoperative evaluation of the patient reveals an absence of metastatic disease, the primary surgical treatment must control the tumor and prevent local recurrence.

The more serious tumors under consideration do not have true capsules. Considerable knowledge and judgment are necessary to resect adequate margins of normal tissue so as to gain this control. Large limb neoplasms usually require that incisional biopsy be planned in a longitudinal orientation. The biopsy must yield adequate tissue for diagnosis without compromising later surgical approaches needed to ablate the neoplasm and to salvage structures beyond the required limits of resection. If possible, definitive surgical procedures are carried out based on frozen section information. This procedure depends on a close working relationship with the specialized pathologist. When additional time or outside consultation is required or additional work-up is needed for surgical planning, the definitive surgical phase of treatment is delayed until these procedures can be accomplished.

Multidisciplinary team assessment of the patient, staging of the tumor, and pooling of efforts to develop the appropriate treatment—frequently surgery alone or in combination with chemotherapy or radiotherapy (or both)—supplies the optimal treatment for these difficult neoplasms.

## MALIGNANCIES PRIMARILY INVOLVING THE SKIN

In our experience, squamous cell carcinomas of the hand are more common than basal cell carcinomas, although both can be found on sun-exposed areas of the upper extremity. In addition, these lesions are found in other settings, e.g., after irradiation and after certain chemical exposures such as to arsenicals (see Fig. 39-2).

Whereas such lesions are relatively simple to treat (by excision with margins of normal tissue and histologic control followed by primary closure) when they are small, large lesions not only pose a challenge with regard to adequate excision and reconstruction but may require regional node dissection [35].

### Basal Cell Carcinoma

Basal cell carcinoma, in my experience, has been seen in older patients as a raised erythematous lesion, a raised erythematous lesion with "pearly" edges and ulcerated center, or a pigmented mass that must be distinguished from melanoma. These lesions have also been seen in the setting of prior irradiation.

One must be concerned with the potential for extensive regional involvement if basal cell carcinomas are untreated or inadequately treated. Therefore recommended treatment is complete excision with a histologically proved margin of normal tissue. Such treatment requires long-term regular follow-up because of the possibility of either missed or skipped areas that were not initially apparent or similar tumor development in surrounding areas of damaged skin [36].

### Squamous Cell Carcinoma

Squamous cell carcinoma, unlike the usual basal cell carcinoma, does have the potential to metastasize. Certain premalignant conditions, e.g., cutaneous horns, keratoses, and possibly even the "keratoacanthoma," may be associated with a subsequent squamous cell carcinoma that is difficult to appreciate on initial examination (Fig. 39-19).

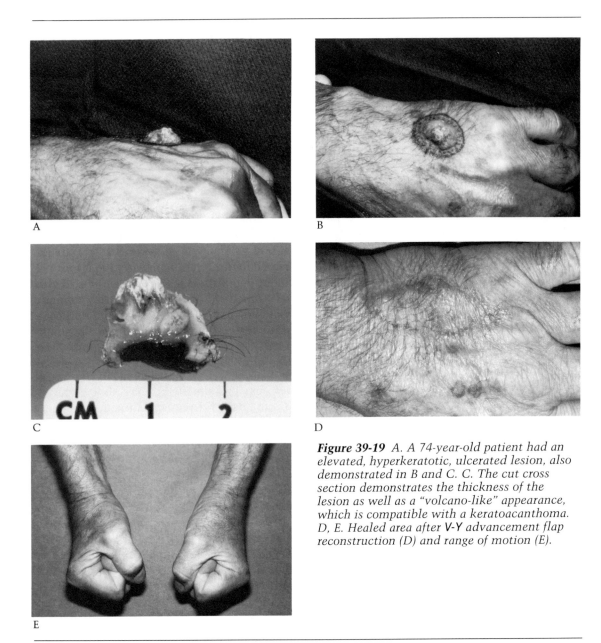

**Figure 39-19** *A. A 74-year-old patient had an elevated, hyperkeratotic, ulcerated lesion, also demonstrated in B and C. C. The cut cross section demonstrates the thickness of the lesion as well as a "volcano-like" appearance, which is compatible with a keratoacanthoma. D, E. Healed area after V-Y advancement flap reconstruction (D) and range of motion (E).*

Squamous cell carcinomas may range from small, erythematous papules to large, hyperkeratotic, scaly, ulcerated exophytic lesions. They usually have less discrete margins than do the basal cell carcinomas. They grow more rapidly and have the capacity not only to invade structures but to metastasize, usually to regional lymph nodes. A special area that is difficult to deal with is the squamous cell carcinoma or even keratoacanthoma in the nail area.

After histologic diagnosis and work-up of the patient, treatment of a nail bed squamous cell carcinoma requires complete removal of the tumor. If regional lymph nodes are involved, regional lymphadenectomy is also recommended. For small (e.g., in situ) nail area lesions, treatment requires at least excision of the surrounding tissue of origin (e.g., the nail bed and adjacent tissue) with skin graft reconstruction. Large or more invasive lesions require distal finger amputation or, on rare occasions, even ray amputation.

The principles involved in treating squamous cell carcinomas of other areas of the skin of the hand require excision of the tumor with margins of normal surrounding tissue established by histologic examination. It is my practice to take greater margins of normal surrounding tissue than would be the case with basal cell carcinomas. However, there is controversy as to just how large to make this excision. In my judgment, such margins result in few recurrent tumors during the follow-up of any group of patients. Although it is possible to close excision areas with local flaps, one must have the ability to repair the area with large local flaps, axial pattern, or myocutaneous flaps (see subsequent discussions), various types of skin grafts, distant flaps, and on rare occasion free flaps.

*Melanoma*
Melanoma refers to a malignant tumor of melanin-producing cells. Except for the unusual melanoma of soft parts, this designation usually refers to melanomas of the skin and nail bed area with regard to the upper extremity. These lesions do not have to contain obvious pigment. Review of the previous descriptions of pigmented lesions helps differentiate them from melanomas by the latter's departure clinically from the orderly arrangement of the pigment, alterations in the surface markings, irregular edges, enlargement in size, and variation in color (especially containing various shades of brown to black and red, white, and blue).

After a careful history and physical examination, diagnosis of these tumors requires appropriate biopsy. When the pathology report defines a malignant pigmented tumor, review of the specimen with the pathologist can help provide additional information that has implications concerning malignant potential and surgical planning. Combining the classification of Clark et al. and Breslow [8, 16] can help the surgeon understand the particular tumor's potential. These malignancies may spread by both lymphatic and hematogenous routes as well as by direct extension. Early treatment, as explained by Clark et al. and others, results in a more predictable outcome [4, 16, 36, 71].

Treatment has become more controversial in recent years with regard to margins of excision of the melanoma. In my experience, wide surgical margins of normal surrounding skin along with the primary tumor are appropriate [83]. It must be added that many authors believe that low risk lesions (i.e., those less than 0.76 mm in thickness and Clark's level I) may be treated by more conservative excision, with smaller margins of normal tissue that may even on rare occasion permit primary closure. In the hand reconstruction of the defect usually requires at least a skin graft. Depth of excision, in my opinion, ought to include the deep fascia when it is present. There is still controversy as to whether prophylactic lymph node dissection is appropriate [3, 7, 62, 80, 81].

MALIGNANCIES OF THE DEEP SOFT TISSUES OF THE UPPER EXTREMITY
Soft tissue sarcomas of the upper extremity are uncommon. This fact, coupled with the appearance of these often highly malignant tumors in young and middle-aged people, makes them a difficult and important area of study.

An excellent review article of the pertinent pathology in this area was compiled by Rosenberg and Schiller [72]. Even in the case of "low grade" sarcomas, appropriate excision is mandatory. Despite the best efforts, local recurrence in this group is not unusual and ultimately may be associated with a decreasing opportunity for cure. Higher grade tumors—which are less differentiated, often are more cellular with significant variation in cellular anatomy, and have increased numbers of mitoses and areas of necrosis—are associated with a less favorable prognosis [72].

### Epithelioid Sarcomas

Epithelioid sarcomas have been reported by some as one of the more common sarcomas of the upper extremity [10, 28]. This tumor is found to occur in the distal extremities, especially the hand in young adults. Epithelioid sarcomas may have a deceptive clinical presentation. Frequently they grow in a nodular or multinodular configuration and may involve the dermis as well as deeper tissues. These deeper tissues include tendon sheaths, tendons, and tissues along fascial planes. The mass is described as being firm and nontender.

On histologic examination this tumor may be a difficult one for the pathologist to interpret. It may be confused with the giant cell tumor, malignant fibrous histiocytoma, squamous cell carcinoma, melanoma, synovial sarcoma, sweat gland carcinoma, and even nodular fasciitis. Radiography may reveal a pattern of speckled calcification, but no truly diagnostic pattern can be described.

The course of this tumor is frequently insidious, and recurrence is common. It often grows along fascial planes or tendons and may metastasize to lymph nodes or lungs [10, 13].

Although treatment recommendations are still developing and are difficult to assess because of the long natural history of this tumor, it appears that at least ray amputation for digital lesions or wide excisions for more proximal lesions are important. Such procedures of course are carried out after complete evaluation and staging of the lesion. When possible, maintenance of at least a muscle group extending from origin to insertion including the tissues surrounding such a tumor may be a worthwhile additional barrier. At present, recurrences suggest that sec-

ondary treatment involves limb amputation. Application of early surgical management is emphasized in the literature.

### Fibrosarcoma

Fibrosarcoma is often a tumor of middle age. Even on histologic examination these tumors can be confused with other collagen-forming, cellular, spindle cell tumors, including fibrous histiocytoma and other sarcomas as well as benign processes [30]. Clinically these tumors are difficult to differentiate from other masses. They are frequently firm and slow growing and may become large before they produce significant symptoms other than physical deformity. Their origin is frequently in deep tissues, and the tumor may even encircle bone.

Pseudocapsules may be seen, but extension of the tumor outside this area is common. Treatment, after biopsy and appropriate workup of the patient, requires consideration of the above-mentioned insidious development and extent of this tumor. Recurrence may occur early or many years later. It must be kept in mind that metastases from this tumor are frequently blood-borne and often proceed to the lung [30].

The difficulty of diagnosis and management is emphasized by the experience of Lafferty et al. with fibrosarcoma arising from a juvenile aponeurotic fibroma [53]. The need for careful assessment, adequate surgery, and continued follow-up of these patients must be emphasized.

### Malignant Fibrous Histiocytoma

The malignant fibrous histiocytoma has been considered an uncommon malignancy, especially of the upper extremity. However, its potential for invasion, metastasis, and death of the patient is now recognized [23]. It has been confused with other tumors including fibrosarcoma. Histologic hallmarks include its composition of cells of both the fibrocytic and histiocytic series [23].

As is true of virtually all the soft tissue sarcomas described, the hand and forearm are not usually the most common sites of occurrence. Therefore these tumors do not seem to be considered in the differential diagnosis of masses of the upper extremity. Although usually described in older patients, our experience includes one patient who was diagnosed as having a malignant fibrous histiocytoma at age 3 [29]. Based on its radiographic appearance, it is occasionally confused with osteosarcoma and other tumors of bone.

When discussing etiologic factors, Enzinger and Weiss [30] included consideration of previous radiotherapy. Therefore although this type of therapy is important for the treatment of many serious malignancies, its choice must be carefully weighed against other treatment alternatives, expected results, and the seriousness of the malignancy (radiation therapy is rarely indicated for benign lesions that have alternative means of treatment) [30]. Evaluation of these patients is as described for any of the patients being considered in the differential diagnosis of malignant tumors. Malignant fibrous histiocytoma, with its high recurrence rate and potential for leading to death of the patient, merits as aggressive an evaluation and treatment as any of the others in this group.

### Rhabdomyosarcoma

Rhabdomyosarcoma, which shows skeletal muscle type differentiation, is one of the more common soft tissue sarcomas in young patients [55]. It is a high grade sarcoma [58] that appears to arise in the skeletal muscles of the limb and may grow rapidly. The lesions are usually divided into three subgroups: embryonal, alveolar, and pleomorphic. The first two groups are those most commonly seen in young patients [72]. Early recognition, in addition to surgical ablation, chemotherapy, and radiotherapy, appears to play a role in the treatment of this tumor [60].

### Synovial Sarcoma of the Hand

Although not necessarily arising from actual joint synovial tissue, the synovial sarcoma of the hand derives its name from a histologic pattern that is similar to that of synovial tissue. It is frequently found in close relation to joints, other ligamentous structures, and fascia.

The literature on this relatively rare tumor describes an aggressive, highly malignant neoplasm that may be seen early as a small, asymptomatic nodule [24]. We have seen it involving the palmar and dorsal aspects of the hand as well as the elbow area (Fig. 39-20).

Radiographic evaluation may reveal some soft tissue calcification as well as areas of radiolucent bone adjacent to the soft tissue mass. Radiographs showing paraarticular calcification with soft tissue masses raise the question of this particular tumor [72]. There appears to be a tendency for synovial sarcoma to invade adjacent bones [68].

These tumors appear to spread by both lymphatic and hematogenous routes. Such spread often becomes detectable within 2 years of the original treatment, although it sometimes does not occur until later. The outlook for synovial sarcoma has been considered poor. Complete extirpation of the tumor must include adjacent bony involvement along with the primary neoplasm. Irradiation and chemotherapy are usually considered.

### MALIGNANT TUMORS OF BONE
### Osteogenic Sarcoma

Osteogenic sarcoma is a rare malignancy of the hand [38]. The tumor is composed of malignant neoplastic cells that produce osteoid [21]. Although these tumors have subcategories, they are all highly malignant and tend to develop blood-borne metastases relatively early. The paraosteal type of osteosarcoma is thought to have a better prognosis but is still prone to local recurrence and eventual metastasis [6]. Along with fibrosarcoma, chondrosarcoma, and other malignancies, there is an increased incidence of these tumors after radiation therapy [21, 59].

Osteosarcomas are frequently found in relatively young individuals (Fig. 39-21). Symptoms include pain and swelling. One must be especially aware of a change in size or the

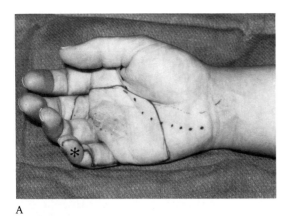

A

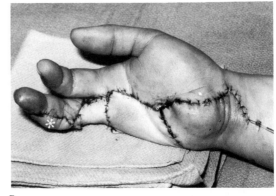

B

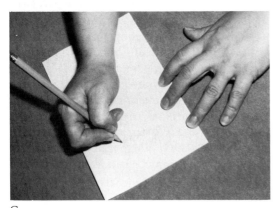

C

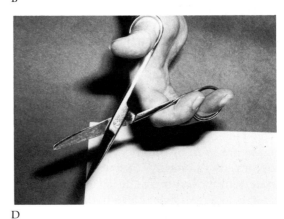

D

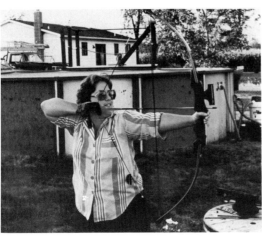

E

*Figure 39-20* A. Dominant right hand of a 28-year-old woman who had noted a soft mass in the distal palm of the hand, proximal to the ring finger, approximately 4 months before coming to our attention. Initial investigation included aspiration followed by an excisional biopsy at another hospital. She was referred for treatment of a "fibrosarcoma." Review of the tissue led to a diagnosis of synovial sarcoma. There were no palpable epitrochlear or axillary nodes and no evidence of disseminated tumor. CT scanning of her chest, abdomen, and hands as well as tomograms of the left lung because of a suspicious area, failed to reveal any evidence of persistent tumor in the hand or metastatic tumor to the lungs. Digital subtraction angiogram of the right hand failed to reveal tumor vascularity but did show that the ulnar artery was dominant. After complete evaluation, the proposed tumor excision is outlined by the solid line. Note: * indicates a vascular island flap outlined on the ulnar side

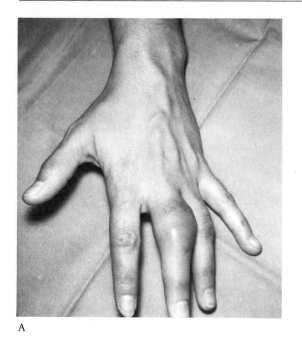

A

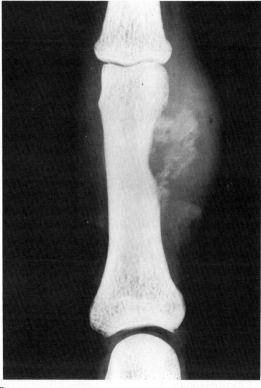

B

◄─────────────────────

***Figure 39-20*** *(continued) of the little finger, which was considered outside the area of tumor resection. B. After ablative surgery and primary reconstruction, the hand had this appearance immediately postoperatively. After the ablative phase of the surgical procedure, all instruments, drapes, and surgeons' and assistants' gowns and gloves were changed. Copious irrigation of the wound with normal saline was carried out. C–E. The patient regained various hand functions. She remains alive, well, and with no evidence of local, regional, or distant tumor at her last follow-up, which was at 7½ years postoperatively. Note that residual synovial sarcoma was found in the pathology specimen despite the above described findings of the scan and digital subtraction angiogram. All soft tissue and bony margins were found to be free of tumor at the time of surgery.*

***Figure 39-21*** *A. A 27-year-old patient presented with a 5-month history of swelling of the left middle finger and a previous biopsy that had not revealed neoplasm. B. Radiographic changes. Biopsy of the tumor revealed that it was osteogenic sarcoma. Treatment included a middle finger ray amputation. Transposition of her index finger for wound closure after the relatively extended ray amputation was carried out, followed by adjuvant chemotherapy. She was alive and well without recurrence of tumor at her 7-year follow-up. (From E. J. Fleegler, K. E. Marks, B. A. Sebek et al. Osteosarcoma of the hand.* Hand *12:316, 1980.)*

above-described complaints in a person who points out change in an area of previous irradiation.

Radiographic findings include lytic, destructive changes. The periosteum may appear elevated in association with a soft tissue mass. Calcification may be present.

Treatment, which may be associated with better results in the hand compared to other sites, includes expeditious patient evaluation followed by wide resection of the area. In the case illustrated (see Fig. 39-21), a ray amputation leaving adjacent soft tissues with the specimen to be removed appeared to be adequate. One must not hesitate to remove adjacent rays in order to obtain adequate barrier tissues. Chemotherapy in the patient presented consisted of adriamycin, vincristine, dacarbazine (DTIC), and cyclophosphamide (Cytoxan). An oncology consultation must be considered, as for other patients with a sarcoma, and the patient's overall treatment individualized. Another patient treated for this disorder underwent what was considered to be adequate resection of an osteosarcoma involving the thumb ray. After discontinuance of his chemotherapy program, the patient developed a recurrence in the remaining ulnar portion of the hand and underwent below-elbow amputation and excision of tumor nodules from his lungs. Further effort at chemotherapy was not successful, and he died 22 months after the original diagnosis.

## Concluding Remarks

Because many of the tumors described are seen infrequently by scattered groups of physicians the "final word" on their treatment is not yet known. However, one must develop principles for approaching these difficult problems. Patient education can provide the opportunity for early tumor recognition. Surgical treatment carried out at an early phase of tumor growth may prevent recurrence [18]. It is difficult to document that amputation is better surgical treatment than extensive, adequate surgery short of amputation [65].

Pathologic grading of malignancies is an important part of each patient's evaluation, planning, and treatment. Follow-up study is most important for helping to arrive at answers to the questions raised [67]. Careful documentation of the history, examination, planning, treatment plan, and follow-up evaluation are important for gathering the needed data on the treatment of these rare tumors.

## References

1. Angelides, A. C. Ganglions of the Hand and Wrist. In D. P. Green (ed.), *Operative Hand Surgery*. Vol. 2. New York: Churchill Livingstone, 1982. Pp. 1635–1650.
2. Averill, R. M., Smith, R. J., and Campbell, C. J. Giant-cell tumors of the bones of the hand. *J. Hand Surg.* 5:39, 1980.
3. Balch, C. M. Surgical management of regional lymph nodes in cutaneous melanoma. *J. Am. Acad. Dermatol.* 3:511, 1980.
4. Balch, C. M., Milton, G. W., Shaw, H. M., et al. *Cutaneous Melanoma: Clinical Management and Treatment Results Worldwide.* Philadelphia: Lippincott, 1985.
5. Bertoni, F., Present, D., and Enneking, W. F. Giant-cell tumor of bone with pulmonary metastases. *J. Bone Joint Surg.* [Am.] 67:890, 1985.
6. Bertoni, F., Present, D., Hudson, T., et al. The meaning of radiolucencies in parosteal osteosarcoma. *J. Bone Joint Surg* [Am.] 67:901, 1987.
7. Blois, M. S., Sagebiel, R. W., Abarbanel, R. M., et al. Malignant melanoma of the skin. *Cancer* 52:1330, 1983.
8. Breslow, A. Thickness, cross-sectional areas and depth of invasion in the prognosis of cutaneous melanoma. *Ann. Surg.* 172:902, 1970.
9. Brizel, H. E., and Raccuglia, G. G. Giant hemangioma with thrombocytopenia radioisotopic demonstration of platelet sequestration. *Blood* 26:751, 1965.
10. Bryan, R. S., Soule, E. H., Dobyns, J. H., et al. Primary epithelioid sarcoma of the hand and forearm. *J. Bone Joint Surg.* [Am.] 56:458, 1974.

11. Campbell, C. J. Invited editorial comment. *J. Hand Surg.* 2:308, 1977.

12. Carroll, R. E. Tumors of the Hand Skeleton. In J. E. Flynn (ed.), *Hand Surgery* (2nd ed.). Baltimore: Williams & Wilkins, 1975. P. 668.

13. Chase, D. R., and Enzinger, F. M. Epithelioid sarcoma. *Am. J. Surg. Pathol.* 9:241, 1985.

14. Chung, E. B., and Enzinger, F. M. Fibroma of tendon sheath. *Cancer* 44:1945, 1979.

15. Clark, W. H., Ainsworth, A. M., et al. The developmental biology of primary human malignant melanomas. *Semin. Oncol.* 2:83, 1975.

16. Clark, W. H., Goldman, L. I., and Mastrangelo, M. J. *Human Malignant Melanoma.* Orlando: Grune & Stratton, 1979.

17. Coleman, B. B., and Anson, B. J. Arterial patterns in the hand based upon a study of 650 specimens. *Surg. Gynecol. Obstet.* 113:409, 1961.

18. Creighton, J. J., Peimer, C. A., Mindell, E. R., et al. Primary malignant tumors of the upper extremity: Retrospective analysis of one hundred twenty-six cases. *J. Hand Surg.* 10A:805, 1985.

19. Culver, J. E., and Fleegler, E. F. Osteoarthritis of PIP joint. *Hand Clin.* 3:385, 1987.

20. Culver, J. E., Sweet, D. E., and McCue, F. Chondrosarcoma of the hand arising from a pre-existent benign solitary enchondroma. *Clin. Orthop.* 113:128, 1975.

21. Dahlin, D. C. *Bone Tumors: General Aspects and Data on 6,221 Cases.* 3rd Ed. Springfield, IL: Thomas, 1978. Pp. 17–27, 99, 226.

22. DeLaey, J. J., DeSchryver, A., et al. Orbital involvement in Ollier's disease (multiple enchondromatosis). *Int. Ophthalmol.* 5:145, 1982.

23. Dick, H. M. Malignant fibrous histiocytoma of the hand. *Hand Clin.* 3:263, 1987.

24. Dick, H. M. Synovial sarcoma of the hand. *Hand Clin.* 3:241, 1987.

25. Elmore, S. M., and Cantrell, W. C. Maffucci's Syndrome. *J. Bone Joint Surg. [Am.]* 48:1607, 1966.

26. Emmett, A. J., and Broadbent, G. D. Shave excision of superficial solar skin lesions. *J. Plast. Reconstr. Surg.* 8:47, 1987.

27. Enneking, W. F., Spanier, S. S., and Goodman, M. A. The surgical staging of musculoskeletal sarcoma. *J. Bone Joint Surg. [Am.]* 62:1027, 1980.

28. Enzinger, F. M. Epithelioid sarcoma. *Cancer* 26:1029, 1970.

29. Enzinger, F. M. Angiomatoid malignant fibrous histiocytoma. *Cancer* 44:2147, 1979.

30. Enzinger, F. M., and Weiss, S. W. Fibrosarcoma. In *Soft Tissue Tumors.* St. Louis: Mosby, 1983. Pp. 103, 106.

31. Feinberg, M. S. Fibroma of a tendon causing limited finger motion: A case report. *J. Hand Surg.* 4:386, 1979.

32. Feldman, F. Primary bone tumors of the hand and carpus. *Hand Clin.* 3:269, 1987.

33. Fitzpatrick, T. B., Arndt, K. A., Clark, W. H., et al. *Dermatology in General Medicine.* New York: McGraw-Hill, 1971. P. 1859.

34. Fitzpatrick, T. B., Arndt, K. A., Clark, W. H., et al. *Dermatology in General Medicine.* New York: McGraw-Hill, 1971. P. 495.

35. Fleegler, E. J. Skin Tumors. Part II. In D. P. Green (ed.), *Operative Hand Surgery.* Vol. 2. New York: Churchill Livingstone, 1982.

36. Fleegler, E. J. Tumors involving the skin of the upper extremity. *Hand Clin.* 3:197, 1987.

37. Fleegler, E. J. In D. Green (ed.), *Soft Tissue Tumors in Operative Hand Surgery* (2nd ed.). New York: Churchill Livingstone, 1988. P. 2323.

38. Fleegler, E. J., Marks, K. E., Sebek, B. A., et al. Osteosarcoma of the hand. *Br. J. Hand Surg.* 12:316, 1980.

39. Gelberman, R. H., and Goldner, J. L. Congenital arteriovenous fistulas of the hand. *J. Hand Surg.* 3:451, 1978.

40. Grabb, W. C., and Smith, J. W. *Plastic Surgery* (3rd ed.). Boston: Little, Brown, 1979. Pp. 646, 648, 649.

41. Greene, T. L., and Strickland, J. W. Fibroma of tendon sheath. *J. Hand Surg.* 9A:758, 1984.

42. Griffin, J. W., Vasconez, L. O., and Schatten, W. E. Congenital arteriovenous malformations of the upper extremity. *J. Plast. Reconstr. Surg.* 62:49, 1978.

43. Grussendorf, E. I., and Gahlen, W. Metaplasia of a verruca vulgaris into spinocellular carcinoma. *Dermatologica* 150:295, 1975.

44. Harris, W. R., and Lehmann, E. C. H. Recurrent Giant Cell Tumor After En Bloc Excision of the Distal Radius and Fibular Autograft Replacement. In J. H. Dobyns and R. A. Chase (eds.), *1985 The Year Book of Hand Surgery.* Chicago: Year Book Medical Publishers, 1985. Pp. 115–116.

45. Hecht, O. A., and Hass, A. Regional multiplicity of a neurilemmoma. *Hand* 14:97, 1982.

46. Huvos, A. G. *Bone Tumors: Diagnosis, Treatment, and Prognosis.* Philadelphia: Saunders, 1979. Pp. 144, 162–169.

47. Iwasaki, H., Kikuchi, M., Taloo, M., et al. Benign and malignant fibrous histiocytomas of the soft tissue. *Cancer* 50:520, 1982.

48. Jaffe, H. L. *Tumors and Tumorous Conditions of the Bones and Joints.* London: Henry Kimpton, 1958.

49. Justis, E. J., and Dart, R. C. Chondrosarcoma of the hand with metastasis: a review of the literature and case report. *J. Hand Surg.* 8:320, 1983.

50. Kaplan, E. N. Vascular Malformation of the Extremities. In H. B. Williams (ed.), *Symposium on Vascular Malformations and Melanotic Lesions.* Vol. 22. St. Louis: Mosby, 1983. Pp. 144–161.

51. Keith, J. E., and Wilgis, S. E. F. Kaposi's sarcoma in the hand of an AIDS patient. *J. Hand Surg.* 11A:410, 1986.

52. Kleinert, H. E., Burget, G. C., Morgan, J. A., et al. Aneurysms of the hand. *Arch. Surg.* 108:554, 1973.

53. Lafferty, K. A., Nelson, E. L., Demuth, R. J., et al. Juvenile aponeurotic fibroma with disseminated fibrosarcoma. *J. Hand Surg.* 11A:737, 1986.

54. Lever, W. F., and Schaumburg-Lever, G. *Histopathology of the Skin.* 6th Ed. Philadelphia: Lippincott, 1983. Pp. 485, 597–600, 682, 683, 697.

55. Linscheid, R. L., Soule, E. H., and Henderson, E. D. Pleomorphic rhabdomyosarcomata of the extremities and limb girdles. *J. Bone Joint Surg. [Am.]* 47:715, 1965.

56. Louis, D. S. Peripheral nerve tumors in the upper extremity. *Hand Clin.* 3:311, 1987.

57. Louis, D. S., Hankin, F. M., Greene, T. L., et al. Lipofibromas of the median nerve: Long-term follow-up of four cases. *J. Hand Surg.* 10A:403, 1985.

58. Mankin, H. J. Principles of diagnosis and management of tumors of the hand. *Hand Clin.* 3:185, 1987.

59. Masuda, S., and Marakawa, Y. Postirradiation parosteal osteosarcoma. *Clin. Orthop.* 184:204, 1984.

60. Maurer, H. M. The Intergroup Rhabdomyosarcoma Study: Update November 1978. *Natl. Cancer Inst. Monogr.* 56:61, 1981.

61. McFarland, G. B., and Morden, M. L. Benign cartilaginous lesions. *Orthop. Clin. North Am.* 8:737, 1977.

62. Milton, G. W., Shaw, H. M., McCarthy, W. H., et al. Prophylactic lymph node dissection in clinical stage I cutaneous malignant melanoma: Results of surgical treatment in 1319 patients. *Br. J. Surg.* 69:108, 1982.

63. Moore, R. J., Curtis, R. M., and Wilgis, E. F. S. Osteocartilaginous lesions of the digits in children: An experience with 10 cases. *J. Hand Surg.* 8:309, 1983.

64. Newmeyer, W. L. Vascular Disorders. In D. P. Green (ed.), *Operative Hand Surgery.* Vol. 2. New York: Churchill Livingstone, 1982. Pp. 1695–1754.

65. Nilsonne, U. Limb-preserving radical surgery for malignant bone tumors. *Clin. Orthop.* 191:21, 1984.

66. Oni, O. O. A. A tendon sheath tumor presenting as trigger finger. *J. Hand Surg.* 9B:340, 1984.

67. Owens, J. C., Shiu, M. H., Smith, R., et al. Soft tissue sarcomas of the hand and foot. *Cancer* 55:2010, 1985.

68. Pack, G. T., and Ariel, I. M., Synovial sarcoma (malignant synovioma): A report of 60 cases. *Surgery* 28:1047, 1950.

69. Palmieri, T. J. Subcutaneous hemangiomas of the hand. *J. Hand Surg.* 8:201, 1983.

70. Pho, R. W. H. Malignant giant-cell tumor of the distal end of the radius treated by a free vascularized fibular transplant. *J. Bone Joint Surg. [Am.]* 63:877, 1981.

71. Roses, D. F., Harris, M. N., and Ackerman, A. B. *Diagnosis and Management of Cutaneous Malignant Melanoma.* Philadelphia: Saunders, 1983. Pp. 7, 13.

72. Rosenberg, A. E., and Schiller, A. L. Soft tissue sarcomas of the hand. *Hand Clin.* 3:247, 1987.

73. Seradge, H. Distal ulnar translocation in the treatment of giant-cell tumors of the distal end of the radius. *J. Bone Joint Surg. [Am.]* 64:67, 1982.

74. Shaw, J. A., and Mosher, J. F. A Giant Cell Tumor in the Hand Presenting as an Expansile Diaphyseal Lesion: Case Report. In J. H. Dobyns and R. A. Chase (eds.), *1985 The Year Book of Hand Surgery.* Chicago: Year Book, 1985. P. 115.

75. Shumer, S. M., and O'Keefe, E. J. Bleomycin in the treatment of recalcitrant warts. *J. Am. Acad. Dermatol.* 9:91, 1983.

76. Smith, J. W., and Guthrie, R. H. Tumors of the Hand. In W. C. Grabb and J. W. Smith (eds.), *Plastic Surgery* (3rd ed.). Boston: Little, Brown, 1979. Pp. 642, 643, 644.

77. Smith, R. J., and Mankin, H. J. Allograft replacement of distal radius for giant cell tumor. *J. Hand Surg.* 2:299, 1977.

78. Spinner, M. *Kaplan's Functional and Surgical Anatomy of the Hand* (3rd ed.). Philadelphia: Lippincott, 1984.

79. Strickland, J. W., and Steichen, J. B. Nerve tumors of the hand and forearm. *J. Hand Surg.* 2:285, 1977.

80. Veronesi, U., Adamus, J., Bandiera, D. C., et al. Inefficacy of immediate node dissection in stage I melanoma of the limbs. *N. Engl. J. Med.* 297:628, 1977.

81. Veronesi, U., Adamus, J., Bandiera, D. C., et al. Delayed regional lymph node dissection in stage I melanoma of the skin of the lower extremities. *Cancer* 49:2420, 1982.

82. Wilgis, S. E. F. *Vascular Injuries and Diseases of the Upper Limb.* Boston: Little, Brown, 1983.

83. Wong, C. K. A study of melanocytes in the normal skin surrounding malignant melanoma. *Dermatologica* 141:215, 1970.

84. Wood, V. E. Hemangioma with bone lesions. *J. Hand Surg.* 7:287, 1982.

85. Wu, K. K., Frost, H. M., and Guise, E. E. A chondrosarcoma of the hand arising from an asymptomatic benign solitary enchondroma of 40 years' duration. *J. Hand Surg.* 8:317, 1983.

86. Zarem, H. A., and Edgerton, M. T. Induced resolution of cavernous hemangiomas following prednisolone therapy. *Plast. Reconstr. Surg.* 39:76, 1967.

# 40

*E. F. Shaw Wilgis*

# Traumatic Aneurysms and Thromboses

Aneurysms and thromboses of the arteries in the hand and upper extremity can be caused by any trauma—open or closed, sharp or blunt—that causes an injury to the intima of the vessel [4]. The intimal rupture serves as a focus for platelet aggregation, eventual clot formation, and thrombosis of the vessel. In the case of an aneurysm, the intimal rupture leads to a dissection within the wall of the vessel, ultimate thinning of the wall, and aneurysm formation.

An open injury to the vessel, if left undetected, leads to an injury through the vessel wall, with subsequent leakage of blood and the development of a pulsating hematoma, which then becomes encapsulated and forms a "false" or pseudoaneurysm. When an open wound is present in the region of a vessel, damage to that vessel must be expected and searched for. If the affected vessel does have a wound, the wound should be closed by arterial repair, using microsurgical technique, in order to prevent the formation of a false aneurysm. When faced with the possibility of a traumatic injury to a vessel, resulting in an aneurysm or thrombosis, several important steps should be taken in management.

## Detection

The clinical assessment must include blood pressure recordings and the palpation of pulses. Specific maneuvers, such as *Adson's test,* which examines the peripheral radial pulse in varying positions of extension and abduction of the shoulder, can be helpful when pinpointing compressive forces that could potentially cause thrombosis of the subclavian artery.

*Allen's test* is a useful clinical test to determine the patency of one of the arteries in a double arterial-supplied system such as the hand. This test consists of compressing both the radial and ulnar arteries and then emptying the hand of all blood by flexion and extension of all digits. The pressure is then removed from the radial artery and the hand is allowed to fill. If one of the two arteries is occluded or the palmar arch is incomplete, the compromised circulation will then become evident. A variant of this test can also be used in the digits, effectively compressing either digital artery and testing the capillary filling of that particular digit. An aneurysm of the arterial supply in the hand can usually be palpated, as the arteries are subcutaneous

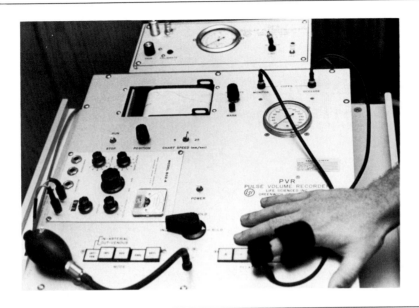

***Figure 40-1*** *Pulse volume recorder.*

in position. Whenever an aneurysm is palpated, Allen's test must be performed to confirm patency of the contralateral artery in the digit or the radial artery at the wrist.

Other noninvasive studies can be employed to further delineate the vascular condition. The *Doppler ultrasonic flow detector* can be used as a diagnostic adjunct [6]. Ultrasound waves are emitted through piezoelectric crystals and are transmitted through the skin and subcutaneous tissue to the superficially located blood vessels. The superficial palmar arch and digital vessels are accessible for monitoring with this instrument. The emitted high-frequency sounds strike the soft tissues and the blood cells moving through the blood vessels. The blood cells, which are in rapid motion, cause an alteration in the pitch of the sound waves on impact, and these waves are then received by the recording part of the probe, are amplified, and are converted to signals. The experienced listener can readily separate arterial and venous flow signals, can differentiate the arterial flow signals through normally patent versus stenotic vessels, and can rec-

ognize arterial flow arriving by collateral vessels that are bypassing a proximal obstruction.

The *plethysmograph* can also be used as a noninvasive technique for evaluating peripheral blood flow. We currently use the pulse volume recorder, developed by Raines [1, 5] (Fig. 40-1). This produces a quantitative, reproducible, segmental plethysmographic recording of the area studied with a minimum of complexities. This device records volume change within a given segment of a digit. The system consists of one or two digital cuffs, which pick up the pressure changes. These cuff pressure changes affect alteration in the cuff volume, which in turn reflects changes in the limb value. The electronic package then transmits and records the data on hard copy paper for the clinician to read (Fig. 40-2). It can be used in conjunction with the Doppler ultrasonic flow detector. The second cuff is added to record the digital perfusion pressure, measured in millimeters of mercury.

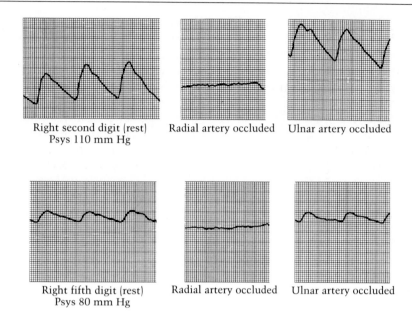

Right second digit (rest)
Psys 110 mm Hg

Radial artery occluded

Ulnar artery occluded

Right fifth digit (rest)
Psys 80 mm Hg

Radial artery occluded

Ulnar artery occluded

*Figure 40-2* Pulse volume recording. Vascular consultation.

Radionuclide, intravenous, dynamic flow studies and static perfusion scans of the extremity have been useful in our experience. Multiple modifications are possible either with the equipment, choice of nuclide, or compounds used for tagging and improving the quality of the image or increasing the diagnostic accuracy, or both. An image or image series is obtained, which provides useful information in a significant number of patients [7] (Fig. 40-3).

In dealing with aneurysms and thromboses, ultimate visualization of the involved vascular segment is a prerequisite to operative correction. *Contrast angiography* has enjoyed a long history as a useful diagnostic method in the evaluation of the vascular status of an extremity. It involves the intraarterial injection of contrast medium and the subsequent visualization of the arterial and venous phase of circulation. This method is invaluable for the location of specific arterial defects such as thromboses or aneurysm.

The femoral is the safest puncture site. Several complications have been reported from the transaxillary route as well as brachial injection sites. However, the discomfort of this method, the requirements for special

*Figure 40-3* Radionuclide angiogram showing ulnar artery thrombosis.

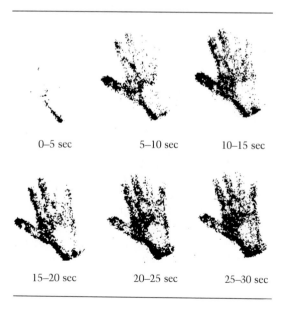

0–5 sec

5–10 sec

10–15 sec

15–20 sec

20–25 sec

25–30 sec

personnel and equipment, the hazards of administration of iodides, and the possible complications at the site of arterial puncture limit its application. It cannot be used routinely or repetitively. One of the disadvantages is that the arteriogram is mainly an anatomic study and gives no information as to the dynamic state of the circulation.

## Treatment

Once the diagnostic evaluation is complete, the clinician must decide whether the affected vessel should have surgical treatment. We believe that most aneurysms, of either the false or true variety, should be resected and replaced by either a vein graft or end-to-end anastomosis. Frequently, digital artery aneurysms can be resected and repaired effectively. Aneurysms will frequently cause local nerve compression and produce paresthesias and pain at the local site.

In a recent series of 30 aneurysms of the upper extremity, Ho and associates [2] reported that 9 were true aneurysms and 18 were false; 2 additional aneurysms were mycotic. By far, the most frequent location was the forearm and wrist. Of those treated by operation, 10 had resection and ligation, since 9 were false aneurysms. The rest were treated successfully by excision and direct repair or by interposition vein grafting. There was 1 case of embolus from an axillary artery aneurysm, with subsequent hand gangrene that was treated by amputation.

Before an aneurysm is approached surgically, the complete preoperative assessment must be accomplished, including a study of collateral circulation. The technique of excision includes operative exposure of the affected vessel under tourniquet control and satisfactory anesthesia. Once the vessel is controlled proximally and distally, the tourniquet can be released to assure the collateral circulation of the hand. The aneurysm can then be resected and replaced with a direct anastomosis or interposition reverse vein graft, using microvascular technique.

An acute thrombosis without circulatory embarrassment of the affected hand can be treated with local measures such as rest and cold compresses. Frequently, the initial episode can be treated in this manner and then elective resection of the thrombosed segment can be undertaken. However, if one determines that arteriotomy would be beneficial, it must be performed within 48 hours after thrombosis. Arteriotomy for a thrombotic embolism to the brachial artery should be done as soon as diagnosis is confirmed. Thrombosis of

**Figure 40-4** A. Ischemia of ring and little fingers secondary to ulnar artery thrombosis. B. Operative dissection of thrombosed ulnar artery. C. Cut section of thrombosed ulnar artery. D. Extraction of distal clot from superficial palmar arch. E. Vein graft reconstruction after verification of proximal and distal flow.

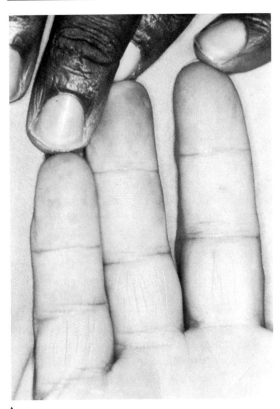

A

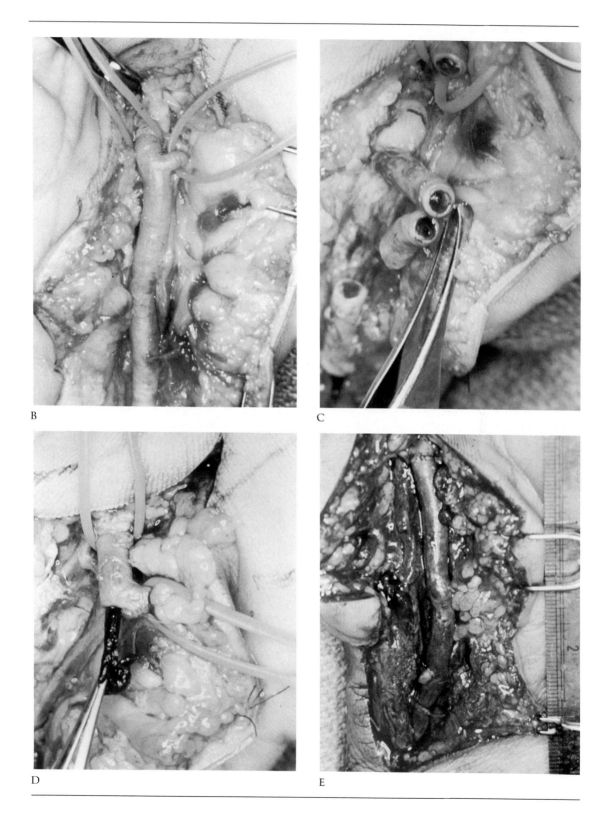

B

C

D

E

the ulnar artery due to blunt trauma is a common incident in the hand. If treated early enough, a local resection with end-to-end anastomosis can sometimes be performed, but this frequently requires excision and interposition vein grafting. Previous reports have indicated that local excision of the thrombosed segment is the treatment of choice; however, the collateral circulation must be confirmed before this manner of treatment is elected. We believe that an effort should be made to restore the bilateral circulation in the hand, if at all possible, since we have seen several cases of late ischemia secondary to prolonged ulnar artery occlusion that had to be reconstructed many years after the thrombotic episode.

The technique for excision of the thrombosed segment of the ulnar artery and interposition vein grafting is illustrated in Fig. 40-4. Thrombosis of digital vessels has been approached surgically but usually is not necessary. An isolated thrombosed digital vessel does not cause ischemic changes in the digit and can be managed conservatively and expectantly.

In cases of a massive thrombosis involving all of the small vessels of the hand, surgical treatment, including thrombectomy, can be attempted. If, however, this is not successful, then administration of thrombolytic agents, as reported by Kartcher and Wilcox [3], has been successful. This technique consists of injecting thrombolytic agents interarterially over a period of time at designated intervals. This is most effective when used in coagulopathy, disseminated intravascular thrombosis, and impending loss of the hand. This technique must be monitored carefully as it causes serious systemic anticoagulation.

In summary, the thromboses and aneurysms in the small vessels of the hand and wrist can be treated in a number of ways. However, the detection and isolation of the specific lesion must be complete before any surgical treatment is attempted. With the advent of microsurgical technique, operation on these vessels, including microvascular reconstructive surgery with interposition vein grafts, is a reality.

## References

1. Darling, R. D., Raines, J. K., Brener, B. J., et al. Quantitative segmental pulse volume recorder: A clinical tool. *Surgery* 72:873, 1972.
2. Ho, P. K., Weiland, A. J., McClinton, M., et al. Aneurysms of the upper extremity. *J. Hand Surg.* 12A:39, 1987.
3. Kartcher, M. M., and Wilcox, W. C. Thrombolysis of palmar and digital arterial thrombosis by intra-arterial thrombolysis. *J. Hand Surg.* 1:67, 1976.
4. Luce, E. A., et al. Compression neuropathy following brachial arterial puncture in anticoagulated patients. *J. Trauma* 12:717, 1976.
5. Raines, J. K., Jaffrin, M. Y., and Rao, S. A noninvasive pressure pulse recorder development and rationale. *Med. Instrum.* 7:245, 1973.
6. Strandness, D. E., Jr., McCutcheon, E. F., and Rushmer, R. F. Application of a transcutaneous Doppler flowmeter in evaluation of occlusive arterial disease. *Surg. Gynecol. Obstet.* 122:1039, 1966.
7. Wilgis, E. F. S., Dragan, J., Stonesifer, G. L., Jr., et al. The evaluation of small vessel flow. *J. Bone Joint Surg.* 6:1199, 1974.

# V
# *Microsurgery*

# 41

*William W. Shaw*
*Kwan Chul Tark*

# Principles of Microvascular Surgery

The invention of the compound microscope by Zacharia Janssen in 1590 generated careful descriptions of every minute structure in the living world. The ensuing disciplines of histology, pathology, and microbiology are among the foundations of modern medicine.

In 1921 Carl-Olof Nylen in Sweden first used the operating microscope for treatment of otosclerosis [16]. Barraquer and Perit employed the operating microscope to suture cornea in 1950, but no tubular structure or blood vessels were repaired. After a long incubation period following the initial work by the Nobel Laureate Alexis Carel in 1902 [4] and his associate Charles Guthrie in 1912 [9], peripheral vascular surgery evolved into a well established discipline involving larger vessels. The results of small blood vessel repairs, however, remained disappointing.

In a monumental work, Jacobson and Suarez reported in 1960 a 100 percent patency rate in vessels 1.6 to 3.2 mm in diameter [11]. This study proved that human hands are capable of immensely more precise work than was previously recognized. Intense experimental work during the 1960s verified the efficacy and refined the technique of microsurgery.

Through the independent works of Chen et al. in China [5], Komatsu and Tamai [13] in Japan, and Buncke et al. [3] and Kleinert et al. [12] in the United States, clinical replantation using microvascular techniques was developed. In 1972 isolated segments of omentum [15] and in 1973 skin flaps [7, 17] were transplanted, establishing the feasibility of microvascular tissue transplantation, the so-called *free flaps.* During the 1980s the applications of microsurgery and free tissue transfer continued to expand, and now these techniques have an impact on nearly every specialty of medicine.

## Basic Microvascular Techniques

Operating on tiny structures under the microscope with sutures that are barely visible seems difficult and almost unimaginable for the novice. In fact, anyone with reasonable technical ability can perform microsurgery, given three prerequisites: (1) suitable magnification; (2) appropriately sized instruments and suture material; and (3) training to acquire hand–eye coordination through the microscope and subsequent experience operating on delicate tissues in a variety of laboratory and clinical situations. As with other complex skills, the eventual level of performance depends on the fundamentals achieved initially.

## MAGNIFICATION

### Loupes

Loupes or surgical telescopes are widely used for magnification, and the quality of these devices has continued to improve. Loupes can be mounted on glasses or headbands, and a custom prescription can be ground into the lenses. In the "wide-field" versions, slightly higher magnification, 3.2× to 4.5×, can be used comfortably, with a working distance of 10 or 20 inches. The loupes are commonly used for dissection of vascular pedicles when preparing them for anastomosis. The microscope is used for the actual repair because of the higher magnification and brighter illumination available.

### Operating Microscope

The main benefit of the operating microscope is improved vision of small structures through optical magnification and brighter illumination. The use of the microscope, however, brings additional new problems of setup time, storage of equipment, position of the scope, posture of the surgeons, limited depth and fields of vision, and maintenance. Currently available operating microscopes represent, by and large, second generation equipment without adequate consideration of the above problems. It is hoped that future microscopes will become more convenient and more flexible. For instance, the use of ceiling-mounted microscopes greatly reduces the problems related to storage convenience, setup time, and positioning (Fig. 41-1).

A *double-headed operating microscope*, with the surgeon and assistant at opposite ends, is essential. Most commonly this setup is achieved through the use of beam splitters, so that the surgeon and the assistant have exactly the same view (e.g., Zeiss microscope). Other times it is achieved through completely separate optical systems between the surgeon and the assistant, allowing independent control of the zoom magnification (e.g., Weck microscope).

*Coaxial illumination* is also important to avoid shadows cast by the hand if the lighting comes too far from the side. Because of the frequent need for changing magnification, most operating microscopes have a continuous *zoom magnification* system operated by the foot pedal. The *focus* is also controlled remotely to free the hands. Many microscopes also have an *X-Y movement* controlled by the foot pedal to permit a smoother scanning. Multiple *adjustable joints* are required to permit various angles of incidence, depending on the part of the body being operated on. Finally, through-the-microscope *photographic or video* capabilities are necessary for documentation and for keeping the entire operating team involved.

## TABLE, CHAIR, AND POSTURE

As pointed out by Acland and others, the most important factors for avoiding fatigue, frustration, and tremor are positioning and comfort [1, 10]. To that end, numerous recommendations have been made in the literature regarding types of seating, table design and height, and microscope design.

The most comfortable position for sitting for long periods is with the feet flat on the floor and the hips and knees at approximately right angles. The height of the chair is therefore determined by the habitus of the surgeon. Chairbacks and arm rests are arranged at the discretion of the surgeon [19]. The most effective *working height* is one that places the surgeon's elbows at or near 90 degrees when the forearm and hands are supported to minimize tremor.

Various objective lens *focal lengths* are available depending on the manufacturer. Focal lengths between 175 and 250 mm are most useful for free flap surgery or hand surgery. Placing a strip of adhesive tape across the brim of the mask and tying the lower drawstrings loosely prevents fogging of the eyepieces and makes operating for long periods more comfortable (Fig. 41-1).

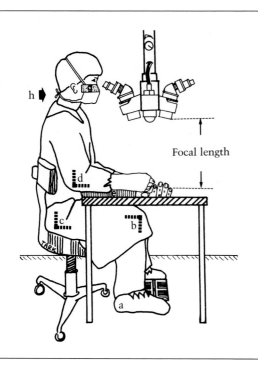

**Figure 41-1** *Most comfortable, stable position for sitting for long periods: (a) feet flat on the floor; (b,c) knees and hips at approximately right angles; (d) elbows at 90 degrees; (e) forearm and hands are supported; (f) 175- to 250-mm focal length; (g) adhesive tape to prevent fogging; (h) loose lower drawstrings.*

Focal length

INSTRUMENTATION

Most microsurgical procedures can be performed using the following set of instruments.

No. 5 jewelers' forceps, 2 pairs
No. 3 jewelers' forceps, 1 pair
Angled forceps, 1 pair
Vessel dilating forceps, 1 pair
Curved tip needle holder, 1
Westcott scissors, 1 pair
Vannas scissors, 1 pair
Rizzuti forceps, 1 pair
Micro-Adson forceps, 1 pair

An assortment of vascular clamps includes at least three sizes of double approx-imating clamps, several angled or straight single clamps, and one or two clamps for large vessels such as the brachial or popliteal artery.

For anastomosis work, most surgeons prefer needle holders without locking mechanisms to avoid the sudden jerking movement when the needle holder is unlocked after each bite. A fine spring-action Castro-Viejo or Barraquer needle holder is satisfactory.

MICROSUTURES
During the 1960s Chinese surgeons [6] used human hair as one of the earliest microsutures. A plethora of microsutures and needles has since become available. It has been shown that the size and type of suture appear to make a significant difference in the patency rate. Silk sutures, for instance, create too much drag through the vessel wall and carry a high risk of thrombosis. Prolene, on the other hand, pulls through the vessel wall well, but the suture material is brittle once it has been manipulated by metal forceps. Currently, the most common micro-needles are hand-honed and swaged onto the respective sutures of 8-0, 9-0, 10-0, and 11-0. There has been some evidence that a partially cutting tip in the needle may be advantageous in minimizing vessel wall injury.

The most important consideration in suture material selection is a practical one, and that is the handling characteristics of the suture. Polyglycolic acid suture has a light color that is difficult to see. It also tends to "float" within the field of view and can become adherent to surrounding tissue when wet. Polypropylene is easily kinked and can become corkscrewed when stretched. It is also difficult to consistently tighten the knots smoothly. Nylon, on the other hand, is easily visible and lacks the other drawbacks of polyglycolic acid and polypropylene sutures. Though it is not as strong as poly-glycolic acid, it remains the material of choice for most applications.

Table 41-1 Sutures used for microvascular surgery

| Application | Suture size and diameter | Needle designation and diameter | | | | |
|---|---|---|---|---|---|---|
| | | Davis & Geck | Ethicon | Xomed | ASSI |
| Vessels > 3 mm: brachial, popliteal | | | | | |
| Epineurium of large peripheral nerves: arm above elbow, lower extremity above ankle | 8–0 45 μm | TE145 140 μm | BV130–3 130 μm | NA | 14V33 140 μm |
| Vessels 2–3 mm: anterior and posterior tibial, radial, ulnar, thoracodorsal, circumflex scapular, inferior epigastric | 9–0 35 μm | TE100 100 μm | BV100 100 μm | 40–22415 100 μm | 10V43 100 μm |
| Epineurium of major forearm nerves: median, ulnar, radial | | | | | |
| Vessels 0.8–2 mm: palmer and digital, gracilis and lateral arm flap pedicles | | | | | |
| Epineurium of digital nerves, epiperineurial sutures, group fascicular repair, large fascicles | 10–0 22 μm | TE70 70 μm | BV75 75 μm | 40–22440 70 μm | 7V43 70 μm |
| Large lymphatics | | | | | |
| Vessels < 0.8 mm: distal digital | | | | | |
| Fascicular sutures | 11–0 18 μm | TE50 50 μm | BV50 50 μm | 40–22445 70 μm | 5V33 50 μm |
| Lymphatics | | | | | |

Source: W. W. Shaw, and D. A. Hidalgo. Microsurgery in Trauma. New York: Futura, 1988. P. 32.

Sutures are available in lengths from 4 to 20 cm. Excessive suture length is commonly a problem when working through the microscope. Long sutures decrease efficiency and cause clutter within the field of view. The ideal suture length is somewhat less than 10 cm in most instances.

The wide variety of needle sizes and tip types, suture types and lengths, and the number of manufacturers contribute to confusion when selecting the appropriate suture for a particular task. In general, it is better to select a few types than stock a large variety of sutures. Suggested sutures are listed in Table 41-1.

## BASIC ANASTOMOTIC TECHNIQUES
### Essentials for a Patent Anastomosis
Aside from the obvious translation of conventional vascular techniques to a microscopic level, there are several essential requirements to ensure a microvascular anastomosis with long-term patency.

1. There must be meticulous *atraumatic dissection* of the blood vessel, with tying or coagulation of branches.
2. The vessel wall and *intima at the site of anastomosis must be normal* when visualized under high power magnification; the injured vessel must be resected back to normal tissue.
3. *Adequate flow* must be demonstrated from the proximal vessel.
4. The anastomosis must be done *without tension,* and, if necessary, the vessel must be mobilized or vein grafts used to ensure a tension-free anastomosis. The incidence of early and late failure is increased by tension on the anastomosis.
5. Adequate *removal of* local overhanging *adventitia* is followed by suture placement *without grasping the intima* (Fig. 41-2A).
6. All traces of blood, air, and foreign body (e.g., cotton or suture threads) are *thoroughly irrigated* away with heparinized

lactated Ringer's solution before completing the anastomosis (Fig. 41-2G).

### Technique of End-to-End Anastomosis
Once the vessel has been prepared and adequate proximal flow ensured, the anastomosis is performed. If proximal flow is impaired, gentle mechanical dilatation with dilating forceps and application of local vasodilating agents (e.g., papaverine, lidocaine) may improve flow. Allowing the vessels to rest undisturbed for several minutes and warming the tissue may also aid in decreasing spasm.

The basic anastomosis procedure described here is a summation of the techniques for arterial anastomosis most widely recommended by several noted authors [2]: The clamps are adjusted so that no tension exists on the anastomosis site. The vessel is divided cleanly and the adventitia trimmed (Fig. 41-2A). The lumen is gently dilated with dilating forceps (Fig. 41-2B). Intraluminal counterpressure with the forceps is useful, but the intima and vessel edge are never grasped by the forceps while inserting the entrance bite (Fig. 41-2C). Only the adventitia is picked up gently by the forceps, and the exit bite suture is placed atraumatically (Fig. 41-2D). Two stay sutures 120 to 180 degrees apart are first placed, and the long ends are anchored either to cleats in the contrast background sheet or in the frame of the vascular clamps (Fig. 41-2E). Two or more coaption sutures are then placed between the stay sutures. The last suture placed in either the front or back wall is critical, as it is difficult to visualize the lumen and prevent inadvertent suturing of the opposite wall (Fig. 41-2F). The vessel is then rotated 180 degrees by releasing the stay sutures and flipping the vessel clamp. The back wall is sutured, and the lumen is thoroughly irrigated and gently distended with heparinized lactated Ringer's solution before tying the final suture (Fig. 41-2G). The final suture is then completed (Fig. 41-2H).

In some situations there is not sufficient

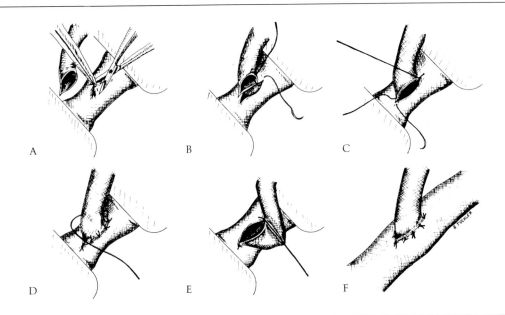

**Figure 41-4** End-to-side anastomosis.
A. Arteriotomy may be done by excising a "wedge" of the vessel wall. B. Place the first stay suture in the more acute angle of the proximal end. C. Repeat the suturing at the opposite side and then bring the long line of the proximal end over and across the anterior surface of the vessel and fasten it to the upper cleat. D. After the first half of the anastomosis is completed, pass the long line of the stay suture under and around the artery and fasten it to the lower cleat. E. This procedure, the Morris maneuver, exposes the posterior edges. F. Place more secondary coaption sutures to finish the anastomosis.

### End-to-Side Anastomosis Technique

If only a single vessel maintains the viability of an extremity, it cannot be sacrificed as the donor vessel for an end-to-end anastomosis, and an end-to-side repair must be used. Marked size discrepancy also demands this method.

The arteriotomy into the donor vessel is the most critical and irreversible step in the procedure. One should master the technique in the laboratory on vessels of varying diameter and wall thickness before using it in clinical practice.

The arteriotomy may be done by excising a "wedge" of vessel wall with straight scissors, or it may be started with a microknife and enlarged carefully to an elliptical or circular defect with microscissors (Fig. 41-4A). Special arteriotomy clamps are available, but they also require practice to achieve consistent results. The arteriotomy must match the size of the vessel to be anastomosed. It may be more convenient to place the first stay suture in the more acute angle of the proximal end (Fig. 41-4B) and then suture the opposite end (Fig. 41-4C). After completing the side facing the surgeon, the first suture, which was left long, can be pulled over the vessel, allowing visualization of the back wall (Figs. 41-4D,E)

### Patency Test

Anastomotic patency may be assessed in several ways. In clinical situations, *return of color, capillary oozing,* or *venous bleeding* from the revascularized tissue signals a competent arterial anastomosis. Engorgement of the tissue indicates compromise of venous drainage.

Direct inspection of both arterial and venous anastomoses under the microscope may reveal signs of patency. Arterial patency is indicated by well dilated vessels showing pulsatile elongation, or *expansile pulsation.* Gently lifting the vessel distal to the anastomosis by placing forceps underneath it demonstrates the *"flicker"* of blood flowing across this area, but it is easily visible only in thin-walled vessels.

The empty and refill patency test, the *milking test,* is traumatic and is performed as gently and as infrequently as possible. Two pair of smooth forceps are used to occlude the vessel distal to the anastomosis. The more "downstream" forceps is then moved gently about 1 cm down the vessel, creating the empty segment between the two forceps. The proximal compression is then released, and rapid filling of the empty segment indicates patency of the anastomosis.

TRAINING

Microsurgical procedures are performed under indirect vision through the operating microscope. The unfamiliar magnification of the hand movements requires a new eye–microscope–hand–instrument coordination, and a specific skill must be acquired. The quality of one's performance depends greatly on the initial training, inherent talents, and continued practice.

Many microsurgical laboratories have evolved for the training of surgeons. In our experience even well trained surgeons require a full week of laboratory training to become comfortable working under the microscope to perform the basic anastomosis confidently. To become expert in the use of end-to-side anastomosis, vein grafts, small vessels (1.0 mm), or anastomosis under awkward conditions generally requires another 2 to 4 weeks of full-time laboratory practice [23].

It is important, however, to recognize that the acquired laboratory microsurgical skill is not automatically translatable to the ability to perform complex clinical reconstructions. Aside from technical differences between

laboratory and operating room, there are several new problems encountered, such as selection of an anastomotic pattern, the design of the microvascular reconstruction, the variation in regional anatomy, and clinical indications for reconstruction. It is essential, therefore, that a period of clinical experience be obtained before one attempts to perform complex reconstructive microsvascular procedures.

## *Pursuit of Small Vessel Patency*

REVIEW OF DATA

Although at the turn of the century Carel and Guthrie had performed successful vascular anastomoses in animals involving relatively small vessels (3 to 4 mm), the procedure was generally thought to be impractical clinically because of the great expertise required. Using various techniques and sutures, the patency rate for vessels 3 mm in diameter remains about 40 to 67 percent. Jacobson's report of 100 percent patency rate in 1.6- and 3.2-mm vessels using 7-0 silk sutures first suggested that improved vision of the small structures produced by optical magnification and better illumination was vitally important for reducing technical errors at the anastomosis. As a result of the intense interest during the 1960s, finer microneedles, sutures, and instruments have become available. A fairly consistent general approach to performing microvascular anastomosis was gradually adopted by most microsurgeons by the early 1970s. Hayhurst and O'Brien, in 1975, described 98 percent long-term patency rates on 0.9-mm arteries. This report became the yardstick for the microvascular patency rate of vessels and was confirmed in subsequent series reported by several other authors. Using a similar technique with 11-0 nylon sutures, 73 to 94 percent patency was described for vessels 0.5 to 0.9 mm in diameter (Table 41-2) [18, 23, 25].

Despite the high patency achieved in the laboratory, in the clinical setting the use of the operating microscope does not automat-

**Table 41-2** *Comparison of patency of microvascular repair reported in the literature*

| Date | Author | Patency (%) | Vessel size (mm) | Technique | Suture |
|---|---|---|---|---|---|
| *Arteries* | | | | | |
| 1960 | Jacobson and Suarez | 100 | 1.4–3.2 | Interrupted | 7-0 silk |
| 1962 | Chase and Schwartz | 100 | 1.2–1.7 | Continuous | 7-0 silk, 9-0 wire |
| 1966 | Green | 90 | 0.8–1.5 | Continuous | 7-0 silk, 9-0 nylon |
| 1967 | Cobbett | 100 | 1.3–1.6 | Interrupted | 8-0 nylon |
| 1975 | Hayhurst and O'Brien | 98 | 0.8–1.0 | Interrupted | 10-0 nylon |
| 1976 | Harashina | 94 | 0.7–0.9 | Interrupted | 11-0 nylon |
| 1977 | Fujimaki | 85 | 0.5 | Interrupted | 11-0 nylon |
| 1981 | Harris and Buncke | 97 | 1.0 | Interrupted | 10-0 nylon |
| *Veins* | | | | | |
| 1965 | Ts'ui | 88 | 1.5–3.5 | Interrupted | 9-0 nylon |
| 1970 | O'Brien | 90 | 1.0–1.2 | Interrupted | 10-0 nylon |
| 1972 | Tamai | 90 | 1.0 | Interrupted | 10-0 nylon |
| 1975 | Hayhurst and O'Brien | 80 | 1.1 | Interrupted | 10-0 nylon |
| 1988 | Tark and Shaw | 94 | 0.7–0.9 | Interrupted | 10-0 nylon |

ically ensure a trouble-free anastomosis. Success with replantation or free flaps generally ranges from 70 to 95 percent depending on the type of cases attempted and the experience of the surgeons. Even among the most experienced groups of microsurgeons, the success rate for microvascular free flaps is about 95 percent [22]. The somewhat lower patency reported clinically points out the necessity for skill and knowledge above and beyond that which can be acquired in the laboratory.

FACTORS INFLUENCING FAILURE
OF PATENCY
For the beginner, the ability to perform a technically adequate vessel anastomosis in the laboratory does not guarantee success in clinical situations. Many factors influence the eventual outcome of the microvascular anastomosis, and the surgeon must favorably influence as many as of them as possible (Table 41-3) [20]. The surgeon's estimation of the technical quality of the anastomosis is the best prediction of patency.

Failure of blood to flow across an anastomosis is usually due to one of four factors: (1) technical errors with the anastomosis; (2) poor flow from the proximal vessel due to

undetected damage more proximally or vasospasm; (3) injury to the vessel wall with resulting micromural thrombi; or (4) a clot or thrombus at the anastomotic site or in an area where a clamp was applied.

The surgeon attempts to discern the cause of failure and proceeds accordingly. If there is sufficient vessel length, reanastomosis can be performed; if not, a vein graft is inserted. Poor proximal flow that does not respond to local vasodilators and warming may require proximal exploration of the vessel, dilation along a proximal length of vessel sufficient to relieve vasospasm, or treatment with local or intraarterial vasodilators. If reapplication of a clamp is necessary, systemic heparin in a bolus of 1000 to 2000 units is given to avoid excessive mural thrombus formation during stasis.

NO REFLOW PHENOMENON
The new reflow phenomenon, which was first described by May et al. in 1978 [14] in the microsurgical field, indicates gradual cessation of flow and eventual anastomotic failure after a well performed anastomosis. Ongoing *arterial obstruction, arteriovenous shunting,* and *alterations of the clotting mechanism related to tissue ischemia* were

*Table 41-3* *Major factors contributing to failure after microsurgery*

*Technical Factors*
  Both walls sutured together
  Traumatic vessel handling
  Apposition of vessel edges
  Disproportional vessel size
  Tension at suture line
  Excessive clamp pressure
  Kinking of vessels
*Reperfusion Factors*
  No reflow
  Blood turbulence
  Spasm
  Hypercoagulability
  Acidosis
  Cold
  Hypovolemia
  Circulating constrictors
*Postoperative Care*
  Infection
  Acidosis
  Environmental factors
  Cold
  Position

suggested as possible factors. Other likely possibilities include (1) edema and swelling of the vascular endothelium and parenchymal cells with resultant narrowing of the capillary lumen, (2) disseminated intravascular thrombosis, and (3) loss of physiologic integrity of the venule or capillary wall.

Other research has implicated reperfusion injury and the production of free radicals as the cause of the no reflow phenomenon. During prolonged ischemia, adenosine triphosphate is broken down to hypoxanthine, and xanthine oxidase is formed by the action of a protease in response to the low oxygen tension. When reperfusion occurs, the presence of molecular oxygen allows hypoxanthine conversion to xanthine and oxygen free radicals. The oxygen free radicals form highly reactive hydroxyl radicals and cause tissue damage. Also, potent vasoactive prostaglandins and thromboxanes appear to play important roles in the postreperfusion microcirculation [8]. The use of allopurinol,

radical scavengers, and various prostaglandins is being investigated to minimize such reperfusion injuries.

PHARMACOLOGIC AIDS
Commonly using pharmacologic agents can be classified as follows.

Anticoagulants
  Heparin
  Aspirin
  Dextran
Fibrinolytic Agents
  Urokinase
Vasodilators
  Lidocaine
  Papaverine

During the early days of clinical microvascular surgery, vasodilators were used frequently, and patients were often given anticoagulants. As our confidence and experience grew, it became clear that in most anastomoses involving healthy vessels no ancillary pharmacologic agents are needed. The reckless use of anticoagulants, particularly heparin, often results in more harm than good. On the other hand, there is strong experimental evidence that anticoagulation is helpful in improving the patency rate, particularly if the anastomosis involves damaged vessels.

Heparin is a complex substance with multiple actions. The most important to the microvascular surgeon is the preferential binding to vascular endothelial cells that replaces the normal negative charge lost in an area of endothelial damage. High local concentration of heparin also inhibits platelet aggregation, decreases fibrinogen clotting, and activates local antithrombin III. Systemic heparin activates serum antithrombin III and lowers blood viscosity.

A common regimen is to use intraoperative heparin during the clamping phase of the anastomosis to prevent excessive luminal clot formation. Postoperatively, the patient is given only aspirin or dextran. Aspirin inactivates circulating platelets by acetylating the enzyme cyclooxygenase present in the platelet wall. The mechanism of action of dextran is not well understood; it appears to have both antiplatelet and heparin-like effects. For digital replantation or when extensive crush is involved, a carefully controlled regimen of heparin, warfarin (Coumadin), or fibrinolytic agent may be indicated [26].

Lidocaine is the most commonly used vasodilating agent but probably in strengths too low to have much beneficial effect. Concentration of 4 to 20% are recommended based on experimental studies. Papaverine at 30 to 60 mg per milliliter is also a potent vasodilator when applied topically.

### POSTOPERATIVE MONITORING

Because of the all-or-none nature of replantation and free-flap surgery, postoperative monitoring is important. Photoplethysmography, cutaneous oxygen tension, laser Doppler, fluorescein concentration, and temperature have all been used for monitoring. At present, the simplest, most effective method appears to be temperature monitoring combined with good clinical observation, although it is likely that more reliable monitoring methods will become available in the near future.

## Vein Grafts

A vein graft was first successfully used by Goyanes in 1906 to bypass a popliteal artery aneurysm [24]. The widespread use of vein grafts did not occur until the advent of aortocoronary bypass procedures during the early 1960s. This development stimulated much of the research that has provided important information on the behavior of transplanted veins.

Autogenous venous interposition grafts are the most useful vascular substitute in microsurgery. Prosthetic materials have been successful for large vessel replacement where flow rates are high, but they have inferior patency rates when a diameter of 4 mm or less is used.

### USES OF VEIN GRAFTS

Vein grafts are frequently used in the following situations.

To prevent tension at an anastomosis
To bridge long gaps
In cases of limited anatomic access
To compensate for marked size discrepancy
For multiple anastomoses from a single source

### FATE OF VEIN GRAFTS

Veins undergo transmural changes when transplanted. Their blood supply is restored in a fashion similar to that for skin grafts. Initially the vasa vasorum dilate with blood, but there is no flow for the first 72 hours. Nutrition occurs by diffusion of nutrients from the vessel lumen during this early period. By 2 weeks the graft receives blood supply from the vessels that have grown into the graft from the surrounding soft tissue [27]. By 2 months there is a return to a predominantly vasa vasorum supply that is connected to a circumferentially oriented capillary network within the media.

Histologic sections of vein grafts have shown that they develop intimal thickening with fibrosis of the media and adventitia. Scanning electron microscopy studies have detailed the process of reendothelialization within vein grafts. Though the endothelium of the graft is intact 1 hour after implantation, most of it has sloughed by 24 hours. There is an extensive migration of leukocytes underneath the endothelium that apparently undermines it. A layer of leukocytes and platelets occupies the denuded areas until remaining islands of endothelium proliferate and restore the surface by the end of the second week. In the region of the anastomosis the process is accelerated, with endothelialization beginning within 2 to 3 days and generally being complete by 1 week.

SOURCES OF VEIN GRAFTS

Vein grafts are generally obtained from the upper and lower extremities. Upper extremity veins have less muscle content than lower extremity superficial veins. They are therefore more flimsy but they have fewer spasm problems as well. The foot and forearm are good sources of 1 to 2 mm diameter veins. Suitable veins can be found with the use of a tourniquet, and their course is marked on the skin for later identification. It is often convenient to harvest the vein near the operative site. However, it may be time-saving to harvest the vein from a distant site when two teams are available. Unsalvageable amputated parts are an excellent source of vein grafts.

Branched veins may be obtained from the dorsum of the foot or, less commonly, the forearm. The presence of valves in these veins is an important consideration when selecting a graft with branches. The direction of the Y graft in situ may be different depending on the application.

TECHNICAL CONSIDERATIONS WITH
THE VEIN GRAFT

*Graft Length*

Experimentally, vein graft length has not yet been shown to be a factor in the patency rates of small diameter vessels. However, clinical experience has suggested a tendency to thrombosis with long grafts that have low flow rates.

When a long segment of vein graft is used, it is best to perform the proximal anastomosis first. The graft is then clamped on the distal end, and flow is reestablished into the graft. This method distends, elongates, and untwists the graft. It is helpful for deciding the proper length prior to final trimming.

*Vessel Size Discrepancy*

In general, diameter discrepancy of any vessel involved in the anastomosis must not exceed a ratio of 2:1. Larger differences are associated with turbulent flow at the anastomosis and lower patency rates.

*Graft Dissection*

It is important to handle the graft minimally during the course of dissection. It is usually possible to dissect it entirely by handling the soft tissue that lies near it and not actually grasping the vein. Side branches must be carefully ligated so as to neither encroach on the lumen nor leave a long stump. Use of the electrocautery to control side branches is not recommended.

*Direction of Flow Marker*

As the graft is harvested, a suture is placed on the proximal end: *Blood flows toward the marker.* This point is an arbitrary convention to help avoid confusion. The suture orients the graft with the understanding that blood flow is always in the direction from the unmarked end of the graft toward the end with the suture. If only a portion of the graft is used, a suture is again placed at the proximal end of the remaining segment to identify the direction of flow. This technique is particularly helpful when multiple teams are participating in a long procedure.

*Vein Graft Preservation*

The best medium for preservation of a harvested graft has been shown experimentally to be a balanced salt solution of pH 7.0 and a temperature of 4°C. Irrigation of vein grafts with heparinized saline is useful only to eliminate gross clot and has not been shown to prevent platelet adhesion [21].

## References

1. Acland, R. D. *Microsurgical Practice Manual.* St. Louis: Mosby, 1980.
2. Ballantyne, D. L., Razaboni, R. M., and Harper, A. D. *Microvascular Surgery: A Laboratory Manual.* New York: Institute of Reconstructive Plastic Surgery, New York University Medical Center, 1980.
3. Buncke, H. J., Buncke, C. M., and Schulz, W. P. Experimental digital amputation and replantation. *Plast. Reconstr. Surg.* 36:62, 1965.
4. Carel, A. La technique operatoire des anastomoses vasculaires et la transplantation des

visceres. *Lyon Med.* 98:859, 1902.

5. Chen, Z. W., Chen, Y. C., and Pao, Y. S. Salvage of the forearm following complete traumatic amputation. *Chin. Med. J.* 82:632, 1963.

6. Chen, Z. W., Yang, D. Y., and Chang, D. S. *Microsurgery.* New York: Springer-Verlag, 1982.

7. Daniel, R. K., and Taylor, G. I. Distant transfer of an island flap by microvascular anastomosis. *Plast. Reconstr. Surg.* 52:111, 1973.

8. Feng, L. J., Berger, B. E., Lysz, T. W., et al. Vasoactive prostaglandins in the impending no-reflow state: Evidence for a primary disturbance in microvascular tone. *Plast. Reconstr. Surg.* 81:755, 1988.

9. Guthrie, C. C. *Blood Vessel Surgery and Its Application.* Pittsburgh: University of Pittsburgh Press, 1959 (1912 reprint).

10. Harwell, R. C., and Ferguson, R. L. Physiologic tremor and microsurgery. *Microsurgery* 4:187, 1983.

11. Jacobson, J. H., and Suarez, E. L. Microsurgery in anastomosis of small vessels. *Surg. Forum* 11:243, 1960.

12. Kleinert, H. E., Kasdan, M. L., and Romero, J. L. Small blood vessel anastomosis for salvage of severely injured upper extremity. *J. Bone Joint Surg.* [Am.] 45:788, 1963.

13. Komatsu, S., and Tamai, S. Successful replantation of a completely cut-off thumb. *Plast. Reconstr. Surg.* 42:374, 1968.

14. May, J. W., Chait, L. A., O'Brien, B. M., et al. The no-reflow phenomenon in experimental free flaps. *Plast. Reconstr. Surg.* 61:256, 1978.

15. McLean, D. H., and Buncke, H. J. Autotransplantation of omentum to large scalp defect with microsurgical revascularization. *Plast. Reconstr. Surg.* 49:268, 1972.

16. Nylen, C. O. The microscope in aural surgery, its first use and later development. *Acta Oto-laryngol.* [Suppl.] *(Stockh.)* 116:226, 1954.

17. O'Brien, B. M., MacLeod, A., Hayhurst, J. W., et al. Successful transfer of a large island flap by microvascular anastomosis. *Plast. Reconstr. Surg.* 52:271, 1973.

18. O'Brien, B. M., and Morrison, W. A. *Reconstructive Microsurgery.* London: Churchill Livingstone, 1987.

19. Sanders, W. E. Principles of Microvascular Surgery. In D. P. Green (ed.), *Operative Hand Surgery.* New York: Churchill Livingstone, 1988.

20. Seaber, A. N. Laboratory design in preparing for elective microvascular surgery. *Hand Clin.* 1:233, 1985.

21. Servant, J. M., Ikuta, Y., and Harada, Y. A scanning electron microscope study of microvascular anastomoses. *Plast. Reconstr. Surg.* 57:329, 1976.

22. Shaw, W. W. Microvascular Free Flap Survival and Applications. In P. Furnas (ed.), *Frontiers of Microsurgery.* St. Louis: Mosby, 1983.

23. Shaw, W. W. Microvascular Surgery. In H. Haimovici (ed.), *Vascular Surgery. Principles and Techniques.* Norwalk, CT: Appleton-Century-Crofts, 1984.

24. Shaw, W. W., and Hidalgo, D. A. *Microsurgery in Trauma.* New York: Futura, 1987.

25. Tark, K. C., Khouri, R. K., and Shaw, W. W. Insert sutures first, tie later new microvascular anastomosis techniques. *Ann. Plast. Surg.*

26. Tark, K. C., Kim, Y. W., Lee, Y. H., et al. Replantation and revascularization of hands: Clinical analysis and functional results of 261 cases. *J. Hand Surg.*

27. Wyatt, A. P., and Taylor, G. W. Vein graft: Changes in the endothelium of autogenous free vein grafts used as arterial replacements. *Br. J. Surg.* 53:943, 1966.

*William W. Shaw*
*Roger K. Khouri*

# 42

# Clinical Microvascular Surgery and Free Tissue Transfers

A *free flap* may be defined as a composite block of tissue that is surgically removed from a donor site in the body and transferred in one stage to a distant recipient site where its circulation is restored via microvascular anastomoses. A detailed knowledge of the regional microvascular anatomy is essential to define the constituents and the boundaries of the donor flaps that can be carried by their respective donor pedicle vessels. The ability to select suitable donor tissues and to transfer them directly to the sites of the defects has permanently altered many reconstructive methods and has expanded the indications for surgery.

## History

Jacobson and Suarez in 1960 showed that 100 percent patency of small vessel anastomoses could be achieved using the operating microscope [35]. Goldwyn et al. in 1963 isolated lower abdominal skin flaps in dogs and showed that the flap could survive on the superficial inferior epigastric artery and vein [26]. Using this technique, Krizek and colleagues in 1965 successfully transferred the lower abdominal groin flap in the dog [42]. Buncke et al. in 1966 experimentally transferred the large toe and second toe as a unit to the hand of rhesus monkeys [9].

During the early 1960s Malt and Mc-Khann [45] and Chen et al. [13] performed the first successful replantation of an amputated arm and hand, thereby establishing the feasibility of restoring the circulation to human tissue parts through the repair of small vessels. The digital revascularization and replantation reported by Kleinert and Kasdan in 1965 [40] and Komatsu and Tamai in 1968 [41] and the first toe to thumb transfer reported by Cobbett in 1969 [15] provided further valuable experience and confidence in clinical microvascular surgery.

Fortuitously, during the same period the concept of axial pattern flaps with identifiable supplying vessels was developed by Bakamjian in 1968 [1], and McGregor and Morgan in 1972 [53], thus setting the stage for the free transfer of skin flaps. In 1972 McLean and Buncke covered a large scalp defect with a revascularized omental flap [54], and Harii et al. transplanted a scalp flap in 1974 [30]. Daniel and Taylor in 1973 reported the transfer of a groin flap based on the superficial epigastric artery and vein and used it to cover an ankle defect [18]. O'Brien et al. in Australia [61] and Yang in Shanghai [96] had similar successes. New donor flaps, reports of large clinical series of free flaps, technical innovations, and new applications quickly followed. Today, microvascular free tissue transfer is an essential part of plastic and reconstructive surgery.

## Principles of Free Flap Surgery

The introduction of free flap surgery to plastic surgery can be aptly compared to the advent of aviation to transportation. There is no longer any question about feasibility, and the advantages of such one-stage transfer are obvious. In fact, when everything goes right, it looks easy. The successes and convenience, however, do not come easily. A slight error in judgment, technique, or planning can result in catastrophe. Also, as a result of more surgery being performed than in previous plastic surgical operations, team work, organization, and complex planning become critical. Although there is no simple cookbook recipe, the surgery can be conceived as a series of steps, each of which must be flawlessly executed to ensure a successful result [34] (Table 42-1).

PREOPERATIVE PHASE
The thoroughness of the preoperative preparation is probably the most important determinant of a successful outcome. The result can only be as good as the plan, and little can be left to chance.

*Problem Assessment*
A careful analysis of the reconstructive problem begins with defining the extent of the defect after débridement or tumor resection. The operation must be optimally timed as well. Exposure of vital structures argues for immediate coverage whereas heavy wound colonization favors a delay. Coverage of traumatic wounds during the "subacute phase" poses a significantly increased risk of infection and vascular thrombosis [72].

*Reconstruction Goals and Priorities*
The possible goals of the surgery can then be identified. Is it to cover exposed vital structures, to provide a vascularized bed for nerve

**Table 42-1** *Surgical plan for free flap surgery*

*Preoperative Phase*
    **P**roblem assessment
    **R**econstruction goals and priorities
    **E**valuate specific surgical considerations
    **P**lan the surgery
    **A**nticipate problems and alternate plans
    **R**ehearse the operation
    **E**ducate the patient
*Operation*
    Coordinate with the anesthesiologist
    Position the operating room table and the patient
    Dissect the donor and recipient sites
    Determine the adequacy of the recipient vessels
    Divide the donor vessels
    Temporarily inset the flap
    Perform the anastomosis
    Close the donor site and check the vascular pedicle
    Inset the flap
*Postoperative Phase*
    Dressings and immobilization
    Systemic management
    Monitor flap circulation
    Reexplore if needed
    Advance activity level
    Secondary procedures

or tendon grafting, to provide muscle power, or to achieve an aesthetic restoration of contour? Priorities must be clearly established beforehand to provide the basis of intelligent decisions during the operation. *Keep it simple.* It is an error to try to accomplish too much and thereby perhaps jeopardize the basic objective.

*Evaluate Specific
Surgical Considerations*
OVERALL MEDICAL STATUS OF THE PATIENT. The presence of two operative sites and the lengthy nature of the surgery impose major surgical stress on the patient. Multiple-trauma victims must have their life-threatening injuries addressed first and their hemodynamic status stabilized. Older patients must have their cardiac, renal, and pulmonary status carefully evaluated preoperatively. Subopti-

mal cardiac function, renal failure, and endocrinopathies are relative contraindications to this type of surgery provided the reason for surgery is vital. The physician's primary axioms of "First do no harm" and "Life before limb or appearance" must be adhered to. Discussion with the anesthesiologist and other specialists may be important for assessing the risk-versus-benefit considerations.

RECIPIENT VESSELS. Preoperative angiography is almost always a requirement for elective extremity cases. The procedure is necessary to identify injured vessels in the traumatized extremity and to rule out significant congenital anomalies or major atherosclerotic changes. This information may influence the choice of recipient vessels and suggest safe areas along the vessel for anastomosis. In the head and neck region, preoperative angiography is generally not needed because of the abundance of recipient vessels. Angiography is also important for the evaluation of certain donor flaps such as the fibula and the ilium.

The status of the *recipient artery* may be unclear owing to either a poorly defined or an extensive "zone of injury." Even an angiogram does not guarantee a dependable recipient artery. Because dissection of the small vessels in the zone of injury is not only technically difficult but also prone to injury and thrombosis, it has become axiomatic that the recipient vessel selected for anastomosis must be situated in a previously undisturbed area.

The status of the *recipient vein* is often difficult to determine preoperatively. However, signs of venous hypertension in the lower extremity or extensive soft tissue trauma with its predisposition to cause venous thrombosis alerts the surgeon to potential problems. It may be best then to plan to first dissect the recipient site to determine if suitable veins are available before initiating dissection of the donor site. The same axiom that the recipient vein should be out of the zone of injury holds true. In the lower extremity, venae comitantes are preferred to

the superficial veins because they are less muscular and thus less prone to spasm.

*Plan the Surgery*

1. The donor flap is selected based on the requirement for tissue type, size, and bulk and after considering from which site the tissue can be best spared. When composite flaps are necessary, a three-dimensional concept of the defect is helpful for determining the degree of freedom each of the components should have to achieve independent insetting at the recipient site. This spatial relation further constrains the choice of composite flap donor sites. Special consideration must also be given to the potential need to reposition the patient to harvest the flap. The technique that provides the best solution with the least difficulty is chosen.

2. The position of the patient during the operation and the placement of the operating table must be carefully planned. The patient is positioned on the operating table in such a way that the best compromise between optimal exposure at the donor site versus that at the recipient site is achieved. The area of the anastomosis must be at a level plane so that neither surgeon is at an awkward angle. In certain cases, it is better to plan to partially dissect the recipient vessels, divide the flap and complete the donor site closure, and then reposition the patient to gain better exposure of the recipient vessels for the anastomosis. If this step is anticipated, usually little effort is required to change position and redrape the patient. However, if it is not planned beforehand, it may take considerable effort and time to reposition the patient in the middle of the operation.

3. Operative guidelines are as follows: To coordinate the multiple aspects of the same operation being performed by the different surgeons, it is generally important to have a single individual designated the "captain." For long cases it is important to plan the reliefs so that the continuity of the procedure is not disrupted. Free flap operations can be-

come significantly prolonged if there is a lack of appreciation for surgical pace. The surgeon must be able to "shift gears" from a relatively quick pace during wound débridement and the initial stages of donor site dissection to a more deliberate and cautious pace when dissecting the donor and recipient vessels. It requires the ability to identify and categorize the various phases of the procedure as they unfold and to then make adjustments accordingly.

*Anticipate Problems and
Alternate Plans*
Coordination with the other specialists involved, and the need for specialized equipment must be anticipated and added to the operative guidelines. Furthermore, a plan of retreat or alternate operative decisions that must sometimes be taken during the course of the surgery must be foreseen and prepared for. For instance, it is far better to use a long vein graft to tap into a normal vessel than to attempt to find a contracted stiff vessel in a densely scarred bed. Similarly, when a technically difficult anastomosis is anticipated because of the nature of the wound topography, the need for vein grafts must be anticipated, and compatible patient positioning during the preparation of a vein graft donor site must be included in the operative plan.

*Rehearse the Operation*
Marking the donor flap design the night before surgery saves time in the operating room and provides an additional opportunity for the members of the team to discuss key anatomic landmarks. At the same time the operative plan is reviewed and special aspects of the dissection are rehearsed. The division of labor is assigned. The most delicate parts of the operation, such as work with the recipient vessels and the vascular pedicle dissection, are usually best done by the most senior member of the team. It is also helpful to review the angiogram at this time.

*Educate the Patient*
Educating the patient is an essential part of the preoperative phase. The patient is asked to actively participate in the decision-making process. The magnitude and the complexity of the operation is explained, and the patient must have a good understanding of the "cost" of the various potential donor sites. It is also wise to offer alternatives to free tissue transfers, such as amputation, prosthesis, or split fistulas. Similarly, the plans of retreat are explained.

Patients must be advised against smoking preoperatively. Both the anesthetic risk and the potential for flap failure are also emphasized.

OPERATION
*Anesthesia*
The anesthesiologist is informed about the operative plan, the patient's positioning, and special surgical problems. This information allows him or her to plan ahead for the setup regarding intubation, intravenous and arterial lines, monitoring, blood replacement, muscle relaxation, and prevention of pressure sores.

Of particular importance is a realistic estimate of the operative time and the expected blood loss. During a long operation involving two sites, a great deal of blood loss can occur insidiously. The anesthesiologist must be informed of the periods of excessive blood loss as they occur so that no lag period develops and no excessive fluid is administered because of a perceived need to "catch up" with the blood loss when in fact the period of significant blood loss is over. A euvolumic state is important for preventing peripheral vasoconstriction and vascular spasm. A hematocrit of 30 to 35 percent is considered adequate for oxygenation while providing optimal viscosity; therefore not all blood loss is replaced.

*Donor and Recipient Site Dissection*
As dissection at both sites proceeds, it is important to periodically step back and reas-

sess the amount of tissue needed and in what configuration. The donor site design may be altered to compensate for an unrecognized deficit in the recipient site. The need to cover a larger than anticipated defect frequently occurs in the extremities when the wound is opened proximally to expose the recipient vessels. To avoid compression of the vascular pedicle from a tight closure, additional flap surface may be needed.

At the recipient site after the débridement to healthy margins or tumor excision, the recipient vessels are exposed and prepared. Extensive skeletonization of the vessels is time-consuming and may cause inadvertent vessel injury.

Most donor site dissections can proceed at a fairly rapid pace until the region of the pedicle is approached. The pace is then slowed, loupes are worn, and finer instruments are used. The pedicle is dissected free from surrounding structures, and skeletonization of the vessels is done only at the level at which they are to be divided. The pedicle vessel is divided only when the recipient vessels are "ready to go."

*Preparation for the Anastomosis*
During the critical step of preparing for the anastomosis, the surgeon must be relaxed and comfortable to concentrate on the procedure. If he or she is struggling, something is wrong. An attempt is then made to correct the difficulty. The microscope is best positioned at the center of the field within optimal reach of both surgeons. Adequate exposure of the recipient vessels is critical. Vascular structures must be clearly visualized before they are manipulated.

After the recipient artery is divided, it is assessed for flow and its lumen examined under magnification. A pulsatile jet of blood in the transected artery is the sine qua non of an adequate recipient vessel. Absence of flow or mere oozing may be due to spasm. If it is not relieved by the topical application of vasodilators, proximal vessel damage is

presumed and an alternate site with good flow is found.

The instrument table is then cleared of large instruments, and the microsurgical instruments and irrigation catheters are arranged within hand reach. Sutures are prepared. At this time the donor pedicle is divided, and the flap is transferred to the recipient site for anastomosis.

*Anastomosis*
Many of the technical considerations of performing the anastomosis are discussed in Chapter 41. The novice is often surprised that the clinical anastomosis is more difficult than those performed in the laboratory even though the vessels may be larger. However, when the anastomosis has been set up properly, this part of the procedure can be relatively easy and pleasurable. The key ingredients are a rested surgeon, a properly positioned microscope, adequate exposure, correct selection of the site of the anastomosis on both donor and recipient vessels, and instruments in good condition.

The flap is first temporarily inset at the recipient site to determine the proper pedicle length that avoids kinking or tension of the vessel. The choice of end-to-side versus end-to-end anastomosis is determined by the vessel size discrepancy and the relative expandability of the recipient vessel. The size of the suture material selected and the method of suturing, whether continuous or interrupted, are reviewed in Chapter 41.

Either the artery or the vein may be anastomosed first. The order of the anastomosis must be such that the first one does not compromise the exposure of the subsequent one. Flow is restored after both vessels are completed. The anastomoses are inspected for leaks. Large leaks are best treated with an additional suture. Small leaks stop spontaneously. Side branches may require ligation.

The artery must remain pulsatile and the vein soft and pinkish blue in color. Most arterial thromboses appear within 15 to 30 minutes of the restoration of blood flow. If there is doubt as to the patency of the anastomosis, it is redone.

The benefits of administering anticoagulants is unproved. However, there is experimental evidence that a single bolus of 2000 to 5000 units of heparin given prior to the clamping step of the anastomosis is helpful in improving patency [28, 37], especially if it involves diseased vessels or vessels clamped for an extended period.

Vein grafts may be required in cases where there is a gap between the recipient vessels and the flap pedicle. The grafts can be sewn to either the recipient vessels or the flap vessels first, depending on the nature of the wound topography. The vessels are chosen to provide the best overall exposure. Long vein grafts, particularly those interposed in the venous drainage of the flap, are subject to external compression during wound closure and may result in thrombosis.

*Closure of the Donor Site*
The closure of the donor site is usually done by the second team during the time of the anastomosis. Though the focus of the operation is elsewhere, donor site closure must be carefully done to avoid the complications of herniation, dehiscence, and poor skin graft take [17].

*Insetting the Flap*
During the flap insetting phase of the procedure, the flap color and the dermal edge bleeding are periodically inspected. The pedicle must lie in a suitable configuration without twisting or kinking. The flap is carefully sutured in the area close to the pedicle to avoid motion and accidental avulsion. The area over the pedicle is closed without any tension, which could compress the pedicle. If insufficient flap tissue is available, a skin graft is in order. Both skin and muscle flaps can be considerably tailored to achieve the optimal aesthetic result. The flap may be partially split, and the various components may be inset separately as needed.

Closed suction drains are placed under the flap but well away from the pedicle.

POSTOPERATIVE CARE
*Dressings, Immobilization, and Activity Level*
Free flaps are usually left exposed for observation and monitoring. Xeroform gauze or an antibiotic ointment may be applied at the suture line or the skin graft sites to prevent desiccation.

Extremities are elevated to promote venous drainage. They must not rest on the flap, nor should the weight of the extremity be borne in the area just proximal to the anastomosis. Suspension with orthopedic equipment may be necessary to achieve this condition.

Minimal motion is recommended at the recipient site to avoid compression or disruption of the pedicle. Patients are kept at bed rest for 5 days or longer for lower extremity flaps before gradual intermittent dependency and ambulation are allowed. The return to normal activities is gauged by the disappearance of swelling and cyanosis with dependency.

*Systemic Management*
Blood pressure and intravascular volume must be carefully regulated. It is critically important to prevent a hypovolemic state, which would predispose the recipient artery to vasospasm thrombosis at the anastomosis. Hypothermia is likewise avoided, as postoperative shivering may cause peripheral vasoconstriction that could contribute thrombosis.

Antibiotics are generally started preoperatively and are discontinued 24 hours later unless specifically indicated. The role of anticoagulants and vasodilators is not established at this time. Reckless use of heparin and other anticoagulants has not only resulted in serious complications but also did not substantially improve the results. Aside from being given as a single intraoperative

**Table 42-2** *Signs of flap distress*

| Sign | Arterial problem | Venous problem |
|---|---|---|
| Color | Pale, white | Purple, cyanotic |
| Capillary refill | Decreased | Rapid |
| Turgor | Decreased | Increased |
| Temperature | Rapid drop | Slow decrease |
| Bleeding on pinprick | Absent | Purple ooze |

bolus, heparin is not used unless there has been a thrombosis of the pedicle requiring revision or long vein grafts have been used. At our microsurgery unit, low-molecular-weight dextran is routinely used on an empiric basis for 5 days at the rate of 40 ml per hour for 12 hours each day. It is preferred because of its contribution to fluid management, its antiplatelet activity, and its relative safety.

Cigarette smoking is absolutely prohibited during the postoperative period. Chemotherapeutic drugs, especially antiestrogens, also seem to predispose to a hypercoagulable state and, if possible, are discontinued during the perioperative period.

*Postoperative Monitoring and Reexploration*

Whereas vascular thrombosis is part of the learning process in the teaching laboratory, it is catastrophic in the clinical setting and must be corrected immediately. Even in experienced hands, up to 10 percent of flaps develop postoperative vascular thrombosis and are salvaged by a timely reexploration.

A pale flap with poor capillary refill usually indicates an arterial inflow problem, whereas a purple flap with rapid refill indicates venous obstruction. This guideline is not foolproof, and the circulation to some flaps may be difficult to assess. When sufficient doubt exists as to the status of the circulation, the flap can be pricked with a needle (away from the pedicle) and the quality of the bleeding observed (Table 42-2). Around-the-clock hourly observation of the

flap by an experienced member of the team for the first several days, although ideal for picking up early thrombosis, is unfortunately not always practical or reliable [71]. A number of monitoring devices that rely on surface temperature recording [38], photoplatysmography, or Doppler effect [81] have been developed and are generally helpful adjuncts. To date no system has proved to be both convenient and consistently reliable.

A review of our experience at Bellevue [38] showed that monitoring with simple surface temperature recording enabled us to save 86 percent of the flaps that developed postoperative vascular thrombosis, and that 71 percent of our flap failures occurred in unmonitored flaps.

When serious doubt persists as to the perfusion of the flap, the patient is taken back to the operating room for an immediate reexploration. The vascular pedicle is quickly exposed, and if a thrombosis is found, a rapid, thorough assessment of the possible cause is made (Table 42-3). Is it due to a tight wound closure (often seen with venous thrombosis as postoperative swelling compounds the problem), poor recipient vessels, a kinked pedicle, or just a technical error? In any event, the segment of vessel immediately adjacent to the thrombosed anastomosis is resected and the flow promptly reestablished by repeating the anastomosis, not hesitating to use an interpositional vein graft if needed to reach a more proximal recipient vessel. Heparinization is by then usually started and continued for a few days. The pedicle must lie comfortably under the flap at the

**Table 42-3**  *Causes of free flap failure*

*Mechanical*
    Anastomosis
        Backwall suture
            Poor intimal contact
            Intimal flap
            Significant vessel size discrepancy
    Pedicle
        Extrinsic: tight skin closure, edema,
            hematoma, external pressure
        Intrinsic: too long (kinked), too short
            (stretched), pinched, twisted
*Hydrostatic*
    Inadequate arterial inflow or venous
        outflow
    Vascular spasm: hypovolemia, hypothermia
*Thrombogenic*
    Traumatic pedicle dissection
    Recipient vessels in "zone of injury"
    Hypercoagulable state (e.g.,
        thrombocythemia, smoking)

time of closure. Skin grafting or a delayed wound closure is performed if there is any tension during the closure. Careful monitoring is resumed. Although unusual, some flaps have suffered more than one thrombotic event and have been saved by a second reexploration.

*Secondary Procedures*
Secondary procedures are often needed for bone, tendon, or nerve grafting and for contour improvement. In general, 6 weeks is a safe period to wait before undertaking a procedure that requires flap mobilization. Suction-assisted lipectomy has proved useful for contouring flaps with excessive subcutaneous fat [29].

## Donor Sites

Any block of tissue with an identifiable arterial inflow and venous drainage can be utilized as a potential free flap. A rebirth of interest in anatomy among plastic surgeons has led to the discovery of many new flap donor sites.

Taylor and Palmer [84], based on extensive anatomic studies, clarified the concept of vascular territories. They advocated that the body could be conceived as a three-dimensional jigsaw puzzle of blocks of tissue, or *angiosomes*. They mapped out 40 separate angiosomes, each perfused by a named artery and venae comitans, the source vessels. Each angiosome has vascular connections to its adjacent angiosomes by way of smaller-caliber vessels called *choke vessels*. These authors found that a source vessel could provide nutritive blood flow to its angiosome proper and, by way of the choke vessels, to the immediately adjacent angiosomes.

The same source vessel can also serve as the pedicle of many flaps: a flap that consists of its angiosome proper plus any of the immediately adjacent ones, including various tissue components. Conversely, the same angiosome may be carried by different vascular pedicles. For example, the skin of the back could be raised either as part of the cutaneous portion of the circumflex scapular vessels or as part of the cutaneous territory of the latissimus dorsi flap. This dynamic concept of tissue perfusion allows virtually unlimited variations in the composition of potential free flaps available in the body.

Some of the characteristic features of the various types of tissue transplanted and the most frequently used flaps are presented in Table 42-4. A discussion of the flap dissection is beyond the scope of this chapter, and the reader is referred to the list of references [62, 70].

SKIN FLAPS
Considered the prototype for all other free tissue transfers, cutaneous flaps are preferred over other forms of coverage in many situations. They provide a reconstruction most compatible with the original skin loss and can be sensate if a cutaneous nerve is included. Their main disadvantage is that there is a limit to the size of flap that can be harvested while still achieving primary wound closure at the donor site [68]. There

*Table 42-4* Tissues used in the various flaps

| Free flap donors | Vascular pedicles | Free flap donors | Vascular pedicles |
|---|---|---|---|
| *Fascial and Fasciocutaneous Flaps* | | *Muscle and Musculocutaneous Flaps* | |
| Scalp and temporalis fascia | Superficial temporal | Extensor digitorum brevis | Dorsalis pedis |
| Scalp and occipital fascia | Occipital | | |
| Postauricular | Postauricular | *Bone Flaps* | |
| Forehead | Superficial temporal | Rib | Posterior intercostal |
| Supraclavicular | Transverse cervical | Rib | Internal mammary |
| Deltopectoral | Internal mammary perforator | Scapula | Circumflex scapular |
| Scapular and parascapular | Circumflex scapular | Iliac crest | Deep circumflex iliac |
| Axillary | Lateral thoracic | Iliac crest | Superficial circumflex iliac |
| Medial upper arm | Ulnar collateral | Fibula | Peroneal |
| Lateral upper arm | Radial collateral | Second metatarsal | Dorsalis pedis |
| Radial forearm | Radial | Serratus muscle with bone | Thoracodorsal |
| Ulnar forearm | Ulnar | Latissimus dorsi muscle with rib | Thoracodorsal |
| Epigastric | Superficial epigastric | Radial forearm with segment of radius | Radial |
| Groin | Superficial circumflex iliac | Lateral arm with segment of humerus | Radial collateral |
| Lower medial thigh | Cutaneous branch of femoral | | |
| Anteromedial thigh | Lateral circumflex femoral | *Visceral Organs* | |
| Posterolateral thigh | Perforator 3 profunda femoris | Omentum | Gastroepiploic |
| Superior posterolateral thigh | Perforator 1 profunda femoris | Omentum and stomach | Gastroepiploic |
| Saphenous | Saphenous | Jejunum | Branch of superior mesenteric |
| Anterior tibial | Anterior tibial | Ileum | Branch of superior mesenteric |
| Peroneal | Peroneal | Colon | Branch of inferior mesenteric |
| Sural | Sural | Appendix | Appendiceal |
| Dorsalis pedis | Dorsalis pedis | Ovary | Ovarian |
| Midsole plantar | Medial plantar | Fallopian tube | Ovarian |
| First toe web | First metatarsal | Testes | Testicular |
| Partial great toe | First metatarsal | Adrenal gland | Adrenal |
| *Muscle and Musculocutaneous Flaps* | | *Specialized Parts* | |
| Latissimus dorsi | Thoracodorsal | Great toe | First metatarsal |
| Serratus anterior | Thoracodorsal | Wraparound toe | First metatarsal |
| Pectoralis major | Thoracoacromial | Second toe | First metatarsal |
| Pectoralis minor | Thoracoacromial | Second and third toes | Second metatarsal |
| Rectus abdominis | Deep inferior epigastric | Second toe PIP joint | First metatarsal |
| Internal oblique | Deep circumflex iliac | Second toe metatarsophalangeal joint | First metatarsal |
| Gluteus maximus | Superior gluteal | Extensor hallucis tendon | Dorsalis pedis |
| Gluteus maximus | Inferior gluteal | Sural nerve | Sural |
| Gracilis | Medial circumflex femoral | Superficial radial nerve | Radial |
| Rectus femoris | Lateral circumflex femoral | Ulnar nerve | Ulnar |
| Tensor fascia lata | Lateral circumflex femoral | | |
| Medial gastrocnemius | Medial sural | | |

is also some experimental evidence that skin flaps may not be as vigorous as muscle flaps in terms of the total blood flow and their ability to defend against bacterial infection when placed over contaminated wounds [10, 11].

Ideally, donor skin flaps are taken from areas that can be closed directly and leave a scar that is well hidden, such as the groin. Donor sites requiring a skin graft for closure in a visible or frequently traumatized area, such as the dorsalis pedis [99] or forearm flaps [76], are less desirable. The size of the pedicle and the ease of dissection also are important factors. The radial artery of the forearm flap, for example, is easier and more reliable compared to the small and variable topography of the superficial circumflex artery of the groin flap. The scapular flap [20] combines these two desirable features and is commonly used. Anatomically, skin flaps are of three types.

1. *Direct cutaneous flaps* are based on axial cutaneous arteries, e.g., the groin flap and the deltopectoral flap. These early flaps were limited by the size and the length of available pedicle. The scapular flaps introduced later circumvent this limitation because the dissection of the vascular pedicle is carried out at a more proximal level where the artery is much larger.
2. *Fasciocutaneous flaps* are based on large and easy to dissect major arteries and the vascularized fascia and skin supplied by them. Examples include the dorsalis pedis flap, the radial and ulnar forearm flaps, and the scalp flap.
3. *Septocutaneous flaps* are based on the arteries that course along the intermuscular septae and the fascia that invests them. These flaps have a vascular pedicle that is intermediate in terms of size and ease of dissection. Examples include the lateral and medial arm flaps [77], the deltoid flap, and the lateral and medial thigh flaps.

FASCIA

Fasciocutaneous and septocutaneous flaps can also be harvested as vascularized fascia alone without the cutaneous component. The donor site disfigurement is thus minimized. These flaps are useful on the hand, for example, where thin coverage is needed. They can also be used to wrap the cartilaginous framework graft needed for auricular and nasal reconstructions [7]. A skin graft, however, needs to be applied over the flap to close the wound, and the donor skin can be chosen to match the color of the recipient site. Fascial flaps also appear to be ideally suited as universal carriers to prefabricate vascularized "spare parts" using the process of staged reconstruction [39].

MUSCULOCUTANEOUS FLAPS

Mathes and Nahai [49], McCraw et al. [52], and others recognized that most muscles are supplied by predictable blood vessels of reasonable size and can be used as attached regional flaps or as free flaps. This recognition has greatly increased the number of flaps available for free tissue transfer. The basic requirement for microvascular transfer is that the portion of muscle transferred be perfused by a pedicle with an adequate size for anastomosis. When transferring muscles with more than one pedicle, the dominant one that perfuses the portion of muscle transferred is used.

In the musculocutaneous flaps, branches of the muscle's vascular pedicle perforate the muscle to supply the overlying skin. Only a small portion of muscle that contains the large cutaneous perforators needs to be included in a flap that could incorporate a wide skin territory. This variation allows the preservation of motor function, minimizing the donor morbidity. Examples of such flaps include the transverse rectus abdominis musculocutaneous flap [62], the superior gluteal musculocutaneous flap [69], and the latissimus dorsi musculocutaneous flap [68]. Because of the vigorous blood supply, the large and long vascular pedicle, and the highly predictable anatomy, many musculocutaneous flaps have become the workhorses of free flap surgery.

## MUSCLE FLAPS FOR COVERAGE

Because the amount of skin surface available for coverage is limited, transplanted muscles are often skin-grafted to provide coverage as well. The latissimus dorsi muscle has a fan-shaped flat origin on the back and is ideally suited to cover large defects [27]. The rectus abdominis muscle is ideally suited for long defects of limited width. The gracilis or the serratus anterior muscles are useful for small defects. Muscular free flaps have some advantages.

1. Muscles can often be harvested through small, well placed incisions less prone to develop into unsightly scars.
2. Because this type of coverage has no subcutaneous fat, the skin tends to be more rigidly adherent. This situation has certain potential advantages when used over the heel or sole [51].
3. There is experimental evidence to suggest that muscle flaps may be more capable of fending off infections and that they could deliver higher levels of antibiotics to the sites of infection [10, 64, 66]. This point renders them the flaps of choice for the coverage of postosteomyelitis débridement defects [50, 94].
4. Muscles are highly pliable and can be divided along their longitudinal fibers into multiple strands that can be placed in irregular defects to obliterate the deadspace [87]. This application has proved useful for coverage of wounds with a complex surface topography where the obliteration of deadspace is critical. A prime example is the postosteomyelitis débridement wound.

A notable problem with skin-grafted muscle flaps is the difficulty of assessing their perfusion postoperatively. The classic signs of color and capillary refill do not apply, and evaporative losses serve to cool the flap, rendering surface temperature recording less reliable.

## MUSCLE FLAPS FOR MOTION

Muscles can be transplanted with their motor nerve to restore motor function. Currently, the principal indications for such a transfer have been for forearm muscle replacement when no tendon transfer is possible [47] and for long-standing facial nerve palsy when the facial muscles have undergone irreversible atrophy [46].

The characteristic features that are important when selecting the appropriate muscle for transfer include the following.

1. A predictable dominant vascular pedicle of good size and length.
2. A single motor nerve, with adequate size and fascicular match with the recipient nerve. It is best to have a long recipient nerve so that the nerve juncture is as close to the muscle as possible, thereby shortening the time lapse before muscle reinnervation.
3. An appropriate power of contraction to achieve the movement desired. It is important to take into account an estimated 50 percent loss of muscle power following the free transfer.
4. An adequate range of excursion to achieve useful motion. This feature is related to the fiber length of the muscle used.
5. The size and shape of the muscle must fit the recipient area and provide a suitable origin and insertion.
6. The potential for partially splitting the muscle into two or more neuromotor units, such as to achieve some degree of independent contraction of the components. It is desirable in the forearm, for example, where it allows some degree of independent thumb and finger motion.

The gracilis muscle is emerging as one of the preferred muscles. It is about 30 cm long and has an effective amplitude of 12 cm. Grip strength of 35 to 40 pounds has been achieved when it is used for digital flexion [47, 48]. On the other hand, when used for facial muscle replacement, only a small segment of the muscle is transferred to restore the excursion needed for a normal smile [46].

BONE

For the free bone flaps transfer, the endosteal and periosteal circulations are maintained. The bone remains alive after its transfer, and its response to biologic and mechanical stress is similar to that of normal bones. The healing at the ends of the graft is similar to that of fractures, and primary bone union occurs between the graft and the recipient bone. In contrast to the nonvascularized grafts, no creeping substitution takes place [5].

The *fibula flap* is the longest and strongest bone transferred by microsurgical techniques. It provides a relatively straight 22- to 25-cm piece of well vascularized cortical bone that readily fits into long bone defects [24]. A few wedge osteotomies may be performed, allowing it to conform to the desired mandibular shape while maintaining its vascularity. Its pedicle, the peroneal artery, may be dissected for a length of 8 to 10 cm and is usually 2 to 3 mm in diameter. A cutaneous component based on the lateral intermuscular septum of the leg may be harvested with the flap [92]. The soleus muscle may also be included when an additional soft tissue component is needed [4]. Although much thinner than the tibia or the femur, when used for their reconstruction the fibula hypertrophies in response to the stresses placed on it.

The *iliac crest* provides a flap rich in cancellous bone. Its arterial supply, the deep circumflex iliac artery, provides branches to the bone, abdominal musculature, and skin. It can also be transferred as bone only, bone and abdominal musculature, or bone, muscle, and skin. The iliac crest has multiple curvatures with ingenious flap design; a bony segment may be harvested such that it could fit into any geometrically complex defect. Meticulous closure of the donor site is important to avoid postoperative herniation of abdominal contents.

The free *scapular bone flap* may be harvested with or without the previously described cutaneous flap [80]. Depending on the size of the patient, a triangular strud of well vascularized strong corticocancellous bone 2.5 cm wide and 10 to 14 cm long may be harvested along the lateral border of the scapula from the glenoid fossa to the scapular tip. The prime advantages of this flap are the length and size of the vascular pedicle and the reliability of the large cutaneous island that can be independently inset. Donor site morbidity is small compared to that seen with other bone flap donors. Although the flap has proved to be most useful for reconstructing small mandibular defects, a drawback is the need to reposition the patient to harvest the flap.

Other vascularized bone donors include the second metatarsal bone based on the dorsalis pedis artery [99], a portion of the distal radius that can be raised with the radial forearm flap, a portion of the distal humerus that can be raised with the lateral arm flap, and the intercostal rib flaps [86] based on the intercostal artery. These donor sites share the disadvantages of potential significant site morbidity and the fact that only a small amount of bone can be harvested.

TOES AND JOINTS

Toes constitute a valuable source of specialized tissue for digital and thumb reconstruction. The presence of a nail, a glabrous pulp with good sensory potential, small joints, and tendons makes the toe a highly versatile donor [23, 44]. In addition to replacing an entire missing digit, various configurations can be taken to replace the pulp, the joint, or the metacarpals as well. Important general considerations that minimize the donor morbidity include the following.

**1.** The foot donor site must be closed primarily. When there is skin deficiency, skin grafts are better tolerated on the hand than on the foot.

2. Plantar dissection must be minimized, and no skin is excised beyond what can achieve a tensionless closure.

3. The first metatarsal head or at least part of it is preserved for its importance in foot function.

Several variations of the donor flap design have been described to meet the specific reconstructive needs while minimizing donor site morbidity [91]. The major reconstructive options include the following.

*1. Great toe transfer* [15, 89]: Although it is larger than the thumb, the great toe resembles the thumb more than the second toe. It also provides a broader, more stable surface for pinch and grasp and is preferred for certain types of manual labor. The limitations are a greater cosmetic and functional defect at the foot and the inability to provide for missing metacarpal length.

*2. Second toe transfer* [43, 91]: With this transfer, the cosmetic foot deformity is minimal as the web space defect is closed by approximating the first and third toes. The aesthetic reconstruction on the hand is usually less attractive than with use of the great toe. The second toe when transferred with its metatarsal bone is a three-joint system. To prevent the associated instability, the metatarsophalangeal (MP) joint is fused. Pinch and grasp power are usually more dependent on the extrinsic motor supply to the transferred digit and less dependent on the choice of donor toe.

*3. Multiple toe transfers* [93]: These transfers are indicated for the severely mutilated hand where the need to restore a functional hand justifies a greater foot defect. It can be done "en bloc" or separately, taking one toe from each foot. A vascular graft to perfuse the ulnar digits may be needed.

*4. Partial toe transfers and variations of*

*the wraparound technique* [56]: These techniques are more refined types of reconstruction that avoid the bulkiness of the total toe transfer [89] while at the same time preserve as much of the toe as possible. These custom-made flaps are preferred for incomplete losses when only specific components such as the nail, the pulp, or a phalanx must be replaced. Often a bone graft is needed either on the thumb or to reconstitute the toe, and the associated problems of graft resorption are encountered.

The transfer of vascularized second toe joints can also be done to replace missing critical joints in the hand or ankylosed temporomandibular joints.

## GASTROINTESTINAL TRACT TRANSPLANTS

Any segment of bowel that can be isolated on a vascular pedicle may serve as a tube to reconstruct the pharynx and the esophagus. Thus the jejunum based on branches of the superior mesenteric artery [65], the sigmoid colon based on the inferior mesenteric artery, and tubed segments of stomach based on the gastroepiploic vessels [3] have been used. The second loop of jejunum remains one of the most popular donor sites because the size of the bowel lumen in this area matches that of the hypopharynx and the cervical esophagus. It also has an accessible vasculature with a pattern of branching suitable for transfer on a single pedicle. Moreover, compared to other gastrointestinal donors, it is associated with less morbidity. Because of the multiple curves of the jejunum, it is difficult to obtain a straight segment that is longer than 12 to 15 cm without separating it from its mesentery at both ends. The second jejunal artery and vein comprise the pedicle that is most often chosen; it can support a 20 cm segment of jejunum. If more length is needed, two vascular pedicles may be necessary. Every effort is made to keep the ischemia time of the gastrointestinal flaps to a minimum lest mucosal slough ensues.

## OMENTAL TRANSPLANTS

The omentum provides a large amount of soft tissue that readily accepts a skin graft for coverage of large cutaneous defects [54]. Either the right or the left gastroepiploic vessels can be used as a pedicle. Because the omentum is malleable, it can fit into any defect and totally obliterates the deadspace with highly vascularized tissue. This point makes it ideally suited to cover postdebridement defects from chronically infected wounds and radiation ulcers. Its use to augment soft tissue defects has been curtailed by its tendency to fall under the effect of gravity, giving a rather jowly appearance. Its major disadvantage is that it requires laparotomy, a decision that is not made lightly. Also, because the omentum cannot be assessed preoperatively, a history of abdominal problems or previous abdominal surgery are contraindications to this choice of flap.

## OTHER SPECIALIZED TISSUES AND ORGANS

Other flaps of specialized tissue have been described, such as vascularized nerves [83] and tendon flaps [90], which are used in cases where the recipient bed is hostile to the revascularization of conventional grafts. Microvascular techniques can be used to transplant many organs perfused by vessels too small for conventional vascular surgery, including autotransplantation of abdominal testis [55, 75] and of fallopian tubes to the contralateral side next to the remaining functional ovary [19, 95] and the temporary transfer of ovaries [98] to protect them from therapeutic radiation damage.

## Applications of Free Flap Surgery
### ADVANTAGES OF AND INDICATIONS FOR FREE FLAPS

The advantages of free flaps and the indications for their use [68, 72] are as follows.

1. *Short reconstruction time.* Single-stage immediate total reconstructions can be achieved leading to earlier mobilization and better restoration of function with a shorter hospital stay. Cross leg flaps and tubed pedicled flaps take 2 to 3 months of hospitalization and involve multiple operative procedures.

2. *Distant donor tissue.* The "borrowing" of tissue is no longer restricted to the immediate vicinity of the defect, which is often also traumatized, scarred, or irradiated. A wider selection of donor flaps is possible, with any area of the body serving as a potential donor.

3. *Specialized tissue.* Conventional methods of transplanting tissue are usually limited to the transfer of skin flaps. Microvascular techniques allow the transfer of specialized tissues (e.g., bone, muscle, nerve) or composite tissues (e.g., intestinal tract segments, toes, and other osteomyocutaneous flaps). These flaps are particularly important when restoring specific functions.

4. *Freedom of design.* The ability to choose the proper tissue, donor site, and orientation of the pedicle allows wider options in the design of the reconstruction for achieving optimal results.

5. *Large, complex defects.* These defects may be reconstructed only with the free tissue transfer of a large flap. Therefore wide debridement or tumor excision may be accomplished without the fear of creating an unreconstructible hole.

6. *Good aesthetic result.* The ability to reconstruct a large defect as a unit, with the possibility of replacing losses in kind, with a freedom of orientation and no bulky pedicle, leads to a good aesthetic result. Furthermore, the donor flap can be obtained from inconspicuous areas where primary closure is possible.

7. *Independent blood supply.* Free flaps bring in their own blood supply and are not dependent on the recipient bed for support. This point allows them to be used in com-

promised wounds, irradiated beds, and over large avascular areas such as bone or foreign bodies.

8. *Applicable all over the body.* Free flaps can be transferred anywhere in the body. The two ends of the body—head and feet—are difficult to cover with pedicled flaps because of a lack of adjacent tissue.

9. *Reliable technique.* A more than 95 percent overall "success" rate can be dependably achieved with free flaps. This rate may vary, however, depending on the constraints of the individual case and the experience of the surgeon.

REGIONAL APPLICATIONS

The regional applications of free flaps [68, 72] are outlined in Table 42-5.

*Head and Neck*

Small defects in the head and neck region are generally best reconstructed with local tissue to achieve the closest color match. For larger defects, distant tissue is usually required. Free flaps were used initially when regional flaps, such as the deltopectoral or the pectoralis major flaps, were unsuitable or had failed. With experience, free flaps are increasingly used preferentially for both difficult and routine reconstructions.

When the expertise to perform free flap surgery is available, the extirpative surgeon is at ease knowing that as much tissue as necessary can be removed to provide a curative cancer operation without worrying about closure of the defect. During the extirpation, and without interfering with the other team, the microvascular surgeons can harvest the flap from a distant site and be prepared to begin the reconstruction immediately after tumor removal. Such direct reconstructions can dramatically improve the patient's quality of life, a factor of great importance considering the poor prognosis of many of these patients. Also, in some cases the achievability of a larger resection may result in higher cure rate and better palliation.

Many recipient vessels are available in the

**Table 42-5** *Applications of free flaps*

*Head and Neck*
  Face: contour and coverage
  Scalp and cranial base coverage
  Intraoral reconstruction
  Mandibular reconstruction
  Esophageal reconstruction
  Facial reanimation
*Trunk*
  Chest and abdominal wall coverage
  Breast reconstruction
  Penile and urethral reconstruction
*Upper Extremity*
  Wound coverage
  Digital replacement and reconstruction
  Functioning muscle transplantation
*Lower Extremity*
  Wound coverage
  Amputation stump salvage
  Bony reconstruction
  Chronic osteomyelitis
  Peripheral vascular disease ulcers

head and neck. The facial, superior thyroid, and transverse cervical arteries are those most commonly used. Irradiation and atherosclerosis do not appear to have a major effect on anastomotic patency in the head and neck region, as is the case elsewhere [57].

FACIAL RECONSTRUCTION. Facial skin defects are best reconstructed with skin flaps taken from above the clavicle because they provide the best color and texture match. Because of their limited availability, larger surface defects require distant skin flaps, including free flaps.

Restoration of facial contour in Romberg's disease, hemifacial microsomia, or posttraumatic and postablative surgery is best achieved with subcutaneous fat from deepithelialized free skin flaps fashioned to fill the defect [88]. Alternatively, a muscle such as the serratus, which may be divided into finger-like strips, can be used to accurately provide the contour needed. However, this procedure is less desirable, as the degree of postoperative atrophy is not predictable.

For nasal reconstructions when the forehead skin is not available, the forearm or dorsalis pedis flaps provide a thin cutaneous cover. Such distant skin flaps, however, lack the refinement, color, and texture match of the forehead flap. Another attractive alternative is the temporalis fascia flap covered with a full-thickness skin graft obtained from the supraclavicular area.

Total ear reconstruction is best performed by a temporalis fascia island flap wrapped around a cartilaginous framework and covered with a skin graft. If the ipsilateral flap is not available (as is not uncommonly the case), the contralateral one can be transferred as a free flap.

SCALP RECONSTRUCTION. When local skin is not sufficient to cover the defect, a free flap is considered the first choice because of the difficulty of getting distant pedicled flaps to reach the scalp. Although reconstruction with a skin flap is ideal, for the large defect the morbidity of skin grafting a skin flap donor is not warranted. Such a reconstruction is best performed with an omental flap or a latissimus muscle flap, which can fan out to cover a large area and can accept a skin graft. Because of the potential morbidity of a laparotomy, most surgeons favor the latissimus muscle, which, if necessary, could be supplemented by the serratus muscle perfused by the same thoracodorsal pedicle.

INTRAORAL RECONSTRUCTION. Pedicled pectoralis major flaps are the most common method of intraoral reconstruction. However, a high complication rate and a bulky pedicle still plague this type of reconstruction. A well planned and executed free flap provides a simpler, reliable alternative. More complex defects, e.g., those that also include other structures such as the external facial skin, the tongue and palate, and the roof and floor of the mouth, can be best reconstructed with a free flap.

The forearm flap provides a thin, hairless skin flap that can be fashioned and folded to fit the defect [78]. It is often the flap of choice in debilitated patients because of its easy dissection. Moreover, its long vascular pedicle can reach across to the intact contra-

lateral neck. Alternatively, the transverse rectus abdominis flap may be used [14]. The cachexia often seen in these patients renders it a thin cutaneous flap that can be folded over to provide both facial coverage and intraoral lining. When intraoral lining alone is needed, a segment of jejunum opened along its antimesenteric border provides a large piece of supple, well-vascularized tissue that produces mucus and may alleviate the post-irradiation dry mouth symptoms.

MANDIBULAR RECONSTRUCTION. In addition to its role in mastication, the mandible is important for speech, swallowing, and the maintenance of facial contour. Mandibular reconstructions with conventional bone grafts and implant materials are often unsuccessful because the soft tissue bed is usually contaminated, is scarred, or has sustained radiation damage. Furthermore, the mandibular bony defect is often compounded by the need to provide intraoral lining and external skin cover. Vascularized composite osteocutaneous or osteomusculocutaneous flaps, by virtue of their capacity to achieve primary healing in a hostile environment, offer a more reliable solution to this difficult problem [21].

For most large bone and soft tissue defects of the mandible, the iliac crest based on the deep circumflex iliac artery, is the flap of choice. It can be harvested simultaneously during the resection. A massive piece of bone can be removed along the curvatures of the ipsilateral ilium such that it conforms best to the desired mandibular shape [82]. The bone may be additionally sculptured without affecting its vascularity. It can also carry a large island of skin for the reconstruction of associated soft tissue defects. Careful preoperative planning is essential owing to the complex three-dimensional nature of the reconstructive challenge.

For large mandibular defects with limited soft tissue requirement, the fibula is a good alternative. The donor site is located well away from the extirpative field so the flap may be comfortably harvested during the tumor resection. A few well-placed partial osteotomies allow the bone to be shaped to the desired configuration while maintaining its vascularity. Plate-and-screw fixation of the osteotomies and of the flap to the mandibular remnant allows solid reconstruction. The long vascular pedicle allows the anastomosis to be performed in the neck away from the radiated field.

For a short defect, the scapular flap [80] has many advantages: It is a large skin island that affords a large freedom of inset, a long and large vascular pedicle, and minimal donor morbidity. The amount of bone available, however, is limited to less than 12 cm. Also, the need to reposition the patient to harvest the flap may preclude simultaneous tumor resection and flap elevation and adds to the operative time.

Other donor sites advocated for small defects are the second metatarsal, which can also provide a temporomandibular joint if taken with the second toe metatarsophalangeal joint, and the osteocutaneous radial forearm flap.

ESOPHAGEAL RECONSTRUCTION. The ability to transfer vascularized segments of the gastrointestinal tract to reconstruct the hypopharynx and the cervical esophagus has largely replaced the notoriously unreliable multiple-stage delayed tubed skin flap procedures. Currently, a segment of the second loop of the jejunum is most commonly used, and its antimesenteric border can be opened to fit the pharyngeal defect [59]. When compared with older methods, the incidence of fistula and stenosis is markedly decreased and the hospital stay significantly shortened.

FREE FLAPS FOR FACIAL REANIMATION. There are 18 muscles that animate each side of the face. Reconstructing this finely tuned neuromuscular system to restore a normal facial expression is presently impossible. Because denervation atrophy develops after 12 to 18 months, every effort must be made to perform an early repair of facial nerve lesions.

When the lesion is intracranial, however, an adequate proximal stump is often not available. Furthermore, microneurorrhaphies of the main trunk, especially when nerve grafts are needed to bridge a gap, frequently result in disorganized axonal regeneration, causing mass contractions or dyskinesis of the facial musculature.

With late reconstructions there is muscle loss due to denervation atrophy. Our present ability to transfer one or two neuromuscular motor units allows rather unsophisticated restoration of facial expression. However, the movement that patients miss the most is the elevation of the corner of the mouth to produce a smile. Free muscle transplantation can produce this active motion as well as a balanced symmetric appearance of the mouth at rest. Voluntary eyelid closure is still not satisfactorily restored by free neuromuscular transfer.

When the proximal facial nerve is available, it provides the best source of motor nerve for the transferred muscle. However, with many long-standing facial nerve palsies, the ipsilateral nerve is not available. A two-stage procedure is thus necessary to reconstruct the normal smile. First, a cross facial nerve graft is placed to tap the impulses that cause the desired motion on the normal contralateral side. After allowing 8 to 12 months for the axons to regenerate along the graft and reach the other side, a second procedure involves the microvascular transfer of a segment of muscle with a microneurorrhaphy of its motor nerve to the nerve graft. The muscle is secured such that its excursion and its direction of pull match the range of motion of the contralateral corner of the mouth during a normal smile [31]. Good results, with close to normal symmetric smiles, have been reported following the microneurovascular transfer of a trimmed segment of gracilis muscle [46].

*Trunk*

Most major defects of the trunk are secondary to surgical ablation for tumor, irradiation, or infectious necrosis. They can usually be covered by local pedicled latissimus dorsi, pectoralis major, serratus anterior, or rectus abdominis muscle or by musculocutaneous flaps for the chest wall. The external or internal oblique, rectus abdominis, rectus femoris, or tensor fascia lata are available for the abdominal wall. Pedicled omentum can also resurface large, distant areas and is particularly useful for postradiation necrosis.

Many recipient vessels are available in the trunk. For the chest wall the subscapular artery and its major branches, the circumflex scapular and the thoracodorsal, are the recipients of choice when available. In cases of postmastectomy irradiation, the transverse cervical vessels are generally uninjured and available. Alternatively, the internal mammary vessels may be dissected from the resected bed of a costal cartilage. For the rarer abdominal recipients, the inferior epigastric is readily dissected from the groin area. Vein grafts to the axillae and groins can always be considered, as well.

CHEST WALL COVERAGE. When the chest wall defect is too large for local pedicle flaps or when surgery or irradiation has made them unavailable, microsurgical transfers are indicated. Even in the presence of available pedicle flaps, large full-thickness chest wall defects may be best treated with the microvascular transfer of a distant composite flap that includes fascia or bone to prevent flailing without resorting to prosthetic implants.

BREAST RECONSTRUCTION. With improvements in the technique and the survival rate, breast reconstruction with free tissue transfers offers many advantages over the pedicled autologous tissue reconstruction [33]. When compared with the pedicled transverse rectus abdominis musculocutaneous flap (TRAM), the free TRAM flap based on the inferior epigastric vessels has consistently better skin perfusion. The lower abdominal skin, being primarily supplied by the inferior epigastric vessels, allows a larger skin flap with less incidence of fat necrosis [6, 85]. Furthermore, because the amount of rectus muscle dissection is limited, the resultant abdominal wall morbidity is minimized. The superior gluteus musculocutaneous free flap also has minimal donor morbidity and is a favored method of reconstruction when the lower abdominal skin is not suitable [69].

PENILE RECONSTRUCTION. The Chinese method of tubed radial forearm free flap is an elegant method for one-stage penile reconstruction [12]. The inner part of the tube provides a urethral conduit and the outer part a cutaneous cover that can be made sensate by connecting the forearm cutaneous nerve to the pudendal nerve stump. The middle segment is deepithelialized and rolled inside. A rib graft or prosthetic implant can be inserted for rigidity.

### Upper Extremity

Free tissue transfers have expanded the reconstructive options for many previously difficult upper extremity problems. Immediate soft tissue coverage has been made more practical, and total early reconstruction with early return of function is now the norm for complex hand injuries. Furthermore, a unique potential to replace lost structures, such as digits, joints, and motor units, has been made possible.

Vascular anastomoses are more reliable in the upper extremity than in the lower. Both ulnar and radial arteries are available within the forearm. On the dorsum of the hand, the radial artery is easily accessible in the first web space. The numerous superficial veins, if not damaged by intravenous medication, are adequate for venous drainage. In contrast to those of the lower extremity, they are less prone to spasm.

UPPER EXTREMITY COVERAGE. Compared to the two-stage abdominal flap procedures, single-stage coverage of upper extremity cutaneous defects with free flaps has the advantage of avoiding prolonged awkward immobilization and allows postoperative hand elevation and early digit mobilization. These features set the stage for better functional recovery.

A skin-only transfer provides a flap with excellent appearance, durability, and the potential for sensibility. The lateral arm flap [77] combines the above advantages. However, flap width is limited to 6 to 7 cm if primary closure of the donor area is to be obtained. Larger cutaneous flaps, such as the scapular flap [20], may be used but have the disadvantage of not being sensate and of being bulky. The temporalis fascia flap with a skin graft provides thin, pliable coverage and appears to have a favored place in hand reconstruction. Muscle flaps conform well to the complex wound topography and have the advantage of a richer blood supply. However, they are usually bulkier, and the aesthetic result is often poorer than with the skin flaps.

DIGITAL REPLACEMENT AND RECONSTRUCTION. Toe to hand transfer is a useful technique for replacing missing thumbs or fingers. It provides a significant cosmetic and functional improvement to the hand that is missing a thumb [44]. For the severely mutilated hand with multiple finger loss, it is a unique way to restore hand function. Partial toe transfers provide the vascularized spare parts needed to improve the function and cosmetic appearance of mutilated digits.

FUNCTIONING MUSCLE TRANSPLANTATION. After Volkmann's ischemic contracture of the forearm, the local muscles are no longer available for transfer. Free microneurovascular muscle transfer has become an effective way of restoring function to such upper extremities.

Most commonly, digital flexion for grasp can be restored. The candidate for such a transfer must have supple joints, good sensibility, and some intrinsic function. Finger and wrist extension must be present. A gracilis muscle transfer could provide a functional grip strength and a full range of flexion, and it would allow full extension [47].

### Lower Extremity

The ability to transfer a large amount of well vascularized tissue to the massively injured extremity has radically changed our management of lower extremity trauma. No longer are patients with severe open tibial fractures being hospitalized for many months for repeated debridement, dressing changes, or skin grafts [67]. All massively injured lower extremities, regardless of their extent, can now be managed by an early generous debridement that converts them to "healthy" wounds, and the resultant large wounds can then be promptly closed by free tissue transfers. This "early definitive reconstruction" allows primary healing of the tissues and markedly decreases the infection rate and the recovery period [25, 32, 36, 97].

Because large bony and soft tissue defects can be reconstructed with vascularized tissue, many severely damaged extremities, previously doomed to amputation, can now be salvaged [36]. The decision to proceed with salvage must be made cautiously to avoid subjecting the patient to a long series of procedures that end with disappointment. However, if the major neurovascular structures are intact, the foot is sensate, and the major joints are functional, salvage is generally worthwhile and must be considered. Alternatively, the distal lower extremity might be used as a source of vascularized tissue to cover the amputation stump, converting to a below-the-knee amputation what would have otherwise been an above-the-knee amputation [74].

For free tissue transfers to the lower leg, either the anterior tibial or the posterior tibial vascular bundles are available for anastomosis. If feasible, the anastomoses can be conveniently done near the ankle where the vessels are easily accessible [73]. Anastomoses done to the more deeply located proximal vessels require a difficult dissection that could cause swelling of the leg musculature between which the pedicle must pass. Compression and venous obstruction to the pedicle must be avoided by using a larger flap that allows a tensionless closure.

In subacute or chronic wounds, there is a surrounding zone of tissue that has undergone an inflammatory response. Anastomoses within this "zone of injury" are hazardous and prone to thrombosis. If the flap pedicle cannot reach beyond the zone of injury, vein grafts are used to tap into more-distant, intact vessels.

End-to-end and end-to-side anastomoses have similar patency rates. The former is technically easier, and the latter is preferred when performed on a lower extremity with only one functioning artery [24].

LOWER EXTREMITY COVERAGE. Attempts to cover a traumatized lower extremity with a local muscle not infrequently result in flap failure because the muscle itself has been injured by the original trauma [58]. Furthermore, it is advantageous to add a healthy muscle from a distant site rather than to sacrifice additional viable muscle left in the traumatized extremity. As the success rate of free flaps has improved to above 95 percent, their indication has changed from a last resource reconstructive option to one that achieves the best reconstruction possible [2].

A soft tissue defect of the lower leg may be covered with many types of free tissue transfer. Skin flaps generally provide the most acceptable surface, color, and consistency. Muscles are preferred when there is a need to fit irregular shapes and cavities and occlude any potential dead space. A skin graft over a well-contoured muscle provides a durable cover for defects of the heel and sole of the foot [51]. There is also less of a chance of infection developing when muscle is used to cover a contaminated bed.

BONE RECONSTRUCTION. Vascularized bone grafts to the lower extremity are indicated when the bony defect after satisfactory débridement is more than 6 to 8 cm in length [79]. Nonvascularized bone grafts have not done well when placed in a scarred, traumatized, contaminated bed. The basic bone flaps—fibula and iliac crest (deep circumflex iliac artery)—can reconstruct most bony defects. Congenital pseudarthrosis of the tibia is now successfully treated with a vascularized fibular transfer [63].

OSTEOMYELITIS. Extensive débridement of the infected bone back to healthy margins seems to produce a significant cure rate in patients with chronic osteomyelitis [50, 94]. This approach is possible only if free muscle flaps are available to cover the large defects thus created.

PERIPHERAL VASCULAR DISEASE ULCERS. Local flaps are notoriously unreliable in the lower extremities with peripheral vascular disease ulcers. After revascularization, foot ulcers overlying bone are best treated with free flaps. By bringing in a new circulation to the ischemic tissues, over and above that afforded by the vascular bypass surgery, free flaps promote wound healing and improve the salvage rate [8, 16].

## Conclusions and Future Directions

Free flap surgery is a complex operation that requires a high level of technical expertise and preoperative preparation. Initially considered by many a radical procedure of last resort, today, in the hands of the experienced microvascular surgeons who can execute it with a low complication rate, its position has shifted to that of being a routine and first choice reconstructive procedure.

Although the major role of free flaps remains coverage of the difficult wound, in the future we are likely to see free flap surgery being performed with increasing complexity and refinement. Prefabricated or recombinant flaps, constructed by adding tissue in situ to a preexisting flap, may further expand our reconstructive limits by allowing restoration of missing functions or body parts with "vascularized spare parts."

## References

1. Bakamjian, V. Y. Total reconstruction of the pharynx with a medially based deltopectoral skin flap. *N.Y. J. Med.* 68:2771, 1968.
2. Banis, J. C., and Acland, R. D. Managing the outer limits of reconstruction with microvascular free tissue transfer. *Arch. Surg.* 119:673, 1984.

3. Baudet, J. Reconstruction of the pharyngeal wall by free transfer of the greater omentum and stomach. *Int. J. Microsurg.* 1:53, 1979.

4. Baudet, J., Panconi, P., Cox, M., et al. The composite fibula and soleus free transfer. *Int. J. Microsurg.* 4:10, 1982.

5. Berggren, A., Weiland, A., and Dorfman, H. Free vascularized bone grafts: Factors affecting their survival and ability to heal recipient bone defects. *Plast. Reconstr. Surg.* 69:219, 1982.

6. Boyd, J. B., Taylor, G. I., and Corlett, R. The vascular territories of the superior epigastric and deep inferior epigastric systems. *Plast. Reconstr. Surg.* 73:1, 1984.

7. Brent, B., Upton, J., Acland, R. D., et al. Experience with the temporoparietal fascial free flap. *Plast. Reconstr. Surg.* 76:177, 1985.

8. Briggs, S. E., Banis, J. C., Kaebnick, H., et al. Distal revascularization and microvascular free tissue transfer: An alternative to amputation in ischemic lesions of the lower extremity. *J. Vasc. Surg.* 2:806, 1985.

9. Buncke, H. J., Jr., Buncke, C. M., and Schultz, W. P. Immediate Nicoladoni procedure in the rhesus monkey or hallux-to-hand transplantation utilizing micro-miniature vascular anastomoses. *Br. J. Plast. Surg.* 19:332, 1966.

10. Calderon, W., Chang, N., and Mathes, S. J. Comparison of the effect of bacterial inoculation in musculocutaneous and fasciocutaneous flaps. *Plast. Reconstr. Surg.* 77:785, 1986.

11. Chang, N., and Mathes, S. J. Comparison of the effect of bacterial inoculation in musculocutaneous and random-pattern flaps. *Plast. Reconstr. Surg.* 70:1, 1982.

12. Chang, T. S., and Hwang, W. Y. Forearm flap in one-stage reconstruction of the penis. *Plast. Reconstr. Surg.* 74:251, 1984.

13. Chen, C. W., Ch'ien, Y. C., and Pao, Y. S. Salvage of the forearm following complete traumatic amputation: Report of a successful case. *Chin. Med. J.* 82:633, 1963.

14. Chicarilli, Z. N., and Davey, L. M. Rectus abdominis myocutaneous free flap reconstruction following a cranio-orbital-maxillary resection for neurofibrosarcoma. 80:726, 1987.

15. Cobbett, J. R. Free digital transfer: Report of a case of transfer of a great toe to replace an amputated thumb. *J. Bone Joint Surg.* [*Br.*] 51:677, 1969.

16. Colen, L. B. Limb salvage in the patient with severe peripheral vascular disease: The role of microsurgical free tissue transfer. *Plast. Reconstr. Surg.* 79:389, 1987.

17. Colen, S. R., Shaw, W. W., and McCarthy, J. G. Review of the morbidity of 300 free flap donor sites. *Plast. Reconstr. Surg.* 76:948, 1986.

18. Daniel, R. K., and Taylor, G. I. Distant transfer of an island flap by microvascular anastomoses. *Plast. Reconstr. Surg.* 52:111, 1973.

19. DeCherney, A., and Naftolin, F. Homotransplantation of the human fallopian tube: Report of a successful case and description of a technique. *Fertil. Steril.* 34:14, 1980.

20. Dos Santos, L. F. The vascular anatomy and dissection of the free scapular flap. *Plast. Reconstr. Surg.* 73:59, 1984.

21. Duncan, M. J., Manktelow, R. T., Zuker, R. M., et al. Mandibular reconstruction in the radiated patient: The role of osteocutaneous free tissue transfer. *Plast. Reconstr. Surg.* 76:829, 1985.

22. Gilbert, A. Vascularized transfer of fibular shaft. *Int. J. Microsurg.* 1:100, 1979.

23. Gilbert, A. Toe transfers for congenital hand defects. *J. Hand Surg.* 7:118, 1982.

24. Godina, M. Preferential use of end to side arterial anastomoses in free flap transfers. *Plast. Reconstr. Surg.* 64:673, 1979.

25. Godina, M. Early microsurgical reconstruction of complex trauma of the extremities. *Plast. Reconstr. Surg.* 78:285, 1986.

26. Goldwyn, R. M., Lamb, D. C., and White, W. L. Experimental study of large island flaps in dogs. *Plast. Reconstr. Surg.* 31:528, 1963.

27. Gordon, L., Buncke, H. J., and Alpert, B. S. Free latissimus dorsi muscle flap with split thickness skin graft cover: A report of 16 cases. *Plast. Reconstr. Surg.* 70:173, 1982.

28. Greenberg, B. M., Masem, M., and May, J. W., Jr. Therapeutic value of intravenous heparin in microvascular surgery: An experimental vascular thrombosis study. *Plast. Reconstr. Surg.* 82:463, 1988.

29. Hallock, G. G. Defatting of flaps by means of suction-assisted lipectomy. *Plast. Reconstr. Surg.* 76:948, 1985.

30. Harii, K., Ohmori, K., and Ohmori, S. Successful clinical transfer of ten free flaps by microvascular anastomoses. *Plast. Reconstr. Surg.* 53:259, 1974.

31. Harii, K., Ohmori, K., and Tori, S. Free gracilis

muscle transplantation with microneurovascular anastomosis for the treatment of facial paralysis. *Plast. Reconstr. Surg.* 57:133, 1976.

32. Harris, G. D., Nagle, D. J., Lewis, V. L., et al. Accelerating recovery after trauma with free flaps. *J. Trauma* 27:849, 1987.

33. Hartrampf, C. R., Scheflan, M., and Black, P. W. Breast reconstruction with a transverse abdominal island flap. *Plast. Reconstr. Surg.* 69:216, 1982.

34. Hidalgo, D. A., and Shaw, W. W. Technical Considerations in Free Tissue Transfer. In W. W. Shaw and D. A. Hidalgo (eds.), *Microsurgery in Trauma.* Mount Kisco, NY: Futura, 1987. Pp. 221–236.

35. Jacobson, J. H., and Suarez, E. L. Microsurgery in the anastomosis of small vessels. *Surg. Forum* 11:243, 1960.

36. Khouri, R. K., and Shaw, W. W. Reconstruction of the lower extremity with microvascular free flaps: A 10 year experience with 304 consecutive cases. *J. Trauma,* 1989.

37. Khouri, R. K., Cooley, B., Kenna, D. M., et al. Thrombosis of microvascular anastomoses in traumatized vessels: Fibrin versus platelets. *Proc. Am. Soc. Reconstr. Microsurg.* 3:102, 1987.

38. Khouri, R. K., Ong, F. D., and Shaw, W. W. Is it helpful to monitor free tissue transfers with surface temperature recordings? *Proc. North Eastern Soc. Plast. Surg.* 5:42, 1988.

39. Khouri, R. K., Tark, K. C., and Shaw, W. W. Prefabrication of flaps using an arteriovenous bundle and angiogenesis factors. *Surg. Forum* 39:597, 1988.

40. Kleinert, H. E., and Kasdan, M. L. Anastomosis of digital vessels. *J. Ky. Med. Assoc.* 63:106, 1965.

41. Komatsu, S., and Tamai, S. Successful replantation of a completely cut off thumb. *Plast. Reconstr. Surg.* 42:374, 1968.

42. Krizek, T. J., Tani, T., DesPrez, J. D., and Kiehn, C. L. Experimental transplantation of composite grafts by microsurgical anastomoses. *Plast. Reconstr. Surg.* 36:538, 1965.

43. Lister, G. Microsurgical transfer of the second toe for congenital deficiency of the thumb. *Plast. Reconstr. Surg.* 82:658, 1988.

44. Lister, G. D., Kalisman, M., and Tsai, T. M. Reconstruction of the hand with free microneurovascular toe to hand transfer: Experience with 54 toe transfers. *Plast. Reconstr. Surg.* 71:372, 1983.

45. Malt, R. A., and McKhann, C. Replantation of severed arms. *J. Am. Med. Assoc.* 189:716, 1964.

46. Manktelow, R. T. Facial Paralysis Reconstruction. In R. T. Manktelow (ed.), *Microvascular Reconstruction.* Berlin: Springer-Verlag, 1986. Pp. 128–144.

47. Manktelow, R. T. Functioning Muscle Transplantation. In R. T. Manktelow (ed.), *Microvascular Reconstruction.* Berlin: Springer-Verlag, 1986. Pp. 151–164.

48. Manktelow, R. T., Zuker, R. M., and McKee, N. H. Functioning free muscle transplantation. *J. Hand Surg.* 9A:32, 1984.

49. Mathes, S. J., and Nahai, F. Classification of the vascular anatomy of muscles: Experimental and clinical correlation. *Plast. Reconstr. Surg.* 67:177, 1981.

50. May, J. W., Jr., Gallico, G., III, and Lukash, F. N. Microvascular transfer of free tissue for closure of bone wounds of the distal lower extremity. *N. Engl. J. Med.* 306:253, 1982.

51. May, J. W., Jr., Hall, M. J., and Simon, S. R. Free microvascular muscle flaps with skin graft reconstruction of extensive defects of the foot: a clinical and gait analysis study. *Plast. Reconstr. Surg.* 75:627, 1985.

52. McCraw, J. B., Dibbell, D. J., and Carraway, J. H. Clinical definition of independent myocutaneous vascular territories. *Plast. Reconstr. Surg.* 60:341, 1977.

53. McGregor, I. A., and Morgan, G. Axial and random pattern flaps. *Br. J. Plast. Surg.* 26:202–213, 1973.

54. McLean, D. H., Buncke, H. J., Jr. Autotransplant of omentum to a large scalp defect with microsurgical revascularization. *Plast. Reconstr. Surg.* 49:268, 1972.

55. McMahon, R. A., O'Brien, B. McB., Aberdeen, J., et al. Results of the use of autotransplantation of the intraabdominal testis using microsurgical vascular anastomosis. *J. Pediatr. Surg.* 15:92, 1980.

56. Morrison, W. A., O'Brien, B. McB., and MacLeod, A. M. Thumb reconstruction with a free neurovascular wrap around flap from the big toe. *J. Hand Surg.* 5:575, 1980.

57. Mustoe, T. A., and Upton, J. Head and neck free flaps: Are they safe in the irradiated or pediatric patient? *Head Neck Surg.* 1(suppl.):S3, 1988.

58. Neale, H. W., Peter, J. S., Kreilein, F. G., et al. Complications of muscle flap transposition

for traumatic defects of the leg. *Plast. Reconstr. Surg.* 72:512, 1983.

59. Nozaki, M., Huang, T. T., Hayashi, M., et al. Reconstruction of the pharyngoesophagus following pharyngoesophagectomy and irradiation therapy. *Plast. Reconstr. Surg.* 76:386, 1985.

60. O'Brien, B. McB., and Morrison, W. A. Free Flaps. In B. McB. O'Brien and W. A. Morrison (eds.), *Reconstructive Microsurgery*. London: Churchill Livingstone, 1987. Pp. 235–324.

61. O'Brien, B. McB., MacLeod, A. M., Hayhurst, J. W., et al. Successful transfer of a large island flap from the groin to the foot by microvascular anastomoses. *Plast. Reconstr. Surg.* 52:271, 1973.

62. Pennington, D. G., Lai, M. F., and Pelly, A. D. The rectus abdominis myocutaneous free flap. *Br. J. Plast. Surg.* 33:277, 1980.

63. Pho, R. W. H., Levack, B., Satku, K., et al. Free vascularized fibular graft in the treatment of congenital pseudarthrosis of the tibia. *J. Bone Joint Surg. [Br.]* 67:64, 1985.

64. Richards, R. R., Orsini, E. C., Mahoney, J. L., et al. The influence of muscle flap coverage of the repair of devascularized tibial cortex: An experimental investigation in the dog. *Plast. Reconstr. Surg.* 79:946, 1987.

65. Robinson, D. W., and MacLeod, A. Microvascular free jejunum transfer. *Br. J. Plast. Surg.* 35:258, 1982.

66. Russell, R. C., Graham, D. R., Feller, A. M., et al. Experimental evaluation of the antibiotic carrying capacity of a muscle flap into a fibrotic cavity. *Plast. Reconstr. Surg.* 81:162, 1988.

67. Serafin, D., Georgiade, N. G., and Smith, D. H. Comparison of free flaps with pedicled flaps for coverage of defects of the leg or foot. *Plast. Reconstr. Surg.* 59:492, 1977.

68. Shaw, W. W. Microvascular free flaps: The first decade. *Clin. Plast. Surg.* 10:1, 1983.

69. Shaw, W. W. Microvascular free flap breast reconstruction. *Clin. Plast. Surg.* 11:333, 1984.

70. Shaw, W. W. Microvascular Free Flaps: Survival, Donor Sites, and Application. In H. Buncke and D. Furnas (eds.), *Symposium on Clinical Frontiers in Reconstructive Microsurgery*. St. Louis: Mosby, 1984. Pp. 3–10.

71. Shaw, W. W. Discussion of direct monitoring of microvascular anastomosis with the 20-MHz ultrasonic Doppler probe: an experimental and clinical study. *Plast. Reconstr. Surg.* 81:159, 1988.

72. Shaw, W. W. General Concepts of Free Tissue Transfer in Trauma. In W. W. Shaw and D. A. Hidalgo (eds.), *Microsurgery in Trauma*. Mount Kisco, NY: Futura, 1987. Pp. 211–220.

73. Shaw, W. W., Baker, D. C., and Converse, J. M. Conservation of major leg arteries when use recipient supply for free flap. *Plast. Reconstr. Surg.* 63:317, 1979.

74. Shenaq, S. M., Krouskop, P. E., Stal, S., et al. Salvage of amputation stumps by secondary reconstruction utilizing microsurgical free tissue transfer. *Plast. Reconstr. Surg.* 79:861, 1987.

75. Silber, S. J., and Kelly, J. Successful autotransplantation of an intraabdominal testes to the scrotum by microvascular technique. *J. Urol.* 115:452, 1976.

76. Song, R., and Gao, Y. The forearm flap. *Clin. Plast. Surg.* 9:21, 1982.

77. Song, R., Song, Y., Yu, Y., et al. The upper arm free flap. *Clin. Plast. Surg.* 9:27, 1982.

78. Soutar, D. S., and McGregor, I. A. The radial forearm flap in intraoral reconstruction: The experience of 60 consecutive cases. *Plast. Reconstr. Surg.* 78:1, 1986.

79. Sowa, D. T., and Weiland, A. J. Clinical applications of vascularized bone autografts. *Orthop. Clin. North Am.* 18:257, 1987.

80. Swartz, W. M., Banis, J. C., Newton, D. E., et al. The osteocutaneous scapular free flap for mandibular and maxillary reconstruction. *Plast. Reconstr. Surg.* 77:530, 1986.

81. Swartz, W. M., Jones, N. F., Cherup, L., et al. Direct monitoring of microvascular anastomosis with the 20-MHz ultrasonic Doppler probe: An experimental and clinical study. *Plast. Reconstr. Surg.* 81:149, 1988.

82. Taylor, G. I. The current status of free vascularized bone grafts. *Clin. Plast. Surg.* 10:185, 1983.

83. Taylor, G. I., and Ham, F. G. The free vascularized nerve graft. *Plast. Reconstr. Surg.* 57:413, 1976.

84. Taylor, G. I., and Palmer, J. H. The vascular territories (angiosomes of the body): Experimental study and clinical applications. *Br. J. Plast. Surg.* 40:113, 1987.

85. Taylor, G. I., Corlett, R. J., and Boyd, J. B. The versatile deep inferior epigastric (inferior rectus abdominis) flap. *Br. J. Plast. Surg.* 37:330, 1984.

86. Thoma, A., Heddle, S., Archibald, S., et al. The free vascularized anterior rib graft. *Plast. Reconstr. Surg.* 82:291, 1988.

87. Tobin, G., Schusterman, M., Peterson, G., et al. The intramuscular neurovascular anatomy of the latissimus dorsi muscle: The basis for splitting the flap. *Plast. Reconstr. Surg.* 67:637, 1981.

88. Tweed, A. E. J., Manktelow, R. T., and Zuker, R. M. Facial contour reconstruction with free flaps. *Ann. Plast. Surg.* 12:313, 1984.

89. Upton, J., and Mutimer, K. A modification of the great-toe transfer for thumb reconstruction. *Plast. Reconstr. Surg.* 82:535, 1988.

90. Vila-Rovira, R., Ferreira, B. J., and Guinot, A. Transfer of vascularized extensor tendons from the foot to the hand with a dorsalis pedis flap. *Plast. Reconstr. Surg.* 76:421, 1985.

91. Wang, W. Keys to successful second toe to hand transfer: A review of 30 cases. *J. Hand Surg.* 8:902, 1983.

92. Wei, F. C., Chen, H. C., Chuang, C. C., et al. Fibular osteoseptocutaneous flap: Anatomic study and clinical applications. *Plast. Reconstr. Surg.* 78:191, 1986.

93. Wei, F. C., Chen, H. C., Chuang, C. C., et al. Simultaneous multiple toe transfers in hand reconstruction. *Plast. Reconstr. Surg.* 81:366, 1988.

94. Weiland, A. J., Moore, J. R., and Daniel, R. K. The efficacy of free tissue transfer in the treatment of osteomyelitis. *J. Bone Joint Surg.* [*Am.*] 66:181, 1984.

95. Wood, C., Downing, B., McKenzie, I., et al. Microvascular transplantation of the human fallopian tube. *Fertil. Steril.* 29:607, 1978.

96. Yang, D. Y. Quoted by F. McDowell: Editorial addendum. *Plast. Reconstr. Surg.* 52:116, 1973.

97. Yaremchuck, M. J., Brumback, R. J., Manson, P. N., et al. Acute and definitive management of traumatic osteocutaneous defects of the lower extremity. *Plast. Reconstr. Surg.* 80:1, 1987.

98. Zhu, J. D., Huang, C. D., Yu, G. Z., et al. Homotransplantation of ovary by microvascular anastomoses. *Microsurgery* 3:200, 1980.

99. Zuker, R. M., and Manktelow, R. T. The dorsalis pedis free flap: Technique of elevation, foot closure, and flap application. *Plast. Reconstr. Surg.* 77:93, 1986.

# 43

*Hanno Millesi*

# Microsurgical Repair of Peripheral Nerves

With the use of fine suture material and proper instruments, the surgery of peripheral nerves has become increasingly less traumatic. For many years magnification was obtained by the use of loupes. Microscopes for operative use have been available since 1963 [67]. The extent of damage to the nerve tissue can obviously be better recognized by magnification; for secondary repairs, for example, when dissecting the neuroma it is easier to achieve a sufficient resection if the surgeon has a better view. The magnifying power of the microscope allows one to proceed with a dissection into tissue layers that can be handled otherwise only with much difficulty. The main advantage is that it is an atraumatic surgical technique that results not only from the magnification but even more from the development of improved instruments. The stable position of the microscope and the excellent illumination, along with the possibility of increasing the magnification, are significant advantages over the use of simple loupes, even if the magnifying power applied during the major part of the operation does not differ greatly.

In addition to the technical refinement of surgery by delicate instruments, microsurgery has changed the surgical approach to peripheral nerve lesions. It has progressed from a rather mechanical procedure with the nerve trunk as the basic unit to a more biologic one with a large fascicle or fascicle group, respectively, as the basic unit.

## Equipment

Rather simple equipment is needed for microsurgery on peripheral nerves. One must have a good microscope that provides magnifications of $4\times$ to $25\times$. It is an added advantage if the microscope provides motorized focusing. A diploscope is not necessary because the assistant can carry out his or her duties without magnification. A set of fine-pointed watchmaker's forceps, a fine forceps with teeth, a needle holder, and scissors that are opened by a spring are all one needs.

There are two ways to transect a nerve, and the methods used involve different equipment. If one end of the nerve is fixed and the nerve can be easily pulled and brought under tension, a sharp knife can be used. A set of forceps to grasp the nerve to be transected and hold it atraumatically permits transection by a special knife along a rim in the nerve holder of the forceps [43]. If the nerve cannot be liberated sufficiently to apply the holding forceps and if it cannot be put under tension without doing harm, the alternative to transecting it or resecting a segment from a stump is to use sharp scissors, having undulated blades. Use of these scissors avoids shifting the nerve tissue, which leads to crushing the tissue. Logically, the transection is performed fascicle by fascicle; it is not done by transecting more tissue at one bite. This technique has proved useful if one has to shorten individual fascicles before attempting coaptation and to shorten nerve grafts that were previously placed in the defect. With the undulated scissors these manipulations can be performed without any pull. In addition, the procedure can be performed layer by layer, starting with the paraneurium and then proceeding through the epineurium and the perineurium of the individual fascicles. After each cut, the related layer is shifted away from the cross section to avoid covering the cross section, e.g., the cutaneous nerve graft, by connective tissue.

For stitches, 10-0 nylon sutures have proved useful. Hemostasis can easily be achieved by bipolar coagulation.

The application of fibrin glues to maintain the coaptation of two nerve stumps was recommended as early as 1972 [38, 39]. It was later reported that in a relatively high percentage of these cases rupture occurred because of increased fibrinolytic activity [27, 28]. The simultaneous application of antifibrinolytic substances were reported either to solve [10] or not solve [28] the problem. In recent years fibrin glues have become available that contain an antifibrinolytic agent, and for this reason gluing of nerves has become more popular. Experts in this field [29, 30] recommend application of the fibrin glue only in cases in which nerve grafting is without tension. The best results have been achieved if, in addition to the glue, some stitches have been applied.

For routine coaptation between a graft and a certain area of a nerve stump, a particular fascicle group, or a particular large fascicle, one or two stitches are used to achieve proper alignment and avoid malrotation. Normal fibrin clotting provides sufficient tensile strength to maintain the coaptation if no shearing forces and no longitudinal stress are acting. An additional application of fibrin glue increases tensile strength, but it is questionable if this practice provides any advantage, as the tension in the longitudinal direction should be zero anyway. To maintain the coaptation after a neurorrhaphy under minimal tension, the fibrin glue is not sufficient [30]. According to experimental data, the results of nerve repair using fibrin glue does not provide superior results [44]. The suggestion to glue individual cutaneous nerve grafts together for easier handling [55] is to go a step back because the advantage of modern nerve grafting by individual skin nerve segments—to be able to unite well-defined points of one cross section with well-defined points of another—is lost. It is therefore questionable if fibrin glue will become a standard technique for peripheral nerve repair, even though it may offer advantages under certain conditions.

## General Considerations of the Surgical Technique

A wide exposure facilitates the whole operation. For secondary repairs the nerve to be repaired is exposed in the same tissue proximal and distal to the site of the lesion. The dissection then proceeds from the scar tissue toward the lesion. If it is known from the preliminary operation that the nerve is not only completely transected but has suffered a long defect, exposure of the whole field can be avoided. Under these conditions it is sufficient to expose the proximal and distal stump and to create a tunnel. Continuity of the nerve is reestablished by putting nerve grafts across the tunnel and performing the proximal and distal coaptation at the separate incisions. In the forearm and hand, the operation is usually performed under tourniquet in a bloodless field. The tourniquet is kept until the exposure is complete and the nerve stumps are prepared. The tourniquet is then released and complete hemostasis is performed using bipolar coagulation. If a nerve graft is needed, the time allotted for hemostasis can be used to obtain the donor graft.

Wound closure is carried out in the usual way. It is imperative to avoid shearing forces that might dislocate the repaired nerves when the skin edges are united. After the operation careful immobilization is essential. In the case of an end-to-end nerve repair, the adjacent joints are immobilized in flexed position for 3 to 4 weeks, after which gradual mobilization is encouraged. If a graft was used and longitudinal tension avoided completely, immobilization is maintained in the exact position of the limb during the operation; this immobilization is continued for 10 days, after which free motion is allowed.

## ANATOMY OF A PERIPHERAL NERVE TRUNK

The macroscopic unit of a peripheral nerve is the fascicle, which consists of the tube-like perineurium and the endoneurium within the tube. The endoneurium is formed by a connective tissue framework consisting of collagen fibrils of small diameter (40 to 65 nm) [15] and nerve fibers. In the endoneurium there are Schwann cells and endoneurial fibroblasts in a ratio of 9:1 [56]. The perineurium, which forms a barrier against the tissue outside the fascicle and maintains a high tissue pressure, consists of an inner layer of mesothelial-like cells that are responsible for the membrane function. A middle layer consists of flat perineurial cells with long cell appendages and a basal membrane. Between these cells are collagen fibrils with the same diameter as in the endoneurium (40 to 65 nm). The more external layer comprises collagen connective tissue with thicker collagen fibrils, similar to the ones in the epineurium. It is a matter of definition whether this tissue is a part of the perineurium or belongs to the epineurium. It occurs in different thicknesses in different parts of the body.

Usually several fascicles are kept together by a rather loose connective tissue, the epineurium, which contains the vessels of the nerve and which surrounds the whole nerve trunk in several layers. It seems, therefore, to be necessary to distinguish between an interfascicular epineurium, which expands between the fascicles, and an epifascicular epineurium, which surrounds the whole nerve. The epineurium consists of collagen fibers with fibrils having a diameter between 60 and 110 nm [15]; consequently, the fibroblasts of the epineurium must be regarded as different from the fibroblasts of the perineurium or the endoneurium. It seems that the fibroblasts of the epineurium are less differentiated than fibroblasts of any connective tissue, in contrast to the perineurial and endoneurial fibroblasts, which are more differentiated for nerve tissue.

The epifascicular epineurium is surrounded by layers of a loose connective tissue that provides a connection with the surrounding tissue. This tissue is comparable to the adventitia of vessels. It provides the ability of the nerve to move in longitudinal direction and to adapt to the motion of the whole limb. A local increase of longitudinal tension can be distributed over the whole length of the nerve, keeping the actual tension of each segment low. This tissue was retained as part of the epineurium [80] or specifically termed conjunctiva nervorum [32] or paraneurium.

The blood supply is provided by segmental vessels that occur in different sizes and numbers at different locations. Briedenbach and Terzis [5] distinguished different types of blood supply, according to the amount of nerve tissue that is dependent on individual vascular pedicles. Knowledge of this difference is important if vascularized nerve grafts are used. Whether a mesoneurium [68, 69] exists that fixes the nerve in its bed and contains the supplying vessels is still a matter of discussion [33]. Probably it is a special manifestation of the paraneurial tissue.

For a nerve trunk it is important that the individual fascicles can move against each other to accommodate to different limb situations and joint positions. This movement is provided by the interfascicular epineurium. If this tissue becomes fibrotic, the ability to move is lost. It is possible that with fibrosis of this tissue the fascicles are fixed in a meander-like shape. Both situations create increased sensibility of the content of the fascicles to longitudinal stress.

The fascicular pattern of a peripheral nerve trunk changes along its course. Studying the number and size of fascicles along a peripheral nerve reveals a striking, rapid change, and only a few millimeters of the nerve consist of the same number of fascicles [76, 79]. Basically we can distinguish three fascicular patterns.

1. *Monofascicular pattern:* The nerve trunk consists of one fascicle only. There is no interfascicular epineurium.
2. *Oligofascicular nerve segment:* A limited number of large fascicles are present.
3. *Polyfascicular nerve segment:* The nerve trunk consists of many fascicles.

For clinical praxis differentiation into five types is more suitable.

1. *Monofascicular nerve segment.*
2. *Oligofascicular nerve segment with two to four fascicles.* Types I and II have in common that there is no or minimal interfascicular epineurium between the fascicles, and optimal coaptation of the fascicles can be achieved by trunk-to-trunk coaptation. In the case of the monofascicular nerve segment, fascicle-to-fascicle and trunk-to-trunk coaptation are the same.
3. *Oligofascicular nerve segment with five to ten fascicles.* In this case there is more interfascicular epineurium between the fascicles, and coaptation of the fascicles in the center of the nerve trunk cannot be controlled by external manipulation. In this case it is much better to separate the fascicles by interfascicular dissection and coapt them individually. The conditions for successful fascicular coaptation are a limited number of fascicles of a certain size, allowing easy surgical manipulation. Five to ten, of course, constitute a compromise; a nerve segment consisting of 12 or 13 fascicles may be handled in a similar way. The second condition is a certain size. Therefore a small nerve branch consisting of five or six fascicles of small diameter must not be treated in the same way because the limited size of the fascicles makes surgical manipulation difficult. These small branches with a limited number of small fascicles are treated as fascicle groups rather than as an oligofascicular nerve segment of type III.

4. *Polyfascicular nerve segment without group arrangement.* In this case the nerve trunk consists of many fascicles of different size; for instance, there might be some large but many small fascicles. The fascicles are equally distributed over the cross section. There is much interfascicular tissue between the nerve trunks (up to 60 percent of the whole cross section). The high number and small size are the reasons why separation of the fascicles by interfascicular dissection is cumbersome, causes surgical trauma, and presents the surgeon with the possibility that the number of fascicles does not correspond. For this reason fascicular repair, as suggested by Tupper [82], is not recommended.

5. *Polyfascicular segment with group arrangement.* Such a nerve segment contains more than ten fascicles of different size. These fascicles are arranged in groups by a different distribution of the interfascicular epineurium. This arrangement is preexistent and the surgeon can detect it by interfascicular dissection, following the vessels that run between these fascicle groups. This pattern is seen frequently in the distal portions of peripheral nerves.

The clinical significance of this group arrangement for the surgical tactics are given in Table 43-1. The fascicular pattern changes for two reasons. First, the nerve fibers deriving from different spinal nerves must be ar-

**Table 43-1** *Clinical significance of groups I to V fascicular patterns*

| Fascicular pattern | Type | No. of fascicles | Preparation of stumps | Ideal coaptation | Alternative | Unfavorable coaptation |
|---|---|---|---|---|---|---|
| Monofascicular | I | 1 | Resection | End-to-end | — | — |
| Oligofascicular | II | 2–4 (5) | Resection | End-to-end | Fascicular | — |
| Oligofascicular | III | 5–6 to 10–12 | Interfascicular dissection | Fascicular | End-to-end | — |
| Polyfascicular without group arrangement | IV | >10–12 large and small fascicles | Resection | End-to-end with guide stitches | Sector–sector | Fascicular |
| Polyfascicular with group arrangement | V | >10–12 large and small fascicles | Interfascicular dissection | Group-to-group | End-to-end | Fascicular |

ranged within the nerve trunk according to the branching of the nerve. Second, a nerve, consisting of many fascicles, is much more able to resist lateral pressure and flexion during limb motion. Therefore nerve trunks along the shaft of an extremity have a mono- or an oligofascicular pattern, but in close proximity to joints they change to a polyfascicular pattern. Intraneural dissection following the group arrangement from the periphery to the center shows, over a long distance, a rather consistent group pattern, followed by a change to a polyfascicular pattern without group arrangement with much fiber exchange; then, after another rather long distance, there is a different but again consistent group pattern. This observation is no contradiction to the rapidly changing fascicular pattern because there certainly is a change of the fascicular pattern within the group. This situation, however, little influences the surgical approach.

## Classification of Nerve Tissue Damage

The various degrees of nerve tissue damage can best be classified by the scheme of Sunderland [75] (Table 43-2). If the amount of damage to a peripheral nerve after an accident must be classified, the reaction of the connective tissue of the nerve trunk is considered as well. The damage of the connective tissue part cannot be recognized at the time of primary repair; the damaged portions later develop a fibrosis that may or may not constrict the fascicular tissue. From the surgical point of view, the following situations may be distinguished.

FIBROSIS OF THE
EPIFASCICULAR EPINEURIUM
In the case of fibrosis of the epifascicular epineurium, the fibrosis is confined to the layers of the epineurium that surround the nerve trunk. Because of shrinkage compression of the whole nerve, like a too-tight stocking, may develop. Such a fibrosis can

**Table 43-2** *Classification of nerve damage (continuity) according to Sunderland*

| Type | Damage |
|------|--------|
| I | Axon intact: no conduction at the site of the lesion; conduction distal to the lesion; no wallerian degeneration |
| II | Axons interrupted: wallerian degeneration |
| III | Endoneurium interrupted but fascicular pattern intact |
| IV | Fascicles interrupted; continuity preserved by connective tissue |
| V | Continuity interrupted |

*Source:* S. Sunderland. A classification of peripheral nerve injuries producing loss of function. *Brain* 74:491, 1951.

develop along with degree I, degree II, or degree III damage according to Sunderland. If we call the circumferential fibrosis "A," we may distinguish damage of degree IA, IIA, or IIIA. After damage of grade I or grade II, according to Sunderland, spontaneous recovery may be expected, although it might be prevented by compression due to the fibrosis of the epifascicular epineurium. If decompression is carried out, the result may be spontaneous recovery.

FIBROSIS OF THE
INTERFASCICULAR EPINEURIUM
With fibrosis of the interfascicular epineurium, there is fibrosis of the epi- and interfascicular epineurium that may extend over the entire cross section or only part of it. Such a fibrosis, type B, also may occur along with a damage of degree I, II, or III, according to Sunderland, and therefore can be termed IB, IIB, or IIIB damage.

FIBROSIS OF THE ENDONEURIUM
If the endoneurial space is obliterated by dense fibrosis, spontaneous regeneration cannot develop. Such fibrosis may be due to severe damage or to obliteration in consequence of a long time interval. This type of

damage (type C) occurs only along with degree III damage of Sunderland and may be called IIIC damage.

If degree IV damage according to Sunderland is present, the fascicular pattern has been lost but continuity is maintained by connective tissue. Two situations occur. The segment with degree IV damage may be completely fibrotic and is said to have IVS damage (S = scar tissue). A neuromatous neurotization produces a neuroma growing slowly along the damaged segment, called IVN damage (N = neuroma).

## Interfascicular Dissection

With brachial plexus surgery, Bateman [3] and Pecinka [57] recommended interneural neurolysis; however, this suggestion has been rejected by most authors because of the tissue trauma and the damage that might be inflicted to the nerve tissue when operating within the nerve. Under microscopic vision and using microsurgical techniques, it is possible to perform dissections within the nerves with minimal tissue trauma. In areas with a high rate of fiber exchange between fascicle groups, some of these connections are transected during interfascicular dissection, but it does not lead to clinically significant functional loss.

The epifascicular epineurium is incised longitudinally; again it is best to start the dissection in healthy tissue and proceed toward the damaged area. The tissue can be reflected easily, following the intraneural vessels as guidelines. The dissection proceeds into the depth of the nerve between the individual fascicles and fascicle groups (Fig. 43-1).

With minor degrees of damage the fibrosis is limited to the epineurium, which may be thickened, compressing the nerve like an overly tight stocking. The fibrosis may involve the interfascicular tissue and, in severe cases, the perineurium and the fascicle itself. The epineurium is incised (starting from healthy tissue), undermined, and re-

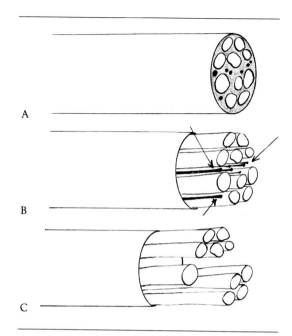

**Figure 43-1** A. Peripheral nerves consist of a number of fascicles, each of which is surrounded by perineurium. The perineurium forms a tube of dense connective tissue that provides tensile strength and maintains the pressure inside the fascicles; this tube acts as a fluid barrier. The fascicles are kept together by the interfascicular epineurium; this tissue expands between the fascicles and the epifascicular epineurium, which surrounds the whole nerve trunk. This tissue layer is covered by a loose connective tissue, the paraneurium. The nerve trunk contains one large fascicle (monofascicular pattern I), a few large fascicles (oligofascicular pattern II), a limited number of middle-size fascicles (oligofascicular pattern III), many fascicles without regular arrangement (polyfascicular pattern IV), or many fascicles arranged in groups (polyfascicular pattern with group arrangement, V). B. The major intraneural vessels are located in the interfascicular spaces (arrows point to vessels). After resection of the epifascicular epineurium, one can dissect between the fascicles, following the course of the vessels. C. In the peripheral sections of the nerves, groups of fascicles can be separated.

sected. If the epineuriectomy brings sufficient relief, one can watch the fascicles expanding after the compression is relieved

**Table 43-4**  Combined classification

| Type | Continuity | Fibrosis | Spontaneous recovery | Surgical treatment |
|---|---|---|---|---|
| I | Axons intact | 0 | Good | — |
| IA | Axons intact | Epifascicular epineurium | Nil, partial, or retarded | Epifascicular epineuriotomy |
| IB | Axons intact | Interfascicular epineurium | Nil, partial, or retarded | Epifascicular epineuriectomy; interfascicular epineuriectomy (partial) |
| II | Axons interrupted | 0 | Good | — |
| IIA | Axons interrupted | Epifascicular epineurium | Nil, partial, or retarded | Epifascicular epineuriotomy |
| IIB | Axons interrupted | Interfascicular epineurium | Nil, partial, or retarded | Epi- or interfascicular epineuriectomy |
| III | Endoneurium interrupted | 0 | Partial | |
| IIIA | Endoneurium interrupted | Epifascicular epineurium | Nil or poor | Epifascicular epineuriotomy |
| IIIB | Endoneurium interrupted | Interfascicular epineurium | Nil or poor | Epifascicular or interfascicular epineuriectomy |
| IIIC | Endoneurium interrupted | Endoneurium | Nil | Resection and grafting |
| IVN | Fascicles interrupted | Neuroma in continuity | Very poor | Resection and grafting |
| IVS | Fascicles interrupted | Fibrosis | Nil | Resection and grafting |
| V | Continuity lost | — | Nil | Grafting |

## INTERFASCICULAR DISSECTION AFTER LOSS OF CONTINUITY

Interfascicular dissection is used in the same way as described above for the repair of two nerve stumps after transection if fascicular coaptation is planned. The dissection is started proximally and distally in healthy tissue and proceeds toward the neuroma and the glioma, respectively. Each fascicle group is transected exactly at the point where it loses normal appearance and disappears in the neuroma. A much more thorough resection of neuroma and scar tissue is achieved compared to the consecutive resection of tissue slices beginning at the end of the stump.

A strip of epineurium is resected to prepare the stumps. This step is done not only to facilitate interfascicular dissection but also to avoid early invasion at the gap between the two stumps by proliferating connecting tissue, which originates to a large extent from the epineurium.

## Restoration of Continuity

### PRIMARY VERSUS SECONDARY NERVE REPAIR

There is a continuing discussion about whether primary or early secondary nerve repair is the treatment of choice.

## Time Factor

It is evident that if primary nerve repair is performed time is gained and a second operation avoided. If satisfactory regeneration occurs, it is a significant advantage; however, if regeneration does not occur, a dilemma develops in terms of time. Sufficient time must elapse before return of function can be expected. On the other hand, it is well known that the chances of good regeneration start to decrease about 6 months after the original injury. If one waits too long, the optimal time for reexploration might be lost. Therefore about 6 months after the primary nerve repair one must decide if sufficient regeneration can be expected or if reinnervation must be considered; this decision is often difficult. In many instances the patient is not aware of the fact that loss of time might be harmful, so it is the responsibility of the surgeon who performs the primary nerve repair to ensure that the patient is seen regularly and the decision about eventual reexploration is made in time.

## Quality of Regeneration

Primary nerve repair does not offer any advantage over secondary repair so far as the quality of regeneration is concerned. On the contrary, there are arguments that the reaction of the neurons and the increase of axon plasma flow favor early secondary repair (during the second or third week after the injury).

## Anatomy

In a clean transection the anatomic relation of the transected part can be easily defined at the time of primary repair because no scar tissue has formed. There is no fibrous retraction of the stumps, and end-to-end nerve repair can be performed more easily because only the elastic retraction of the nerve tissue has to be overcome. However, if the nerve stumps have retracted because of elasticity of the nerve tissue, additional incisions may be necessary to locate the retracted stumps; this situation leads to a danger of spreading an eventual infection. In the case of second-ary repair one always starts the dissection from the healthy tissue, where the anatomy is still well preserved. If fibrous retraction has already occurred within the nerve stumps, nerve grafting offers a good solution to the problem, which means that nerve grafts are being used often for secondary repairs.

## Evaluation of Stumps

The forces acting on the nerve during the injury cause certain damage to the nerve stumps. The damaged parts become fibrotic, and this fibrosis impedes nerve regeneration in both the proximal and the distal stump. The key to proper nerve repair is sufficient resection of the damaged part. With secondary nerve repairs the amount of damage can be easily recognized because the damaged part has already become fibrotic. With primary nerve repair this evaluation is difficult, and thus there is the risk of uniting two potentially fibrotic stumps.

## Local Factors

If the injury causes not only transection of the peripheral nerve but also other injuries to muscles, tendons, and bone, or if a skin defect is present, there is an increased risk of postoperative complications that might interfere with proper nerve regeneration. It is evident that in such a case early secondary nerve repair offers a safer solution.

## General Condition of the Patient

The general status of the patient is an important factor when making the decision of whether to perform primary nerve repair or a delayed repair.

## Factors Regarding Personnel and Equipment

The chances of good regeneration after nerve repair are increased if the nerve repair is performed by an experienced surgeon with modern equipment and sufficient time to perform the repair as exactly as possible. If experienced personnel and equipment are not available or if the operation must be performed under time pressure in an emergency situation, it is better to delay the repair until a later date.

*Other Factors in the Decision Between Primary and Secondary Repair*
Whether to perform primary nerve repair is an individual decision based on local and general factors regarding the patient. The training and experience of the surgeon also influence the decision. The surgeon who is generally involved with emergency surgery tends to perform primary repairs. Another surgeon who does reconstructive surgery and thus tends to see cases of failed primary nerve repairs decides more often in favor of early secondary repair.

The main guideline for handling the case is the principle of not inflicting additional damage on the patient. If there is a clean cut without further complications and without nerve tissue defect, primary nerve repair can save time and does not cause much harm. In such a case primary nerve repair is performed and the patient is followed closely so that in case of failure the decision for reexploration is made in time. If there is a loss of nerve substance or a skin defect, it is wise to delay the nerve repair. In such a case the optimal time for early secondary repair is when the original wound has healed well, the edema has disappeared, and the general status of the patient is good. It could be after as little as 2 weeks or as much as 6 weeks after the injury; 2 to 3 weeks after the original injury is the optimal time from the theoretical point of view regarding nerve regeneration. However, more important are the local and general conditions of the patient: If these factors are not favorable, the theoretical arguments are not strong enough to force an earlier date for the secondary repair.

## END-TO-END NERVE REPAIR VERSUS NERVE GRAFT

There is no question that an end-to-end nerve repair offers the best chance of nerve regeneration. If there is no nerve defect, the fascicular pattern of the two stumps is compatible and the corresponding fascicles can be reunited. With end-to-end repair the regenerating axons have to cross only one suture line to reach the peripheral stumps. There is also no question that end-to-end nerve repair has its limits, however. If there is a loss of nerve substance, the structure of the fascicular pattern is different. The two stumps must be approximated under tension, and coaptation has to be maintained against tension. It is true that by flexing the adjacent joints tension can be relieved so long as immobilization is maintained. When mobilization commences, however, the suture site is exposed to longitudinal tension; even if the flexed position is relieved gradually, the permanent tension has its consequences on the suture site. As is the case with scar reaction in other tissues, hypertrophy of scar tissue or stretching of the scar tissue might develop. There is clinical and experimental evidence that these changes at the suture site can damage axons that have already crossed the suture line and have reached the distal stump. In such cases it is better to avoid tension through the use of nerve grafts. The disadvantage of the nerve graft—having two suture lines—is compensated for by the fact that these suture lines are in optimal shape. Regenerating axons are able to cross two optimal suture lines more easily than one poor suture line.

In the past most surgeons regarded grafts as not particularly useful. However, thanks to modern techniques, especially microsurgical techniques, the results of nerve grafting have been improved, although the value of nerve grafts is not generally accepted. The discussion continues as to what size of defect would be an indication to perform a nerve graft rather than to force an end-to-end nerve repair. There are surgeons who are confident that a median nerve defect of 3 to 4 cm could be easily overcome by mobilizing and flexing the adjacent joints. Other surgeons, including me, regard a defect of 1.5

to 2.0 cm large enough to consider nerve grafting. Of course there are individual differences because some patients have much laxer tissues and a defect can be overcome more easily than in other patients. Age plays a role: A longer gap can be closed by an end-to-end nerve repair with likelihood of recovery in children than in adults.

The result of an end-to-end nerve repair depends on the ability of the patient to restore mobility in the longitudinal direction by regenerating paraneurial tissue. A transected nerve repaired by end-to-end coaptation under a certain tension—protected by flexion of the adjacent joints—is exposed to tension when mobilization is started. The suture site and a segment of the nerve (the segment length depending on the extent of the damage) become adherent to the surrounding tissue in consequence of the original trauma and the surgical trauma. If the lesion is close to a joint, the tension exerted on the site of nerve repair is distributed over only a short segment of the nerve and therefore is high for each segment. Only after the mobility of the site of repair has been regained are the forces distributed over a longer segment and therefore more equally. Without doubt certain patients have greater potential for regeneration of loose connective tissue. The amount and velocity of regeneration of this tissue depends on the amount of damage, which is minor with a clean-cut injury and major with a blunt injury.

INTRANEURAL TOPOGRAPHY AS IT
RELATES TO NERVE REPAIR
At proximal levels the fibers of individual functions are distributed diffusely over the cross section of the nerve. More distally the fibers tend to be arranged according to the division into the branches. Even in monofascicular nerves, sectors with preference for fibers of certain functions can be defined. For example, the facial nerve at the stylomastoid foramen represents a monofascicular nerve, but by studying the fiber distribution

using serial sections [42] it is possible to distinguish sectors of preference for fibers going to the forehead, eyelids, cheek, upper lip, lower lip, and neck. At the root level of the brachial plexus and in the proximal portions of the peripheral nerves, the structure is monofascicular, oligofascicular, or polyfascicular, without group arrangement.

In the periphery—which is the area where most nerve lesions occur—the nerves have a polyfascicular structure with group arrangement. As discussed above, it is this peripheral zone in which the definition of corresponding fascicles is important because in the peripheral segments the individual fascicle groups already carry fibers for a certain function. In more proximal portions of the nerves, the fibers for certain functions are distributed over a larger area of the cross section. This diffuse distribution at proximal levels is so marked that the peripheral nerve trunk can be transected for one-third of its cross section without a clinically detectable loss of function [66].

To define the corresponding fascicle group at operation, a sketch is made of the fascicular pattern of two cross sections. If there is a clean transection, by comparing the size and the arrangement of the fascicles the corresponding fascicle can be recognized. Observation of the longitudinal vessels on the surface of the nerve stumps helps to avoid malrotation. If there is even a small defect, the number of fascicles does not correspond. It is then much easier to define the corresponding fascicle groups. Exposing the two nerve stumps to the next branching is helpful. The location of the branches helps to define the correct orientation of the stump in space. With a peripheral lesion the exposure is extended to the division of the nerve, where the individual branches can be defined easily. Retrogradely, the fascicles of the individual branches are followed until the distal stump is reached. Using such retrograde dissection, the exact location of the fascicles in the distal stump of the median nerve, which forms the motor thenar branch, can be defined. Having defined the fascicular pattern of the distal stump, it should be possible, by comparing the two sketches, to achieve a good guess about which fascicles or fascicle groups of the proximal stump correspond with the distal stump.

It is possible to differentiate between motor and sensory nerves by direct stimulation [20]. So long as no wallerian degeneration has occurred within the first days after injury, stimulation of motor fibers of the distal stump produces a muscle contraction, whereas stimulation of sensory fibers does not provoke a response. Stimulation of motor fibers of the proximal stump are not registered by the patient, but stimulation of sensory fibers of the awake patient, operated under local anesthesia, causes certain feelings depending on the fibers stimulated [16]. Motor and sensory fibers can also be differentiated using special staining techniques based on acetylcholine esterase [14, 19], acetylcholine transferase [11], or carboanhydrase [61]. An evaluation of long-term results demonstrates that in most of the author's cases clinical selection regarding which group of the proximal stump corresponded to which group of the distal stump was correct.

## Technique of End-to-End Nerve Repair

The classic epineurial nerve repair achieves coaptation of the two stumps by suturing the epifascicular epineurium without touching the fascicles or interfascicular tissue. Another advantage is that the epineural sutures are able to accept some tension (Fig. 43-3). When the epineurial suture was developed during the 1870s it was a great advance because before that time the surgeons did not dare to touch the nerve. They attempted indirect coaptation of the trunks by adjusting the surrounding tissue because they feared "convulsiones" after manipulating the nerve itself. From this fact derived the practice of designating the procedure according to the tissue layer where the stitches are located, e.g., epineurial or perineurial repair if individual fascicles were coapted and epiperineural repair if both layers were caught by the stitches. In reality this point is only one aspect (and probably not the most important one) of a repair procedure. Four basic steps can be distinguished that describe the technical aspects of a peripheral nerve repair.

*1. Preparation of the stumps.* The nerve stumps can be prepared in two ways: (1) resection until normal tissue is reached; or (2) interfascicular dissection, starting in normal tissue and dissecting toward the lesion. With the oligofascicular type III pattern, the individual fascicles are separated; with the polyfascicular pattern with group arrangement (type V), the individual fascicle groups are separated. Using this procedure, a large amount of epineurial tissue is removed that occupies a large proportion of a cross section. Without this removal the epineurial fibroblasts, which multiply faster than the endoneurial fibroblasts or the Schwann cells [6, 7], have a better chance of occupying the space between the two stumps. If the epineurial tissue is resected, these cells have a longer way to travel before they reach the site of coaptation, and therefore the chances of Schwann cells and endoneurial fibroblasts occupying the space is improved. The same is true for separation of the fascicle groups after resection of the epineurial tissue and coapting the stumps of each corresponding group individually. If we must deal with a monofascicular pattern (type I) or an oligo-

*Figure 43-3* Epineurial suture. Nerve repair under tension. A. Each stitch approximates the area where the stitch is located. The remaining cross section tends to separate. B. Many stitches are necessary. C. In an oligofascicular nerve, epineural repair provides satisfactory fascicular alignment. D, E. In polyfascicular nerves, buckling of the fascicles (D) or inner separation (E) can occur.

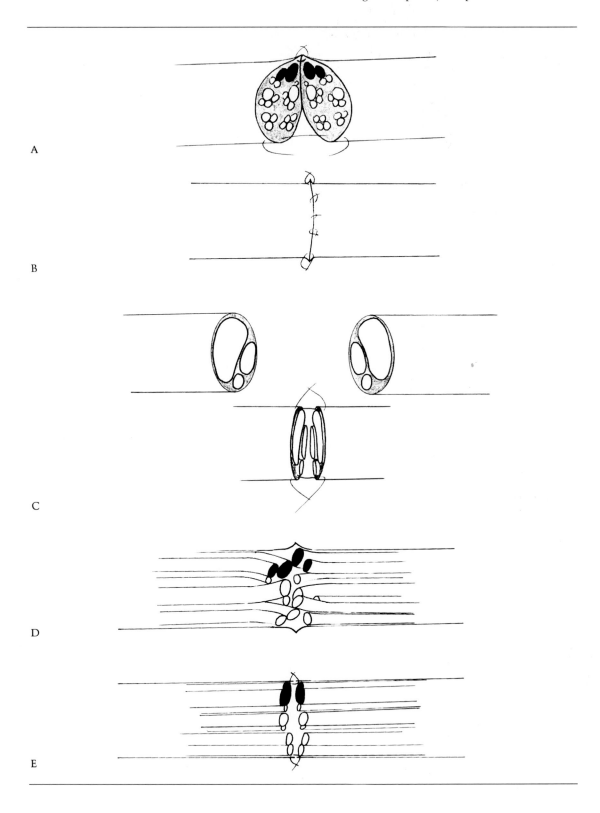

A

B

C

D

E

fascicular pattern with only a few large fascicles (type II), an exact coaptation can easily be achieved by external manipulation, and the interfascicular epineurium does not play an important role. For this reason, resection of the interfascicular and epifascicular connective tissue in these cases does not offer any advantage; rather, it would cause additional damage. Therefore experiments to investigate the relative value of epineurial or fascicular (perineurial) nerve repair without taking into account the fascicular pattern do not provide reliable information. In the case of the monofascicular or the oligofascicular pattern type II, trunk-to-trunk coaptation is the treatment of choice. If we have to deal with a polyfascicular pattern without group arrangement (type IV), we are in a dilemma. From what was stated above about oligofascicular pattern type III and polyfascicular pattern with group arrangement (type V), resection of the epifascicular epineurium and individualization of the fascicles would be desirable, as suggested by Tupper [82]. Clinical experience has demonstrated that the theoretical advantage is outweighed by the difficulty of defining the corresponding fascicles. In this situation, as with mono- and oligofascicular patterns, type II coaptation of the stumps by dissection is advisable.

*2. Approximation.* The two stumps must be approximated, which can be achieved with one or two stitches. Even if the use of tissue glue is intended, the approximation must be achieved in some way, and it can be done (in most cases) simply by approximation stitches or by touching the stumps with an instrument, if there is some tension in the longitudinal direction.

*3. Coaptation.* The bringing together of two structures is described by the term *coaptation.* In our case, coaptation refers to the two stumps of a nerve trunk (trunk-to-trunk coaptation), individual fascicles (fascicular coaptation), fascicle groups (fascicle group coaptation), or sectors of two cross sections. With peripheral nerve repair the main point in each of these coaptations is to coapt the fascicular tissue as well as possible.

*a.* In a nerve segment with monofascicular pattern, trunk-to-trunk coaptation is the same as fascicular coaptation because the trunk consists of only one fascicle.

*b.* In an oligofascicular nerve segment with a few large fascicles (type II), trunk-to-trunk coaptation ensures exact coaptation of the few fascicles.

*c.* With an oligofascicular pattern (type III) that has a large number of large fascicles, each fascicle is coapted with the corresponding fascicle (fascicular coaptation), and a large amount of interfascicular and epifascicular epineurium is removed.

*d.* With a polyfascicular pattern without group arrangement (type IV), individualization of the fascicles is not a realistic procedure, as outlined above, therefore trunk-to-trunk coaptation is recommended. To avoid malrotation, interfascicular guide stitches have been adopted [24, 70] (Fig. 43-4). Intrafascicular stitches, which end across the skin and can be removed, as suggested by Hakstian [20], never became popular.

*e.* For polyfascicular segments with group arrangements (type V) individual fascicle groups are coapted with the stitches anchored in the interfascicular epineurial tissue or in the perineurium of one or the other fascicle (Figs. 43-5 and 43-6).

*4. Maintaining the coaptation.* If there is tension in the longitudinal direction, stitches in addition to the approximation stitches must be used. The problem of the application of tissue glues has already been discussed. If there is no tension at all, as in cases of nerve grafting, normal fibrin clotting would be appropriate.

WRAPPING THE SUTURE SITES
Wrapping the suture site with foreign material (Silastic membrane, collagen membrane, millipore) to avoid invasion of the suture site by proliferating connective tissue from the surrounding tissue has not proved successful. Despite the good external appearance of the suture sites, invasion of the suture line by connective tissue cannot be avoided. One of the main sources of prolif-

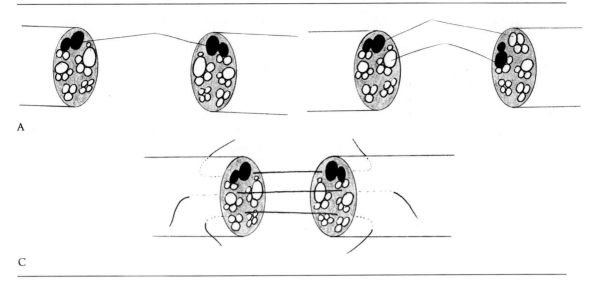

A

C

**Figure 43-4** *Epineurial repair with guide sutures. A. Exact alignment of the corresponding fascicles is essential in polyfascicular nerves containing many nerve fibers of many functions. B. Malrotation brings the motor fibers in the fascicles (black) into contact with sensory fascicles (white) or with interfascicular tissue. C. Guide sutures prevent malrotation.*

**Figure 43-5** *Interfascicular coaptation. After resection of a strip of epineurium and interfascicular dissection in a nerve with group arrangement of the fascicles, the fascicle groups are isolated and coapted with the corresponding fascicle group. Approximation is achieved by one or two fine stitches (nylon 10-0), which are anchored in the remaining interfascicular tissue. Coaptation is maintained by natural fibrin clotting. No tension can be accepted. Further separation is not favorable. In nerves with a few major fascicles, the individual fascicles are isolated and coapted (fascicular coaptation).*

erating connective tissue is the epineurium, which remains inside the tube. Foreign body reaction against the tube may occur, especially if the site of the nerve repair is located in an area of constant motion.

## Management of Nerve Defects
Nerve defects can be managed in three ways.

***1.*** *Shortening the distance between the two stumps.* This goal can be achieved by resecting a bone segment with osteosynthesis, as suggested by Goldner [17, 18]. Another possibility is to relocate the nerve into a shorter bed, e.g., transposition of the ulnar nerve to the volar side of the elbow joint. If the elbow joint is not flexed, approximately 2 cm can be gained. Flexing the elbow joint

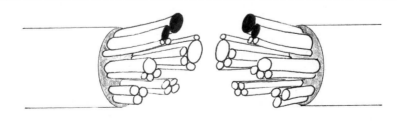

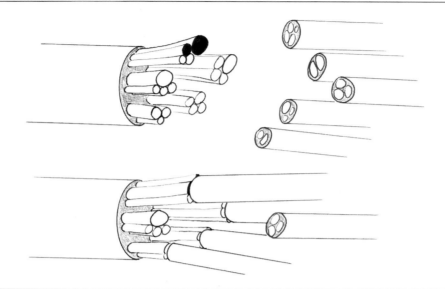

does increase the gain, but the nerve must later be elongated, as discussed below.

**2.** *Elongation of nerve tissue.* Without a nerve defect, a cleanly transected nerve retracts because of its elasticity. At primary repair the nerve tissue can be elongated easily to its original length. The nerve then regains its original basic tension. So long as the gliding capacity in longitudinal direction is not disturbed, the tension is equally distributed along the whole length of the nerve and remains below the critical level.

If the same nerve after clean transection is repaired several weeks after the accident, the elastic retraction may have become fixed by fibrosis. In this case, elongation to the original length is not possible by simply overcoming the elastic retraction; unchanged segments of the nerve must elongate to a greater degree to make up for the loss of elasticity of the fibrotic segment.

A nerve defect can be compensated for by further elongation of the normal segments of the nerve. If this elongation passes a critical level, irreversible damage develops [21, 22, 35, 47–49, 53, 54]. The distribution of the required elongation over a longer segment of the nerve can be achieved by mobilizing the nerve in both directions. This maneuver

**Figure 43-6** *Polyfascicular nerve with group arrangement. After resection of the epineurium and interfascicular dissection, each fascicle group is coapted with one graft (interfascicular grafting).*

may decrease the vascularization of the nerve—not in the sense that there is any danger of necrosis, but the circulation might be less than optimal. Starkweather et al. [71] observed that vast mobilization had a negative influence on nerve regeneration. The nerve becomes adherent along the entire length of the mobilized segment with unpredictable influence on the distribution of forces. The elongation can be distributed over a longer time interval by flexing the adjacent joints for the period of healing and gradual mobilization. In this case the early phase of wound healing and nerve regeneration occurs without tension at the site of coaptation. After 3 to 6 weeks according to the immobilization, the whole nerve and especially the site of coaptation are gradually exposed to increased tension. Because the site of coaptation has become adherent to the surrounding tissue, equal distribution of tension is not possible, and the nerve segment between the axis of motion and the site of coaptation is exposed to extensive elongation. The unfavorable conditions at the suture site cause degeneration of the axons that have already crossed the site of coaptation and reached the distal stump [46–49].

3. *Adding new tissue.* New tissue can be added in two ways: (1) nerve grafting (discussed later); and (2) neuromatous neurotization. Free-ending proximal stumps form a neuroma that can proceed over some distance in a distal direction. If it meets a distal stump by chance, spontaneous healing occurs. Such neuromas can grow along a nerve segment, having suffered fourth-degree damage, with a few fibers reaching the distal stump (damage grade IVN). Schröder and Seiffert [62] observed that such neuromas proceed, or grow, along a certain segment of preserved nerve graft [25], and they devised the term *neuromatous neurotization.* Lundborg and Hansson [34] described the formation of nerve tissue between two stumps connected by a mesothelial chamber. These various investigators all described the growth of a neuroma which is able to enlarge because there is no obstacle within the chamber. Similarly, neuromatous neurotization may occur along an empty perineurial tube [59] and along arterial and venous segments [60, 73].

## *Classification of Nerve Grafts*
### MECHANICAL ASPECTS
Regarding the length of nerve graft required to bridge a given defect, the surgeon is faced with two possibilities. First, he or she can determine the length of the graft after attempting to approximate the two stumps as closely as possible. This measurement is then the *minimal length* of the graft. In this case, the disadvantages of nerve grafting— the axon sprouts must cross two sites of coaptation—are combined with the disadvantages of a coaptation under tension. This technique was used extensively in the past because it was (wrongly) assumed that the result of nerve grafting depends on the length of a graft, which is not the case. There is a relation between the length of a graft and the result. With increasing length, the result to be expected deteriorates. The result, however, does not depend on the length of the graft but, rather, on the length of the nerve defect—which may require a long graft. As the length of the defect increases, the chance of coapting corresponding nerve fibers significantly decreases. With any given defect, the result does not change if a graft of 4 cm or one of 6 cm is used, for example. To the contrary, the nerve graft 6 cm long, situated in a suitable recipient site does better than a graft of 4 cm implanted into scar tissue.

The second possibility is to select a length of graft based on the neutral or even extended position of the adjacent joints *(maximal length).* If the graft is allowed to heal in this situation, it is not exposed to any tension when the limb is later mobilized. However, even a graft with maximal length must accept tension forces at the site of coaptation if the limb was flexed during healing and the graft has formed adhesions to the surrounding tissue in relaxed position, according to the state of flexion. It is obvious that the graft must form adhesions in order to obtain a blood supply and to survive.

### SOURCE OF NERVE GRAFTS
Autogenous nerve grafts do not cause immunologic problems, and their application is the method of choice. The same is true for isogenic grafts. Allogenic and xenogenic nerve grafts cause an immunologic response that must be suppressed to avoid rejection. Such grafts may have a chance in the future if, by proper matching, fresh allogenic nerve grafts are used that cause a minimal reaction, or if the immunologic response is suppressed until the axon sprouts have crossed the graft. If the Schwann cells, fibroblasts, and mesothelial cells of the donor are then gradually replaced by the recipient tissue without destroying the axon basal membrane unit, such grafts may be functional.

Preserved allogenic or xenogenic grafts do not cause a significant immunologic reaction because they contain only the collagen framework, without cells. For the same reason, they were neuroticized by neuromatous neurotization, which in itself is a great disadvantage and works only over a limited distance. Grafts have been preserved by lyophilization [83], preservation in cialite solution [1], and irradiation [23, 26, 36, 37, 84]. Lyophilized nerve grafts have also been wrapped in lyophilized dura [25], but these grafts did not work satisfactorily [31].

Experimental attempts have been made to combine an allogenic or xenogenic framework with Schwann cells from the recipient and multiplied by cell culture [2].

DONOR NERVE

The question was raised whether intact or predegenerated nerve grafts are preferable. At present there is no convincing evidence that predegenerated grafts yield better results.

Trunk grafts do not survive free grafting without some central anoxic damage, which produces fibrosis [4]. Such nerves are used as grafts only by maintaining or immediately restoring the circulation. If a nerve trunk is to be used as a free graft, the epifascicular epineurium must be removed, and the nerve, according to the fasicle groups, is divided into smaller units, which survive free grafting much better than larger ones (split nerve graft).

Cutaneous nerves of the diameter (e.g., of the sural nerve) survive free grafting well [13]. Because these grafts are thinner than the nerve trunks to be repaired, several segments of the cutaneous nerves are combined by stitches or gluing to form a graft of the same size as the nerve being repaired (cable grafting) [63, 64, 76]. Cable grafts have major disadvantages: A great portion of the surface of each graft is in contact with another free graft and has no chance of making contact with the recipient bed to become vascularized. It is not possible to connect well defined spots of the two cross sections. The use of individual cutaneous nerves [45, 50, 51] does allow these possibilities, and their use has proved superior to cable grafts. To avoid contact of the grafts with nonfascicular tissue in the cross section, the stumps are prepared by interfascicular dissection if the

stump has an oligofascicular pattern of type III or a polyfascicular pattern with group arrangement (type V). The interfascicular dissection has provided the possibility of solving the difference of caliber between the nerve trunk and the cutaneous nerve graft. Therefore, use of this term for this grafting procedure is justified.

CIRCULATION

With free grafting, the graft is deprived of a blood supply. If the relation between the surface and the diameter of the graft favors the surface and the recipient site is suitable, spontaneous revascularization occurs within a short time. The grafts have an excellent circulation after only a few days [9, 85].

Under certain conditions nerve grafts can be transplanted with preservation of blood supply. In such cases the diameter of the graft is unimportant. Strange [72] restored the continuity of the median nerve using a pedicled graft from the ulnar nerve. With better knowledge of the blood supply of particular nerve segments, it has become possible to use segments of a nerve, e.g., an island flap, on its vascular pedicle. Therefore the ulnar nerve has been used to bridge a defect of the brachial plexus by transferring it as an island flap with the collateralis ulnaris superior artery as a pedicle.

The third possibility is the immediate restoration of blood supply by microvascular anastomosis, as suggested by Taylor and Ham [77, 78]. These grafts are independent of the recipient site because they have their own blood supply. They do not require adhesions with the surrounding tissue, and probably the paraneurium survives better. The median and ulnar nerves, the peroneal nerve, and the sciatic nerve or parts of it have been used. Fachinelli et al. [12] and Townsend and Taylor [81] developed techniques to graft the sural nerve as a vascularized nerve graft. By grafting the superficial branch of the radial nerve with the radial artery, a vascular pedicle was provided in combination with a free cutaneous nerve graft.

Originally it was expected that nerve grafts with preserved or immediately restored circulation would be neurotized rapidly and would yield good results. At the moment there is neither clinical nor experimental evidence that nerve regeneration is significantly better along these grafts than for other grafts [40, 58].

## Technique of Nerve Grafting

The technique of nerve grafting is basically the same as with end-to-end nerve repair, except that proximal and distal coaptations are performed. If a monofascicular nerve segment is coapted with cutaneous nerve grafts, several such nerve grafts are necessary to satisfy the cross section of the one large fascicle *(fascicular nerve grafting 1:3, 1:4 . . .).* In an oligofascicular nerve segment the individualized fascicles may have a diameter similar to that of the cutaneous nerve grafts, and one graft is used for one fascicle *(fascicular nerve grafting).* If the stump consists of a polyfascicular segment with group arrangement, one cutaneous nerve graft is needed for each group *(group fascicular nerve grafting* or *interfascicular nerve grafting).* In the case of a polyfascicular nerve segment, each nerve graft is coapted with a particular sector of the cross section *(sector nerve grafting).* With long defects the type of coaptation might be different at the proximal or distal site of coaptation.

Approximation of the graft to the desired spot of the stump is achieved with the help of one stitch. If this stitch is placed in an optimal position, there is excellent coaptation, and because there is no tension aerial contact is achieved. Normal fibrin clotting helps to maintain the coaptation. If the first stitch was not placed ideally, the graft rotates against the stump and a second or third stitch becomes necessary. During repair of a nerve trunk, several cutaneous nerve segments are necessary. If the fascicle groups or fascicles of the stump have been transected at different levels, interdentation and side-to-side contact are achieved, which permit using a minimal number of stitches. Small nerves, such as digital nerves, are regarded as one fascicle group and thus are coapted with one cutaneous nerve graft. Because there is no side-to-side contact with other nerve structures, several stitches (preferably three) are required.

DONOR NERVES
There are many nerves available as donors for nerve grafting.

*Sural Nerve*
The sural nerve is my first choice. It is easily defined by a small transverse incision behind the lateral ankle. With a gentle pull, the course of the nerve can be palpated; the whole nerve can be excised with several additional transverse incisions. One must keep in mind that in the area of the lateral ankle the sural nerve divides into several branches. All these branches must be transected; if this step is taken, the nerve can then be extracted easily. Other surgeons prefer a longitudinal incision to excise the whole nerve under vision. Nerve strippers must not be used, as they destroy the source from the peroneal nerve. At proximal levels the sural nerve may be monofascicular, but during its course it becomes more and more polyfascicular. Therefore it offers the possibility of selecting an optimal portion if only a short graft is needed.

*Nervus Cutaneus Antebrachii Medialis*
The medial cutaneous nerve of the forearm provides a rather thick graft at its proximal level. It divides into two branches in the distal part of the upper arm. This nerve is not used if the ulnar nerve of the same extremity must be repaired.

*Nervus Cutaneus Antebrachii Dorsalis*
The use of the dorsal cutaneous nerve of the forearm was suggested by McFarlane and Mayer [41].

## Ramus Superficialis Nervi Radialis

The superficial radial nerve is known for its association with frequent painful neuromas after traumatic lesions; therefore its use is not recommended. It must not be used if the median nerve of the same extremity is involved because of the overlapping of sensory function. However, with a brachial plexus lesion, when the nerve is already not functioning and many grafts are needed, its use may be necessary.

## Ramus Dorsalis Nervi Ulnaris

A rather short but thick graft of the dorsal ulnar nerve can be utilized. Such a graft is not used in a median or ulnar nerve lesion of the same extremity in order to avoid a large sensory loss resulting from possible overlapping.

## Intercostal Nerves

The intercostal nerves contain motor fibers, which was an argument in favor of their use. However, they have extensive branching, which might lead to a loss of axons.

## Nervus Cutaneus Femoris Lateralis

The lateral cutaneous nerve of the thigh is easily found below the iliac spine. It can be exposed into the pelvis, which has the advantage that the proximal neuroma is buried deep within the pelvis. For this reason this nerve is used when the indication for nerve grafting is a painful neuroma. Any neuroma formed at the site of transection of this nerve would not be exposed to mechanical irritation.

## Nervus Saphenus

The saphenous nerve must not be excised as a graft if the sural nerve of the same site is used.

## Nerves of the Cervical Plexus

The nerves of the cervical plexus are easily available and are often used to graft defects of the facial nerves.

COMMENT

The functional loss after excision of a donor nerve is minimal and can be neglected. However, it is evident that the patient must be warned about possible complications and must agree to excision of the donor nerve.

DISTAL SUTURE SITE

After nerve grafting the regenerating axons must cross two suture lines. It is possible that at the distal end of the graft a dense scar has formed by the time the regenerating axons arrive. Further progress of the axons may thus be impeded. This situation can be recognized by the fact that the Tinel Hoffmann sign, which advances from the proximal stump along the graft, stops at the distal end of the graft. If the Tinel Hoffmann sign's failure to progress persists for several months, exposure of the distal suture site is indicated. The problem might be external compression, which can be corrected; if scar tissue blocks the distal suture site, this segment is resected and an end-to-end nerve repair is performed. Among the first 50 cases of my series, this problem occurred in seven (14 percent). With increasing technical skill the incidence of blockage at the distal suture site has dropped considerably.

## Reexploration After Failure of Conventional Nerve Repair

One of the problems associated with primary repair is the fact that, in cases of failure, reexploration must be undertaken at the proper time. If there is no return of function, the decision to explore and resect the suture site is easily made. If there is some indication that function might return but in an unsatisfactory way, the surgeon who performs the reexploration accepts great responsibility; on the other hand, waiting might mean that all chances of a useful recovery are lost.

A painful neuroma at the suture site and paresthesias are good arguments in favor of reexploration. After exposure, thickening at the suture site is usually seen, mostly as a result of proliferation of epineural tissue. The operation starts with an epineurectomy proximal and distal to the coaptation site and then resection of the epineurium at the site. The stitches from the first operation are usually found underneath this epineural thickening. An interfascicular dissection is performed starting from the healthy tissue. Fascicles or fascicle groups that are in good contact with the corresponding fascicles of the distal stump are isolated and saved. Fascicles or fascicle groups forming a neuroma without contact are resected and are then reunited by nerve grafts.

## References

1. Afanasieff, A. Premieres résultats de 20 homogreffes de nerfs conservés par le cialit (main et avant-bras). *Presse Med.* 27:1409, 1967.
2. Aguayo, A. J. Construction of Graft. In A. Gorio, H. Millesi, and S. Mingrino (eds.), *Posttraumatic Peripheral Nerve Regeneration (Experimental Basis and Clinical Implications)*. New York: Raven, 1981. P. 365.
3. Bateman, J. E. An operative approach to supraclavicular plexus injuries. *J. Bone Joint Surg. [Br.]* 31:34, 1949.
4. Bielschowsky, M., and Unger, E. Die Überbrückung grosser Nervenlücken: Beiträge zur Kenntnis der Degeneration und Regeneration peripherer Nerven. *J. Physiol. Neurol.* 22:267, 1916–1918.
5. Breidenbach, W. B., and Terzis, J. K. The anatomy of free vascularized nerve grafts. *Clin. Plast. Surg.* 11:65, 1984.
6. Bunge, R. P. Contributions of Tissue Culture Studies to Our Understanding of Basic Process in Peripheral Nerve Regeneration. In A. Gorio, H. Millesi, and S. Mingrino (eds.), *Posttraumatic Peripheral Nerve Regeneration (Experimental Basis and Clinical Implications)*. New York: Raven, 1981. P. 105.
7. Bunge, R. P. Construction of Grafts. In A. Gorio, H. Millesi, and S. Mingrino (eds.), *Posttraumatic Peripheral Nerve Regeneration (Experimental Basis and Clinical Implications)*. New York: Raven, 1981. P. 366.
8. Curtis, R. M., and Eversman, W. W. Internal neurolysis as an adjunct to the treatment of the carpal tunnel syndrome. *J. Bone Joint Surg. [Am.]* 55:733, 1973.
9. Daly, P. J., and Wood, M. B. Endoneural and epineural blood flow: Evaluation with vascularized and conventional nerve grafts in the carina. *J. Reconstr. Microsurg.* 2:45, 1985.
10. Duspiva, W., Blümel, G., Haas-Denk, G., and Wreid Lübke, I. Eine neue Methode der Anastomisierung der peripheren Nerven. *Langenbecks Arch. Chir.* Suppl. 100, 1977.
11. Engel, J., Ganel, J., Melamed, R., et al. Choline acetyl transferase for differentiation between human motor and sensory nerve fibers. *Ann. Plast. Surg.* 4:376, 1981.
12. Fachinelli, A., Masquelet, A., Restrepo, J., et al. The vascularized sural nerve: Anatomy and surgical approach. *Int. J. Microsurg.* 3:57, 1981.
13. Foerster, O. Communication held at Ausserordentliche Tagung der Deutschen Orthopaedischen Gesellschaft, Berlin, February 2–9, 1916. *Munch. Med. Wochenschr.* 63:283, 1916.
14. Freilinger, G., Gruber, H., Holle, J., and Mandl, H. Zur Methodik der sensomotorisch differenzierten Faszikelnaht peripherer Nerven. *Handchirurgie* 7:133, 1975.
15. Gamble, H. J., and Eames, R. A. An electron microscope study of the connective tissue of human peripheral nerves. *J. Anat.* 95:655, 1964.
16. Gaul, J. S., Jr. Electrical fascicle identification as an adjunct to nerve repair. *J. Hand Surg. [Am.]* 8:289, 1983.
17. Goldner, L. Discussion at Symposium: Peripheral Nerves of the Upper Extremity. Durham, N. C., 14–16, September 1978.
18. Goldner, L. Personal communication at the 5th American Orthopaedic Association International Symposium: Limb Reconstruction: Micro- or Macrosurgery. Boca Raton, 7–11, November 1984.
19. Gruber, H., and Zenker, W. Acetylcholinesterase: Histochemical differentiation between motor and sensory nerve fibres. *Brain Res.* 51:207, 1973.
20. Hakstian, R. W. Funicular orientation by direct stimulation: An aid to peripheral nerve repair. *J. Bone Joint Surg. [Am.]* 50:1178, 1968.

21. Highet, W. B., and Holmes, W. Traction injuries to the lateral popliteal nerve and traction injuries to peripheral nerves after suture. *Br. J. Surg.* 30:212, 1943.

22. Highet, W. B., and Sanders, F. K. The effect of stretching nerves after suture. *Br. J. Surg.* 30:355, 1943.

23. Hiles, R. W. Freeze dried iradiated nerve homograft: A preliminary report. *Hand* 4:79, 1972.

24. Ishikawa, F. Experimental studies on nerve suturing, especially in peripheral nerves. *Med. J. Hiroshima Univ.* 1966.

25. Jacoby, W., Fahlbruch, R., and Mackert, B. Indikation und Technik der Überbrückung von Nervendefekten mit homologen lyophilisierten Nerven. *Melsunger Med. Mittl.* 116:209, 1972.

26. Jacoby, W., Fahlbruch, R., Mackert, B., et al. Überbrückung peripherer Nervendefekte mit lyophilisierten und desantigenisierten Transplantaten. *Munch. Med. Wochenschr.* 112: 586, 1970.

27. Kuderna, H. Discussion at the Symposium: Indication, Technique and Results of Nerve Grafting, Vienna, May 21–23, 1977. *Handchirurgie* Suppl. 2, 1977.

28. Kuderna, H. Ergebnisse und Erfahrungen in der klinischen Anwendung des Fibrinklebers bei der Wiederherstellung durchtrennter peripherer Nerven. Presented at the 17th Annual Meeting of the Deutsche Gesellschaft für Plastische und Wiederherstellungschirurgie. Heidelberg, 1–3 November 1979.

29. Kuderna, H. Erfahrungen mit der Fibrinklebung peripherer Nerven Communication held at the Gesellschaft der Ärzte in Wien, 13 April 1984.

30. Kuderna, H. Die Fibrinklebung peripherer Nerven. In H. Nigst (ed.), *Nervenwiederherstellung nach traumatischen Läsionen.* Stuttgart: Hippokrates, 1985. P. 78.

31. Kuhlendahl, H., Mumenthaler, M., Penzholz, H., et al. Behandlung peripherer Nervenverletzungen mit homologen Nervenimplamtaten. *Z. Neurol.* 202:252, 1972.

32. Lang, J. Über das Bindegewebe und die Gefässe der Nerven. *Z. Anat. Entwicklungsgesch.* 123:61, 1962.

33. Lundborg, G. Ischaemic nerve injury. *Scand. J. Plast. Reconstr. Surg.* Suppl. 6, 1970.

34. Lundborg, G., and Hansson, H. A. Regeneration of a peripheral nerve through a preformed tissue space. *Brain Res.* 178:573, 1979.

35. Lundborg, G., and Rydevik, B. Effect of stretching the tibial nerve of the rabbit. *J. Bone Joint Surg.* [Br.] 55:390, 1973.

36. Marmor, L. Regeneration of peripheral nerve defects by irradiated homografts. *Lancet* 1: 1911, 1963.

37. Marmor, L. Regeneration of peripheral nerves by irradiated homografts. *J. Bone Joint Surg.* [Am.] 46:383, 1964.

38. Matras, H., and Kuderna, H. The principle of nervous anastomosis with clotting agents. In: *Transactions of the 6th International Congress of Plastic and Reconstructive Surgery, Paris, 1975.* Paris: Masson, 1976. P. 134.

39. Matras, H., Dinges, H. P., Lassmann, H., and Mamoli, R. Zur nahtlosen interfaszikulären Nerventransplantation im Tierexperiment. *Wien. Med. Wochenschr.* 122:517, 1972.

40. McCullogh, C. J., Gagay, O., Higginson, D. W., et al. Axon regeneration and vascularisation of nerve grafts: An experimental study. *J. Hand. Surg.* [Br.] 9:323, 1984.

41. McFarlane, R. M., and Mayer, J. R. Digital nerve grafts using the lateral antebrachial cutaneous nerve. *Hand. Surg.* 1:81, 1976.

42. Meissl, G. Die intraneurale Topographie des extrakraniellen Nervus fascialis. *Acta Chir. Aust.* [Suppl.] 28:1, 1979.

43. Meyer, V. E., and Smahel, J. The surgical cutsurface of peripheral nerves. *Int. J. Microsurg.* 2:187, 1980.

44. Smahel, J., Meyer, V. E., and Bachem, U. Gluing of peripheral nerves with fibrin: An experimental study. *J. Reconstr. Microsurg.* 3:211, 1987.

45. Millesi, H. Zum Problem der Überbrückung von Defekten peripherer Nerven. *Wien. Med. Wochenschr.* 118:182, 1968.

46. Millesi, H. Clinical Aspects of Nerve Healing. In T. Gibson and J. C. Van der Meulen (eds.), *Wound Healing.* Montreux: Foundation International Cooperation in the Medical Sciences, 1975. P. 882.

47. Millesi, H. Healing of nerves. *Clin. Plast. Surg.* 4:459, 1977.

48. Millesi, H., Berger, A., and Meissl, G. Razvoj Reparatorno-Operativnih Postupaka Kod Ozljeda Periferinih Zivaca. Drugi Simpozija Bolestima O Ozljedema Sake, Zagreb, 1970. P. 161.

49. Millesi, H., Berger, A., and Meissl, G. Experimentelle Untersuchung zur Heilung durchtrennter peripherer Nerven. *Chir. Plast. (Berl.)* 1:174, 1972.

50. Millesi, H., Ganglberger, J., and Berger, A. Erfahrungen mit der Mikrochirurgie peripherer Nerven. *Chir. Plast. (Berl.)* 3:47, 1966.

51. Millesi, H., Ganglberger, J., and Berger, A. Interfasciculäre Nerventransplantation mit Hilfe der mikrochirurgischen Technik. *Excerpta Med. Int. Congr. Ser.* 174:56, 1967.

52. Miyamoto, Y. Experimental study of results of nerve tissue under tension versus nerve grafting. *Plast. Reconstr. Surg.* 64:540, 1979.

53. Miyamoto, Y. End-to-End Coaptation Under Tension on Repair of Peripheral Nerves. In A. Gorio, H. Millesi, S. Mingrino (eds.), *Posttraumatic Peripheral Nerve Regeneration (Experimental Basis and Clinical Implications).* New York: Raven, 1981. P. 281.

54. Miyamoto, Y., Watari, S., and Tsuge, K. Experimental studies on the effects of tension of intraneural microcirculation in sutured peripheral nerves. *Plast. Reconstr. Surg.* 63:398, 1979.

55. Narakas, A. Personal communication at the XI Meeting of the Groupe d'Avancement de Microchirurgie, Sitges, 31 May 1985.

56. Ochoa, A. J., and Mair, W. G. P. The normal sural nerve in man. *Acta Neuropathol. (Berl.)* 13:197, 1969.

57. Pecinka, H. Die operative Behandlung der traumatischen Lähmungen des Plexus brachialis. *Zentrabl. Chir.* 85:1678, 1960.

58. Pho, R. W. H., Lee, Y. S., Rujiwetpongstorn, V., and Pang, M. Histological studies on the vascularised nerve graft and conventional nerve graft. *J. Hand Surg. [Br.]* 10:45, 1985.

59. Restrepo, Y., Merle, M., Michon, J., et al. Fascicular nerve graft using an empty perineurial tube: An experimental study in the rabbit. *Microsurgery* 4:105, 1983.

60. Rigoni, G., Smahel, J., Chiu, D. T. W., and Meyer, E. Veneninterponat als Leitbahn für die Regeneration peripherer Nerven. *Handchirurgie* 15:277, 1983.

61. Riley, D. A., and Lang, D. H. Carbonic anhydrase activity of human peripheral nerves: Possible histochemical aid to nerve repair. *J. Hand Surg. [Am.]* 9:112, 1984.

62. Schröder, J. M., and Seiffert, K. E. Die Feinstruktur der neuromatösen Neurotisation von Nerventransplantaten. *Virchows Arch. Pathol. Anat.* 5:219, 1970.

63. Seddon, H. J. Restoration of function in peripheral nerve injuries. *Lancet* 1:418, 1947.

64. Seddon, H. J. The use of autogenous grafts for the repair of large gaps in peripheral nerves. *Br. J. Surg.* 35:151, 1947.

65. Seddon, H. J. *Surgical Disorders of the Peripheral Nerves.* Edinburgh: Churchill Livingstone, 1972.

66. Sherren, J. *Injuries of Nerves and Their Treatment.* New York: Wood, 1907.

67. Smith, J. W. Microsurgery of peripheral nerves. *Plast. Reconstr. Surg.* 33:317, 1964.

68. Smith, J. W. Factors influencing nerve repair. I. Blood supply of peripheral nerves. *Arch. Surg.* 93:335, 1966.

69. Smith, J. W. Factors influencing nerve repair. II. Collateral circulation of peripheral nerves. *Arch. Surg.* 93:433, 1966.

70. Smith, J. W. Injuries of Nerves. In W. C. Grabb and J. W. Smith (eds.), *Plastic Surgery.* Boston: Little Brown, 1968. P. 705.

71. Starkweather, R. J., Neviaser, R. J., Adams, J. P., et al. The effect of devascularization on the regeneration of lacerated peripheral nerves: An experimental study. *J. Hand Surg.* 3:163, 1978.

72. Strange, F. G. St. C. An operation for nerve pedicle grafting: Preliminary communication. *Br. J. Surg.* 34:423, 1947.

73. Strauch, B., Rosenberg, B., Brunelli, G., et al. Autogenous vein graft substitute in long segment nerve defects. Presented at the Inaugural Meeting of the American Society for Reconstructive Microsurgery, Las Vegas, 17–19 January, 1985.

74. Sunderland, S. Blood supply of the nerves of the upper limb in man. *Arch. Neurol. Psychiatry* 53:91, 1945.

75. Sunderland, S. A classification of peripheral nerve injuries producing loss of function. *Brain* 74:491, 1951.

76. Sunderland, S. *Nerves and Nerve Injuries.* Baltimore: Williams & Wilkins, 1968.

77. Taylor, G. I., and Ham, F. J. The free vascularized nerve graft. *Plast. Reconstr. Surg.* 57:413, 1976.

78. Taylor, G. I. Nerve grafting with simultaneous microvascular reconstruction. *Clin. Orthop.* 133:56, 1978.

79. Terzis, J. K., Felker, B. L., and Sismour, E. M.

A computerized study of the intraneural organization of the median nerve. Presented at the 39th Annual Meeting of the American Society for Surgery of the Hand, 6–8 February 1984.

80. Thomas, P. K. The connective tissue of peripheral nerve: An electron microscope study. *J. Anat.* 97:35, 1963.

81. Townsend, P. L. G., and Taylor, G. I. Vascularised nerve grafts using composite arterialised neuro-venous systems. *Br. J. Plast. Surg.* 37:1, 1984.

82. Tupper, J. W. Fascicular Nerve Repair. In D. L. Jewett and H. R. McCarrol, Jr. (eds.), *Nerve Repair and Regeneration: Its Clinical and Experimental Basis.* St. Louis: Mosby, 1980. P. 320.

83. Weiss, P. Functional nerve regeneration through frozen dried nerve grafts in cats and monkeys. *Proc. Soc. Exp. Biol. Med.* 54:277, 1943.

84. Weiss, P., and Taylor, A. C. Repair of peripheral nerves by grafts of frozen dried nerves. *Proc. Soc. Exp. Biol. Med.* 52:326, 1943.

85. Wood, M. B. Neovascularization of nerve grafts: A quantitative study in canines. Presented at the 7th Symposium of the International Society of Reconstructive Microsurgery, New York, 13–19 June 1983.

*Graham D. Lister*

# 44

# *Replantation*

The first successful replantation of an amputated arm was reported in 1962 by Malt and McKhann [48], and Komatsu and Tamai [38] performed the first successful digital replantation in 1968. Since then a large number of replantations have been undertaken [77], and the number of centers equipped to perform revascularizations [33, 35] and replantations [8, 34, 61, 62, 67, 87] has increased greatly. Successful replantation has also been reported for other parts of the body, including lower limb [31, 42, 50, 84], scalp [9, 11, 21, 26, 27, 55, 57, 73, 80, 85], penis [16, 78, 86], and ear [68]. Most replantations are of amputated upper extremity parts, however, and are the sole concern of this chapter. When the improved techniques that are detailed here are employed, and when cases are selected properly, it is possible to achieve a survival rate of over 95 percent in ideal digital replantations and over 40 percent in salvage cases. With an increased number of parts surviving, the surgeon has rightly turned his or her attention to function, the foremost consideration in all surgery of the hand [15, 22, 36, 43, 49].

## Selection

Although the number of surgeons willing to attempt replantation is increasing, they are still geographically removed, in most cases, from the potential beneficiary of their skills. Clear rules regarding suitability for replantation are necessary if undue hope and unnecessary expenditure are to be avoided. Ideally, these rules are known to all emergency physicians, but it is impossible to follow them always in practice. It is obviously best that the referring physician speak directly to the replantation surgeon, and it is imperative that whoever takes the referring call be well versed in the rules of patient selection [63].

ABSOLUTE CONTRAINDICATIONS
*Significant Associated Injuries*
There are rarely other major injuries in cases of digital amputation, but injuries involving the trunk and head frequently occur in conjunction with loss of an arm. These other injuries may have been overlooked in the understandable preoccupation with the more dramatic amputation. Time must be taken to eliminate or treat such injuries, as they may be life-threatening. In some rare instances, this care precludes replantation.

*Extensive Injury to the Affected Limb*
Successful repairs are uncommon when injuries involve multiple levels. Extensive degloving and crush injuries involving much of the extremity are even less likely to be repaired successfully.

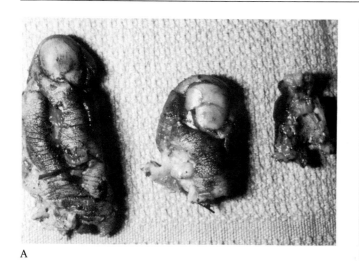

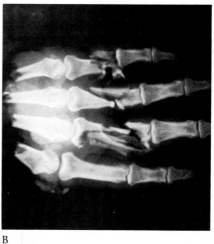

A

B

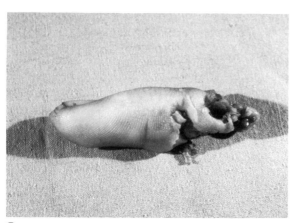

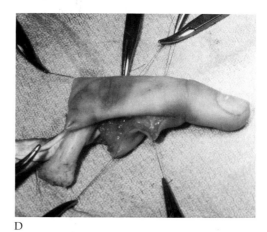

C

D

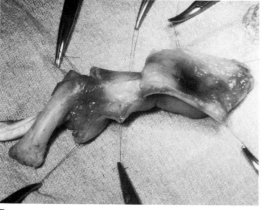

E

**Figure 44-1** *A. Parts evidently crushed are unsatisfactory for replantation. B. Radiographic evaluation of digits, to which the extent of injury is uncertain, can frequently help when assessing soft tissue injury, as it corresponds to, or exceeds, the bounds of comminuted fractures. C. A red streak, seen here as dark bruising along the line of the neurovascular bundle, is evidence of avulsion of branches and therefore likely to preclude successful replantation. D,E. Bruising underneath the skin is often revealed to be more extensive when the skin is reflected in the course of preparing an amputated part.*

Success of replantation after severe crush or multiple injuries of the amputated part depends on blood flow, which cannot be achieved without adequate "runoff." Major injuries to the amputated part, such as crush injuries (Fig. 44-1A), compromise this runoff. Radiographic studies of the part may reveal multiple fractures, which can be used as a measure of the severity of the crush injury (Fig. 44-1B). Avulsion of the branches of the digital arteries may be suspected in the presence of "red streaks"—patches of bruising along the sides of the fingers due to extravasation of blood (Fig. 44-1C–E). These streaks usually indicate that attempts at vascular repair will fail. Final evaluation of avulsion may come with preparation of the part under the microscope, when careful inspection may reveal avulsed branches or intramural thrombi extending distally far enough to preclude success even using interposition vascular grafts.

*Chronic Illness*
Chronic illness sufficient to make transportation or prolonged surgery hazardous is a contraindication. We have had one potential candidate for replantation admitted from an intermediate airport in left heart failure and two other patients who developed myocardial infarction during replantation.

RELATIVE CONTRAINDICATIONS
Relative contraindications are often encountered in combination, in which case the bar to replantation is proportionately greater.

*Single-Digit Amputations*
The functional results have thus far made the replantation of a single digit proximal to the proximal interphalangeal joint an unrewarding exercise [83]. The index finger, unless it functions almost perfectly, cannot be used, and poor function in any of the ulnar three digits hampers motion in the others owing to the common origin of the profundus tendons. Nonetheless, sensory return is predictably satisfactory after microscopic

digital nerve repair following a clean injury [22]. Therefore replantation is justifiable if the amputation of a single digit is through the middle phalanx or beyond [54, 83, 92] and if the patient or relatives still want to proceed after being made aware of the problems of replantation. Such distal single-digit replantations commonly take only 2 to 3 hours of operating time and can be done on an outpatient basis (Fig. 44-2).

*Age of the Patient*
The amount of degenerative change in the vascular tree is variable, but if the degeneration is advanced the survival rate is reduced. More important, recovery of function is not as good in the older patient. When this factor is considered in conjunction with the greater likelihood of stiffness in the uninjured fingers, the surgeon must be circumspect when choosing the course to follow.

Infancy is no contraindication to replantation; indeed microsurgery in the very young has been found to be successful and free of complications [66]. Cooperation during postoperative therapy is lacking, however, which may result in tendon adhesions that are difficult or impossible to overcome with secondary tenolysis.

*Avulsion Injuries*
With avulsion injuries the damage done to both vessels and nerves usually is not limited to the site of amputation but often extends for some distance both proximally and distally. The extent of injury due to avulsion has been shown to be 4 cm on electron microscopy, in contrast to 8 mm on optical microscopy [58]. Such damage may result in vascular failure or poor nerve regeneration. The mechanism of injury often signals this type of avulsion, an obvious example of which is the ring degloving injury. In other instances the less experienced examiner may believe initially that the amputation has been fairly sharp but on closer inspection of the part may discover structures dangling from its cut end (Fig. 44-3A). These struc-

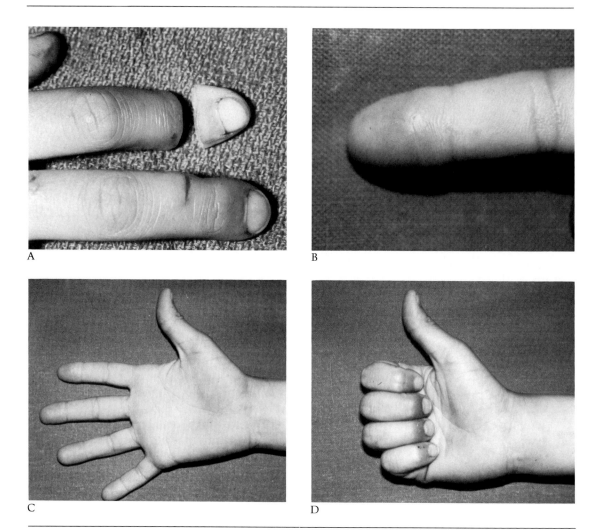

tures may be tendons or (more commonly) nerves, but they are rarely vessels. Although this finding suggests that the vessels at least are in good condition, it is usually not the case; the reason for the absence of the vessels is that they are more commonly avulsed distally (Fig. 44-3B). Sometimes an apparently suitable distal stump can be found. In other instances viability may be successfully restored with the use of vascular grafts, but sensory return is less than ideal. In thumbs from which the vessels have been avulsed, revascularization and reinnervation

**Figure 44-2** *Single-digit replantation. Amputations distal to the proximal interphalangeal joint are frequently satisfactory for replantation. A. An adolescent sustained a relatively clean amputation just distal to the distal interphalangeal joint. B. Replantation was undertaken. C, D. There was a satisfactory result with complete retention of normal function. (Case courtesy of Dr. L. R. Scheker.)*

may be achieved by transposing the neurovascular bundle from the ulnar side of the middle or index finger [47, 69] (Fig. 44-4).

*Ring avulsion* has been classified into three groups.

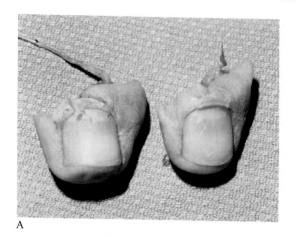

A

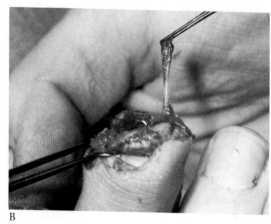

B

**Figure 44-3** *A. Two amputated tips, from which dangle structures. The presence of a long segment of avulsed nerve suggests not only that eventual sensory recovery would be unsatisfactory were replantation attempted but also that it is likely that the arteries were avulsed from the pulp distally. B. This phenomenon is shown in which the artery is held out to length from the corresponding stump.*

**Figure 44-4** *A, B. Following avulsion of the thumb, no satisfactory vessels or nerves were found proximally. A neurovascular transfer was undertaken from the ulnar aspect of the middle and the radial aspect of the ring fingers, thereby restoring not only flow but also sensation.*

Class I: circulation adequate
Class II: circulation inadequate
Class III: complete degloving or complete
amputation

In developing this classification, Urbaniak and others [82] pointed out that complete ring avulsion amputations have potentially poor function, and complete deglovings are difficult or impossible to revascularize. They therefore recommend amputation for class III injuries, a view that has been disputed [81]. As with many other replantation decisions, this one requires careful discussion of the potential problems with the patient.

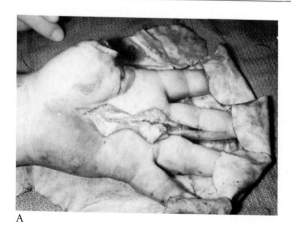

A

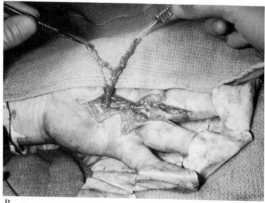

B

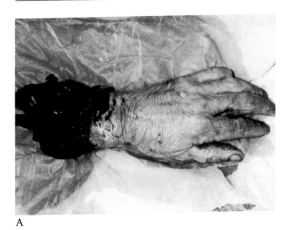

A

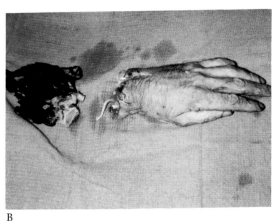

B

*Figure 44-5* *A, B. Replantation offers an unique opportunity for satisfactory debridement.*

*Lengthy Warm Ischemia Time*
Muscle undergoes irreversible changes after 6 hours at room temperature, whereas connective tissues, nerves, tendon, skin and bone remain viable for varying periods in excess of 12 hours. With immediate cooling of the part, we have successfully restored circulation to a digit 27 hours after injury. Others have successfully replanted extremities after longer ischemia [12, 53]. Even when flow is successfully reestablished, the more muscle and the longer the warm ischemia time, the poorer the muscle recovery is likely to be.

*Extreme Contamination*
Extreme contamination rarely prevents replantation because amputations present an unusual opportunity for radical surgical debridement (Fig. 44-5). However, occasionally oil or grease is driven into the tissues to an extent that makes debridement impossible.

*Previous Injury or Surgery*
On occasion a digit has been previously injured, which might be evident from old scars or radiographic changes, or it might not be noted initially. If not recalled by the patient when the history is taken, such as injury might be suspected only when the surgeon encounters a thrombosed artery, scarred veins, or a digital neuroma.

*Psychological Disturbance*
Patients with psychological problems, especially those who have amputated their own limbs, have done poorly in our experience. The decision to replant parts in such cases is made only after due consultation [74] (Fig. 44-6).

SALVAGE REPLANTATIONS
If the surgeon follows these rules of selection, the patient whose case he or she believes should be undertaken is called an *ideal replantation* candidate. In three instances (described below) relative contraindications are disregarded. Such cases, undertaken despite the presence of such contraindications, are termed *salvage replantations.*

*Children*
Relative contraindications may be set aside in children [30], not only because the results of primary repair are so much better but also (and more important) because the eventual vocation of any child is unknown and his or her skills may require all the digits that can be saved. Furthermore, if function remains impaired, he or she can select an appropriate occupation. Finally, the child has more time

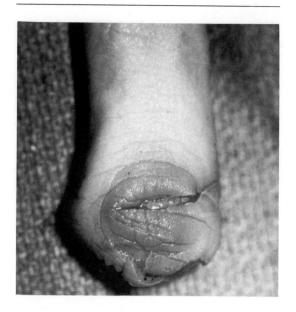

**Figure 44-6** *Amputations that occur under suspicious circumstances are always viewed as possible self-inflicted injuries. The amputated part shown here was supposedly the result of a wood-chopping injury while the patient was alone in the woods. Examination of the part revealed the additional laceration distal to the point of amputation, which was suggestive of a hesitation cut. Further questioning revealed this case to be a self-amputation. In this instance, replantation was not undertaken.*

available for rehabilitation and secondary surgery. Normal growth in replanted extremities can be anticipated [20].

*Multiple Digit Loss*
When faced with loss of a patient's hand or arm, or loss of more than two digits, the surgeon must attempt replantation except when the prospects are hopeless (Fig. 44-7). If several digits have been amputated in an unsuitable fashion, replantation is attempted on each of them, as the surgeon cannot predict which of the digits is likely to survive. The replantations are not, however, done in a slavishly anatomic fashion. Rather, the operator must recall the prime concern of restoring function, which may be best

achieved by putting one digit on a different stump to maintain appropriate length or important joint motion or to restore significant sensation [13]. Furthermore, parts from a nonreplantable digit can be used for reconstructing the hand, even to the degree of using the skin as a small free flap [5].

*Thumb*
The thumb is of much greater functional importance than any other digit and must be replaced [14, 18, 72]. It functions well even when it is deprived of all interphalangeal joint motion and has only protective sensation (Fig. 44-8).

## Transportation
Having decided that both patient and part are fit for transfer, the replantation surgeon gives clear instructions regarding transportation. Customary precautions for the evacuation of any patient are necessary, including the following.

1. Appropriate management of other injuries or illnesses.
2. Arrest of hemorrhage. Arrest can usually be achieved by application of a pressure dressing and elevation of the involved extremity. No further treatment of the stump is needed. Time spent on meticulous cleaning and debridement is time lost for restoring circulation.
3. Ensurance of normovolemia and normotension during travel. This point may require preliminary transfusion but can usually be achieved by starting an intravenous infusion.
4. Adequate analgesia. There is no cause to deny the patient relief from pain, provided a record is kept and passed on to the receiving anesthesiologist.
5. Preventive antibiotics. Although not favoring prophylactic antibiotics as a general rule, we believe they have benefit for the patient being moved over long distances for lengthy surgical procedures. Cephalothin intravenously is appropriate.

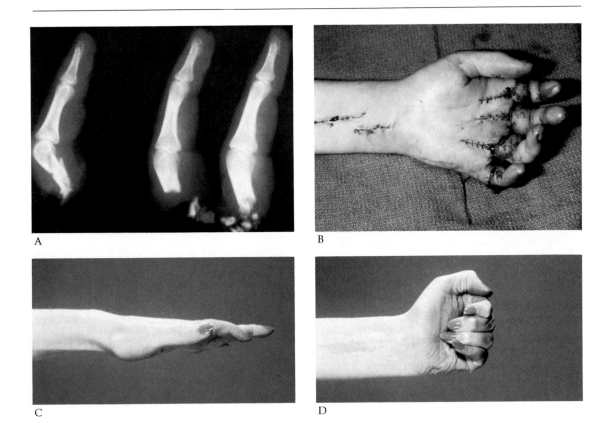

A    B

C    D

*Figure 44-7 Multiple digit loss. Despite some comminution of the parts shown on radiographic examination (A), loss of all four fingers in this patient dictated replantation of all four amputated digits (B). C, D. A satisfactory functional result was achieved in the long term.*

6. Qualified company on the journey is highly desirable; it is mandatory for patients in whom intravenous fluids are being administered.

The amputated part requires little treatment. Any gross contaminant can be washed off, but lengthy irrigation of the exposed tissues is *not* done because it can make the identification of structures more difficult. The amputated part is placed *dry* in a dry polyethylene bag, and the bag is placed in a mixture of regular ice and water, which gives a temperature of approximately 4°C.

## Preparation for Surgery
### HISTORY
A patient comes to replantation only after a full evaluation. The history taken from the patient or relatives includes not only details of the injury but (even more important) information about other injuries and preexisting illness.

### Mechanism of Injury
The patient is often accompanied by someone who knows about the circumstances of the amputation. When it was the result of an instrument other than a straightforward sharp edge, a detailed description of the mechanism can be of assistance in determining the degree of shortening necessary to eliminate all damaged tissue.

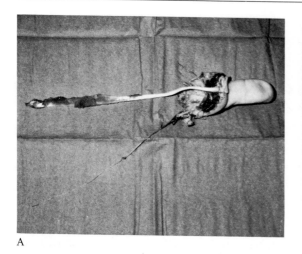

A

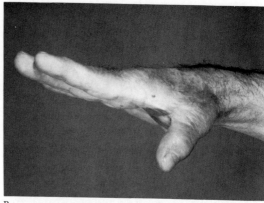

B

**Figure 44-8** *A. Avulsion of this thumb resulted in the flexor pollicis longus being pulled out of the muscle belly and both digital nerves being damaged over a significant length. B, C. Replantation was satisfactorily undertaken and the resultant thumb was superior to a prosthesis despite poor sensation and no significant motion. (From G. D. Lister.* The Hand: Diagnosis and Indications. *Edinburgh: Churchill Livingstone, 1984.)*

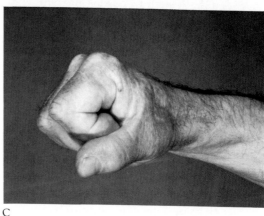

C

### Associated Injuries
Because the amputated extremity understandably captures the attention of emergency personnel other injuries may have been missed. The receiving surgeon must pursue any other complaints and conduct a swift but complete physical examination.

### Preexisting Illness
It must be remembered that the patient is about to spend a long time on an operating table and that replantation is never justified if it risks the patient's general health. Standard investigations include electrocardiography and chest radiography, depending on the patient's age and general health, and a complete blood count. Consultation with specialists may be necessary if there is any doubt about the patient's fitness for surgery. The anesthesia department is always encouraged to take part in this assessment.

### MONITORING AND MAINTENANCE OF THE PATIENT
The patient should come to replantation with the following aids to his or her continued general health: (1) blood pressure monitor; (2) precordial or esophageal stethoscope; (3) electrocardiography; (4) pulse monitor; (5) intravenous therapy, with antibiotics and transfusion when indicated; (6) urinary catheter (with volume recorded hourly); (7) central venous pressure catheter, again depending on the patient's age and general health; and (8) rectal thermometer.

Preoccupation with restoring circulation to the amputated part may cause the surgeon to overlook the welfare of the patient during a lengthy procedure. Resulting problems can be avoided by the presence of a competent anesthesiologist.

*Cardiovascular Status*
Some estimate of blood loss prior to arrival may be obtained from observers, but it is most reliably indicated by the usual compensatory mechanisms of tachycardia, sympathetic overactivity (as evidenced by peripheral vasoconstriction and sweating), and hypotension. If such trends are present, they must be reversed by typing and crossmatching, intravenous therapy, and transfusion. Circulating blood volume can be assessed during surgery by measuring the *hourly urinary output* through the catheter, frequent estimation of the *microhematocrit*, and use of a *pulse monitor*. The height of the wave on a pulse monitor is an index of pulse pressure and therefore of peripheral perfusion. Excess transfusion can be as great a problem as hypovolemia in children and the elderly; it can best be avoided by placing a *central venous pressure line*. The pulse monitor and central venous pressure line, together with continuous *electrocardiography*, aid in observing the patient who has preexisting cardiac problems or who develops them during surgery.

*Temperature*
Euthermia should be maintained by the use of a heating/cooling blanket. Temperature is monitored using a rectal probe.

ANESTHESIA AND SEDATION
Most of our replantations are performed under axillary block using bupivacaine (Marcaine) 0.5% with epinephrine. The block lasts 12 to 16 hours and may thereafter be supplemented by further block or by the induction of general anesthesia. Sedation is given as required in the form of diazepam (Valium) and pentobarbital (Nembutal).

PREPARATION OF THE PART
Once the patient arrives at the replantation center, the replantation surgeon confirms that the criteria for selection have been met. Then, while another physician readies the patient for surgery, the replantation surgeons take the amputated part and the radiographic studies to the operating room and immediately commence preparation. This preparation involves several steps.

*Skeletal Management*
The radiographs are studied, and decisions are made.
BONE SHORTENING. Whenever bone shortening can be achieved without sacrificing function, it is done (Fig. 44-9). The surgeon decides from the radiographs and from subsequent inspection of the part in what proportion the shortening can be done on the part and on the patient. Although efficient osteosynthesis is a major consideration when deciding whether the bone to be excised is to be taken primarily from the stump or the part, of equal importance is the preservation of joints and tendon insertions. If shortening in either direction would destroy salvageable and significant function, vascular grafts may be employed. It must be borne in mind, however, that the damaged vessel replaced by the graft is to some degree a measure of the injury sustained by all soft tissues. If such tissues are retained, healing and function may be impaired.
PRIMARY ARTHRODESIS OR ARTHROPLASTY. When the amputation passes through a joint and damages the articular surfaces, immediate fusion in the correct position with respect to the joint and the digit produce the required bone shortening and result in the quickest return to maximum function. Where bone resection required by the injury is such that arthrodesis would produce an unacceptably short digit, or where the amputation is through the metacarpophalangeal joint, immediate Silastic arthroplasty may in the first instance maintain length and in the second useful motion [90]. In our experience, sepsis and instability have

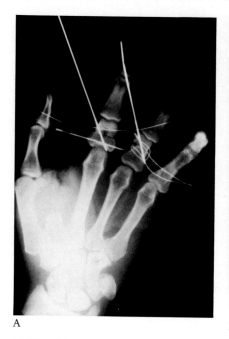
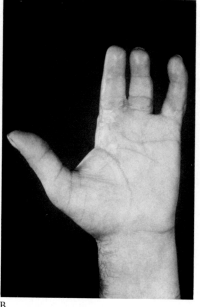
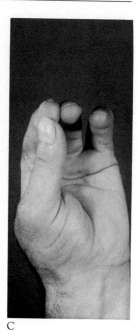

A      B      C

*Figure 44-9* *This patient sustained amputation of the three radialmost fingers in a punch press. The extent of injury to the proximal phalanx was wide, and the index finger was damaged at multiple sites. A. Ray amputation of the index finger was therefore performed and significant bone shortening undertaken as shown preoperatively. B, C. The resultant digits were short and had a relatively small range of motion but provided a satisfactory grip. Sensation was excellent because good nerves could be repaired owing to the bone shortening.*

not been problems with immediate arthroplasty.

CHOICE OF FIXATION. To prepare the skeleton appropriately, the surgeon selects the means of fixation after studying the radiographs. Firm internal fixation ensures bony union and permits early motion. Thus wherever possible, compression plates are used for the humerus, radius, ulna, and metacarpals, and type A intraosseous wiring is used for the phalanges [44] (Fig. 44-10).

*Inspection of the Part*
Having made these decisions, the surgeon commences work on the amputated part, which is laid on a sterile sheet with an operating microscope available. The amputated part is inspected to ensure that replantation is appropriate.

*Skin Incisions*
In the arm or forearm, extensile incisions are made to expose the neurovascular structures for dissection. They are not placed directly over the nerves and vessels, as swelling may prevent direct closure and skin grafts are better placed over adjacent muscle. By staggering the incisions in the stump and the part, the flaps are prepared for Z-plasty transposition during closure. With such high amputations, fasciotomies are performed during preparation of the part (see Fig. 13E and F, below). They are placed over anterior and dorsal compartments and over the second and fourth metacarpals to give access to all intrinsic muscle groups.

For the digit, various incisions have been recommended, including the Bruner and the triple incision mentioned in the last edition of this text. We have employed two midlat-

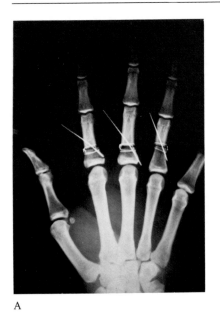

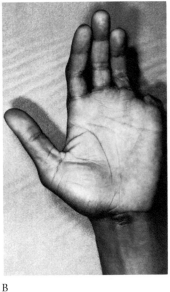

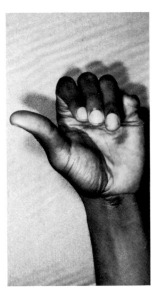

A                                                    B                                                    C

**Figure 44-10** *A. Replantation of these three digits was performed using type A intraosseous wiring. A 0.045 Kirschner wire and 0 monofilament wire were used to achieve stability to the extent that early motion could be undertaken. B, C. The eventual motion was satisfactory.*

eral incisions [59] (Fig. 44-1D,E). These incisions give excellent access to all structures while not exposing vessels or nerves if left unsutured. With ring avulsion injuries, in which almost the full length of the digital arteries may have to be replaced, a single dorsal midline incision out to and even beyond the distal interphalangeal joint gives good exposure (Fig. 44-11). If the incision cannot be closed directly, a small venous flap from an adjacent digit may restore both venous continuity and skin cover.

It is often beneficial to incorporate Z-plasties in the closure around the part; this practice lengthens the circumferential scar, which may otherwise become constrictive, and takes up the tissue made redundant by skeletal shortening. Certainly, at no time prior to closure should any potentially viable skin be excised. Edema can cause a remarkable reduction in available skin, and there are few more difficult situations for the surgeon than when faced with a circumferential defect overlying vascular repairs.

*Preparation of Neurovascular Structures*
The dissection is performed under the operating microscope, the amputated part being held by an assistant or by stay sutures attached to the table. As for all dissections, structures are mostly easily identified away from the site of injury. Hence the longitudinal incisions enable the surgeon to identify the arteries and nerves and to trace them back to the site of amputation. What is also important is that the tissues can be inspected away from the primary wound for evidence of extravasation of blood or avulsion of branches. For avulsive injuries it is good practice to perform the vessel repair beyond the first intact branch, that is, proximal to that branch proximally and distal to it distally. This technique often dictates the use of a vascular graft but gives excellent

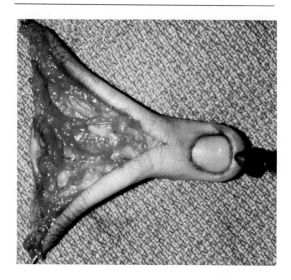

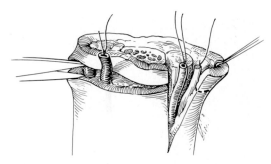

**Figure 44-12** *Veins can best be exposed by making a small incision 1 to 2 mm from the margin of amputation. The dissection in this incision reveals the veins, which can then be marked for subsequent repair. The incision also serves to débride the wound satisfactorily.*

**Figure 44-11** *Exposure of the arteries, veins, and distal interphalangeal joint in a ring avulsion injury can best be achieved using a single midline incision.*

prospects for establishing flow. Such damage indicates significant crush or avulsion, which probably has damaged the main vessels; in such cases vascular grafts may well be required.

As each neurovascular structure is dissected out and identified, a marking suture of 8-0 nylon is placed in its end. The vessels and nerves can be easily seen at this stage; however, hours later, when the part has been replanted and the tissues are blood-stained, the structures will have retracted into an amorphous mass of soft tissue. It is our practice to tag each vessel with two ends of equal length, whereas the nerve is tagged with only one long end. Microvascular clamps are not used for identification for three reasons: (1) they may slip off in the course of subsequent manipulations; (2) if left on for a considerable time, they can cause intimal damage; (3) if the vessel is for some reason not used, the clamp may be forgotten over the course of a long case with several changes of scrub nurse, only to be revealed (to the sur-

geon's embarrassment) on the postoperative radiographic studies. The veins in a digit are exposed by an incision running parallel to the skin margin and 1 to 2 mm from it (Fig. 44-12). This method also serves to débride the wound. Taking the rim of skin to be removed with forceps and having the remaining skin margin held with hooks by an assistant, the surgeon can extend the exposure of the veins by dissecting with a knife in the plane between the veins and the skin to be retained. The skin flap so created can be held back with a stay suture, taking care not to kink the veins. If the skin flap is first raised from the extensor tendon, the veins can be peeled off the undersurface of the flap.

In larger parts, the cut end of the vessels are inspected after the limb has been wrapped with an Esmarch bandage as if for exsanguination (Fig. 44-13A, B). Blood clots may be extruded by this maneuver, and they are entirely removed [79]. Rarely, fragments remain beyond reach in the artery. A Fogarty catheter may then be gently used.

*Tendon Exposure*
Depending on the position of the hand at the time of injury, the distal tendon ends may lie

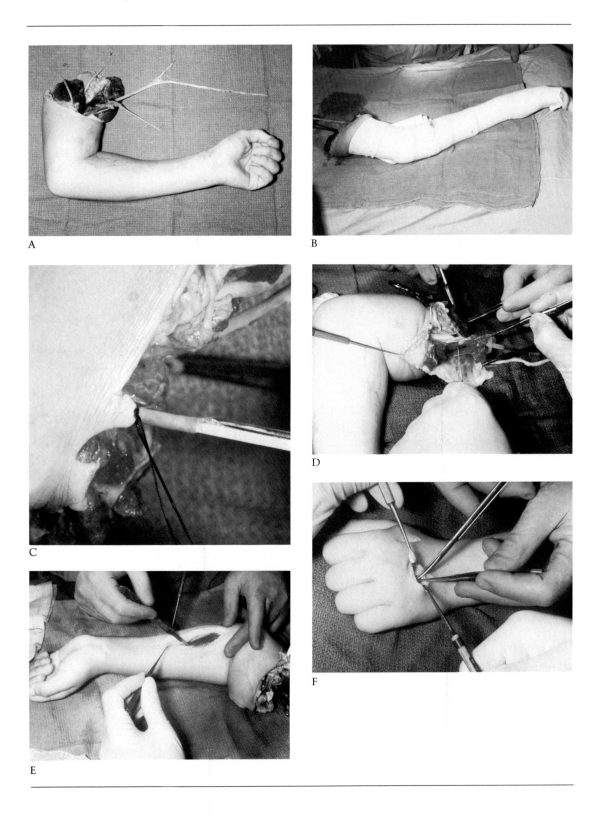

A

B

C

D

E

F

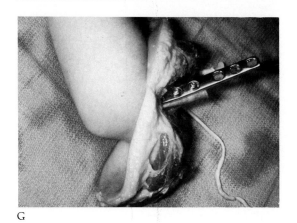

G

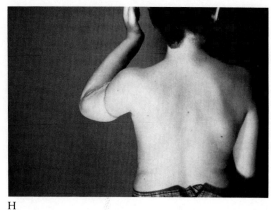

H

**Figure 44-13** *A. Avulsion amputation of the upper extremity at the level of the midhumerus was sustained by a 12-year-old boy. B. The limb was wrapped with an Esmarch bandage and the artery inspected for the presence of clots. C. The artery was then cannulated and the limb perfused with heparinized Ringer's lactate. D. All muscle that did not "weep" fluid was excised on the presumption that this muscle would not be perfused once circulation was reestablished. Appropriate bone shortening was then performed. E, F. Fasciotomy of the forearm and the interosseous compartments was undertaken prior to replantation, and a six-hole compression plate (G) was applied to the part, all before the patient was anesthetized. H. Promising early function was achieved.*

at the amputation site or further distally. Appropriate incisions are made in the sheath to display the tendon ends, taking special care to preserve the pulleys over the proximal and middle phalanges and to leave a cuff of sheath attached to bone for subsequent closure.

### Debridement, Especially of Muscle

Debridement requires removal of all contaminated and nonviable tissue. Contaminated tissues can be identified as easily as in any wound and can be excised with unusual freedom, as bone shortening can ensure wound closure. By contrast, to determine what tissue will *eventually* have no circu-

lation presents a problem unique to the amputated part because, of course, there is no blood flow whatsoever at the time of debridement. Removal of such tissue is vital to the success of the procedure, as later intercalated necrosis may lead to infection, septicemia, and secondary amputation. The problem is most pronounced where the muscle content of the part is significant. A catheter of appropriate size is inserted into the main artery(ies) and the part perfused with heparinized Ringer's lactate (Fig. 44-13C). Any tissue that does not "weep" lactate is radically excised, as it will not be perfused after replantation (Fig. 44-13D).

### Bone Resection

In those cases in which the surgeon has chosen to shorten the amputated part, the periosteum is carefully stripped away from the bone end for subsequent closure and the bone resected with a power saw. To avoid any possibility of damage to the soft tissues during this resection, a rubber dam is placed over the bone end (Fig. 44-14). It can be prepared by cutting a 5-mm hole in a piece taken from the Esmarch bandage. Although in rare instances the bone cut differs, in most it is absolutely transverse in both the part and the stump, thus avoiding any malalignment. For arm and forearm replanta-

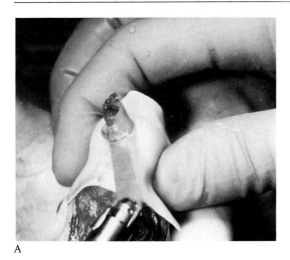

A

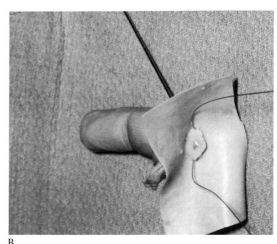

B

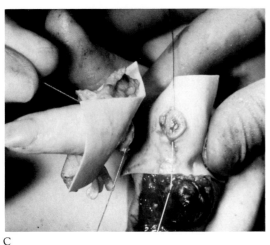

C

**Figure 44-14** *Bone resection in a phalanx can be accomplished without damage to vital soft tissue structures using a rubber dam constructed from a small segment of Esmarch bandage. Osteotomy can be undertaken (A), skeletal fixation is prepared in the part (B), and the two parts are brought together (C). Osteosynthesis is thus achieved knowing that the soft tissues have been well protected.*

tion, sufficient bone must be resected to ensure that sound, viable muscle closure is achieved (Fig. 44-15). The surgeon working on the part must also undertake any other preparation for fixation that can be done, such as application of a plate (Fig. 44-13G) or retrograde insertion of a Kirschner wire and the drilling of transverse holes for intraosseous wiring.

*Hemostasis*
It is strange to write of hemostasis in an amputated part, but bleeding after replantation can be a significant problem that can be re-

duced by bipolar coagulation of vessels encountered while preparing the amputated part. Such vessels may be obscured after replantation and may be difficult to locate without the risk of damage to the vascular anastomoses. Of particular importance are the vessels in a transmetacarpal amputation (Fig. 44-16). The metacarpal arteries, which are the branches of the deep palmar arch, are of significant size but are rarely if ever used for revascularizing the extremity. They connect, more often than not, with the common digital arteries at the point of their bifurcation. Herein lies their importance, because

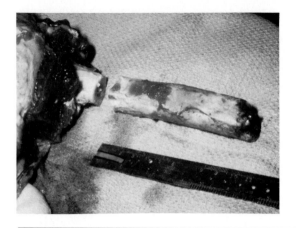

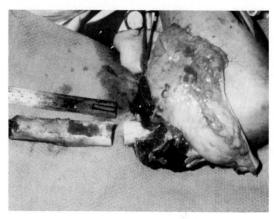

*Figure 44-15* Bone shortening in a case of macroreplantation at the level of the humerus. After débridement of the nonperfused muscle and damaged muscle (see Fig. 44-13), 20 cm of bony shortening was necessary to achieve satisfactory soft tissue approximation after osteosynthesis. (From J. Matiko and G. D. Lister. Fixation of Fractures in Reattachment of Amputated Parts. In N. J. Barton (ed.), The Hand and Upper Limb: Fractures of the Hand and Wrist. *New York: Churchill Livingstone, 1986.)*

hematoma further reduces flow distally by both pressure and inducing vascular spasm. These vessels must therefore be sought on the amputated part and ligated.

By the time the amputated part has been prepared, the patient is usually ready. The extremity is returned to the ice pack while the surgeon is attending to the stump.

PREPARATION OF THE STUMP
When preparing the stump the same techniques are used (as detailed above, under Preparation of the Part) with respect to skeleton, periosteum, skin incisions, and identification of nerves and veins. Two structures require additional attention.

after the superficial arch and its branches have been repaired back bleeding may occur along the metacarpal arteries; this bleeding reduces digital perfusion and often causes a significant hematoma in the palm. Such a

*Figure 44-16* With transmetacarpal amputation, the metacarpal arteries are not customarily repaired; therefore after bone fixation and repair of the common digital artery, back flow occurs through the anastomosis to the metacarpal artery, particularly, in the presence of heparinization. This sequence is likely to lead to poor peripheral flow, which progressively decreases as the hematoma in the palm enlarges. (From A. Godfrey, G. D. Lister, and H. E. Kleinert. Replantation of the Digits of the Hand. In H. Dudley and D. C. Carter (eds.), Rob and Smith's Operative Surgery. *Borough Green, Kent: Butterworths, 1984.)*

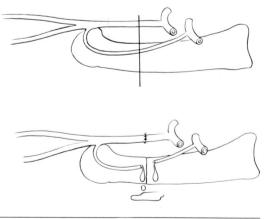

## Tendons

The flexor tendons will have retracted proximally and must be retrieved by flexing the wrist. Once retrieved they are held out at a level suitable for later repair by transfixing them proximally with 23-gauge hypodermic needles. If left until after bony fixation has been performed, retrieval is more difficult.

## Arteries

By seeking out the arteries before elevating the tourniquet, the surgeon can often locate them all simply by inspecting the stump through operating loupes for the telltale pulsations. The arteries, like the nerves and veins, are tagged with 8-0 nylon as previously described. However, before this step is done, the presence of adequate proximal flow is confirmed by gripping the end of the vessel with jeweler's forceps, drawing the vessel out to length, and cutting through three-fourths of the vessel circumference with microsurgical scissors. If good flow is not encountered, steps are taken to improve the flow. As a crude guide, flow from a digital artery should reach the end of the hand table, and flow from the ulnar or radial artery should reach the near side of the scrub nurse's table. Steps to be taken are as follows.

DILATATION OF THE VESSEL. Much has been made in the past of the sanctity of the vessel lumen. Certainly the lumen must be treated with delicate respect, but dilatation performed as described below not only confirms the presence of flow but also overcomes vascular spasm for some time. In larger vessels, dilatation can be performed using loupes and plastic intravenous cannulas of increasing dimension—a bouginage of the vessel. In smaller vessels, this step must await introduction of the microscope; the initial dilatation is performed with carefully selected jeweler's forceps or specially designed dilatation forceps [1].

MORE PROXIMAL SECTION OF THE VESSEL. By choosing to resect more vessel to obtain acceptable flow the surgeon often commits to the use of vascular grafts.

RELEASE OF PROXIMAL COMPARTMENTS. Flow may be poor even when the vessel appears entirely normal and there is a strong proximal pulse. It may be due to posttraumatic swelling in tight compartments—for example, in Guyon's canal. These swellings must be released by proximal incision and fasciotomy.

Commonly, good flow is achieved initially only to abate even if the vessel is held out to appropriate length. This sign often indicates physiologic spasm. Anastomosis and a period of warmth often overcomes this problem more satisfactorily than further manipulation of the vessel. It must certainly be tried if the vessel appears in all other respects to be good. On rare occasions further resection and grafting are required for persistent absence of flow.

## Hemostasis in the Stump

Having identified appropriate vessels carrying good flow, the surgeon takes time with the tourniquet released to achieve hemostasis. Bleeding is deliberately provoked by mechanical débridement. Otherwise, after replantation when vessel spasm abates, significant hemorrhage may ensue. This problem is especially likely with transmetacarpal amputations; in such cases, the branches of the deep palmar arch must receive particular attention.

## Replantation

When the preparation of all structures in the stump and the amputated part (or parts) is complete, the amputated part can be taken off ice and replantation commenced [10, 36, 37, 45, 61, 64, 65]. For amputations of the arm or forearm the replantation can be performed with the distal part still encased in ice packs, which gives a better chance of preserving muscle viability.

USE OF A TOURNIQUET
If continued oozing obscures the surgeon's view, the tourniquet is used after exsanguination of the extremity. The tourniquet

must be released after a maximum of 120 minutes but can be reapplied without hesitation [41] provided that (1) it has been left off for 20 minutes, (2) flow has been observed in any anastomoses for 20 minutes before reapplication, and (3) the patient has received aspirin (650 mg as a suppository at least 30 minutes before reapplication).

SEQUENCE OF REPAIR
Structures are repaired in the following sequence under normal circumstances.

*Bone*
Firm skeletal fixation by internal methods is desirable because it promotes early union [29, 56]. Joints are not fixed, thereby permitting early motion. Thus compression plates are recommended for humerus, radius, ulna, and metacarpals, and type A intraosseous wiring is recommended for phalanges. As for all osteosyntheses, attention must be given to alignment, rotation, and angulation because subsequent correctional osteotomy is a tiresome and unnecessary procedure. For multiple digital replantations, the skeleton of all digits can be fixed at this stage except (1) when ischemia time has been long (in excess of 6 hours at the stage of osteosynthesis) or (2) when arthrodesis of one digit is necessary because appropriate angulation may impede the access to adjacent digits during the microsurgical stages.

*Periosteum*
When the bone has been shortened and the periosteum carefully preserved, the periosteum can be repaired with benefit because its presence speeds union and also probably helps to prevent tendon adhesions. A 5-0 absorbable suture is usually employed.

*Flexor Tendons*
All flexor tendons are repaired by the technique we have described [46]. The tendons are sutured with as much care as in a straightforward laceration to give the best chance of good functional return. Committed as we now are to early active motion fol-lowing replantation, particular care is taken to ensure the strength and hold of the core suture, even to the length of placing two at right angles to one another. The sheath is closed, as this method has been shown to decrease the incidence of tendon adhesions [52].

*Extensor Tendons*
The extensor tendons are repaired with 4-0 or 5-0 synthetic nonabsorbable suture using a series of interrupted figure-of-eight stitches.

INTRODUCTION OF THE MICROSCOPE
At this juncture, if the tourniquet has been in use, it is released. The microscope is now introduced. The instrument employed must have the following capabilities: (1) magnification from 3.5 × to 16 × or 25 × ; (2) powerful independent lighting with a reserve lamp; (3) controls for zoom magnification and focusing; and (4) two binocular operating positions, the angles of which can be adjusted.

The microscope is positioned by the surgeon in such a way that it can be swung into place over the hand when required with no further handling. Such positioning is done immediately after the patient is prepared and draped. The surgeon at that time makes a final check that the instrument is functioning properly and ensures that the eyepieces are correctly positioned and focused for both himself or herself and the assistant.

POSITIONING FOR MICROSURGERY
The patient's hand is held immobile by some device (e.g., a lead hand) in a position that gives clear exposure of the vessels to be repaired. This position is most difficult to achieve in the case of the ulnar digital artery of the thumb over the metacarpal and proximal phalanx. To display it properly, the patient would be best placed prone, but this position is not practical. In this circumstance, as with type III ring avulsion injuries, it is best to anastomose a vascular graft to the amputated part *before* replantation. The proximal anastomosis is then done at

the usual juncture in the operation, in the case of the thumb either to the princeps pollicis or end-to-side to the radial artery. The hand must be sufficiently far away from the microsurgeon to permit the surgeon to rest his or her forearms comfortably on the hand table. The surgeon's wrists and ulnar border of the hands must also be supported, often by placing stacked towels underneath them. Tremor is thus largely eliminated. We do *not* subscribe to the view that the microsurgeon should eschew coffee, alcohol, nicotine, or whatever other pleasurable pursuits may take his or her fancy; what little tremor these substances provoke can be overcome. Nor do we consider it necessary for the experienced microsurgeon, on hearing of a pending replantation, to hasten to the animal laboratory to sharpen his or her skills. This practice seems only to add to the burden and to accelerate the onset of fatigue. It would be better to sleep as well as possible on a nearby stretcher.

VESSEL REPAIR

Looking through the microscope, the surgeon relocates the vessel ends previously tagged with 8-0 nylon. When the view of them is perfect, any adjustments or additional incisions or skin stay sutures that are required are performed. Repair can then be undertaken in the following order.

*Preparation of the Vessel*
A length of vessel on either side of the division sufficient to permit application of the approximating microvascular clamp is prepared, stripping off the adventitia by gripping the extreme end of the vessel (later to be excised) and peeling back the adventitia and attached fat with jeweler's forceps and microsurgical scissors. Any tethering branches are coagulated with bipolar microforceps.

*Excision of the Vessel End*
The end of the vessel that has been handled is excised with scissors. After the walls have

been eased apart with microforceps, a clean, smooth lumen should be revealed. Dilatation as previously described is repeated if necessary, and the vessel end thoroughly irrigated with warm heparin solution. Never again should the vessel end be gripped with forceps.

*Correction of Tension*
The surgeon must ensure that no undue tension is necessary to bring the vessel together. Vessel ends that cannot be approximated by double microvascular clamps or by the use of a 10-0 nylon suture are under excessive tension. To repair them despite such tension, by either traction on the vessel or use of a large suture, results in an unsatisfactory, difficult, leaking anastomosis that, if left uncorrected, leads to a failed replant. Undue tension can be easily overcome by use of a vascular graft.

*Suturing the Vessel*
The technique for microvascular repair has been described in Chapter 42.

*Veins*
We now repair all veins of suitable caliber. To do so before arterial repair has several advantages: reduced edema and blood loss, a field relatively clear of obscuring hemorrhage, ease of skin closure, and an appropriate "structure" to the whole performance, as the denouement after the climax of achieving flow by arterial repair is thus made brief. There are three exceptions to this sequence: when ischemia is thought to be already excessive, when serious doubt exists regarding one's ability to achieve arterial flow in a salvage replant, and when there is considerable bulk of devascularized muscle. In the last instance flow must be restored as quickly as possible. There is also considerable danger of uncontrolled acidosis if venous drainage is permitted to freely enter the circulation from that bulk of muscle. Locally, perfusion has been shown to be reduced by persistent systemic acidosis [17].

If the surgeon later ensures good arterial inflow by repairing all arteries, the only potential cause of failure in an ideal replant is congestion due to venous insufficiency, with a resultant rise in resistance to arterial runoff and later arterial thrombosis. The more veins that are repaired, therefore, the greater is the chance of survival. All veins that can be found are repaired. If insufficient veins are found dorsally during digital replantation, palmar veins are adequate, especially distal to the proximal interphalangeal joint. Whereas previously we recommended repair of a minimum of four per digit, our anatomic studies have demonstrated that the optimal number of veins varies according to the level. For example, over the proximal phalanx either one or both of the ends of the proximal venous arcade provide adequate drainage.

*Arteries*
All available arteries are now repaired using the technique described above. The vessel is observed for a period of 20 minutes after it has been sutured to ensure that flow continues [3]. The criteria for continued flow are as follows.

1. Bleeding from the amputated part, especially its veins.
2. Swift refill of the artery. It is tested by carefully emptying a segment distal to the anastomosis, which involves moving two forceps apart while they occlude the vessel and then releasing the proximal forceps (Fig. 44-17).
3. Pinkness of the extremity. This sign is not necessarily present immediately in digits replanted after a long cold ischemia time; such digits may remain pale for up to 45 minutes in the face of good flow as assessed by the first two criteria.

Poor or absent flow may be due to (1) a lack of proximal flow, (2) technically incorrect anastomosis, (3) poor runoff, or (4) spasm. The first three of these problems

have already been discussed. Spasm is a normal homeostatic mechanism that is always encountered; it must be overcome before repair by dilatation. After repair, spasm may recur, most commonly as the result of one or more of three causes [4].

1. Unhealthy vessel. The cure is resection and reanastomosis or insertion of a graft.
2. Whole blood in contact with the vessel.
3. Cold.

*Irrigation*
The second and third causes of spasm can be avoided by thorough irrigation with warm fluids after completion of the anastomosis. The irrigating fluids must be kept in a warming bath; we have found either a blood warmer with a sterile liner or regular heating lamps over the instrument table to be most useful. The choice of irrigating fluid [76] has in the past included the following.

1. Magnesium sulfate [60]. Acland [2] demonstrated the merits of this solution for preventing platelet aggregation in *experimental animals*, but he frequently denied that it has any value in thicker-walled human vessels.
2. Bupivacaine (Marcaine). Used in high doses, this agent induces bleeding from vessels adjacent to the repaired artery and thereby increases hematoma formation.
3. Heparin. Heparin has no drawbacks when used for irrigation, but it does not have advantages when applied to the outside of the vessel.
4. Papaverine.

For irrigation we currently use heparin inside the lumen before the anastomosis and warm Ringer's lactate externally after vessel repair. While the artery is being observed, any open veins are permitted to bleed freely. It is especially true with arm or forearm amputations and when there is associated crush of the part because perfusion of the part by arterial blood that does not recirculate re-

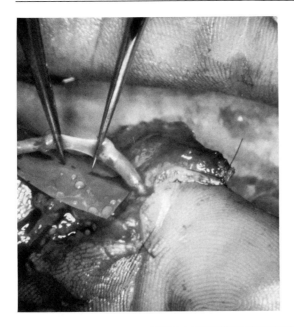 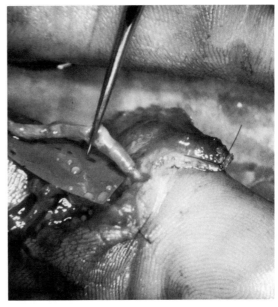

**Figure 44-17** *The sweeping test for flow. See text for explanation.*

verses lactic acidosis in the extremity while avoiding a sudden fall in systemic pH [79]. The adjacent nerve can be repaired during the period of observation.

NERVE REPAIR

The arguments for and against fascicular and epineurial repair have been presented elsewhere [45]. Suffice it to say that we believe that the best results are obtained when the fascicles are aligned without distortion or strangulation or excess use of suture material. It is possible to achieve either good or bad results according to these criteria using either technique. Attention is therefore directed less at the choice of technique than at its execution with respect to the fascicles on completion of the repair. We repair groups of fascicles on forearm major nerves and perform either fascicular or epineurial repair on digital nerves.

SKIN CLOSURE

The skin is closed in such a way as to avoid all compression that would compromise venous return. This goal can usually be achieved, especially if Z-plasties have been incorporated. In all cases, however, a critical eye is kept on the color of the digital pulps. Any duskiness or increase in speed of refill after blanching is corrected by releasing appropriate skin sutures. Occasionally, significant skin defects are left, especially with crush amputations or after prolonged ischemia. In such instances, free split-thickness skin grafts are applied. Exposure of any of the repaired vessels, even of vein grafts, do not cause concern because skin grafts take well in such circumstances. However, in the long term the scar contracture that occurs in the bed of the skin graft reduces or occludes flow, so grafts on vessels are to be avoided unless absolutely necessary.

## Special Operative Considerations
VASCULAR GRAFTS

Failure to employ vascular grafts when they are indicated is usually due to inexperience and often causes more technical difficulty for the surgeon than does their use.

### Indications for Vascular Grafts

RELUCTANCE TO SHORTEN THE SKELETON. Such reluctance may result from the need to preserve a significant joint such as the metacarpophalangeal joint of any of the digits.

FAILURE TO SHORTEN THE SKELETON ADEQUATELY. Even if skeletal shortening has been done in an attempt to avoid the need for grafts, the surgeon must not stubbornly persist in attempting anastomoses under tension.

RESECTION OF A DAMAGED VESSEL. As emphasized previously, only ideal vessels should be repaired; the operator must remember, however, that resection of long segments involves sacrificing their branches as well, which may result in loss of skin overlying the graft or in localized ischemia in bones, joints, or tendons, with effects that are still to be determined.

SHUNTING OF FLOW. Although rarely necessary, shunting of the flow may be indicated when one artery to the limb or digit is damaged proximally and the other distally. This situation is encountered only with salvage replantation following previous trauma or multiple level injuries.

DESIRE TO LENGTHEN THE COURSE OF THE ARTERY. The surgeon may wish to avoid an obvious skin defect, especially over a bed unlikely to take a free skin graft. Such defects require flap cover, but a delay of a few days may be prudent after replantation.

NEED TO IMPROVE EXPOSURE FOR MICROSURGICAL REPAIR. Such a situation arises in the thumb amputation just distal to the metacarpophalangeal joint. Often the princeps pollicis is the only important artery at this level, but it is difficult to position the hand to allow a good view of the vessel through the microscope, as the vessel lies on the ulnar aspect of the thumb. This problem can be overcome by placing a graft between the radial artery on the dorsum of the first web space and the digital artery over the proximal phalanx. These positions are both relatively accessible to the microscope. If the radial artery of the index finger is to be sacrificed in this procedure, it is first occluded with a vascular clamp; the tourniquet is then released, and flow to the index finger is confirmed.

### Vein Grafts

Veins have a remarkable capability to vary their caliber, far exceeding that of arteries. Within reason, they can often therefore be dilated enough that they almost exactly match the vessel to which they are being attached. However, if they are thereafter subjected to arterial pressure, they assume their maximum diameter, which may be disproportionately large. A vein of roughly equivalent dimension in the undisturbed state must therefore be selected from the following sites [6].

1. For digital vessels: Veins of the anterior forearm in its distal half are used (Fig. 44-18).
2. For forearm vessels: Dorsal forearm veins are used, or if it appears unwise to harvest veins from the injured arm, those from the opposite arm or from the lower part of the

**Figure 44-18** *The veins of the forearm are marked out prior to replantation as a source of satisfactory vein grafts to replace digital arteries.*

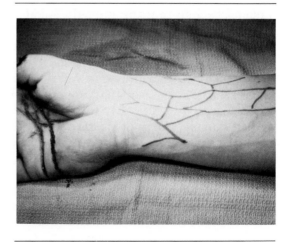

leg are used. Leg veins, if not varicose, are particularly suitable for major artery repairs, as their walls are somewhat thicker than those of the arm.

HARVESTING VEIN GRAFTS. Vein grafts are harvested under tourniquet control, as only then can small tributaries be identified and coagulated with bipolar forceps. When it is intended to use a vein graft to join one artery proximally to two or more distally, as for injuries to the superficial palmar arch, a vein with an adequate number of proximal branches is selected. These branches may be difficult to find, and if so arterial grafts are then considered (see below). Because an incision directly over the vein increases the possibility of inadvertent injury, a lazy S cut is made with the vein as its axis. The caliber of the vein is checked immediately after skin incision, because the vein goes into spasm during dissection. All branches are ligated or coagulated. Because of the great elasticity of veins, the necessary length of graft (as previously measured) is marked off before sectioning either end; it is most conveniently done with 10-0 nylon sutures in the wall. If a great length is required, the sutures are placed on the same aspect of the vein to aid in avoiding torsion. Some convention is employed to indicate the direction of flow so that the venous valves are not an impediment. We place a ligature on the proximal end of the vein and none on the distal end. More graft than is required is taken. The graft must be correctly oriented for flow.

ANASTOMOSIS. The technique of anastomosis is similar to that described above; only a few additional points need to be made. The first end to be anastomosed must be that from which flow is to come. Note that the double clamp holds the vessels for repair, but the vessels can be further stabilized by applying distal traction to the graft.

SIZE DISCREPANCY. There is often a discrepancy in caliber between graft and vessel. If it does not exceed 2:1, it presents few problems. Sutures are inserted as already de-

scribed, first dividing the circumference of each side of the repair into thirds, and then dividing each third into thirds. The discrepancy is thus distributed evenly around the repair. When such a discrepancy exceeds 2:1, a new graft of better fit must be taken.

BLOOD FLOW IN THE GRAFT. After the first anastomosis is completed, there are benefits in allowing flow through the graft.

1. Torsion is avoided, as the flow straightens out the graft.
2. Flow can be confirmed: If the anastomosis is faulty, it must be revised. Using this method, the revision can be done before the graft is cut to length.
3. The length of graft required can be more accurately judged. Vein grafts lengthen marvelously under the influence of arterial pressure.
4. Leaks can be repaired at the proximal anastomosis and along the graft, allowing the surgeon to concentrate on distal leaks after the second repair.

If the surgeon is concerned about leaving blood static in the graft while the second repair is done, a clamp can be reapplied proximal to the first anastomosis and the graft washed out with heparin saline. However, we find this step unnecessary.

CHECKING GRAFT SIZE. Despite all efforts to prevent it, the graft may be too long once flow is fully established through a vein graft. This situation results in kinking, with a significant reduction in perfusion. The surgeon must not hesitate to take out a segment of vessel at the site of repair and redo it; 15 to 20 minutes spent on another anastomosis seems especially inconsequential when one is faced with an underperfused replantation on the following day.

*Arterial Grafts*
When long segments of an artery are to be replaced, and especially when one proximal vessel is to be joined to several distally, vein grafts have two major shortcomings. First,

it is impossible to obtain a good match in caliber at both ends. Second, sufficient branches without valves are difficult to find. In such circumstances arterial grafts present a much superior solution [23]. Although the superficial temporal artery can be used (Fig. 44-19), the subscapular tree with its many scapular, thoracodorsal, and serratus branches presents an ideal source of spare parts, familiar to the microsurgeon. When the need is anticipated, the chest wall can be prepared and opened by a second team to display a major portion of the subscapular system. Segments of the correct length and caliber and having sufficient branches can be selected by the replantation surgeon once the exact needs have been determined.

When a long graft with, at most, one branch is required, the posterior interosseous artery is ideal and readily accessible. It is now my practice to use this artery routinely for all thumb replantations distal to the metacarpophalangeal joint, performing the first anastomosis to the unattached thumb.

*Composite skin and vein grafts* may be used where both are required on the dorsum of the finger. Such composites, which have been called "venous flaps" by some, can be taken from an adjacent finger or from the dorsum of the foot [28].

LEVELS OF AMPUTATION
Certain factors are peculiar to replantations at different levels of amputation.

*Arm and Forearm*
There is a significant bulk of ischemic muscle in the arm and forearm. For this reason, arterial repair in most cases follows bone fixation in order to reestablish circulation at the earliest moment. The vessels are sturdy and can be repaired with 8-0 nylon, which can withstand the disturbance caused by subsequent muscle and nerve repair. During the period of bone fixation, metabolism in the extremity can be lowered by keeping it packed in ice. Even with these precautions,

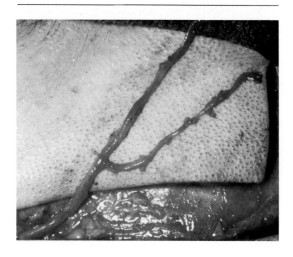

**Figure 44-19** *The superficial temporal artery provides a satisfactory arterial graft for replacement of long arterial segments.*

fasciotomy of the forearm and intrinsic muscular compartments is performed.

After bone fixation it is beneficial if two surgeons can work simultaneously; one starts with the ulnar artery repair and works across the anterior aspect of the arm, while the other commences with the radial artery and then moves on the tendons of the thumb, the radial nerve, and the extensors.

*Wrist*
In addition to the considerations discussed above, the wrist (Fig. 44-20) presents the problem of bone shortening at the level of an important joint. It can be resolved by any one of three methods.

1. Excision of the joint and primary arthrodesis: This procedure is particularly appropriate when the joint surfaces have been damaged, and it has distinct merit in the person who does heavy manual labor.
2. Proximal row carpectomy: Most appropriate in sedentary workers, this procedure has drawbacks that are well recognized.
3. Shortening osteotomy of the radius and a Darrach procedure: Described in Japan,

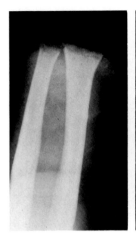 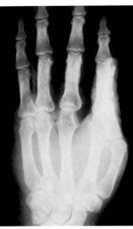 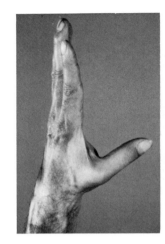 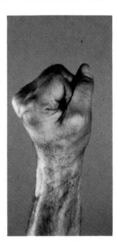

**Figure 44-20** *Disarticulation amputation through the wrist can be replanted with satisfactory restoration of function. (Case courtesy of Dr. L. R. Scheker.)*

this technique is a modification that preserves function while facilitating the repair of all structures.

*Transmetacarpal Area*
As stated already, the prevention of hematoma is of great importance in the transmetacarpal area; consequently, special precautions must be taken before replantation. Here most of all, postoperative anticoagulant therapy is probably contraindicated.

*Proximal Phalanx*
In the proximal phalanx (the "no man's land" of Bunnell), tendon repairs are all-important. The consequences of prolonged ischemia are much less devastating with digital replantation; therefore time can be devoted to a careful primary tendon repair. Whenever possible the joints are left free, and active and gentle passive motion is commenced on the first day after replantation (Fig. 44-21). Rubber band traction is not indicated because of the extensor tendon repair.

*Proximal Interphalangeal Joint*
If the proximal interphalangeal joint is destroyed, the arthrodesis must be in the most

functional position. In the index finger, it is in this position that the pulp can be most readily approximated to that of the thumb: 0 to 20 degrees, according to the amount of shortening. In the other fingers, it is the greatest angle that can be achieved at the joint while still allowing the tip of the finger to extend to the plane of the palm of the hand by hyperextension of the metacarpophalangeal joint. It is usually an angle of 30, 40, and 50 degrees in the middle, ring, and small fingers, respectively.

*Middle Phalanx*
Beyond the superficialis insertion in the middle phalanx, sensation is all-important, and the chances of excellent sensory recovery are high. Although apparently unnecessary, replantation at this level is relatively straightforward and gives good functional results [54, 83, 92].

*Distal Phalanx*
Replantation at the level of the distal phalanx [25] is largely cosmetic (and none the worse for that), with the notable exception

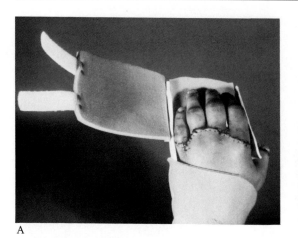

A

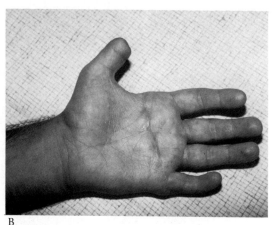

B

**Figure 44-21** *A. After replantation of all four digits at the level of the metacarpophalangeal joint, a palmar support splint with the wrist in flexion was fitted. Active motion was undertaken commencing on the first postoperative day with a relatively satisfactory range of motion on review 1 year later (B, C).*

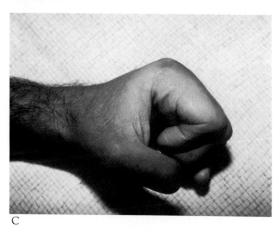

C

of the thumb; in the thumb the absence of the nail seriously hinders the ability to pick up thin, flat objects. If the amputation is through the nailbed, the sequence of repair is unique. The tip of the nail is stabilized by both a Kirschner wire placed retrogradely through the amputated phalanx and suture of the palmar skin. Vessel repair is performed looking from the dorsal view past the unreduced bone; there are five or six vessels, both arteries and veins, on the palmar periosteum, any one of which requires only three to six 10-0 sutures. The bone is reduced and pinned, and the nailbed is repaired. Replantation at the level of the distal phalanx usually takes less than 2 hours and can be done on an outpatient basis (Fig. 44-22).

## Dressing

Although understandably fatigued, the replantation surgeon can ensure better results if he or she applies or supervises the dressing of the hand (Fig. 44-23).

**1.** The initial dressing of paraffin gauze is laid in longitudinal strips onto the wound, with fluffed dry gauze applied in abundance over it, again longitudinally. No circumferential dressings are applied below the next layer, which is of plastic sponge.

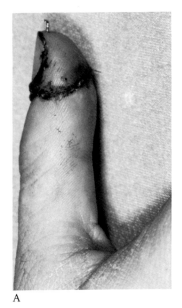
A

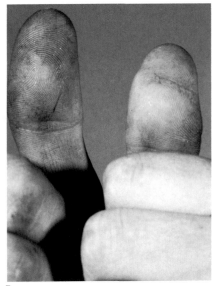
B

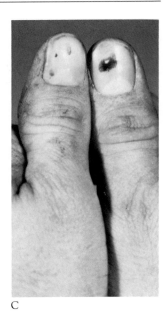
C

2. A plastic sponge 1 to 3 cm thick is wrapped once around the entire limb, leaving a gap down one side; it is held in place by a circumferential stretch gauze bandage. The sponge extends out as far as the tips of the fingers.

3. Plaster of Paris is then applied over the customary paper felt bandage. This plaster is again laid on longitudinally; it must pass around the flexed elbow in "sugar tong" fashion and incorporate a plaster sling beyond the fingertips, from which the limb is suspended.

4. The fingers are checked on one final occasion for circulation and for the absence of constrictive dressings.

5. The arm is elevated above the elbow using the plaster sling or a 15-cm stockinette.

## Postoperative Care
### SMOKING
We do not permit cigarette smoking after microsurgical procedures, although we concede that the evidence to support this rule is contradictory [89, 91].

*Figure 44-22* *A. Replantation at the level of the nail bed of the thumb is a worthwhile procedure especially if undertaken as an outpatient. B, C. The outcome is superior to any other form of thumb tip reconstruction.*

### MEDICATION
We have at various times employed all the drugs that have been recommended to assist microvascular repairs. We have dispensed with most of them and will probably discard the remainder in the near future. Antibiotics are given until 2 days after replantation unless some indication exists to continue therapy. The other medications we use are detailed below.

*Ideal Replantation*
Aspirin, 650 mg, is given every second day.

*Salvage Replantation*
DEXTRAN 40. This agent is the additive therapy most often used, in doses of 500 ml every 12 hours.

HEPARIN. In certain cases, especially when it has not been possible to ensure that all vessels employed are in perfect condition (as in crush injuries), we still administer hepa-

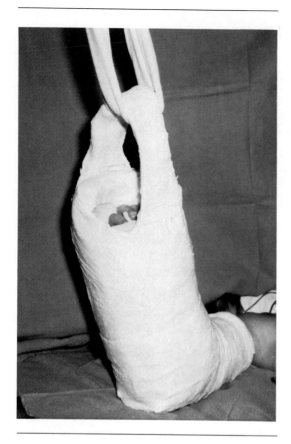

**Figure 44-23** *The dressing used after replantation must support the patient under the elbow. Circumferential compressive dressings on the hand that may hinder satisfactory circulation are avoided.*

rin by continuous intravenous infusion. The initial dose, given before flow is permitted to pass through the first anastomosis, is 100 mg (or 10,000 IU) in the adult. Thereafter doses are titrated against 6-hour estimations of the activated partial thromboplastin time, which is kept at a level two and one-half times that of the control. As our confidence in the technique of replantation has increased, however, we have used heparin less because of its disadvantages [7, 70]. It can cause allergic reactions, internal hemorrhage, and uncontrolled bleeding from the extremity. The patient may require transfusion (with its attendant dangers) and protamine neutral-

ization (with a possibility of increased clotting by the elimination of endogenous heparin). Hemorrhage at the site of replant may cause acute vasospasm, with resultant failure and chronic fibrosis, which in turn reduces function.

PROTHROMBIN DEPRESSANTS. In those cases in which heparin had been employed, prothrombin depressants are substituted; they are introduced on the third day in doses sufficient to reduce prothrombin activity to 20 to 30 percent of normal.

OTHER TREATMENTS. Venous congestion, when no further venous repairs can be accomplished, can be relieved by (1) removal of the nail plate and application of a heparin pledget [24]; (2) a "fish-mouth" incision and similar local anticoagulant; (3) the use of leeches [26]; or (4) employing custom-made "milking" devices [39].

OBSERVATION
*Circulation Checks*
Initially, circulation checks [41] are performed at hourly intervals.

COLOR OF THE NAILBED AND RETURN OF BLOOD AFTER BLANCHING. If the color is pale, with slow return, arterial insufficiency is present; if the color is dark red, with swift return, there is venous congestion. The perfect response exists when the color is pink, with return comparable to that in adjacent digits. The pinkness of a good replantation tends to diminish after 4 to 5 days and should not cause concern.

DRESSING CHECKS. Even when circumferential dressings are not used, dressings soaked in blood that has congealed can be a potent source of constriction. When dressings are adherent or heavily blood-stained, they must be carefully removed and replaced. With the dressing described above, it can be done easily without changing the outer sponge and plaster casting. Heavy bloodstaining of dressings is a clue to the presence of venous insufficiency. Replanted parts with good hemostasis and good venous outflow bleed little.

TEMPERATURE. Using a thermocouple, temperature is a useful guide [64, 75], especially when the adjacent fingers were not injured and can be used for comparison. A fall of temperature below 30°C is an indication for immediate exploration.

*Other Methods of Checking Flow*

DIGITAL PULSE MONITOR AND ULTRASONOGRAPHY. When these aids are required because there is doubt regarding color and refill, reexploration is usually already indicated.

TRANSCUTANEOUS PO$_2$. See references 32 and 51 for a discussion of transcutaneous PO$_2$.

REEXPLORATION

Like fasciotomy and tracheostomy, exploration of a replantation is necessary if the surgeon even considers it. The situation invariably proves to be worse than anticipated. Provided it is undertaken in good time, reexploration is a worthwhile procedure, often necessitating the use of vascular grafts. With experience, our rate of reexploration has fallen steadily.

## Late Problems

NONUNION AND MALUNION

Originally not uncommon, skeletal problems such as nonunion and malunion have been virtually eliminated by the use of greater care when obtaining rigid internal fixation of congruous bone ends. Prolonged ischemia appears to increase the chances of nonunion [40].

MUSCLE CONTRACTURES

Wherever significant muscle bulk has remained ischemic for more than 6 hours, contractures are probable. Intrinsic contractures can be released, and when necessary their function can be taken over by tendon transfers. Ischemic contracture of the forearm muscles presents a much greater problem, which is dealt with elsewhere.

INADEQUATE SENSATION

The higher the amputation, the more does inadequate sensation become a problem. However, if adequate shortening has been performed and the limb is well vascularized, we have found the results of nerve repair during replantation to be at least as good as those of a conventional primary repair [22, 88, 93].

JOINT STIFFNESS

Every effort is made to avoid transfixing joints with the internal fixation necessary for replantation. If it has been successfully avoided, limited range-of-motion exercises are commenced on the first postoperative day. The joints are then passively manipulated when the dressing is first changed at 5 days.

TENDON ADHESIONS

The single greatest cause of poor function with replantation—tendon adhesions—can be somewhat reduced by meticulous repair and early active exercise. Active exercise is commenced despite the obvious hazard of possible rupture, as the latter danger is outweighed by the problem of adhesion. When adhesions have occurred, tenolysis or tendon graft (with or without preliminary rods) has thus far produced only limited improvement.

Secondary procedures, most often tenolysis, are required with some 50 percent of replantation procedures [19]. The eventual functional outcome is related to the level and mechanism of injury [71].

## Organization

Successful replantation requires organization.

SURGEONS

Replantation is undertaken by the lone surgeon only after careful consideration of the consequences. It is not the single-digit amputation on any given day that seriously disrupts a surgical practice but the three-finger amputation in yet another patient on the following day. Regular replantation requires at least three surgeons capable of such work, with skilled assistance.

NURSES

In the emergency and operating rooms, smooth progress is possible only with the presence of nurses knowledgeable in the management of amputated parts, operating microscopes, and microsurgical instruments. In the ward, nurses practiced in evaluation of circulation and handling of dressings are essential if otherwise salvageable extremities are not to be lost.

PLANNING

When confronted with a multiple-digit replantation, the surgeon must plan the procedure to ensure maximum efficiency. With the involvement of three or four surgeons and assistants, the operation can proceed swiftly in stages, each done by different pairs. Thus no surgeon need operate for more than 4 to 6 hours without rest during a case that may take more than 24 hours.

## *References*

1. Acland, R. New instruments for microvascular surgery. *Br. J. Surg.* 59:181, 1972.
2. Acland, R. Prevention of thrombosis in microvascular surgery by the use of magnesium sulphate. *Br. J. Plast. Surg.* 25:292, 1972.
3. Acland, R. Signs of patency in small vessel anastomosis. *Surgery* 72:744, 1972.
4. Acland, R. Thrombus formation in microvascular surgery: An experimental study of the effects of surgical trauma. *Surgery* 73:766, 1973.
5. Alpert, B. S., and Buncke, H. J. Mutilating multidigital injuries: Use of a free microvascular flap from a nonreplantable part. *J. Hand Surg.* 3:196, 1978.
6. Alpert, B. S., Buncke, H. J., and Brownstein, M. Replacement of arteries and veins with vein grafts when replanting crushed, amputated fingers. *Plast. Reconstr. Surg.* 61:17, 1978.
7. Ariyan, S., and Stansel, H. C. Further hazards of heparin therapy in vascular surgery. *Arch. Surg.* 111:120, 1976.
8. Biemer, E., Duspiva, W., Herndl, E., et al. Early experiences in organizing and running a replantation service. *Br. J. Plast. Surg.* 31:9, 1978.
9. Biemer, E., Stock, W., Wolfensberger, Ch., et al. Successful replantation of a totally avulsed scalp. *Br. J. Plast. Surg.* 32:19, 1979.
10. Buncke, H. J., and Schultz, W. P. Experimental digital amputation and reimplantation. *Plast. Reconstr. Surg.* 36:62, 1965.
11. Buncke, H. J., Rose, E. H., Brownstein, M. J., et al. Successful replantation of two avulsed scalps by microvascular anastomoses. *Plast. Reconstr. Surg.* 61:666, 1978.
12. Chiu, H. Y., and Chen, M. T. Revascularization of digits after thirty-three hours of warm ischemia time: A case report. *J. Hand Surg.* 9A:63, 1984.
13. Chiu, H. Y., Lu, S. Y., Lin, T. W., et al. Transposition digital replantation. *J. Trauma* 25:440, 1985.
14. Chow, J., Bilos, J., and Chumprapaph, B. Thirty thumb replantations: Indications and results. *Plast. Reconstr. Surg.* 64:626, 1979.
15. Chow, J. A., Bilos, Z. J., Chunprapaph, B., et al. Forearm replantation—long-term functional results. *Ann. Plast. Surg.* 10:15, 1983.
16. Cohen, B. E., May, J. W., Daly, J. S., et al. Successful clinical replantation of an amputated penis by microneurovascular repair. *Plast. Reconstr. Surg.* 59:276, 1977.
17. Dell, P. C., Seaber, A. V., and Urbaniak, J. R. The effect of systemic acidosis on perfusion of replanted extremities. *J. Hand Surg.* 5:433, 1980.
18. Earley, M. J., and Watson, J. S. Twenty-four thumb replantations. *J. Hand Surg.* [Br.] 9:98, 1984.
19. Frey, M., Mandl, H., and Holle, J. Secondary operations after replantations. *Chir. Plast.* 5:235, 1980.
20. Furnas, D. W. Growth and development in replanted forelimbs. *Plast. Reconstr. Surg.* 46:445, 1970.
21. Gatti, J. E., and LaRossa, D. Scalp avulsions

and review of successful replantation. *Ann. Plast. Surg.* 6:127, 1981.

22. Gelberman, R., Urbaniak, J., Bright, D., et al. Digital sensibility following replantation. *J. Hand Surg.* 3:313, 1978.

23. Godina, M. Arterial autografts in microvascular surgery. *Plast. Reconstr. Surg.* 78:293, 1986.

24. Gordon, L., Leitner, D. W., Buncke, H. J., et al. Partial nail plate removal after digital replantation as an alternative method of venous drainage. *J. Hand Surg. [Am.]* 10:360, 1985.

25. Grandis, C., and Mantero, R. Replantation of small segments of the distal phalanx of the digits. *Ann. Chir. Main* 2:283, 1983.

26. Henderson, H. P., Matti, B., Laing, A. G., et al. Avulsion of the scalp treated by microvascular repair: The use of leeches for postoperative decongestion. *Br. J. Plast. Surg.* 36:235, 1983.

27. Hentz, V. R., Palma, C. R., Elliott, E., et al. Successful replantation of a totally avulsed scalp following prolonged ischemia. *Ann. Plast. Surg.* 7:145, 1981.

28. Honda, T., Nomura, S., Yamauchi, S., et al. The possible applications of a composite skin and subcutaneous vein graft in the replantation of amputated digits. *Br. J. Plast. Surg.* 37:607, 1984.

29. Ikuta, Y. Method of bone fixation in reattachment of amputations in the upper extremities. *Clin. Orthop.* 133:169, 1978.

30. Jaeger, S. H., Tsai, T. M., and Kleinert, H. E. Upper extremity replantation in children. *Orthop. Clin. North Am.* 12:897, 1981.

31. Jupiter, J. B., Tsai, T. M., and Kleinert, H. E. Salvage replantation of lower limb amputations. *Plast. Reconstr. Surg.* 69:1, 1982.

32. Keller, H. P., and Lanz, U. Objective control of replanted fingers by transcutaneous partial $O_2$ ($PO_2$) measurement. *Microsurgery* 5:85, 1984.

33. Kleinert, H. E., and Kasdan, M. L. Restoration of blood flow in upper extremity injuries. *J. Trauma* 3:461, 1963.

34. Kleinert, H. E., Jablon, M., and Tsai, T. An overview of replantation and results of 347 replants in 245 patients. *J. Trauma* 20:390, 1980.

35. Kleinert, H. E., Kasdan, M. L., and Romero, J. L. Small blood vessel anastomosis for salvage of severely injured upper extremity. *J. Bone Joint Surg. [Am.]* 45:788, 1963.

36. Kleinert, H. E., Kutz, J. E., Atasoy, E., et al. Replantation of nonviable digits—ten years' experience. *J. Bone Joint Surg. [Am.]* 56:1092, 1974.

37. Kleinert, H. E., Serafin, D., Kutz, J. E., et al. Reimplantation of amputated digits and hands. *Orthop. Clin. North Am.* 4:957, 1973.

38. Komatsu, S., and Tamai, S. Successful replantation of a completely cut-off thumb. *Plast. Reconstr. Surg.* 43:374, 1968.

39. Kotani, H., Kawai, S., Doi, K., et al. Automatic milking apparatus for the insufficient venous drainage of the replanted digit. *Microsurgery* 5:90, 1984.

40. Kuwata, N., Kawai, S., and Doi, K. Clinical and experimental studies of bone union in reimplantation of digits: A preliminary report on ischemic interval. *Microsurgery* 5:30, 1984.

41. Lendvay, P. G. Replacement of the amputated digit. *Br. J. Plast. Surg.* 26:398, 1973.

42. Lesavoy, M. A. Successful replantation of lower leg and foot, with good sensibility and function. *Plast. Reconstr. Surg.* 64:760, 1979.

43. Lister, G. D. Mikrochirurgisch probleme der replantation. *Handchirurgie* 9(2):45, 1977.

44. Lister, G. D. Intraosseous wiring of the digital skeleton. *J. Hand. Surg.* 3:427, 1978.

45. Lister, G. D. Microsurgery in Nerve Repair. In D. Lamb and K. Kuczynski (eds.), *A Practice of Hand Surgery*. London: Blackwell, 1981. Pp. 192–199.

46. Lister, G. D., Kleinert, H. E., Kutz, J. E., et al. Primary flexor tendon repair followed by immediate controlled mobilization. *J. Hand Surg.* 2:441, 1977.

47. Lobay, G. W., and Moysa, G. L. Primary neurovascular bundle transfer in the management of avulsed thumbs. *J. Hand Surg.* 6:31, 1981.

48. Malt, R. A., and McKhann, C. F. Replantation of severed arms. *J.A.M.A.* 189:716, 1964.

49. Malt, R. A., Remensnyder, J. P., and Harris, W. H. Long-term utility of replanted arms. *Ann. Surg.* 176:334, 1972.

50. Mamakos, M. S. Lower extremity replantation—two and a half-year follow-up. *Ann. Plast. Surg.* 8:305, 1982.

51. Matson, F. A., Bach, A. W., Wyss, C. R., et al. Transcutaneous $PO_2$: A potential monitor of the status of replanted limb parts. *Plast. Reconstr. Surg.* 65:732, 1980.

52. Matthews, P., and Richards, H. Factors in the

adherence of flexor tendon after repair. *J. Bone Joint Surg. [Br.]* 58:230, 1976.

53. May, J. W. Digit replantation with full survival after 28 hours of cold ischemia. *Plast. Reconstr. Surg.* 67:566, 1981.

54. May, J. W., Toth, B. A., and Gardner, M. Digital replantation distal to the proximal interphalangeal joint. *J. Hand Surg.* 7:161, 1982.

55. McGrouther, D. A., Chan, T. S., Downie, P. A., et al. Reconstruction of a scalp avulsion injury by replantation and a local skin flap. *Br. J. Plast. Surg.* 34:44, 1981.

56. Meuli, H., Meyer, V., and Segmuller, G. Stabilization of bone in replantation surgery of the upper limb. *Clin. Orthop.* 133:179, 1978.

57. Miller, G. D. H., Anstee, E. J., and Snell, J. A. Successful replantation of an avulsed scalp by microvascular anastomoses. *Plast. Reconstr. Surg.* 58:133, 1976.

58. Mitchell, G. M., Morrison, W. A., Papadopoulos, A., et al. A study of the extent and pathology of experimental avulsion injury in rabbit arteries and veins. *Br. J. Plast. Surg.* 38:278, 1985.

59. Nissenbaum, M. A surgical approach for replantation of complete digital amputations. *J. Hand Surg.* 65:58, 1980.

60. Nomoto, H., Buncke, H. J., and Chater, N. L. Improved patency rates in microvascular surgery when using magnesium sulfate and a silicone rubber vascular cuff. *Plast. Reconstr. Surg.* 54:157, 1974.

61. O'Brien, B. McC. Replantation surgery. *Clin. Plast. Surg.* 1:3, 1974.

62. O'Brien, B. McC. Replantation and reconstructive microsurgery surgery. Part 1. *Ann. R. Coll. Surg. Engl.* 58:87, 1976.

63. O'Brien, B. McC. Replantation and reconstructive microvascular surgery. Part 2. *Ann. R. Coll. Surg. Engl.* 58:171, 1976.

64. O'Brien, B. McC. *Microvascular Reconstructive Surgery.* Edinburgh: Churchill Livingstone, 1977.

65. O'Brien, B. McC., and Miller, G. D. H. Digital reattachment and revascularization. *J. Bone Joint Surg. [Am.]* 55:714, 1973.

66. O'Brien, B. McC., Franklin, J. D., Morrison, W. A., et al. Replantation and revascularisation surgery in children. *Hand* 12:12, 1980.

67. O'Brien, B. McC., MacLeod, A. M., and Miller, G. D. H. Clinical replantation of digits. *Plast. Reconstr. Surg.* 52:490, 1973.

68. Pennington, D. G., and Pelly, A. D. Successful replantation of a completely avulsed ear by microvascular anastomosis. *Plast. Reconstr. Surg.* 65:820, 1980.

69. Pho, R., Chacha, P., and Yeo, K. Rerouting vessels and nerves from other digits in replanting an avulsed and degloved thumb. *Plast. Reconstr. Surg.* 64:330, 1979.

70. Poole, M. D., and Bowen, J. E. Two unusual bleedings during anticoagulation following digital replantation. *Br. J. Plast. Surg.* 30:267, 1977.

71. Russell, R. C., O'Brien, B. McC., Morrison, W. A., et al. The late functional results of upper limb revascularisation and replantation. *J. Hand Surg. [Am.]* 9:623, 1984.

72. Schlenker, J. D., Kleinert, H. E., and Tsai, T. Methods and results of replantation following traumatic amputation of the thumb in sixty-four patients. *J. Hand Surg.* 5:63, 1980.

73. Spira, M., Daniel, R., and Agris, J. Successful replantation of totally avulsed scalp, with profuse regrowth of hair: Case report. *Plast. Reconstr. Surg.* 62:447, 1978.

74. Stewart, D. E., and Lowrey, M. R. Replantation surgery following self-inflicted amputation. *Can. J. Psychiatry* 25:143, 1980.

75. Stirrat, C., Seaber, A., Urbaniak, J., et al. Temperature monitoring in digital replantation. *J. Hand Surg.* 3:342, 1978.

76. Swartz, W. M., Brink, R. R., and Buncke, H. J. Prevention of thrombosis in arterial and venous microanastomoses by using topical agents. *Plast. Reconstr. Surg.* 58:478, 1976.

77. Tamai, S. Twenty years' experience of limb replantation—review of 293 upper extremity replants. *J. Hand Surg.* 7:549, 1982.

78. Tamai, S., Nakamura, Y., and Motomiya, Y. Microsurgical replantation of a completely amputated penis and scrotum. *Plast. Reconstr. Surg.* 60:287, 1977.

79. Tamai, S., Tatsumi, Y., Shimizu, T., et al. Traumatic amputations of digits: The fate of remaining blood. An experimental and clinical study. *J. Hand Surg.* 2:13, 1977.

80. Tantri, D. P., Cervino, A. L., and Tabbal, N. Replantation of the totally avulsed scalp. *J. Trauma* 20:350, 1980.

81. Tsai, T. M., Manstein, C., DuBou, R., et al. Primary microsurgical repair of ring avulsion amputation injuries. *J. Hand Surg. [Am.]* 9A; 68, 1984.

82. Urbaniak, J. R., Evans, J. P., and Bright, D. S. Microvascular management of ring avulsion injuries. *J. Hand Surg.* 6:25, 1981.

83. Urbaniak, J. R., Roth, J. H., Nunley, J. A., et al. The results of replantation after amputation of a single finger. *J. Bone Joint Surg. [Am.]* 67:611, 1985.

84. Usui, M., Minami, M., and Ishii, S. Successful replantation of an amputated leg in a child. *Plast. Reconstr. Surg.* 63:613, 1979.

85. VanBeek, A. L., and Zook, E. G. Scalp replantation by microsurgical revascularization: Case report. *Plast. Reconstr. Surg.* 61:774, 1978.

86. Wei, F. C., McKee, N. H., Huerta, F. J., et al. Microsurgical replantation of a completely amputated penis. *Ann. Plast. Surg.* 10:317, 1983.

87. Weiland, A. J., Villarreal-Rios, A., Kleinert, H. E., et al. Replantation of digits and hands: Analysis of surgical techniques and functional results in 71 patients with 86 replantations. *J. Hand Surg.* 2:1, 1977.

88. White, J. C. Nerve regeneration after replantation of severed arms. *Ann. Surg.* 170:715, 1969.

89. Wilson, G. R., and Jones, B. M. The damaging effect of smoking on digital revascularisation: Two further case reports. *Br. J. Plast. Surg.* 37:613, 1984.

90. Wray, R. C., Young, V. L., and Weeks, P. M. Flexible-implant arthroplasty and finger replantation. *Plast. Reconstr. Surg.* 74:97, 1984.

91. Yaffe, B., Cushin, B. J., and Strauch, B. Effect of cigarette smoking on experimental microvascular anastomoses. *Microsurgery* 5:70, 1984.

92. Yamano, Y. Replantation of the amputated distal part of the fingers. *J. Hand Surg. [Am.]* 10:211, 1985.

93. Yamauchi, S., Nomura, S., Yoshimura, M., et al. A clinical study of the order and speed of sensory recovery after digital replantation. *J. Hand Surg.* 8:545, 1983.

# 45

Luis O. Vásconez
John B. McCraw
Alberto G. Camargos

# Muscle, Musculocutaneous, and Fasciocutaneous Flaps

Present anatomic knowledge as well as increasing clinical experience demonstrates that the blood supply to the skin comes from multiple sources, including distinct arteries that course under the skin and supply it. Examples include the superficial temporal, dorsalis pedis, and superficial circumflex iliac arteries supplying the forehead, dorsum of the foot, and "groin flap." Flaps based on these vessels are called *axial flaps.* The demonstration that the overlying skin remains alive so long as the underlying muscle and major vascular supply is maintained intact indicates that the skin is supplied from vessels that emanate through the muscle and perforate the fascia toward the skin (musculocutaneous flaps). A third source of blood supply to the skin are the septocutaneous vessels that perforate and course on top of the fascia. These vessels could be direct branches from the major arteries or segmental branches from larger arteries that course through the intermuscular septum, perforate the fascia, and arborize on top of it to supply the skin. They are the basis for the so-called fasciocutaneous and septocutaneous flaps that have been described for the trunk and lower legs.

There may be other sources of blood supply, and even more important, the same piece of skin may be supplied from multiple sources so that if one ligates or destroys one vessel the overlying skin does not necessarily die. A clear example is to make an incision in the anterior thigh and ligate the major vessel that supplies the rectus femoris muscle. Neither the muscle nor the overlying skin would necrose.

This multifactorial source of blood supply is important to remember and helps in the understanding and design of successful flaps based on a reliable source of blood supply. Although this chapter describes specifically our knowledge and guidelines of the various musculocutaneous and fasciocutaneous flaps, it is emphasized that the student must always remember the multifactorial sources of blood supply to the skin and thus be able to evaluate new knowledge as it is described.

## Terminology
The *muscle flap* consists of muscle detached from its normal origin or insertion and transposed to another location. The flap may remain attached to its intact blood supply or be completely detached and transferred as a "free" muscle flap.

A *musculocutaneous flap* is a composite of muscle and overlying skin, the cutaneous

*1113*

segment. Whereas the blood supply to a simple skin flap is either random or axial, the muscle of this flap is a carrier for the skin, providing a blood supply via perforators. Most muscles have several vascular pedicles. The dominant vascular pedicle is capable of providing nutritional support to a large segment of muscle when other adjacent vascular pedicles are ligated. The point of entry of the dominant vascular pedicle into the musculocutaneous flap is pivotal for rotation and thus determines the mobility of the flap. This point is the *axis of rotation*. The *arc of rotation*, or *reach*, is the area the flap covers when elevated on its dominant vascular pedicle. The exact reach varies with the person's build and in general is greater for thin individuals. It must be emphasized that the arc of rotation is greater in the cadaver because the muscles are flaccid and free of scarring.

The *fasciocutaneous flap* includes the skin, subcutaneous tissue, and underlying fascia, which may be distinct from the fascia covering the underlying muscle. The sources of blood supply to the fasciocutaneous flap are varied and may include a perforating vessel from the underlying muscle or direct or longitudinal vessels coursing on top of the fascia. Clinical experience has demonstrated a number of anatomic territories of safe fasciocutaneous flaps. In some of them the blood supply has not been completely delineated.

A *septocutaneous flap* refers to flaps in the lower leg that are supplied through segmental branches from the three major arteries of the leg, which usually course along the intermuscular septum, perforate the fascia, and supply the overlying subcutaneous tissue and skin. Each septocutaneous artery supplies a segment of overlying skin, arborizes, and forms anastomoses with the adjacent superior and inferior septocutaneous vessels. If one maintains intact one of these vessels, one can design a flap superiorly or inferiorly as an island or as a turnover flap. Although studied in the leg, it is likely that this system of septocutaneous vessels may also be present in other parts of the body, particularly the arm.

## Muscle and Musculocutaneous Flaps

In 1906 Ombredanne of Paris [17] published the first report of a planned muscle flap using the pectoralis minor muscle to recreate a breast mound following mastectomy. Tanzini introduced the latissimus dorsi muscle and its overlying skin for postmastectomy chest wall reconstruction. In 1912 D'Este also described the use of the latissimus dorsi musculocutaneous flap. In 1918 Cole described the use of flaps for the treatment of wounds involving the mucous membrane of the mouth and nose [4]. Owens described a compound neck pedicle for repairing large facial defects in 1955 [18], and in 1965 Bakamjian employed this same compound skin and sternocleidomastoid flap to close large palatal defects resulting from radical maxillectomy for cancer [1]. The principle of musculocutaneous flaps was again reported in 1968 by Hueston and McConchie when they described the compound pectoral flap [9]. However, it was not until Orticochea in 1972 [18] reported his work with compound muscle and skin flaps that the principle became popular and widely accepted. He used the term *musculocutaneous* flap when he reported a cross-thigh gracilis musculocutaneous flap. Later the term *myocutaneous* flap was introduced for the sake of brevity [14, 15]. During the mid-1970s, Ger [5, 6] further developed the understanding of muscle flaps with numerous descriptions of their use to close complicated skin defects. Vasconez expanded the applications of the muscle flap [23, 24] and introduced the concept of variable vascular dominance, as well as the possibility that cutaneous regions have blood supplies from multiple systems. The latter understanding led to classic publications by McCraw et al. [13–15] and others

[11, 12] describing many new muscle and musculocutaneous flaps and their independent vascular territories.

## CLASSIFICATION OF MUSCULOCUTANEOUS FLAPS

Several authors have attempted classifications for muscle and musculocutaneous flaps. As our understanding of skin and muscle vascular anatomy evolves so does our need for a better system. Mathes and Nahai [11] reported one of the earlier systems based on anatomic variables: (1) regional source of arterial pedicles entering the muscle; (2) size of the pedicles; (3) number of pedicles; (4) location in relation to origin and insertion; and (5) angiographic patterns of muscle vasculature. Based on such variables these authors defined five patterns of muscle circulation.

Bonnel in 1985 [3] described another classification based on two criteria: (1) the type of main arterial pedicle penetrating the muscle; and (2) the presence or absence of intermuscular anastomotic accessory arteries or osteoperiosteal anastomotic arteries. Although the classification adds further detail to the understanding of vascular anatomy, it, as well as the one of Mathes and Nahai, is cumbersome to memorize. As our knowledge of skin and muscle vascular anatomy expands, these classifications are often restrictive without adding major clinical benefit to the practicing plastic surgeon.

## GUIDELINES ON THE SELECTION OF FLAPS

Success and safety of transposed flaps is based on a sound knowledge of the surgical anatomy, blood supply, and arc of rotation of the flap. The modern goal for reconstruction is no longer mere flap survival in coverage of the defect but optimum refinement of function and form. The available tools to obtain this goal include skin flaps, fasciocutaneous flaps, muscle flaps with or without skin grafts, musculocutaneous flaps, osteocutaneous flaps, fascial flaps, and myoadipose flaps. Each method has its functional and aesthetic advantages as well as its limitations. The plastic surgeon needs to select the correct flap for the individual problem from this vast number of options.

A skin flap, possibly adequate for coverage of bare bone, tendon, or cartilage, may be totally inadequate for more complicated defects, e.g., exposed abdominal viscera, dura, brain, vascular prosthesis, major blood vessels, or radionecrosis of bone. Many of the latter serious problems, hidden in the chest, abdomen, or mediastinum, require the *most reliable* available solution, i.e., a richly vascularized muscle or musculocutaneous flap.

When flap *bulk* is desirable, as for breast reconstruction, resurfacing a contour defect, or coverage of a deep defect, the musculocutaneous or myoadipose flap may be the method of choice. The subcutaneous layer of fat in the gluteus maximus, rectus abdominis, and gracilis musculocutaneous flaps are particularly thick and are good choices for bulk. For coverage of a shallow defect where bulk is not desirable (e.g., intraorally, lower leg), the choices may include movement of only muscle without subcutaneous tissue or possibly a thin free flap (radial forearm). Denervated muscle further reduces its bulk by 50 percent of its original size.

The *durability* of a flap is an important criterion in areas subjected to repeated wear and tear. Skin-grafted muscle may be as durable as the intact skin of the musculocutaneous flap, but the latter has the additional problem of hair growth and functional adnexal glands when used in some areas (intraoral). On the palms and soles, the glabrous skin is especially adapted to serve prehensile function. The presence of fibrous septae holding the skin down to the subcutaneous fatty layer makes such tissue suitable for gripping and holding; one must aim for resurfacing these areas with skin of a similar glabrous nature.

The *pliability* of a flap is another important criterion. Pliability is inversely proportional to the thickness of the subcutaneous layer. Muscle alone is most pliable and a thick musculocutaneous flap is least pliable. When muscle alone or muscle with fat (myoadipose tissue) is used, there is usually enough pliability to transpose it without tension.

*Sensibility* of a flap is essential for the hands, feet, and other weight-bearing areas. It is possible to transpose innervated musculocutaneous flaps such as a tensor fascia lata neurosensory flap. In muscle flaps that are skin-grafted the sensibility is diminished, but if the underlying muscle remains innervated pressure sensibility may be preserved. In weight- and pressure-bearing areas such as the feet the two main requirements are adequate padding and sensate skin. On the foot, the padding must be adequate but not excessive enough to cause problems with foot wear. In the pressure areas sensate skin is essential to avoid further breakdown.

Protective sensibility has *not* been achieved consistently even in innervated muscle and musculocutaneous flaps. Skin flaps reinnervate best from the surrounding area if free of scar [21].

*Donor site morbidity* is another major factor when selecting the best flap. Donor defects of muscle flaps are almost always closed directly with a resulting cosmetically acceptable scar. Donor defects for musculocutaneous flaps, especially when the cutaneous segment is large, commonly require skin grafting of the secondary defect.

*Expendability of muscle function* must be considered when choosing which muscle to harvest. Some muscles may be harvested without compromising significant function. Loss of specific muscle function may be only relatively important and dictated in part by the gain of the reconstructive objective. Removal of the latissimus dorsi muscle may compromise the function of a swimmer; transference of the gastrocnemius and soleus muscles may affect running ability.

The general status of the tissue of the proposed flap must be considered. Previous ir-

radiation or trauma to the site of a musculocutaneous flap inevitably increases the chance of failure. Although major vascular pedicles may not be significantly affected, peripheral vessels supplying the dermal and subdermal plexus may be obliterated. In such a case a free flap from a distant source would be a better solution provided the anastomosis is made with healthy vessels out of the field of injury.

*Understanding anatomy* is the basis for successful surgery. Although surgeons are often familiar with the anatomy of the region they operate on, variations may occur and may pose technical problems; for example, the vessels for an anterior thigh flap may have pedicles arising at a lower level than usual, thus lowering the flap's pivot point. The understanding of basic embryologic principles is useful for anticipating their occurrence. Knowing anatomic variability is particularly important for musculocutaneous flaps, where some muscles have segmental blood supply, e.g., sartorius and bicep femoris.

WHEN TO USE MUSCLE IN THE
COVERAGE OF WOUNDS

Plastic surgeons are called on to cover or manage wounds throughout the body. Open wounds, by definition, are contaminated and are covered by granulation tissue. Some of these wounds may have exposed prostheses that are essential and cannot be removed, e.g., a knee or vascular prosthesis. In addition, there may be infected wounds, as in the mediastinum, where adequate debridement cannot be performed because essential structures such as major blood vessels may be injured. Postradiation ulceration poses a great management challenge for which guidelines have now been established.

From experimental and clinical evidence it appears that contaminated wounds should be covered, after adequate debridement, with muscle or omentum. Infected bone of long standing, as in the case of osteomyelitis, is best treated by debriding the defect and then filling it with muscle. For the management of pressure sores muscle is used after adequate debridement not only to counteract the persistent infection but also to fill the deadspace that is produced by the excision. When covering an exposed knee joint a muscle flap is preferable to a fasciocutaneous flap, not only to overcome infection but to avoid the ugly secondary defect, which necessitates a skin graft over the leg.

Postradiation ulcerations are best managed by following the principle of wide excision of the irradiated ulcer and the surrounding skin to include the area of telangiectasia and skin pigmentation. The large defect is immediately covered with muscle or omentum.

There is no evidence to indicate that muscle covered with a skin graft used in a weight-bearing area such as the sacrum or the heel provides greater protection against reulceration than skin alone. In fact, there is evidence that skin is much more resistant to pressure and to reulceration than the "padding of muscle."

## SPECIFIC MUSCLE AND MUSCULOCUTANEOUS FLAPS

A description of the major muscle and musculocutaneous flaps follows, indicating their anatomic basis, arc of rotation, and clinical usefulness. Along with the usefulness we indicate the precautions as well as the possible complications of each unit.

### Temporalis Muscle

The temporalis muscle originates from the temporal fossa and inserts into the coronoid process of the mandible. It aids in mastication, but its function is expendable because of the other jaw muscles. It is supplied by two deep temporalis branches of the maxillary artery that enter the undersurface of the muscle just above its insertion and run longitudinally toward the superior portion of the muscle. The parallel arrangement of these vessels allows safe separation of the temporalis muscle into segments, which

maintains its vascularity. The superficial temporal artery located superficial to the muscle supplies the galea and may communicate with the deep temporal vessels.

The most common use of this muscle unit has been in the active muscle transfer for cases of facial paralysis. There the muscle is divided into segments that are rerouted to activate the eye, the corner of the mouth, and the upper and lower lips. The nerve supply, which comes from branches of the deep temporal nerve, is maintained.

The temporalis muscle is also useful for coverage of defects within a radius of 8 cm from the coronoid process. It is applicable as well to the obliteration of defects in the orbit as well as coverage of intraoral defects in the cheek, pharynx, and palate.

The muscle and its overlying fascial layers as well as the deep and superficial temporal vessels have been studied extensively for the design and determination of vascularized split calvarial bone flaps, which are being used for reconstruction of the facial skeleton. The temporalis fascia, which is supplied by the superficial temporal artery, has been used as the source of free fascial flaps for coverage of defects in the leg and the hand.

### Sternocleidomastoid Muscle

The sternocleidomastoid muscle arises from two tendinous bands on each side of the head of the clavicle. It inserts into the mastoid process.

The sternocleidomastoid muscle has three sources of segmental blood supply. The upper two-thirds of the muscle is supplied by the occipital artery, and the lower one-third is supplied by the thyrococervical trunk. The central segment is also supplied by branches of the superior thyroid artery, which by necessity are divided as the muscle is transposed either superiorly or inferiorly. The *motor nerve* for this muscle is the accessory nerve.

Owens and Bakamjian first used this musculocutaneous unit to cover intraoral defects, including those of the palate. At the present time the sternocleidomastoid muscle is used, based on the occipital artery, for coverage of exposed mandible, particularly in the presence of plates or prosthetic mandibular replacements. With an island of skin in the distal end, it has been used for intraoral mucosal coverage as well as for resurfacing defects near the corner of the mouth.

Based inferiorly on the thyrocervical trunk with or without an island of skin on the superior end, it can be used to cover tracheostomy defects or postradiation esophageal or pharyngeal fistulas. The muscle has also been used with limited success as a "filler" for patients with Romberg's disease involving the lower face.

The sternocleidomastoid muscle and musculocutaneous unit is presently used sparingly because patients who would be candidates for its use have usually had a radical neck dissection or have undergone radiation treatment for intraoral cancer. Just as important in the design of either the superiorly or inferiorly based unit is the fact that the eleventh cranial nerve (CN XI) is usually injured, producing paralysis of the trapezius muscle. The reliability of the skin paddle, if extended beyond the clavicle, is low.

*Platysma Muscle*
The platysma muscle originates in a broad front from the manubrium to the acromion. The insertion covers the lower margin of the mandible, and it has connections with the rhysorius and angular depressor muscles of the lower lip. The vascular supply of the platysmal has been extensively studied, and it appears that the muscle is supplied from small branches of the facial artery as well as the superior thyroid arteries. The *motor nerve* is mostly the cervical branch of the facial nerve. A branch of the marginal mandibular nerve innervates the upper medial platysma.

The platysma is used as a musculocutaneous unit with its island of skin outlined on top or near the clavicle. It is pivoted at the angle of the mandible maintaining the tenuous vessels from the facial artery. Ideal for intraoral use to resurface the buccal mucosa as well as the mucosa of the lower lip, it has also been used with some success to provide filling of the atropic tissue in patients with Romberg's disease involving the lower face.

The tenuous blood supply makes it a difficult unit to dissect. One could easily injure the mandibular branch of the facial nerve, and even if the latter is preserved, some asymmetry of the lip results. If the dissection extends laterally CN XI could also be injured.

*Trapezius Muscle*
The trapezius muscle is triangular and originates from a broad aponeurosis from the twelfth thoracic spine, to the cervical vertebrae, to the occiput of the cranium. Its insertion is also broad, extending from the spine of the scapula to the tip of the clavicle. Its function is mainly to elevate and retract the scapula and shoulder.

The dominant blood supply to the trapezius is the transverse cervical artery (Fig. 45-1). The artery courses at the root of the neck, being a branch of the thyrocervical branch, and enters the deep surface of the deep trapezius muscle where it divides into an ascending and a descending branch. The ascending branch parallels the anterior border of the trapezius, and the descending branch parallels the vertebral column. The upper trapezius muscle in the neck is supplied by branches of the occipital artery. The *motor nerve* is the accessory nerve.

The unit is most often used as a musculocutaneous flap vertically designed parallel to the vertebral column. The skin can be an island or a paddle with its base at the root of the neck. The skin portion can be extended beyond the tip of the scapula into the territory of the latissimus dorsi with relative safety. Its dissection is done with care, staying superficial to the paravertebral fascia and the scapula. About 6 to 8 cm of skin can be

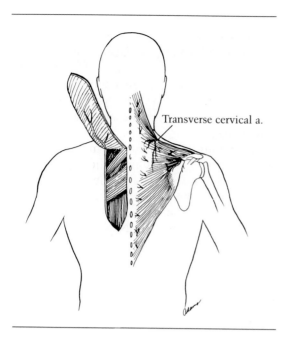

Transverse cervical a.

**Figure 45-1** *Trapezius myocutaneous muscle with the transverse cervical artery arborizing at the root of the neck. On the left the trapezius myocutaneous flap has been elevated and usually includes branches that descend inferiorly.*

included with the secondary skin defect still closing primarily (Fig. 45-2). When pivoted at the root of the neck, the flap can cover dural defects in the upper dorsal or thoracic spine, and its superior reach is to the occiput as well as to the frontotemporal area.

As a transposition flap it is an ideal flap for coverage of defects in the upper thoracic and cervical spine. It has also been used for intraoral coverage and for coverage of defects of the face and skull. It has been helpful for coverage of postradiation defects in the frontotemporal and parietal area in patients with postradiation or postsurgery ulcerations in the scalp due to brain tumors. Less popular is the use of the trapezius unit with an island of skin over the shoulder and, with inclusion of the scapular spine, as a bone substitute for coverage of defects in the lower face.

Proper positioning or repositioning of the

patient may be necessary for adequate access to the donor and recipient sites. This point is particularly important in cases of primary reconstruction following extirpation of head and neck tumors. Under normal circumstances CN XI is not injured during this procedure, although it is possible to do so, producing shoulder droop. If the secondary defect has been closed with considerable tension, the wound is likely to disrupt, producing delayed healing. The use of a skin graft on the back is unsightly.

*Pectoralis Muscle*
The pectoralis major muscle covers an extensive area over the anterior chest wall and originates from the sternum, clavicle, and first five ribs (Fig. 45-3A). The clavicular portion of the muscle can be thought of as having a separate secondary origin from the upper three ribs and the full length of the clavicle. The muscle fibers are horizontal in the upper portion and oblique in the lower portion of the muscle (Fig. 45-3B). It inserts into the anterior lip of the humeral bicipital groove just lateral to the insertion of the latissimus dorsi. The muscle has anatomically been divided into clavicular, sternal, and costochondral portions.

The pectoralis muscle has multiple sources of blood supply that anastomose freely one with the other. The major blood supply comes from the thoracoacromial artery, a branch of the subclavian, but just as important are the perforating arteries from the internal mammary artery (Fig. 45-4). There are also branches from the highest intercostal artery and the lateral thoracic artery. The thoracoacromial artery supplies the entire muscle, and the other vessels supply segments of the pectoralis major. The thoracoacromial artery exists on the medial border of the pectoralis minor muscle and pierces the clavipectoral fascia to divide into four arterial branches: pectoral, acromial, clavicular, and deltoid. The pectoral branch is the largest of these vessels; it supplies the pectoralis major and minor muscles and

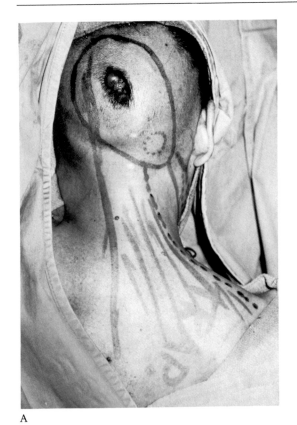

A

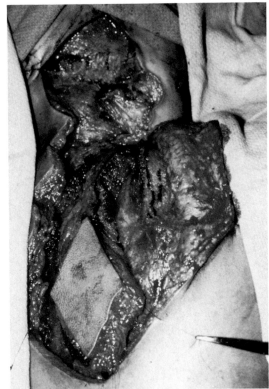

B

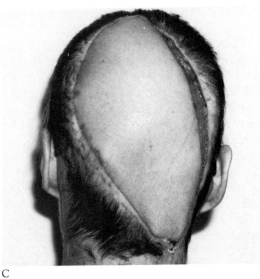

C

**Figure 45-2** Trapezius myocutaneous flap. The patient had a postradiation persistent and recurrent angiosarcoma. The lesion was excised and covered immediately with a trapezius myocutaneous flap that contained an island of skin on its distal portion. A. Preoperative plan. B. After tumor excision and elevation of trapezius musculocutaneous flap. C. Postoperative results.

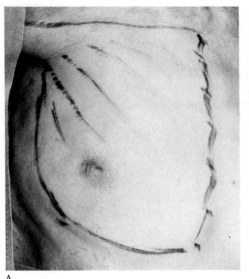
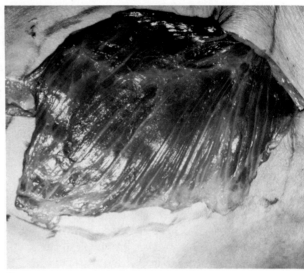

A                                              B

**Figure 45-3**  *The pectoralis major muscle topographic anatomy (A). After removal of the skin, the underlying muscle is evident (B).*

**Figure 45-4**  *Pectoralis major muscle, demonstrating its dual blood supply. On the left side the muscle has been elevated, demonstrating the thoracoacromial vessel that exits just medial to the pectoralis minor muscle. On the left side are the segmental perforating branches from the internal mammary artery. Note that the pectoralis major muscle has the semblance of three components: clavicular, sternal, and axillary portions.*

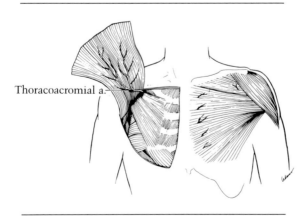

Thoracoacromial a.

has an extensive intramuscular course with branches and anastomoses with the perforating vessels from the internal mammary artery and the lateral thoracic artery. This segmental and multiple blood supply has been used for the segmentation of the pectoralis major muscle, when indicated.

The upper half of the pectoralis major muscle is innervated by the lateral pectoral nerve and the lower or lateral half by the medial pectoral nerve. This terminology is used because the nerves are branches of the lateral or medial cords of the brachial plexus; it has no relation to the position of the muscle itself.

The muscle alone can be used to cover defects over the shoulder when used as a turnover flap. Smaller defects over the clavicle can be covered by the adjacent clavicular portion of the pectoralis major muscle. Because of its proximity the muscle can be freed from its insertion along the humerus and from its sternal and rib attachments, and it can be transposed to the midline in unilateral or bilateral fashion to cover defects following excision of the sternum or for partial coverage of mediastinal wound infections. It is not sufficient for coverage of an entire mediastinal wound because it does not reach the lower one-third of the sternum and upper abdomen.

It is the most common flap in use for head and neck reconstruction, particularly intraorally, because of its safety. It is used with an island of skin that can be outlined in the lower one-third, extending down to the costal margin (if necessary including a portion of the anterior rectus sheath) or elegantly with a skin paddle at the submammary area. It is the flap of choice for coverage of pharyngeal fistulas and reconstruction of the esophagus. The muscle has also been used as a turnover flap based on the perforating branches of the internal mammary artery for coverage of mediastinal wounds.

When designing the cutaneous segment the territory of the deltopectoral flap is first marked and preserved. The cutaneous segment is then designed such that it avoids malplacement of the breast and nipple during direct closure. The flap is raised from inferiorly upward and may be tunneled subcutaneously. The clavicular portion of the muscle is spared, although it can be incised to free the pedicle if necessary. In the turnover pectoralis major muscle flap the muscle is divided at the junction of the medial two-thirds and the lateral one-third. The lateral border of the pectoralis minor muscle is used as a landmark. The medial segment is perfused by the internal mammary artery and the lateral segment by the thoracoacromial artery. This lateral one-third of the pectoralis muscle is then sutured to the remaining pectoralis minor muscle and rib periosteum to preserve the anterior axillary fold.

The muscle alone is also ideal for intrathoracic purposes, particularly plugging pleurocutaneous fistulas and as a "salvage" patch for the heart.

Disadvantages include the fact that the aesthetic deformity is significant, particularly in men. If a bulky pedicle that has not been denervated is transferred into the neck, it produces bothersome contractures of the muscle. For intraoral resurfacing the flap is safe, but it is bulky and at times makes swallowing difficult.

In women the dissection is cumbersome because of the overlying breast, and in men the nipple may be malpositioned upon primary closure of the defect. The safety, reliability, and ease of elevation of the flap outweigh a good number of the disadvantages, and in fact the flap has become the most popular musculocutaneous unit for head and neck reconstruction.

### Latissimus Dorsi Muscle

The latissimus dorsi, a rectangular muscle that extends from the tip of the scapula to the midline of the back posteriorly and to the iliac crest inferiorly, has its anterior border approximating the posterior axillary line. The muscle originates from the iliac crest and the surface of the external oblique inferiorly to the thoracolumbar fascia and the spines of the lower six vertebrae posteriorly. It inserts into the lesser tubercle and the intertubercular groove of the humerus in front of the teres major muscle. Its function is to act primarily as an abductor and medial rotator of the arm.

The thoracodorsal artery, a branch of the subscapular artery, is the dominant blood supply. These proximal vessels can supply the entire muscle with the exception of the most distal aspects of the latissimus muscle. The distal muscle is predominantly supplied by the paravertebral posterior perforating vessels, which are seen as two rows of segmental vessels, respectively, lying 5 to 10 cm from the midline of the back (Fig. 45-5). The motor nerve is the thoracodorsal nerve.

This versatile muscle or musculocutaneous unit is useful for reconstruction of the breast, chest wall, head and neck region, shoulder and arm, axilla, back, and abdomen. These applications are based on the relatively long proximal vascular pedicle, which allows the muscle or musculocuta-

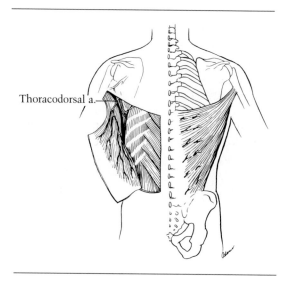

*Thoracodorsal a.*

**Figure 45-5** *Latissimus dorsi flap with its dual blood supply consisting of the thoracodorsal artery as well as the segmental paravertebral perforators, of which there are two rows.*

neous unit to swing as a pendulum and to cover defects within its reach.

The latissimus dorsi can cover the upper part of the sternum but not the distal part. It is ideal for coverage of defects along the scapula and shoulder, and although used less commonly than the pectoralis major muscle, it can cover defects intraorally. Used as a musculocutaneous unit, it can resurface large losses of muscle and skin in the deltoid region and arm. When used as muscle alone, it is an admirable unit to provide flexion of the elbow. Because of its reliable long and relatively large (2.5 mm) vascular pedicle, it is one of the most popular free flap donor sites.

The latissimus dorsi has been used extensively for breast reconstruction where two-thirds of the muscle is transferred as a pendulum to the anterior chest to replace the lost or atropic pectoralis major muscle. An island of skin is strategically placed that adds skin to the anterior chest to provide an increase in the vertical and transverse diameters, which are responsible for the ptosis

and projection, respectively, of the reconstructed breast. Clinical experience, however, has demonstrated that the best placement of the skin island is transversely below the scapula in the form of an ellipse, wide enough to allow primary closure of the secondary defect (Fig. 45-6).

The advantages of this unit are its ease of elevation as well as its safety and reliability. If the thoracodorsal artery has been ligated as part of the radical mastectomy procedure, the muscle still survives with reverse flow from the branch to the serratus anterior or through smaller branches from the circumflex scapular vessels.

Among its disadvantages is the fact that transfer of the latissimus dorsi muscle produces a slight, but noticeable, winging of the scapula even though the serratus anterior is intact. Patients also exhibit some flattening of the back, and the large area of dissection is prone to develop seromas and occasionally hematomas. If a skin graft is needed because an overly large skin island has been included with the flap, the secondary defect is most unattractive. Additionally, reconstruction of the breast with the latissimus dorsi musculocutaneous unit in obese patients has been unsatisfactory and inadequate because of the inability to obtain symmetry with the opposite breast.

### Serratus Anterior Muscle

The serratus anterior muscle originates from the anterior surface of the seventh through the tenth ribs and inserts on the costal surface of the vertebral border of the scapula. The muscle is supplied by two vessels that enter proximally and that arise in the axilla: the lateral thoracic artery, which is visible on the lateral surface of the serratus anterior muscle, and a branch of the thoracodorsal artery, which enters the posterior aspect of the muscle before it terminates in the latissimus dorsi muscle. The thoracodorsal branch is the larger of the two vessels, and it is easily seen as one elevates the latissimus dorsi

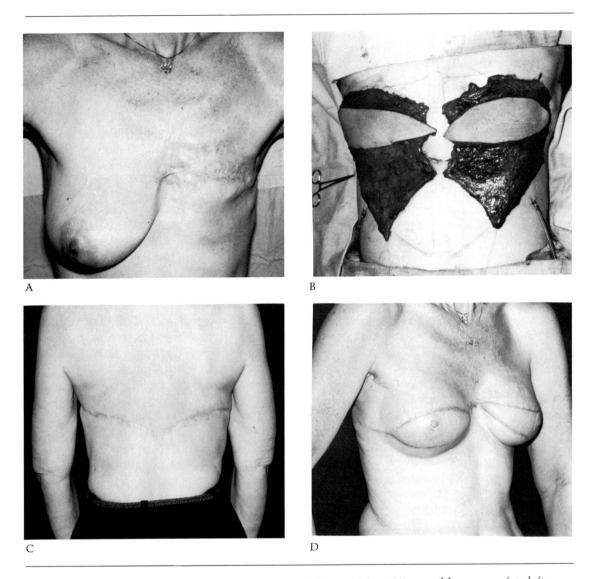

A

B

C

D

**Figure 45-6** *A 46-year-old woman after left mastectomy for carcinoma of the breast. At this time she presented with carcinoma of the right breast. The right mastectomy was performed at the same time as the bilateral reconstruction was done with bilateral latissimus dorsi myocutaneous flaps. A. Preoperative status. B. After the mastectomy the patient was burned, and the bilateral latissimus dorsi flaps were elevated. C, D. Postoperative views.*

on its vascular leash. Its motor nerve is the long thoracic nerve.

The unit is used as a muscle alone relatively sparingly. Its widest application has been for intrathoracic coverage of bronchopleural fistulas and rarely for primary reconstructions of the trachea and bronchi for which there are considerable experimental data. Microvascular teams have also made use of the multiple slips of this muscle as a free flap muscle transfer to reanimate the paralyzed face and for coverage of defects in the hand.

Its major disadvantage is that one usually has to retract the latissimus dorsi and portions of the pectoralis major muscle to obtain adequate access to it. Moreover, there is usually a large area of dissection that is prone to hematoma and seroma. Winging of the scapula is usually marked.

### Rectus Abdominis Muscle and Musculocutaneous Units

The rectus abdominis muscle inserts into the pubic tubercle and the pubic crest. It originates from the lower chest wall over a broad area that encompasses the cartilage of the sixth, seventh, and eighth ribs. The muscle is encased by the anterior and posterior rectus sheath and has loose attachments to the confluence of the sheaths laterally with the oblique musculature as well as to the linea alba medially. It has three to five subdivisions called intersectiones tendineae, which are usually vascular and show secure attachments to the rectus sheath medially and laterally.

The rectus abdominis muscle is supplied by the superior as well as the deep inferior epigastric vessels that form the epigastric arcade. In addition, it has segmental blood supply through the segmental intercostal vessels, which enter the muscle on its posterior surface and anastomose freely with the epigastric arcade. The deep inferior epigastric vessel is approximately twice the caliber of the superior epigastric vessel. The entire muscle can survive on either the su-

perior or the inferior deep epigastric vessels, and relatively large segments of the muscle survive on single intercostal branches.

The epigastric arcade sends two rows of perforating vessels that are located paramedially; they perforate the anterior rectus fascia and supply the overlying skin. These perforators are concentrated around the umbilicus and are absent near the pubic region. Venae comitantes are present with the epigastric arcade, and the venous flow is unidirectional toward the liver; backflow is impeded because of the presence of venous valves. Anastomotic connections have been demonstrated on the arterial and venous side from the superficial inferior epigastric system toward the deep epigastric arcade, again unidirectionally. This point has clinical importance in that the skin of the abdominal wall has a dual blood supply and is clinically applicable to thinning of the transverse island abdominal flap for breast reconstruction. The motor nerves are the intercostal nerves five through twelve.

The unit can be used as a muscle or a musculocutaneous flap based on either the superior or the deep inferior epigastric vessels. Transverse or vertical islands of skin can be outlined superiorly or inferiorly—or in fact anywhere along its length.

The muscle alone is admirably suited for use on its superior pedicle for coverage of mediastinal wound infections following aortocoronary bypass procedures (Fig. 45-7). It can be used as a complement to mobilization of the pectoralis major muscle, which covers the upper two-thirds of the wound, with the rectus abdominis muscle covering the inferior one-third; or it may be used as the sole treatment for the entire mediastinal wound from the suprasternal notch to the xiphoid. The superior epigastric vessel supplies the entire muscle, which is divided from the pubic tubercle and is turned over to fill the mediastinal cavity. It has also been used to cover smaller defects in the lower chest wall and to cover large pacemakers inserted in the abdominal wall.

Based on the *superior epigastric vessel,* the most popular use of the unit is as the transverse island abdominal flap for breast reconstruction. The skin island is placed at the level of the umbilicus with the defect to simulate a well done abdominoplasty (Fig. 45-8). As an upper rectus flap, a skin island is outlined at the inframammary level; it includes a small segment of rectus muscle, which contributes the perforators to supply the skin, which is then turned 180 degrees for reconstruction of the breast.

The most elegant use is with the Hartrampf lower rectus flap method of breast reconstruction, which usually provides enough bulk in the form of subcutaneous tissue to allow breast reconstruction without the use of an implant. The upper rectus flap outlined in the contralateral submammary line is more difficult to use and necessitates use of an implant in most cases. The skin island is totally reliable on the ipsilateral hemiabdomen just past the midline. Attempts to extend it to zone 4 beyond the contralateral rectus muscle result in necrosis.

Based on the *inferior epigastric vessels* and with an island of skin ideally placed in the submammary fold of such dimensions to allow primary closure and extended to the anterior axillary line *(Flag flap)* the wide arc of rotation of this unit provides a versatile unit superior to all other musculocutaneous flaps except for a free flap (Fig. 45-9). This unit provides coverage to the entire trochanter and anterior thigh down to the knee as well as the flanks.

Other outlines of musculocutaneous units have been described including the vertical rectus, which is a safe unit that can be based on either the superior or the deep inferior epigastric vessels. Additionally, Taylor et al. described a musculocutaneous unit outlined from the umbilicus toward the tip of the scapula that includes the inferior epigastric vessels and a relatively small portion of the rectus abdominis muscle.

The loss of one rectus abdominis muscle appears to be fairly well tolerated. When

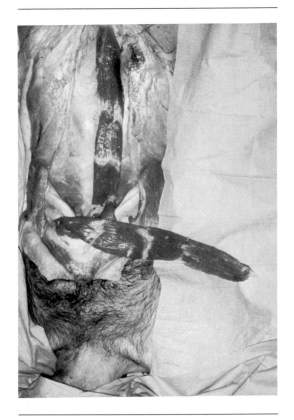

**Figure 45-7** *The rectus abdominis muscle is freed from its origin along the costal margin and is pivoting on the deep inferior epigastric vessel. Note the wide arc of rotation.*

both muscles are used, however, there may be some loss of pelvic tilt in the supine position. The major disadvantage of this unit is related to the weakness that may result, particularly in the inferior portion of the abdomen distal to the linea semicircularis. By necessity, segments of anterior rectus fascia are included with the musculocutaneous unit, and there may be an asymmetric bulging if not frank hernia in the lower abdomen. The incidence of hernias as well as bulging areas have been decreased in the Hartrampf type of breast reconstruction by dividing the muscle at the linea semicircularis and removing only small segments of anterior rectus sheath; this method allows primary closure of the remnants of the rectus sheath as

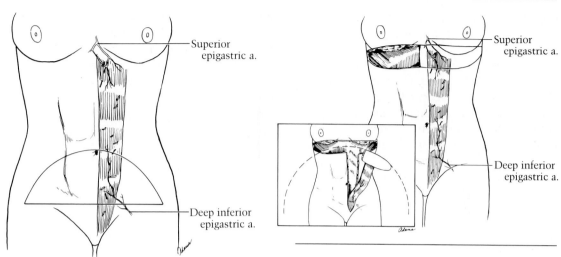

**Figure 45-8** *Rectus abdominis muscle with the epigastric arcade, which is composed of the superior and the deep inferior epigastric artery. The lower transverse island abdominal flap has been outlined at the level of the umbilicus.*

**Figure 45-9** *"Flag flap," which includes skin usually outlined at the inframammary level (the flag) and uses the rectus abdominis muscle with the inferior epigastric vessel as the carrier. The flag has a wide range of rotation, reaching almost to the knee, particularly if the inguinal ligament is divided.*

well as external oblique muscle mobilization to centralize the umbilicus and provide inferior abdominal symmetry. With the use of one rectus unit the umbilicus is usually eccentric, and it can be brought to the midline with varying degrees of success by suturing it (if it has a long pedicle) as well as by plication of the opposite anterior rectus fascia.

### Gluteus Maximus Muscle

The gluteus maximus, an important muscle that is the strongest external rotator and extensor of the hip, takes its origin from the lateral margin of the sacrum and the posterior superior iliac crest. It has origins to a lesser extent from the coccyx and along the sacrotuberous ligament. The muscle, which is quadrilateral in shape, passes over the greater trochanter and inserts into it and also along the iliotibial tract.

The gluteus maximus is supplied by su-perior and inferior gluteal vessels that arise from the internal iliac vessels. The piriform muscle divides the location of the superior and inferior vascular bundles (Fig. 45-10). It is clinically important to note that the inferior gluteal nerve, which innervates the muscle, travels along the inferior gluteal vessels. Although less studied, the muscle also receives blood supply along its insertion from the iliotibial tract and greater trochanter most likely from unnamed vessels along the cruciate anastomosis. Multiple perforating vessels supply the overlying skin. The motor nerve is the inferior gluteal nerve, which includes components of L5, S1, and S2.

The gluteus muscle alone or with a skin island has been used extensively for coverage of sacral or ischial defects in paraplegics. In these patients the loss of function of the muscle is a minor consideration. The simplest way to cover the sacrum is as a turnover flap, dividing its insertion from the iliotibial tract and turning it over like a page in

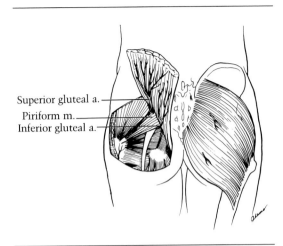

Superior gluteal a.

Piriform m.

Inferior gluteal a.

**Figure 45-10** *Gluteus maximus with the superior and inferior gluteal arteries supplying it and the piriform muscle separating the two arterial systems. On the left side the muscle has been divided near its insertion along the greater trochanter. There is also a fairly dominant blood supply that enters through the trochanteric insertion and anastomoses with the superior and inferior gluteal vessels. On the right side perforating branches from the gluteal system supply the overlying skin, making it possible to move the overlying gluteal skin in a V-Y fashion without disturbing the underlying muscle.*

a book to cover the sacrum while the superior and inferior gluteal vessels are maintained intact.

If muscle is not considered necessary to cover a defect in the sacrum, the second simplest way would be to outline V-Y-type skin advancement flaps bilaterally without interfering with the underlying muscle. The skin islands are outlined in the form of a V with the base along the sacrum, and because of the mobility of the gluteal skin it can be advanced immediately for approximately 5 to 8 cm on each side, long enough to cover defects in the sacrum without disturbing the underlying gluteus maximus. The skin does advance and maintains its blood supply because of the multiple perforating vessels from the underlying muscle. Musculocuta-

neous skin islands based on either the superior or the inferior vascular pedicle and outlined near the trochanter can serve as rotation or transposition flaps to cover defects along the ischium as well as portions of the sacrum. They have the disadvantage that one is dealing with a relatively short vascular pedicle that prohibits the mobility of the skin islands and makes a relatively bloody dissection.

The use of the gluteus maximus muscle with or without a skin island in ambulatory patients is possible and advisable utilizing the modifications of Ramirez [20]. It is best suited to cover postradiation ulcers in the sacrum. Ramirez et al. [16] advised its use by making a V incision over the skin to gain access to the origin of the muscle from the iliac crest, the sacrum, and along the sacrotuberous ligament. The muscle is freed from those origins completely, maintaining intact the superior and inferior gluteal vessels and over the gluteus medius muscle down to its insertion along the trochanter and iliotibial tract. Leaving the insertion intact, the freed muscle advances medially toward the sacrum for approximately 5 to 8 cm. Bilateral advancements are necessary for larger defects. The muscles are then sutured to each other over the sacrum, and a V-Y advancement of skin is performed. This approach has the advantage of maintaining the function of the muscle in ambulatory patients. The procedure is difficult and relatively bloody, particularly as one frees the muscle along the sacrotuberous origin.

The use of the superior half of the gluteus muscle is not advised in ambulatory patients because it is the superior portion that is the more important contributor to abduction of the thigh at the hip joint. Other uses include employment of the superior gluteal vessels and the overlying skin and fat as a free flap donor site for breast reconstruction.

In the paralyzed patient the use of musculocutaneous units are limited by the relatively short length of the superior and inferior vascular pedicles. Attempts to rotate islands of skin outlined near the trochanter for more than 90 degrees may result in kinking of the venous return and necrosis of the flap. The main disadvantage in the ambulatory patient is the difficulty of the dissection, particularly freeing the origin along the sacrum and the sacrotuberous ligament. The plane between the gluteus maximus and medius is best found as one dissects along the posterior iliac crest, and it is identified because of the finer texture of the muscle fibers of the gluteus medius.

*Gracilis Musculocutaneous Flap*

The gracilis muscle originates from the pubic tubercle and the inferior ramus of the pubis; it inserts into the pes anserinus at the medial knee (Fig. 45-11). It aids in thigh abduction and knee flexion, but it is a totally expendable muscle.

The muscle has three to five vascular pedicles supplying it along its length. The largest and most important is the proximal one, which is a branch of the profunda femoris. The other vascular pedicles travel along the intermuscular septi and are smaller. The entire muscle can survive on its most proximal pedicle, which is the largest. The viability of the muscle based on the distal blood supply, which is a branch of the saphenous artery, is less likely beyond its distal one-third. The gracilis musculocutaneous unit has been used extensively to reconstruct perineal defects. It was first advocated and it is still useful for resurfacing defects and reconstructing the vagina after pelvic exenteration. It is less useful, however, for reconstruction of the agenic or hypoplastic vagina.

The unit has also been used for coverage of ischial pressure sores as well as for reconstruction of the labia majora. Muscle alone or as a musculocutaneous unit has also been used to resurface perineal defects after resection for granulomatous colitis. Penile reconstruction has been done with the musculocutaneous unit. The use of the muscle alone for penile reconstruction has been unsatisfactory because of the eventual shrinkage of

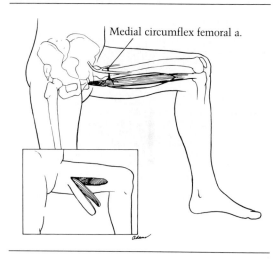

**Figure 45-11** *Gracilis muscle, demonstrating its origin and insertion. It is always lower than one envisions it.*

the muscle. Microsurgeons have used the gracilis muscle alone extensively as a free flap muscle, particularly for resurfacing defects in the lower extremity where the length and relative flatness of the muscle have made it ideally suited.

Among the disadvantages of this muscle is its location. The proximal vascular pedicle is sometimes too low to allow the unit to pivot widely. The skin island is totally unreliable in its distal one-third. In addition, it is difficult to determine the skin island territory over the gracilis muscle, particularly in patients who are relatively obese, because of the flabbiness of the overlying skin. Even more important, it has been determined that the skin and fascial territory over the gracilis muscle can be elevated on its proximal base just as safely as can a fasciocutaneous flap without the underlying gracilis muscle (Fig. 45-12).

Although strongly advocated for obliteration of fistulous tracts in the presacral space, the relatively small and narrow gracilis muscle is unable to do so, and the recurrence rate of the fistulas is high. A preferred approach for perineal fistulas is the use of the gluteus

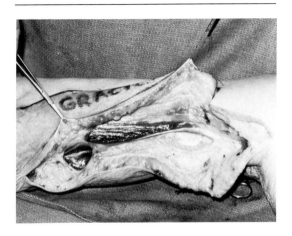

**Figure 45-12** *Gracilis muscle and overlying fasciocutaneous flap, which can be used independently of each other.*

muscle. Aggressive use of the gracilis musculocutaneous unit for reconstruction of the hypoplastic or aplastic vagina has led to complications in some cases.

*Tensor Fascia Lata Muscle*
The tensor muscle originates from the anterosuperior iliac spine but mainly from the greater trochanter of the femur. It is a relatively small muscle with a long fascial extension that inserts into the lateral aspect of the knee and acts as a lateral knee stabilizer.

The lateral circumflex femoral artery, which is a branch of the profunda femoris, sends terminal vessels that supply the tensor fascia lata, the rectus femoris, and the vastus lateralis muscles (Fig. 45-13). These branches enter the respective muscles at approximately the same level, 8 to 10 cm below the inguinal ligament. The cutaneous portion of the distal two-thirds of the tensor fascia lata unit receives direct intermuscular vessels from the third and fourth branches of the profunda femoris. The muscle is innervated from the inferior branch of the gluteal nerve L4-L5.

The tensor fascia lata has a wide arc of rotation although not as large as is demonstrated on the cadaver. It is the flap of choice for coverage of trochanteric pressure sores; it has also been used to reconstruct the abdominal wall and for defects in the medial thigh. When used in its reverse fashion, i.e., freeing the origin from the iliac spine, it can cover defects along the anterosuperior iliac spine, particularly with an extended skin island.

The inclusion of the lateral femoral cutaneous nerve in the territory of the tensor fascia lata has been advocated for use as a sensory flap with variable success. The unit is also used as a free microvascular donor site, but this use is less popular now.

Its disadvantages include the following. The skin over the distal one-third of the flap near the knee is unreliable because of its different blood supply through the profunda femoral artery. In an athletic person removal of the tensor fascia lata may cause some lateral instability to the knee. During reconstruction of the abdominal wall the pivot point located laterally makes it difficult to

**Figure 45-13** *Tensor fascia lata with its blood supply from the lateral circumflex artery. It is a relatively short muscle that has a long fascial extension.*

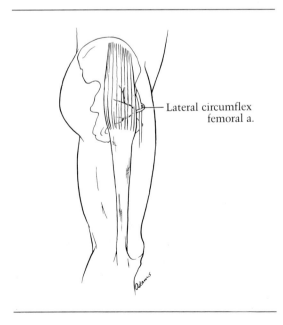

Lateral circumflex
femoral a.

reach defects beyond the lower abdomen. The lack of muscle over most of this unit is a disadvantage when covering postradiation defects over the lower abdomen, pubis, and medial thigh. The tensor fascia lata flap, when used to cover defects of the medial thigh, is likely to necrose in its distal portion perhaps owing to dependency. Although it can reach the ischium, its routine use is not advisable because the distal portion of the flap is likely to necrose.

### Rectus Femoris Muscle

The rectus femoris originates from the anteroinferior iliac spine and the upper border of the acetabulum; it inserts into the patellar tendon. In the distal one-third of the thigh the rectus femoris is densely fused with the vastus lateralis and vastus medialis muscles, which form part of the quadriceps mechanism. Its function is extension of the knee, particularly in the terminal 15 to 20 degrees.

The rectus femoris is supplied from a branch of the lateral circumflex femoral vessels. Just before entering the muscle the artery branches into two parts, one to supply the upper portion of the muscle and the other the lower portion. The proximal branch seems to be adequate to supply the entire muscle if the distal branch is ligated (Fig.45-14). The motor nerve is the femoral nerve.

The rectus femoris muscle alone or as a myocutaneous unit is being used increasingly for reconstruction of lower abdominal defects, particularly postradiation ulcers over the pubis or when the abdominal defect extends below the umbilicus. It is also preferable to resurface postradiation ulcerations in the perineum or after groin dissections, but it is not appropriate for vaginal reconstruction. Occasionally the muscle alone has been transferred intraabdominally through a lower abdominal incision to provide support and coverage for the pelvic floor.

The loss of terminal knee extension has been cited as a disadvantage, but it does not occur if one reapproximates the fascia of the

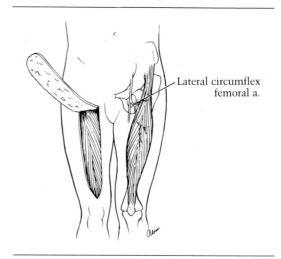

Lateral circumflex femoral a.

**Figure 45-14** *The rectus femoris muscle is demonstrated on the left side. On the right side the fasciocutaneous flap has been elevated, leaving the underlying rectus femoris muscle intact. The blood supply to the fasciocutaneous flap is from a true musculocutaneous perforator located proximally.*

vastus medialis and vastus lateralis. The remaining three muscles of the quadriceps mechanism are usually more than adequate to provide strong terminal knee extension in most patients. There is some difficulty dissecting the muscle, particularly in freeing it with its intermuscular attachments to the vastus medialis and lateralis. Consequently, the suggested approach to elevating this flap consists in dividing the central portion of the patellar tendon and then finding the rectus femoris muscle proximally at the midthigh, followed by dissection to free the rectus femoris from the adjacent two muscles.

### Gastrocnemius Muscle

The gastrocnemius muscle is composed of two heads that are partially fused in the midline of the calf. The sural nerve traverses the midline between the two heads.

The muscle originates from the femoral condyle and inserts into the achilles tendon. The latter is further reinforced by the insertion of the soleus muscle. The medial or lat-

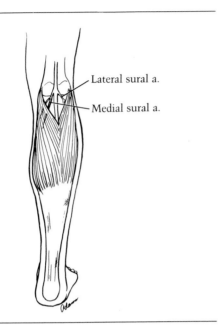

***Figure 45-15*** *The two heads of the gastrocnemius muscle are shown with the vascular supply branching from the popliteal artery.*

eral head of the gastrocnemius muscle can be expended with little or no deficit when walking or in normal running.

Each head of the gastrocnemius is supplied by the sural artery, which is a branch of the popliteal artery. The sural artery passes directly into the proximal portion of both heads, where it arborizes and then travels longitudinally along the length of the muscle (Fig. 45-15). There are also direct fasciocutaneous arteries arising from the popliteal artery as well as septocutaneous vessels arising from the trifurcation of the popliteal artery in the leg. The motor nerve is the popliteal nerve.

The gastrocnemius muscle is best used as a muscular unit alone, rather than as a musculocutaneous unit, to avoid the secondary donor site in the posterior calf, which requires skin grafting. For defects over the knee, the medial head of the gastrocnemius covers the knee joint and even the patella, particularly if the origin from the medial

femoral condyle is also divided. The lateral head is appropriate when covering the exposed lateral aspect of the knee joint; it is shorter in length, however, and one has to exercise caution to preserve the peroneal nerve, which lies superficial and near the head of the fibula.

The medial head of the gastrocnemius is ideally suited to cover exposed bone over the proximal one-third of the tibia. There the muscle can be transferred as a transposition flap, or it can be turned over the deep surface, becoming superficial to cover bony defects with an immediate skin graft over the fascia. (It is not necessary to remove the fascia for the skin graft to take.)

The skin and fascial territory of the medial head of the gastrocnemius can be elevated with the underlying muscle or as a separate fasciocutaneous flap (the "super flap" of Ponten—because it has a double blood supply). For small defects over the middle one-third of the tibia, a fasciocutaneous flap is appropriate without disturbing the underlying gastrocnemius muscle.

Among the disadvantages of the muscle flap is that a portion of the proximal achilles tendon must be divided to free the medial or lateral head of the gastrocnemius muscle. This maneuver, though, usually poses no difficulty. At times it is difficult to find the midline raphe between the medial and lateral head of the gastrocnemius muscle; identifying the sural nerve is helpful. Finally, a skin graft of the posterior calf is unsightly.

MUSCLE FLAPS
A number of useful muscles have been described and are used clinically as pure muscle flaps without skin territory. They include the external oblique, the biceps femoris, the vastus lateralis, and vastus medialis, as well as the muscles in the lower leg.

*External Oblique Muscle*
The external oblique is one of the largest and strongest of the flat abdominal wall muscles. It originates from the posterior aspects

of the sixth to the twelfth ribs and runs obliquely downward to its broad attachment at the linea semilunaris and the inguinal ligament.

The blood supply to the external oblique comes from the sixth through the twelfth intercostal vessels, which are segmentally arranged and enter the undersurface of the muscle near the posterior axillary line, diffusely arborizing throughout the muscle. The *motor nerves* are the sixth through twelfth intercostal nerves.

Although the overlying skin can be carried through muscular perforators, the unit is used mainly alone for reconstruction of the abdominal wall and in efforts to decrease the waist during an aesthetic abdominoplasty. The muscle is freed from its insertion along its juncture with the anterior rectus sheath and is advanced medially, either bilaterally or unilaterally. It has been most helpful for reconstruction of the abdominal wall following use of the Hartrampf flap and for the closure of abdominal hernias.

Its disadvantage is that the ilioinguinal and iliofemoral nerves can be injured, producing parasthesia.

### Biceps Femoris Muscle

As its name indicates the biceps femoris muscle has two heads. The long head of the muscle originates from the ischial tuberosity along with the semitendinous and semimembranous muscles. The short head has a deeper origin from the linea aspera of the femur and the lateral supracondylar line of the femur. It inserts into the head of the fibula and the lateral condyle of the tibia.

The muscle is supplied by multiple segmental vessels. These vessels arise from the profunda femoris and travel through the intermuscular septum, supplying the upper two-thirds of the muscle; the lower one-third is supplied by direct vessels from the popliteal artery (Fig. 45-16). The *motor nerve* is the sciatic nerve.

Although a musculocutaneous unit has been used as a V-Y advancement flap divid-

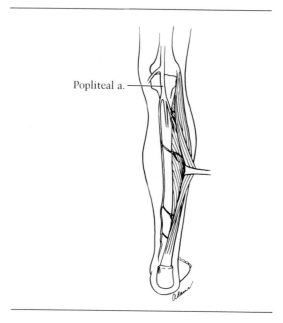

Popliteal a.

**Figure 45-16** *The soleus muscle has been retracted to show the vascular supply, which is partly segmental. The proximal arterial pedicle supplies the entire soleus muscle, and a portion of the soleus muscle can be based on one of the smaller distal branches.*

ing the origin and insertion for coverage of ischial pressure sores, it is the muscle alone that can be advanced, also as a V-Y flap. Alternatively, it can be used as a turnover flap to fill defects along the ischium.

Unfortunately, because of the segmental blood supply and the limited intermuscular vascular connections, the turnover flap is limited, as is the V-Y type of advancement.

### Vastus Lateralis Muscle

The vastus lateralis muscle originates anteriorly from the greater trochanter and the trochanteric line of the femur and posteriorly from the lateral lip of the linea aspera and the intermuscular septum. It inserts into the tendon of the rectus femoris, the upper border of the patella, and the lateral condyle of the tibia. Thus it forms a part of the lateral patellar retinaculum. It is part of the quadriceps mechanism that serves to extend the knee and to stabilize it.

The proximal vastus lateralis muscle is supplied by the lateral circumflex femoral artery, a branch of the profunda femoris. The distal one-third of the muscle is also supplied by septocutaneous arteries arising from the superficial femoral vessels. The *motor nerve* is the femoral nerve.

The primary use of the vastus lateralis muscle is for situations that require muscle coverage to fill a deep cavity, usually at the level of the trochanter. It can be used in combination with the tensor fascia lata or as a second line of repair for trochanteric defects where the tensor fascia lata flap has failed or (as is most likely) when a trochanteric ulcer has recurred in a paraplegic patient.

Its disadvantages are that the dissection is deep, the most distal portion of the muscle is unreliable, and its use is limited to paraplegic patients with recurrent trochanteric pressure ulcers.

### Vastus Medialis Muscle

The vastus medialis has a broad origin from the distal one-half of the intertrochanteric line, the medial lip of the linea aspera, and a portion of the medial femoral condyle. It inserts into the medial border of the patella and the tendon of the quadriceps femoris. It is also a component of the quadriceps mechanism.

The proximal one-half of the vastus medialis is supplied by branches of the profunda femoris artery. The distal one-half of the muscle is supplied by intermuscular vessels branching from the superficial femoral artery. The *motor nerve* is the femoral nerve.

The vastus medialis has been described for possible use as an advancement or a rotation flap to cover defects in the distal anterior thigh down to the level of the midpatella. There is also a documented report of using the muscle to aid in the reconstruction of the extensor mechanism of the knee. The unit, however, has not received wide clinical application.

There has been limited clinical use of this unit to recommend it for widespread use.

## COVERAGE OF THE LEG WITH MUSCLE FLAPS

Coverage of exposed bone on the lower leg has changed considerably. The medial head of the gastrocnemius muscle remains the flap of choice for coverage of the exposed tibia in its proximal one-third. For smaller defects in the midtibia, the soleus muscle provides sufficient and lasting coverage. For the distal one-third of the tibia as well as for larger defects, the facility and reliability of microsurgical techniques have made free muscle flaps the method of choice for coverage of defects, not only in the distal one-third but in fact for larger defects of the entire leg.

We must keep in mind, however, the use of the soleus muscle and one of the peroneal muscles from the lateral aspect of the leg, which can help in the coverage of defects in the medial and occasionally the distal one-third of the tibia.

### Soleus Muscle

Soleus muscle is a bipiniform (double feather) shaped muscle. Its width encompasses the posterior two-thirds of the calf. It originates from the upper one-third of the dorsum and the medial surface of the fibula and mid-posterior tibia. It inserts into the achilles tendon over a 5-cm area just anterior and distal to the insertion of the gastrocnemius muscle.

The muscle has a mixed blood supply. The proximal vasculature arises directly from the popliteal vessels and can reliably carry all but the distal 4 to 5 cm of the muscle. The distal muscle is supplied by several segmental perforating vessels arising from the posterior tibial artery. The *motor nerve* is the tibial nerve.

The soleus muscle, when freed from its insertion on the achilles tendon and based proximally, covers defects into the midtibia. Because its most distal portion is narrow the coverage is smaller than one would like.

The reverse distal soleus based on the segmental distal vessels has been described but is not completely reliable. However, one could use one-half or one-fourth of the muscle based on a distal vessel and turn it down to cover small defects over the ankle.

Its main disadvantage is the limited amount of coverage it provides. Sometimes one has to stretch the muscle considerably, which results in partial disruption of the wound and reappearance of the exposed bone. On other occasions the soleus muscle must be supplemented by the use of the extensor digitorum communis muscle. However, when successful it avoids the need for a free flap.

*Peroneus Brevis Muscle*
Occasionally when defects occur on the lateral aspect of the tibia, on the distal one-third, one can explore the lateral musculature; among the three peroneal muscles, the peroneus brevis is usually the most fleshy and can be freed from its tendinous insertion. The tendon of insertion is anastomosed to the adjacent tendons, and the muscle can be transposed to cover a small defect. On occasion the peroneus bevis muscle can be stretched to provide coverage over the exposed bone without freeing the distal attachment.

The extensor digitorum communis, which has a segmental blood supply through the septocutaneous vessels, has been described as a flap that can be stretched to cover a defect on the lateral aspect of the tibia or as a distally based muscle flap to cover the ankle. The extensor digitorum communis originates from the lateral border of the upper two-thirds of the tibia and the medial border of the fibula. Its blood supply comes from multiple deep segmental perforating vessels from the anterior tibial artery.

There is limited clinical experience to make general recommendations on these two muscle flaps.

MUSCLES FROM THE FOOT
Three muscles from the foot have been used to provide coverage as muscle flaps. They include the abductor hallucis, the flexor digitorum brevis, and the extensor digitorum brevis.

*Abductor Hallucis Brevis*
The abductor hallucis originates from the medial aspect of the calcaneum and is adherent to the first metatarsal bone throughout this length. The muscle inserts into the medial condyle of the proximal phalanx of the great toe.

The abductor hallucis muscle is supplied by a branch from the medial plantar vessel, which enters at the proximal portion of the muscle. There is a secondary vascular leash that penetrates the midportion of its muscular belly but that can be sacrificed without harming its viability. The *motor nerve* is the medial plantar nerve.

The abductor hallucis muscle can be freed from its insertion and rotated 90 percent to cover defects over the medial malleolus. The relative small size of the muscle, however, limits its use to small defects.

*Flexor Digitorum Brevis*
The flexor digitorum brevis muscle originates from the medial process of the calcaneum as well as from the plantar fascia. It consists of four small muscles that insert into the second through the fifth toes.

The flexor digitorum brevis muscle belly is supplied by small branches from the medial and lateral plantar vessels, which enter at the proximal one-third of the muscles. The *motor nerve* is the medial plantar nerve.

The flexor digitorum brevis has been used as a turnover flap for coverage of defects on the heel.

There are disadvantages to its use. The dissection can be difficult, as one must divide the plantar fascia as well as the tendinous insertions. In doing so, the underlying digital nerves, which can be confused with the tendons, may be injured. The incisions needed to dissect the flexor hallucis or the flexor digitorum brevis muscle through the medial aspect of the foot or the midfoot are inconsequential. Although a musculocutaneous flap of the flexor digitorum brevis muscle has been described, the dissection is difficult and the flap of limited use.

*Extensor Digitorum Brevis*

The extensor digitorum brevis, a relatively flat muscle, has a proximal blood supply and covers the dorsum of the foot. It has been used as a transposition muscle flap to cover defects over the ankle. The dissection requires exposure in the dorsum of the foot with retraction of the long extensor tendons. It may be considered for small defects, although its clinical use is limited.

Fasciocutaneous flaps have been described for the foot, including the medial plantar foot, as well as from the medial and lateral aspect of the sole of the foot to cover defects of the heel. These flaps appear to have considerable potential and await further clinical experience. The student is referred to the original articles of Hidalgo and Shaw [8] and Baker [2], which provide an erudite exposition of the anatomy and the clinical uses of fasciocutaneous flaps on the foot.

## Fasciocutaneous Flaps

Early reconstructive plastic surgery evolved around the waltzing tube pedicle flap, the flap width/length ratio, and the delay procedure. It was emphasized that the flap length must not be longer than the width of the carrying pedicle. Early in this century flaps were raised in the subcutaneous plane, although occasionally it was advised to include at least part of the fascia if possible. McGregor [16] also observed that the deltopectoral flap might be extended if the fascia was included in the flap. Still, for most of the century skin flaps were raised at varying depths of the subcutaneous tissue with strict adherence to the length/width ratio principle. The delay procedure likewise was a major necessary principle for ensuring the success of a skin flap. By partially raising a flap from its bed, immediately replacing it in its bed, and reharvesting the tissue layer for its reconstructive purpose, it was thought that the blood supply would be enhanced and the nonvital portion would demarcate. The delay procedure was haphazard and in effect consisted in trial and error.

It was Ponten [26] who demonstrated the reliability of a flap elevated without the underlying muscle. This flap consisted of skin, subcutaneous tissue, and fascia; and Ponten first described it in the territory of the medial head of the gastrocnemius. We now know that this fasciocutaneous flap has a source of blood supply that could be a direct vessel from the sural artery or a musculocutaneous perforator from the gastrocnemius muscle that perforates the fascia and arborizes on top of the fascia to supply the overlying skin. Since then, other territories where one could outline and elevate a skin and fascial flap have been described and found to be reliable without need for a delay. The sources of blood supply to these fasciocutaneous flaps are several. The source could be distinct, i.e., perforating vessels from the underlying muscles such as with the Ponten flap; it could be septocutaneous vessels, which branch periodically from the major arteries such as in the leg; or it could be a major artery that supplies the overlying fascia and skin, as in the radial forearm flap. We do not have a unifying concept to group these fasciocutaneous flaps into categories; and it is likely, as indicated at the beginning of this chapter, that the sources of blood supply are multiple and if one remains it is sufficient to supply the fascia and overlying skin.

The most common fasciocutaneous muscle flaps with what is known of their blood supply are described in the following sections.

GASTROCNEMIUS FASCIOCUTANEOUS FLAP (PONTEN SUPER FLAP)

The gastrocnemius fasciocutaneous flap corresponds to the medial head of the gastrocnemius muscle, and it can be extended down to approximately 10 cm from the medial malleolus. It is elevated, with the skin and the fascia dividing a portion of the achilles tendon. It can be used to cover defects in the mid and proximal tibia. Its blood supply is most likely through the septocutaneous system of vessels described by Carriquiry et al.

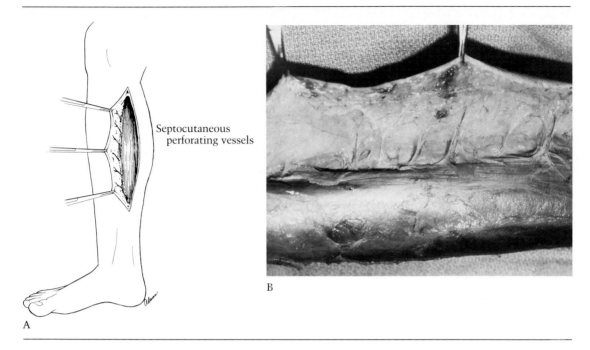

***Figure 45-17*** *Septocutaneous perforators*
*A. Anatomic dissection of septocutaneous*
*vessels is shown in B. Each of the vessels from*
*the trifurcation has segmental septocutaneous*
*perforators, which have clinical importance in*
*the design of fasciocutaneous flaps in the leg.*

[20], although a distinct branch from the sural artery has also been found as well as perforating branches from the gastrocnemius muscle. A similar flap can be outlined on the lateral aspect of the leg, again based on the septocutaneous vessels.

FASCIOCUTANEOUS FLAPS BASED ON SEPTOCUTANEOUS VESSELS
The work of Carriquiry and Vásconez [25] demonstrated segmental branching from the three major arteries of the leg that travel through the intramuscular septum and perforate the fascia, arborizing on top of it to anastomose with the superior and inferior arteries while supplying the subcutaneous tissue and the skin (Fig. 45-17). If one of these vessels is preserved, a fasciocutaneous flap of sufficient size can be elevated by a variety of methods. The flap can be a turn-

over flap, as demonstrated by Thatte and Talwar [27] from the medial and lateral aspect of the leg, or it can be a distally based flap from the midcalf, which can be helpful for coverage of defects over the ankle. The three vessels in the lower leg have this segmental branching, and consequently fasciocutaneous flaps can be outlined in the medial, lateral, and posterior calf. Fascial flaps alone have also been reported to be transposed to cover the bone.

*Fasciocutaneous Flaps in the Anterior and Medial Thigh and Lower Abdominal Wall*
At the level of the inguinal ligament there is considerable arterial branching that resembles the spokes of a cart wheel. Superiorly, the superficial inferior epigastric artery supplies the lower abdominal wall; extending laterally, the superficial circumflex iliac artery supplies the well known territory of the groin flap; medially it is the superficial medial circumflex artery; and there are unnamed branches that extend inferiorly like the spokes of a cart wheel. These vessels can

be used to outline territories of skin and fascia, leaving intact the underlying muscle on well known territories of the musculocutaneous flaps.

### Fasciocutaneous Flap on the Anterior Thigh

The entire skin and fascia of the anterior thigh from midlateral to midlateral line can be elevated as a fasciocutaneous unit, leaving intact the underlying musculature. As this unit is elevated one finds intermuscular septal vessels that are divided and are not true muscular perforators. Proximally there is a distinct muscular perforator at the same level as the major blood supply to the rectus femoris muscle that perforates the muscle and the overlying fascia to supply the skin. In addition, there is a distinct unnamed inferiorly directed vessel originating from the profunda femoris at the level of the inguinal ligament that is the most likely source of arterial supply to this fasciocutaneous territory. This fasciocutaneous flap has been used alone or in combination with a separate rectus femoris muscle for reconstruction of lower abdominal defects. Although the entire anterior thigh can be taken as a fasciocutaneous flap, it is advised that this fasciocutaneous flap be of a limited width so that the donor defect can be closed primarily; moreover, it must be centered over the rectus femoris muscle.

### Gracilis Territory Fasciocutaneous Flap

The skin and fascial territory over the gracilis muscle, which can also be elevated without the underlying muscle in the form of skin and fascia, has been used to cover defects in the ischium. The blood supply is most likely from a true proximal perforator at the level of the proximal pedicle of the gracilis muscle as well as direct vessels from the "cart wheel" arrangement of the femoral artery branching.

The tensor fascia lata fasciocutaneous flap, already discussed, is a combination of muscle and fasciocutaneous territory.

### Posterior Thigh Fasciocutaneous Flap

Hurwitz [10] described an area on the posterior thigh over the biceps femoris territory that can be elevated with skin and fascia; it had a distinct longitudinal running vessel along the posterior cutaneous nerve that was included in the flap. This vessel is a branch of the inferior gluteal artery and is present in most patients. Even when this vessel is not present, the same territory can be outlined and elevated with skin and fascia owing to the branching from the cruciate anastomosis, which supplies the posterior thigh. The flap is usually outlined between the greater trochanter and ischial tuberosity, and the width is limited by what can be closed primarily.

## FASCIOCUTANEOUS FLAPS IN THE CHEST

The lateral scapular flap has been described in the posterolateral chest; it extends from the tip of the scapula inferiorly for approximately 20 cm, with its anterior border along the posterior axillary line. The blood supply is a direct branch from the posterior scapula artery, which also supplies the well known scapular flap utilized for free flap surgery. This vertically oriented flap has been useful for coverage of defects along the axilla, particularly burn scars that produce axillary contractures. The presence of skin grafts over the fascia have not precluded its use.

## FASCIOCUTANEOUS FLAPS IN THE ARM

The segmental septocutaneous arrangement described for the lower leg has not been studied in the arm. It is likely that this system also prevails in the upper extremity.

In the arm there are distinct fasciocutaneous territories based on distinct vessels such as the posterior arm flap over the triceps and the less reliable medial arm flap. The deltoid flap is also a fasciocutaneous flap, and it is used as a free flap donor site.

Less well known are fasciocutaneous flaps that can be outlined in the forearm for coverage of defects in the antecubital fossa and elbow. These fasciocutaneous flaps are usually outlined on the dorsum or the volar aspect of the forearm for coverage of burn contractures in the antecubital fossa (dorsal fasciocutaneous forearm flap) and for coverage of the elbow joint (volar fasciocutaneous flaps). They are transposition flaps that include the skin, subcutaneous tissue, and if possible the thin fascia covering the forearm musculature. The blood supply probably comes from intermuscular vessels that are branches of the brachial artery.

The radial forearm (Chinese) flap, another fasciocutaneous flap, has gained considerable interest because of its use as a free flap territory. It includes all of the radial artery and accompanying fascia, and it supplies the overlying fascia and skin territory over the forearm, which may include a portion of the radial bone; it can be used as a free flap followed by reconstruction of the radial artery with a vein graft or as a distally based flap for coverage of defects in the dorsum or volar aspect of the hand.

There are other territories that perhaps fall into the classification of fasciocutaneous flaps, e.g., forehead, deltopectoral muscle, dorsalis pedis muscle. These flaps are discussed elsewhere in this book, and their classification is not important. Rather, they help us to understand the blood supply, which allows us to elevate and transpose a flap that is reliable and accomplishes the objective of the reconstruction.

Acknowledgment
Our thanks go to Drs. Rexon Ngim and Thomas O. Rumley, who reviewed our manuscript.

## *References*
### MUSCLE AND MYOCUTANEOUS FLAPS

1. Bakamjian, V. Y. A technique for primary reconstruction of the palate after radical maxillectomy for cancer. *Plast. Reconstr. Surg.* 31:103, 1963.
2. Baker, G. L., Newton, E. D., and Franklin, J. D. Fasciocutaneous island flap based on the medial plantar artery: Clinical applications for leg, ankle, and forefoot. *Plast. Reconstr. Surg.* 85:47, 1990.
3. Bonnel, S. New concepts on the arterial vascularisation of skin and muscle. *Plast. Reconstr. Surg.* 75:552, 1985.
4. Cole, P. P. Treatment of wounds involving the mucous membrane of the mouth and nose. *Lancet* 1:11, 1918.
5. D'Este, S. La technique de l'amputation de la mamelle pour carcinome mammaire. *Rev. Chir. (Paris)* 45:164, 1912.
6. Ger, R. The technique of muscle transposition in the operative treatment of traumatic and ulcerative lesions of the leg. *J. Trauma* 11:502, 1971.
7. Ger, R. The management of chronic ulcers of the dorsum of the foot by muscle transposition and free skin grafting. *Br. J. Plast. Surg.* 29:199, 1976.
8. Hildago, D. A., and Shaw, W. W. Anatomical basis of plantar flap design. *Plast. Reconstr. Surg.* 78:627, 1986.
9. Hueston, J. T., and McConchie, I. H. A compound pectoral flap. *Aust. N. Z. J. Surg.* 38:61, 1968.
10. Hurwitz, D. J., Swarts, W. M., and Mathes, S. J. The gluteal thigh flap: A reliable sensate flap for the closure of buttock and perineal wounds. *Plast. Reconstr. Surg.* 68:521, 1981.
11. Mathes, S. J., and Nahai, F. Classification of the vascular anatomy of muscles: Experimental and clinical correlation. *Plast. Reconstr. Surg.* 67:177, 1981.
12. Mathes, S. J., and Nahai, F. (ed.). *Clinical Applications for Muscle and Musculocutaneous Flaps.* St. Louis: Mosby, 1982.
13. McCraw, J. B., and Vasconez, L. O. Musculocutaneous flaps: Principles. *Clin. Plast. Surg.* 7:9, 1980.
14. McCraw, J. B., and Dibbell, D. G. Experimental definition of independent myocutaneous vascular territories. *Plast. Reconstr. Surg.* 60:212, 1977.
15. McCraw, J. B., Dibbell, D. G., and Carraway, J. H. Clinical definition of independent myocutaneous vascular territories. *Plast. Reconstr. Surg.* 60:341, 1977.
16. McGregor, I. A., and Morgan, G. Axial and random pattern flaps. *Br. J. Plast. Surg.* 26:202, 1973.
17. (Ombredanne, L.) Teimourian, B., and Ad-

ham, M. N. Louis Ombredanne and the origin of muscle flap use for immediate breast mound reconstruction. *Plast. Reconstr. Surg.* 72:905, 1983.

18. Orticochea, M. The musculocutaneous flap method. *Br. J. Plast. Surg.* 25:106, 1972.

19. Owens, N. A compound neck pedicle designed for repair of massive facial defects: Formation, development and application. *Plast. Reconstr. Surg.* 15:369, 1955.

20. Ramirez, Q., Orlando, J. C., and Hurwitz, D. J. The sliding gluteus maximus myocutaneous flap: Its relevance in ambulatory patients. *Plast. Reconstr. Surg.* 74:68, 1984.

21. Rantio, J., et al. Suitability of the scapular flap for reconstruction of the foot. *Plast. Reconstr. Surg.* 85:922, 1990.

22. Taylor, G. I., Corbett, R., and Boyd, J. B. The extended deep inferior epigastric flap: A clinical technique. *Plast. Reconstr. Surg.* 72:751, 1983.

23. Vásconez, L. O., Bostwick, J., and McCraw, J. Coverage of exposed bone by muscle transposition and skin grafting. *Plast. Reconstr. Surg.* 53:526, 1974.

24. Vásconez, L. O., McCraw, J. B., and Hall, E. J. Complications of musculocutaneous flaps. *Clin. Plast. Surg.* 7:123, 1980.

## FASCIOCUTANEOUS FLAPS

25. Carriquiry, C., Costa, M. A., and Vasconez, L. O. An anatomic study of the septocutaneous vessels of the leg. *Plast. Reconstr. Surg.* 76:354, 1985.

26. Ponten, S. The fasciocutaneous flap: Its use in soft tissue defects of the lower leg. *Br. J. Plast. Surg.* 34:215, 1983.

27. Thatte, R., and Talwar, P. De-epithelialized "turn over" axial-pattern flaps in the lower extremity. *Br. J. Plast. Surg.* 36:327, 1983.

## *Suggested Reading*

### MUSCLE AND MYOCUTANEOUS FLAPS

Ariyan, S. The pectoralis major myocutaneous flap. *Plast. Reconstr. Surg.* 63:73, 1979.

Bostwick, J., III. Latissimus dorsi flap: Current applications. *Ann. Plast. Surg.* 9:377, 1982.

Carriquiry, C. Heel coverage with a deepithelialized distally based fasciocutaneous flap. *Plast. Reconstr. Surg.* 85:116, 1990.

Coleman, J. J., and Jurkiewicz, M. J. Methods of providing sensation to anesthetic areas. *Ann. Plast. Surg.* 12:177, 1984.

Fong, P. H., Casanova, R., and Vasconez, L. O. Myocutaneous and fasciocutaneous flaps in the upper limb. *Hand Clin.* 1:759, 1985.

Ger, R., and Duboys, E. The prevention and repair of large abdominal wall defects by muscle transposition: A preliminary communication. *Plast. Reconstr. Surg.* 72:170, 1983.

Hagerty, R. C., Bostwick, J., and Nahai, F. Denervated muscle flaps: Mass and thickness changes following denervation. *Ann. Plast. Surg.* 12:171, 1984.

Hill, H. L., Hester, R., and Nahai, F. Covering large groin defects with the tensor fascia lata musculocutaneous flap. *Br. J. Plast. Surg.* 32:12, 1979.

Hill, H. L., Nahai, F., and Vasconez, L. O. The tensor fascia lata myocutaneous free flap. *Plast. Reconstr. Surg.* 64:517, 1978.

Hodgkinson, D. J., and Shepard, G. H. Muscle, musculocutaneous and fasciocutaneous flaps in forearm reconstruction. *Ann. Plast. Surg.* 10:400, 1983.

Lewis, V. L., et al. The fasciocutaneous flap: A conservative approach to the exposed knee joint. *Plast. Reconstr. Surg.* 85:252, 1990.

Luce, E. A., and Gottlieb, S. F. The pectoralis major island flap for coverage in the upper extremity. *J. Hand Surg.* 7:156, 1982.

Mathes, S. J., and Buchanan, R. T. Tensor fascia lata: Neurosensory musculocutaneous free flap. *Br. J. Plast. Surg.* 32:184, 1979.

Mathes, S. J., McCraw, J. B., and Vasconez, L. Muscle transposition flaps for coverage of lower extremity defects: Anatomic considerations. *Surg. Clin. North Am.* 54:1337, 1974.

Mathes, S. J., Vasconez, L. O., and Jurkiewicz, M. J. Expansions and further applications of muscle flap transposition. *Plast. Reconstr. Surg.* 60:6, 1977.

McCraw, J. B. The recent history of myocutaneous flaps. *Clin. Plast. Surg.* 7:3, 1980.

McCraw, J. B., and Arnold, P. G. *Atlas of Muscle and Musculocutaneous Flaps.* Norfolk, VA: Hampton Press, 1986.

Nahai, F., and Mathes, S. J. Musculocutaneous flap or muscle flap and skin graft. *Ann. Plast. Surg.* 12:199, 1984.

Nahai, F., Morales, L., Bone, D. K., and Bostwick,

J. Pectoralis major muscle turnover flaps for closure of the infected sternotomy wound with preservation of form and function. *Plast. Reconstr. Surg.* 70:471, 1982.

Nakajima, H., Fujino, T., and Adachi, S. A new concept of vascular supply to the skin and classification of skin flaps according to their vascularisation. *Ann. Plast. Surg.* 16:1, 1986.

Orticochea, M. History of the discovery of the musculocutaneous flap method as a substitute for the delay method. *Ann. Plast. Surg.* 11:63, 1983.

Plaza, de la R., Arroyo, J. M., and Vasconez, L. O. Upper transverse rectus abdominis flap: The Flag Flap. *Ann. Plast. Surg.* 12:410, 1984.

Scheflan, M., Nahai, F., and Bostwick, J. Gluteus maximus island musculocutaneous flap for closure of sacral and ischial ulcers. *Plast. Reconstr. Surg.* 68:533, 1981.

Soutar, D. S., Sheker, L. R., Tanner, N. S. B., et al. The radial forearm flap: A versatile method for intraoral reconstruction. *Br. J. Plast. Surg.* 36:1, 1983.

Strauch, B., Vásconez, L. O., and Hall-Findlay, E. J. (eds.). *Grabb's Encyclopedia of Flaps.* Boston: Little, Brown, 1990.

Tanzini. Spora 11 nito nuova processo di aupertozione della menuelle. *Riforma Med.* 22:757, 1906.

Tobin, G. R. Vastus medialis myocutaneous and myocutaneous-tendinous composite flaps. *Plast. Reconstr. Surg.* 75:677, 1985.


## FASCIOCUTANEOUS FLAPS

Amarante, J., Costa, H., Reis, J., et al. A new distally based fasciocutaneous flap of the leg. *Br. J. Plast.* 39:338, 1986.

Barclay, T. L., Cardoso, E., Sharpe, D. T., et al. Repair of lower leg injuries with fasciocutaneous flaps. *Br. J. Plast. Surg.* 35:127, 1982.

Barclay, T. L. Sharpe, D. T., and Chisholm, E. M. Cross-leg fasciocutaneous flaps. *Plast. Reconstr. Surg.* 72:843, 1983.

Bonnel, F. New concepts of the arterial vascularisation of skin and muscle. *Plast. Reconstr. Surg.* 75:552, 1985.

Bunkis, J., Ryu, R. K., Walton, R. L., et al. Fasciocutaneous flap coverage for periolecranon defects. *Ann. Plast. Surg.* 14:361, 1985.

Chase, R. A. Historical review of skin a soft tissue coverage of the upper extremity. *Hand Clin.* 1:599, 1985.

Cormack, G. C., and Lamberty, B. G. H. The anatomical vascular basis of the axillary fasciocutaneous pedicled flap. *Br. J. Plast. Surg.* 36:425, 1983.

Cormack, G. C., and Lamberty, B. G. H. The blood supply of thigh skin. *Plast. Reconstr. Surg.* 75:342, 1985.

Donski, P. K., and Fogdestam, I. Distally based fasciocutaneous flap from the sural region: A preliminary report. *Scand. J. Plast. Reconstr. Surg.* 17:191, 1983.

Fisher, J. External oblique fasciocutaneous flap for elbow coverage. *Plast. Reconstr. Surg.* 75:51, 1985.

Fong, P. H., Casanova, R., and Vasconez, L. O. Myocutaneous and fasciocutaneous flaps in the upper limb. *Hand Clin.* 1:759, 1985.

Haertsch, P. The surgical plane in the leg. *Br. J. Plast. Surg.* 34:464, 1981.

Haertsch, P. A. The blood supply to the skin of the leg: A post-mortem investigation. *Br. J. Plast. Surg.* 34:470, 1981.

Hazarika, E. Z. An inadvertent test of the robustness of a 5:1 fasciocutaneous flap. *Br. J. Plast. Surg.* 38:522, 1985.

Lamberty, B. G. H., and Cormack, G. C. The antecubital fascio-cutaneous flap. *Br. J. Plast. Surg.* 36:428, 1983.

Maruyama, Y. Bilobed fasciocutaneous flap. *Br. J. Plast. Surg.* 38:515, 1985.

Maruyama, Y., Ohnishi, K., and Chung, C. C. Vertical abdominal fasciocutaneous flaps in the reconstruction of chest wall defects. *Br. J. Plast. Surg.* 38:230, 1985.

Moscona, A. R., Govrin-Yehudain, J., and Hirshowitz, B. The island fasciocutaneous flap; a new type of flap for defects of the knee. *Br. J. Plast. Surg.* 38:512, 1985.

Nakajima, H., Maruyama, Y., and Koda, E. The definition of vascular skin territories with prostaglandin E: The anterior chest, abdomen and thigh-inguinal region. *Br. J. Plast. Surg.* 34:258, 1981.

Tolhurst, D. E., Haeseker, B., and Zeeman, R. J. The development of the fasciocutaneous flaps. *Ann. Plast. Surg.* 13:495, 1984.

Tolhurst, D. E. Surgical indications for fasciocutaneous flaps. *Ann. Plast. Surg.* 13:495, 1984.

# VI
## Breast

# 46

*Thomas M. Biggs*
*David H. Humphreys*

# Augmentation Mammaplasty

From prehistoric times the female breast has represented a life-engendering structure and has been one of the primary features symbolizing feminine attributes. Despite diversity in ancient or modern cultures, the body image of the modern woman is adversely affected by the unaesthetic breast. From the mastectomy amputee to the spectrum of deviations from an aesthetic norm of breast shape and size, unhappiness and poor self-image are sustained. The task of augmentation mammaplasty, then, is to improve the self-esteem and thus improve the lives of those women desiring fuller, more shapely breasts.

Augmentation of the breast has been attempted with a number of techniques during the past century. Czerny reconstructed a volume defect in a breast after removal of a benign tumor in 1895 by using autogenous fat. Percutaneous injections of paraffin were performed by Gersuny in 1899. They were unstable biologic implants that resulted in granulomatous tissue reactions as well as poor cosmetic contour. Free fat grafts, glass bead implants, and fat dermal grafts have all been attempted and reported but have proved less than satisfactory. Dermal fat grafts and dermal fat flaps were utilized with some degree of success prior to the development of a reliable prosthetic implant. In 1951 Pangman described a synthetic implant of a polymer of polyvinyl alcohol and formaldehyde—the Ivalon sponge. Severe firmness secondary to ingrowth of scar tissue into the sponge, along with a high incidence of infection and seroma formation, produced a less than sustained and enthusiastic use of this implant. Injection of silicone fluid to augment the breast was practiced by some during the 1950s and 1960s. Aside from unnatural-appearing breasts, numerous untoward complications were seen. Granulomas, migration of silicone, chronic swelling, and even embolic phenomena and death have been linked with silicone injection for augmentation.

The modern era of breast augmentation began with the introduction of the silicone gel prosthesis in 1963 by Cronin and Gerow. The senior author of this chapter was privileged as a resident to be present at the placement of the first silicone gel prosthesis at the initial clinical trial. The original prosthesis had a Dacron patch at the back that was used to "fix" the implant to the chest wall, as motion of the implant was considered undesirable. A small retromammary pocket was created just large enough for the implant. With the development of seamless implants and the appreciation of the normal sequela of fibrous encapsulation of the implants, the concept of the "large pocket–

smaller implant," maintained through continued manipulation of the implant, produced superior, more natural long-term results. Concomitant with surgeons' experience, the prosthesis underwent design modifications. The Dacron patch was removed, the shell made thinner, and the shape altered.

A befuddling assortment of prostheses and a variety of approaches now confront the surgeon and patient in their mutual quest for the optimum result. Presently, there are three general types of implantable augmentation breast prosthesis: Two have a smooth outer envelope, or shell, of silicone elastomer, and the third has a fuzzy outer envelope of polyurethane. Of the two with the shell of smooth silicone elastomer, one comes prefilled with a soft silicone gel, and the other combines the gel in one compartment with an inflatable compartment for saline. Various designs for increased or decreased projection with varying base diameters and volumes are manufactured by several companies. The polyurethane-covered implant contains a core of soft silicone gel. Silicone for medical uses takes protean forms. By manipulation of the cross-linking of the dimethylsiloxane units, substances from a nonviscous fluid to a hard rubbery block can be created. The silicone gel-filled implants most closely mimic the palpable softness of normal breast tissue.

### Initial Interview

The candidate for augmentation mammaplasty is evaluated in an empathic and unhurried manner. The patient may have a friend or relative who has undergone the procedure and so is knowledgeable about the postoperative appearance and potential sequelae attendant to the procedure, or she may be medically naive and have no idea what to expect. Our approach is to begin the initial interview with a probe into the patient's knowledge of the procedure of augmentation mammaplasty in general. One avoids condescension to the well informed and intelligent patient as well as erroneous assumption of basic knowledge on the part of the less informed candidate about this technique. Communication, as always, must effectively begin with this nondirective approach to the patient. We ascertain at this time the patient's expectations of the procedure along with her prejudices, fears, and illusions with regard to augmentation of her breasts. The emotional stability of the patient can usually be evaluated well by a skillful and patient surgical interview. If serious psychopathologic tendencies are discovered, deferral of surgery and appropriate counseling are recommended.

The patient's history is obtained, with careful questioning regarding occupation and recreational life-style being most important. If the appearance of the breasts during dynamic athletic activity such as bodybuilding or swimming is of particular concern to the patient, it is opportune to note that the appearance of breasts during excessive contraction of the pectoralis muscle may be somewhat altered when the implant is submuscular. A complete history for benign or malignant breast disease, previous biopsies, cysts, pain, or tenderness is necessary. Particular and pointed questioning on the use of salicylates is advised. If aspirin or a similar coagulant-altering drug is being taken by the patient, she is urged to discontinue it at least 2 weeks prior to the anticipated date of surgery.

After obtaining the history and before having the patient draped for physical examination, the surgeon discusses the history of the operation. It is important to go far back into history describing the breast as a mythical symbol of femininity and how a desire to improve the appearance of one's breasts is not an expression of psychopathology or even vanity but simply a desire to conform to one's own self-image, which is the creation of our own culture.

During the history discussion, the appearance on the scene of the Silastic prosthesis is described, and the subsequent evolution in breast enhancement operations is explained. This method gives the opportunity to discuss early problems such as firmness, infection, and hematoma and the fact that through an evolution of the prosthesis and a refinement of technique, these complications have been markedly diminished—*but not totally eliminated.* It is preferable to finish this discussion by frankly stating that despite these complications, which have been considerably decreased, this operation yields perhaps as high a degree of patient happiness as any performed.

A physical examination is conducted with scrupulous evaluation of the breasts. Studied observation of symmetry, noting the extent or lack of breast tissue and subcutaneous fat along with the elasticity of the skin, is mandatory. The chest wall characteristics, bony prominences, and presence of scoliosis or kyphosis are noted. Particular attention is paid to the inframammary fold and the angle the breast makes with the chest, anticipating the effect an implanted and thus heavier breast will have on this fold. Congenital deformities of the breasts, such as tuberous herniation or "Snoopy" shape, are noted. If ptosis is present, it is pointed out to the patient, and the possibility of concurrent mastopexy is entertained. Finally, the breasts are examined for any masses, suspicious thickening, or presence of any hypertrophic scars. Should the breast examination reveal a mass or other focal abnormality, or should the history arouse suspicion of pathology, a xeromammagram is obtained prior to performing the augmentation.

After the physical examination, discussion of individual patient goals regarding size and shape is made more meaningful. If the patient is flat-chested with tight skin, she must understand that only a moderate augmentation is possible at initial operation. Similarly, an obese patient may lack the dramatic change she desires even after a large implant is placed. Cup size, per se, is not promised, although patient desires re-

garding the larger or smaller choices in augmentation must be fully ascertained and agreed on. The surgeon's aesthetic judgment is often the decisive element in final selection of size. Many patients have implicit faith in the plastic surgeon's sense of artistry and duty to its execution. A sense of moderation with regard to overall body proportion guides the surgeon in the ultimate selection of implant size.

The surgeon now explains the operative procedure in detail to the patient. Incisions, anesthesia, operative facilities, office follow-up, and continued patient maintenance of the megapocket are discussed. We have discarded the term "massage" as inaccurate and misleading. Vigorous squeezing of the breast and implant may, in fact, disseminate bacteria around the breast tissue and implant, causing potential problems.

The surgeon mentions again the potential sequelae commonly associated with the procedure of augmentation mammaplasty: hematoma, infection, asymmetry, postoperative discomfort, dysesthesia (hypoesthesia, hyperesthesia, or numbness), hypertrophic scar formation, and firmness from excessive capsule formation. We attach great importance to the extended discussion of capsular formation, which we believe not to be a complication but a normal aspect of healing with the use of the silicone implant or any foreign material. We demonstrate the "normal" capsule surrounding the implant by using the patient's drape sheet loosely holding a real implant. We show the patient how spherical contracture of the capsule surrounding the implant makes the once soft gel feel firm by tightening the drape sheet around the implant. We also discuss the potential need for capsule release following augmentation should an undesirable firmness result at any time after the surgery.

After the extended discussion and the physical examination, it is imperative that the patient is encouraged to ask all the questions she can possibly be concerned about, and they must be answered with frankness.

The inevitable question about size is impossible to answer specifically, and it must be so stated; a general response can be given, and the patient must be made to understand that it is just that—a general response.

Before the initial interview is completed, the patient, if she is a smoker, is advised to discontinue the use of tobacco 1 week before surgery and to refrain for 1 week following the operation. Details regarding coughing and intermittent hypertension with potential bleeding are explained.

Preoperative photographic documentation using direct frontal and right and left oblique views completes the presurgical evaluation of the augmentation mammaplasty patient. A thorough explanation of her costs, including surgeon's fee, hospital fees, and anesthesia fee, is given so that she may leave the surgeon's office fully prepared to proceed, having been advised on all aspects of the endeavor.

In a survey of American Society of Plastic and Reconstructive Surgeons (ASPRS) members, augmentation mammaplasty was the single most commonly performed aesthetic procedure in 1984. It may be done successfully in the hospital as an inpatient procedure or as an outpatient procedure in a hospital, surgicenter, or office. Local or general anesthesia may be used. A variety of approaches are used worldwide with pleasing results. Our approach has evolved over the past quarter-century. Retromammary placement of the implant under local anesthesia was our standard operation during the 1960s and 1970s. We changed techniques to subpectoral placement under general anesthesia in 1981 and continue to believe that this technique works best for us. With regard to the postoperative complications of hematoma and infection, our present technique has virtually eliminated them. The incidence of capsular contracture in our patients has declined significantly since using the submuscular placement. The number of patients requiring operative fibrous capsule re-

lease after augmentation has become distinctly smaller and is less than 5 percent.

We prefer general anesthesia for augmentation mammaplasty. The safety of general anesthesia, with control of the airway at all times and careful monitoring of vital signs, frees the surgeon from anxiety about the overly sedated and perhaps hypoxic patient in a semicooperative state. It also allows complete muscular relaxation necessary for creation of the appropriate submuscular pocket by bloodless dissection with electrocautery. With skillful anesthesia, the problems of postoperative nausea are rarely encountered.

## Operative Technique

The patient is placed on the table in the supine position with the arms at the side. The "break" in the table is in such a position as to allow for fluid intraoperative assessment of the patient in a near-vertical position as the table "flexes." The shoulders are level. After induction of anesthesia, the elbows are flexed at 90-degree angles, and foam protectors are placed at the bony prominences. The hands are taped to the iliac spines in a symmetric and stable manner (Fig. 46-1). The patient's chest and upper abdomen are prepped with povidone-iodine (Betadine) or chlorhexidine gluconate (Hibiclens), painted with alcohol, and dried. Plastic Steri-Drapes are placed horizontally across the chest above the clavicles and across the costal margins, with vertical drapes overlapping them at the anterior axillary line or just posterior to it. Lint-free disposable drapes cover the remainder of the patient. All talc and cornstarch are wiped meticulously off the gloves of the surgeons and all scrubbed assistants with alcohol-moistened sponges. A bright fiberoptic headlight is important equipment for the operating surgeon. We have found it to provide superior illumination and better visibility of the operative field than any of the variety of illuminated retractors that are

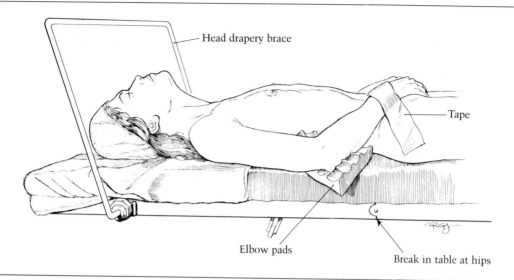

Head drapery brace

Tape

Elbow pads

Break in table at hips

**Figure 46-1** *The positioning of the patient on the operating table is shown. Note the break in the table at the level of the hips to allow intraoperative flexion for aesthetic assessment in near-vertical attitude.*

offered. The midline of the chest is determined and marked for reference.

An incision is planned in the inframammary fold. This incision allows direct visualization of the entire subpectoral pocket and meticulous incremental dissection of such a pocket with electrocautery. It allows control and maintenance of the curvilinear inferior lateral soft tissues and ultimate control over placement of the inframammary fold. It has the advantage of being a truly extraglandular operation for placement of the implant, with no breast parenchyma or ducts violated. It also allows capsule release through the identical incision should the need arise at a later time. It heals as a barely perceptible thin ivory scar in most patients. The single disadvantage is individual patient preference for another area.

Other incisional approaches produce many fine results for many plastic surgeons (Fig. 46-2). With the periareolar approach, an incision at the periphery of the areola is made,

usually from the three o'clock to the nine o'clock position. The dissection then proceeds inferiorly either subcutaneously or transglandularly until the inferior border of the pectoralis major muscle is identified. The subpectoral or retromammary pocket is then dissected and the implant inserted. The advantages of the periareolar incision are individual patient preference and the natural camouflage of the scar using the areolar skin interface in color transition. The potential disadvantages are several. Patients with small

**Figure 46-2** *The three incisional approaches used for augmentation are shown: inframammary, periareolar, and transaxillary.*

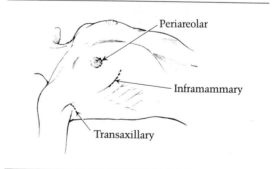

Periareolar

Inframammary

Transaxillary

areolae are not suitable, as the resulting incision may not allow insertion of the implant. Ductal and parenchymal tissue of the mammary gland are traumatized with entrance into potential "nonsterile" tissue, which may predispose to scarring within the breast itself and nodule formation. Hemostasis is more difficult to achieve, and there is poor visualization of the megapocket. Excessive surgical retraction may contribute to postoperative ecchymosis over the skin in the inferior quadrants of the breast. With exposure through the periareolar incision, precise delineation of the new inframammary fold is more problematic and uncontrolled than with more direct access.

A third approach for augmentation of the breasts utilizes a transaxillary incision and a superior to inferior dissection of the pocket. Retromammary or retropectoral placement of the prosthesis may be effected. Although this approach has its advocates for the advantages of a small and topographically favorable scar obscured by the normal axillary folds, we believe the disadvantages and potential problems encountered in this technique make it the least desirable approach. Complications associated with the transaxillary approach are in part due to the capriciousness of axillary anatomy and in part to lack of control of the formation of the pocket, notably in the inframammary area. The anatomy of the axilla is variable with respect to the course of the intercostobrachial and medial brachial cutaneous nerves. These important sensory nerves may lie superficially and be damaged when making the skin incision, leaving anesthetic or dysesthetic areas in the upper arms. Medium-sized veins may be encountered with regularity, and lateral thoracic vein thrombosis and even subclavian vein thrombosis have been described with this approach. The abundance of lymphatics in the axilla can produce an untoward lymphangitis of the upper arm, clearly a dangerous and unacceptable complication for an elective cosmetic procedure.

Aesthetic technical difficulties also make this approach problematic. The necessary reliance on blind, blunt dissection at the inframammary fold may result in poor delineation of the new fold, inadequate contouring in a "tight" chest, and an unacceptably high incidence of asymmetry. Use of larger implants is hampered through the transaxillary approach, and inflatable implants are often necessary because of the shorter incisions. It is axiomatic that exposure is the key to strict hemostasis. With the limited visual access afforded by the transaxillary route, bleeding may be difficult to control.

Should the need arise with either the axillary or the periareolar technique, adequate open capsular release requires an inframammary approach for maximal success, creating the unhappy situation of further scars.

### Surgical Technique

With the patient supine and prepared for operation as described above, determination of the new inframammary fold is the first step in surgical planning. The exact midline of the chest is marked with methylene blue from the sternal notch to the xiphoid. The surgeon then grasps the breast at the areola with the thumb and fingertips and exerts firm inferior and gentle anterior traction (Fig. 46-3). The curvilinear skin crease that rises up from the lower chest wall with this maneuver is the new inframammary fold and is also drawn with methylene blue. We have found this simple technical aid to be consistently useful for planning the inframammary incision on virtually all types of breast, from those with normal volumes to the most minimal. It allows for the postoperative settling and skin stretching that occur with gravity and time. If measured, this line reproducibly falls 5 to 6 cm inferior to the areola, depending on the case. The inner extent of the incision begins no more medial than a line tangent to the nine o'clock position of the left areola or the three o'clock position of the right areola. The length of the

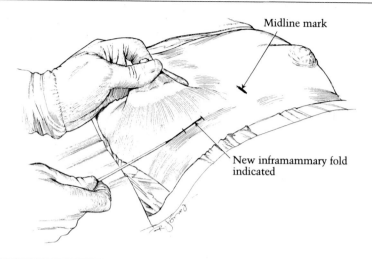

Midline mark

New inframammary fold indicated

**Figure 46-3** *Determination of the new inframammary fold is shown. The breast is pulled anteriorly with gentle inferior traction, and the line is drawn in the true inframammary fold.*

incision is 5 cm. A scalpel is used to incise the skin through the deep dermis only. Electrocautery is used from this point on in the procedure. As soon as the subcutaneous fatty layer is reached, the incision is immediately beveled upward, which maintains a shelf of soft tissue on the chest wall (Fig. 46-4). This maneuver reinforces the inframammary crease area and prevents unwanted postoperative descent of the prosthesis. It is an error to raise any portion of the subcutaneous inferior skin flap, as it may perceptibly lower the new inframammary crease. The inferior edge of the pectoralis major muscle is then identified (Fig. 46-5). The obliquity, thickness, and position of the muscle edge show great variability and must be ascertained with adequate exposure and thoughtful restraint. With proper upward traction by the assistant using a Dever retractor, the cobwebs from the muscle edge to the ribs and pectoralis minor are carefully taken down with the cutting current. The retractor is repositioned on the undersurface

of the muscle, and the broad medial origin of the pectoralis major muscle is released from its costosternal attachments (Fig. 46-6). Often these attachments are broad and highly vascular. Laterally, the muscle is freed to a point midway between the anterior and midaxillary lines. It is important to maintain a rounded contour of the soft tissue attachment at the lateral inferior areas, as too great a dissection here causes the implant to assume too posterior and lateral a position.

**Figure 46-4** *The incision is beveled upward as electrocautery dissection proceeds.*

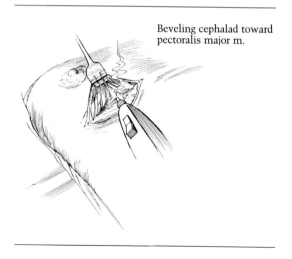

Beveling cephalad toward pectoralis major m.

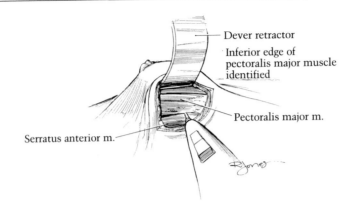

Dever retractor

Inferior edge of pectoralis major muscle identified

Pectoralis major m.

Serratus anterior m.

*Figure 46-5* The inferior edge of the pectoralis major muscle is identified at its confluence with the serratus anterior muscle.

Because of the conjoined origin of the pectoralis major and serratus anterior muscles, great care must be taken to identify precisely the lateral edge of the pectoralis major lest great confusion arise later. Once this edge is determined, the entirety of the origin of the pectoralis major is elevated. Differentiation of the pectoralis major and minor muscles is usually not difficult because of the more cephalad origin of the minor muscles. The dissection medially extends to near the midline, with care being taken to avoid dividing the vessels that enter the muscle in this area. With good light and retraction, these

vessels can be seen, dissected around, and avoided. If they are divided, great care is taken to achieve hemostasis. If the origin of the pectoralis major is not dissected medially to a sufficient extent, the implant cannot descend properly into the inferomedial area, and a contracted, displaced look results within a few weeks, if not on the operating table. As the dissection proceeds superiorly, the full origin of the pectoralis minor is left undisturbed and the thoracoacromial vessels are visualized from below, cradled in yellow fat on either side. Superiorly, the dissection stops just below the clavicles and only 1 to 2 cm from the suprasternal notch medially (Figs. 46-7 and 46-8). The intense illumination from the headlight allows immediate recognition and coagulation of any bleeding. With completion of the dissection, a generous volume of saline is irrigated, and the return of the solution is carefully scrutinized. A pale pink color confirms the initial impression of requisite hemostasis.

Intraoperative aesthetic decisions as to proper implant size are then made. A tray of sterile sizer implants is prepared routinely on all augmentations, and a trial sizer is then placed within the pocket. The attitude of the implant as it lies within the newly

*Figure 46-6* The medial costosternal attachments of the pectoralis major muscle are released. Note the extension on the electrocautery.

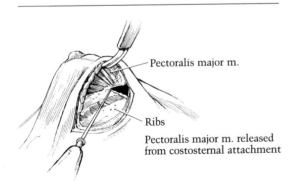

Pectoralis major m.

Ribs

Pectoralis major m. released from costosternal attachment

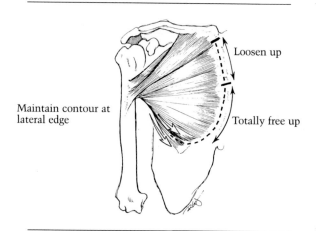

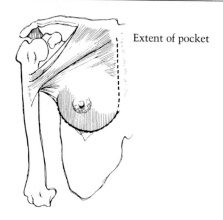

**Figure 46-7** *The lateral contour is maintained in the dissection as indicated by the arrows, and the medial attachments are liberally released.*

**Figure 46-8** *The extent of the submuscular dissection is shown. It is necessary to create a "megapocket" to the extent indicated for the result to look natural.*

created subpectoral megapocket is assessed as it is manipulated in all four directions. If further release is indicated in any portion of the pocket, the implant is removed and the release is now accomplished. The two sides are carefully compared: They should appear as mirror images medially and laterally, both high and low. This being the case, the patient is then raised to the vertical position on the table; she is assessed then from the foot of the table, with the overhead lights aimed at the nipples on either side. Any subtle asymmetry may be noted and accounted for at this time. Intrinsic anatomic asymmetry may be adjusted for by the use of implants of varying volumes, but usually prostheses of the same size are used. Slight asymmetry of the chest wall and breast volumes is neither an unusual nor an unaesthetic circumstance. Significant asymmetry may be corrected by an "implant-only reconstruction," i.e., an augmentation, with possibly concomitant adjustment of the opposite side. Occasionally, at a later time, the implant may need to be exchanged up or down a size for a more critical and demanding result. Infrequently, a patient may ask to be made larger months or years after the ini-

tial augmentation. Our use of the Silastic gel-filled implant during the initial procedures has allowed secondary adjustments and revisions to be effected with ease and predictability. We advise, therefore, extreme caution with the use of polyurethane-coated implants for augmentation because, once implanted, elective removal may be difficult.[*] The polyurethane coating becomes melded to the patient's tissues in an adhesive manner. These implants may have a tertiary role, however, in the salvage of intransigent capsule formers and in selective breast reconstructions. The permanent implants are then chosen as the patient is returned to the supine position. They are opened, moistened with saline, and immediately inserted with delicate fingertip manipulation. The label on the undersurface of the implant is palpated to make certain the implant has not

[*]During the period of time between acceptance of this manuscript and its publication, the authors have had greater experience with the polyurethane-coated implant and feel it has much to offer, not only in breast reconstruction and secondary mammaplasties but in primary augmentation as well. Their experience in over 300 patients suggests that the polyurethane implant has a negligible rate of fibrous contracture with minimal complications.

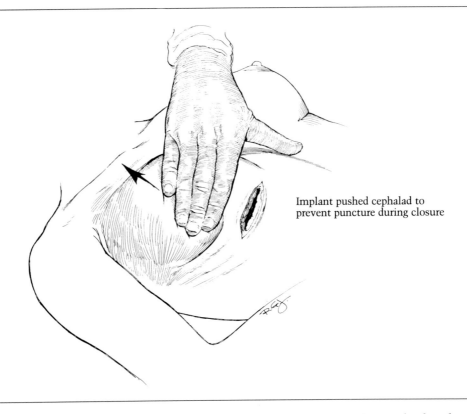

Implant pushed cephalad to
prevent puncture during closure

**Figure 46-9** *The implant is displaced to avoid
puncture during closure.*

been inadvertently turned during the insertion.

Closure of the wounds is done with interrupted 3-0 Vicryl for the deep fascial layer. The implant rests high within the megapocket to avoid accidental puncture during closure (Fig. 46-9). The deep dermis is closed with 4-0 buried interrupted Vicryl suture. We believe it important that this layer not be placed at all superficially in the dermis, as prolonged reddening of the scar may result owing to a too shallowly situated absorbable suture. A subcuticular 3-0 Prolene pullout suture is placed in the final skin layer. Steri-strips may be used for further wound reinforcement, but occasional unpleasant skin blistering has caused us to abandon their use. A mild supportive dressing of gauze and microfoam tape completes the procedure.

Perioperative cephalosporin is administered by intravenous bolus prior to the skin incision as soon as the intravenous line has been placed. This antibiotic is the only one given, and no further postoperative antibiotics are needed. We use no steroids of any sort for augmentation mammaplasty. The use of steroids has not been proved to enhance the softness of the healing process surrounding the implant. We have seen numerous undesirable side effects from steroid use, notably alteration of the dermis and altered inframammary contouring, which can compromise an otherwise acceptable augmentation.

## Postoperative Care
All dressings are removed at 24 hours, and the patient is free to bathe as usual. We ad-

vise the patient against vigorous physical exercise for 3 weeks, but no specific prohibitions are made concerning arm use. The patient may wear a soft brassiere according to preference, or she may go braless, whichever is more comfortable. The patient is instructed on maintenance of the megapocket by restrained movement of the implant upward and medially only once or twice a day. No vigorous manipulation, "massage," or squeeze tactics are taught. We believe that overly aggressive and compulsive manipulation of the implant and the overlying breast may actually have a nonsalutary effect on capsular formation. Incessant squeezing of the breast tissue may shower bacteria into the surgically traumatized tissues and possibly cause a low grade inflammatory response, producing an adverse effect on the capsule. The Prolene suture is removed at 7 to 10 days after surgery.

The operation is commonly a joyful event for both the patient and surgeon. Postoperatively, however, the patient may need reassurance as to her new size prior to the event of the implant's becoming incorporated into her body image.

## Ptotic Breasts

The patient with ptotic breasts and the "deflated" appearance subsequent to involutional changes may present special problems. If the ptosis is mild, augmentation alone may correct both the volume and the contour defect. In these cases, subpectoral placement of the implant is less than ideal; a suprapectoral pocket allows the implant to fill up the excess skin envelope more aesthetically. If the ptosis is moderate to severe, a mastopexy augmentation is discussed with the patient from the outset. Moderate ptosis may be corrected with augmentation initially, followed by skin markings in the vertical position with judicious vertical and horizontal tacking. Skin removal with nipple repositioning may be called for to produce a desirably aesthetic breast. If the

patient has vehement objections to the incisions, the limitations of an augmentation must be forthrightly presented.

## Long-Term Follow-Up

Whereas the problem of infection and hematoma are rare early on and even more rare later, the problem of firmness from fibrous contracture occurs most frequently during the sixth to twelfth months. The cause of early contracture is probably hematoma or operative inflammatory changes, whereas the cause of late firmness is still unknown (possibly low grade infection). We believe operative correction of fibrous capsule contracture should rarely be done before the third postoperative month, with an interval of at least 6 months a preferable waiting period. The capsulotomy can then be done under general anesthesia in an operating room setting. The technique of manual compression and rupture of the capsule has been effective for retromammary placement (rarely for retropectoral placement), but it is generally ineffective for a contracture developing within the first few weeks of surgery.

The patient is evaluated periodically for at least 1 year. If follow-up is less than 12 months, the accuracy of the determination of satisfactory results is lessened, and the surgeon is less able to give patients who are considering this surgery an informed consultation.

## Suggested Readings

Baker, J. L., Jr. Classification of spherical contractures. Presented at the Aesthetic Breast Symposium, Scottsdale, Arizona, 1975.

Barker, D. E., Retsky, M. I., and Schultz, S. "Bleeding" of silicone from bag-gel breast implants and its clinical relation to fibrous capsule reaction. *Plast. Reconstr. Surg.* 61:836, 1978.

Biggs, T. M., Cukier, J., and Worthing, J. F. Augmentation mammaplasty: A review of 18 years. *Plast. Reconstr. Surg.* 69:445, 1982.

Burkhardt, B. R., et al. Capsules, infection, and

intraluminal antibiotics. *Plast. Reconstr. Surg.* 68:43, 1981.

Capozzi, A., and Pennisi, V. R. Clinical experience with polyurethane-covered gel-filled mammary prostheses. *Plast. Reconstr. Surg.* 68:512, 1981.

Carrico, T. J., and Cohen, I. K. Capsular contracture and steroid-related complications after augmentation mammaplasty. *Plast. Reconstr. Surg.* 64:377, 1979.

Courtiss, E. H., and Goldwyn, R. M. Breast sensation before and after plastic surgery. *Plast. Reconstr. Surg.* 58:1, 1976.

Cronin, T. D. The voice of polite dissent—"Augmentation mammaplasty by the transaxillary approach" by J. H. Wright and A. G. Bevin. *Plast. Reconstr. Surg.* 58:621, 1976.

Cronin, T. D., and Gerow, F. J. Augmentation mammaplasty: A new "natural feel" prosthesis. Proceedings of the Third International Congress of Plastic and Reconstructive Surgery. *Excerpta Medica Int. Cong. Ser.* 66, 1963.

Dempsey, W. C., and Latham, W. D. Subpectoral implants in augmentation mammaplasty: Preliminary report. *Plast. Reconstr. Surg.* 42:515, 1968.

Ellenberg, A. H. Marked thinning of the breast skin flaps after the insertion of implants containing triamcinolone. *Plast. Reconstr. Surg.* 60:755, 1977.

Hetter, G. P. Satisfactions and dissatisfactions of patients with augmentation mammaplasty. *Plast. Reconstr. Surg.* 64:151, 1979.

Hoehler, H. Breast augmentation: The axillary approach. *Br. J. Plast. Surg.* 26:373, 1973.

Jones, F. R., and Tauras, A. P. A periareolar incision for augmentation mammaplasty. *Plast. Reconstr. Surg.* 51:641, 1973.

McGrath, M. H., and Burkhardt, B. R. The safety and efficacy of breast implants for augmentation mammaplasty. *Plast. Reconstr. Surg.* 74:550, 1984.

Oneal, R. M., and Argenta, L. C. Late side effects related to inflatable breast prostheses containing soluble steroids. *Plast. Reconstr. Surg.* 69:641, 1982.

Regnault, P. Partially submuscular breast augmentation. *Plast. Reconstr. Surg.* 59:72, 1977.

Shah, Z., Lehman, J. A., Jr., and Tan, J. Does infection play a role in breast capsular contracture? *Plast. Reconstr. Surg.* 68:34, 1981.

Tebbetts, J. B. Transaxillary subpectoral augmentation mammaplasty: Long-term follow-up and refinements. *Plast. Reconstr. Surg.* 74:636, 1984.

Worton, E. W., Seifert, L. N., and Sherwood, R. Late leakage of inflatable silicone breast prostheses. *Plast. Reconstr. Surg.* 65:302, 1980.

# 47

*John W. Little III*
*Scott L. Spear*
*Sharon Romm*

# Reduction Mammaplasty and Mastopexy

Reduction mammaplasty represents one of the clearest examples of the interface between reconstructive and aesthetic plastic surgery. Although the avowed goals of this procedure are weight and volume reduction of the breast, aesthetic enhancement remains equally important. This point is especially true in recent years, as the techniques of breast reduction have been refined and the safety of the procedure improved. With an increasing uniformity of techniques, emphasis has shifted to technical refinements for improved aesthetic results. At the same time, greater importance has been placed on preservation of both sensation and physiologic function. Although there remains a fundamental difference between reduction mammaplasty and mastopexy, both operations can follow the design of the techniques to be described for reduction mammaplasty alone.

## Anatomy and Physiology

The adult breast is composed of 16 to 18 lobes consisting of ducts, ductules, and lobular-alveolar units in a fibrofatty stroma. The boundaries of the normal female breast extend from the second rib superiorly to the seventh rib inferiorly and from the sternal edge medially to beyond the anterior axillary line laterally. Additional breast tissue extends toward the axilla as the tail of Spence. In cases of substantial breast hypertrophy, the breast may be continuous with other areas of subcutaneous fat around the mid-axillary and posterior axillary regions. The major ducts of the underlying breast tissue extend into the nipple and form milk ampullae. Most of the glands of the nipple-areola are sebaceous and apocrine. The milk duct ampullae open into the nipple separately and in the lactating breast serve as a milk reservoir. The skin of the breast is thick in the region of the areola but thins beyond the areola and is at its thinnest in the region of the axilla. In its superior portion, the breast overlies the pectoralis fascia and may extend through the fascia into the pectoralis muscle. In its inferior portion the breast overlies the fascia of the serratus anterior muscle, the external oblique abdominis muscle, and the rectus abdominis muscle [9, 10, 18, 26].

Sensory innervation to the superior portion of the breast is supplied by the supraclavicular nerves formed from the third and fourth branches of the cervical plexus. The medial breast skin is supplied by the anterior cutaneous divisions of the second through seventh intercostal nerves. The dominant innervation to the nipple appears to derive from the lateral cutaneous branch of the fourth intercostal nerve, whereas lateral cutaneous branches of other intercostal nerves travel subcutaneously to the areola and the skin of the breast to and beyond the midclavicular line. Independent confirmation of the importance of the lateral cutaneous branch of the fourth intercostal nerve has led to greater acceptance of techniques that include its course in the vascular pedicle to the nipple [9].

There are three chief sources of blood supply to the breast. The internal thoracic or internal mammary artery supplies the medial portion through medial perforators near the sternal border. The variable lateral thoracic artery supplies the lateral portion. The anterior and lateral branches of the intercostal vessels supply the remainder. Although there is a substantial degree of collateralization between these vessels in the breast parenchyma, it has been estimated that the internal thoracic artery provides approximately 60 percent of the total. The lateral thoracic artery is thought to supply an additional 30 percent, primarily to the upper, outer, and lateral portions. The anterior and lateral branches of the third, fourth, and fifth posterior intercostal arteries supply the remaining lower outer breast quadrant. The variability and overlap between these vascular networks accounts for the remarkable safety of nipple-bearing pedicles of diverse design based on different vascular supplies.

The breast has two major venous drainage systems: one superficial, the other deep. The superficial drainage system is divided into two types: transverse and longitudinal. The transverse veins run medially in the subcutaneous space and empty into the internal thoracic veins by multiple perforating vessels. The longitudinal drainage ascends to the suprasternal area to connect with the superficial veins of the lower neck. There are anastomotic connections across the midline, but only between the superficial systems. The major portion of the deep drainage is through perforating branches of the internal thoracic vein. Additional venous drainage is in the direction of the axillary vein. A remaining route of drainage is posteriorly through perforators into the intercostal veins, which carry blood posteriorly to the vertebral veins.

The lymphatic pathways draining the breast parallel closely the venous pathways and include cutaneous, internal thoracic, posterior intercostal, and axillary routes. Although most lymph flow is through the axillary region, the internal thoracic channels may carry 3 to 20 percent of it [9, 10, 18, 26].

The macroscopic and microscopic appearances of the mammary gland change dramatically with hormonal manipulation. Normal development occurs as a response to rising levels of estradiol during puberty. With the onset of ovulatory cycles and the appearance of progesterone and pituitary prolactin, ductal, lobuloalveolar, and stromal elements develop. Growth proceeds and stops abruptly for unknown reasons, despite an absence of measurable changes in hormone levels. The cessation of growth is thought to be specific to the breast tissue itself and related to a finite number of available hormonal receptor sites. During pregnancy and the arrival of human placental lactogen there is a dramatic growth in breast size and increased differentiation of the lobuloalveolar elements. This change is related to a concomitant rise in estrogen and progesterone levels. With the completion of pregnancy the prolactin level remains elevated, although the other hormonal levels fall abruptly. The breast continues to manufacture milk, but growth and differentiation cease. With the end of lactation, a substantial involutional process occurs, leaving the breast with greater or lesser quantities of many elements than were present prior to the pregnancy.

A similar pattern of breast activity is seen during the menstrual cycle. During the first week there is epithelial proliferation in response to rising levels of estrogen. During the second week increased differentiation of epithelial cells occurs in relation to increased follicular differentiation. With ovulation and increasing progesterone and prolactin levels the breast tissue enters the luteal phase, characterized by secretion into the lobuloalveolar lumens but without further proliferation of cellular elements. During the final week of the cycle, under the influence of estrogen, progesterone, and prolactin the secretory phase occurs. It is demonstrated by apocrine secretion from the luminal cells and a change in the stroma of the breast, from dense compactness to an edematous appearance with prominent fluid buildup in the interstitial spaces coincident with venous congestion. During the final days of the cycle and falling levels of estrogen and progesterone, the stroma of the breast returns to its compact, well demarcated state.

For many women, postpartum breast involution results in loss of shape and volume, prompting a request for augmentation mammaplasty, mastopexy, or both. In a similar fashion, menopausal diminution of estrogen and progesterone is associated with involution of the breast. Late in menopause alveolar tissue almost disappears, leaving a vestigial ductal system similar to that in the prepubescent breast. Fat and connective tissue now predominate about small epithelial islands [10].

Despite an extensive search for underlying metabolic causes of breast hypertrophy and gigantomastia, these conditions remain poorly understood local phenomena, the products of end-organ hormonal sensitivity, genetic background, and overall body weight [55].

## Reduction Mammaplasty
### INDICATIONS
Women seek to reduce the size of their breasts for reasons both physical and psychological. Heavy, pendulous breasts cause physical discomfort. Common complaints are neck and back pain and irritating grooves cut in the skin of the shoulders by the pressure of brassiere straps. The breasts themselves may be chronically painful, and the skin in the inframammary region is subject to maceration and dermatoses. From a psychological point of view, excessively large breasts can be a troublesome focus of embarrassment for the teenager as well as the woman in her senior years. Unilateral hypertrophy with asymmetry heightens embarrassment and may prompt undesirable behavioral changes in the teenager.

Reduction mammaplasty is best performed when breast growth is complete, with the ideal patient in her late teens or early twenties. There are, however, exceptions. Surgery may be indicated in young individuals before the completion of growth, where the prospect of reoperation is outweighed by the benefits of more normal psychosocial development. Neither is advanced age a contraindication to surgery. Women in their sixties and seventies may appreciate an ultimate, if delayed, resolution of a lifelong problem, with particular benefit to a demineralized skeletal system. Whereas planned preoperative weight reduction is encouraged in the obese individual, the recalcitrant patient still benefits from reduction mammaplasty. Frequently, where previous attempted weight loss has appeared futile to such patients, the achievement of reduced breast size becomes a first-time stimulus to committed weight loss. Certainly, overly large breasts encourage a sedentary life style at odds with modern concepts of exercise and fitness. As with any elective surgery, motivation for breast reduction and enhanced harmony of body proportions must be sufficient to balance issues of scarring as well as decreased sensation and physiologic functioning.

### HISTORY
Large breasts have been considered throughout history a sign of femininity, a symbol of woman's ability to nurture. Yet a woman who has breasts significantly larger than the aesthetic standard of her time may be seen as grotesque rather than sensuous. An attrib-

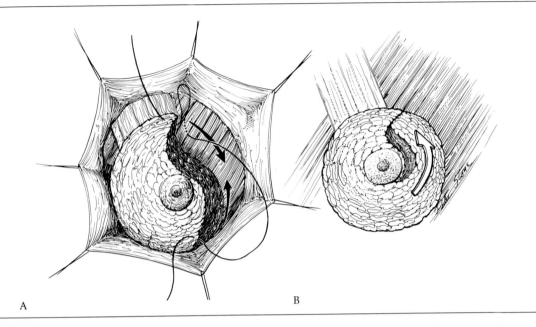

A   B

ute becomes a deformity. Thus an operation to reduce the size of the breast and fashion a normal shape has been sought for centuries.

Even though early surgeons showed concern with altering the appearance of many body features, no mention is made of changing breast proportions until relatively late. A first and isolated hint of interest in camouflaging the bulk of an overly large breast was given by Guido Lanfranchi, an Italian working in France during the thirteenth century, when he designed special dressings that, bound against the patient's chest, compressed the breasts and provided the illusion of smaller proportions [28]. The first true surgical reduction of the female breast probably dates from 1669 and was performed by William Durston of England [30]. During the early years of the twentieth century, Morestin, expanding on the work of Thomas [62] and Guinard [20], described the prevailing reduction mammaplasty technique of the day [41]. Through an incision in the inframammary fold he elevated the gland from the underlying muscle and removed a thick disk of breast tissue with inframammary skin. He

also employed this procedure to achieve symmetry when one breast was significantly larger than the other [40]. Lexer, in 1912, described a method for the correction of mammary hypertrophy [31]. A modified technique, published in 1923, excised a wedge of breast tissue and skin from above and below the nipple. The nipple was elevated to an appropriate position, and support for the breast was provided by a sling of pectoralis major muscle [27].

Biesenberger [5] in 1928, expanding on the work of Axhausen [2], proposed an approach in which skin flaps were widely undermined from the subjacent breast tissue, which was then reduced through lateral excision. The remaining breast with its attached nipple-areola was rotated laterally and superiorly, forming a breast cone (Fig. 47-1). Despite prevailing problems with flap ischemia and skin necrosis, this procedure remained a popular operation in Europe and America for the next 20 years.

As new techniques for reduction mammaplasty were developed over the following decades, inconsistent survival of the nipple-areola complex remained a major concern. Thorek, who devised a number of procedures to improve body contour and was the first to amputate a gigantic, overhanging abdominal panniculus, is credited with reporting the first reduction mammaplasty in which the nipple was removed and replaced as a free graft, although Lexer may have accomplished it 10 years earlier [34]. In 1922 Thorek presented his work illustrated with photographs of pleasing results. The breasts were amputated, retaining sufficient tissue to reshape a smaller form. The shaved nipple-areola complex was replaced at the breast apex as a free graft [63, 64] (Fig. 47-2). Despite Thorek's success, opponents, including Maliniac, maintained that free nipple grafting was "out of the question" [33]. Nonetheless we find today, almost half a century later, continued reliance on breast amputation and free nipple graft for treatment of many cases of gigantomastia.

In 1930 Schwarzmann [56] proposed the concept of a subdermal blood supply to the nipple. Although not entirely correct, it fostered the deepithelialized dermal pedicles of the modern era, including those of Strömbeck [60], Skoog [58], and McKissock [36]. Wise [67] in 1956 expanded on concepts of Aufricht [1] and Penn [44] when presenting his pattern of preoperative marking. The resulting T-closure is a component of most techniques in common usage today. Exceptions to this pattern include the lateral resection technique of Mouly and Dufourmentel presented in 1971 [42]. A wedge of breast tissue and skin was removed from the lateral aspect of the breast according to a prescribed pattern, with results predictably better in patients who required a lesser resection. A later modification is Regnault's "B" technique [50], so named because the skin resection follows the pattern of the capital letter B. The resultant scar curves laterally from areola to inframary crease toward the axilla, avoiding the medial component of

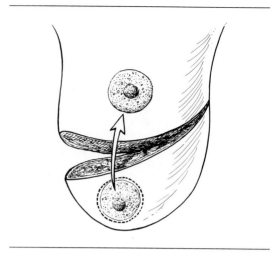

***Figure 47-2*** *Thorek technique. Breast amputated and nipple transposed as a free graft.*

the traditional inframammary incision (Fig. 47-3).

Resection of the central, inferior pole of the breast, the very portion retained in the vertical and inferior pedicle procedures of today, culminated in the Aries-Pitanguy technique [45, 46] (Fig. 47-4). Strömbeck [60] in 1960 was the first to use a pedicle of dermis and subcutaneous tissue on which the nipple could be transposed superiorly with consistent safety. Breast tissue was resected from above and below a horizontal bipedicle, with skin undermining kept to a minimum to avoid complications of skin necrosis (Fig. 47-5). Skoog [58] modified the technique from a bipedicle to a monopedicle base. Despite initial wide acceptance, resulting breasts suffered from a tendency toward a boxy shape, with a retracted nipple-areola complex.

More recently, McKissock described transposing the nipple on a vertically oriented, dermoglandular bipedicle flap folded on itself [36]. Such orientation avoided the tethering problems of the horizontal procedures. He emphasized the importance of preoperative planning, opposing unplanned resection. His procedure has remained, until

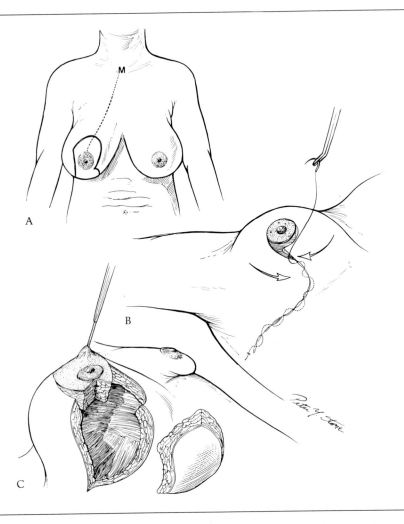

**Figure 47-3** *Regnault "B" technique.*
*A. Preoperative "B" markings. B. Infralateral*
*resection. C. Closure avoids medial scar.*

recently, the most frequent technique performed in the United States. Ribeiro [52] first suggested transposing the nipple on an inferiorly based dermoglandular flap. This technique, subsequently modified and improved by Courtiss and Goldwyn [6] and Georgiade et al. [12], encouraged the preservation of sensation to the nipple-areola. Weiner et al. [65], on the other hand, described a single, superiorly based dermal pedicle for nipple transposition. Finally, a central-mound technique without a conventional, directional pedicle has been described by Balch [3].

Modifications of early techniques largely concerned improved safety and survival of the transposed nipple-areola and skin flaps. Subsequent concerns focused on the aesthetic shape and balance of the reduced breasts. More recently, attention has been directed to preservation of sensation, especially to the nipple-areola, and physiologic functioning, as typified by breast-feeding [21, 68]. Current concerns include efforts to limit the pattern and extent of scarring, as in the Regnault technique [50] and others reported from Europe and South America [35].

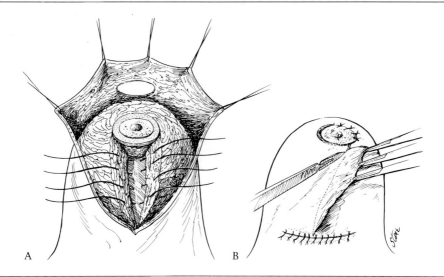

**Figure 47-4** *Aries-Pitanguy technique.*
*A. Inferior central resection. B. Tailored closure*
*"cut-as-you-go."*

Although inventive, these techniques appear less appropriate for the major reductions commonly performed in the United States and, in any case, have fewer adherents here. The future evolution of reduction mammaplasty will surely include continued efforts for still better sensation and physiology in breasts meeting the highest aesthetic standards with the least scarring.

**Figure 47-5** *Strömbeck technique.*
*A. Horizontal bipedicle. B. Inverted-T closure.*

## CURRENT TECHNIQUES

Current methods of breast reduction can be differentiated by their pattern of skin resection and resulting scar. In one group the scar pattern is kept lateral and oblique to the areola, avoiding a medial component. In the other, an inverted-T scar is used with a medial extension in the inframammary line. The lateralizing techniques may be less appropriate to the major reductions performed commonly in the United States and are not addressed in this section. The popular techniques with inverted-T scars have performed well in terms of predictability, versatility,

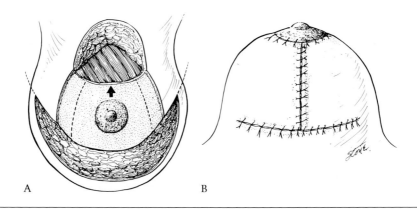

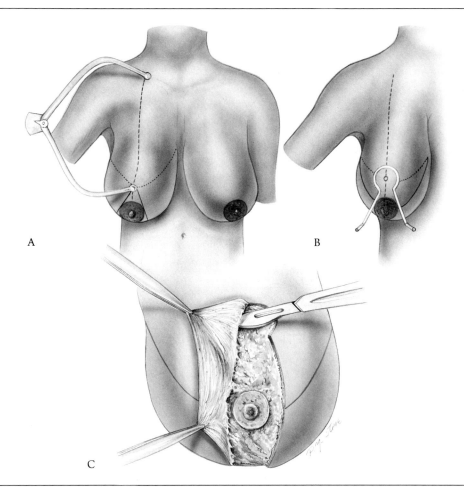

A

B

C

***Figure 47-6*** *McKissock technique. A. Nipple positioned at inframammary line. B. Wire pattern completes preoperative markings. C. Vertical pedicle deepithelialized.*

and reliability in large, as well as moderate and small, reductions. Most commonly performed among these procedures are the vertical pedicle technique, the inferior pedicle technique, and, most recently, the central mound technique.

*Vertical Pedicle Technique*
McKissock [39] first described his vertical bipedicle technique for nipple transposition during reduction mammaplasty in 1972, and it has evolved in subsequent publications [37, 38]. A superior dermoglandular bridge is left primarily for structural support, with the blood supply to the nipple derived largely from subdermal and retained parenchymal vessels inferior to the nipple-areola. With this technique the central breast is reduced to a vertically oriented bipedicle flap based superiorly on the upper margin of the new areolar window and inferiorly on the inframammary line and chest-wall musculature. The flap carries the nipple-areola and, although deepithelialized, depends primarily on inferior parenchyma for blood supply. Planned preoperative skin marking is a critical aspect of this technique.

With the patient erect, the breast meridian

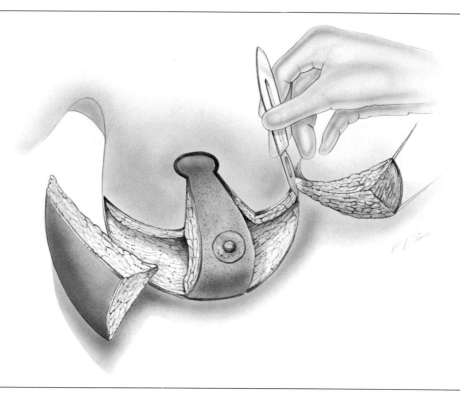

*Figure 47-7* *McKissock technique. Medial and lateral dermoglandular resections.*

is established by dropping a line from the midclavicle through the nipple and continuing inferiorly across the inframammary line (Fig. 47-6). The inframammary level is measured in relation to the clavicle using obstetric calipers. This distance is transposed to the anterior breast and marked on the breast meridian. Whereas the initial descriptions set the nipple some 2 cm higher, more recent reports indicate this point as the appropriate site for the new nipple position [39]. Diverging lines are drawn from this key point and pass as tangents to either side of the dilated areola. A wire keyhole pattern is then adjusted to a similar angle of divergence and superimposed on the lines, indicating the proper size and location of the new areolar window. A distance of 5 to 6 cm is measured down from the window to establish the length of the limbs of the pattern.

From these extremities lines are directed medially and laterally in a subtle lazy S fashion to intersect the inframammary fold, which has also been indicated. More recent reports deemphasize the lazy S design, especially medially [39].

The areola is circumscribed at a diameter of 37 mm. The vertical flap is outlined by extending the lines of the vertical limbs inferiorly as two parallel lines straddling the breast meridian line down to the inframammary fold. The entire flap, except the reduced nipple-areola, is deepithelialized. The vertical pedicle is then cut along its medial and lateral margins down to the fascia of the underlying musculature, and medial and lateral dermoglandular wedges are resected to either side (Fig. 47-7). McKissock more recently recommended retention of a thin layer of breast over the lateral musculature to favor preservation of sensation to the nipple-areola [39]. Additional breast tissue is re-

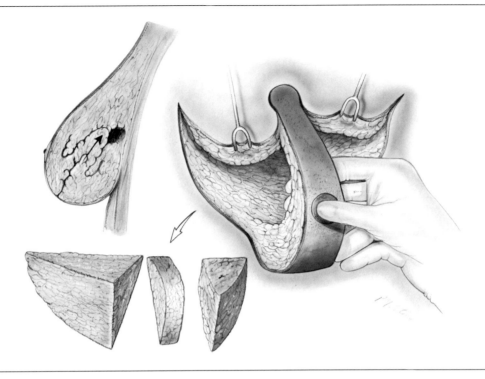

**Figure 47-8** *McKissock technique. Central glandular resection produces bucket-handle flap for infolding.*

sected from the remaining medial and lateral elements: little to none medially, but a considerable amount, including the axillary tail, laterally. A window of breast tissue is removed from the upper portion of the bipedicle flap, from the level of the nipple to the height of the keyhole pattern, creating a bucket-handle effect (Fig. 47-8). This resection must not extend above the upper limit of the areolar window in order to avoid loss of superior breast volume. The flap is folded superiorly upon itself, bringing the areola into position within the keyhole pattern. The medial and lateral flaps are brought together over the pedicle, and closure is begun working from the extremities toward the center (Fig. 47-9). Any central excess of skin is excised at the vertical closure. A Penrose drain is left across the full width of the breast, exiting through the lateral inframammary closure.

*Inferior Pedicle Technique*

The inferior pedicle technique of breast reduction is credited to Robbins [53], Courtiss and Goldwyn [6], and Georgiade et al. [11, 12]. Their methods are modifications and derivations of the techniques of McKissock and Ribeiro [36–38, 52]. The planning of the operation is essentially the same as for the McKissock procedure with the desired nipple location determined in the same manner. An inferiorly based dermoglandular pedicle is planned with a base of 4 to 9 cm at the inframammary line that gradually tapers as it ascends to encompass the nipple-areola complex. Deepithelialization with this technique is limited to the zone immediately about and inferior to the nipple-areola (Fig. 47-10). Skin and parenchymal resections are performed medial and lateral to the pedicle,

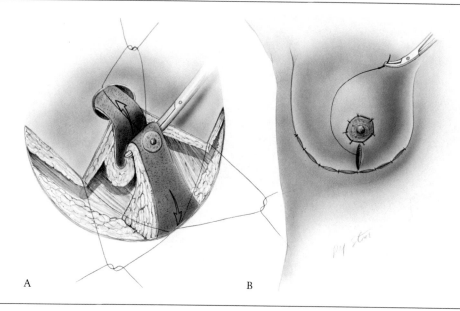

A                                                    B

**Figure 47-9** *McKissock technique. A. Vertical bipedicle folded on itself as key sutures tied. B. Closure.*

**Figure 47-10** *Inferior pedicle technique. A. Preoperative markings with inferior pedicle deepithelialized. B. Medial dermoglandular resection.*

as for the vertical pedicle technique, but also superior to the nipple-areola, up to the level of the keyhole pattern. These excisions are performed leaving a beveled carpet of breast tissue over the muscular fascia, especially laterally. Immediately superior to the 1-cm

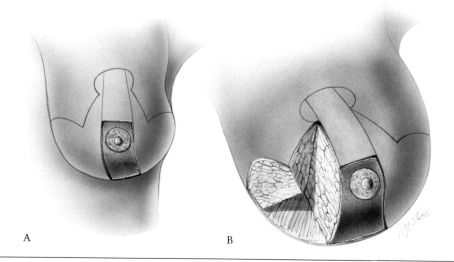

A                                                    B

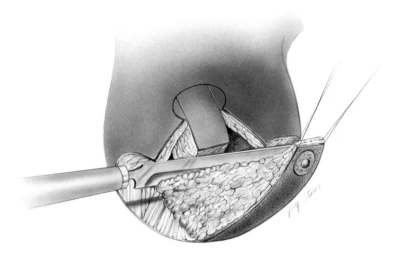

*Figure 47-11* Inferior pedicle technique. Pedicle developed.

deepithelialized cuff about the nipple-areola, the pedicle is terminated and divided down to muscle fascia, taking care not to undercut the inferior vascular base (Fig. 47-11). A pyramidal pedicle of dermis and parenchyma is thus left subjacent and inferior to the nipple-areola, based on the chest wall musculature and inframammary line. In the vicinity of the areola it measures 2 to 4 cm in thickness and near the base it is 4 to 10 cm. After com-

pletion of the breast resection, the nipple-areola is brought to the desired position in the keyhole pattern, and the medial and lateral flaps are brought together as with the McKissock technique (Fig. 47-12). The infe-

*Figure 47-12* Inferior pedicle technique. A. Nipple-areola positioned. B. Closure.

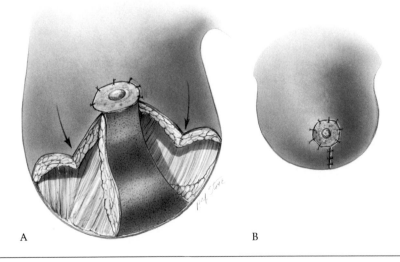

A                                                    B

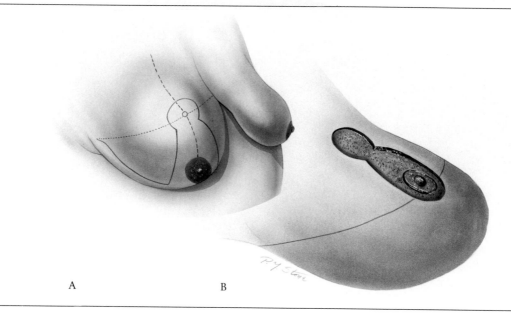

**Figure 47-13** *Central mound technique. A. Preoperative markings. B. Limited central deepithelialization.*

rior pedicle design is likely the most popular technique in use today in the United States.

*Central Mound Technique*

The central mound technique, described by Balch [3] and endorsed by others [22], can be seen as a further evolution of the prior two designs. The pedicle is based on central chest wall musculature alone and is not contiguous with any skin boundary. Hence it has no directional base in the sense of traditional skin pedicles that may be classified as superior, inferior, transverse, or the like. So too is it the least structured in terms of the surgical technique, representing a "cut-as-you-go" approach to breast reduction.

Preoperative marking is again performed as for the McKissock technique. The skin is deepithelialized within the entire keyhole pattern, a process continued inferiorly to include the reduced nipple-areola complex (Fig. 47-13). An incision is placed in the inframammary crease and is carried down per-

pendicularly to the pectoralis fascia. Incisions are now made and beveled around the margins of the keyhole pattern at its medial and lateral limbs. This incision is continued below the level of the limbs to circumscribe the deepithelialized pattern, including the nipple-areola, and is beveled in a caudal direction toward the inframammary fold. The limb incisions, both medial and lateral, are made in the standard fashion, developing flaps of thickness similar to those in other techniques. Now the medial and lateral inferior quadrants of skin and breast, as well as the central inferior tissue intervening between the nipple-areola and the inframammary fold, are excised as a single curvilinear, ellipsoid unit that includes the axillary tail (Fig. 47-14). A skin incision at the superior aspect of the keyhole is deepened only enough to allow comfortable transposition of the central mound pedicle with its nipple-areola into the keyhole position. The skin flaps are brought about the pedicle as in other techniques, and closure is undertaken again from the extremities centrally (Fig. 47-15).

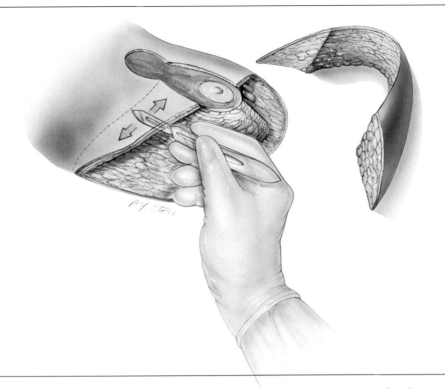

**Figure 47-14** *Central mound technique. Dermoglandular resection.*

**Figure 47-15** *Central mound technique. A. Nipple-areola advanced superiorly. B. Closure.*

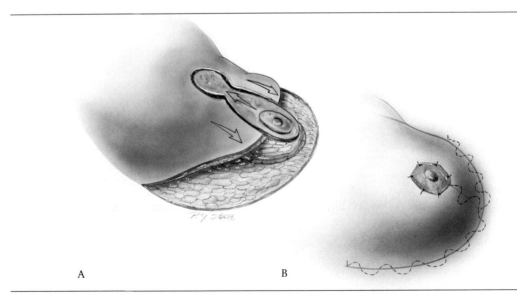

A                                    B

## AUTHORS' TECHNIQUE

The vertical pedicle technique of reduction mammaplasty was the first that offered consistently safe transfer of the nipple-areola complex on a pedicle that was itself unencumbered by mechanical restrictions, unlike those of transverse design. There has continued a natural evolution beyond this popular technique to that of inferior pedicle design and, most recently, central mound design. The latter designs have developed through our better understanding of the parenchymal blood supply and lateral intercostal innervation to the area of the nipple-areola complex. Rather than existing as fundamentally different techniques, however, these three approaches to reduction mammaplasty represent a spectrum of design, the modifications of one blending into another. The authors have continued to prefer the proven vertical pedicle design, incorporating modifications that recognize some of the advantages of the more recent approaches. Although the retention of the superior dermoglandular bridge of the bipedicle is readily acknowledged by them to represent a "belt and suspenders" redundancy where blood supply to the areola is concerned, their cumulative clinical experience with this technique remains without a single instance of nipple-areola loss, giving them the greatest possible confidence in this time-honored design. So too is it a straightforward technique to teach to beginning surgeons, making it appropriate for the training environment in which they practice. In this regard, it offers the comfort of a structured resection, with less of the "cut-as-you-go" approach of the other two, especially the central mound technique. Once mastered, it lends itself to easy modification into either of the other techniques. Therefore we continue to perform and to teach the vertical bipedicle technique of reduction mammaplasty, incorporating modification of its pedicle base toward a lateralized origin to favor nerve and blood supply to the nipple-areola and adding suction-assisted lipectomy to limit the extent of lateral, inframammary scarring [61].

### Preparation

In all patients preoperative low-dose screening mammography is recommended to help rule out occult pathology; it is repeated at 1 year as a postoperative baseline. In addition, 2 units of autologous whole blood donation are routinely scheduled at appropriate preoperative intervals.

### Preoperative Marking

Markings are determined with the patient sitting on the operating table immediately prior to anesthesia induction. In practice, this step requires no more than 3 to 4 minutes and avoids the possibility that markings placed earlier might become indistinct by the time of surgery. Furthermore, the entire resident and student team is more likely to be present at the markings when they are done as an integral part of the procedure. Easily the most important educational lessons involve the determination of such markings. Indeed, it can be argued that attendance at a reduction mammaplasty operation by a trainee who has not witnessed or taken part in the determination of preoperative markings is, in fact, a vain exercise. As McKissock stressed, such planning is the most important step in the execution of the procedure. Significant deviations from the preoperative plan are ill-advised and likely to result in unpredictable postoperative results.

The initial marking is a vertical line down the central breast meridian from clavicle to inframammary fold (Fig. 47-16). This line follows the aesthetic axis of the breast and specifically ignores the occasional nipple-areola complex that may fall medially or laterally off this line. Such "cross-eyed" or "wall-eyed" nipples are then corrected during the ensuing reduction technique as they are brought to the true meridian of the breast cone (Fig. 47-17).

The most critical determination remains

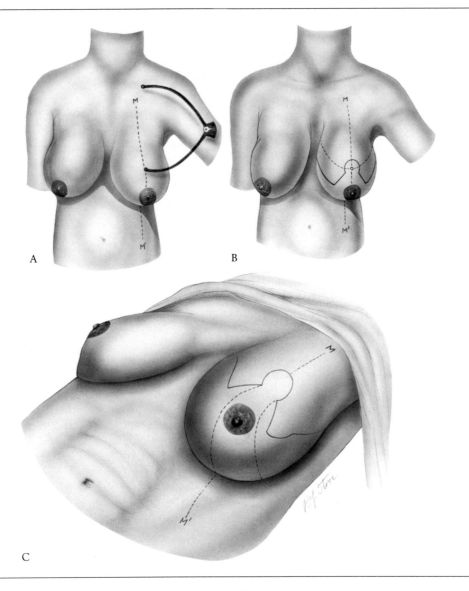

**Figure 47-16** *Authors' technique. A. Positioning the nipple. B. Preoperative markings completed. C. Vertical pedicle positioned with lateralized base.*

that of the desired level for the nipple-areola. If but a single concept from this chapter is embraced by the beginning surgeon, let it be the admonition *not to mark the new nipple-areola position too high,* advice equally important for reduction mammaplasty and mastopexy. Such superior malpositioning of the complex is easily the most common significant error during reduction mammaplasty by any technique and remains the most difficult to correct secondarily. Determinations of nipple position that have relied on fixed measurements from body landmarks, including any given distance from the sternal notch, as well as those that relate the position to, for example, the midhumeral point, have proven treacherous and

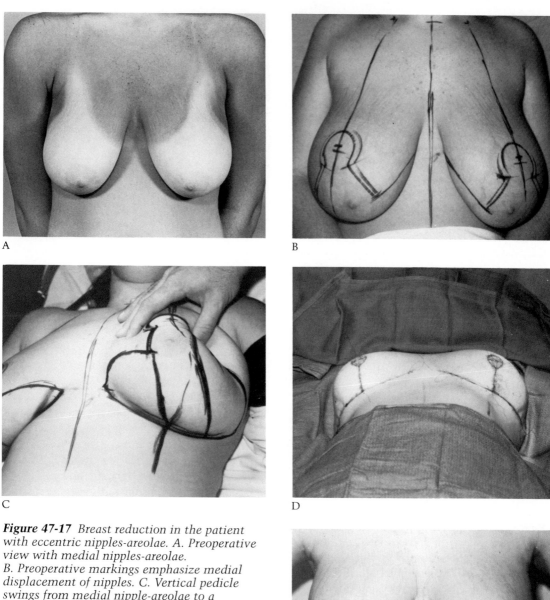

A

B

C

D

**Figure 47-17** *Breast reduction in the patient with eccentric nipples-areolae. A. Preoperative view with medial nipples-areolae. B. Preoperative markings emphasize medial displacement of nipples. C. Vertical pedicle swings from medial nipple-areolae to a lateralized base. D. Closure. E. Early postoperative view with nipples-areolae centralized.*

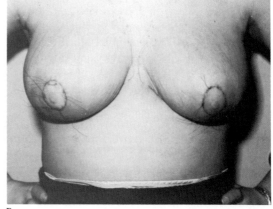

E

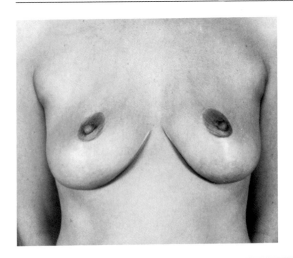

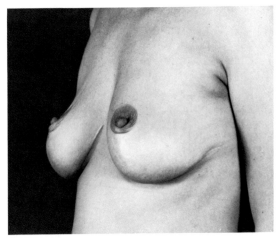

**Figure 47-18** *Typical late "dropout" secondary to superior malpositioning of the nipples-areolae in a patient referred for revision. Late result, 5 years after the initial surgery.*

unreliable in avoiding such malposition. The overwhelming majority of cases of late "dropout," where the breast parenchyma descends below the nipple-areola complex over time, can be attributed to initial markings set too high (Fig. 47-18).

The one acceptable landmark for use in the determination of nipple-areola position remains the inframammary fold itself, as emphasized by McKissock. Using an obstetric caliper, the distance is measured from the intersection of the breast meridian line with the clavicle to the intersection of the same line with the inframammary fold, and this distance is transposed to the anterior breast at the same meridian line. The new nipple position falls most commonly at this point of intersection, although in some circumstances it may be adjusted superiorly to a limit of 2 cm. The greater the final retained volume of breast tissue following any reduction or mastopexy procedure, the more important it is that the nipple position fall at the lower mark. The most notable exception to this rule occurs when performing mastopexy on a single breast to encourage symmetry with an opposite breast that has been reconstructed with a submuscular prosthesis, in which the breast contour is unnatu-

rally round and high compared to the normal, ptotic breast. In the case of modest level disparity between the inframammary folds of asymmetric breasts, the higher position is selected; for greater disparity, a compromise setting is recommended.

Subsequent markings are then facilitated by readily available marking devices from surgical supply houses. Although a simple hardware store washer and bent wire can adequately substitute, the authors prefer the commercially available Freeman cookie cutter areolar marker (Padgett Instruments, Kansas City, MO) with diameters of 38 or 42 mm and the keyhole-pattern bent wire designed specifically for marking the McKissock technique (Padgett Instruments). Whereas McKissock preferred to mark the limbs of the areolar pattern at the narrowest angle permissible by the width of the pigmented areola, the authors routinely set the limbs of the wire device wider than that dictated by the areola. In their hands, the final medial adjustments during closure are thereby kept to a minimum. The arms are invariably set between 60 and 90 degrees, in most cases closer to the former than the latter. The more round and dense the gland, the narrower the angle is set within this range, whereas the arms are opened for the more lax and ptotic breast which undergoes proportionately less reduction in volume. With the new nipple position at the center of the keyhole areolar pattern, the areolar keyhole and limbs are indicated. Limb length varies between 5 and 6 cm, averaging 5.5 cm.

The inframammary fold is now marked from its medial to lateral extent. In the broad breast, the lateral aspect of the inframammary fold is marked in a transverse fashion, rather than swinging superiorly to follow the true sweep of the fold in this area of common scar hypertrophy. It is thought that such transverse orientation in this troublesome zone is less likely to encourage scar hypertrophy than does a curvilinear design that rises obliquely. More important still is the actual limitation of the lateral extent of the scar, embracing what would otherwise produce dog-ear formation at closure. Vigorous suction-assisted lipectomy is then applied to this area of accumulation, depressing the bulge into a more acceptable contour. So too is the typical subaxillary fold of obese women routinely contoured by this helpful adjunct near the completion of reduction mammaplasty.

The superior lines of resection are then drawn from the termini of the keyhole pattern limbs to their intersections at the inframammary fold. It is important that these lines intersect at a right angle to the pattern limbs. Whereas the lateral line inscribes a subtle curvilinear arc, the medial line is drawn more or less straight to its intersection with the inframammary line. If the breasts are large and there is near confluence of the two inframammary folds, the pattern is further modified by blunting or short-circuiting the medial angle and removing the resultant skin excess with a V-Y plasty, avoiding continuity of the inframammary scars.

Finally, the vertical pedicle is indicated by dropping parallel lines from three and nine o'clock at the keyhole pattern to the inframammary fold. Pedicle width varies between two and four fingerbreadths, depending on the desired final breast volume as well as the total pedicle length in terms of maintaining adequate blood supply to the nipple. Although the pedicle must, of course, encompass the nipple-areola, below this level it is swung laterally such that its medial border abuts the meridian line of the breast at the inframammary fold, creating a lateralized base.

### Technique

The patient is placed supine on the operating table and inducted under general intubation anesthesia. Her arms are placed in the akimbo position with padded hands behind the buttocks and padded elbows abducted away from the body, allowing access for lateral lipectomy and closure. After preparation and draping, the areolar cookie cutter is used to indicate a 42-mm or, less commonly, 38-mm disk on the dilated areola.

The authors endorse the selective use of vasoconstrictive agents during reduction mammaplasty as a proved technique for reducing blood loss during this procedure [38]. When using such solutions, however, we studiously avoid instillation into the nipple-bearing vertical pedicle. The ready clinical assessment of the pattern of dermal bleeding in the periareolar portion of the deepithelialized pedicle has, in our opinion, contributed to an absence of nipple-areola complications. The invalidation of such clinical assessment by indiscriminate instillation of vasoconstrictive agents in an effort to further limit blood loss, we believe, is an imprudent trade-off. All patients donate one or two units of autologous blood preoperatively, which is reinfused at the time of surgery.

The procedure is begun by deepithelialization of the dermal pedicle. Although newer techniques have confirmed that dermis is a nonessential component of the pedicle in terms of nipple-areola survival, such treatment requires little more time than deskinning alone and preserves a better bleeding surface to assess pedicle blood supply. The vertical bipedicle is then developed. This maneuver can be difficult for the beginning surgeon, who frequently finds that the resultant vascular base of the pedicle has been undercut in the area of its important attachment to the underlying chest-wall musculature. The key to a successful vertical flap lies in the proper positioning of the breast on the chest wall. If the pedicle is cut with the breast hanging freely under the influence of gravity, rolling off the thoracic barrel in a lateral oblique fashion, a uniform pedicle may be difficult to achieve. If, on the other hand, the breast is gathered into a spherical mound and is balanced on the chest wall by the assistant, and if initial cuts are made perpendicular to the curvilinear chest-wall barrel rather than to the operating table itself, the maneuver is rendered straightforward. The medial border of the pedicle is incised down to the fascia of the medial chest-wall musculature (Fig. 47-19). The lateral incision, however, is developed only to a depth of two-thirds the distance to its muscle fascia. The flap is confirmed to be of uniform and adequate thickness, especially toward its base.

The medial resection is performed next. The medial inframammary incision is cut perpendicularly through the subcutaneous tissue to the muscle fascia, and the parenchyma of the medial inferior quadrant is elevated from this layer to a level above the planned superior line of resection. This freed inframedial quadrant is taken in hand, and with inferior traction the superior incision is begun. The incision is placed perpendicularly into the parenchyma some 1 to 2 cm and then is tapered in an upward direction, removing additional gland from the medial breast. A similar tapering maneuver is begun at the medial limb of the keyhole pattern and is treated in the same way, leaving 1 to 2 cm of gland at the skin margin and taper-

ing in a medial direction. In general, much less medial parenchyma is removed from underneath the intact medial breast element than is the case with the lateral component. Excessive resection here may produce an empty look in the medial portion of the breast. In many breasts, then, no such additional medial breast is removed.

Attention is now turned to the lateral resection, which is begun by incising the inframammary incision lateral to the pedicle down perpendicularly to the chest wall muscular fascia, clearly identifying this level only at this point, so that it otherwise remains unexposed during the subsequent resection. The inferior lateral quadrant of the breast is then elevated from below up, with one critical difference from the previous medial resection: The pedicle base is broadened laterally from the two-thirds depth of the initial pedicle cut, such that a significant breast component covers the chest-wall muscle. Thus the lateral margin of the vertical pedicle is an outward tapering slope rather than the clean vertical wall of the medial margin. This execution of the lateral wall of the pedicle, along with the lateralized design of the pedicle base, helps to ensure inclusion of intact lateral innervation and blood supply to the nipple-areola.

Taking the large infralateral quadrant in hand, again with inferior traction, the superior incision is developed to a thickness of 1 to 2 cm, at which level a considerable tapering and undercutting maneuver is performed to remove significant volume from underneath the lateral breast skin. This undercutting maneuver is again performed in a second plane beginning at the lateral limb of the keyhole pattern and tapering laterally. The major part of the axillary tail is included in the resection specimen.

The residual vertical pedicle is now suspended between paired skin hooks where the pedicle intersects the keyhole pattern at three and nine o'clock and the assistant's fingers at the nipple-bearing portion of the pedicle. The superior glandular window is

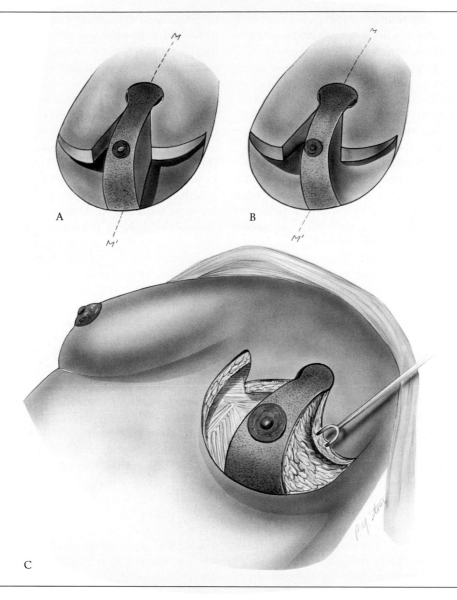

*Figure 47-19* Authors' technique.
*A. Conventional pedicle centered on meridian line (M to M¹). B. Modified pedicle with the base lateral to the meridian line and the lateral margin of flap tapered outward. C. Medial and lateral dermoglandular resections completed.*

now removed from the pedicle, creating a bucket-handle bipedicle flap. This excision is seen as roughly rectangular. The superior cut is made from twelve o'clock at the areolar window to twelve o'clock at the areola, leaving 1 to 2 cm of parenchyma with the dermal bridge. Near the superior, or twelve o'clock, margin of the areola the dissection abruptly turns vertically and drops to the chest wall in a perpendicular fashion, taking care not to undercut the nipple-areola complex or remove any of its subjacent glandular support and innervation. A similar vertical incision is dropped from the superior aspect of the resection at twelve o'clock on the areolar window and is again carried perpendicularly down to the chest wall. Finally the glandular specimen is removed from the muscle fascia. This maneuver produces significant additional reduction in glandular volume, but its further purpose is to allow a comfortable infolding of the superior aspect of the pedicle, avoiding internal tension that might otherwise compromise circulation within the flap. If the superior glandular bridge is left thicker than 2 cm, such an infolding maneuver becomes awkward and forced.

Careful hemostasis by electrocoagulation is reconfirmed, and a soft silicone suction catheter that traverses the inferior pedicle parenchyma is brought out through a stab wound in the hair-bearing axilla. The catheter is removed on the first or second postoperative day. At this point the modified vertical pedicle with its lateralized base and sloping lateral wall can be equally considered a conventional inferior pedicle flap with attached superior dermoglandular bridge or stabilizing element. In the increasingly frequent case of the patient wishing a maximal reduction to breasts as small as possible, we consider the superior blood supply a desirable, if not critical, addition to an inferior parenchyma of perhaps minimal thickness.

Closure is begun by three key sutures (Fig. 47-20). The first suspends the nipple-areola at its twelve o'clock point to the corresponding point on the keyhole pattern, infolding the superior pedicle. A second suture brings the subcutaneous and deep dermal tissues of the two superior points of the vertical limbs together. The third suture brings the two inferior points together and fixes them to the extension of the meridian breast line on the chest wall at the medial margin of the pedicle base.

Inferior closure is begun laterally and worked medially using wide-spaced sutures in the deep dermis and subcutaneous tissue to approximate the margins of the closure, thereby preventing further lateral extension of the scar. Invariably, the length of the superior margin proves longer than that of the inferior margin. Some of this discrepancy is consumed by stepwise closure. Any remaining excess is removed medially at the line of vertical closure. In practice, it rarely exceeds 1 to 2 cm of additional skin resection.

Medial closure is begun in the same way, working medially to laterally. If the medial exicision has been blunted rather than followed out to a full tapered ellipse in the inframammary fold, this area is left for later V-Y plasty. The entire inframammary closure, along with the lower two-thirds of the vertical closure, are completed in their entirety with two additional layers of closure: one by fine, inverted absorbable sutures in the deep dermis and the second by a running intradermal monofilament suture for later pullout. Both such closures are completed before any sutures are added around the nipple-areola.

Thus as the closure progresses bilaterally, the surgeon is able to discern subtle differences in remaining volume when comparing the two sides. Although it is important to weigh the specimen for comparison purposes, and more important still to segregate right-sided and left-sided tissues because of the possibility of occult malignancy, it must be remembered that what is retained is the ultimate determinant of size and final symmetry. As the closure progresses, if it becomes apparent that one breast is fuller than the other, the vertical pedicle may be delivered through the keyhole pattern by removing only the single twelve o'clock key suture, and central reduction is accomplished by further reduction of the pedicle itself. It is done under strict visualization of the pattern of dermal bleeding in the periareolar region so that devascularization of the nipple-areola does not occur through such additional resection.

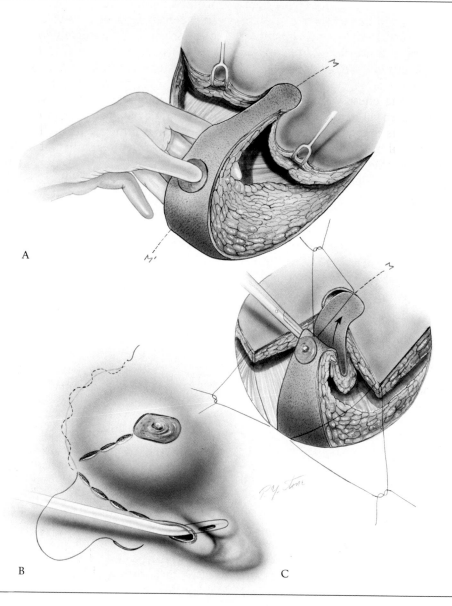

**Figure 47-20** *Authors' technique. A. Central glandular window resected. B. Pedicle infolded as key sutures are placed. C. Closure with lateral liposuction.*

Finally, if there are additional areas of discrepancy toward the lateral or medial aspects of the breast, they are addressed with the suction-assisted lipectomy cannula. It is our routine practice in heavy women to use this adjunct in the region of the subaxillary lateral fold. Aggressive lipectomy in this area achieves better contour blend in such

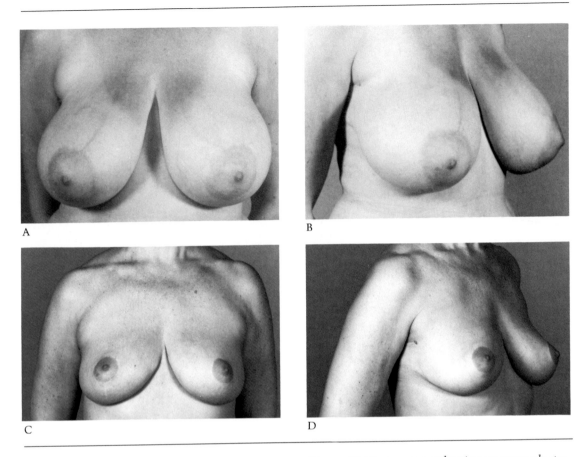

*Figure 47-21* Average reduction mammaplasty (650 gm each side). A, B. Preoperative views. C, D. Postoperative views at 6 years.

individuals and reduces the need for lateral extension of the scar to remove dog-ear fullness, a practice notoriously productive of hypertrophic scar in this region.

Before the circumareolar closure is begun, the nipple-bearing portion of the vertical bipedicle flap is delivered through the aperture of the areolar window so that it is bulging slightly above the plane of the breast. As the areolar margins are sewn to the skin at the keyhole pattern, the nipple-areola complex is pulled down into the plane of the breast. This simple maneuver has served to avoid the problem of the depressed nipple-areola complex that has been associated by some with this and other bipedicle techniques. On the other hand, if when placing the periareolar stitches the surgeon must pull the pigmented tissues up to the level of the sur-

rounding skin, a depressed or retracted complex may result. Again, two-layer closure is accomplished with fine buried dermal sutures and running intradermal monofilament brought out though the areolar side of the closure. Adhesive strips further reinforce the closure, and greasy dressings are placed over the nipple-areola complex and the region of the intersection of the vertical and inframammary incisions. A bulky circumferential pressure dressing is added.

Later that day in the patient's room, the two nipples-areolae are examined for appropriate blanch and refill. If there had been any question at the completion of the procedure about the viability of these structures, intra-

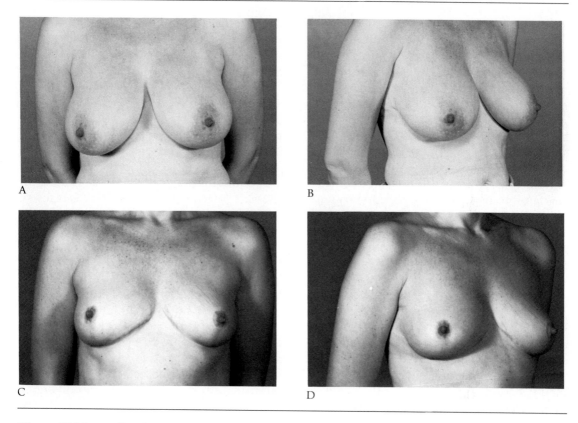

**Figure 47-22** *Small reduction mammaplasty (350 gm each side). A, B. Preoperative views. C, D. Postoperative views at 4 years.*

venous fluorescein dye would have been administered to reassure the surgeon on this point. If this test had shown an absence of fluorescence on either side, inadequate blood supply to that nipple-areola would have been assumed. Such an unstained areola is removed as a full-thickness skin graft and the superior portion of the dermal pedicle sutured around the areolar window. The defatted nipple-areola is then replaced as a full-thickness graft on the dermal bed. The authors have not found need to perform this maneuver to date. Patients are routinely discharged from the hospital in a brassiere on the first or second postoperative day, with the admonition to continue round-the-clock brassiere support for 2 weeks (Figs. 47-21 and 47-22).

## Breast Amputation with Free Nipple Graft: Authors' Technique

An excellent, if often maligned, alternative to reduction mammaplasty with a nipple-bearing pedicle remains the time-honored procedure of breast amputation with free nipple graft. This technique is consistently productive of well shaped breasts with excellent aesthetic appeal. In large women, in particular, an attractive breast contour is more easily accomplished than with conventional approaches. Its disadvantage lies only in a limited unnaturalness to the nipple-areola complex: specialized sensation is certainly lost, as well as some degree of nipple projection, especially erectile nipple projection; lactation is similarly sacrificed; and occasional spotty survival of the grafted areola produces areas of depigmentation that can be troublesome in dark-skinned individuals.

This rapid technique is especially indicated for women with gigantomastia, presenting 2500 gm or more of breast tissue per side, as well as patients with other complicating factors, such as increased age or systemic disease where significant reduction in blood loss and operating time is desired. It remains perhaps the preferred alternative for many elderly patients who present for reduction mammaplasty because of increasing symptoms involving a demineralized skeletal system. With respect to the patient with extremely large breasts, the authors consider this alternative whenever the nipple-areola complex is to be elevated more than 6 inches. This guideline remains a loose rule of thumb that is modified by any number of factors, especially the age of the patient. We remain reluctant to use this alternative in young or unmarried patients, for example. Although concern for ischemic injury to the retained nipple-areola complex in such greatly enlarged breasts remains a major indication for this alternative, it may not be the sole or even primary reason to recommend it. Rather, the technical reality of breast reduction for such large breasts may prove unwieldy when a pedicle is maintained for the sole purpose of bearing the nipple-areola complex; the execution of surgery may be complicated and the resultant shape and form disappointing. Additionally, specialized sensation to the nipple-areola of such massive breasts is commonly diminished preoperatively, thereby dismissing the major objection to the use of this facile alternative.

PREOPERATIVE MARKING
The breast markings remain similar to those for the vertical pedicle technique (Fig. 47-23). The meridian line of the breast is drawn and the inframammary fold transferred to it with calipers. The wire keyhole pattern is not used for this technique, however. Instead, two diverging arms are drawn from the selected nipple point at an angle approximating 90 degrees. Limb length is measured at 7.5 to 8.5 cm (average 8 cm). The infra-

mammary line is marked, and the medial and lateral extensions from the limbs are indicated as for the standard technique. The areola is marked for reduction with the areolar marker.

TECHNIQUE
The procedure is begun by removing the nipple-areola complex rapidly with attached subjacent breast tissue and setting it aside in a moist saline sponge, clearly indicating the side of origin, right or left. We do not follow the skin markings as some have suggested when performing the glandular resection because we find it too frequently productive of inadequate central projection of the breast. Far better is Rubin's alternative of retaining inferior parenchyma at the inframammary line to be covered by the superior skin flaps [54]. We prefer, however, to retain superiorly based parenchyma between the diverging limbs of the pattern, as well as an additional amount dropping below this area. This retained tissue is designated with a single curvilinear line placed below the diverging arms, and the enclosed area is rapidly deskinned. The breast is now ready for amputation. It is critical here that the pendulous gland be gathered in a spherical fashion and balanced on the curving barrel of the thoracic cage before the amputation is undertaken. Clearly, the greatest pitfall in this otherwise straightforward procedure is the amputation of excessive breast tissue, leaving only superior flaps with subcutaneous tissue and little breast. If the breast is allowed to hang pendulously, gravity pulls virtually the entire gland below the level of the amputating blade, presenting the surgeon with a regrettable surprise when refashioning an inadequate breast from the remaining superior flaps. When, on the other hand, the gland is gathered and presented in a spherical fashion by an assistant, the amputating blade leaves a significant amount of parenchyma superiorly. The dictum that more can always be removed later prevails here.

The amputating incision is carried per-

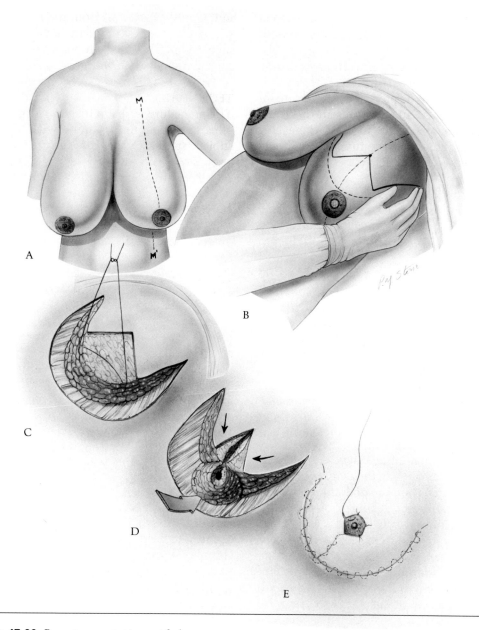

**Figure 47-23** *Breast amputation with free nipple-areola graft: authors' technique. A. Breast meridian marked. B. Preoperative markings completed. C. Amputation completed. D. Central tissue coned and rotated into retromammary space. E. Free nipple-areolar graft added at closure.*

pendicularly down to the chest-wall musculature. The inframammary incision is similarly carried perpendicularly to the musculature. The large intervening wedge of gland is then dissected progressively from medial to lateral away from the muscle fascia, maintaining exact hemostasis as the resection pro-

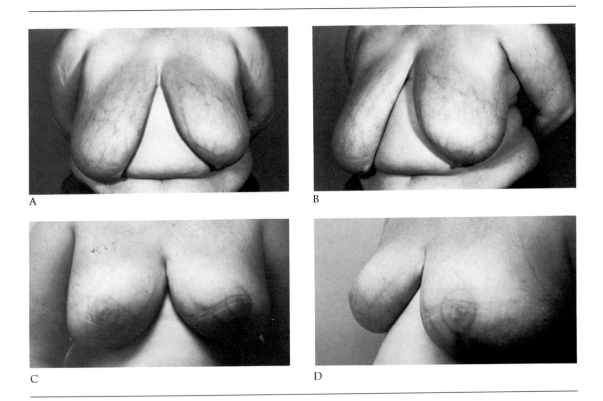

A

B

C

D

**Figure 47-24** *Large reduction mammaplasty by amputation with free nipple-areola grafts (2500 gm each side). A, B. Preoperative views. C, D. Postoperative views at 6 months.*

gresses. The central portion of the remaining superior gland, including the deskinned portion between and below the diverging limbs, is now dissected from the underlying muscle fascia superiorly the distance of a hand's-breadth, creating a subglandular pocket. A single absorbable suture is used to infold the central deskinned parenchyma. This tissue is then rotated into the subglandular pocket and fixed to the pectoralis fascia with an additional suture. With closure of the remaining skin margins, a pleasing conical shape is created, with the infolded central breast tissue forcing an impressive projection. Closure is completed in the standard fashion working from the extremities centrally.

Finally, the site for the nipple-areola complex is determined and measured upward from the inframammary fold on either side. It may or may not fall precisely at the supe-

rior extent of the vertical closure. The area is marked with the areolar marker and is deepithelialized. The defatted nipple-areola complex is sutured in place and secured with a tie-over dressing. It is important not to thin the areolar portion of the graft excessively during the defatting process, so that the resulting areolar graft has a more natural appearance. Similarly, ductal tissue is left within the papilla, to favor nipple projection. A greasy dressing with wet cotton bolus is then tied in place over the complex and is removed at 4 days. Because the dissection surfaces are limited and hemostasis is straightforward, a drain is not used under routine circumstances (Fig. 47-24).

## Modified Reduction Mammaplasty Following Contralateral Breast Reconstruction

Of the four common alterations to the remaining breast after contralateral breast reconstruction—dermal mastopexy, submuscular augmentation mammaplasty, prophylactic mastectomy with reconstruction, and reduction mammaplasty—only the latter presents significant potential interference to follow-up examination of that structure. The authors therefore follow the strict policy of discussing this option preoperatively with the patient's oncologist and surgeon. When reduction mammaplasty is elected to modify the remaining breast, every effort is made to limit intraparenchymal scarring that might interfere with subsequent examination of the breast for neoplasm, whether by palpation, mammography, or other technique. At the same time, retention of a sensate, responsive nipple-areola remains a major justification for this alternative over prophylactic mastectomy with reconstruction. A compromise technique addresses both goals—of limited glandular scarring and retained nipple-areola sensation in such breasts undergoing less than massive reduction.

After conventional markings, the keyhole pattern is set, in this instance some 2 cm or more above the traditional level corresponding to the inframammary fold. A modified inferior wedge of skin and breast is then resected from the lower pole of the breast, between the superior and inframammary markings (Fig. 47-25). This wedge is modified from that of a simple amputation by retaining a portion of the central parenchyma in line with what would otherwise be the base of a conventional vertical pedicle, thereby avoiding undue flattening centrally. A degree of flattening, of course, is desirable to better match the contralateral breast, especially if the reconstruction was by submuscular prosthesis. The dermis of the upper keyhole pattern is divided to either side of the nipple-areola only enough to allow sufficient upward mobility of that structure. Thus is deep intraparenchymal dissection and scarring avoided, as is major infolding of dermoglandular elements. The flatter result with less conical projection thus better compares with the contralateral reconstructed breast.

### Mastopexy

Whereas reduction mammaplasty involves uplift of the breast with significant reduction of mass and volume, mastopexy connotes uplift alone, with little or no such reduction. Most patterns of skin reduction described for reduction mammaplasty are therefore applicable to mastopexy. Despite these similarities, fundamental differences exist between the two. Whereas reduction mammaplasty is primarily invoked to restore balance to a distorted physique and bring relief to a strained musculoskeletal system, it brings with it a clear, if secondary, aesthetic benefit. Mastopexy, on the other hand, must be seen to be essentially aesthetic in nature. Although the pattern and extent of scarring, for example, remain important considerations with reduction mammaplasty, they present as the major and critical trade-offs with mastopexy. At least a mild degree of ptosis is factored into the final result of a well done reduction mammaplasty, but such residual ptosis may be less acceptable to the small-breasted woman with primary aesthetic motivation for undergoing mastopexy.

If the goal of resuspending and reshaping a high, round, firm, and in fact immature breast from a fallen, elongated, lax, and mature one has eluded all techniques to date, surely that of maintaining such a profile against the persistent effects of time and gravity must remain unfulfilled, at least in the gravitational field of Earth as we know it. Mastopexy therefore represents an aesthetic operation in which the primary goal must be seen as compromised from the beginning.

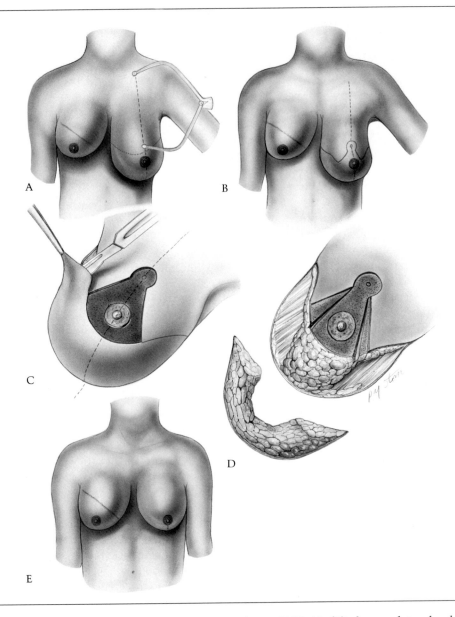

**Figure 47-25** *Modified contralateral reduction mammaplasty following breast reconstruction. A. Nipple positioned. B. Preoperative markings completed. C. Upper pedicle deepithelialized. D. Modified inferior dermoglandular wedge resection. E. Closure.*

## HISTORY

Techniques for elevating ptotic breasts, improving breast shape, and repositioning the nipple-areola have evolved over the past century [29]. Early procedures involved the removal of skin and fat, leaving behind substantive breast tissue. Later procedures, to maintain the higher form, attached a portion

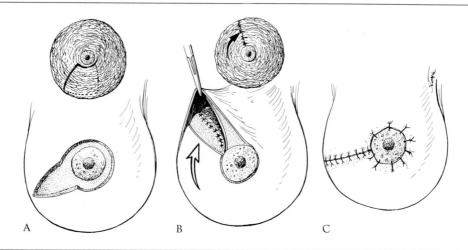

A          B          C

*Figure 47-26* *Dufourmentel mastopexy technique. A. Infralateral skin reduction. B. Lateral gland rotated superiorly. C. Closure.*

of the gland to an elevated position on the anterior chest wall. More recently, a silicone prosthesis has been inserted during or after mastopexy to enhance the final appearance.

The first description of mastopexy was offered by Pousson [47], who removed large crescents of skin and fat from the superior portion of the breast and then fixed the gland with sutures to the pectoralis major muscle. Girard in 1910 described an operation performed through the inframammary crease. He dissected breast from the pectoralis fascia, rolled it upon itself, and suspended it from the cartilage of the second rib. No skin, fat, or gland was removed [14]. In 1923 Lotsch, in an important precedent to the modern mastopexy, elevated the nipple-areola complex to an aesthetic level [32]. He excised a circle of skin from around the nipple-areola and undermined the skin margins to allow superior transposition. Loose skin was tightened about the inferior aspect of the breast, and redundant skin was excised. Early patterns of excision varied from surgeon to surgeon. Dufourmentel excised a lateral crescent of skin from around the are-

ola [8] (Fig. 47-26). Noel in 1928 proposed excision of multiple crescents of skin from above the nipple-areola, thereby elevating that structure [43]. Weinhold [66] excised skin from above and below the areola. In 1958 Gillies and Marino [13] improved the small, lax breast by elevating and rotating the ptotic gland, folding it on itself to enhance projection in "periwinkle" fashion. More recently Goulian [17], in his "dermal mastopexy," supported the elevated breast through a "skin brassiere" fashioned without undermining (Fig. 47-27). Hinderer [24] recommended dermal strips to fix the gland to the pectoralis muscle. After acceptance that the nipple-areola could move safely on a pedicle of dermis, procedures designed to reduce large breasts were found suitable for correcting ptosis alone. The skin was tailored by the reduction pattern, with the glandular tissue retained to provide volume and projection. Gonzalez-Ulloa [15] was the first to recommend concomitant subglandular augmentation of the breast during mastopexy to correct the ptotic, hypoplastic gland.

INDICATIONS

Patients request mastopexy to improve an unaesthetic appearance and fallen position

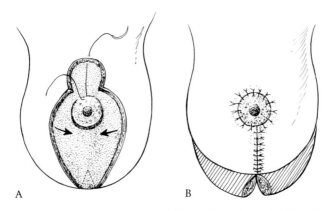

A      B

*Figure 47-27* *Dermal mastopexy technique of Goulian. A. Central deepithelialization. B. Tailored closure "cut-as-you-go."*

of their breasts caused by stretching of the skin and loss of parenchymal volume. This natural aging process may be accelerated by weight loss, pregnancy, lactation, and menopause. The appearance of laxity and flaccidity may be heightened by the presence of striae.

Regnault [49] classified ptosis by degree: *First degree ptosis* occurs when the nipple descends to the level of the inframammary fold; *second degree ptosis* pertains when the nipple falls below the fold but remains above the lowest contour of the breast; and *third degree ptosis* occurs when the nipple reaches the lowest contour of the breast. *Pseudoptosis* describes the loose, lax breast whose nipple remains above the inframammary fold.

### AUTHORS' TECHNIQUES
#### Mastopexy Alone
Mastopexy is performed under local anesthesia on an outpatient basis. For significant (i.e., second or third degree) ptosis the authors utilize the same markings as for reduction mammaplasty. Again the meridian line of the breast is determined and the inframammary fold transferred to that line. It is equally important during mastopexy not to elevate the nipple-areola complex unduly. It may surprise the inexperienced surgeon to learn how little objective elevation is required to bring the nipple to the proper level

in a breast that may appear lax. Again, one must have a good reason to elevate the complex to a level above the transposed inframammary line—and the bigger the breast, the better the reason. The most common exception remains an effort to match an opposite breast reconstructed with a submuscular prosthesis, where additional elevation may be appropriate. Here, especially, the addition of a submuscular implant may be desirable to imitate the superior fullness, often to an unnatural degree, of the opposite reconstructed breast.

After selecting the proper nipple site, the wire keyhole pattern is spread to an appropriate divergence to encourage a decided tightness to the closure of the underpanel of breast skin, such that the immediate result has a flattened appearance. With mastopexy accurate preoperative confirmation of the skin pattern can be undertaken by infolding the central and inferior skin and bringing together the key points to assess tension (Fig. 47-28). Early side-to-side tension is necessary to some degree to compensate for the inevitable postoperative relaxation of skin and support. One must not create so much tension, however, that ischemia or unnatural tightness results.

After marking the areola for reduction, the

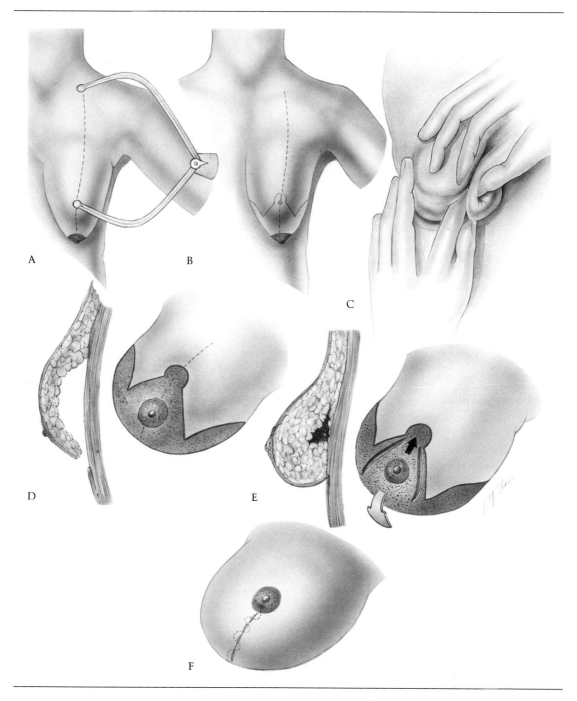

**Figure 47-28** *Mastopexy: authors' technique. A. Nipple positioned.*
*B. Preoperative markings. C. Breast infolded to confirm markings.*
*D. Deepithelialization complete and breast freed from muscle fascia.*
*E. Dermoglandular flap rotated into retromammary space and fixed to*
*chest wall. F. Closure.*

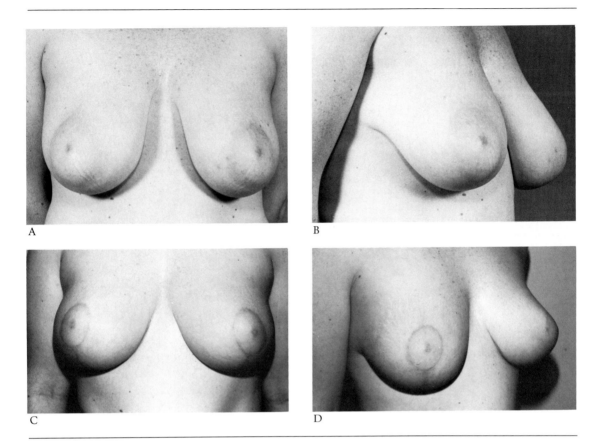

A

B

C

D

**Figure 47-29** *Mastopexy alone in the large breast. A, B. Preoperative views. C, D. Postoperative views at 6 months.*

area within the pattern is rapidly deepithe-lialized. This step has less to do with concerns of vascularity than it has the attractive, if unsubstantiated, theory of Goulian that dermal-to-dermal healing fortifies the skin brassiere and resists redescent [16, 17]. Incisions are placed through the dermis along the upper portion of what would be the vertical bipedicle flap of a reduction mammaplasty such that the nipple-areola complex may elevate to the keyhole without undue distortion to the lateral limbs. Clearly, the greater the elevation, the greater is the need for development of the central portion of the vertical flap. In further agreement with Goulian, the authors avoid undermining the skin, preferring instead to maintain the skin–parenchyma relations undisturbed in an effort to resist downward settling.

When a considerable portion of the deepithe-lialized breast hangs below the level of the new inframammary fold, this redundant portion of the gland is suspended as a superior dermoglandular pedicle, rolled under the breast and fixed to the chest wall musculature. This technique is readily accomplished by dividing through the dermoglandular bed at the inframammary line and undermining the gland at the muscular level. The resulting subglandular pocket must be large enough to accommodate the inferior gland excess. This dermoglandular redundancy is folded behind the breast and fixed with a single suture to the muscle fascia at a height sufficient to eliminate gross redundancy.

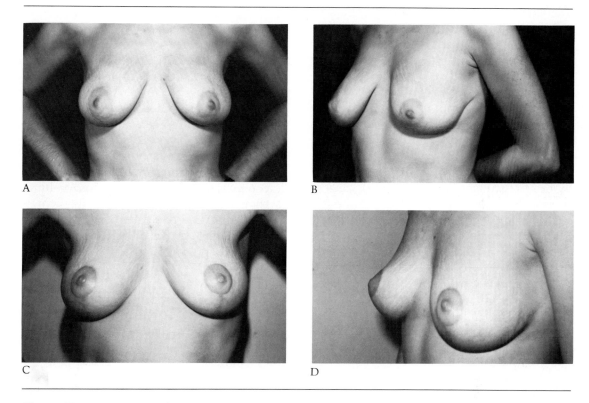

**Figure 47-30** *Mastopexy alone in the small breast. A, B. Preoperative views. C, D. Postoperative views at 2 years.*

This technique may be deemed inappropriate when lifting the opposite breast to improve symmetry with a breast reconstructed after mastectomy for cancer. Here intraparenchymal scarring must be minimized or avoided, including subglandular dissection. If this maneuver is omitted, however, when the skin is closed, redundant glandular volume may distribute itself on either side of the inframammary line, presenting an inferior bulge below the line. Should it occur, proper dressing can correct the situation. Firm, folded dressings are stacked on top of the inferior bulge up to the exact inframammary line and are held in place with tape. An underwire brassiere reinforced with an elastic bandage is added over the dressing material. The infraglandular excess is thus forced above the inframammary fold into the breast

proper, where it heals and remains. Such dressings are discontinued within 5 days.

Skin closure is then performed in standard fashion with little or no undermining. Every effort is made to limit the length of the inframammary scar, even at the price of small dog-ear accumulations. The brassiere is the postoperative bandage, and its support is continued for 6 weeks (Figs. 47-29 and 47-30).

Patients are counseled before mastopexy that unnatural flatness to the inferior aspect of the breast and a downward point to the nipple correct themselves within the first few months after surgery. They are further told that some recurrence of ptosis is inevitable by 6 months and finally that a minor revision is available in the office if early relaxation is significant. Here rapid retightening of the inferior skin panel is performed by ellipsoid reexcision of the vertical closure. If this routine of primary overcorrection and secondary, if minor, revision is seen as a weakness in the overall design of mastopexy, the authors willingly concede this point and, more important, insist that their patients understand it as well.

*Mastopexy with Augmentation*
Concomitant augmentation mammaplasty with mastopexy was a natural evolution in the treatment of the ptotic, hypoplastic breast [15]. A further development became the practice of subglandular augmentation alone for the correction of lesser degrees of ptosis, substituting the brief scar of the former for the extensive scar pattern of the latter. Unfortunately, symptomatic capsular contracture, a frequent problem with subglandular conventional prostheses, became even more frequent in the unsupported soft tissue environment of the ptotic breast. This difficulty has been greatly reduced, at least in the hands of the authors, by the total submuscular positioning of these same conventional prostheses.

McKissock emphasized improvement in long-term aesthetic results when submuscular augmentation mammaplasty becomes a component of routine mastopexy, the major benefit deriving from restoration of superior fullness in the breast [39]. It is the loss of such fullness that is the presenting concern of many women exhibiting little formal ptosis in terms of nipple-areola descent. Restoration and maintenance of superior fullness remains the elusive goal of mastopexy repair over time. Efforts to create such fullness with transposition of breast parenchyma have largely failed. Techniques that roll up inferior redundancy, as just described, fail to restore volume at a sufficiently superior level. Effective superior translocation of autogenous gland requires major dissection within central, not inferior, portions of the breast, creating fundamental disruption of the gland, along with likely alterations in nipple-areola sensitivity.

The authors concur, therefore, with the expedience of submuscular prosthetic augmentation for pursuing this goal. Their personal

evolution along these lines now recommends inferior excision in addition to superior prosthetic augmentation as components of breast uplift and tightening through mastopexy [51]. In breasts with significant inferior redundancy, a transverse dermoglandular wedge is excised and discarded rather than retained and forced superiorly into the tightened skin brassiere. As for modified reduction mammaplasty in the high risk breast, such inferior amputation avoids intraparenchymal scarring. The lost volume is then replaced and typically augmented through insertion of a submuscular prosthesis, producing enhanced aesthetic results with superior fullness.

*Concentric Mastopexy*
In the authors' opinion, concentric or doughnut mastopexy [4, 19] alone offers insufficient correction to justify its routine use in mastopexy. Furthermore, it may produce three undesirable changes: There is a decided tendency toward postoperative enlargement of the areola, often to unnatural and unattractive dimensions; the circumareolar scar is not infrequently spread and occasionally hypertrophies; and there follows a flattening of the breast contour at the apex. In two specific situations, however, this technique may be of special help: in the constricted or tuberous breast and in the breast with mild to moderate laxity undergoing submuscular augmentation mammaplasty.

CONSTRICTED BREAST. Constricted [53] or tuberous [48] breasts are widely spaced breasts of narrow or constricted base or origin from the chest wall, with enlarged and pouting or protruded areolae. Always a challenge to correction, this deformity is especially troublesome in a unilateral, asymmetric situation.

The mainstay of correction remains aggressive concentric reduction of pigmented tissues to reduce the areola into the plane of the breast. The undesirable areolar flattening that occurs in conventional breasts undergoing doughnut mastopexy becomes advantageous in the constricted breast with a protuberant areola. The constricted base may, however, defy uniform expansion through prosthetic augmentation, demanding relief through inferior radial release and soft tissue augmentation by local interpolation from the inframammary fold, an aggressive solution proposed by Dinner [7] but probably unacceptable to most patients with lesser forms of the condition.

MICROMASTIA WITH MILD PTOSIS. Hypomastia with significant ptosis requires formal mastopexy with attendant scarring as an adjunct to augmentation. When ptosis is mild, on the other hand, subglandular augmentation with conventional prostheses has given excellent early correction but has too frequently progressed to distortion from significant capsular contracture. Subglandular treatment with textured implants may diminish this problem [23]. Whereas submuscular augmentation with conventional implants has also tended to avoid this contractile complication, so has it been prone to its own problem in the lax breast—the double silhouette. Although the muscle brassiere maintains the prosthesis in a relatively high, round form on the chest wall, the ptotic breast may hang below this point, creating a double-bubble profile. Although this disappointment improves with time as the muscle relaxes and the implant settles inferiorly, an unacceptable profile may persist.

The limited skin tightening available through concentric mastopexy is frequently effective in preventing this deformity following submuscular augmentation in the moderately ptotic breast. The principle to keep in mind when planning the two concentric circles defining the excision is that the areolar complex has a marked tendency to expand after this procedure. Designs that retain the entire pigmented areola and remove only a peripheral zone of skin invariably produce a large, even hideous "dinner plate" areola. Instead, after placing the skin of the areolar region under appropriate tension, a central diameter of 3 cm or less is indicated for the first

(inner) circle; the second (peripheral) circle is then added at two or, maximally, two and one-half times the diameter of the first (6 to 7 cm).

After deepithelializing the intervening segment, which involves significant amounts of areola, the submuscular augmentation mammaplasty is undertaken through the inferomedial dermal bed. Closure of the concentric defect is undertaken by a meticulous, if tiresome, halving procedure with fine absorbable sutures until the discrepancy has been bunched centripetally (Fig. 47-31). Although effective in the circumstances described, efforts to apply this technique to breasts with greater degrees of ptosis remain inadvisable.

## The Periareolar "Round Block" Technique for Reduction Mammaplasty and Mastopexy

In all types of mammaplasty, a main concern is to limit the scar. This is particularly true of operations for ptosis and hypertrophy, which usually leave substantial scars. Ideally the scarring would be confined to the periareolar area where the scar is generally inconspicuous.

Until recently, periareolar mammaplasty techniques were limited to moderate ptosis in small breasts because of the risk of enlarging or distorting the areola by excessive tension on the areolar skin [9a]. The problem seems to have been solved by the Benelli "round block" technique [5a, 5b, 5c, 5d, 5f], which eliminates tension, postoperative enlargement, and/or distortion. The technique can be used to reduce large areolas and for the treatment of ptosis and hypertrophies. The resulting periareolar scar is good. Furthermore, no postoperative enlargement of the areola or scar results.

The keystone of the "round block" technique is a supra- and subdermal periareolar blocking suture that is nonresorbable and fixed (Figs. 47-32, 47-33, 47-34). In the technique, a woven nylon fiber (0 or 1 according

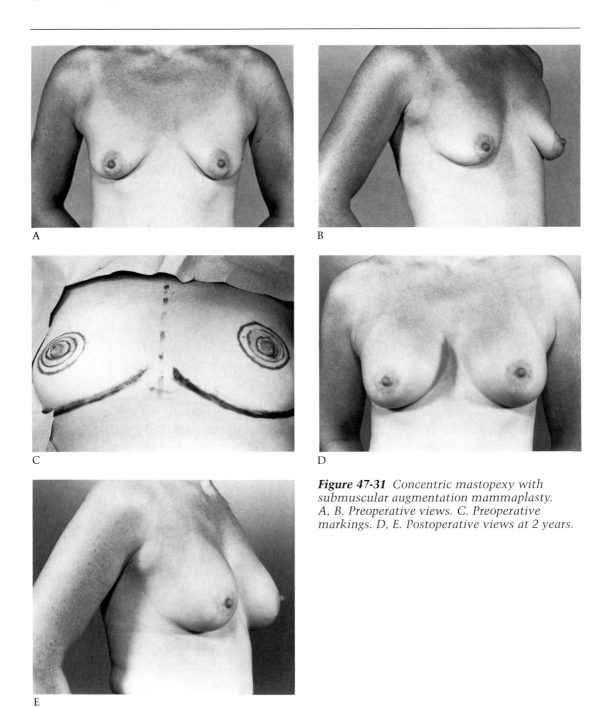

**Figure 47-31** *Concentric mastopexy with submuscular augmentation mammaplasty. A, B. Preoperative views. C. Preoperative markings. D, E. Postoperative views at 2 years.*

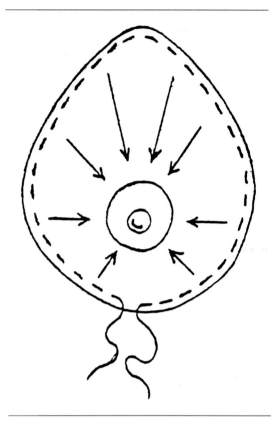

**Figure 47-32** *The periareolar blocking suture of heavy woven nylon fiber produces a solid, circular dermo-dermic scar. This eliminates excessive tension on the areola and preserves its desired size and shape.*

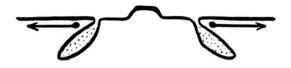

**Figure 47-33** *The periareolar blocking suture creates a dermal to dermal fixation by its method and level of insertion.*

Then mark point B, the base of the new areola. Outline on the surrounding surface of the breast the area of skin to be de-epithelialized, taking into account the amount of cutaneous excess. There is no need to be concerned with de-epithelializing large surface areas because the fixed nature of the "round block" avoids all postoperative areolar deformity. Excess skin associated with ptosis commonly requires de-epithelialization of 14 cm vertically (point A to point B) and 12 cm transversely (point C to point D). If necessary, more skin can be removed. Outline the circumference of the new areola. The diameter, usually determined according to the size of the breast, is commonly about 4 cm. Carefully, de-epithelialize the area between the areola and the peripheral outline keeping the underlying dermis intact.

In performing a mastopexy, make a horizontal incision in the dermis on the lower side of the de-epidermized area (Fig. 47-36). Use the incision to perform a deep subcutaneous dissection of the lower and median parts of the mammary gland. The dissection should extend to, but not below, the submammary fold. Establish hemostasis—a hematoma could easily form where dissection has taken place.

For ptosis, a criss-cross periosteal mastopexy can be used to increase the breast projection, refine the lower quadrants, and add to the upper quadrants. Start by detaching the inferior portion of the gland from the prepectoral area above the submammary fold to create a glandular flap with a superior

to the amount of traction expected) is used to encircle the areola and fix its diameter by the tension under which it is tied. This, along with two crossed sutures of 2–0 braided nylon (one in the horizontal diameter of the areola and the other in the vertical diameter), avoids a protrusion of the areola and maintains it in a solid, circular dermo-dermic scar.

TECHNIQUE

Preoperatively, draw a line along the breast meridian (Fig. 47-35). On it, identify point A, which will be the top of the new areola.

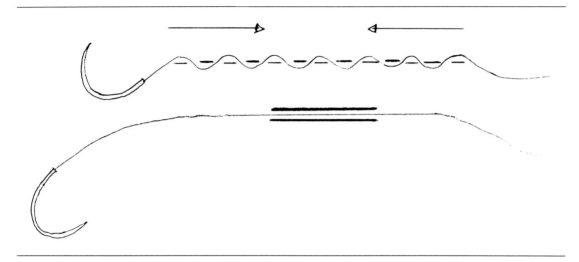

**Figure 47-34** *Upper sketch demonstrates the placing of the heavy nylon suture so it passes alternately through the supradermal and subdermal layers. Lower sketch demonstrates how the suture appears as the excess skin slides along the gather or folds before it is tied.*

**Figure 47-35** *Preoperative planning for surgery. Points A and B are the new locations for the top and bottom of the reduced areola. The outline of the area to be de-epithelialized is carefully marked on the surrounding skin.*

**Figure 47-36** *Incision for performing a mastopexy is just beneath the areola. Dissection is carried out to create criss-cross flaps that will support the elevated and improved breast contours.*

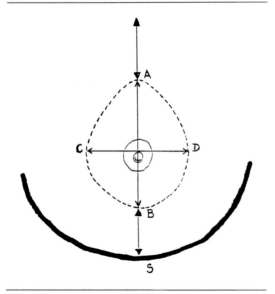

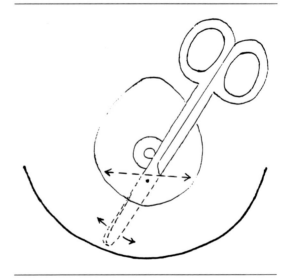

base. This glandular flap is separated into two parts, the external and the internal, by a vertical incision in the center of the flap (Fig. 47-37). A criss-cross periosteal mastopexy is then performed by attaching the medial part of the external flap to the presternal periosteum over the submammary fold. The periosteum is secured with a large curved needle that is pushed to the bone through the sternal insertion of the large pectoral muscle. In this way, the external glandular flap is strongly fixed in the paramedial position under the internal glandular flap. The internal glandular flap is then fixed to the costal periosteum laterally over the submammary fold. Several inverted stitches are placed along the line where the glandular flaps cross. The suture used for all of these points is a 2–0 monofilament nylon. This criss-crossed periosteal mastopexy constitutes a very strong support of the mammary cone. The anterior projection of the breast is guaranteed by this maneuver.

In cases of moderate or minor mammary hypertrophy, an excision of glandular volume can easily be performed by resection of glandular tissue on the external or internal glandular flaps or both before performing the mastopexy.

In the case of major hypertrophy, the excision can be extended to the upper pole of the gland by splitting the flap into a superficial and a deep component and resecting the deep portion. The superficial portion then can be turned back on itself and anchored at the level of the second intercostal space. In this way the flap supporting the areola is lifted, lessening the ptosis and augmenting the superior portion of the breast.

The periareolar suture is begun under the dermis at the lower edge of the incision made to perform the mastopexy. This suture is a nonresorbable, woven thread of strong quality (0 or 1) that is started at the edge of the de-epithelialized area and passed alternately from the supra to the subdermal position and back again (Fig. 47-34), finishing at its starting point. Then, an even distribu-

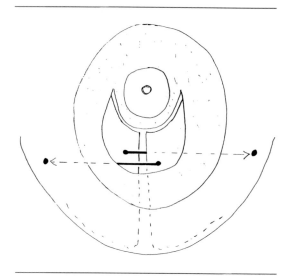

**Figure 47-37** *Criss-cross flaps increase breast projection, refine lower quadrants, and add bulk to the upper quadrants.*

tion of the skin pleats or gathers can be achieved by sliding the excess skin along the suture. The suture can be blocked in the position that will achieve the desired areolar diameter. An aspiration drain is placed inferiorly.

In order to avoid a protrusion of the areola due to intramammary pressure, place two crossed sutures—one in the horizontal diameter of the areola and the other in the vertical diameter (Fig. 47-38). The ends of the braided nylon 2–0 are threaded onto a straight needle and crossed under the nipple in the center of the areola. These stitches are simply put into place and should not be tied tightly. They have a passive role of fixation to prevent tuberous protrusion of the areola.

Use a cutaneous suture to position the four cardinal points of the areola. No dermodermic uniting suture is necessary since the "round block" ensures the fixed state of the structure. A cutaneous suture can be made very easily and without tension. A continuous horizontal mattress suture with a resorbable suture permits an eversion of the

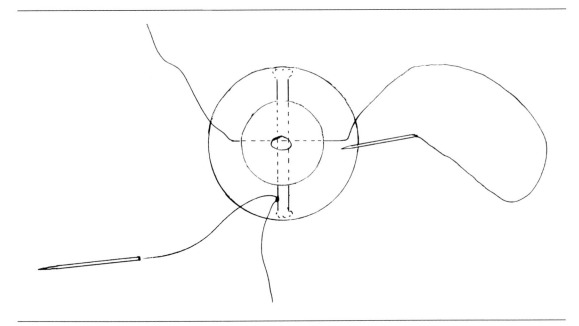

*Figure 47-38* *Two crossed sutures, one horizontal and one vertical, aid in positioning the areola and prevent tuberous protrusion of its contents.*

edges, resulting in a better hygiene of the scar. Dressings are held in place by a well-supporting brassiere.

*Postoperative Care*
Support the breast by wearing a brassiere day and night for a month.

Clean the suture every day with antiseptic and cover with dressing.

*Postoperative Development*
The periareolar skin pleats will disappear in some weeks. Bruising is common on the lower part of the breast and exposure to the sun is not advised until its complete disappearance. The periareolar diameter is well-fixed, the suture encircling the areola at a depth.

## Complications

Breast reduction and mastopexy are associated with a number of complications that may be divided into errors of planning, errors of execution, and nonspecific postoperative mishaps. As previously emphasized,

the cornerstone of excellence in breast reduction technique is accurate preoperative planning and marking to ensure adequate, symmetric, and aesthetic reduction of the breast. The most grievous and common error of planning is placing the nipple too high. In nearly all situations the nipple must be situated at or near the level of the inframammary fold, with vertical limb length from areola to fold limited to less than 6 cm. Adherence to these guidelines for nipple placement minimizes the all-too-common late complication of glandular "dropout" with upward-gazing areola. The nipple may also be misplaced to either side of the breast meridian. Accurately defining the true breast meridian and moving the nipple along this line is crucial and may require a transverse shift of the nipple located aberrantly off the aesthetic axis of the breast. With proper planning, the breast immediately acquires a pleasing, if somewhat inferiorly flattened, conical shape.

Inadequate skin resection in general or inadequate glandular resection at the periphery of the breast may produce a boxy, unattractive, amorphous, or irregular-looking breast. On the other hand, overly ambitious resection, especially centrally, may leave insufficient gland and skin to fashion a breast of suitable size or projection. Although to some extent unavoidable, especially in scar-prone individuals, scar hypertrophy may be aggravated by excess skin resection with increased skin tension or injudicious placement of incisions either outside or beyond the inframammary fold. Exaggerated "lazy-S" resections are especially inadvisable in this regard. Suction-assisted lipectomy beyond limited, well placed incisions helps keep hypertrophic scars to a minimum.

Asymmetry may occur when symmetric breasts are reduced disparately or when insufficient care is given to achieve symmetry in breasts initially asymmetric. In the former case, appropriate planning and execution, including recording of specimen weights during the procedure, yield a balanced result. In the latter case, it may not be always or even frequently possible to achieve desired symmetry where there exists significant preoperative disproportion, especially with breasts of fundamentally different shape [25]. The larger breast, however, clearly requires a greater volume reduction and may also require adjustment of the keyhole pattern to match the change in breast dimensions. Careful comparative evaluation of the breasts during closure with fine tuning by liposuction or serial glandular paring helps keep asymmetry to a minimum.

Symmastia, or loss of cleavage between the breasts, may be seen either as part of the initial problem of breast hypertrophy left uncorrected by the operation or as a postoperative result of confluence of the medial inframammary scars presenting as a transverse scar band across the sternum. Every effort must be made to avoid joining the scars from either side across the midline to prevent the formation of such a band. Shorter inframammary scars with the possible help of a V-Y plasty may aid in this endeavor. Patients presenting with glandular symmastia may be helped by aggressive midline suction-assisted lipectomy. Vertical Y-V plasty has been proposed to alleviate this problem [59] but necessitates an oblique scar, which violates the midline and may itself favor scar hypertrophy.

Despite appropriate preoperative planning, faulty execution of the plan can lead to difficulties. An overly narrowed pedicle may create nipple-areola ischemia, producing a range of sequelae from areolar depigmentation and scar hypertrophy to possible total nipple-areola loss. Attempts to transfer the nipple on a pedicle in cases of massive hypertrophy are at increased risk for such complications. When misjudgment or poor execution lead to an ischemic nipple-areola, there is evidence that the complex may be salvaged by conversion to a free graft within the first 24 hours after surgery [57]. Although not entirely avoidable, nipple-areola denervation is a complication that can be minimized by proper planning and execution. Maintaining support for the nipple-areola on a central-lateralized dermoglandular base maintains circulation and innervation in most cases. In cases of free nipple grafting, sensation is impaired, lactation is lost, and pigment changes are possible, especially in dark-skinned individuals. Evidence suggests that most of the currently popular techniques of reduction mammaplasty with nipple transfer on a subjacent glandular pedicle are compatible, if not uniformly associated, with subsequent successful nursing [21, 68].

Devascularization of skin or parenchyma by inexpert resection or excessive skin tension may lead to fat necrosis with drainage and sinus formation, skin flap slough, and nipple-areola injury. Minor skin flap necrosis is not uncommon, however, at the suture line junction of skin closures of inverted-T design.

Infection is appropriately rare following reduction mammaplasty and is probably not traceable to any specific error. Most surgeons do not employ antibiotic prophylaxis with this surgery. Postoperative bleeding or hematoma is similarly uncommon, although many practitioners do employ routine, if brief, postoperative drainage. Late cyst formation, occasionally seen, is related to retained epithelial elements in buried dermoglandular structures infolded within the breast.

Whereas the most serious error of planning remains superior malposition of the nipple, the most common postoperative disappointment is unfavorable or hypertrophic scarring. Seen in its most basic guise, reduction mammaplasty represents a trade-off of disproportionate, cumbersome, unaesthetic breasts for attractive, proportionate ones marred, however, by a significant pattern of visible, if not offensive, scarring. Although in most cases the trade-off proves worthwhile with scars that politely fade with time, there are many exceptions where spread, thickened, reddened, or symptomatic scars remain unhappy reminders of the operative experience. Unfortunately, it is especially true in the younger segment of the patient population. Appropriate patient selection with candid informed consent remain the best approach to the scarring problem associated with reduction mammaplasty. The well selected and informed patient with unfavorable scarring, of course, voices disappointment concerning this aspect of her outcome but inevitably reaffirms, immediately thereafter, the correctness of her decision for surgery and her gratitude for its other considerable benefits.

## References

1. Aufricht, G. Mammaplasty for pendulous breasts: Empiric and geometric planning. *Plast. Reconstr. Surg.* 4:13, 1949.
2. Axhausen, G. Plastic surgery of breast. *Med. Klin.* 22:1437, 1926.
3. Balch, C. The central mound technique for reduction mammoplasty. *Plast. Reconstr. Surg.* 67:305, 1981.
4. Bartels, R. J., Strickland, D. M., and Douglas, W. M. A new mastopexy operation for mild or moderate breast ptosis. *Plast. Reconstr. Surg.* 57:687, 1976.
5. Biesenberger, H. Eine neue methode der mammaplastik. *Zentralbl. Chir.* 55:2382, 1928.
5a. Benelli, L. A new periareolar mammaplasty: Round block technique. In Proceedings of the Congress of the International Society of Aesthetic Plastic Surgery. Zurich, Switzerland, September 11–14, 1989.
5b. Benelli, L. Periareolar mammoplasty tecnica round block. International Symposium Recent Advances in Plastic Surgery. Sao Paulo, Brazil, March 3, 1989.
5c. Benelli, L. Technique de plastie mammaire le round block. *Revue francaise de Chirurgie Esthetique.* No. 50, Tome XIII, March, 1988.
5d. Benelli, L. Traitement des ptoses mammaires par voie periareolaire: Technique personnelle: Le "round block." Symposium de Chirurgie Esthetique, College d'Enseignement et de Recherche de Chirurgie Esthetique. Paris, November 6, 1987.
5e. Benelli, L., Faivre, J. Traitement chirurgical des lesions inesthetiques de l'areole et du mamelon. Chirurgie Esthetique, 1984, Maloine Editeur.
5f. Benelli, L. A new periareolar mammoplasty: The "round block" technique. *Aesth. Plast. Surg.* 14:93–100, 1990.
6. Courtiss, E., and Goldwyn, R. M. Reduction mammoplasty by the inferior pedicle technique. *Plast. Reconstr. Surg.* 59:500, 1977.
7. Dinner, M. I. Management of the tubular breast syndrome by a submammary transposition flap. Presented at the Annual Meeting of the American Society for Aesthetic Plastic Surgery. Washington, D.C., 1984.
8. Dufourmentel, L. L'incision areolaire dans la chirurgie du sein. *Bull. Mem. Soc. Chir.* 20:9, 1928.
9. Edwards, E. A. Surgical Anatomy of the Breast. In R. M. Goldwyn (ed.), *Plastic and Reconstructive Surgery of the Breast.* Boston: Little, Brown, 1976.
9a. Faivre, J., Carissimo, A., Faivre, J. M. La voie periareolaire dans le traitement des petites ptoses mammaires. Chirurgie Esthetique,

1984, Maloine Editeur.

9b. Felicio, Y. Periareolar reduction mammaplasty, a single incision technique. International Symposium Recent Advances in Plastic Surgery. Sao Paulo, Brazil, March 3, 1989.

10. Georgiade, N. *Reconstructive Breast Surgery.* St. Louis: Mosby, 1976.

11. Georgiade, N., et al. Is there a reduction mammoplasty for "all seasons"? *Plast. Reconstr. Surg.* 63:765, 1979.

12. Georgiade, N. G., et al. Reduction mammoplasty utilizing an inferior pedicle nipple-areola flap. *Ann. Plast. Surg.* 3:211, 1979.

13. Gillies, H., and Marinom, H. The "periwinkle" shell principle in the treatment of the small ptotic breast. *Plast. Reconstr. Surg.* 21:1, 1958.

14. Girard, C. Uber mastoptose und mastopexie. *Arch. Klin. Chir.* 92:829, 1910.

15. Gonzalez-Ulloa, M. Correction of hypotrophy of the breast by means of exogenous material. *Plast. Reconstr. Surg.* 25:15, 1960.

16. Goulian, D. Dermal mastopexy. *Clin. Plast. Surg.* 3:171, 1976.

17. Goulian, D., Jr. Dermal mastopexy. *Plast. Reconstr. Surg.* 47:105, 1971.

18. Gray, E. *Anatomy of the Human Body*, edited by C. M. Gross. Philadelphia: Lea & Febiger, 1959.

19. Gruber, R. P., and Jones, H. W. The "donut" mastopexy: Indications and complications. *Plast. Reconstr. Surg.* 65:34, 1980.

20. Guinard, M. Comment on: Rapport de l'ablation esthetique des tumeurs de sein, par M. H. Morestin. *Bull. Mem. Soc. Chir.* 29:568, 1903.

21. Hatten, M., and Keleher, C. Breast feeding after reduction mammoplasty. *J. Nurs. Midwif.* 28:19, 1983.

22. Hester, T. R., Bostwick, J., Miller, L., et al. Breast reduction utilizing the maximally vascularized central breast pedicle. *Plast. Reconstr. Surg.* 76:890, 1985.

23. Hester, T. R., Nahai, F., Bostwick, J., et al. A five-year experience with polyurethane-covered mammary prostheses for treatment of capsular contracture, primary augmentation mammaplasty and breast reconstruction. *Clin. Plast. Surg.* 15:569, 1988.

24. Hinderer, U. T. The dermal brassiere mammaplasty. *Clin. Plast. Surg.* 3:349, 1976.

25. Hoffman, S. Recurrent deformities following reduction mammoplasty and correction of breast asymmetry. *Plast. Reconstr. Surg.* 78:55, 1986.

26. Hollinshead, W. H. *Anatomy for Surgeons.* Philadelphia: Harper & Row, 1982.

27. Kraske, H. Die Operation der atrophischen und hypertrophisches Hangerbrust. *Munch. Med. Wochenschr.* 70:671, 1923.

28. Fleischhacker, R. V. (ed.), *Lanfranco of Milan: Lanfranco's "Science of Chirurgie."* London: Kegan Paul, 1894.

29. Letterman, G., and Schurter, J. History of the Surgical Correction of Mammary Ptosis. In J. Owsley and R. Peterson (eds.), *Symposium on Aesthetic Surgery of the Breast.* St. Louis: Mosby, 1978. P. 72.

30. Letterman, G., and Schurter, M. Will Durston's "mammaplasty." *Plast. Reconstr. Surg.* 53:48, 1974.

31. Lexer, E. Hypertrophie bei der Mammae. *Munch. Med. Wochenschr.* 59:2702, 1912.

32. Lotsch, F. Uber Hangebrustplastik. *Zentrabl. Chir.* 50:1241, 1923.

33. Maliniac, J. W. Critical analysis of mammectomy and free transplantation of the nipple. *Med. J. Rec.* 134:474, 1931.

34. Maliniac, J. Harmful fallacies in mammaplasty. Abstract, International Congress of Plastic Surgery, London, 1959. As quoted in T. D. Rees. *Plastic Surgery of the Breast.* In J. M. Converse (ed.), *Reconstructive Plastic Surgery* (2nd ed.), Vol. VII. Philadelphia: Saunders, 1977. P. 3662.

35. Marchac, D., and de Olarte, G. Reduction mammoplasty and correction of ptosis with a short inframammary scar. *Plast. Reconstr. Surg.* 69:45, 1982.

36. McKissock, P. K. Reduction mammoplasty with a vertical dermal flap. *Plast. Reconstr. Surg.* 49:245, 1972.

37. McKissock, P. K. Reduction mammoplasty by the vertical bipedicle flap technique. *Clin. Plast. Surg.* 3:309, 1976.

38. McKissock, P. K. Reduction mammoplasty. *Ann. Plast. Surg.* 2:321, 1979.

39. McKissock, P. K. Personal communication, 1986.

40. Morestin, H. Hypertrophic mammaire. *Bull. Mem. Soc. Anat.* 80: 682, 1905.

41. Morestin, H. La reduction graduella des difformites tegumentaires. Translation and comments by J. M. Converse. *Plast. Reconstr. Surg.* 42:163, 1968.

42. Mouly, R., and Dufourmentel, C. Mamma-

plasty by the Lateral Method. In J. T. Hueston (ed.), *Transactions of the Fifth International Congress of Plastic and Reconstructive Surgery.* Sydney, Australia: Butterworths, 1971. P. 1173.

43. Noel, A. Aesthetische Chirurgie der weiblichen Brust: ein neues Verfahren zur Korektur der Hangerburst. *Med. Welt.* 2:51, 1928.

44. Penn, J. Breast reduction. *Br. J. Plast. Surg.* 7:357, 1955.

45. Pitanguy, I. Breast Hypertrophy. In *Transactions II International Congress of Plastic and Reconstructive Surgeons.* London: E & S Livingstone, 1960.

46. Pitanguy, I. Surgical correction of breast hypertrophy. *Br. J. Plast. Surg.* 20:78, 1967.

47. Pousson, J. De la mastopexie. *Bull. Mem. Soc. Chir.* 23:507, 1897.

48. Rees, T. D., and Aston, S. J. The tuberous breast. *Clin. Plast. Surg.* 3:339, 1976.

49. Regnault, P. Breast ptosis. *Clin. Plast. Surg.* 3:193, 1976.

50. Regnault, P. Breast reduction: B technique. *Plast. Reconstr. Surg.* 65:840, 1980.

51. Regnault, P., Daniel, R. K., and Tirkanits, B. The minus-plus mastopexy. *Clin. Plast. Surg.* 15:595, 1988.

52. Ribeiro, L. A new technique for reduction mammoplasty. *Plast. Reconstr. Surg.* 12:110, 1975.

53. Robbins, T. H. A reduction mammoplasty with the areola-nipple based on an inferior dermal pedicle. *Plast. Reconstr. Surg.* 59:64, 1977.

54. Rubin, L. R. Surgical Treatment of the Massive Hypertrophic Breast. In N. G. Georgiade (ed.), *Reconstructive Breast Surgery.* St. Louis: Mosby, 1976.

55. Ryan, R. F. Virginal hypertrophy. *Plast. Reconstr. Surg.* 75:737, 1985.

56. Schwarzmann, E. Die technik der mammaplastik. *Chirurg* 2:932, 1930.

57. Singer, R., and Krant, S. M. Intravenous fluorescein for evaluating the dusky nipple-areola during reduction mammoplasty. *Plast. Reconstr. Surg.* 67:534, 1981.

58. Skoog, T. A technique of breast reduction. *Acta Chir. Scand.* 126:453, 1963.

59. Spence, R. J., Feldman, J. J., and Ryan, J. J. Symmastia: The problem of medial confluence of the breasts. *Plast. Reconstr. Surg.* 73:261, 1984.

60. Strömbeck, J. O. Mammaplasty: Report of a new technique based on the two pedicle procedure. *Br. J. Plast. Surg.* 13:79, 1960.

61. Teimourian, B., Massac, E., and Wiegering, C. E. Reduction suction mammoplasty and suction lipectomy as an adjunct to breast surgery. *Aesthetic Plast. Surg.* 9:197, 1985.

62. Thomas, T. G. On the removal of benign tumors of the mamma without mutilation of the organ. *N.Y. Med. J. Obstet. Rev.* 35:337, 1882.

63. Thorek, M. Histological verification of efficacy of free transplantation of the nipple. *Med. J. Rec.* 134:474, 1931.

64. Thorek, M. Possibilities in the reconstruction of the human form. *N.Y. Med. J.* 116:572, 1922.

64a. Toledo, S. Periareolar mammoplasty with syringe liposuction. International Symposium Recent Advances in Plastic Surgery. Sao Paulo, Brazil, March 3, 1989.

65. Weiner, D. L., et al. A single dermal pedicle for nipple transposition in subcutaneous mastectomy, reduction mammoplasty or mastopexy. *Plast. Reconstr. Surg.* 51:115, 1973.

66. Weinhold, E. Discussion zum vortrag kuster: operation bei Hangebrust und Hangebauch. *Zentrabl. Gynaekol.* 50:2581, 1926.

67. Wise, R. J. A preliminary report on a method of planning the mammaplasty. *Plast. Reconstr. Surg.* 17:367, 1956.

68. Zacher, J. B. Breast feeding after reduction mammoplasty. Presented at the American Society of Aesthetic Plastic Surgeons, New Orleans, April 1986.

*G. Patrick Maxwell*

# 48

# *Breast Reconstruction Following Mastectomy and Surgical Management of the Patient with High-Risk Breast Disease*

## Breast Reconstruction Following Mastectomy

Breast reconstruction may be one of the most significant female surgeries of this era, and one which may reverse the dread that has been associated with the loss of one's breast.—*Schain et al.* [83]

During the last 25 years, breast reconstruction has evolved from a rarely performed surgical venture to a daily occurrence that has become an important part of the rehabilitation process following mastectomy. The aesthetic quality of these reconstructions, fostered by technical advances, has emerged from that of amorphous blobs appearing as breast mounds to nearly normal anatomic-appearing breasts. Symmetry, which was hardly possible and seldom achieved, is now the standard for which we strive.

In 1895 Czerny published the first article on breast reconstruction wherein he transplanted a large lipoma to reconstruct a breast removed for benign disease [17]. Tansini in 1906 described a little appreciated procedure utilizing a latissimus dorsi musculocutaneous flap for immediate coverage of a radical mastectomy defect [53, 93]. Kleinschmidt in 1924 designed an axillary-based flap that was rotated on itself for mastectomy coverage and mound formation [47]. The following year Sauerbruch described a breast-sharing procedure utilizing a flap from the remaining breast for mastectomy coverage [14], and Reinhard in 1932 described a staged procedure of splitting and transferring one-half of the opposite breast for breast mound formation [78]. Longacre in 1953 suggested the use of local rotation flaps to enhance soft tissue coverage in breast reconstruction [52], and Gillies and Millard in 1957 advocated the use of a tubed pedicle flap from the abdomen wherein the umbilicus was extroverted to substitute as the nipple [31]. Another tubed pedicle technique using the lower portion of the opposite breast was described by Holdsworth in 1956 [42]. In 1973 Pontes refined the breast-sharing approach with a single-stage procedure [76]. Orticochea also in 1973 used buttock skin and subcutaneous tissue on a forearm carrier to supply distant tissue for breast reconstruction [74].

Modern breast reconstruction has been fostered by several developments: the trend from radical to modified radical mastectomies, the improvement in silicone breast prostheses, the advent of tissue expanders, the submuscular placement of these devices, and the predictable transfer of vascularized tissue, especially via musculocutaneous flaps and microsurgery. With general surgeons performing more modified radical mastectomies, soft tissue coverage became less difficult, and more attention could be focused on breast mound creation. Snyderman and Guthrie in 1971 first suggested subcutaneous placement of a silicone prosthesis for breast reconstruction [92]. Custom prostheses [7] were developed for infraclavicular fill when needed. The placement of breast prostheses in the submuscular position [16, 43] lessened considerably the incidence of extrusion and perhaps capsule contracture. The use of tissue expanders, advocated by Radovan [77], enabled chest skin and muscle to be expanded into a breast mound.

Although previous efforts at tissue transfer for breast reconstruction were useful, the development of arterialized flaps made this transfer consistently predictable. Kiricuta suggested omental coverage of implants for reconstruction in 1963 [45], and Bohmert [8] and Cronin et al. [16] utilized the thoracoepigastric flap in 1977. Olivari [73], Mulbauer and Olbrish [68], and Schneider et al. [87] advocated the use of latissimus dorsi musculocutaneous flaps for breast reconstruction, and Robbins [80] suggested the vertically oriented rectus abdominis musculocutaneous flap for the same purpose. Hartrampf et al. [39] refined the latter flap to incorporate a transverse island of abdominal skin (TRAM flap), thus resulting in an abdominal lipectomy-type donor site. The use of microsurgical tissue transfers for breast reconstruction has also been advocated by Fujino et al. [27] and Serafin et al. [88]. All of these developments provide plastic surgeons a number of reasonable alternative solutions for reconstruction of the most severe radical mastectomy patient, as well as that of the relatively easier thin, small-breasted woman who has undergone modified radical mastectomy. These surgical techniques may be used for either delayed (secondary) reconstruction or immediate reconstruction at the time of mastectomy.

## Comprehensive Patient Management

During the last several years a comprehensive individualized approach to women with breast cancer has developed. This approach involves the general surgeon, oncologist, radiotherapist, plastic surgeon, and female support groups, and it centers on the patient. The comprehensive approach also includes public education and awareness of the incidence and treatment of breast cancer combined with preventive screening and self-breast examinations, all of which have led in many situations to early detection and diagnosis.

The first step in the therapeutic comprehensive approach is the breast biopsy, usually performed by a general surgeon and done as a primary, isolated procedure (in the appropriate clinical setting). When the biopsy is found on permanent section to be malignant, a treatment plan is formulated by the patient under the guidance of her general surgeon. Consultations with a plastic surgeon and radiotherapist may be in order prior to selecting the treatment plan. Treatment options include lumpectomy and radiotherapy, modified radical mastectomy with immediate reconstruction, or mastectomy (modified or radical) alone, which can be followed by delayed reconstruction if clinically appropriate and if the patient so chooses. The oncologist is usually brought into the picture in the immediate postoperative setting, depending on axillary lymph node involvement and tumor hormonal assay. Patient support organizations may also contribute during the perioperative period.

Although proper eradication of the cancer is the obvious primary focus, the importance of the breast to the self-image and sexuality of the female patient is acknowledged and respected. Breast reconstruction has thus become an integral part of the comprehensive management of the patient with breast cancer [81].

## Psychological Considerations

The emotional morbidity associated with mastectomy is significant [83], and "the stress from it causes considerable upset in virtually all areas of a patient's life" [65]. The psychological problems resulting from mastectomy include depression and other mood disturbances [67], loss of sexual interest [91], a negative body image and loss of femininity [94], fears of recurrence [72], and self-consciousness in terms of clothing. Breast reconstruction has been shown to lessen these psychological disturbances [32], and the number of women who have undergone reconstruction has increased dramatically.

Although not every woman who has had a mastectomy elects to undergo reconstruction, studies have focused on the factors that influence the sizable percentage of women who do [83] (Table 48-1). Other studies that have focused on timing seem to indicate that women who undergo immediate reconstruction may have less distress than those who have delayed reconstruction [98].

## Selection of Candidates

All women who are about to undergo or have had a mastectomy are potential candidates to be informed of breast reconstruction; however, not every woman elects, and therefore must not be pushed, to pursue it. There is perhaps no other area of reconstructive surgery where patient individualization is more important [55]. The plastic surgeon must therefore listen carefully to each patient's expressed needs and desires and juxtapose them with her emotional status, clinical staging, and technical reconstructive possibilities.

The two main considerations when selecting candidates for reconstruction are patho-

**Table 48-1** *Factors influencing the decision to have breast reconstruction*

| Motives | % Mentioned |
|---|---|
| To be able to wear more clothing styles | 83 |
| To eliminate external prosthesis | 79 |
| To be less occupied with physical state | 78 |
| To feel more balanced | 72 |
| To feel "whole again" | 72 |
| To feel more feminine | 69 |
| To be less occupied with cancer | 59 |
| To improve sexual relations | 39 |
| To improve marital relations | 16 |

*Source:* W. S. Schain, E. Jacobs, and D. K. Wellisch. Psychosocial issues in breast reconstruction. *Clin. Plast. Surg.* 11:237, 1984.

logic and motivational. Obviously, patients with favorable prognoses are better candidates for reconstruction than patients with poor prognoses. There are patients, however, with more guarded prognoses who, because of their particular situation, may be acceptable candidates. Strongly motivated patients are generally good candidates for breast reconstruction and derive significant benefit from surgery.

All patients require a lengthy initial consultation to allow the surgeon to assess their goals and to explain the alternatives with the reasonable expectations and possible complications of each. Photographs and diagrams are especially helpful, as are educational brochures. A second consultation (frequently with both patient and husband) may be desirous. The patient must understand that everyone who undergoes mastectomy is unique in terms of family history, pathology of the tumor, status of the contralateral breast, and technical reconstructive considerations. Her thorough understanding and acceptance of the necessary surgical steps, potential complications, and appropriate expectations is mandatory [33].

## Selection of Technique

Millard's statement, "There is not now, and probably never will be one method that is best for all cases of breast reconstruction. . . ." [66] remains accurate. The determinative factors that must be evaluated with each patient include the patient's overall health and body habitus, the mastectomy site, the contralateral breast, and the patient's preference.

### MASTECTOMY SITE

The type of mastectomy performed has a major bearing on the selection of the procedure. A radical mastectomy may have left an infraclavicular depression, loss of anterior axillary fold, and inadequate soft tissue cover, whereas a modified radical mastectomy, which does not alter the upper chest, may have left ample soft tissue in the lower chest area. The amount of pectoralis muscle present, the amount of skin present, the quality of these tissues, and the quality of the mastectomy scar must be evaluated. Based on this evaluation, one can determine if an implant alone would work, if the skin and muscle present can be adequately expanded, or if a flap is required. Once these factors have been assessed, consideration is given to which of these potential procedures would actually produce the best aesthetic result in the given case and weigh it against the other relevant factors.

### PATIENT'S HEALTH AND BODY HABITUS

Healthy patients may be candidates for any type of reconstruction, whereas older patients or those in compromised health are probably best suited for the simpler procedures, e.g., submuscular implantation or tissue expansion. Healthy patients with a flabby (but not pendulously obese) abdomen may be good candidates for a transverse rectus abdominis flap (TRAM) reconstruction. Previous subcostal incisions that have divided the rectus muscle, paramedian incisions that have injured the perforators, and

midline and lower quadrant incisions that may alter TRAM flap viability must also be considered. Most surgeons consider heavy smoking and diabetes contraindications to a TRAM flap procedure.

Upper abdominal laxity makes lowering of the abdominal apron easier, allowing a lower placed donor site lipectomy closure with a TRAM reconstruction. Innervation of the latissimus dorsi muscle must be clinically evaluated in consideration of a latissimus flap. The texture and color of the back skin are also observed during the evaluation for a latissimus flap. Hypertrophic or keloid scars present at the mastectomy site or elsewhere mean that new scars from rectus or latissimus procedures may not be preferable. A tissue expander, however, may improve mastectomy scar hypertrophy through internal compression and thus avoids the creation of new scars. Microsurgical procedures are generally considered when none of the above-mentioned operations are appropriate, but there are those who advocate this technique as the preferred one [34].

### CONTRALATERAL BREAST

Because symmetry is the goal in breast reconstruction, the size and shape of the contralateral breast must be evaluated and a determination made as to which reconstructive procedure can best match it. Consideration may also be given to altering the contralateral breast to better match the planned reconstructed breast. This alteration might be a reduction, augmentation, or mastopexy. Because the opposite breast is at increased risk to develop breast cancer [70, 79] consideration must be given to this point. If a contralateral prophylactic procedure (total mastectomy or subcutaneous mastectomy) is planned, it may alter the reconstructive technique used on the mastectomy site. Thus the contralateral breast plays a major role in the selection of the reconstruction technique.

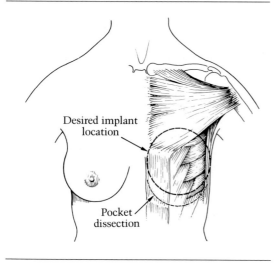

**Figure 48-1** *The desired location of the silicone implant is shown. The dissection must be carried 2 cm lower to achieve the desired result when smooth-walled implants are used.*

## Surgical Techniques for Secondary Reconstruction

SUBMUSCULAR RECONSTRUCTION

When planning a submuscular reconstruction, the inframammary fold on the contralateral side is marked and the mark is transposed to the side of the reconstruction (Fig. 48-1). A second mark is made approximately 2 cm below the first mark, which becomes the lower extent of the pocket dissection. If the submuscular pocket is not made lower initially, the implant generally ends up too high (if smooth-walled implants are used). The pocket that is created may be truly submuscular by dissecting deep to the pectoralis major muscle, rectus abdominis fascia, and serratus anterior muscle, or it may be only subpectoral with the dissection passing to the subcutaneous plane inferior to the origin of the pectoralis major muscle (Fig. 48-2).

Access for this type of reconstruction may be through a new incision in the inframammary fold area or through the lateral aspect of the old mastectomy scar. Pocket dissec-

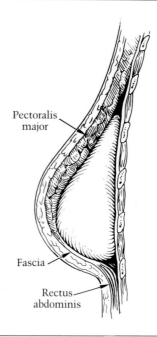

**Figure 48-2** *Although the implant is said to be submuscular, the lower one-third of the prosthesis is frequently covered by the fascial connection between the pectoralis major and rectus abdominis muscles. For secondary reconstruction, the lower dissection (inferior to the pectoralis major) may be subcutaneous.*

tion is easy superiorly but may be difficult inferiorly at the junction of the pectoralis major, rectus abdominis, and serratus anterior muscles and fascia. The pocket must be made large but is limited laterally just past the anterior axillary fold. Suction drainage is usually necessary.

Adequate wound closure is important, especially if the incision is placed in the dependent inferior position. If the pocket is truly submuscular, the muscle layer is closed followed by closure of the subcutaneous and cutaneous layers. If the dissection is subcutaneous inferiorly, it is especially important to achieve a competent two- or three-layer closure. It is important to keep the implant down in the pocket initially with an upper breast dressing. Ace bandage circumferential

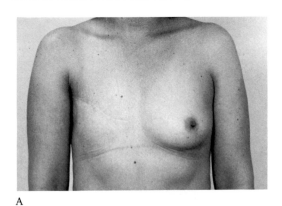

A

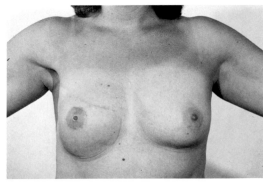

B

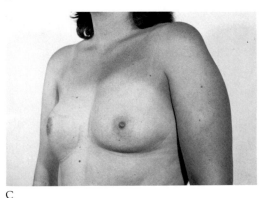

C

**Figure 48-3** *A. Following right modified radical mastectomy. B. Result after subpectoral insertion of a silicone prosthesis. C. Note the lack of definition of the inframammary fold on the reconstructed breast.*

wrap of the upper breast may be necessary for several weeks.

Implant displacement "exercises" within the pocket are begun several days postoperatively and continued aggressively to help establish a large pocket and therefore minimize capsule contracture when a smooth-walled implant is used. Textured-surface implants do not require displacement exercises. If double-lumen implants are used, a steroid solution with or without antibiotics may be added to the outer lumen.

*Implant Selection*
Surgeons differ in their preference of prostheses for breast reconstruction. The options include smooth-walled silicone gel, saline, double-lumen adjustable implants, and those containing a central projectile column. Textured-surface implants of silicone

and polyurethane-covered silicone are also available. The prostheses come in a wide variety of sizes (generally 100 to 600 ml) and shapes (low and high profile, round, and teardrop). Custom sizes and shapes may also be ordered from any manufacturer. Sterilized "sizer" implants are useful intraoperatively for choosing the correct size and shape of the permanent implant.

Today most surgeons decide between smooth-walled implants and textured-surface implants. The issues of silicone safety and the possibility of breast implants obscuring cancer detection have been raised and carefully studied. The unknown fate of a biodegradable coating (polyurethane) has also been questioned. To date no known deleterious effects have been seen with either smooth or textured silicone breast implants or polyurethane-covered implants. The only

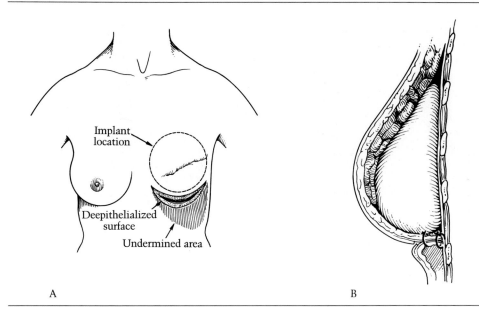

A                                                                    B

*Figure 48-4* A. *The external approach for inframammary fold creation utilizes abdominal advancement with deepithelialization. B. The deepithelialized flaps are attached directly to themselves and the chest wall.*

acknowledged problem is the increased difficulty of evaluating mammograms. Polyurethane implants have been rather conclusively shown to have a lesser incidence of capsule contracture [13, 24, 40, 41, 84]. Although the same may be true of textured silicone, it has not been clinically confirmed.

After pocket dissection, the operating table is changed to an upright sitting position, and various sizes and shapes of sizer implants are inserted before selecting the prosthesis to be used. In general, high profile implants are used for most submuscular reconstructions, whereas low profile implants are occasionally necessary to match a small contralateral breast. Polyurethane implants may be stacked one on another to give a better breast shape [60]. An adjustable implant (or expander implant) [4] is another device that may be useful for this type reconstruction, as its volume may be altered postoperatively.

### Inframammary Fold Creation

The contour and symmetry of the inframammary fold is important for obtaining an aesthetically pleasing result from breast reconstruction. Although it is possible to obtain this shape after dissection of a pocket and insertion of an implant alone, certain patients require the surgical establishment of an inframammary fold (Fig. 48-3). Advanced abdominal soft tissue is attached to the prethoracic wall either through a skin incision with deepithelialized flaps [82, 97] or by internal suturing [60].

The correct location for the inframammary fold is marked preoperatively with the patient in the upright position. Another mark is made about 2 cm below this one and is brought laterally and medially into a crescent. A third mark is made 8 to 10 cm lower, which is the extent to which the abdominal undermining can be carried out. When the external approach is utilized (Fig. 48-4), the crescent area is deepithelialized and an incision made into its central portion. Dissection is carried out in the subcutaneous plane at the level of the rectus abdominis fascia superiorly until the originating fibers of the

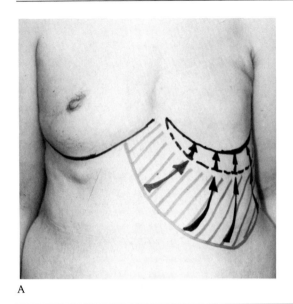

A

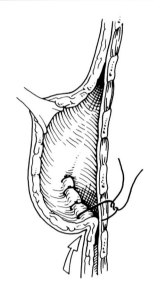

B

**Figure 48-5** *A. For internal inframammary fold creation, the desired location of the fold is marked (solid line), and another mark is made several centimeters below it (dotted line). After undermining, the deep surface of the skin below the dotted line is sutured to the prethoracic fascia at the level of the solid line.*
*B. Interrupted internal sutures are carefully placed to ensure the desired location and curvature.*

pectoralis major muscle are encountered. These fibers are elevated to allow entrance to the subpectoral space above. The upper abdominal tissue is undermined at the level of the rectus abdominis fascia, and it is advanced superiorly, suturing the deepithelialized edge to the prethoracic chest wall fascia to establish the inframammary fold. The prosthesis is placed in the subpectoral position, and the inferior deepithelialized edge is then closed and sutured in a layered fashion to its inferior counterpart. Careful closure of this suture line is important to prevent inferior implant extrusion.

When internal suturing is utilized, the preoperative markings are similar, except an inferolateral mark is made in the midcrescent area (Fig. 48-5) where the incision is placed. The incision may also be made in the lateral area as part of the original mastectomy scar. The advanced soft tissue is sutured on its deep surface to the prethoracic chest-wall fascia to establish the inframammary fold (Fig. 48-6). These sutures (usually of 2-0 vicryl or silk) must be carefully placed through the subcutaneous tissue, just catching the deep dermis. Their spacing must also

be exact, as is the tension under which they are tied. As the upper abdominal tissue is advanced superolaterally, it is occasionally necessary to excise a lateral (midaxillary) skin roll.

*Complications*
The most frequently reported complications have been infection (which could necessitate implant removal), capsule contracture, lack of inframammary fold definition, and implant misplacement with subsequent asymmetry.

TISSUE EXPANSION
The use of tissue expanders allows the stretching (or expansion) of qualitatively adequate but quantitatively deficient prethoracic soft tissue to ample volume for

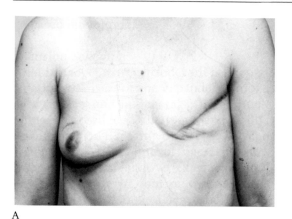

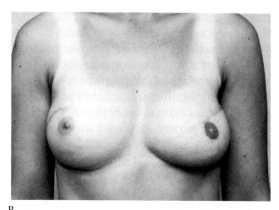

A

B

**Figure 48-6** *A. After left modified radical mastectomy. B. After subpectoral reconstruction on the left with internal inframammary creation. C. Note the contour of the inframammary fold created by internal suturing. A subcutaneous mastectomy with reconstruction has been performed on the right through an old biopsy scar.*

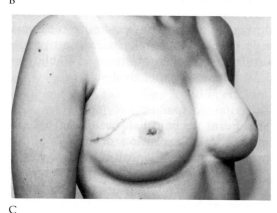

C

insertion of a submuscular implant. This technique has become one of the most popular for breast reconstruction [2, 48, 57, 75, 96], as it has the distinct advantage of combining lesser operative procedures that have less postoperative recuperation time with the capability of achieving excellent results. Other advantages include a resultant breast mound with skin of identical color and texture and few additional scars. The disadvantages of tissue expansion include more frequent office visits for percutaneous expansion, some discomfort (due to pressure) after the expansions, and asymmetry during overexpansion seen in the later stages of the expansion process. It also requires a relatively "patient patient" to accept the inexact

appearance of the expanded mound for a number of months prior to insertion of the permanent prosthesis.

When planning insertion of a smooth surface expander, the contralateral inframammary fold is transposed to the reconstructed side by appropriate markings. Another mark is then made approximately 2 cm below this point, and the pocket dissection is carried to this lower mark (Fig. 48-7). Surgical access for pocket creation may be through a new lateral inframammary fold incision or through the lateral aspect of the old mastectomy scar. The pocket may be subpectoral (usual technique) or truly submuscular, as discussed above. Expanders are designed with the self-sealing, self-contained valve on

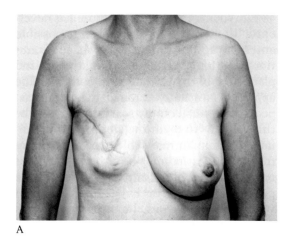

A

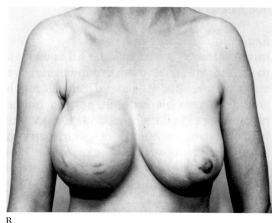

B

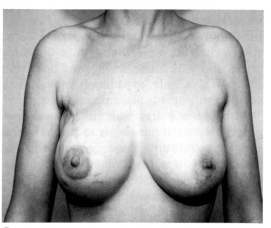

C

**Figure 48-8** *A. After right modified radical mastectomy. B. Tissue expander has been filled to 800 ml for a 6-month interval. C. Result after replacement of the expander with a 580-ml prosthesis and internal inframammary fold creation.*

pander malpositioning, remote port injection malfunction, capsular contracture, and patient pain and deformity following expansion.

## LATISSIMUS DORSI RECONSTRUCTION

The latissimus dorsi musculocutaneous flap has provided a consistently reliable method of breast reconstruction [6, 9, 10, 15, 54]. Its main advantage is its ability to supply additional vascularized muscle and skin to the breast mound in a predictable fashion during a single operative procedure. Its primary disadvantage is the creation of new chest scars plus a back donor scar.

### Flap Anatomy and Preoperative Considerations

The latissimus dorsi muscle, which is the mirror image of the pectoralis major, arises from the lower thoracic vertebrae, the lumbar and sacral spinal processes, and the iliac crest. Its large, flat muscle belly converges into a flat tendon that inserts into the lesser tubercle of the humerus. The thoracodorsal artery provides the dominant vascular supply to the flap. The subscapular artery originates from the axillary artery, gives off the scapular circumflex artery, and terminates in the thoracodorsal artery. This vessel, lo-

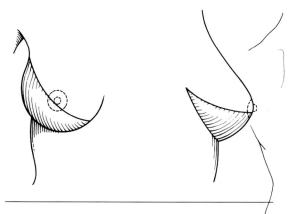

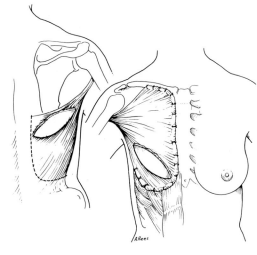

**Figure 48-9** *Two views of the preferred location of a latissimus dorsi skin island in the inferolateral position defining the inframammary fold.*

**Figure 48-10** *For the radical mastectomy reconstruction, the chest defect requires all possible muscle to be located superior to the skin island, assuming the latter is to be in the inferolateral position. Thus the skin island is designed high on the back in a more transverse orientation.*

cated in the posterior aspect of the axilla, gives off one or two serratus branches before entering the anterior undersurface of the latissimus dorsi muscle. The thoracodorsal artery is accompanied on its course by the thoracodorsal nerve and veins.

Because the thoracodorsal structures might be injured during axillary dissection, one must carefully examine the patient preoperatively to determine if the latissimus dorsi muscle is innervated. Retrograde flow through the serratus branch allows the flap to still be safely utilized following thoracodorsal artery ligation [25, 61]. Muscle atrophy after thoracodorsal nerve division, however, diminishes the bulk of the flap, which may make it less useful.

*Chest Incision*
The first step in designing a latissimus dorsi flap is to determine where on the chest the skin island should be positioned. Initially, the old mastectomy scar was excised and the skin island placed in the defect. Experience, however, has shown that in most cases the resultant breast mound looks best when the skin island is positioned in the inferolateral

pole of the breast and its inferior margin defines the inframammary fold (Fig. 48-9). This technique can be utilized only when the quality of the old mastectomy scar is acceptable and is retained. Thus in some situations the latissimus skin island is placed inferolaterally, ignoring the old mastectomy scar, whereas in other cases the scar is excised and replaced by the flap.

*Location and Design of the Skin Island*
The location of the skin island on the back is determined by two factors: (1) the chest requirement of skin to muscle position for the reconstruction, and (2) the patient's preference for the site of the back scar. With radical mastectomy reconstructions the chest requires muscle superiorly with the skin island inferiorly; thus the skin island must be designed high on the back muscle (Fig. 48-10). With modified radical mastectomy re-

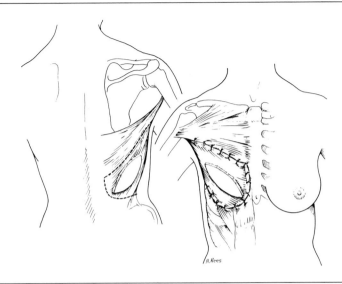

**Figure 48-11** *For modified radical mastectomy reconstruction, there is no upper muscle deficiency. Thus the skin island can be placed in a lower oblique position on the back, and only a portion of the latissimus dorsi muscle has to be taken.*

constructions, the chest requirements are for both skin island and muscle to be located inferiorly, which allows the skin island to be designed in a lower oblique position on the back (Fig. 48-11). Juxtaposed against the above are the patient's wishes and acceptance of a higher transverse back scar in the brassiere line or a low oblique scar that allows her to wear a low-back one-piece bathing suit or evening dress without a visible scar.

There are two schools of thought on the shape of the latissimus skin island drawn on the back. Most favor an elliptical design that allows the back to be closed in a straight line [15, 54]. This ellipse may be used as is or tailored for breast mound needs. Others prefer to design the skin island on the back in various shapes to conform individually to the patient's breast mound requirements [66]. This method results in back donor scars of various configurations. A recent innovation, especially applicable in obese women, is to design the skin island in a fleur-de-lis pattern in the posterior axillary skin fat roll and transfer this larger bulk to the chest perhaps without the need for an implant [62].

*Technical Detail*

After careful preoperative markings in the upright position, the procedure is begun with the patient in the lateral decubitus position. The flap is elevated from distal to proximal. Care is taken to not injure the serratus branch unless one is absolutely certain the thoracodorsal artery is intact. The latissimus dorsi tendinous insertion into the humerus may be left or severed. Some believe this tendon may be resecured anteriorly to give better anterior axillary fold configuration. A tunnel is made across the apex of the axilla to pass the flap from the back to the front. Drains are inserted in the back, and after donor site closure the patient is turned to the supine position.

A subpectoral pocket is then created, and the flap is redraped in the desired position. The upper latissimus muscle is sutured to the lower pectoralis muscle. For radical mastectomy reconstructions it is necessary to

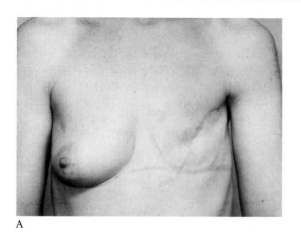
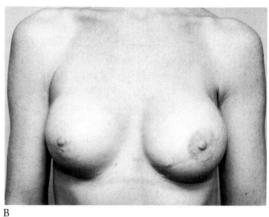

A                                    B

**Figure 48-12** A. After left modified radical mastectomy. B. Result after left latissimus dorsi reconstruction. Note inferolateral placement of the skin island.

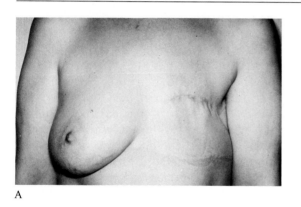
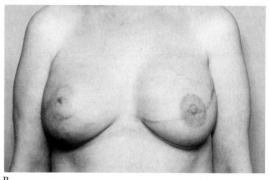

A                                    B

**Figure 48-13** A. Patient with a marked modified mastectomy defect. B. After left latissimus dorsi reconstruction and right subcutaneous mastectomy with reconstruction.

secure the latissimus muscle superiorly to the periosteum of the clavicle to obliterate the infraclavicular defect. The skin island is carefully tailored and the inframammary fold formed by suturing it in position (or by dissection alone). An appropriately sized implant, expander-implant, or expander is selected, utilizing sizer prostheses, with the patient now in the upright position. Because

the long-term incidence of capsular contracture has been thought by some to be high with latissimus reconstructions [64], a textured or expander-implant expander may be appropriate, especially as more ptosis may be created and a second operation follows regardless. Suction drains are placed in the wound prior to closure and remain there for 4 to 5 days (Figs. 48-12 and 48-13).

## Complications

Flap viability complications are rare with this hearty flap, but if it is overextended they can occur. The combination of a denervated latissimus muscle, axillary irradiation, and aggressive dissection injuring or tinting the serratus branch constitute "overextension." Hematoma, infection, early implant slippage, capsule contracture, and donor site seromas have been reported. Involuntary flexion of the transposed latissimus muscle can occur. Shoulder and arm donor morbidity is minimal but present, as is some depression in the back donor area.

### TRANSVERSE RECTUS ABDOMINIS FLAP

The transverse rectus abdominis flap (TRAM flap, transverse abdominal island flap) has the tremendous theoretical advantages of (1) creating a breast mound composed of autogenous tissue without the need of silicone prostheses [20, 38, 39, 85, 86] and (2) producing an abdominal lipectomy in the donor area. It probably produces the best long-term results of all the techniques of breast reconstruction [37]. Its disadvantage is that it is an operation of greater magnitude with a longer postoperative recuperation time than other techniques [30].

## Flap Anatomy and
## Preoperative Considerations

The paired rectus abdominis muscles originate from the cartilage of the sixth, seventh, and eighth ribs and insert into the pubic tubercle and pubic crest [63]. The blood supply to the rectus abdominis muscle comes from the superior epigastric artery above and the deep inferior epigastric artery below. Within the muscle these main vascular sources are connected by a watershed area. Although the deep inferior epigastric system has been shown to have higher perfusion pressures, the superior epigastric artery and vein carry the lower abdominal soft tissue and comprise the vascular basis for the transverse rectus abdominis flap. The blood supply is also enhanced by the posterior perforating vessels, which accompany the eight through twelfth sensory and motor nerves as they enter the upper lateral rectus sheath and the subfascial plexus, which runs underneath the anterior rectus fascia. The musculocutaneous perforators that supply the flap are centered in the periumbilical area and emerge through the medial half of the rectus muscle to supply the subdermal plexus superficial to it.

Patient selection is important for this operation. Patients with an obese, pendulous abdominal panniculus carry a much higher risk of flap loss and thus are not good operative candidates. Likewise, heavy smokers and diabetics are probably not good candidates. Any previous abdominal incision that transected the rectus abdominis muscle or interrupted its perforators precludes use of a flap based on that particular muscle. The ideal candidate is the patient with the loose, "poochy," fatty lower abdomen who would profit from an abdominal lipectomy and is properly motivated.

## Design

The "ideal" design of the transverse skin island is identical to that which one would design for an abdominal lipectomy. The flap must survive on its vascular blood supply, however, such that these alterations must be made. Because the dominant vascular perforators are located in the periumbilical area, the umbilicus must always be included, and on some occasions the skin island must be located more superiorly than one would wish. The looser the upper abdominal skin, the easier it is to place the flap in the "ideal position."

## Muscle Selection

Four zones have been arbitrarily identified on the single muscle flap based on predictability of flap survival (Fig. 48-14). This numerical sequence has not proved to be correct. The arterialized one-half of the flap virtually always survives, whereas there is much less certainty as the midline is crossed and the random side is entered. This finding has led to greater utilization of the double muscle flap [44], especially with the more

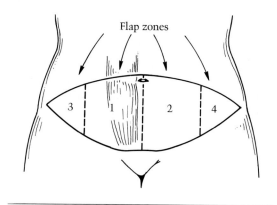

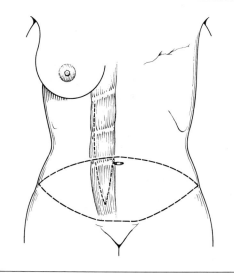

**Figure 48-14** *Vascular zones of the TRAM flap. Zones 1 and 3 are on the arterialized one-half, and zones 2 and 4 are on the random one-half.*

**Figure 48-15** *Standard single-pedicle TRAM flap design utilizing the contralateral muscle. Only that portion of the muscle noted is raised with the flap.*

obese panniculus, when a vertical lower midline scar is present, or when larger flap tissue requirements are present. For the standard single muscle flap, the contralateral muscle is preferred by most, as there seems to be less twist in the tunneled vascular pedicle, and flap contouring seems easier (Figs. 48-15 and 48-16). When previous abdominal scars preclude the use of contralateral muscle, the ipsilateral side suffices.

*Abdominal Wall Reconstruction*
It is imperative that a competent abdominal wall be maintained after this procedure [36]. Use of fascial flaps and grafts and of relaxation incisions has proved unsatisfactory. With careful technical attention and proper intraoperative patient relaxation, primary sound abdominal closure is always possible with single muscle flaps and most double muscle flaps. Many surgeons use overlay synthetic mesh for reinforcement or place mesh within the fascial sheath from which the muscle was removed.

*Flap Tailoring*
There are a number of techniques for tailoring the flap into a breast mound. The most frequently utilized approach is to orient the flap vertically with the random portion lo-

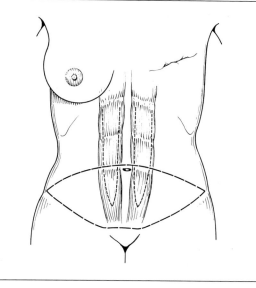

**Figure 48-16** *Design for the double-pedicle TRAM flap. Note the portion of the muscles that are raised with the flap.*

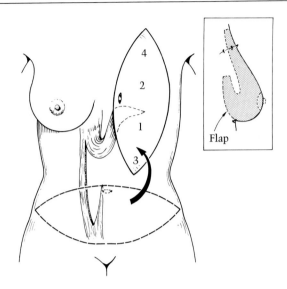

**Figure 48-17** *Vertical orientation for breast mound contouring using a contralateral single-muscle TRAM flap: applies to single- or double-pedicle flaps. (From Maxwell, G. P., Technical alternatives in transverse rectus abdominis breast reconstruction. Persp. Plast. Surg. 1:1, 1987.)*

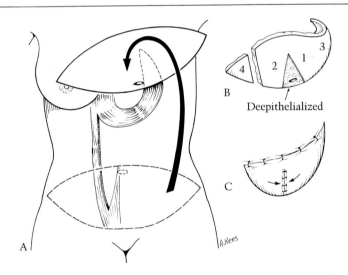

**Figure 48-18** *Transverse orientation of a TRAM flap removing a deepithelialized wedge (B) gives more breast mound projection (C). This shaping technique is limited to double-pedicle flaps. (From Maxwell, G. P., Technical alternatives in transverse rectus abdominis breast reconstruction. Persp. Plast. Surg. 1:1, 1987.)*

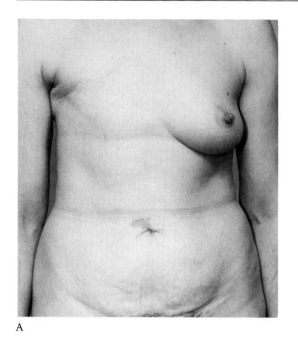

A

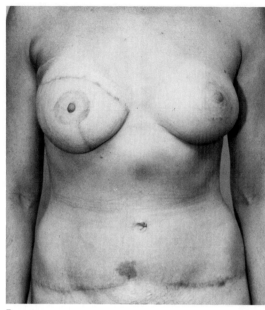

B

*Figure 48-19* *A. After right modified radical mastectomy. B. Result after contralateral single-pedicle TRAM flap tailored with a transverse orientation and a deepithelialized wedge. (From Maxwell, G. P., Technical alternatives in transverse rectus abdominis breast reconstruction. Persp. Plast. Surg. 1:1, 1987.)*

cated superiorly and the umbilicus at the medial border [21] (Fig. 48-17). The inferior arterialized portion is then folded under on itself. This method is the safest maneuver with the least flap folding. Its limitations are the lateral width of the flap and hence the lateral width of the resultant breast as well as the amount of projection the resultant breast may have. Turning the flap slightly more obliquely aids in gaining more lateral breast fullness. When a larger breast with more projection is desired, the flap may be turned transversely (180 degrees) with the umbilicus pointed downward [56]. A triangular area around the umbilicus is deepithelialized and sutured to itself to give central breast projection. This folding technique *must be restricted to double pedicle flaps for safety* (Figs. 48-18 and 48-19). When the

ipsilated muscle is used, a vertical orientation is preferred. Bilateral TRAM flap reconstructions also are done best using vertically oriented flaps (hemiflaps) (Fig. 48-20).

*Technical Detail*
With the patient sitting, preoperative marks are made. Measurements of the tissue deficits and necessary flap dimensions may be helpful. The upper portion of the transverse abdominal skin island is marked just above the umbilicus, and the desired lower transverse mark is similar to that for an abdominal lipectomy. The existing inframammary fold is transposed to the opposite side. The chest skin may be opened by a new incision made 1 to 2 cm above this mark and accepting the original mastectomy scar or by excising the existing scar and recreating the original defect. The quality and location of the original scar influence this determination.

Under general anesthesia with the patient in the supine position, the upper incision of the transverse skin island is made, and

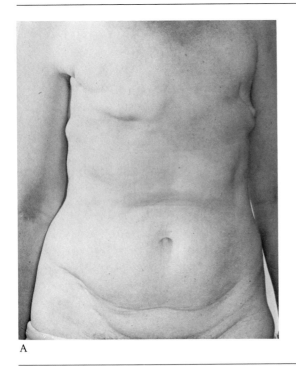

A

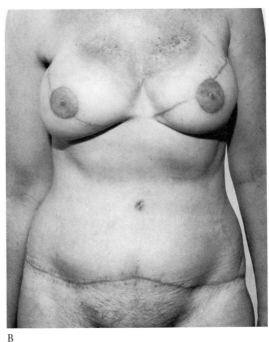

B

**Figure 48-20** *A. After bilateral modified radical mastectomies. B. Result after bilateral TRAM reconstruction using an ipsilateral pedicle and a vertical flap orientation.*

the upper abdominal panniculus is elevated above the costochondral cartilages. The operating table is then flexed to an angle of approximately 60 degrees, and the upper skin apron is pulled down to determine how far it will reach and thus the exact location of the inferior incision. In many patients it coincides with the preoperative desired mark, whereas in others a compromise in the superior direction must be made. The chest incision and inframammary fold dissection are confirmed while the panniculus is held taut.

With the patient back in the supine position, the inferior abdominal incision is made, and the random side of the flap is elevated to the midline, noting the location of the perforating vessels as they emerge through the anterior rectus fascia. The arterialized side of the flap is then elevated to half-way across the anterior rectus fascia. A transverse incision is made in the midportion of the anterior rectus sheath, approximately one-third of the way from the pubis to the umbilicus; the muscle is divided; and the

deep inferior epigastric vessels are identified, sutured, and divided. A sterile Doppler probe is then utilized to determine the location of the superior epigastric blood vessels along the deep surface of the rectus muscle above the lower abdominal flap. Using these parameters, the lateral 30 percent (or more) of the rectus muscle and fascia can be preserved as well as a portion medial to the umbilicus. After incision around the umbilical stalk, the remaining central portion of the rectus abdominis muscle with its overlying fascia is delivered from the sheath to allow the flap to be suspended on its superior epigastric blood supply. Some surgeons prefer to remove the entire muscle rather than follow the technique described here.

The chest skin flaps are elevated to create an adequate pocket, and a connecting wide tunnel is made medially with the abdominal dissection over the sternum. The flap is carefully passed through this tunnel to the chest wall. Care is taken to avoid any undue tension or torque on the vascular pedicle. Abdominal reconstruction can be accomplished by primary closure of the remaining medial anterior rectus muscle and sheath to the remaining lateral muscle and sheath. No. 2 Neurilon figure-of-eight sutures from xiphoid to pubis are used for this closure. Some prefer a double-layer running suture of similar strength. Prolene mesh overlay for reinforcement in the lower abdominal area can also be applied. The same muscle-harvesting approach and abdominal closure technique is used for double-pedicle flaps and bilateral flaps (hemiflaps).

The table is then flexed, and abdominal closure and umbilical inset are accomplished concomitant with breast mound contouring. As cited above, there are several techniques for this aspect, and one's preferences must be tailored to the requirements of the mastectomy defect. A "tailor-tack" technique of temporary sutures is used until the desired shape has been reached. At that point, after appropriate marks have been made, peripheral tissue is deepithelialized, and the flap is sutured back into the desired position for completion. Suction drains are used in both the breast and the abdomen.

## ALTERNATIVE RECTUS ABDOMINIS FLAP TECHNIQUES

Although the transverse rectus abdominis flap is the most popular type of breast reconstruction utilizing the rectus abdominis muscle, there are other possible options. A skin island may be vertically oriented over the rectus abdominis muscle to provide additional tissue for the reconstructed breast [19]. Also, various combinations of vertical plus transverse skin islands have been described [18]. Another option is the use of a transversely oriented skin island located high on the contralateral rectus muscle just

underneath the inframammary fold of the existing breast [49, 95].

### Complications

Without exact anatomic knowledge, clinical experience, and attention to surgical detail, one may expect more postoperative complications from this procedure. In addition to these considerations, careful patient selection is probably the single most important factor in minimizing complications.

Potential complications are postoperative superficial or deep vein thrombosis due to patient immobilization. This problem is avoided by compressive hose, calf exercises, and early ambulation. Flap necrosis or subsequent fat necrosis are avoided by patient selection and liberal use of double-pedicle flaps. Abdominal flap slough, abdominal wall weakness, or hernia must be avoided by careful operative technique. Abdominal seromas occasionally occur.

## MICROVASCULAR BREAST RECONSTRUCTION

Microvascular breast reconstruction has served as a backup procedure for more difficult or unusual situations for at least a decade. Generally, this approach has been employed only when other less technically demanding techniques were not applicable. There has been a growing number of surgeons who have taken another position: Microsurgical breast reconstructions are superior to other techniques and so must be given primary consideration [34, 89]. The theoretical advantages are an enhanced blood supply to the autogenous breast tissue, more ease in shaping this tissue, and aesthetically acceptable, nonfunctionally compromised donor sites; that is, the abdomen may be stronger following a free TRAM reconstruction than a double-pedicle TRAM.

Whereas these theoretical advantages have not yet been confirmed clinically, there are some obvious disadvantages: longer operative time, increased hospital expense, the need for postoperative monitoring, potential surgical "take-backs" for reexploration, and a failure rate approaching 10 percent in the hands of the most expert microsurgeons.

Even while the debate over the indications of microsurgical breast reconstructions continues, one must be knowledgeable about the potential donor flaps and recipient vessels available. The inferior transverse rectus (TRAM) flap based on a single deep inferior epigastric vascular lease is currently the most popular free flap [26]. Other donor flaps are the superior gluteal flap [89], the inferior gluteal flap [69], the lateral thigh flap [22], and the latissimus dorsi flap. The surgical design for the reconstructed breast utilizing any of these flaps is similar to that when a pedicled flap is used. Standard microsurgical planning, instrumentation, technique, and monitoring are necessary in these cases. The recipient vessels are usually those in the thoracodorsal, thoracoacromial, or intercostal areas. Occasionally, it is necessary to enter the neck vasculature as well.

Microsurgical technique may also be applied to breast reconstruction to augment a pedicled TRAM flap [5, 90]. It may be done in one of two ways: a planned vascular augmentation to a single-pedicle flap hooked into the contralateral deep inferior epigastric vessels retained in a cuff of inferior rectus muscle, or an emergency "supercharged" TRAM flap where the inferior epigastric vessels on the pedicled side are utilized to save a flap during the immediate postoperative period. There is some evidence that a single venous hookup may be adequate in the latter situation.

SKIN FLAPS

Although once occupying a major portion of the surgeon's armamentarium for breast reconstruction, the use of skin flaps is now much less frequent. The thoracoepigastric flap is the single flap that might still be applicable [8, 16]. This flap is transversely oriented with its base medial, overlying the rectus abdominis musculocutaneous perforators. The flap is designed in the lower tho-

racic upper abdominal area. Whereas primary rotation of the flap has been advocated by some, others have suggested a delay procedure for more flap length. The flap is rotated superiorly into the prethoracic area, with primary donor site closure being achieved after extensive abdominal undermining.

## Surgical Techniques for Immediate Breast Reconstruction

SUBMUSCULAR IMPLANT RECONSTRUCTION

It is helpful to mark the inframammary fold preoperatively for later orientation. The orientation and design of the mastectomy scar must be discussed with the general surgeon. The preferred placement of the resultant scar is in the low oblique position, which can be done for many breast cancers but not for those located in the upper medial quadrants.

When the general surgeon has completed the mastectomy, the wound is carefully assessed for flap viability, tension on flap closure, and pectoralis major muscle and fascial integrity. Intravenous fluorescence may be helpful for assessing flap viability. An implant is placed only if these factors are favorable [28, 29, 71].

Total muscle coverage of the implant must be obtained. The submuscular pocket is created by elevating the lateral edge of the pectoralis major and dissecting the space underneath this muscle. The pectoralis minor is then split, and a lateral muscle flap consisting of pectoralis minor in continuity with serratus anterior is elevated. The inferior aspect of the pocket is prepared by elevating the fascial (or submuscular) interface between the pectoralis major and the rectus abdominis. Inferolaterally, the dissection elevates slips of the external oblique muscle. The inferior extent of this submuscular pocket is about 2 cm below the inframammary fold when a smooth-walled implant is used. This pocket can also be created by a transversely placed incision placed low in

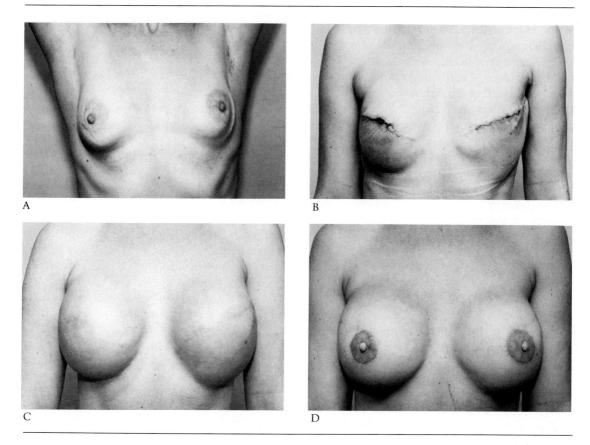

**Figure 48-21** *A. Patient with a recent biopsy of the left breast in the axillary tail area confirming duct cell cancer. B. Two weeks after left modified radical mastectomy and right total mastectomy with insertion of 800 ml of tissue expanders filled with 200 ml of saline. C. Expanders filled to total volume while patient undergoes chemotherapy. D. Result after placement of 650-ml implants bilaterally.*

the mastectomy wound over the fifth or sixth rib.

A silicone prosthesis of appropriate size and shape is inserted, and the integrity of the muscular cover is assessed. Appropriate suction drains are placed, the muscle edges are sutured together, and the skin is closed.

TISSUE EXPANDER RECONSTRUCTION

Tissue expansion is the most frequently used technique for immediate breast recon-

struction today. It allows placement of a thin (partially expanded) prosthesis underneath the muscle and thus minimal increased tension on the healing skin flaps. Once they have healed, however, it allows the flexibility of increasing the expander to the desired volume (Fig. 48-21).

Preoperative markings and technique are similar to those outlined for insertion of a submuscular implant. The dissection is carried below the existing inframammary fold, whereas the expander is placed exactly at the desired fold level when an immobile, textured silicone expander is used. Total muscle coverage has been shown to minimize the complication rate of immediate expander reconstruction. Integrated valves allow easier expander positioning. When a remote valve is used, a subcutaneous pocket must be created in the midaxillary area for valve placement. The volume of saline placed in the expander at this time is variable. It must be adequate to fill out the base of the prosthesis but not enough to put undue tension on the skin flap closure. Drainage and closure are performed as discussed above. Expansion is then begun at 1 week postoperatively, and every effort is made to establish the desired volume during the first 6 to 8 weeks. This volume is held or increased further during the next 4 to 6 months. Chemotherapy has not been detrimental to expansion, but the second operation must await its completion.

LATISSIMUS DORSI RECONSTRUCTION
The latissimus dorsi muscle can be valuable for immediate breast reconstruction either as a preoperative planned skin muscle flap or an intraoperatively necessary island muscle flap "pitch." A replacement for the skin to be removed with the mastectomy can be designed on the back and transferred with the underlying muscle. Either an implant or an expander may be placed underneath the flap. When the general surgeon removes a portion of the pectoralis major or excises the pectoral fascia, it is impossible to obtain total muscle coverage of an expander. In these cases it is prudent to utilize access to the anterior edge of the latissimus dorsi muscle obtained through the lateral aspect of the mastectomy incision. A small island muscle flap can be designed on the thoracodorsal blood supply, which is sutured to the lower pectoralis muscle above and the rectus abdominis fascia below, giving a secure muscle cover. A tissue expander is then safely placed in this submuscular pocket and the operation completed in the usual fashion.

RECTUS ABDOMINIS RECONSTRUCTION
A TRAM flap can be utilized for immediate breast reconstruction. The design of the skin island, flap elevation, and abdominal reconstruction are performed just as for a secondary reconstruction. The flap is placed in the subcutaneous pocket from which the breast has been removed. After appropriate shaping utilizing the "tailor-tuck" technique, all infolded flap portions are deepithelialized and the wounds reclosed.

A major advantage to immediate TRAM flap reconstruction is the ability to preserve the intact inframammary fold [58], to place the autogenous tissue in the subcutaneous position (rather than underneath muscle), and to replace abdominal skin in the exact location of the removed breast skin. This procedure allows the oncologic and reconstructive surgeon much more leeway during preoperative planning and has therefore produced some of the best surgical results of the various operative techniques.

MICROVASCULAR RECONSTRUCTION
Immediate reconstruction using a free flap poses another dilemma. On the one hand, the complexity of the operative procedure and monitoring is increased, as is the operative time. On the other hand, the thoracodorsal vessels are exposed by the axillary dissection, making this aspect of the procedure easier than the delayed setting with a scarred axilla. The other advantages to an immediate pedicled TRAM flap reconstruction are also present here.

NIPPLE-AREOLA RECONSTRUCTION
Nipple-areola reconstruction is usually performed with a second operative procedure, although it may be deferred to a third procedure. Either local or general anesthesia may be used, and it may be done on an in- or outpatient basis. There are several technical options available for nipple and areola creation. The method selected depends on the size and color of the opposite nipple and areola, the type of breast mound on which it is placed, and the patient's and surgeon's preference.

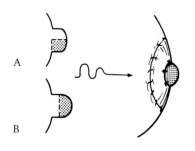

**Figure 48-22** *Composite grafts for nipple reconstruction are taken from either the lower (A) or distal (B) aspect of the donor nipple.*

## Nipple Creation

When the contralateral nipple is of adequate size and the patient is accepting, a composite graft can be taken from the opposite nipple [9, 101]. It may come from the lower one-half of the nipple or the tip, depending on its shape. This graft is sutured to the central portion of the deepithelialized areola site and generally "takes" well (Fig. 48-22). Other composite graft donor sites, such as ear lobule [11] and toe pulp [46], have been reported, but they are generally not as satisfactory.

The other popular technique for nipple creation utilizes local flaps. The quadripod flap has a pinwheel design [3, 51]. The four radiating wings are elevated as medially based dermal cutaneous flaps. As the center of the pinwheel is approached, the dermis is incised in a circular fashion, and the underlying fat is teased out. The wings of the flap are then sutured to themselves (Fig. 48-23).

The "skate" flap technique [50] gives a projectile nipple. This flap is designed in a linear configuration radiating from the central base with large wings on each side. The wings are elevated at the level of the deep dermis, and the linear portion includes deep fat. It is held at a 90-degree angle and wrapped with the wings themselves (Fig. 48-24). Other flaps have also been described that are similar in principle.

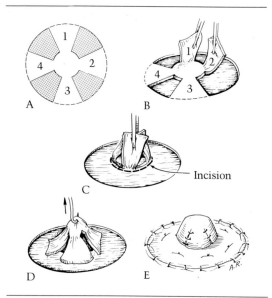

**Figure 48-23** *Quadripod nipple reconstruction. A. Deepithelialization of stippled area. B. Elevation of medially based dermocutaneous flaps. C. Incision through the dermis. Flaps are teased out on their subcutaneous base (D) and sutured to themselves (E).*

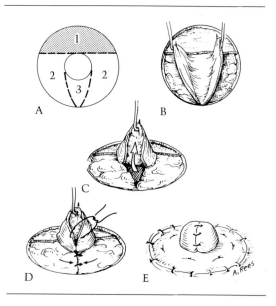

**Figure 48-24** *A. "Skate" nipple reconstruction. Deepithelialization of stippled area. B. Dermocutaneous flaps are elevated. C. Full-thickness elevation with underlying fat. D, E. Flaps are wrapped and closed.*

### Areola Creation

The areola is usually created by a grafting technique. The entire marked circular area is deepithelialized in nipple graft situations, whereas only the residual area within the circle is deepithelialized for flap nipple techniques. The donor site for the areola graft is based on the color required to match the opposite areola unless tattooing is part of the primary technique. When a tan areola is needed (as is generally the case in Caucasians), the upper inner thigh is the most frequent donor site [12]. It is closed primarily to give a scar that is hidden in the perineal crease. The graft may also be taken more posteriorly toward the inner gluteal crease for a similar tan color. For dark brown to black areola color (as for black patients), the labia minora is used [1]. Axillary dog ears, abdominal redundant skin, or any other easily accessible area may be used regardless of color if another tattooing is to be done. In all these situations, the graft is defatted to a thick split-thickness graft and sutured to the deepithelialized area on the breast mound [35]. A small hole is made in the center through which the nipple is pulled. A bolster dressing is generally placed over the graft for several days.

### Tattooing

Tattooing has become increasingly popular [50]. Intradermal pigmentation placed by traditional tattoo methods and equipment may be used for nipple coloration, for areola adjustments and coloration over previously placed grafts, or for areola creation directly on the breast mound without using a grafting technique as described above.

# Surgical Management of the Patient with High-Risk Breast Disease

Because of the high incidence of breast cancer in women (approximately 10 percent of all women who live until age 70), public attention has focused on preventive breast screening measures and self breast awareness. Most women have a palpable nodularity to their breasts that is created by the lobules and glandular elements. These elements go through proliferative changes during the normal menstrual cycle that may cause the glandular elements to feel more discrete or tender. As result of these factors, women frequently seek medical evaluation of their breasts.

Approximately 50 percent of women who see a physician with a breast complaint have a marked degree of "physiologic nodularity." The term *fibrocystic breast disease* is frequently used in these situations. This term is thought to be inappropriate by some authorities [117, 134] because of its general grouping of a spectrum of histologically distinct conditions and its referral to all of them as disease processes.

The most common benign breast lesions are listed in Table 48-2. These conditions may present as palpable masses that, although benign, must be distinguished from malignancies. The factors associated with cancer risk, e.g., strong family history [130], invasive carcinoma in the opposite breast [116, 120, 127, 133], and in situ lobular carcinoma in the opposite breast, may not have palpable breast masses.

Table 48-3 summarizes these breast cancer risk factors. Because these factors do exist cancer "preventive" or prophylactic surgical procedures have been described [106, 126, 132] and advocated with varying degrees of enthusiasm. Although every patient and condition must be carefully individualized and conservatism is stressed, Woods

**Table 48-2** *Common benign breast lesions*

*Lesions associated with cancer risk*
    Hyperplasia without atypia
        Moderate
        Severe
    Atypical hyperplasia
        Ductal
        Lobular

*Lesions not associated with cancer risk*
    Cysts (with or without apocrine change)
    Blunt duct adenosis
    Duct ectais/scarring/fat necrosis
    Sclerosing adenosis
    Fibroadenoma
    Physiologic mild epithelial hyperplasia

*Source:* K. S. McCarty, P. Bernhardt, M. Fabian, et al. Medical Management of Patients with High-Risk Disease of the Breasts. In N. G. Georgiade et al. (ed.), *Essentials of Plastic, Maxillofacial, and Reconstructive Surgery.* Baltimore: Williams & Wilkins, 1987. P. 703.

[136] has suggested that the following situations may be appropriate for consideration of prophylactic mastectomy.

**1.** A patient at increased risk for breast cancer based on her maternal family history (Table 49-2).
**2.** A patient who has (or has had) cancer of the opposite breast of a type known to have a high incidence of bilaterality.
**3.** A patient with extensive nodularity to her breasts to the degree that evaluation is virtually impossible.
**4.** A patient who has undergone multiple previous biopsies, especially if their histopathology indicated potential increased risk of malignancy.
**5.** A patient with severe, disabling mastodynia—and incapacitated to the extent that she is willing to accept the possibility of failure from the procedure.

**Table 48-3** *Summary of breast cancer risk factors*

| Factor | Increased risk* |
|---|---|
| *Family history: primary relative with breast cancer* | 1.2–3.0 |
|     Premenopausal | 3.1 |
|     Premenopausal and bilateral | 8.5–9.0 |
|     Postmenopausal | 1.5 |
|     Postmenopausal and bilateral | 4.0–5.4 |
| *Menstrual history* | |
|     Age at menarche: 12 | 1.3 |
|     Age at menopause: 55 with 40 menstrual years | 1.48–2.0 |
| *Pregnancy* | |
|     First child after age 35 | 2.0–3.0 |
|     Nulliparous | 3.0 |
| *Other neoplasms* | |
|     Contralateral breast cancer | 5.0 |
|     Cancer of the major salivary gland | 4.0 |
|     Cancer of the uterus | 2.0 |
| *Benign breast disease* | |
|     Atypical lobular hyperplasia | 4.0 |
|     Lobular carcinoma in situ | 7.2 |
| *Previous biopsy* | 1.86–2.13 |

*General population risk = 1.0.
*Source:* S. M. Love, R. S. Gelman, and W. Silen. Sounding board: Fibrocystic "disease" of the breast—a nondisease? *N. Engl. J. Med.* 307:1010, 1982.

6. A patient with chronic suppurative mastitis failing to respond to persistent conservative therapy.
7. The rare patient with overwhelming cancer phobia who is resistant to counseling.
8. Select patients with lobular carcinoma in situ.

The two operations that have been suggested for such conditions are total mastectomy (simple mastectomy, total mammary adenectomy) and subcutaneous mastectomy. There is disagreement and controversy among experts as to the appropriateness of these procedures. Both sides of this controversy are presented below.

## Subcutaneous Mastectomy

Because simple mastectomy with its resultant chest deformity was considered an aggressive approach to benign breast disease, less disfiguring operations have been described since the turn of the century [126, 132]. In 1962 Freeman described a subcutaneous mastectomy with immediate or delayed reconstruction for benign disease [106]. The procedure was performed through an inframammary incision and the prosthesis placed in the subcutaneous space. This operation was conceptually and emotionally attractive to many surgeons; and with the introduction of the silicone prosthesis the following year [102], it received immediate clinical evaluation [105, 115, 122, 123]. As might be expected, the initial complication rate was high [125, 129]. During the ensuing 25 years the operation improved substantially owing to careful patient selection [136], submuscular implant placement [114], selective use of skin envelope reduction [108, 110, 113], secondary reconstruction, autogenous tissue transposition [100], and tissue expansion [124].

The operation today is thought by many to be an appropriate surgical prophylactic procedure for the removal of approximately 90 to 95 percent of breast tissue in the carefully selected candidate. In general, the resultant reconstructed breast is aesthetically more acceptable than that following total mastectomy with reconstruction. Breast skin and the nipple-areola complex remain intact, and scarring is minimized. An opposing knowledgeable group of physicians do question the procedure, however.

CRITICISMS OF
SUBCUTANEOUS MASTECTOMY

*1. Because all of the breast tissue is not removed, it is not a cancer-preventing operation.* Previous anatomic studies have documented the presence of breast tissue penetrating the pectoral fascia, extending onto the sternum and laterally to the latissimus dorsi muscle. Therefore it is probable that neither a subcutaneous nor a total mastectomy removes 100 percent of the breast tissue. The presence of breast tissue within subcutaneous mastectomy skin flaps has also been shown [109], but the careful surgeon creates subcutaneous mastectomy flaps in the correct plane of the breast capsule and does not simply "shell out" the breast tissue. The flaps must be similar in thickness to those of a total mastectomy. There is breast tissue left underneath the nipple-areola complex, so the patient must continue to be carefully followed.

Despite occasional isolated reports of breast cancer occurring in the subcutaneous mastectomy patient [101, 112, 119], the largest reported series with long-term follow-up seem to confirm that relative cancer "prevention" has been achieved: (1) Jarrett et al. [113] reported 276 subcutaneous mastectomy patients followed for 6 years with no cases of breast cancer. (2) Woods [135] reported that, of 1400 patients who had undergone subcutaneous mastectomy at the Mayo Clinic over 20 years, only three eventually developed breast cancer. (3) Pennisi reported a collective review [121] of 1500 patients who had undergone subcutaneous mastectomy with a median follow-up of 2 years, among whom six patients developed breast cancer.

**2.** *The complication rate is unjustifiably high.* Through the late 1970s when silicone prostheses were placed in the subcutaneous position, the complication rate was high, with skin necrosis, nipple-areola slough, and implant extrusion being the most offensive complications, followed by capsule contracture. The placement of implants in the submuscular position (obtaining total muscle coverage) greatly facilitated the procedure and is probably the single most important development in its evolution. In the small to moderate-size breast, the operation now has an acceptable complication rate. The large breast is more difficult, requiring either skin envelope reduction, tissue expansion, or a TRAM flap. Even in these cases, however, the complication rate is generally acceptable.

**3.** *The aesthetic results are not acceptable.* The key to patient satisfaction with this operation is preoperative education. The patient must understand that the procedure is a mastectomy with reconstruction and not an aesthetic breast procedure. With this point clarified, it is generally possible to achieve relatively good aesthetic results in small to moderate-size breasts. Although large breasts are more difficult, careful selection technique allows acceptable results here as well.

## Total (Simple) Mastectomy

With the high complication rate associated with subcutaneous mastectomies of the early 1970s and the lack of long-term benefits from the procedure yet to be evaluated, a move toward a more straightforward procedure developed. This position, advocated by Horton and Carraway [111] and others [99, 103, 107, 128], held that the general surgeon could perform a standard simple mastectomy, theoretically removing "all" breast tissue, and the plastic surgeon could then perform an immediate submuscular recon-

struction. Nipple-areola reconstruction was accomplished by its replacement on the newly created breast mound as a free graft. The technical aspects of this operation have evolved to include minimizing and selectively orienting the skin excision, skin envelope reduction as necessary, consideration of tissue expansion, and secondary nipple-areola reconstruction in most instances. These procedures, which may be performed by the plastic surgeon alone or in conjunction with the general surgeon, offer the theoretical advantage of near-total breast removal and its projected improved prophylactic results. It is argued by some that its complication rate is substantially lower than that of subcutaneous mastectomy. The negative side of the argument is that a woman with a benign breast condition is subjected to bilateral (or unilateral) mastectomies that, at best, result in reconstructed breasts with greater scarring and less than "normal" nipple-areola complexes fashioned from other parts of the body. It also remains to be confirmed that "all" of the breast tissue has been removed and that this operation gives better long-term prophylaxis than a subcutaneous mastectomy. The controversy continues, but it is probably accurate to say that each operation has its place in the management of patients with problematic breasts.

### OPERATIVE TECHNIQUE: TOTAL MASTECTOMY WITH IMMEDIATE RECONSTRUCTION

An ellipse is designed to include the nipple-areola complex, preferably in the gently sloping oblique orientation (Fig. 48-25). The inframammary fold is marked, and another mark is made approximately 2 cm below it. The total mastectomy is carried out through the elliptical incision. The plane of the skin flaps is the same as that of a modified radical mastectomy. The pectoral fascia should be preserved. Although axillary dissection is not a part of this operation, the lower axillary lymph nodes may be removed. At the completion of the extirpative portion of the

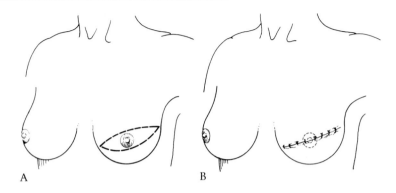

A                              B

*Figure 48-25* Total mastectomy. A. Preferred orientation of skin ellipse is in the gently sloping oblique orientation. B. Mastectomy with submuscular reconstruction.

procedure, the skin flaps are carefully assessed by evaluating dermal bleeding and using intravenous fluorescein as indicated.

A submuscular pocket is then created. Entrance to this plane is either through the inferolateral border of the pectoralis major or by direct incision over the fifth or sixth rib (Fig. 48-26). When the former approach is used, dissection is carried out in the areolar plane deep to the pectoralis major over the pectoralis minor (Fig. 48-27). A laterally based muscle flap deep to the serratus anterior is then elevated, and the connection between the two is completed. This total muscle cover consists of pectoralis major, rectus abdominis fascia, external oblique, and serratus anterior muscles. The extent of the dissection is the infraclavicular border superiorly, the lateral sternal border medially, the lower preoperative inframammary mark made preoperatively inferiorly, and the anterior axillary fold laterally. Sizer prostheses are placed, and the appropriate implant is selected. Muscle closure is achieved such that there is no exposure of the prosthesis in the subcutaneous space. Submuscular and subcutaneous drains are utilized. The nipple-areola complex may be discarded, defatted, and replaced primarily as nipple-areola grafts or, in occasional situations, banked and replaced during a secondary procedure (Fig. 48-28).

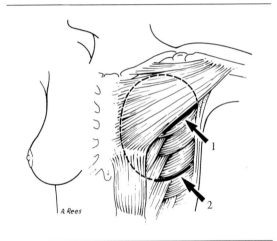

*Figure 48-26* The submuscular pocket is entered around the inferolateral border of the pectoralis major (1) or through a direct incision over the fifth or sixth rib (2). The limits of the pocket are demonstrated.

## SKIN ENVELOPE REDUCTION AND IMMEDIATE RECONSTRUCTION

In the patient with mammary ptosis in whom total mastectomy is indicated, a skin envelope reduction must be utilized. Any of the standard skin envelope reduction tech-

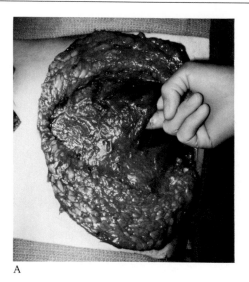
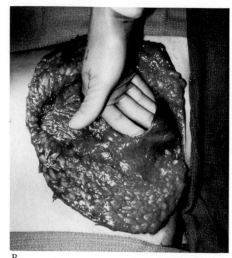

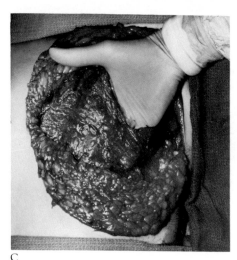

*Figure 48-27* A. The submuscular space is entered around the inferolateral border of the pectoralis major. B. A lateral serratus anterior muscle flap is elevated. C. The connection between the two spaces is made by elevating the external oblique muscle and rectus abdominis fascia.

niques may be considered. The markings for the skin envelope reduction are made preoperatively in the upright position. The mastectomy is then performed within these marks. In most cases a broadly based dermal flap is preserved for reinforcement of the weakened lower muscular cover. The remainder of the procedure is performed as above, and when the implant has been secured in the submuscular position, skin flaps are closed in the usual inverted-T configuration (Fig. 48-29).

TISSUE EXPANSION RECONSTRUCTION
In selected patients, tissue expansion is utilized for the reconstructive process. Selection of expansion utilization is generally in situations where a question of skin flap viability occurs or where a larger postoperative breast is desired. The expander is placed in

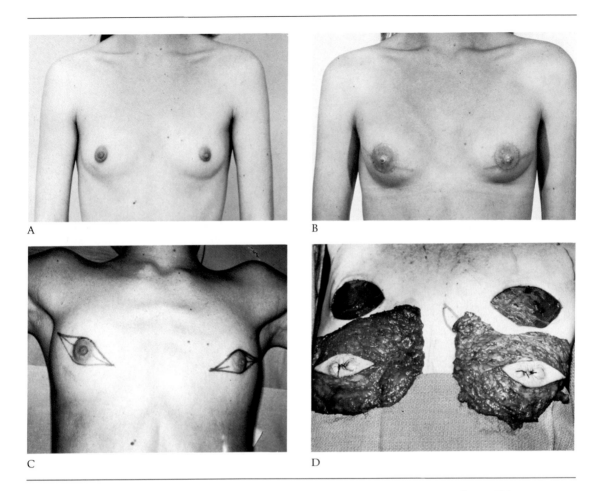

A

B

C

D

**Figure 48-28**  *A. Patient with small breasts preoperatively. B. Postoperatively, following total mastectomy with submuscular reconstruction and nipple-areola reconstruction in a secondary procedure. C. Preoperative markings of skin ellipse. D. Mastectomy specimen.*

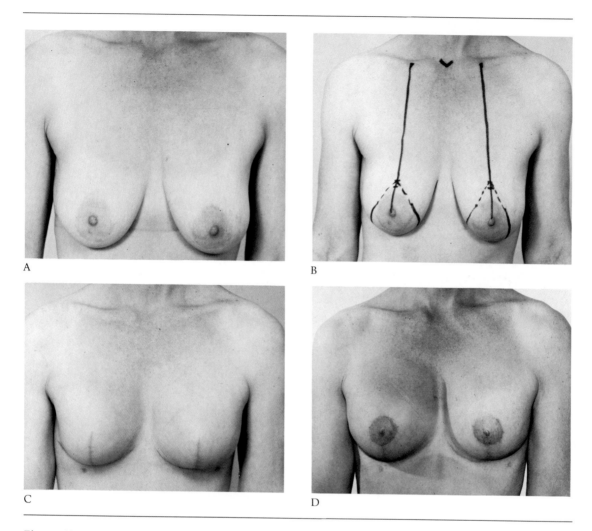

**Figure 48-29**  *A. Candidate for total mastectomy with ptotic breasts shown preoperatively. B. A standard skin envelope reduction is designed. C. Result after total mastectomy with submuscular implants. D. Result after secondary nipple-areola reconstruction.*

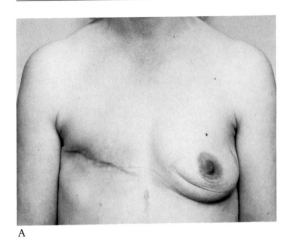

A

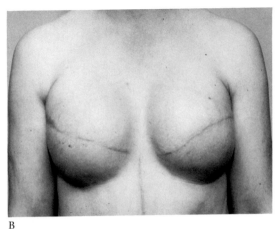

B

*Figure 48-30* A. *After right modified radical mastectomy. Total mastectomy is planned for the opposite breast. B. Result after left total mastectomy with bilateral insertion of tissue expanders. C. Result after expander replacement with permanent prostheses and right nipple-areola reconstruction.*

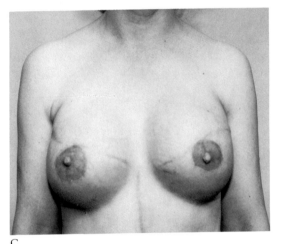

C

the submuscular position, as described above. When textured surface expanders are used, the inferior edge of the expander is placed at the desired level of the inframammary fold. Expansion is begun several weeks after operation, and eventual reconstruction is completed by exchanging the expanders with permanent prostheses (Fig. 48-30). An expander implant is another option.

OTHER TECHNIQUES

Most total mastectomy reconstructions employ one of the above techniques, but the oc-

casional patient requires additional tissue. When the lower pectoral fascia is removed and total muscle coverage of a prosthesis is not possible, an island of latissimus dorsi muscle may be utilized as a muscle patch to achieve total muscle cover over the prosthesis. This procedure is easily performed through the lateral aspect of the mastectomy incision. In rare instances, a latissimus dorsi skin muscle flap is useful for completing the total mastectomy reconstruction.

Autogenous tissue may be used for reconstruction of the total mastectomy. In those cases, either a standard TRAM flap tech-

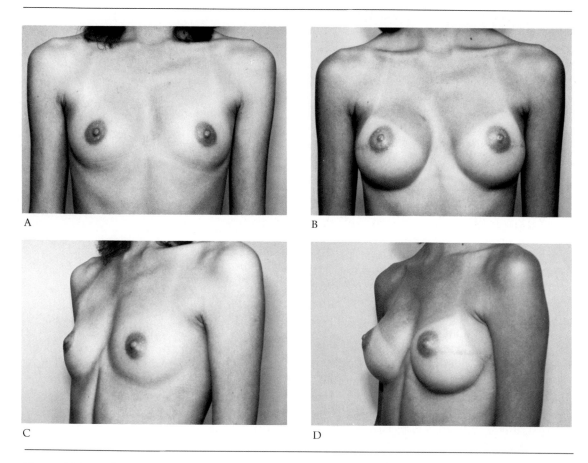

A

B

C

D

**Figure 48-31** *Subcutaneous mastectomy in a small-breasted woman. A, C. Preoperative views. B, D. Postoperative views demonstrating the excellent aesthetic results that can be achieved.*

nique is used, or a deepithelialized TRAM flap is buried underneath the skin envelope.

## Subcutaneous Mastectomy
IMMEDIATE RECONSTRUCTION
Subcutaneous mastectomy with immediate reconstruction is a fairly straightforward operative procedure in the small-breasted woman that generally gives acceptable aesthetic results (Fig. 48-31). The operation can be performed either through an inframammary approach or a straight lateral transverse incision (Fig. 48-32). Preoperatively, in the upright position, the inframammary fold is marked, and another mark is made several centimeters below it. The desired skin incision is also marked. Previous breast scars must be taken into account. Intraoperatively, the incision is made through skin and subcutaneous tissue and is carried down to the level of the breast capsule. The plane at the juncture of the subcutaneous tissue with the breast tissue is easily identified. Flap elevation is accomplished in this plane without difficulty, although occasionally it is somewhat bloody. Approximately 1 cm of breast tissue is left underneath the nipple-areola complex during the initial flap dissection. When flaps have been completely elevated, the entire breast specimen is removed, preserving the pectoralis fascia. The

axillary tail of the breast is marked and sent to the pathology laboratory for gross evaluation. The flaps are checked, and any possible residual breast tissue is removed. The breast tissue underneath the nipple-areola complex is then thinned to leave only a minimal amount. Skin flap viability is assessed in the usual fashion.

The submuscular pocket is formed in the manner described above. The submuscular pocket dissection is carried to the lower of the two inframammary marks made preoperatively. Total muscle coverage is important. Sizer prostheses are utilized, and the patient is placed in an upright position to determine the exact size and shape of the prosthesis to be used. After selection of the prosthesis, muscular closure is carried out, drains are inserted submuscularly and subcutaneously, and the procedure is completed (Figs. 48-33 and 48-34).

Pressure is avoided on the skin flaps during postoperative dressing. In small-breasted women the skin is left to redrape itself, whereas with larger breasts with slight ptosis skin may be relocated by taping. With this technique, described by Jarrett et al. [113], the nipple-areola complex is placed in the desired position and held there by tape. The tape is changed postoperatively over the

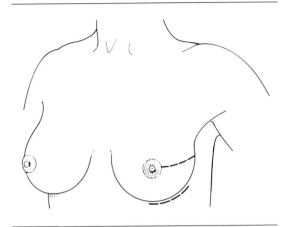

*Figure 48-32* *Alternative skin incisions for subcutaneous mastectomy in the small to moderate-size breast.*

following weeks to allow skin shrinkage and nipple-areola relocation (Fig. 48-35).

Although most patients who undergo subcutaneous mastectomy are reconstructed during the same operative procedure, there are some situations in which secondary reconstruction is preferable. Chronic suppurative mastitis, diabetics or heavy smokers with

*Figure 48-33* *Subcutaneous mastectomy with submuscular implants in a patient with moderate-size breasts. A. Preoperatively. B. Result.*

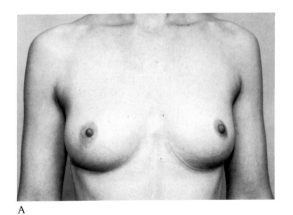

A

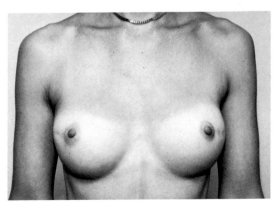

B

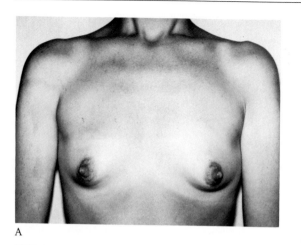
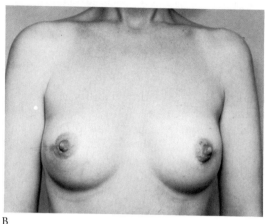

A

B

*Figure 48-34* *Subcutaneous mastectomy with submuscular implants in a woman with small breasts with skin redundancy. A. Preoperatively. B. Result.*

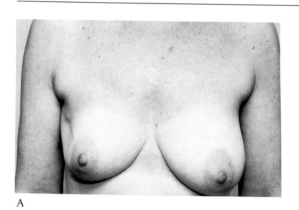
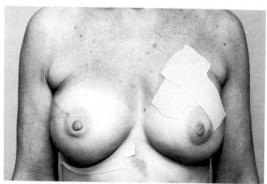

A

B

*Figure 48-35* *Subcutaneous mastectomy with submuscular reconstruction. A. Patient with a ptotic breast after a large right upper quadrant biopsy. B. Postoperative taping is utilized to shrink the skin envelope and relocate the nipple-areola. C. Result.*

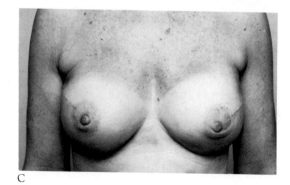

C

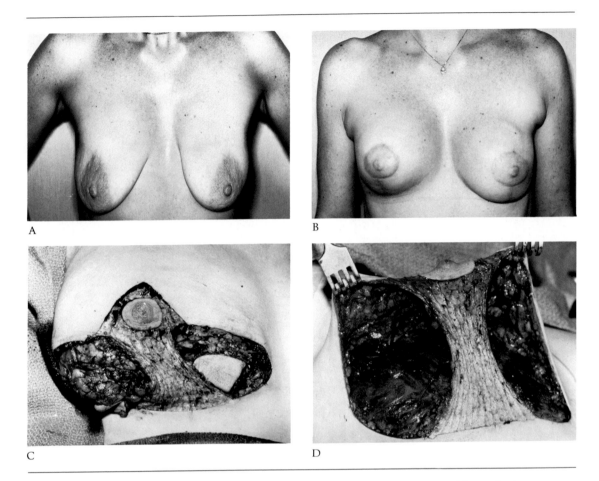

A

B

C

D

*Figure 48-36* A. Patient with marked mammary ptosis in whom subcutaneous mastectomy is indicated. B. Result after subcutaneous mastectomy with skin envelope reduction and submuscular reconstruction. C. Intraoperatively, demonstrating preservation of the dermal pedicle. D. Subcutaneous mastectomy carried out around the pedicle with excellent exposure.

tenuous skin flaps, and extreme breast size are examples of such situations [131].

TISSUE EXPANSION RECONSTRUCTION
Although the patient with slight mammary ptosis and small to moderate-size breasts may be a candidate for subcutaneous mastectomy with submuscular reconstruction and skin taping, as indicated, the patient with large breasts or more moderate ptosis might be a better candidate for immediate insertion of a tissue expander [104]. With this technique, preoperative markings are the same as discussed above. Rather than inserting a submuscular implant, however, a tissue expander is used. Although there might be some initial skin redundancy, over

time the skin can be expanded until it has a smooth surface and pleasing breast mound appearance. At a secondary procedure, the expander is removed and the permanent prosthesis inserted. The results with silicone-textured expanders followed by polyurethane-covered implants have been excellent. The use of tissue expanders may also be prudent in the patient with tenuous skin

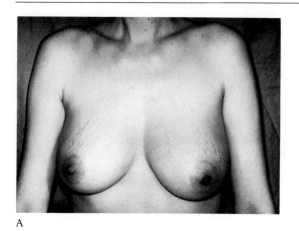

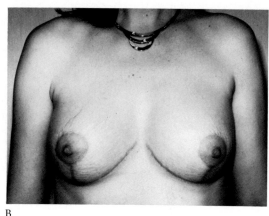

A                                                                     B

*Figure 48-37  A. Large breasts in a patient with silicone granulomas. B. Result after subcutaneous mastectomies, skin envelope reduction, and submuscular reconstruction.*

flaps seen at the conclusion of the subcutaneous mastectomy procedure or simply as a safer two-staged approach that may yield better results.

An alternative to the use of a tissue expander for subcutaneous mastectomy reconstruction is the use of an adjustable implant. This implant is similar to an expander except that the remote fill site and tubing can be pulled out after adequate expansion, and the self-sealing valve prevents the need for implant removal. The adjustable implants come with smooth or textured silicone surfaces.

### SKIN ENVELOPE REDUCTION WITH IMMEDIATE RECONSTRUCTION

The patient with marked mammary ptosis requires skin envelope reduction. It can be carried out at the same time as the subcutaneous mastectomy (Fig. 48-36). Preoperatively, in the upright position, the skin envelope reduction pattern is marked on the breast. Any standard type of skin reduction employing dermal pedicles may be utilized. The subcutaneous mastectomy is carried

through the inferior, medial, and lateral spaces, where the skin is to be removed. Submuscular reconstruction is carried out in the standard fashion with primary closure of the tailored skin envelope (Fig. 48-37). Assessment of skin and nipple-areola viability is important intraoperatively. In cases of questionable viability of the nipple-areola complex, conversion to a free graft nipple-areola technique may be considered. This combined approach carries a higher complication rate and is being used less often with permanent implants. Its combination with tissue expansion or TRAM flaps in the large or ptotic breast, however, has been quite useful.

### TRANSVERSE RECTUS ABDOMINIS FLAP RECONSTRUCTION

Autogenous tissue may be used for subcutaneous mastectomy reconstruction. It has great theoretical appeal in that fatty tissue is utilized to reconstruct the breasts, thus producing the breasts and alleviating the possible complications with silicone prostheses. It is especially attractive in large-breasted women, in whom it is more difficult to perform reconstruction with prostheses. With this technique the deepithelialized TRAM flaps from each side of the lower abdomen are passed on their respective rectus muscle

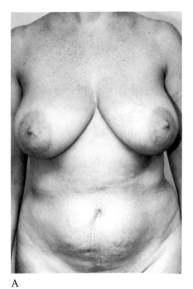
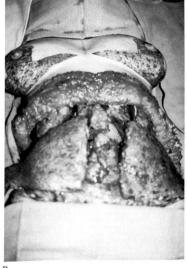
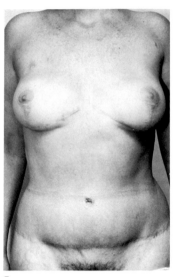

A                                    B                                    C

*Figure 48-38* A. Patient with large, pendulous breasts in whom subcutaneous mastectomy is indicated. B. Bilateral skin envelope reduction, subcutaneous mastectomy, and deepithelialization of TRAM flaps were carried out simultaneously. C. Postoperative result.

and vascular pedicle to fill in the subcutaneous space [118]. Thus all technical considerations for transverse rectus abdominis flap reconstruction outlined in the previous chapter are applicable.

With the patient standing upright in the preoperative position, the desired breast incisions are marked. The procedure may either incorporate skin envelope reduction or maintain the current integrity of the breast skin envelope. A lower transverse flap is outlined on the abdomen. Intraoperatively, subcutaneous mastectomies are performed. Concomitantly, deepithelialization can be carried out on each side of the TRAM flap. The flap is then split and each side elevated in the usual hemiflap fashion (Fig. 48-38).

## Conclusion

Despite controversy, collective data indicate that prophylactic mastectomy procedures are appropriate in many clinical situations. Furthermore, there appear to be appropriate clinical indications for both total mastectomy and subcutaneous mastectomy.

## References

BREAST RECONSTRUCTION
FOLLOWING MASTECTOMY

1. Adams, W. M. Labial transplant for correction of loss of the nipple. *Plast. Reconstr. Surg.* 4:245, 1949.
2. Argenta, L. C., Marks, W. C., and Grabb, W. C. Selective use of serial expansion in breast reconstruction. *Ann. Plast. Surg.* 11:188, 1983.
3. Barton, F. E. Latissimus dermal-epidermal nipple reconstruction. *Plast. Reconstr. Surg.* 70:234, 1982.
4. Becker, H. Breast reconstruction using an inflatable breast implant with a detachable reservoir. *Plast. Reconstr. Surg.* 73:678, 1984.
5. Beegle, P. H., and Hartrampf, C. R. Microvascular augmentation of the transverse abdominal flap in chest wall reconstruction. Presented at the Annual Scientific Meeting of the American Society of Plastic and Reconstructive Surgeons, Los Angeles, October 1986.
6. Biggs, T. M., and Cronin, E. D. Technical as-

pects of the latissimus dorsi myocutaneous flap in breast reconstruction. *Ann. Plast. Surg.* 6:381, 1981.

7. Birnbaum, L., and Olsen, J. A. Breast reconstruction following radical mastectomy using custom designed implants. *Plast. Reconstr. Surg.* 61:355, 1978.

8. Bohmert, H. Personal communication as reported in N. G. Georgiade. *Reconstructive Breast Surgery.* St. Louis: Mosby, 1976. P. 302.

9. Bostwick, J. *Aesthetic and Reconstructive Breast Surgery.* St. Louis: Mosby, 1983.

10. Bostwick, J., Vasconez, L. D., and Jurkiewicz, M. E. Breast reconstruction after a radical mastectomy. *Plast. Reconstr. Surg.* 61:682, 1978.

11. Brent, B., and Bostwick, J. Nipple-areola reconstruction with auricular tissue. *Plast. Reconstr. Surg.* 60:353, 1977.

12. Broadbent, T. R., Metz, P. S., and Woolf, M. Restoring the mammary areola by a skin graft from the upper thigh. *Br. J. Plast. Surg.* 30:220, 1977.

13. Capozzi, A., and Pennisi, V. R. Clinical experience with polyurethane-covered gel-filled mammary prosthesis. *Plast. Reconstr. Surg.* 68:512, 1981.

14. Cocke, W. M. *Breast Reconstruction.* Boston: Little, Brown, 1977. P. 4.

15. Cohen, B. B., and Cronin, E. D. Breast reconstruction with the latissimus dorsi musculocutaneous flap. *Clin. Plast. Surg.* 11:287, 1984.

16. Cronin, T. D., Upton, J., and McDonough, J. M. Reconstruction of the breast after mastectomy. *Plast. Reconstr. Surg.* 59:1, 1977.

17. Czerny, V. Plastic replacement of the breast with lipoma. *Chir. Kong, Verhandl.* 2:216, 1895.

18. Dinner, M. I., and Dowden, R. V. The L-shaped combined vertical and transverse abdominal island flap for breast reconstruction. *Plast. Reconstr. Surg.* 72:894, 1983.

19. Dinner, M. I., Labandter, H. P., and Dowden, R. V. The role of the rectus abdominis myocutaneous flap in breast reconstruction. *Plast. Reconstr. Surg.* 69:209, 1982.

20. Drever, J. M. The lower abdominal transverse rectus abdominis myocutaneous flap for breast reconstruction. *Ann. Plast. Surg.* 10:179, 1983.

21. Elliot, L. F., and Hartrampf, C. R. Tailoring of the new breast using the transverse abdominal island flap. *Plast. Reconstr. Surg.* 72:887, 1983.

22. Elliott, L. F., Beegle, P. H., and Hartrampf, C. R. The lateral thigh free flap in breast reconstruction. Presented at the American Association of Plastic Surgeons Annual Meeting, Scottsdale, Arizona, 1989.

23. Elliott, M. P., and Dubrul, W. Magna-site tissue expander: An innovation for injection site location. *Plast. Reconstr. Surg.* 81:605, 1989.

24. Eyssen, J. E., Von Werssowetz, A. J., and Middleton, G. D. Reconstruction of the breast using polyurethane-coated prosthesis. *Plast. Reconstr. Surg.* 73:415, 1984.

25. Fisher, J., Bostwick, J., and Powell, R. W. Latissimus dorsi blood supply after thoracodorsal vessel division: The serratus collateral. *Plast. Reconstr. Surg.* 72:502, 1983.

26. Friedman, R. J., Argenta, L. C., and Anderson, R. Deep inferior epigastric free flap for breast reconstruction after radical mastectomy. *Plast. Reconstr. Surg.* 76:455, 1985.

27. Fujino, T., Harashina, T., and Enomoto, K. Primary breast reconstruction after a standard radical mastectomy by a free flap transfer: Case report. *Plast. Reconstr. Surg.* 58:371, 1976.

28. Georgiade, G. S., Georgiade, N. G., McCarty, K. S., et al. Modified radical mastectomy with immediate reconstruction for carcinoma of the breast. *Ann. Surg.* 193:565, 1981.

29. Georgiade, G. S., Riefkohl, R., Cox, E., et al. Long-term clinical outcome of immediate reconstruction after mastectomy. *Plast. Reconstr. Surg.* 76:415, 1985.

30. Georgiade, G. S., Voci, V. E., Riefkohl, R., et al. Potential problems with the transverse rectus abdominis myocutaneous flap in breast reconstruction and how to avoid them. *Br. J. Plast. Surg.* 37:121, 1984.

31. Gillies, H., and Millard, D. R. *Principles and Art of Plastic Surgery.* Vol. 1. Boston: Little, Brown, 1957. P. 413.

32. Goin, J. M., and Goin, M. K. Breast Reconstruction after Mastectomy. In *Changing the Body: Psychological Effects of Plastic Surgery.* Baltimore: Williams & Wilkins, 1981.

33. Goldwyn, R. M. Consultation for breast re-

construction. *Plast. Reconstr. Surg.* 73:818, 1984.

34. Grotting, J. C., Urist, M., Maddox, W. A., et al. Conventional TRAM flap versus microsurgical TRAM flap for immediate breast reconstruction. *Plast. Reconstr. Surg.* 83:828, 1989.

35. Gruber, R. P. Nipple-areola reconstruction: A review of techniques. *Clin. Plast. Surg.* 6:71, 1979.

36. Hartrampf, C. R. Abdominal wall competence in transverse abdominal island flap operations. *Ann. Plast. Surg.* 12:139, 1984.

37. Hartrampf, C. R. The transverse abdominal island flap for breast reconstruction: A seven-year experience. *Clin. Plast. Surg.* 15:703, 1988.

38. Hartrampf, C. R. *Transverse Abdominal Island Flap Technique for Breast Reconstruction After Mastectomy.* Baltimore: University Park Press, 1984.

39. Hartrampf, C. R., Scheflan, M., and Black, P. W. Breast reconstruction with a transverse abdominal island flap. *Plast. Reconstr. Surg.* 69:216, 1982.

40. Herman, S. The Meme implant. *Plast. Reconstr. Surg.* 73:411, 1984.

41. Hester, T. R., Jr., Nahai, F., Bostwick, J., et al. A five-year experience with polyurethane-covered mammary prostheses for treatment of capsular contracture, primary augmentation mammaplasty, and breast reconstruction. *Clin. Plast. Surg.* 15:569, 1988.

42. Holdsworth, G. W. A method of reconstructing the breast. *Br. J. Plast. Surg.* 9:161, 1956.

43. Horton, C. E., Rosato, F. A., McCraw, J. B., et al. Immediate reconstruction following mastectomy for cancer. *Clin. Plast. Surg.* 6:37, 1979.

44. Ishii, C. H., Bostwick, J., Raine, T. J., et al. Double pedicle transverse rectus abdominis myocutaneous flap for unilateral breast and chest wall reconstruction. *Plast. Reconstr. Surg.* 76:901, 1985.

45. Kiricuta, I. L'emploi du grand epiploon dans la chirurgie du sein cancereux. *Presse Med.* 71:15, 1963.

46. Klatsky, S., and Manson, P. N. Toe pulp free grafts in nipple reconstruction. *Plast. Reconstr. Surg.* 68:245, 1981.

47. Kleinschmidt, O. Mammary plastics. *Zentralbl. Chir.* 51:653, 1924.

48. Lapin, R., Daniel, D., Hutchins, H., et al. Primary breast reconstruction following mastectomy using a skin expander-prosthesis. *Breast* 6:20, 1980.

49. Lejour, M., and DeMay, A. Experience with 33 epigastric rectus flaps in breast reconstruction. *Handchir. Mikrochir. Plast. Chir.* 15:257, 1983.

50. Little, J. W., and Spear, S. L. The finishing touches in nipple areola reconstruction. *Perspect. Plast. Surg.* 2:1, 1988.

51. Little, J. W., Munasifi, T., and McCulloch, D. T. One-stage reconstruction of a projecting nipple: The quadripod flap. *Plast. Reconstr. Surg.* 71:126, 1983.

52. Longacre, J. T. The use of local pedicle flaps for reconstruction of the breast after subtotal or total extirpation of the mammary gland. *Plast. Reconstr. Surg.* 11:380, 1953.

53. Maxwell, G. P. Iginio Tansini and the origin of the latissimus dorsi myocutaneous flap. *Plast. Reconstr. Surg.* 65:686, 1980.

54. Maxwell, G. P. Latissimus dorsi breast reconstruction: an aesthetic assessment. *Clin. Plast. Surg.* 8:373, 1981.

55. Maxwell, G. P. Selection of secondary breast reconstruction procedures. *Clin. Plast. Surg.* 11:253, 1984.

56. Maxwell, G. P. Technical alternatives in transverse rectus abdominis breast reconstruction. *Perspect. Plast. Surg.* 1:1, 1988.

57. Maxwell, G. P. The use of a silicone textured tissue expander in immediate breast reconstruction. Presented at the American Society of Plastic and Reconstructive Surgeons Annual Meeting, San Francisco, October 1989.

58. Maxwell, G. P., and Fisher, J. Alternatives in immediate breast reconstruction. Presented at the American Association of Plastic Surgeons Annual Meeting, Nashville, May 1987.

59. Maxwell, G. P., and Fisher, J. The use of immediate intraoperative expansion in plastic surgery of the breast. Presented at the American Society for Aesthetic Reconstructive Surgeons Annual Meeting, San Francisco, 1987.

60. Maxwell, G. P., Craig, D., and Fisher, J. The use of polyurethane-covered implants as building blocks in plastic surgery of the breast. Presented to the American Society of Plastic and Reconstructive Surgeons Annual Meeting, San Francisco, October 1989.

61. Maxwell, G. P., McGibbon, B. M., and Hoopes, J. E. Vascular considerations in the use of a latissimus dorsi myocutaneous flap after a mastectomy with an axillary dissection. *Plast. Reconstr. Surg.* 64:771, 1979.

62. McCraw, J. B. Fleur-de-lis latissimus dorsi breast reconstruction. Presented at the American Association of Plastic Surgeons Annual Meeting, Scottsdale, Arizona, May 1989.

63. McCraw, J. B., and Arnold, P. G. *McCraw and Arnold's Atlas of Muscle and Musculocutaneous Flaps.* Norfolk: Hampton Press, 1986.

64. McCraw, J. B., and Maxwell, G. P. Early and late capsular "deformation" as a cause of unsatisfactory results in latissimus dorsi breast reconstruction. *Clin. Plast. Surg.* 15:717, 1988.

65. Meyerowitz, B. E. Psychosocial correlates of breast cancer and its treatments. *Psychol. Bull.* 8:108, 1980.

66. Millard, D. R., Jr. Post-mastectomy breast reconstruction: How to choose the best method for the specific case. *Plast. Reconstr. Surg.* 71:783, 1983.

67. Morris, T., Greer, S., and White, P. Psychosocial and sexual adjustment to mastectomy: A two-year follow-up study. *Cancer* 40:2381, 1979.

68. Muhlbauer, W., and Olbrish, R. The latissimus dorsi myocutaneous flap for breast reconstruction. *Chir. Plast.* 4:27, 1977.

69. Nahai, F. Personal communication.

70. Nielson, M., Christensen, L., and Anderson, J. Contralateral cancerous breast lesions in women with clinical invasive breast carcinoma. *Cancer* 57:897, 1986.

71. Noone, R. B., Murphy, J. B., Spear, S. L., et al. A six-year experience with immediate reconstruction after mastectomy for cancer. *Plast. Reconstr. Surg.* 76:258, 1985.

72. Northouse, L. L. Mastectomy patients with the fear of recurrence. *Cancer Nurs.* 3:213, June 1981.

73. Olivari, N. The latissimus flap. *Br. J. Plast. Surg.* 29:126, 1976.

74. Orticochea, M. Use of the buttock to reconstruct the breast. *Br. J. Plast. Surg.* 26:304, 1973.

75. Paul, M. D. Primary breast reconstruction with a subpectoral silicone tissue expander. *Ann. Plast. Surg.* 15:404, 1985.

76. Pontes, R. Single stage reconstruction of the missing breast. *Br. J. Plast. Surg.* 26:377, 1973.

77. Radovan, C. Breast reconstruction after mastectomy using the temporary expander. *Plast. Reconstr. Surg.* 69:195, 1982.

78. Reinhard, W. Total mastoneoplasty following amputation of breast. *Dtsch. Z. Chir.* 236:309, 1932.

79. Ringberg, A., Palmer, B., and Linell, F. The contralateral breast at reconstruction surgery after breast cancer operation—a histopathological study. *Breast Cancer Res. Treat.* 2:151, 1982.

80. Robbins, T. H. Rectus abdominis myocutaneous flap for breast reconstruction. *Aust. N. Z. J. Surg.* 49:527, 1979.

81. Rosat, F. E., Horton, C. E., and Maxwell, G. P. Postmastectomy breast reconstruction. *Curr. Probl. Surg.* 17:585, 1980.

82. Ryan, J. J. A lower thoracic advancement flap in breast reconstruction after mastectomy. *Plast. Reconstr. Surg.* 60:523, 1977.

83. Schain, W. S., Jacobs, E., and Wellisch, E. K. Psychosocial issues in breast reconstruction. *Clin. Plast. Surg.* 11:237, 1984.

84. Schatten, W. E. Reconstruction of breasts following mastectomy with polyurethane-covered gel-filled prosthesis. *Ann. Plast. Surg.* 12:147, 1984.

85. Scheflan, M., and Dinner, M. I. The transverse abdominal island flap. I. Indications, contraindications, results and complications. *Ann. Plast. Surg.* 10:24, 1983.

86. Scheflan, M., and Dinner, M. I. The transverse abdominal island flap. II. Surgical technique. *Ann. Plast. Surg.* 10:120, 1983.

87. Schneider, W. J., Hill, H. L., Jr., and Brown, R. G. Latissimus dorsi myocutaneous flap for breast reconstruction. *Br. J. Plast. Surg.* 30:277, 1977.

88. Serafin, D., Georgiade, N. G., and Given, K. S. Transfer of free flaps to provide well-vascularized thick cover for breast reconstructions after radical mastectomy. *Plast. Reconstr. Surg.* 62:527, 1978.

89. Shaw, W. W. Breast reconstruction by superior gluteal microvascular free flaps without silicone implants. *Plast. Reconstr. Surg.* 72:490, 1983.

90. Shaw, W. W., and Fong, L. J. A comparison of the superior vs. inferior blood supply of the

TRAM flap by arterial perfusion pressure measurements. Presented at the Annual Scientific Meeting of the American Society of Plastic and Reconstructive Surgeons, Los Angeles, October 1986.

91. Silberfarb, P. M., Maurer, L. H., and Crouthamel, C. S. Psychosocial aspects of neoplastic disease. I. Functional status of breast cancer patients during different treatment regimens. *Am. J. Psychiatry* 137:450, 1980.

92. Snyderman, R. K., and Guthrie, R. H. Reconstruction of the female breast following radical mastectomy. *Plast. Reconstr. Surg.* 47:565, 1971.

93. Tansini, I. Sopra il mio nuovo processo di amputazione della mamella. *Gaz. Med. Ital.* 57:141, 1906.

94. Thomas, S. G. Breast cancer: The psychosocial issues. *Cancer Nurs.* 1:53, February 1978.

95. Vasconez, L. O., Psillakis, J., and Johnson-Gieheik, R. Breast reconstruction with contralateral rectus abdominis myocutaneous flap. *Plast. Reconstr. Surg.* 71:668, 1983.

96. Versaci, A., and Balkovich, M. E. Breast reconstruction by tissue expansion for congenital and burn deformities. *Ann. Plast. Surg.* 16:20, 1986.

97. Versaci, A. D. A method of reconstructing a pendulous breast utilizing the tissue expander. *Plast. Reconstr. Surg.* 8:387, 1987.

98. Wellisch, D. K., Schain, W. S., Noone, R. B., et al. Psychosocial correlates of immediate versus delayed reconstructions of the breast. *Plast. Reconstr. Surg.* 76:713, 1985.

## SURGICAL MANAGEMENT OF THE PATIENT WITH HIGH RISK BREAST DISEASE

99. Bland, K. I., O'Neal, B., Weinder, L. J., et al. One stage simple mastectomy with immediate reconstruction for high risk patients. *Arch. Surg.* 121:221, 1987.

100. Bostwick, J. *Aesthetic and Reconstructive Breast Surgery.* St. Louis: Mosby, 1983.

101. Bowers, D. G., and Radlauer, C. B. Breast cancer after prophylactic subcutaneous mastectomy and reconstruction with Silastic prostheses. *Plast. Reconstr. Surg.* 44:541, 1969.

102. Cronin, T. D., and Gerow, F. Augmentation mammaplasty—a new "natural feel" prosthesis. In *Transactions of the Third International Congress of Plastic Surgeons.* Amsterdam: Excerpta Medica, 1964.

103. Dinner, M. I., and Lebandter, H. P. Total mammary adenectomy with histological evaluation and immediate reconstruction. *Plast. Reconstr. Surg.* 68:505, 1981.

104. Fisher, J., Maxwell, G. P., and Woods, J. Surgical alternatives in subcutaneous mastectomy reconstruction. *Clin. Plast. Surg.* 15:667, 1988.

105. Fredericks, S. A 10 year experience with subcutaneous mastectomy. *Clin. Plast. Surg.* 2:347, 1975.

106. Freeman, B. S. Subcutaneous mastectomy for benign breast lesions with immediate or delayed prosthetic replacement. *Plast. Reconstr. Surg.* 30:676, 1962.

107. Freeman, B. S., and Widner, D. R. Total glandular mastectomy. *Plast. Reconstr. Surg.* 62:167, 1978.

108. Georgiade, N. G., and Hyland, W. Technique for subcutaneous mastectomy and immediate reconstruction in the ptotic breast. *Plast. Reconstr. Surg.* 56:121, 1975.

109. Goldman, L. D., and Goldwyn, R. M. Some anatomical considerations of subcutaneous mastectomy. *Plast. Reconstr. Surg.* 51:501, 1973.

110. Harley, J. H., Schatten, W. E., and Giffin, J. M. Subcutaneous mastectomy—the excess skin problem. *Plast. Reconstr. Surg.* 56:5, 1975.

111. Horton, C. E., and Carraway, J. H. Total Mastectomy with Immediate Reconstruction for Premalignant Disease. In R. M. Goldwyn (ed.), *Plastic and Reconstructive Surgery of the Breast.* Boston: Little, Brown, 1976. P. 459.

112. Humphreys, L. Subcutaneous mastectomy is not a prophylaxis against carcinoma of the breast: Opinion or knowledge. *Am. J. Surg.* 145:311, 1983.

113. Jarrett, J. R., Cutler, R. G., and Teal, D. F. Aesthetic refinements in prophylactic subcutaneous mastectomy with submuscular reconstruction. *Plast. Reconstr. Surg.* 69:624, 1982.

114. Jarrett, J. R., Cutler, R. G., and Teal, D. G. Subcutaneous mastectomy in small, large or ptotic breasts with immediate submuscular placement of implants. *Plast. Reconstr. Surg.* 62:702, 1978.

115. Kelly, A. P., Jacobson, H. S., Fox, J. I., et al.

Complications of subcutaneous mastectomy and replacement by Cronin Silastic mammary prosthesis. *Plast. Reconstr. Surg.* 37:438, 1966.

116. Leis, H. P., Mersheimer, W. L., and Black, N. N. The second breast. *N.Y. J. Med.* 62:2460, 1965.

117. Love, S. M., Gelman, R. S., and Silen, W. Sounding board: Fibrocystic "disease" of the breast—a nondisease? *N. Engl. J. Med.* 307:1010, 1982.

118. Maxwell, G. P., and Tornambe, R. Management of mammary subpectoral implant distortion. *Clin. Plast. Surg.* 15:601, 1988.

119. Mendez-Fernandez, M. A., Henley, W. S., et al. Paget's disease of the breast after subcutaneous mastectomy and reconstruction with a silicone prosthesis. *Plast. Reconstr. Surg.* 65:683, 1980.

120. Nielsen, M., Christensen, L., and Anderson, J. Contralateral cancerous breast lesions in women with clinical invasive breast carcinoma. *Cancer* 57:897, 1986.

121. Pennisi: Letter to the editor. *Plast. Reconstr. Surg.* 74:153, 1984. Also personal communication.

122. Pennisi, V. R. Subcutaneous mastectomy and fibrocystic disease of the breast. *Clin. Plast. Surg.* 3:205, 1976.

123. Pennisi, V. R., and Capozzi, A. Treatment of chronic cystic disease of the breast by subcutaneous mastectomy. *Plast. Reconstr. Surg.* 52:520, 1973.

124. Radovan, C. Breast reconstruction after mastectomy using the temporary expander. *Plast. Reconstr. Surg.* 69:195, 1982.

125. Redfern, A. B., and Hoops, J. E. Subcuta-

neous mastectomy: A plea for conservatism. *Plast. Reconstr. Surg.* 62:706, 1978.

126. Rice, C. O., and Strickler, J. R. Adenomammectomy for benign breast lesions. *Surg. Gynecol. Obstet.* 93:759, 151.

127. Ringberg, A., Palmer, B., and Linell, F. The contralateral breast at reconstructive surgery after breast cancer operation—a histological study. *Br. Cancer Res. Treat.* 2:151, 1982.

128. Rosato, F. E., Horton, C. E., and Maxwell, G. P. Postmastectomy breast reconstruction. *Curr. Probl. Surg.* 17:586, 1980.

129. Schlenker, J. D., Bueno, R. A., Ricketson, G., et al. Loss of silicone implants after subcutaneous mastectomy and reconstruction. *Plast. Reconstr. Surg.* 62:853, 1978.

130. Settin, R. W., Rubin, G. L., Webster, L. A., et al. Family history and the risk of breast cancer. *J.A.M.A.* 253:1908, 1985.

131. Slade, C. L. Subcutaneous mastectomy: Acute complications and long-term follow-up. *Plast. Reconstr. Surg.* 73:84, 1984.

132. Thomas, T. G. On the removal of benign tumors of the mamma without mutilation of the organ. *N.Y. Med. J. Obstet. Rev.* 35:337, 1982.

133. Urban, J. A., Papachriston, D., and Taylor, J. Bilateral breast cancer. *Cancer* 40:1968, 1977.

134. Winchester, D. P. The relationship of fibrocystic disease to breast cancer. *Bull. Am. Coll. Surg.* 71:29, 1986.

135. Woods, J. E. Detailed technique of subcutaneous mastectomy with and without mastopexy. *Ann. Plast. Surg.* 18:51, 1987.

136. Woods, J. E. Subcutaneous mastectomy: Current state of the art. *Ann. Plast. Surg.* 11:541, 1983.

# 49

*Peter McKinney*
*Victor L. Lewis, Jr.*

# Gynecomastia

Gynecomastia (literally, *woman breast*) is caused by an increase in ductal tissue and stroma in the male breast. The term was introduced by Galen during the second century AD, and a description of a surgical reduction followed during the seventh century AD by Paulis of Aegina, who described it as an effeminacy of men [5, 10]. Gynecomastia is a benign condition most likely caused by a variety of hormonal changes, most of which are reversible (e.g., during puberty), but it may also be idiopathic [2]. Some authors have suggested that the breast must be enlarged more than 2 cm for a diagnosis of gynecomastia [5]. However, in the largest series reported (1800 men) 0.5 cm was used to classify grade I gynecomastia [4]. Depending on the build of the chest, the mere perception of a swelling can be called gynecomastia. The image of the hermaphrodite explains why it is so objectionable to the male subject, especially to the emerging adolescent.

## Etiology

Although often appearing transiently at birth, puberty is the main cause of gynecomastia, with an incidence as high as 65 percent in boys in the 14- to 15-year age group. Within 2 to 3 years the incidence drops precipitously, so that the condition virtually disappears during the late teens (7.7 percent at age 17) [4] only to rise again with progressive age, reaching an incidence of 30 percent in older men. These numbers can be misleading, as the diagnosis depends on whether one uses the 0.5 cm or the 2.0 cm criterion for the diagnosis. Suffice it to say that the condition is present in a high percentage of boys, most of whom have it at puberty, and it almost completely disappears within several years. A study done in a World War II naval hospital found the incidence to be as low as 8 per 100,000. The important thing to remember is that the condition is often a normal finding, but it can also be associated with a more serious disease at any age. The common cause is an increase in estrogens, a decrease in androgens, or a deficit in androgen receptors [4]. Systemic causes to be excluded other than puberty may include the following: liver—hepatitis, cirrhosis; lung—carcinoma or inflammatory disease; testes—carcinoma or malfunction; adrenal tumors; pituitary tumors; carcinoma of the colon or prostate; thyroid disease; testosterone imbalance; congenital syndromes, e.g., Kleinfelter syndrome; excess estrogens from carcinoma of the lung or carcinoma of the testes; drugs (marijuana or heroin); familial and idiopathic causes; and debilitating diseases such as severe burns [6].

Hence although it is important to recognize gynecomastia as a possible normal condition, one must not overlook other possibilities such as drugs or organ disease. Both problems must be ruled out in pubertal boys, and if gynecomastia is diagnosed, when psychologically possible it is best to wait as long as 2 years to see if spontaneous regression occurs [10].

## Pathology

There does not appear to be a relation between the cause of gynecomastia and the histologic appearance. Three types of gynecomastia—florid, fibrous, and intermediate—have been described that appear to be related to the duration of the condition [1]. There is increase in ductal tissue and hypervascularity in the florid type, whereas acellular fibrous stroma and few ducts are seen in the fibrous type. The intermediate type is a mixture of the other two. True acinar lobules are not seen in gynecomastia [5]. Florid gynecomastia is usually of less than 4 months' duration, the intermediate-type gynecomastia 4 to 12 months, and the fibrous type of more than 12 months [3, 4].

## Diagnosis

The condition is obvious but the etiology must be ascertained by the history, physical examination, and appropriate laboratory evaluation. A review of systems is made, especially looking for organ changes in the liver, testes, prostate, adrenal, pituitary, lungs, and thyroid. A history of drug intake (e.g., marijuana, antihypertensive drugs, or steroids) must be sought. Physical examination includes checking the above organs and the breasts. Laboratory studies may need to include liver function studies or urine studies for 17-ketosteroids, androgens, and gonadotropic hormones. Consultation with an endocrinologist may be valuable for evaluating these patients. For instance, if a 30-year-old man has a 6-month history of unilateral gynecomastia, a more thorough investigation is indicated. Mammography has been men-

tioned as necessary by some [3, 7, 8], but we have not found it helpful as the amount of tissue available is usually small and easily palpable and the tissue is going to be removed in toto anyway for pathologic examination.

## Classification

Classification can be made in a variety of ways, such as etiology, age, and pathologic type. From a surgical viewpoint a classification based on the surgical requirement is best. Hoffman and Simon divided gynecomastia into four grades: grade I, small enlargement, no skin excess; grade IIA, moderate enlargement, no skin excess; grade IIB, moderate enlargement with extra skin; and grade III, marked enlargement with extra skin [5]. In their opinion grades IIB and III require some skin excision. However, any classification is subjective, and excess skin depends on the shape of the breast, i.e., a tubular "Snoopy" type breast with a narrow base in an older patient is more likely to have excess skin than a greatly enlarged breast in a young patient. Letterman and Schurter [8] simplified the classification into three types of gynecomastia based on the required correction: (1) intraareolar incision with no excess skin; (2) intraareolar incision with mild skin redundancy corrected with excision of skin through a superior periareolar scar only; and (3) excision of chest skin with or without shifting the nipple. In our practice, we have seen gynecomastia that required external skin excisions only once in 30 cases (Table 49-1). We prefer to reduce the gland through a periareolar incision and perform a skin correction at a later date if necessary because with the passage of time most skin envelopes shrink to an acceptable condition, and in the adolescent boy growth may further correct this condition. This choice, of course, is personal preference to avoid a scar on the chest wall if possible.

On rare occasions there is a need for external incisions, and the surgeon must have a battery of choices available. Such choices may include Letterman and Schurter's su-

**Table 49-1** *Synopsis of 30 patients seen by the authors: 1967–1985*

| Parameter | Data |
|---|---|
| Number of patients | 30 |
| Age (years) | 13–55 (average 24) |
| Tissue resected | Bilateral 27 |
| | Unilateral 3 |
| Number of patients, by grade | |
|   Grade I | 9 |
|   Grade II | 20 |
|   Grade III | 1 |
| Etiology | |
|   Cancer of the testicle | 1 |
|   Low testosterone | 2 |
|   Growth hormone | 1 |
|   Kleinfelter syndrome | 1 |
|   Undescended testes | 1 |
|   Estrogen administered for scalp hair growth | 1 |
|   Marijuana usage | 1 |
|   Idiopathic | 22 |
| Complications | |
|   Operative hematoma | 1 |
|   Depression deformities | 3 |
|   Nipple irregularity | 1 |
|   Secondary skin retraction | 1 |

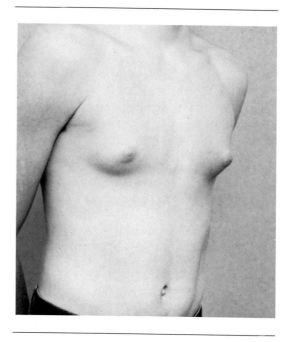

**Figure 49-1** *Grade I gynecomastia in an adolescent. The tissue is mostly underneath the nipple, and the chest wall is thin. The condition had been present for 3 years.*

perior areolar reduction or their repositioning of the nipple through a lateral oblique incision [7, 8]. Again, however, we emphasize that we believe it is better to wait for the skin to shrink or the patient to grow, and we do the skin excision as a secondary procedure. To date, we have had only one patient in whom the secondary procedure was necessary.

For the surgical planning, the authors prefer to consider three classifications of gynecomastia.

*Grade I:* a localized button of tissue in a thin-chested young boy that is concentrated around the areola. These buttons are usually easy to remove; the chest is not fatty; there is no dishing and waviness of the skin to worry about; and the button is a hard, isolated piece of tissue that is easily defined without skin excess (Fig. 49-1).

*Grade II:* diffuse gynecomastia on a fatty chest where the edges of the tissue are indistinct. This tissue is difficult to taper and get smooth (Fig. 49-2A). Dishing was common before the addition of suction lipectomy, which has helped reduce this deformity considerably.

*Grade III:* diffuse gynecomastia with excessive skin. These patients require external skin excisions, or nipple repositioning, or both (Fig. 49-3A).

## Surgical Technique

The selection of local or general anesthesia is a personal preference and depends in part on the size of the excision. In an older male with grade I gynecomastia, local anesthesia

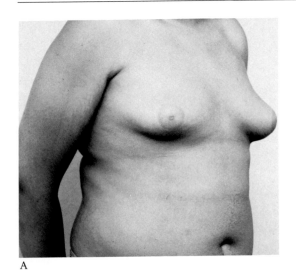

A

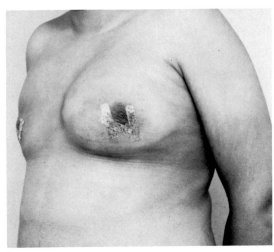

B

is easy. With grade II disease it is more difficult, and general anesthesia is usually more
comfortable.

Preoperative markings are done with the
patient in a sitting position, arms at the
sides and the back slightly arched forward. A
felt-tipped pen marks the area to be resected,
leaving a button of tissue under the nipple.
The edges of the gynecomastia where resection begins and where suction will begin, if
required, are also marked.

The introduction of suction lipectomy has
changed the treatment of gynecomastia. It
has improved our ability to taper the edges
and avoid the "dishing" effect. Some conditions, such as grade II gynecomastia, can be
corrected with a suction lipectomy technique alone [9]. However, most patients
with gritty, hard, fibrous gynecomastia require an open surgical procedure. Because
suction lipectomy is relatively new, it is necessary to explore its possibilities. Perhaps
the sharp curet technique of Ulrich Kesselring can broaden the indications for suction
lipectomy in gynecomastia. To date, the authors have treated several patients with mild
grade II gynecomastia using suction lipectomy alone, with good results.

*Figure 49-2* A. A 16-year-old boy with
gynecomastia. Note the "tone" to the breast
skin, i.e., massive enlargement but no drooping
of the breast per se. B. The same patient
developed a hematoma that required
evacuation despite hemostasis, suction
drainage, and pressure dressing. Note
particularly, however, that the skin has
retracted already, and skin resection was not
necessary in this patient.

## Incisions

Since Dufourmantel in 1928 and Webster in
1946 [5] described the periareolar incision,
there is rarely a reason to do otherwise. This
incision must be placed at the junction of
the areolar and skin. If placed in the pigmented area the scar shows as a white line
especially on a dark areola, and if placed on
the skin the thicker dermis produces more
scar. This exact position is not so easy to
find and may explain why some surgeons do
not use this approach. However, when done
correctly and after appropriate healing the
scar is virtually invisible. We still see the inframammary incision being used in some
patients, and this scar, to us, negates the purpose of the operation. A bright operating
room light or the use of epinephrine may
"wash out" the area and make the junction

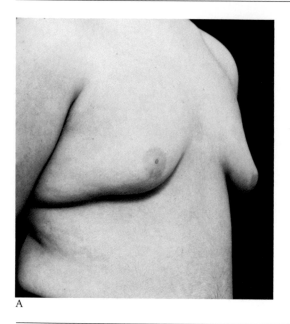

A

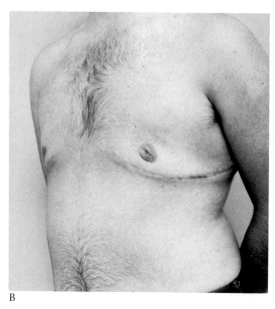

B

*Figure 49-3* *A. A 15-year-old boy with grade III gynecomastia. Note the ptosis of the chest skin. B. This patient is the only one who required skin resection. It was done secondarily, however, and the nipple was not shifted but the ptotic skin merely resected underneath. Most youngsters' skin retracts satisfactorily without resection.*

indistinct. It is helpful to scratch the area before epinephrine injection in a not-too-bright light. Marcaine 0.25% with 1:400,000 epinephrine is utilized even under general anesthesia, as it aids in hemostasis and reduces pain upon awakening. The incision is made in the described periareolar area 5 to 10 mm deep, and the areolar-nipple is undermined at this level to leave a button of tissue to prevent the nipple from sticking on the chest wall and retracting (Fig. 49-4). Note that the nipple normally protrudes slightly from the chest wall so that in thin individuals less tissue is needed under the areola to effect this protrusion. Again, having the arms at the side of the chest is a more natural position for assessing it. The chest skin

is undermined between the subcutaneous fat and the breast to the extent of the preoperative markings, and tapering is begun with scissors. This plane usually separates easily, much as during rhytidectomy, even in the grade II gynecomastia patient. If the tissue mass is large, the tissue can be split in two segments down to the pectoral fascia and then dissected off the fascia either with blunt or sharp dissection. Usually there are some areas in the inframammary crease in the grade II patient that require sharp dissection. All edges of resection must be tapered.

Correction of grade I (localized) gynecomastia is usually a simple surgical procedure. The major problem is not leaving enough tissue under the nipple to prevent retraction. The surgical plane is distinct, and adequate subcutaneous tissue can be left on the thin skin of the chest wall so that it does not stick down. Grade II is more difficult and presents several problems. The nipple button may be difficult to leave because much of it is fat rather than fibrous tissue. The plane is more indistinct, and waviness of the

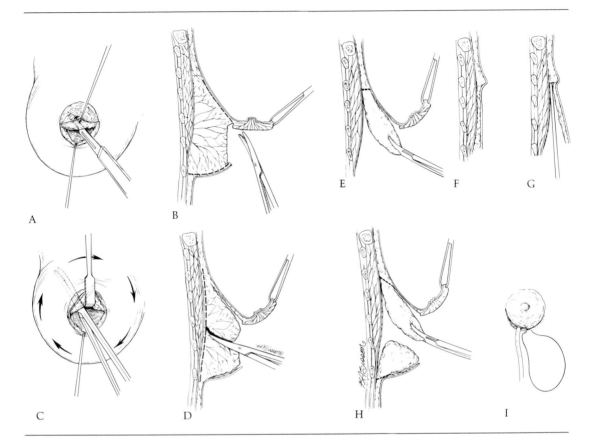

**Figure 49-4** *A. An infraquadrant periareolar incision is utilized and the nipple undermined. B. When the nipple is undermined, extra tissue is left underneath the nipple so that it protrudes slightly above the surrounding skin. If the undermining is too thin, the nipple may "stick" to the chest wall. C. The undermining is then contoured under the skin of the chest wall. There is usually a distinct plane between the gynecomastia tissue and the subcutaneous plane of the chest skin. D. After the undermining is accomplished and if the breast is large, the tissue can be split by dissecting through the breast to the loose areolar tissue between the breast and the pectoral fascia (dotted line). E–H. Dissection on the loose areolar plane reduces bleeding, which may occur if the muscle is entered. There is usually one perforator from the muscle in the center of the field. The dissection is tapered at the edges; otherwise a ridge or "dishing" is noticeable (E, F). This problem can be treated with suction lipectomy at the time to flatten the edges (G). Tapering the resection (H, dotted line) avoids this problem. I. Closure is done after hemostasis is complete and a drain is brought out through the wound. Placing the drain here avoids "stab" wound scars on the chest wall. A Penrose or a suction drain is utilized.*

chest skin can occur after healing. Care must be taken to cut parallel to the chest skin. The position of the arms and the direction of the surgical assistant's retraction must be taken into account as the skin flaps are dissected. Waviness may occur on the fatty chest because of fat necrosis after surgery and may leave a depression in the center or at the edges of the resection. Tapering at the edges is important. A combination of surgical resection and suction lipectomy at the edges gives the best results. The grade III gynecomastia patient provides an easier dissection because of the exposure, especially if the nipple is moved at the same time. We have only one patient in this group, and in this case we waited for the skin to shrink and then made an inframammary excision *only,* without moving the nipple (see Fig. 49-3). A headlight or fiberoptic retractor makes it easier to obtain hemostasis. Drains (Penrose or suction) are brought out through the periareolar incision. Bringing drains out through the chest wall skin may leave a hypertrophic scar that is always visible. If a large drain is required we prefer to use the axilla, although it is more uncomfortable initially. A pressure dressing helps to get the flaps to stay down and reduces seroma formation.

## Complications

A surgical problem is fluid shift. Schurter and Letterman reported cardiac arrest due to fluid shift in a large resection. Infection is not common and is rarely reported. We do not use "prophylactic" antibiotics. Small hematomas are common following correction of grade II gynecomastia. In one patient we had to evacuate surgically a large hematoma despite the use of suction drain and pressure dressing (see Fig. 49-2). Nipple retraction can be avoided in the grade I patient, but it is more difficult to avoid in the grade II patient because of the fatty nature of the tissue. A wavy appearance of the skin depends on the surgical plane encountered and how carefully one stays parallel to the skin. Dishing at the edges depends on how carefully one tapers the resection. Loose skin is more likely in the older patient than in the young one. If present, it is corrected secondarily, not primarily, as most patients' skin retracts satisfactorily.

## Summary

Gynecomastia is in most instances a benign, self-limiting condition. However, organic causes must be considered. If the condition persists, surgical correction is undertaken through a periareolar incision with satisfactory reduction in most patients. Suction lipectomy is helpful for tapering the edges of the resection, and in some patients it may be used for the entire procedure. Only rarely is it necessary to perform an external skin incision on the chest wall to reduce the skin envelope.

## References

1. Bannayan, G. A., and Ajdu, S. I. Gynecomastia: Clinicopathologic study of 351 cases. *Am. J. Clin. Pathol.* 57:431, 1972.
2. Chrichlow, R. W. Diseases of the Male Breast. In H. S. Gallagher (ed.), *The Breast.* St. Louis: Mosby, 1978. P. 508.
3. Georgiade, N. G. *Reconstructive Breast Surgery.* St. Louis: Mosby, 1976.
4. Georgiade, N. G. *Aesthetic Breast Surgery.* Baltimore: Williams & Wilkins, 1983. P. 334.
5. Goldwyn, R. *Plastic and Reconstructive Surgery of the Breast.* Boston: Little, Brown, 1976. Pp. 93 and 305.
6. Kernahan, D., and Thomson, H. (eds.). *Symposium Pediatric Plastic Surgery.* St. Louis: Mosby, 1982. P. 200.
7. Letterman, G., and Schurter, M. The surgical correction of gynecomastia. *Am. Surg.* 35:322, 1969.
8. Letterman, G., and Schurter, M. Surgical correction of massive gynecomastia. *Plast. Reconstr. Surg.* 49:259, 1972.
9. Lewis, C. M. Lipoplasty: Treatment for gynecomastia. *Aesthetic Plast. Surg.* 9:287, 1985.
10. Rees, T. D., and Aston, S. J. Mammary Augmentation, Correction of Asymmetry and Gynecomastia. In *Aesthetic Plastic Surgery.* Vol. 2. Philadelphia: Saunders, 1980.

# VII
# Trunk and Lower Extremity

# 50

*Donald Serafin*
*Christopher P. Demas*

# Reconstructive Procedures for the Lower Extremity Soft Tissues

Reconstructive surgery of the lower extremity has been revolutionized by advances in surgical techniques. Detailed anatomic dissections have demonstrated numerous muscle and musculocutaneous flaps that can be used to treat complicated lower extremity wounds. Subsequent dramatic advances in composite tissue transplantation have prevented numerous amputations and aided more rapid ambulation in countless other patients. With increased use of these techniques, the reconstructive surgeon no longer needs to resort to older, conventional methods of wound treatment such as cross-leg flaps. Although muscle and musculocutaneous flaps have been described for use on all locations of the lower extremity, the best application of this method of reconstruction is for extensive wounds in the proximal two-thirds of the lower extremity. Extensive wounds in the distal one-third of the extremity, specifically the foot, present more difficult reconstructive problems. It is in this area that large wounds are best treated with a microsurgical method.

## Soft Tissue Coverage

Damage to soft tissue with resultant exposure of underlying structures can result from vascular disease, trauma, or prolonged pressure. The goal of this chapter is to outline the approach to these wounds and offer choices for restoring the soft tissue envelope.

When a plastic surgeon is confronted with a lower extremity wound, he or she must make a thorough assessment of the damaged structures, carefully determining the quality of the vascular supply and the extent of nerve injury. It is senseless to attempt coverage in an extremity with a tenuous blood supply. To perform reconstruction in a totally anesthetic limb is also unwise. After neurovascular assessment, the skeletal integrity must be evaluated for fractures, bone loss, and infection. (A detailed discussion of the treatment of fractures and segmental bone loss is beyond the scope of this chapter.) Finally, the extent of soft tissue loss and the quality of neighboring tissue must be analyzed. The soft tissue injury is usually less complicated in wounds secondary to pressure and low velocity trauma. Wounds associated with open fractures or resulting from high velocity trauma, however, tend to have a full spectrum of severity (Table 50-1). The severity of soft tissue injury is clearly the most important factor for predicting infection and nonunion of the fracture.

Upon completion of the initial assessment, sequential steps for restoration of function must be determined and executed as needed: angiography, revascularization, fasciotomy, external fixation, jet lavage, sharp

**Table 50-1** *Gustilo classification of open fractures*

| Type | Criteria |
|------|----------|
| I | Open fracture with clean laceration < 1 cm long |
| II | Open fracture with clean laceration > 1 cm long without extensive soft tissue injury, flaps, or avulsions |
| III | Open fracture with extensive damage to soft tissue including muscle, skin, and neurovascular structures |
| | Adequate coverage available despite extensive damage |
| | Extensive injury with periosteal stripping, bone exposure, and/or massive contamination |
| | Open fracture with arterial injury requiring repair |

debridement, possible neurorrhaphy, and control of infection. After these steps have been executed, the planning and timing of coverage must be determined. If the degree of soft tissue injury is clearly demarcated, aggressive soft tissue coverage is indicated primarily. For high-energy wounds such as those associated with motorcycle accidents, the zone of injury is not always evident at the initial debridement, and serial debridement of devitalized tissue may be required. Nonetheless, early coverage is essential to control infection and promote bony union. The ultimate goal prior to coverage is to have a clean, thoroughly debrided wound with healthy, uncontaminated tissue surrounding the defect. The type of coverage required depends on the location, neurovascular exposure, presence of osteomyelitis, bone in the depth of the wound, and size of the defect.

Once the extremity is prepared and the method of coverage is chosen, there are a few final considerations that must be made. In the case of muscle and musculocutaneous flaps, one must consider if there is adequate uninjured or undiseased blood supply and venous drainage to support the flap. Second, the arc of rotation must be adequate to inset the flap without tension. Finally, any disad-

vantages in the choice of flap selection must be evaluated. Will it cause significant loss of locomotor function? Is the donor defect cosmetically acceptable? Is the method of reconstruction chosen the best one, or is a vascularized flap necessary? If the choice is vascularized flaps, similar questions must be addressed: Is there an adequate, easily accessible recipient blood supply? Is the donor defect cosmetically and functionally acceptable?

## *Groin and Thigh Reconstruction*

If there is no exposure of vital structures, wound defects in the groin and thigh region can be simply managed with split-thickness skin grafts. When vessels and nerves are exposed after radical groin dissection or posttraumatic reconstructive vascular surgery, there are numerous local muscle or musculocutaneous flaps that can be used. Occasionally the defects are extensive, and local tissue is inadequate or has been destroyed, as with an electrical injury. Rarely, one may have to manage osteomyelitis of the femur. In this setting reliance on composite tissue transplantation is necessary to satisfy the needs of wound coverage.

### MUSCLE OR MUSCULOCUTANEOUS FLAPS

#### *Tensor Fascia Lata Muscle*

The tensor fascia lata makes an excellent musculocutaneous flap that can be used to cover the entire ipsilateral groin and the upper one-half of the thigh anteriorly and posteriorly. The tensor fascia lata is a type I muscle whose origin is the anterior iliac crest; it inserts on the iliotibial tract. The single dominant pedicle is the transverse branch of the lateral femoral circumflex artery, which enters the deep surface of the muscle 8 to 10 cm below the anterosuperior iliac spine (Fig. 50-1). In this region it is most frequently indicated for coverage after radical groin dissection. It is an expendable muscle and is easily elevated. The donor defect can be closed in most circumstances. Al-

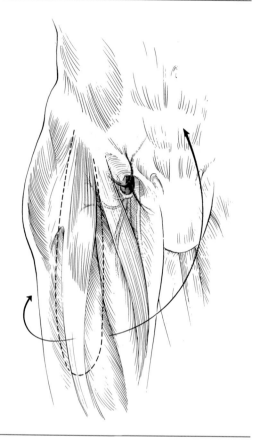

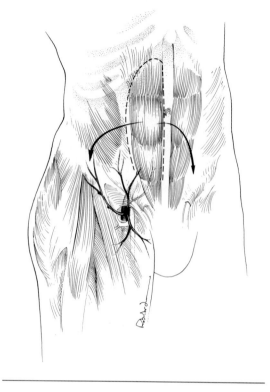

**Figure 50-2** *Anterior view of the abdomen, demonstrating a rectus abdominis muscle flap. One can see the deep inferior epigastric vascular pedicle.*

**Figure 50-1** *Oblique view of the leg, demonstrating a tensor fascia lata flap. The vascular pedicle is demonstrated entering the muscle belly approximally 8 to 10 cm below the anterior iliac spine.*

though there is a paucity of well vascularized muscle, when large amounts of tissue are needed the skin paddle can be as large as 25 × 40 cm, precluding easy closure without skin grafts. A distal delay is often required. If bulk is needed to fill a defect or muscle is required for vessel coverage, the tumor fascia lata flap is not the best solution in this area.

### Rectus Abdominis Muscle
The rectus abdominis is a hearty type I muscle that can provide a muscle or musculocutaneous flap. It can safely cover both

groins in its inferior arc of rotation based on the inferior epigastric artery. It provides excellent muscular bulk and coverage for exposed vessels while carrying a relatively large skin paddle (Fig. 50-2). It also has utility when osteomyelitic defects of the hip require vascularized coverage. The donor defect can usually be closed primarily. The muscle is not truly expendable. There is little morbidity, however, as the other rectus muscle can compensate for its loss. If skin is required, a transverse paddle can be outlined in the periumbilical region. Care must be taken to preserve the periumbilical perforators. Alternatively, a vertical skin paddle can be employed. There have been reports of herniation of the abdominal wall with the flap.

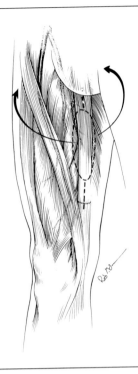

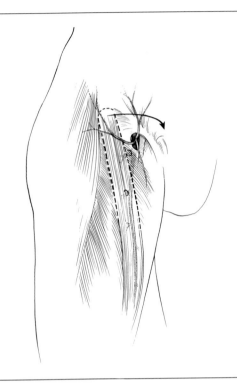

**Figure 50-3** *Medial oblique view of the thigh, demonstrating the gracilis myocutaneous flap. The medial femoral circumflex artery enters the muscle proximally. The wide arc of rotation is indicated by the arrows.*

**Figure 50-4** *The sartorius muscle is demonstrated with multiple pedicles coming off the superficial femoral artery. The close proximity to the femoral triangle is demonstrated, as are the proximal pedicles, which can be ligated for transfer of the flap to a distal location.*

*Gracilis Muscle*
The gracilis is an expendable type II muscle that is thin and flat. The origin is the pubic symphysis, and the insertion is the medial tibial condyle. The single dominant pedicle (medial femoral circumflex artery) enters the medial one-third of the muscle about 10 cm inferior to the pubic tubercle (Fig. 50-3). The donor defect can be closed primarily, but the dissection is difficult in obese individuals. The arc of rotation makes it useful for ipsilateral groin and anterior or posterior thigh coverage. It is particularly useful for covering a large groin defect with exposed vessels. The donor defect can always be closed primarily. The major drawback of use of the gracilis muscle is an unreliable skin paddle distally. Rather than creating a cutaneous island, proximal skin can be left intact and deepithelialized if necessary. The skin paddle has been extended by using the sartorius muscle concomitantly.

*Sartorius Muscle*
An expendable muscle of the thigh, the sartorius muscle is most useful for covering groin vessels because of its type IV blood supply via the superficial femoral artery (Fig. 50-4). This segmental blood supply limits the arc of rotation. It takes origin from the anterosuperior iliac spine and inserts on the medial tibial condyle. It requires minimal dissection to detach the proximal origin of this muscle, ligate one or two proximal pedicles, and transpose the muscle belly medially. There is no proximal skin paddle.

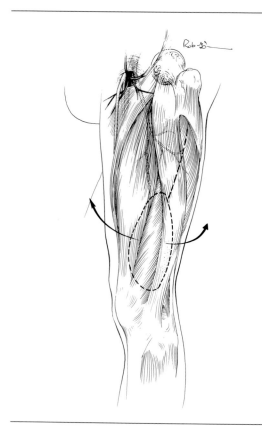

***Figure 50-5*** *Lateral view of the leg demonstrating the vastus lateralis muscle with its wide arc of rotation. Note the intimate attachments of this muscle to surrounding musculature. The vascular pedicle is seen proximally.*

## Vastus Lateralis Muscle

A large muscle on the posterlateral thigh, the vastus lateralis muscle lies underneath the tensor fascia lata (TFL) and between the vastus intermedius and biceps femoris muscles. The wide origin of this muscle is the greater trochanter, gluteal tuberosity, and lateral intermuscular septum. It inserts on the patella. It is a type V muscle whose dominant pedicle is a branch of the lateral femoral circumflex artery. It enters the muscle belly 10 cm inferior to the anterior iliac crest. The vastus lateralis has a wide arc of rotation, similar to that of the TFL.

Original reports describe it as being used for a muscle flap only or combined with the TFL flap as a conjoined musculocutaneous flap. More recent clinical experience has demonstrated that it can support a relatively large skin paddle over its distal portion (Fig. 50-5). It is used when other reconstructive alternatives are not possible. It is a large muscle mass and can fill a deadspace well in the groin or after extirpative surgery in the proximal thigh.

There are some technical points that must be highlighted regarding its elevation. Care must be taken when dissecting it distally so that the suprapatella bursa is not entered. When the muscle is dissected off the vastus intermedius, the vascular pedicle can be interrupted. The donor defect is significant, as this muscle is one of the important stabilizers of the knee. However, late postoperatively there is minimal dysfunction, as the other muscles compensate.

## Rectus Femoris Muscle

The rectus femoris muscle provides a flap of last choice for coverage in this area, especially in ambulatory patients. It is a type II muscle whose dominant pedicles arise from the lateral circumflex femoral artery. Flap elevation is relatively easy. The arc of rotation is similar to those of the TFL and vastus lateralis muscles (Fig. 50-6). Its use is indicated only when all other reconstructive options are impossible. As a strong extensor of the leg and a thigh flexor, there is functional disability following its use. The donor defect can usually be closed but may require a skin graft.

### VASCULARIZED FLAPS

Virtually any composite free tissue transfer can be used in the groin and thigh region. The latissimus dorsi muscle with split-thickness skin graft is most commonly indicated if multiple rotation flaps cannot fill a relatively large defect. It can close a massive defect up to 40 × 20 cm. This flap is most commonly indicated when soft tissue injury accompanies open fracture of the fe-

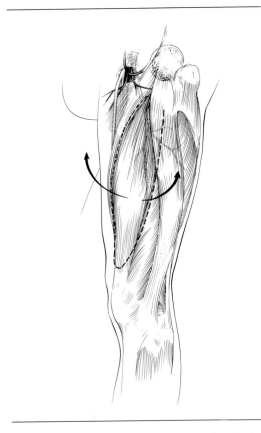

**Figure 50-6** *Lateral oblique view of the thigh demonstrating the large rectus femoris muscle. The arc of rotation is similar to those of the tensor fascia lata and vastus lateralis flaps.*

mur. A large mass of tissue can be brought in to fill the defect. Major disadvantages are that the athletic patient has noticeably weakened arm extension. Alternative free transfers are the scapular/parascapular flap for soft tissue coverage only and the omental flap for large cavities associated with osteomyelitis of the femur following débridement. The advantage is well vascularized tissue, bulk, and a lengthy pedicle that removes the anastomosis from the zone of injury or infection.

## Knee

Reconstruction of defects around the knee presents a number of requirements that

must be met. Most often, soft tissue coverage is required, which can be accomplished with a split-thickness skin graft provided there are no exposed osseous-tendinous structures. If there is an exposed joint, vessel, or prosthetic device, however, a thin, pliable fasciocutaneous or cutaneous flap is indicated. Scar contracture is minimized, joint motion is facilitated, and padding is provided to bony prominences. Fortunately, there are local flaps that can satisfy these requirements of reconstruction. A local rotation musculocutaneous flap can also be used for functional patella tendon repair. If local tissue is inadequate, the large vessels in the area can be easily exposed for vascularized composite tissue transplantation.

## MUSCLE OR MUSCULOCUTANEOUS FLAPS

### Gastrocnemius Muscle

The medial and lateral heads of the gastrocnemius muscles are reliable as both muscle and musculocutaneous flaps. They are the first choice for reconstruction around the knee joint when bulk and new blood supply are required. They are used to cover exposed bone, joints, prosthetics, and vital structures after contracture release. These type I muscles each have a sural artery pedicle and can be used singly or together. The medial head is larger and is used more often, especially when defects extend to the contralateral side (Fig. 50-7). It can also be used as an island or turnover flap to cover popliteal vessels (Fig. 50-8). The medial head has the advantage of a larger cutaneous territory extending to within 5 cm of the medial malleolus. If both muscles are used, there is significant loss of plantar flexion with only the soleus muscle left to assume this function; but if one head is not used, the other muscle hypertrophies along with the soleus. If the gastrocnemius is used as a musculocutaneous flap, the bulk may be extreme and the donor site unsightly, as primary closure is not possible. Using these muscles as muscle flaps only with a split-thickness skin graft alleviates

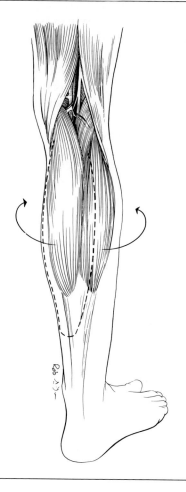

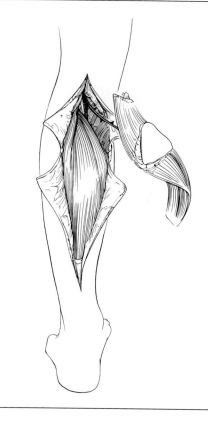

**Figure 50-8** *Posterior view of the leg demonstrating the gastrocnemius musculocutaneous island flap. The sural artery is shown dissected free of surrounding structures and branches. This donor defect can be closed primarily.*

**Figure 50-7** *Posterior view of the leg, demonstrating the medial head of the gastrocnemius muscle being used as a musculocutaneous flap with a long skin paddle extending to within 2 to 5 cm of the medial malleolus. Note that the vascular pedicle is entering the muscle proximally. The wide arc of rotation is demonstrated.*

this problem. When dissecting the cutaneous territory of the medial head distally, one must be cautious to dissect the fascia carefully as the vessels on its anterior surface supply the skin distally. When dissecting the lateral head, one must take care to avoid damaging the peroneal nerve.

### Vastus Medialis Muscle

The vastus medialis is a type IV muscle lying on the anteromedial aspect of the thigh underneath the sartorius and medial to the rectus femoris. It has a broad origin from the distal one-half of the intertrochanteric line, the medial lip of the linea aspera, and the medial intermuscular septum. The aponeurosis inserts on the medial border of the patella and quadriceps femoris tendon (Fig. 50-9). This flap is indicated when the gastrocnemius is not available or when transfer of the quadriceps femoris tendon is desired. It has a small arc of rotation and is useful

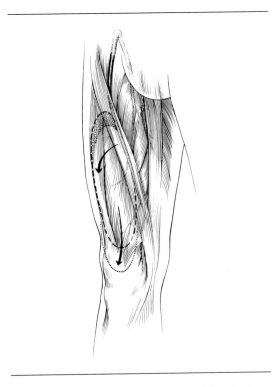

**Figure 50-9** *Medial oblique view of the thigh demonstrating the vastus medialis flap employed as a rotation flap for wound cover of the anterior upper knee. Note that the cutaneous paddle is not created as an island.*

when there is an anterior or upper knee defect and one desires a better cosmetic result than that associated with the gastrocnemius flaps. The greatest advantage is that a myocutaneous-tendinous defect can be closed primarily. Knee function is not impaired. It can cover a large defect by detaching its proximal origin, but this maneuver sacrifices function of the muscle. It is recommended that one does not create this flap as an island, as venous drainage may be impaired and it does not improve the rotation. Care must be taken when elevating this flap that the femoral neurovascular bundle is not endangered as one approaches the medial border.

### Vastus Lateralis

If there is no alternative other than composite free tissue transfer, a vastus lateralis turn-down flap is a consideration for knee coverage. The advantage is avoidance of the potential complications and lengthy surgery associated with free tissue transfer. This flap is not entirely reliable, however; it is based on geniculate artery perfusion of the distal one-third to one-half of the muscle, which must be preserved during dissection. Superficial muscle necrosis may occur after transfer and mandates delayed skin grafting. The alternatives are those discussed above, including free tissue transfers.

### POSTERIOR CALF FASCIOCUTANEOUS FLAP

The posterior calf fasciocutaneous flap is indicated when skin and subcutaneous tissue can provide needed coverage, i.e., for impending prosthetic exposure or large soft tissue defects down to bone. It was a wide arc of rotation, and it can cover the entire anterior knee (Fig. 50-10). It is most useful when employed as an island flap, thereby eliminating exposure of the popliteal area and improving its arc of rotation. However, it does not bring in an abundant blood supply in cases of infection, it lacks bulk, and the donor defect is often unacceptable.

### VASCULARIZED FLAPS

Virtually any composite tissue can be utilized in the knee region depending on the requirements of the recipient site. The most reliable flap when local tissue is inadequate is the latissimus dorsi muscle or musculocutaneous flap. The rectus abdominis flap is also applicable if less muscle is needed. If muscle and bulk are not needed, the scapular flap serves reliably. The third attractive alternative is the lateral thigh septocutaneous free flap, which is good for durable yet pliable soft tissue coverage.

The dissection is relatively easy, the vessels are 3 to 4 mm in size, and it does not require prepping and draping a separate field. The only disadvantage is that the double team approach may be hindered with the two fields of operation in close proximity unless the contralateral leg was chosen as a donor site. There is also the possibility of limited donor site availability when a flap is raised from the side of the injury.

## *Leg*
### PROXIMAL TO MIDDLE ONE-THIRD OF THE LEG
Soft tissue defects involving the proximal one-third of the leg are accessible to conventional musculocutaneous and fasciocutaneous flaps. Anteromedial defects can best be reconstructed with a medial head gastrocnemius muscle flap and skin graft. The donor defect is closed primarily and limited to a single scar. The soleus muscle flap is most useful for reconstruction of middle one-third soft tissue defects. Fasciocutaneous flaps can also be employed. A secondary deformity of the donor site, however, is a significant consideration. Usually, fasciocutaneous flaps are employed when conventional muscle flaps cannot be.

Vascularized flaps are indicated when conventional flaps are not suitable. Indications include (1) extensive defects, (2) composite tissue loss, (3) trauma or disease that precludes use of conventional flaps, (4) restoration of function, and (5) aesthetic considerations.

### *Muscle or Musculocutaneous Flaps*
GASTROCNEMIUS MUSCLE. The gastrocnemius is a type I muscle whose medial head has its origin in the medial condyle of the femur. The lateral head originates from the lateral condyle. The vascular pedicle is usually single, originating from the popliteal artery and entering the medial and lateral heads at the condyles. The medial and lateral heads are separated by a raphe, joining the achilles tendon at the junction of the middle one-third and distal one-third of the

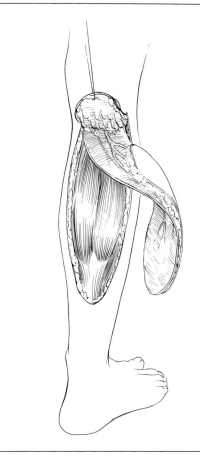

**Figure 50-10** *Posterior view of the leg demonstrating the fasciocutaneous posterior calf flap. Note that the superficial branch of the popliteal artery enters proximally. The large size of this flap enables one to cover a large area of tissue loss at a significant distance from the donor site.*

leg. The arc of rotation encompasses the proximal leg, knee and distal thighs. Usually the medial head is employed following separation from the lateral head at the raphe. The lateral head may be employed either singly or in combination. Injury to the peroneal nerve must be avoided. The muscle, or a portion thereof, may be employed alone and covered with a skin graft, or a cutaneous flap may be employed. In the latter instance the donor site often requires a skin graft. Sacrifice of the entire muscle results in weakened plantar flexion.

Middle one-third and proximal distal one-third defects can be reconstructed with a distally based medial gastrocnemius muscle flap. The vascular pedicle to the medial head is ligated and separated from the lateral head, dividing the proximal vascular branches from the lateral head. Distal branches remain. Problems may ensue because the medial vascular pedicle is usually larger and dominant.

SOLEUS MUSCLE. The soleus is a type II muscle, originating from the upper one-third of the fibula and middle one-third of the tibia. The long origin and segmental blood supply from the posterior tibial artery limits the arc of rotation to the middle one-third of the leg. The muscle fibers extend distally to the calcaneal region, farther than the gastrocnemius (Fig. 50-11). The soleus can be separated distally and is usually rotated laterally and grafted. A cutaneous paddle cannot be employed. The soleus muscle can be pedicled distally, but the posterior tibial artery and vein must be ligated just below the knee. Distal leg and ankle defects can be covered, but a major limb vessel is sacrificed. Furthermore, venous return must overcome the valve system, making congestion more likely. Persistent edema of the leg is also common.

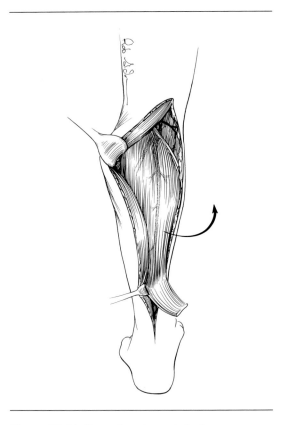

**Figure 50-11** *Posterior view of the leg demonstrating the soleus muscle elevated distally to the calcaneal region. Note that this muscle can be easily transposed laterally. The major pedicles from the peroneal and posterior tibial arteries are demonstrated, as are the minor posterior tibial artery pedicles. These pedicles limit the amount of movement unless one ligates them.*

*Fasciocutaneous/Fascial Flaps*

At the midportion of the lower leg several perforating branches from the posterior tibial, anterior tibial, and peroneal artery pierce the deep fascia and send longitudinal branches on its anterior surface. In addition, on the posterior surface of the leg, 4 cm distal to the crease, a branch of the popliteal artery pierces the deep fascia and courses distally. A fasciocutaneous flap, proximally based in the middle one-third of the leg, can be constructed with a length/width ratio of 2.5:1.0 to 3.0:1.0.

Defects of the middle and proximal distal one-thirds of the leg can be reconstructed. A fasciocutaneous flap is usually employed with a skin graft placed at the donor site. To facilitate rotation, the fascia may be incised proximally, taking care not to injure the longitudinal blood supply on the anterior surface of the fascia. Fascia alone may be transposed, but dissection is more difficult and prolonged, as the vascular plexus on the anterior surface of the fascia must be preserved with a thin layer of subcutaneous tissue. The posterior calf fascial free flap has been described.

Vessels perforating the deep fascia have also been described 8 to 10 cm proximal to the malleoli on the medial and lateral surface of the distal one-third of the leg. Distally based flaps overlying the peroneal artery laterally and posterior tibial artery medially have been described for wound coverage of the heel and ankle.

### Vascularized Flaps

Vascularized flaps (free flaps) are most indicated when conventional methods cannot be readily utilized. Extensive trauma may preclude the use of the gastrocnemius or soleus flaps. Extensive areas of soft tissue loss with bone devoid of periosteum or tendon exposure may mandate coverage with the microsurgical methods. Chronic osteomyelitis may require débridement and wound closure with well vascularized tissue. Vascularized muscle and omentum have been employed successfully. The restoration of function following compartment exenteration subsequent to electrical burns, tumor excision, or ischemia (Volkmann's) may mandate replacement with vascularized muscle to include a neural coaptation. Finally, aesthetic requirements may dictate the use of a microsurgical method for concealment of a donor deformity. Musculocutaneous and fasciocutaneous flaps have a significant donor deformity, whereas muscle flaps and skin grafts have less.

When skin alone is required, the scapular flap is the donor tissue of choice. If the recipient defect is extensive and avascular, a vascularized latissimus muscle flap and a skin graft are usually selected. Depending on recipient site requirements, the latissimus dorsi or rectus abdominis muscle provides suitable wound closure following débridement of osteomyelitic bone in the proximal or middle one-third of the leg. If the reconstructive goal is to restore compartment function, the contralateral gastrocnemius, latissimus dorsi, or sartorius may be selected.

### Miscellaneous Flaps

CONVENTIONAL FLAPS. Cutaneous direct distant (cross-leg) and indirect distant (Jump or Gilles) flaps are rarely employed for proximal or middle one-third soft tissue defects. Flap morbidity is great, as are patient morbidity, cost, and hospitalization.

MUSCULOCUTANEOUS (GASTROCNEMIUS) AND FASCIOCUTANEOUS (MEDIAL) CROSS-LEG FLAPS. These flaps have limited use, particularly when ipsilateral musculocutaneous units are not available and microsurgical expertise is lacking. The flap can be made longer, facilitating placement and recipient site coverage. Furthermore, the delays necessary for conventional random flaps can be avoided.

VASCULARIZED CROSS-LEG FLAP. Rarely, there is an indication for a vascularized cross-leg flap. During the course of a reconstructive procedure, a problem of the recipient site vasculature may preclude anastomosis of the dissected donor flap. The cross-leg concept can be employed utilizing the healthy contralateral recipient vasculature.

PERONEAL ISLAND FLAP. An island of skin as large as 16.5 × 14.0 cm or as small as 5.0 × 2.5 cm can be transferred on the proximal peroneal artery and vena comitans to defects about the knee and the proximal and middle one-third of the leg (Fig. 50-12). Based distally, with the proximal artery ligated, the flap can cover the distal leg and foot. The latter depends on retrograde venous return with problems of congestion similar to those outlined previously. Many times the donor defect from a flap of smaller dimensions can be closed primarily without a skin graft.

MUSCLE SPLITTING AND TRANSPOSITION. Defects in the middle one-third of the leg overlying the tibia may be closed with a portion of the anterior tibial muscle split longitudinally and folded over (Fig. 50-13). This procedure is made possible because the anterior tibial muscle is circumpenate and has an internal tendon throughout much of its length. Function is not diminished significantly. The turned-over muscle is grafted.

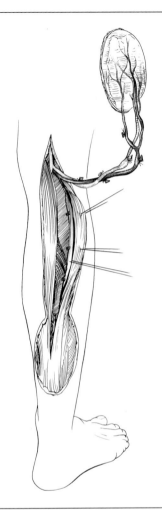

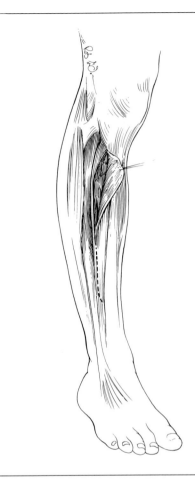

**Figure 50-12** Posterior view of the leg, demonstrating the peroneal island flap. Note the extensive dissection required for splitting the gastrocnemius muscle as well as the soleus muscle in order to gain a lengthy pedicle of artery and vein.

**Figure 50-13** Anterior view of the leg, demonstrating the split anterior tibialis muscle folding over to cover a defect of the tibia.

Obviously, this technique cannot be employed if there has been significant injury to the muscle in the anterior compartment.

DISTAL ONE-THIRD OF THE LEG

The distal one-third of the leg presents unique problems to the reconstructive surgeon. This region is characterized by the scarcity of muscle. Conversely, bone, tendons, and connective tissue predominate. Soft tissue loss, when it occurs, cannot be replaced easily with a skin graft. Furthermore, at this distal location the muscle mass is limited and the blood supply, comparatively, is reduced. The relative scarcity of soft tissue and diminished blood supply limits the amount of tissue available for wound coverage. Conversely, there is a high concentration of large vessels suitable for microsurgical access in this small cross-sectional area. As a consequence, vascularized composite tissue transplantation is often preferred to other methods of reconstruction of this distal location.

*Muscle Flap*

EXTENSOR DIGITORUM LONGUS. The extensor digitorum longus muscle arises from the upper three-fourths of the medial surface of the fibula and adjacent lateral condyle of the tibia. It is a type II muscle with segmental arterial supply from the anterior tibial artery along the length of the muscle. Approximately 20 cm from the ankle four or five perforating pedicles can be seen entering this muscle. The muscle is innervated segmentally by the deep peroneal nerve. The muscle extends the toes and dorsiflexes the ankle. It is an expandable muscle that works synergistically with the tibialis anterior and extensor hallucis longus.

The proximal muscle belly can be detached from its origin and the segmental blood supply interrupted. Perforators approximately 20 cm from the ankle are left intact. The muscle is folded over to cover distal defects of the lower leg and ankle. The muscle surface is grafted. Although a cutaneous paddle nourished by septocutaneous perforators can be employed, there is little added advantage to using muscle alone. Venous congestion is not a problem as intermuscular channels accommodate to increased flow, which continues through the remaining perforators in a normal antegrade fashion.

SOLEUS MUSCLE. A distally based soleus muscle flap has been described for coverage of the lower one-third of the leg. A concept similar to that described above exists. The soleus muscle fibers extend distally to the calcaneal region with perforators noted distally. The muscle can be freed proximally and turned around to cover distal defects. Disadvantages relate to the bulk of the turned-down muscle and venous congestion. A cutaneous paddle usually is not employed.

## GASTROCNEMIUS MUSCLE

A distally based medial head of the gastrocnemius muscle can be "turned down" to cover distal one-third defects. The surface of the muscle is grafted.

*Fasciocutaneous Flaps*

Distally based fasciocutaneous flaps have been previously described. A flap from the sural region based on perforating branches of the peroneal artery, piercing the deep fascia of the posterior border of the lateral compartment, can be employed for lateral defects of the lower leg, heel, and ankle. Similarly, a medial flap based on perforating arteries of the posterior tibial artery can be employed for medial lower leg and ankle defects. The donor site of the flap is usually grafted. Interestingly, fascial flaps without a cutaneous paddle have not been employed, perhaps because of a significant decrease in blood supply with loss of the dermal plexuses and mechanical problems related to compression and twisting of the pedicle, accentuated by the loss of cutaneous support.

*Vascularized Flaps*

Soft tissue defects of the distal one-third of the tibia and ankle are usually the result of trauma or osteomyelitis/osteitis. If the recipient blood supply is adequate, reconstruction can often be best accomplished with vascularized tissue. Chronic, contaminated wounds are best reconstructed with muscle. The proximity of the recipient blood supply to the wound permits greater selection of donor composite tissue, as the length of the vascular pedicle is not the most important variable limiting donor tissue selection. Small wounds can be covered with a portion of the gracilis muscle, larger wounds with the rectus abdominis muscle, and extensive areas with latissimus dorsi muscle. The muscle is usually grafted, limiting bulk and providing a more normal contour of the reconstructed area.

If chronic contamination of osteomyelitis is not a problem, tendon gliding and joint mobility with satisfactory contour can be reconstructed with a vascularized fascial flap from either the temporal region or the posterior calf. Like muscle, the surface is grafted.

Vascularized cutaneous flaps can also be

provided but are usually less desirable because of bulk. Reconstructed contours are less adequate, and often defatting procedures are required in addition.

*Miscellaneous Flaps*
Conventional flaps, musculocutaneous cross-leg flaps, vascularized cross-leg flaps, and peroneal island flaps (based distally) have been described. Each has limitations, and use must be restricted to specific indications.

An anterior tibial artery flap similar to the peroneal artery flap can also be employed. Limitations include venous insufficiency and footdrop due to injury to the deep peroneal nerve, which supplies the foot extensors. This problem can be minimized by the flap design below the midpoint of the extensor muscles. Venous insufficiency occurs because venous return is retrograde. Furthermore, a dominant leg artery is sacrificed. This method has applicability only when other methods cannot be employed.

## Ankle and Dorsal Foot
Vascularized composite tissue transplantation is clearly the preferred method of reconstruction, provided the necessary skills, support, and facilities are available. Selection of the appropriate donor tissue is described above (see Distal One-Third of the Leg). If this method cannot be utilized, a limited number of alternatives are available.

MUSCLE
*Extensor Digitorum Longus*
Use of the extensor digitorum longus is outlined above (see Proximal to Middle One-Third of the Leg). The turned-over muscle can be used to cover soft tissue defects of the lower leg and ankle. The muscle is grafted and the donor site closed primarily.

*Extensor Digitorum Brevis*
The extensor digitorum brevis is a fleshy muscle consisting of four slips located on

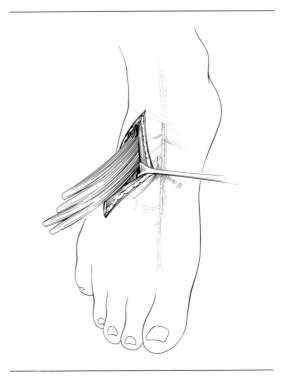

**Figure 50-14** *View of the dorsum of the foot, demonstrating the extensor digitorum brevis muscle flap. To maximize mobility of this flap the dorsalis pedis artery must be ligated distally.*

the dorsum of the foot underneath the tendons of the extensor digitorum longus and extensor hallucis longus. It takes origin from the calcaneus and talus laterally and inserts laterally into the extensor mechanism of the second, third, and fourth toes. It is supplied on its medial surface usually by two vascular pedicles, 1 and 3 cm distal to the lower edge of the extensor retinaculum. The muscle has the shape of a rectangular trapezoid with an approximate dimension of 5 × 8 cm (Fig. 50-14). The muscle is supplied by the deep branch of the peroneal nerve. After isolation on its pedicle(s), the muscle can be rotated laterally, medially, or posteriorly to cover moderate-size skin defects. The surface is grafted.

During the course of dissection and mobilization the dorsalis pedis artery is ligated

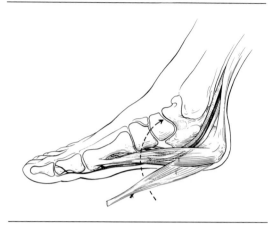

**Figure 50-15** *Lateral view of the foot, demonstrating the abductor digiti minimi. Note its small size and limited arc of rotation.*

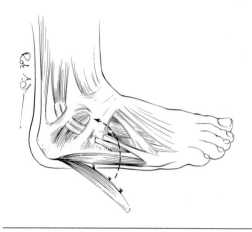

**Figure 50-16** *Medial view of the foot, demonstrating the abductor hallucis muscle. Note its small size and limited arc of rotation.*

distally with an attempt to preserve the branch to the deep plantar arch. The arc of rotation is centered on the dorsalis pedis—anterior tibial artery complex.

Disadvantages include sacrifice of the dominant blood supply to the dorsum of the foot and ankle, which is usually not a problem unless there is an associated injury to the posterior tibial artery at the ankle. Skin graft healing is usually complete, without tendon exposure noted in the dorsalis pedis flap.

*Abductor Digiti Minimi*
Transfer of the abductor digiti minimi muscle based proximally can be employed to cover small defects in the region of the lateral malleolus and heel. The donor defect is closed primarily. The surface of the transferred muscle is grafted (Fig. 50-15). Distal defects in the region of the fifth metatarsal can also be reconstructed with a distally based abductor digiti minimi muscle. Transfer is possible only if communication with the dorsalis pedis system via the deep plantar artery exists.

*Abductor Hallucis*
Transfer of the abductor hallucis muscle based proximally can be employed to cover small defects in the region of the medial

malleolus (Fig. 50-16). A distally based transfer is usually not advocated because of poor vascular communication with the deep plantar artery. The surface of the transferred muscle is grafted.

### FASCIOCUTANEOUS FLAPS
The distally based fasciocutaneous flaps described earlier in the chapter can also be employed to cover ankle and heel defects. Similar indications and restrictions are applicable.

### AXIAL CUTANEOUS FLAPS
*Dorsalis Pedis Artery Flap*
The dorsalis pedis artery flap was one of the first arterialized flaps described to cover calcaneal, medial, and lateral ankle defects. It is based on the anterior tibial-dorsalis pedis artery system and has a long arc of rotation, providing coverage to the distal one-third of the tibia as well (Fig. 50-17). It can be employed as a true neurosensory flap if the deep peroneal nerve is included. A relatively large segment of skin (8 × 15 cm) can be transferred. It has two significant disadvantages if selected for reconstruction as a cutaneous island. First, a major artery must be sacrificed, which is of particular importance if the pos-

terior tibial artery is injured at the ankle. Second, the donor site frequently presents a problem, with areas of delayed healing in the skin graft of the donor site.

*Lateral Calcaneal Artery Flap*

The lateral calcaneal artery flap, designed as an island, can be employed for wound coverage of small defects of both malleoli and the posterior heel region. A skin paddle (3 × 5 cm) located just below and anterior to the lateral malleolus is designed over the lateral calcaneal artery, demonstrated by Doppler pulse. The cutaneous paddle remains attached to its neurovascular pedicle consisting of the lateral calcaneal artery, lesser saphenous vein, and branch(es) of the sural nerve (Fig. 50-18). The length of the pedicle determines the arc of rotation. The donor site is covered with a skin graft. This flap, which has potential as a neurosensory flap, has applicability for reconstruction of small defects, especially of the achilles region and lateral malleolus.

VASCULARIZED FLAPS

Defects of the dorsum of the foot can be reconstructed with a fascial flap from either the temporalis or posterior calf. The former is more easily harvested in the supine position by a second team of surgeons working concurrently. The donor site deformity is minimal, having special applicability in the female patient. The fascial flap permits tendon gliding; it lacks bulk and provides a pleasing contour to the dorsum of the foot. Selection of the microsurgical method is particularly suited if the dorsalis pedis and anterior tibial arteries are intact. The entire dorsum of the foot can be reconstructed. A skin graft is applied to the surface of the fascial flap.

Vascularized cutaneous flaps can also be employed but are bulky. Extensive defects or chronically contaminated wounds are usually treated with cutaneous flaps or muscle flaps covered with a skin graft.

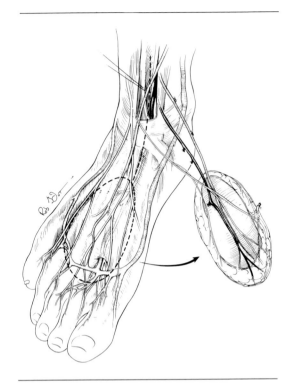

**Figure 50-17** *Dorsum of the foot, demonstrating the dorsalis pedis neurosensory island flap. Note the long pedicle and wide arc of rotation.*

MISCELLANEOUS FLAPS

The variety of flaps described in the section on miscellaneous flaps for the leg can also be employed. These flaps, however, are secondary considerations, employed only when other methods are not suitable.

## Plantar Foot

The plantar aspect of the foot consists of specialized skin. It is glabrous and, including the palmar skin, accounts for less than 4 percent of the total body surface area. In contrast to dorsal skin, which has a protective function, glabrous skin on the plantar aspect of the feet supports the weight of the body, facilitates ambulation, and serves as a mechanism for communication with the en-

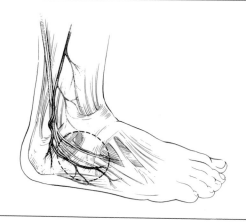

**Figure 50-18** *Lateral view of the foot, demonstrating the lateral calcaneal artery flap. Note that the pedicle can be long, enabling one to reach the contralateral side of the heel cord if necessary.*

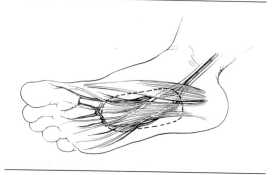

**Figure 50-19** *View of the sole of the foot demonstrating the plantar fasciocutaneous flap, which is shown here as an island. This flap is usually employed to cover a defect of the heel. Note the undisturbed plantar skin on the lateral plantar surface and overlying the metatarsal heads.*

vironment. Soft tissue reconstruction is dictated by the satisfaction of these special functional requirements. The ideal reconstructive goal is achieved when sensibility is restored and soft tissue coverage is provided with adequate padding over bony prominences with limited tangential motion. Special attention must be directed to the weight-bearing aspect of the foot, i.e., the region of the metatarsal heads, lateral instep, and heel. In general, the medial instep is non-weight-bearing and can be transposed to weight-bearing areas.

FASCIOCUTANEOUS FLAP

Fasciocutaneous flaps can be designed to consist of plantar skin and fascia; they are based on the medial plantar vessels and cutaneous nerve branches. The lateral plantar vessels and cutaneous nerves can also be included, but it is usually not necessary. A suitable amount of lateral plantar skin and fascia must remain undisturbed in the weight-bearing area (Fig. 50-19). Both medial and lateral plantar arteries can also be dissected proximally underneath the abductor hallucis to their common origin from the posterior tibial artery. The entire unit can be transferred or transplanted as a vascularized flap. To facilitate transposition, an intraneural dissection of the cutaneous nerve branches from the medial (or lateral) plantar nerve is required. Sensibility to the flap is preserved but may be altered. Sacrifice of the medial plantar artery does not adversely affect the blood supply to adjacent tissue. The lateral plantar artery is dominant. It may also be transferred in the flap, provided the dorsalis pedis artery with its deep plantar branch is intact.

The medial plantar artery can be sectioned proximally, isolating the medial plantar skin on the blood supply from the plantar arch. The flap can be transposed to cover defects over the metatarsal heads. Sensibility is significantly reduced, as cutaneous nerve branches are severed.

ARTERIAL CUTANEOUS FLAP

An arterial cutaneous flap based medially can be transposed to cover heel defects. The fascia does not have to be included. During dissection it is necessary to identify cutaneous branches of the medial or lateral cutaneous nerves (or both) and separate them from the medial and lateral plantar nerves for several centimeters. This maneuver preserves sensibility and facilitates rotation.

## VASCULARIZED FLAPS
### Fasciocutaneous Flap
As indicated previously, the goal of reconstruction of weight-bearing plantar soft tissue defects must include restoration of sensibility, provision of soft tissue cover over bone and tendons, and minimization of bulk and tangential movement. These goals are best accomplished with a plantar fasciocutaneous flap from the contralateral foot. Isolation of the flap on the medial plantar artery and cutaneous nerve branches is preferred, but the distal posterior tibial artery or the lateral plantar artery (or both) may also be included. Anastomosis and neural coaptation to appropriate recipient vessels and nerves are then accomplished.

### Muscle Flaps
Extensive plantar defects require cover with either vascularized muscle or cutaneous flaps. The latissimus dorsi muscle is the preferred donor tissue after transplantation, as muscle bulk is reduced with fibrosis and atrophy. As a result of this contracture, tangential stress is reduced. A cutaneous paddle is not included; rather, the surface of the muscle is grafted. The restoration of sensibility is limited. Long-term follow-up, however, demonstrates limited neurotropic ulcerations. This point emphasizes the importance of bulk reduction and limitation of tangential movement as important considerations for successful reconstruction.

### Cutaneous Flap
Vascularized cutaneous flaps can be employed to cover various-size plantar defects. A limited number of true donor neurosensory flaps are available, but nonneurosensory cutaneous flaps are employed most frequently. The vascularized scapular flap is often the donor tissue of choice. Dependent on many variables, especially age, sensibility returns within 4 to 6 months as a result of peripheral neurotization rather than from the relatively avascular and scarred deep bed. Consequently, if a nonneurosensory cutaneous flap is selected, wide excision of the scar and the poor quality skin adjacent to the recipient defect is recommended. Peripheral neurotization is facilitated from healthy surrounding tissue. The single disadvantage of a cutaneous flap is its bulk. After transplantation this bulk is often increased as a result of flap relaxation with absence of edema and surrounding wound margin contraction. Secondary operations are thus often necessary to reduce bulk and minimize tangential stress. Surgical attachment of the flap to the underlying fibrous tissue is attempted, as it serves as a substitute to the fibrous septae seen in normal plantar glabrous skin, which functions to limit tangential movement.

## Suggested Reading
### GENERAL INFORMATION
Godina, M. Early microsurgical reconstruction of complex trauma of the extremities. *Plast. Reconstr. Surg.* 78:285, 1986.

Gustilo, R. B., Mendoza, R. M., and Williams, D. N. Problems in the management of type III (severe) open fractures: A new classification of type III open fractures. *J. Trauma* 24:742, 1984.

Yaremchuk, M. J., Brumback, R. J., Manson, P. N., et al. Acute and definitive management of traumatic osteocutaneous defects of the lower extremity. *Plast. Reconstr. Surg.* 80:1, 1987.

### GROIN AND THIGH RECONSTRUCTION
Bostwick, J., Hill, L., and Nahai, F. Repairs in the lower abdomen, groin, or perineum with myocutaneous or omental flaps. *Plast. Reconstr. Surg.* 63:186, 1979.

Dowden, R. V., and McCraw, J. B. The vastus lateralis muscle flap: Technique and applications. *Ann. Plast. Surg.* 4:396, 1980.

Drimmer, M. A., and Krasna, M. The vastus lateralis myocutaneous flap. *Plast. Reconstr. Surg.* 79:460, 1987.

Irons, G. B. Rectus abdominis muscle flaps for closure of osteomyelitis hip defects. *Ann. Plast. Surg.* 11:469, 1983.

Mathes, S. J., Alpert, B. S., and Chang, N. Use of the muscle flap in chronic osteomyelitis: Experimental and clinical correlation. *Plast. Reconstr. Surg.* 69:815, 1982.

Nahai, F. Muscle and musculocutaneous flaps in gynecologic surgery. *Clin. Obstet. Gynecol.* 24:1277, 1981.

KNEE

Arnold, P. G., and Mixter, R. C. Making the most of the gastrocnemius muscle. *Plast. Reconstr. Surg.* 72:38, 1983.

Arnold, P. G., and Prunes-Carrillo, F. Vastus medialis muscle flap for functional closure of the exposed knee joint. *Plast. Reconstr. Surg.* 68:69, 1981.

Gryskiewicz, J. M., Edstrom, L. E., and Dibbell, D. G. The gastrocnemius myocutaneous flap in lower extremity injuries. *J. Trauma* 24:539, 1984.

Moscona, A. R., Gorrin-Yehudain, J., and Hirshowitz, B. The island fasciocutaneous flap; a new type of flap for defects of the knee. *Br. J. Plast. Surg.* 38:512, 1985.

Tobin, G. R. Vastus medialis myocutaneous and myocutaneous-tendinous composite flaps. *Plast. Reconstr. Surg.* 75:677, 1985.

LEG

*Proximal to Middle One-Third of the Leg*

Barclay, T. L., Cardoso, E., Sharpe, D. T., et al. Repair of lower leg injuries with fasciocutaneous flaps. *Br. J. Plast. Surg.* 35:127, 1982.

Barford, B., and Pers, M. Gastrocnemius-plasty for primary closure of compound injuries of the knee. *J. Bone Joint Surg. [Br.]* 52:124, 1970.

Hirshowitz, B., Moscona, R., Kaufman, T., et al. External longitudinal splitting of the tibialis anterior muscle for coverage of compound fractures of the middle third of the tibia. *Plast. Reconstr. Surg.* 79:407, 1987.

Mathes, S. J., and Nahai, F. *Clinical Applications for Muscle and Musculocutaneous Flaps.* St. Louis: Mosby, 1982.

Mathes, S. J., and Nahai, F. *Clinical Atlas of Muscle and Musculocutaneous Flap.* St. Louis: Mosby, 1979.

Maxwell, G. P., and Dibbel, D. G. Experimental definition of independent myocutaneous vascular territories. *Plast. Reconstr. Surg.* 63:176, 1979.

McCraw, J. B., Fishmann, J. H., and Sharzer, L. A. The versatile myocutaneous flap. *Br. J. Plast. Surg.* 62:15, 1978.

Ponten, B. The fasciocutaneous flap: Its use in soft tissue defects of the lower leg. *Br. J. Plast. Surg.* 34:215, 1981.

Yoshimura, M., Shimada, T., Imura, S., et al. Peroneal island flap for skin defects in the lower extremity. *J. Bone Joint Surg. [Am.]* 67:935, 1985.

*Distal One-Third of the Leg*

Amarante, J., Costa, H., Reis, J., et al. A new distally based fasciocutaneous flap of the leg. *Br. J. Plast. Surg.* 39:338, 1986.

Arnold, P. G., and Hodgkinson, D. J. Extensor digitorum turn-down muscle flap. *Plast. Reconstr. Surg.* 66:599, 1980.

Bashir, A. H. Interiorly-based gastrocnemius muscle flap in the treatment of war wounds of the middle and lower third of the leg. *Br. J. Plast. Surg.* 36:307, 1983.

Fogdestam, I., and Donski, P. K. Distally based fasciocutaneous flap from the sural region. *Scand. J. Plast. Reconstr. Surg.* 17:191, 1983.

Wee, J. T. K. Reconstruction of the lower leg and foot with the reverse-pedicled anterior tibial flap: Preliminary report of a new fasciocutaneous flap. *Br. J. Plast. Surg.* 39:327, 1986.

ANKLE AND DORSAL FOOT

Gang, R. K. Reconstruction of soft tissue defect of the posterior heel with a lateral calcaneal artery flap. *Plast. Reconstr. Surg.* 79:415, 1987.

Grabb, W. C., and Argenta, L. C. The lateral calcaneal artery skin flap (the lateral calcaneal artery, lesser saphenous vein and sural nerve skin flap). *Plast. Reconstr. Surg.* 68:723, 1981.

Hidalgo, D. A., and Shaw, W. W. The anatomic basis of plantar flap design. *Plast. Reconstr. Surg.* 78:627, 1986.

Hidalgo, D. A., and Shaw, W. W. The anatomic basis for plantar flap design: clinical applications. *Plast. Reconstr. Surg.* 78:637, 1986.

Holmes, J., and Rayner, C. R. W. Lateral calcaneal artery island flaps. *Br. J. Plast. Surg.* 37:402, 1984.

Landi, A., Soragni, O., and Monteleone, M. The extensor digitorum brevis muscle island flap for soft-tissue loss around the ankle. *Plast. Reconstr. Surg.* 75:892, 1985.

Leitner, D. W., Gordon, L., and Buncke, H. J. The

extensor digitorum brevis muscle island flap. *Plast. Reconstr. Surg.* 76:777, 1985.

McCraw, J. B. Selection of alternative local flaps in the leg and foot. *Clin. Plast. Surg.* 6:227, 1979.

McCraw, J. B., and Furlow, L. T. The dorsalis pedis arterialized flap: A clinical study. *Plast. Reconstr. Surg.* 55:177, 1975.

Scheflan, M., and Nahai, F. Foot Reconstruction. In S. J. Mathes and F. Nahai (eds.), *Clinical Applications for Muscle and Musculocutaneous Flaps.* St. Louis: Mosby, 1982.

PLANTAR FOOT

Harrison, D. H., and Morgan, B. D. G. The instep island to resurface plantar defects. *Br. J. Plast. Surg.* 34:315, 1981.

Morrison, W. A., Crabb, D. McK., O'Brien, B. McC., et al. The instep of the foot as a fasciocutaneous island and as a free flap for heel defects. *Plast. Reconstr. Surg.* 72:56, 1983.

Serafin, D., and Pederson, W. C. Philosophy of Restoration of Weight Bearing Area. In G. Brunelli and J. Steichen (eds.), *Reconstructive Microsurgery.* Italy: Brescia, 1987.

Serafin, D., and Ruff, G. Glabrous and Hairy Skin Free Flaps. In G. Brunelli and J. Steichen (eds.), *Reconstructive Microsurgery.* Milan: Brescia, 1987.

# 51

*John E. Sherman*

# Pressure Sores

The management of pressure sores is one of the few domains of plastic surgery that is not contested by the expanding dimensions of other surgical subspecialties. Accordingly, treatment of pressure sores is one of the most difficult challenges of reconstructive plastic surgery. Knowledge of epidemiology, pathophysiology, and prevention are essential for the successful treatment of these patients.

The terms *decubitus ulcer* and *pressure sore* are often used interchangeably. The *decubitus ulcer* is a pressure sore that develops over bony prominences when a patient is in the recumbent position. Thus pressure sores of the sacrum, heel, trochanter, and patella are decubitus ulcers. To avoid confusion, it is preferable to call ulcers that develop after prolonged and excessive pressure *pressure sores.*

## Epidemiology

Approximately 3 to 4 percent of patients hospitalized in acute care facilities and almost 40 to 50 percent of those in chronic care facilities develop pressure sores. Treatment advances in spinal cord injury with the resultant decrease in mortality has increased the population of paraplegics. The incidence of pressure sores in this group is approximately 5 to 8 percent yearly.

The sites of occurrence of these sores vary depending on the series reported. The largest series are from the Veterans Administration hospitals, comprised predominantly of paraplegics. In 1964 Dansereau and Conway tabulated the incidence of pressure sores by anatomic area among 649 patients with 1604 pressure sores (Table 51-1).

## Pathophysiology

Pressure sores almost invariably form over bony prominences (Figs. 51-1 and 51-2). The clinical sign of necrosis at the skin level is usually small compared to that of the necrotic area over bone and resembles an inverted cone. A staging system for grading pressure sores has been developed by Edberg et al. (Table 51-2). Knowledge of the early signs of ischemia is essential to the treatment of pressure sores. Several theories have been proposed to account for the development of pressure sores.

A *neurogenic trophic factor* was first proposed by Charcot in 1879. He believed that injury to the central nervous system caused decreased tissue tolerance to local pressure. This theory has not been proved.

*Shear forces* have also been implicated in

**Table 51-1** *Incidence of 1604 pressure sores by anatomic area*

| Location of ulcer | No. of lesions | Occurrence (%) |
|---|---|---|
| Ischial tuberosity | 447 | 28 |
| Trochanter | 310 | 19 |
| Sacrum | 278 | 17 |
| Heel | 138 | 9 |
| Malleolus | 85 | 5 |
| Pretibial area | 76 | 5 |
| Patella | 65 | 4 |
| *Total* | 1399 | 87 |
| Other sites | 205 | 13 |

*Source:* J. G. Dansereau and H. Conway. Closure of decubiti in paraplegics. *Plast. Reconstr. Surg.* 33:474, 1964.

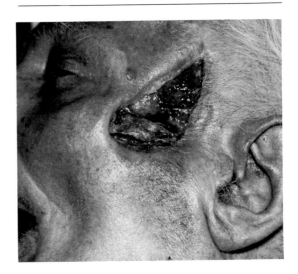

**Figure 51-1** *Pressure sore over the left zygoma in a patient after a cerebrovascular accident.*

the formation of pressure sores. By the movement of the skin and compression of small perforating blood vessels, ischemic necrosis has been implicated in the formation of sores. Dinsdale has shown that shear forces also increased the amount of pressure applied directly to the epidermis.

*Malnutrition and anemia* are contributing factors to the development of pressure sores. Any chronic systemic illness that impairs blood supply and delays wound healing can also be implicated. A debilitated, compromised patient seemingly develops pressure sores more rapidly than a patient who is in positive nitrogen balance and is healthy.

The most important factor in the development of ulcers is *direct pressure*. Unrelieved pressure that is maintained above the normal end-capillary arterial pressure of 32 mm Hg over a bony prominence results in an ulcer. Groth has shown that an inverse relation exists between time and pressure. The effect of this time and pressure depends on the patient's ability to restore blood flow and heal the damage after the ischemic episode.

It has also been shown that fat and muscle are more susceptible than skin to the effects of pressure. These areas are also closer to the underlying bone—hence the appearance of

**Table 51-2** *Stages of pressure sore development*

| Stage | Criteria |
|---|---|
| I | *Hyperemia.* Observed within 30 minutes or less, manifested by redness of the skin, which disappears within 1 hour after pressure is removed. |
| II | *Ischemia.* Develops if pressure is continuous for 2 to 6 hours. In contrast to hyperemia, redness from ischemia requires at least 36 hours to disappear after pressure is relieved. |
| III | *Necrosis.* Pressure not relieved within 6 hours may produce necrosis which is detected clinically by blueness of the skin or a hard lump similar to a boil. The necrosis does not disappear at a definite time interval after pressure is relieved. |
| IV | *Ulceration.* Within 2 weeks a necrotic area may become ulcerated and infected. If pressure sore progresses to this stage, bony prominences may become involved and destroyed. |

*Source:* E. L. Edberg, K. Cerny, and E. S. Stauffer. Prevention and treatment of pressure sores. *Phys. Ther.* 53:246, 1973. Reprinted with the permission of the American Physical Therapy Association.

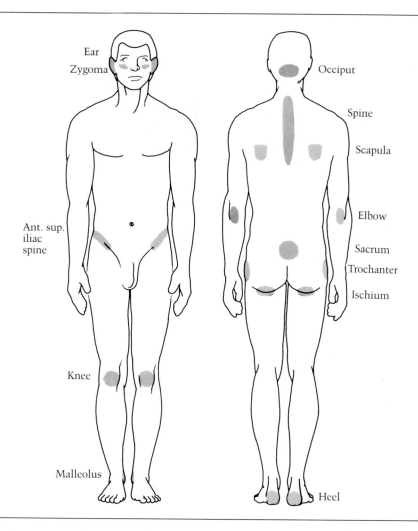

**Figure 51-2** *Most common locations of pressure sores.*

the "inverted cone" of damage, with the base of the cone near the bone.

Understanding the relation between time and pressure is essential. Pressures of 70 mm Hg applied for more than 2 hours causes irreversible tissue damage. If these pressures are relieved intermittently, the damage is significantly less. Lindan et al. quantitated the pressures of the adult man in the prone and supine positions (Fig. 51-3). They showed that these pressures are significantly higher than the end-capillary pressures—hence the potential for tissue damage.

## Bacteriology

Most wounds, especially in the hospital environment, are colonized. Granulating wounds are not clean wounds. Granulation tissue is the body's response to inflammation and bacteria.

To assess the degree of bacterial involvement and possible infection, a culture biopsy must be performed. Simple swab cultures have no place in the care of pressure sores. One gram of tissue is removed from the wound, and a quantitative culture is prepared. If the number of organisms exceeds $10^5$ per gram of tissue, infection exists and

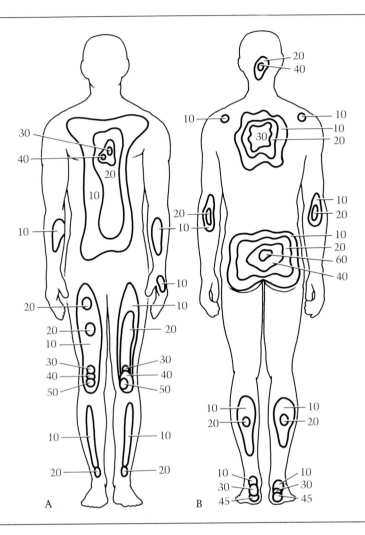

**Figure 51-3** *Distribution of pressures in a normal man. A. Prone. B. Sitting. (From O. Lindan, R. M. Greenway, and J. M. Piazza. Pressure distribution on the surface of the human body. I. Evaluation in lying and sitting positions using a "bed of springs and nails." Arch. Phys. Med. Rehabil. 46:378, 1965.)*

treatment, consisting in antibiotics and débridement, is essential. Antibiotics are helpful for treating the periphery of the wound where perfusion still exists. Considering the pathophysiology of the ischemic pressure sore, it would be naive to believe that systemic antibiotics could reach the center of the infected wound.

Wound cultures usually show a mix of gram-positive and gram-negative bacteria. Anaerobic cultures often show *Bacteroides fragilis.* Other organisms that are often involved are *Staphylococcus aureus, Proteus mirabilis, Pseudomonas aeruginosa,* and *Escherichia coli.*

## Prevention

*Avoidance of pressure* is the guiding principle to the treatment and prevention of pressure sores. Alternating pressure can minimize the development of pressure sores, even in the event of high pressures (Fig. 51-4).

Ideally, the patient is turned every hour. Patients who are able to do so must change their positions frequently. Sleeping in the prone po-

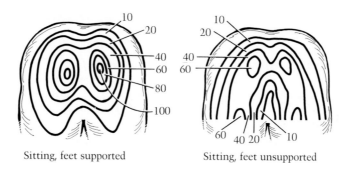

Sitting, feet supported          Sitting, feet unsupported

**Figure 51-4** *Distribution of pressures in a normal man, sitting. (From O. Lindan, R. M. Greenway, and J. M. Piazza. Pressure distribution on the surface of the human body. I. Evaluation in lying and sitting positions using a "bed of springs and nails." Arch. Phys. Med. Rehabil. 46:378, 1965.)*

sition is preferable, as the abdomen tolerates pressure better than the back. Attention is then directed to the anterosuperior iliac spines, which are not well protected.

When the patient is sitting, he must raise himself every half-hour to allow reperfusion of ischemic tissues. Uninterrupted sitting must not exceed 2 hours, at which time the patient may return to bed in the prone or supine position.

However, all of these remedies are not practical in most institutions, so a variety of devices have been designed to reduce the delivered pressure. Air-fluidized beds, such as the Clinitron, have been developed to reduce the pressures over the bony prominences. In these beds, air is pumped through a bed of Silicone-coated beads. Low air loss (LAL) beds have also been developed, in which the patient is supported by a column of air through cushions. In the LAL beds the patient can be in a sitting or recumbent position, and the shearing force is minimized. It also facilitates transfer of the ambulatory patient. Each of these beds reduces the pressure in the range of 15 to 30 mm Hg when they are properly used. Therefore these pressures maintain a level below that of the end-capillary arterial pressure over the bony prominences except in the areas of the heels, where pressures

have been recorded at 70 mm Hg. Therefore the heels must be padded even when these beds are employed.

## Treatment
PREOPERATIVE CARE

The surgeon must look beyond the pressure sore for initial management of the patient. Evaluation of the patient's nutritional status is essential. Laboratory studies include a complete blood count, assays for total proteins and albumin, and coagulation profiles. Urine cultures are routinely ordered. Treatment of any concomitant urinary tract infection is performed prior to surgery. Restoration for positive nitrogen balance is mandatory, which may require hyperalimentation or total parenteral nutrition. If the hemoglobin is less than 12 gm per deciliter, the patient is transfused. Prior to débridement, the ulcer is carefully examined. Radiographs of the bones often aid in determining the condition and thickness of the underlying bone.

Manual examination of the wound is done to assess the amount of undermining present. Ischial wounds are carefully evaluated to judge the proximity of the rectum. Patients are started on a high-protein, low-residue diet. Mechanical bowel preparation is started 1 day prior to surgery. Diphenoxylate (Lomotil) is also started preoperatively and maintained until 5 days after surgery.

In elderly patients who are incontinent of feces or in patients with massive ischial wounds impinging on the rectal area, a temporary or permanent diverting colostomy may be considered. Patients with sacral and ischial wounds are mechanically cleansed with enemas preoperatively and placed on diphenoxylate to reduce the possibility of fecal contamination.

Appropriate antibiotics are started in the presence of positive culture biopsies. If no organism is present in higher than $10^5$ concentration, prophylactic broad-spectrum antibiotics may be used during the pre- and perioperative periods.

After debridement and flap closure, avoidance of pressure on the operative site is essential. Patients are maintained on Clinitron beds for 1 week postoperatively to minimize pressure over other bony prominences that may appear during positioning.

Relief of spasticity in the paraplegic with a trochanteric or ischial sore is necessary prior to surgery. Spasms generally make positioning difficult, and the patient may be unable to rest supine or prone. In the past, surgical rhizotomy was performed for relief of spasms. However, only when the patient's spasm cannot be controlled with drugs should rhizotomy or cordotomy be undertaken.

## SURGICAL MANAGEMENT
### Debridement
Excision of the ulcer and necrotic tissue with the underlying bursa is necessary prior to closure. With severely contaminated wounds, debridement is not performed at the time of closure. Pharmacologic and enzymatic debridement is not often effective for the large, open wound. Debridement is performed in the operating room where exposure is maximal and control of bleeding is facilitated. Bedside debridement is ineffective and can result in uncontrolled bleeding.

After debridement, dressings are changed every 8 hours or at each nursing shift. Kerlex or gauze rolls are placed with silver sulfadiazine cream or povidone in the wound. Only silver sulfadiazine has been shown to reduce and maintain bacterial colony counts below $10^5$. The mechanical action of the gauze causing debridement is helpful. Small $4 \times 4$ gauze pads are avoided, as they can be lost in the periphery of the wound.

### Ostectomy
As noted above, the underlying bone plays a major role in the formation of the pressure sore. Consideration of partial or total ostectomy is necessary, as the exposed bone is often osteoporotic and osteomyelitic. This construction can serve as a nidus of infection if not removed. If total ostectomy is performed, careful attention is directed to the presacral venous plexus, which, if entered, could result in rapid, profuse bleeding.

The question of ostectomy for ischial ulcers is more involved. With partial ischiectomy, Conway and Griffith noted a reduction of the recurrence rate to 38 percent and with total ischiectomy 3 percent. However, after total ischiectomy the patient shifts his or her weight to the contralateral ischium, often developing a pressure sore over that site. In patients on whom bilateral ischiectomy is performed, development of peroneal ulcers and urethrocutaneous fistulas are also potential problems.

### Closure of Pressure Sores
The basic principles of closure are (1) debridement or excision of the ulcer with scar bursa and, if present, heterotopic calcifications; (2) partial or total ostectomy; and (3) closure of the wound with regional rotation flaps. As a master chess player must plan several plays in advance, so must a plastic surgeon when planning a flap. Considering the incidence of recurrence, there are two tenets to be observed when choosing a flap. (1) No matter how small a defect, a large flap is planned. It enables elevation and rerotation of the flap in the event of recurrence. (2) The choice of a local regional flap and closure of the secondary defect does not preclude the future use of adjacent flaps.

### Surgery
The choice of flap (i.e., random skin versus

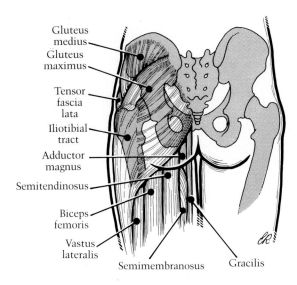

Gluteus medius
Gluteus maximus
Tensor fascia lata
Iliotibial tract
Adductor magnus
Semitendinosus
Biceps femoris
Vastus lateralis
Semimembranosus
Gracilis

**Figure 51-5** *Reginal anatomy of the sacrum and ischium.*

myocutaneous) is individualized for each patient. The use of a myocutaneous flap often prevents the use of adjacent flaps with overlapping skin territories. The increased bulk of the muscle protects the overlying skin by diffusing pressure. Mathes showed that the myocutaneous flap has a greater resistance to bacterial inoculation than random pattern flaps. However, Kosiak and Keane have each shown that the muscle is more susceptible to the effects of pressure than either skin or subcutaneous tissue. Isolated myonecrosis may occur, even with intact overlying skin.

## Closure of Specific Ulcers

### SACRAL ULCERS

As outlined above, ostectomy and débridement are performed either separately or in conjunction with flap closure of the defect. For closure of the moderate-size sacral ulcer, an inferiorly based random flap or gluteus maximus myocutaneous flap is preferred. The regional anatomy of the sacrum is shown in Figure 51-5.

The gluteal random flap, as originally described by Conway and Griffith, is designed to be as large as possible, so that if the ulcer recurs the flap can be elevated and reused. The length/width ratio should be no greater than 2:1 (Figs. 51-6 and 51-7). The donor site of the flap can be closed primarily or skin-grafted. Careful hemostasis is essential, and the use of several large Hemovac or Jackson Pratt drains is mandatory; these drains are brought out laterally through stab wound incisions.

The inferiorly and medially based gluteus maximus myocutaneous flap is also effective for closure of sacral ulcers (Fig. 51-8). In nonambulatory patients the entire gluteus can be used for coverage. In patients who are ambulatory the segmental use of the muscle is preferred to prevent hip instability. The superior portion of the muscle, based on the superior gluteal artery at the level of the piriformis muscle, is then rotated into the defect.

For large defects of the sacrum, two flaps can be used. A useful combination comprises two gluteus maximus myocutaneous flaps, one based inferiorly and the other based superiorly (Fig. 51-9). This "yin-yang"

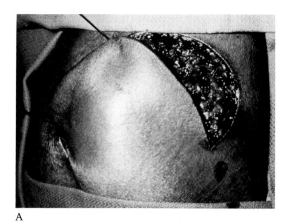

A

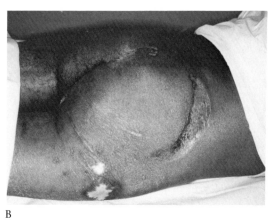

B

**Figure 51-6** *A. Sacral defect closed with a random gluteal flap. B. Postoperative result with skin graft of a donor defect.*

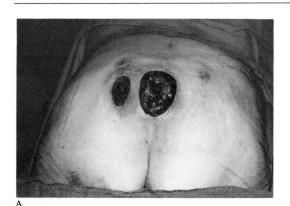

A

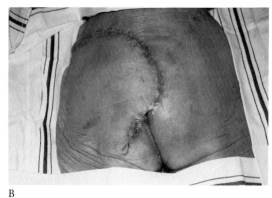

B

**Figure 51-7** *A. Defect of the sacral and parasacral area. B. Random gluteus flap covers both ulcers. C. Late result.*

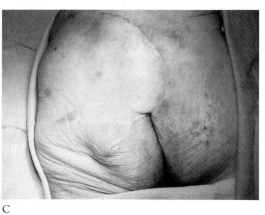

C

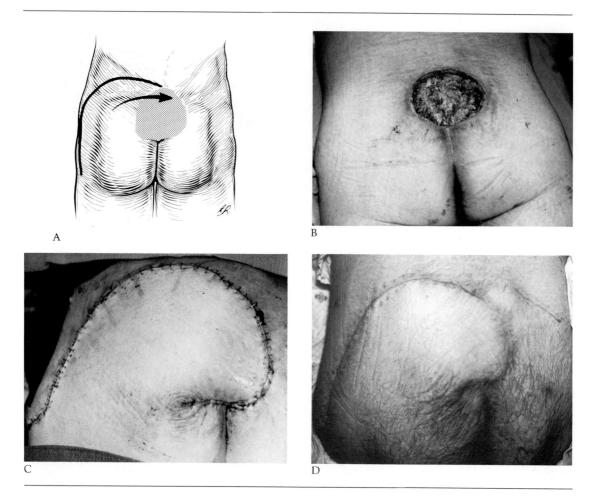

A

B

C

D

**Figure 51-8** *A. Defect of the sacrum closed with a gluteus maximus myocutaneous flap. B. Defect. C, D. Flap secured, late postoperative result.*

flap allows large defects to be readily closed but results in a suture line over the sacrum. Recurrences of the ulcer are treated with the elevation rotation of either or both of these flaps. Other flaps for closure of sacral defects include the transverse lumbosacral flap, bilateral gluteus advancement flaps, and the expansive gluteus maximus flap.

Sensation can be brought to nonsensate areas during flap closure with the use of sensory island flaps (Fig. 51-10). The upper quadrant flap is easier to use because of its simplified elevation and insertion.

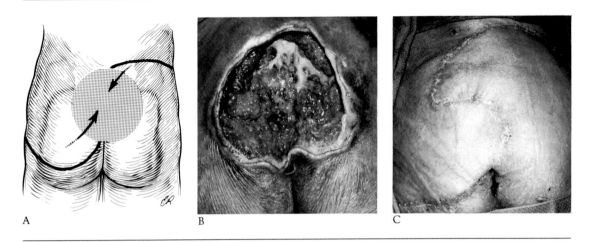

A          B          C

**Figure 51-9** *A. Bilateral gluteus maximus myocutaneous flaps for a large sacral defect. B. Sacral defect. C. Late healed result.*

**Figure 51-10** *Flaps for closure of the sacrum.*

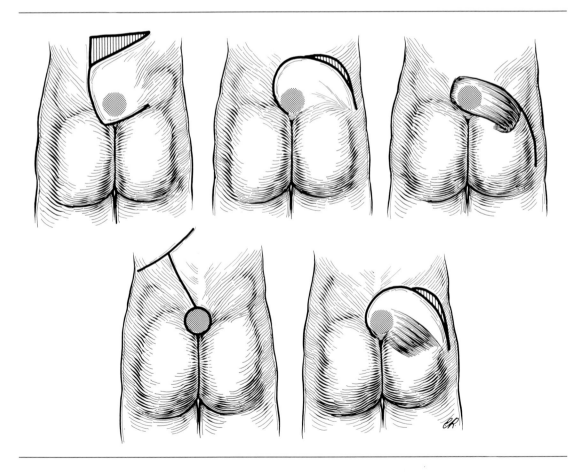

## TROCHANTERIC ULCERS

Debridement, bursectomy, and resection of the greater trochanter (Fig. 51-11) must be performed prior to closure. Of the many choices of flaps for closure of the trochanteric ulcer (Fig. 51-12), the most versatile is the tensor fascia lata (TFL) myocutaneous flap (Fig. 51-13). This flap is based on the lateral circumflex femoral branch of the profunda femoris artery. It can be elevated as either a rotation flap, an island flap, or a bipedicle flap. In debilitated patients after ostectomy, a vastus lateralis muscle flap can be used for additional bulk underneath the TFL flap (Fig. 51-14). If the TFL flap is wider than 9 cm, a skin graft can be used to cover the donor defect. This procedure is preferable to wide undermining of the adjacent skin for closure, which would impinge on adjacent skin flap territories.

Anteriorly based random thigh flaps and random bipedicle flaps (see Fig. 51-12) have also been employed for closure of these defects. After closure, suction drains are placed at the site of the greater trochanter and are brought out separately through stab wound incisions.

## ISCHIAL ULCERS

As discussed above, the effects of partial and total ischiectomy must be carefully considered. The regional anatomy of the ischium is shown in Figure 51-5. The flaps used for closure of ischial ulcers are outlined in Figure 51-15.

For small ischial wounds, closure can be effected with simple excision and closure of the defect. However, the recurrence rate of this simple closure is high. The random posterior thigh flap with skin graft of the donor site, as outlined by Campbell and Converse and by Conway and Griffith, is still a useful technique for closure of these defects (Fig. 51-16).

Closure can also be facilitated by the use of the island TFL flap (Fig. 51-17), the inferior gluteus maximus myocutaneous flap (Fig. 51-18), or the gracilis myocutaneous flap (Fig. 51-19). The bulk of the gracilis is carefully considered in paraplegics, as this muscle is often atrophic and difficult to dissect. Other flaps useful in this area are gluteal thigh flaps, as described by Hurwitz et al.

**Figure 51-11** *Regional anatomy of the trochanter.*

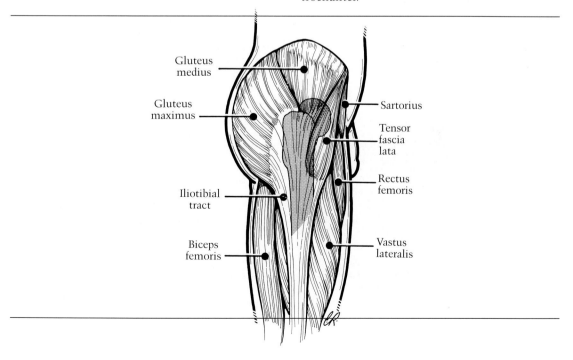

Gluteus medius

Gluteus maximus

Iliotibial tract

Biceps femoris

Sartorius

Tensor fascia lata

Rectus femoris

Vastus lateralis

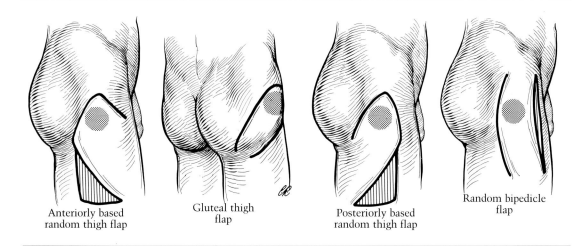

Anteriorly based
random thigh flap

Gluteal thigh
flap

Posteriorly based
random thigh flap

Random bipedicle
flap

**Figure 51-12** *Flaps for closure of trochanteric pressure sores.*

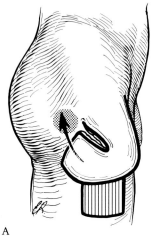

A

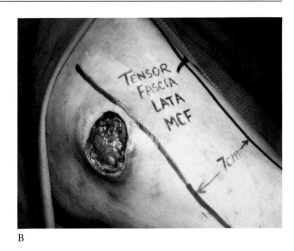

B

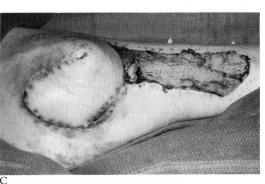

C

**Figure 51-13** *A. Rotation of tensor fascia lata (TFL) myocutaneous flap. B. Defect of trochanter. C. TFL flap rotated, donor site skin grafted.*

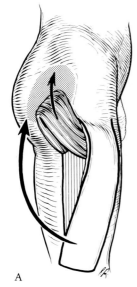

A

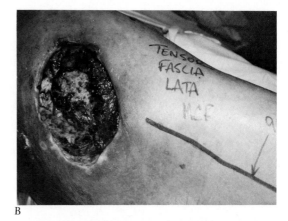

B

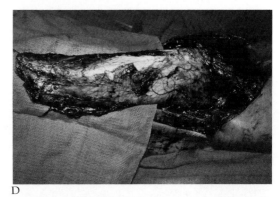

D

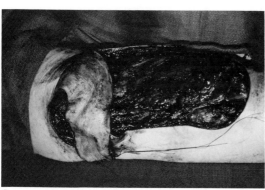

C

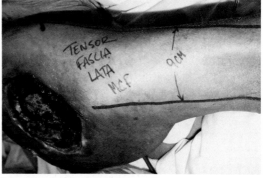

E

**Figure 51-14** *A. TFL and vastus lateralis flaps for closure of a trochanteric defect. B. Defect of the trochanter. C. TFL flap dissected and elevated. D. Vastus lateralis elevated. E. Flaps rotated into the defect. Skin graft closure of donor site.*

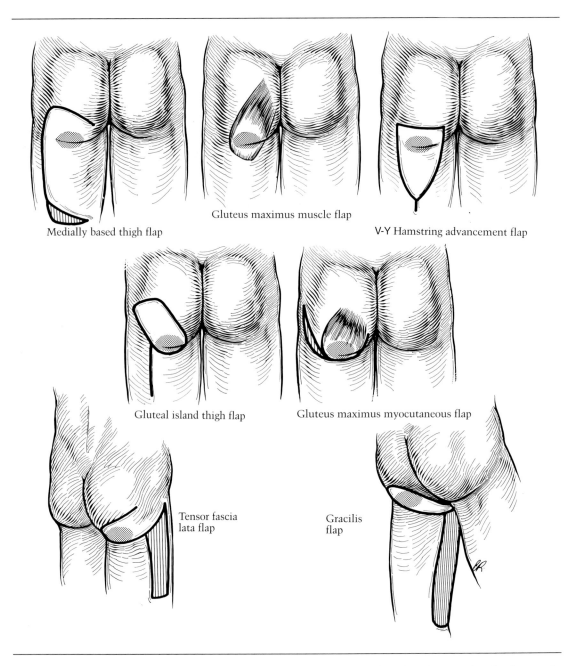

Medially based thigh flap

Gluteus maximus muscle flap

V-Y Hamstring advancement flap

Gluteal island thigh flap

Gluteus maximus myocutaneous flap

Tensor fascia
lata flap

Gracilis
flap

**Figure 51-15** *Flaps for closure of ischial wounds
(see flaps for trochanteric wounds).*

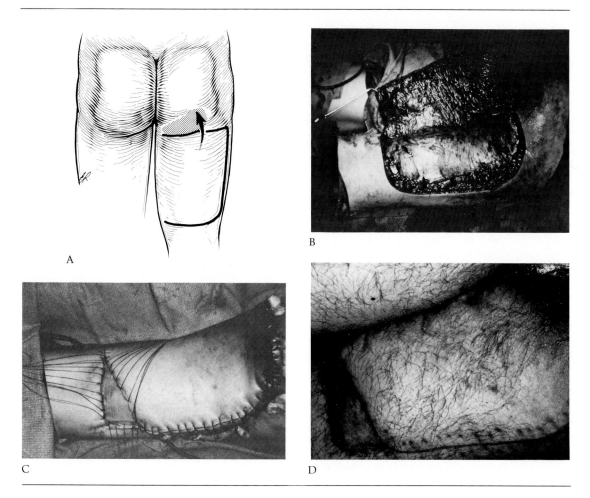

**Figure 51-16** *A. Random posterior thigh flap for ischial defect. B. Flap elevated. C. Donor site grafted. D. Healed, late result.*

## Amputations

Amputations are reserved for severe end-stage disease. They are performed only when there is untreatable infection of the hip or inadequate tissue for soft tissue closure over a joint. The hip is disarticulated, and resurfacing is accomplished with a total anterior thigh flap. As described by Georgiade and co-workers, the complexity of the operation is self-evident: These authors reported an average blood loss of 3000 ml, and there were 34 complications in 28 patients.

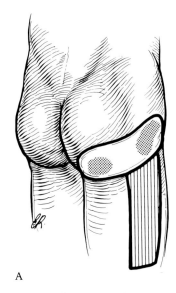

A

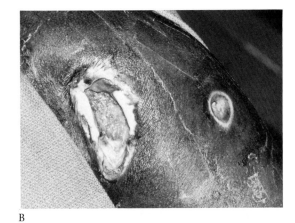

B

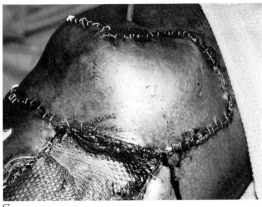

C

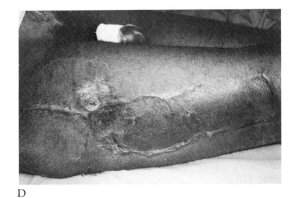

D

**Figure 51-17** *A. Island TFL flap for closure of an ischial and trochanter defect. B. Defect. C. Flap rotated and skin graft. D. Closure.*

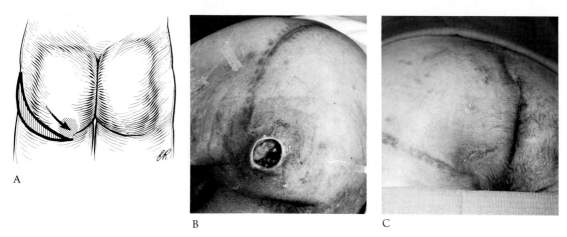

**Figure 51-18** *A. Inferiorly based gluteus maximus myocutaneous flap for closure of ischial defect. B. Defect. C. Late result healed.*

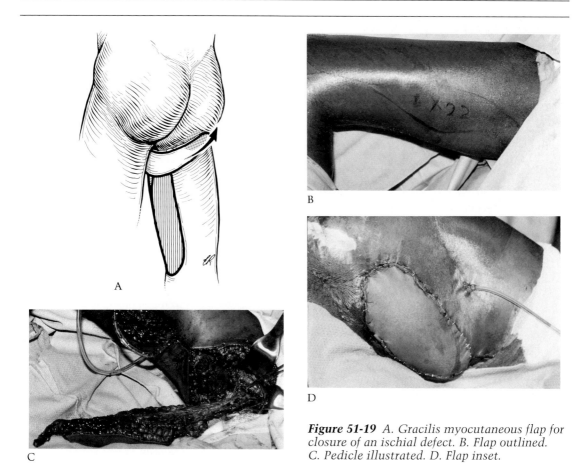

**Figure 51-19** *A. Gracilis myocutaneous flap for closure of an ischial defect. B. Flap outlined. C. Pedicle illustrated. D. Flap inset.*

## Suggested Reading

Bovet, J., et al. The vastus lateralis musculocutaneous flap in the repair of trochanteric pressure sores: Technique and indications. *Plast. Reconstr. Surg.* 69:830, 1982.

Calderon, W., Chang, N., and Mathes, S. J. Comparison of the effect of bacterial inoculation in musculocutaneous and fasciocutaneous flaps. *Plast. Reconstr. Surg.* 77:785, 1986.

Campbell, R. M., and Converse, J. M. The saddle flap of ischial decubitus ulcers. *Plast. Reconstr. Surg.* 14:442, 1954.

Chang, N., and Mathes, S. J. Comparison of the effect of bacterial inoculation in musculocutaneous and random-pattern flaps. *Plast. Reconstr. Surg.* 70:1, 1982.

Charcot, M. *Lectures on the Diseases of the Nervous System.* (2nd ed.). Translated by G. Sigerson. Delivered at La Saltpetriere. Philadelphia: Henry C. Lea, 1879.

Chase, R. A., and White, W. L. Bilateral amputation in rehabilitation of paraplegics. *Plast. Reconstr. Surg.* 24:445, 1959.

Constantian, M. *Pressure Ulcers: Principles and Techniques of Management.* Boston: Little, Brown, 1980.

Conway, H., and Griffith, B. H. Plastic surgery for closure of decubitus ulcers in patients with paraplegia: Based on experience with 1000 cases. *Am. J. Surg.* 91:946, 1956.

Daltrey, D. C., Rhodes, B., and Chattwood, J. G. Investigation into the microbial flora of healing and nonhealing decubitus ulcers. *J. Clin. Pathol.* 34:701, 1981.

Daniel, R. K. Muscle coverage of pressure points: The role of myocutaneous flaps. *Ann. Plast. Surg.* 8:446, 1982.

Dansereau, J. G., and Conway, H. Closure of decubiti in paraplegics. *Plast. Reconstr. Surg.* 33:474, 1964.

Dibbell, D. G. Use of a long island flap to bring sensation to the sacral area of young paraplegics. *Plast. Reconstr. Surg.* 54:220, 1974.

Dinsdale, S. M. Decubitus ulcers: Role of pressure and friction in causation. *Arch. Phys. Med. Rehabil.* 55:147, 1974.

Edberg, E. L., Cerny, K., and Stauffer, E. S. Prevention and treatment of pressure sores. *Phys. Ther.* 53:246, 1973.

Georgiade, N., Pickrell, K., and Maguire, C. Total thigh flaps for extensive decubitus ulcers. *Plast. Reconstr. Surg.* 17:220, 1956.

Ger, R. The surgical management of decubitus ulcers. *Surgery* 69:106, 1971.

Griffith, B. H., and Schultz, R. C. The prevention and surgical treatment of recurrent decubitus ulcers in patients with paraplegia. *Plast. Reconstr. Surg.* 27:248, 1961.

Groth, K. E. Experimental studies in decubitus ulcer. *Nord Med.* 15:2423, 1942.

Hauben, D. J., et al. The use of the vastus lateralis musculocutaneous flap for the repair of trochanteric pressure sores. *Ann. Plast. Surg.* 10:359, 1983.

Hill, H. L., Brown, R. G., and Jurkiewicz, M. J. The transverse lumbosacral back flap. *Plast. Reconstr. Surg.* 62:177, 1978.

Hurwitz, D. J., Swartz, W. M., and Mathes, S. J. The gluteal thigh flap: A reliable, sensate flap for the closure of buttock and perineal wounds. *Plast. Reconstr. Surg.* 68:521, 1981.

Kosiak, M. Etiology and pathology of ischemic ulcers. *Arch. Phys. Med. Rehabil.* 40:62, 1959.

Kosiak, M. Etiology of decubitus ulcers. *Rehabil. Rec.* 2:8, 1961.

Kosiak, M. Etiology of decubitus ulcers. *Arch. Phys. Med. Rehabil.* 42:19, 1961.

Kostrubala, J. G., and Greeley, P. W. The problem of decubitus ulcers in paraplegics. *Plast. Reconstr. Surg.* 2:403, 1947.

Kronskop, T., et al. The effectiveness of air flotation beds. *Care Sci. Pract.* November 1984.

Landis, D. M. Studies of capillary blood pressure in human skin. *Heart* 15:209, 1930.

Lindan, O., Greenway, R. M., and Piazza, J. M. Pressure distribution on the surface of the human body. I. Evaluation in lying and sitting positions using a "bed of springs and nails." *Arch. Phys. Med. Rehabil.* 46:378, 1965.

Linder, R. M., and Upton, J. Prevention of pressure sores. *Surg. Rounds* 23:42, 1983.

Minami, R. T., Mills, R., and Pardoe, R. Gluteus maximus myocutaneous flaps for repair of pressure sores. *Plast. Reconstr. Surg.* 60:242, 1977.

Nahai, F., et al. The tensor fascia lata musculocutaneous flap. *Ann. Plast. Surg.* 1:372, 1978.

Paget, J. Clinical lectures on bed-sores. *Students J. Hosp. Gaz. (Lond.)* 1:44, 1873.

Parry, S. W., and Mathes, S. J. Bilateral gluteus maximus myocutaneous advancement flaps: Sacral coverage for ambulatory patients. *Ann. Plast. Surg.* 8:443, 1982.

Royer, J., et al. Total thigh flaps for extensive decubitus ulcers: A 16-year review of 41 total thigh flaps. *Plast. Reconstr. Surg.* 44:109, 1969.

Schulman, N. H. Primary closure of trochanteric decubitus ulcers: The bipedicle tensor fascia lata musculocutaneous flap. *Plast. Reconstr. Surg.* 66:740, 1980.

Snively, S. L., and Tebbetts, J. B. Pressure Sores. In *Selected Readings in Plastic Surgery.* Vol. 3, No. 39, 1986.

Snyder, G. B., and Edgerton, M. T. The principles of the island neurovascular flap in the management of ulcerated anesthetic weightbearing areas of the lower extremity. *Plast. Reconstr. Surg.* 36:518, 1965.

Tribe, C. R. Causes of death in the early and late stages of paraplegia. *Paraplegia* 2:19, 1963.

Vasconez, L. D., Schneider, W. J., and Jurkiewicz, M. J. Pressure sores. *Curr. Probl. Surg.* 24:23, 1977.

Wingate, G. B., and Friedland, J. A. Repair of ischial pressure ulcers with gracilis myocutaneous island flaps. *Plast. Reconstr. Surg.* 62:245, 1978.

# 52

# Lymphedema

Timothy A. Miller
Andrew E. Turk

Lymphedema is a chronic condition involving the extremities that is characterized by the accumulation of protein-rich fluid within the intercellular space of the subcutaneous tissue and skin. For reasons that are not entirely clear, the deep muscle compartment is not involved in the edematous process. Lymphedema can be caused by surgical removal or destruction by disease of regional lymph nodes (acquired lymphedema), or it can result from an inborn error in the anatomy or function (or both) of the lymphatic vessels (primary lymphedema).

## Anatomy

Some embryologic aberration exists in the development of lymphatics in patients afflicted with primary lymphedema. It is generally agreed that lymphatics and lymph nodes arise from endothelial sprouting of the primordial venous system [3, 10]. This development begins in four areas: the paired jugular and iliac systems, the cisterna chyli, and the retroperitoneal system. These sacs develop peripherally and invade almost all tissues of the body with the major exceptions of the central nervous system, bone marrow, and coats of the eye. The thoracic duct results from fusion of the cisterna chyli and left jugular buds. Lymphatic channels and regional nodes of each extremity are eventually formed by the peripheral growth and drain to either the cisterna chyli (lower extremities) or directly into the thoracic ducts (upper extremities), which return lymph to the venous system. Variations in the communications between the major lymphatic trunks and the subclavian veins are relatively common [2].

LEG LYMPHATICS

Lymphedema occurs in the subcutaneous compartment. Under normal conditions this area is drained by three groups of lymphatics: a dermal plexus, collecting channels, and superficial lymphatic trunks. Intradermal lymphatics (which do not have valves) drain into a valved system lying in the deepest dermal level at the subcutaneous junction [3]. This portion of the lymphatic system would therefore be preserved in any pedicle flap. By means of collecting channels, the dermal plexus drains into main lymphatic trunks located in the superficial surface of the investing muscle fascia. It is these lymphatics that are seen in lymphangiograms.

In 1957 Kinmonth et al. introduced lymphangiography as a radiologic means for visualizing the lymphatic system [4]. Information about lymphatic drainage, evidence of obstruction, and characteristics of the number and quality of lymphatics has largely been obtained by this method. There is general agreement that the superficial (subcutaneous) and deep (muscle) lymphatic systems are separate and communicate only under abnormal conditions, e.g., proximal obstruction [6, 13].

The deep lymphatic system consists of several channels located adjacent to the bone [5]. In the leg, vessels can be cannulated posterior to the medial malleolus [8]. The superficial lymphatic system drains into two pathways closely corresponding to the venous drainage of the leg. As lymphatic vessels are seen on lymphangiograms they ascend in the deep subcutaneous area and maintain a constant diameter. Valves can be seen at relatively regular intervals (1 cm), creating a lymphatic lumen that does not increase in diameter as it ascends. For routine lymphangiography a soluble blue dye is injected into the web space of the toes. The dye enters the dermal lymphatics and eventually outlines the superficial mesial and lateral trunks, which are identified through a small incision, cannulated, and injected with contrast material. Approximately five vessels are usually seen along the medial aspect of the extremity, generally following the course of the greater saphenous vein to drain into the superficial inguinal nodes. A drainage system posterior to the lateral malleolus and paralleling the lesser saphenous system can also be seen along the lateral aspects of the leg. Approximately four vessels normally drain the subcutaneous tissue and skin into the popliteal lymph nodes located in the posterior knee. The collecting vessels ascend the thigh medially through the deep femoral trunk to drain into the deep inguinal nodes. Some of the posterior trunks may bypass the popliteal nodes and enter the superficial inguinal nodes. These valved trunks in the anterior and posterior subcutaneous systems bifurcate and rejoin, maintaining the same diameter as they ascend the extremity. In the normal system approximately eight

vessels are seen along the medial aspect of the thigh.

Some evidence exists that lymphatic channels draining the lower leg do not receive tributaries from the thigh. Lymphangiographic studies have shown that the thigh drains into the superior inguinal lymph nodes, whereas those from the lower leg drain into the more inferior inguinal nodes [7]. Therefore some patients present with acquired lymphedema and swelling that is limited to the lower leg.

The inguinal nodes are divided into two groups: (1) superficial (around the fossa ovalis) and (2) deep (within the fatty tissues of the femoral sheath). These nodes (approximately 15) drain into the nodes surrounding the iliac vessels. Although virtually all lymphatic flow passes through the inguinal nodes, it has been shown that lymph drainage can bypass these nodes and drain directly into the iliac area [11].

ARM
The superficial lymphatic channels of the arm appear anatomically similar to those in the leg, coursing along the general pattern of the basilic veins (medial aspect) and cephalic veins (lateral aspect). At times they join each other, but they normally course separately until they drain into the axillary nodes.

## Physiology

The lymphatic system serves a number of functions: drainage of a fraction of the macromolecular protein loss from the capillary circulation, removal of bacteria and foreign material, and transport of specific substances (vitamin K, long-chain fatty acids) from the gastrointestinal tract.

Lymphatics at the capillary level have no basement membrane and are therefore permeable [11, 15]. Because of this permeability, the low hydrostatic pressure within lymphatics (compared to interstitial fluid), and valves that encourage unidirectional flow, lymph passes proximally and does not normally accumulate within the interstitium. Lymph is essentially an ultrafiltrate somewhat similar to plasma. It forms as a transudate resulting from the relatively high hydrostatic pressure of the arterial system. According to Starling's law, the osmotic pressure within the blood partially balances this loss. The protein loss is substantial. During any 24-hour period, more than 50 percent of the circulating albumin is lost [15]. Although the major portion of that loss is resorbed into the venules by a combination of osmotic and hydrostatic forces, a minimal amount (approximately one part per thousand) is not resorbed [8]. The lymphatic system is responsible for the return of this fraction of the macromolecular capillary loss.

Lymph normally contains 0.1 to 0.5 gm of protein per deciliter in the extremities (compared to 6 gm per deciliter in blood). In this more dilute protein concentration, there is a disproportionately high albumin/globulin ratio owing to the higher molecular weight of globulin, which emphasizes the fact that lymph results from an ultrafiltration process across a semipermeable membrane. Once lymph enters a lymphatic space it is not appreciably altered or concentrated [12].

Lymph flow is comparatively slow and results from a combination of factors: interstitial pressure, the negative and positive fluctuation in intraabdominal and intrathoracic cavities, as well as the adjacent compression of arterial pulsation and muscular activity. The valves promote proximally directed flow. It is likely that the latter two extrinsic forces particularly influence the flow within the deep lymphatic system.

There have been some questions as to whether lymphatic flow is also due to an intrinsic contractile mechanism within the vessels themselves. One study demonstrated the presence of adrenergic receptors on the smooth muscle of the lymphatics, suggesting that spontaneous lymphatic contractility is an important force for the transportation of lymph [14]. Several investigators have shown that lymphatics respond to a variety of hormonal and chemical influences, and it seems likely that some peristalsis-like function does exist [1, 9, 17, 28]. If so, it would most critically affect the subcutaneous lymphatics that are not surrounded by muscle, as in the deep compartment.

Clinical lymphedema probably results from some etiologies involving impaired transcapillary fluid exchange or transport of lymph. Although different factors obviously characterize the primary (congenital) and acquired types of this condition, in both lymph drainage fails to keep up with production, generating the accumulation of relatively protein-rich interstitial fluid. Edema due to cardiac failure rarely contains more than 0.9 gm total protein per deciliter, whereas in chronic lymphedema total protein may be as high as 5 gm per deciliter [29]. According to the concept of Donnan's equilibrium, the resultant high osmotic pressure secondary to the high protein concentration attracts and obligates even greater amounts of fluid. It has also been observed that in lymphedematous extremities there is a 20 to 30 percent increase in venous flow, presumably as a compensatory mechanism [24].

With lymphedema a new balance of pressures is established, and the increase in interstitial pressure and surrounding tissue compliance tends to increase lymph flow. Wearing elastic stockings encourages this aspect of lymphatic drainage.

## Symptoms

The severity of symptoms can vary from mild extremity swelling to seriously disabling or life-threatening complications such as recurrent cellulitis and lymphangiosarcoma. Early edema fluid accumulation causes a soft, pitting type of edema usually beginning in the ankle and gradually ascending. Although measurement may reveal only a modest increase in extremity diameter, the associated weight increase can be substantial (e.g., an increase of 9 cm around the thigh results in an approximately 2-kg increase in weight). Such patients typically complain of fatigue in the involved extremity. As swelling increases, normal function can be compromised, and there is significant discomfort, presumably due to distention of the tissues. Corresponding with the duration of the process, the protein concentration of the edema fluid gradually increases [29]. This situation, combined with lymphatic stasis, provides an ideal culture medium for bacteria. As many as 25 percent of patients have recurrent episodes of lymphangitis [26]. Typically, these attacks are not preceded by trauma and have a rapid onset. Such attacks account for significant morbidity in some patients and can occur several times in a year. It is important to place these patients on bed rest and antibiotics immediately and to continue treatment for at least 10 days.

In time, fibrosis of the connective tissue elements within the subcutaneous tissue and skin increases, a process that accelerates if episodes of infection also occur. With chronic lymphedema (elephantiasis) the skin is thick and hyperkeratotic, and the entire extremity is indurated with a nonpitting edema. Knight et al. demonstrated that lymphedematous fluid had a biochemical imbalance in favor of collagen deposition in the skin and reduced lysis, which may explain, in part, the hypertrophic changes that can mimic elephant skin [22].

*Lymphangiosarcoma* is a rare, highly malignant endothelial tumor that can occur in any patient with lymphedema [18], although it is most common in the acquired form, particularly in postmastectomy patients. Similar to Kaposi sarcoma, it is characterized by the appearance of papular bluish lesions that often ascend the extremity. It occurs infrequently and usually only after lymphedema has been present for several years. Although it can be treated by a combination of surgery, radiotherapy, and chemotherapy, the condition is rarely cured. Early radical amputation of the affected limb appears to offer the best chance for survival [27, 30].

## Primary Lymphedema

Perhaps more accurately termed *idiopathic*, the classification *primary lymphedema* can be subdivided by age of onset or by lymphangiographic findings. In general, these two considerations are related.

Milroy's disease is a specific congenital form of lymphedema first described in 1892 [23]. A hereditary form of extremity edema that is present at birth, it is characterized by marked hypoplasia of the lymphatic trunks and a familial, sex-linked incidence [19].

There is general agreement that primary lymphedema stems from some anatomic developmental or functional abnormality of the lymphatics (or both). This category probably encompasses several conditions with varying and incompletely understood etiologies. Edema may appear at any time, from birth (lymphedema congenita) to middle age (lymphedema tarda), but the highest incidence occurs during adolescence (lymphedema praecox), accounting for approximately 80 percent of patients. The remaining 20 percent of cases are equally divided between the other two groups.

Three general lymphatic patterns have been described in primary lymphedema: aplasia, hypoplasia, and hyperplasia (varicose) [4]. The most common lymphangiographic finding is hypoplasia, seen in 70 percent of patients with primary lymphedema. After initial injection of blue dye into the web space, there is slow spread over the dorsum of the foot. Occasionally a single superficial lymphatic channel can be visually identified after injection of one of the blue dyes. On radiographic examination there is typically a single, slightly enlarged lymphatic vessel. In the aplastic form (approximately 15 percent) the blue dye diffuses readily through the dermal plexus but remains confined to the dorsum of the foot and rarely extends above the ankle. Upon exploration no lymphatic trunk can be identified. The blue dye can remain for months in these patients. In the hyperplastic or varicose pattern (15 percent), blue dye diffuses over the dorsum of the foot, and several trunks can be visualized along the anterior aspect of the ankle. Numerous dilated, tortuous channels filling easily with contrast medium can be seen radiologically. Moreover, dermal backflow (retrograde filling of the dermal plexus) is almost always evident. The varicose type is thought to be the consequence of incompetent lymphatic valves [4]. Also seen in other forms of lymphedema, dermal backflow is considered evidence of some form of lymphatic obstruction.

Lymphangiographic findings generally correlate with the age of onset [28]. In those individuals who have congenital or early-onset edema, the aplastic lymphangiographic form is likely, but when the onset occurs during adolescence the hypoplastic form predominates.

The uncertainties regarding the etiology of primary lymphedema derive from its many unusual, unexplained features: Women are afflicted at least three times more frequently than men; the left leg is affected significantly more often than the right one; and the upper extremity is rarely involved. No single pathophysiologic concept seems to encompass the spectrum of this condition. The tendency for symptoms to appear during the menarche and pregnancy suggests a hormonal cause, yet there is no explanation for the significant incidence in men. A particularly difficult aspect is identification of a precipitating factor. It is unclear why normal, middle-aged adults would develop lymphedema with no known predisposing cause.

Although most evidence seems to indicate that some anatomic abnormality is likely to be present in patients who have lymphedema, it is becoming apparent that this correlation is not absolute. In a lymphangiographic study of 200 patients, it was impossible to correlate radiographic results with the clinical severity of the condition [24]. In patients who have unilateral lymphedema, abnormal lymphangiographic findings on the clinically normal side are characterized [16].

Although a substantial number of these patients eventually develop bilateral swelling, others do not [21, 25]. It is therefore possible that, in addition to an anatomic abnormality, some functional derangement within the lymphatics may exist.

## Acquired Lymphedema

Whereas the basic pathology inherent in primary lymphedema undoubtedly resides in the lymphatics, the regional lymph nodes are the pathologic site in the acquired form. The axillary or inguinal nodes can be destroyed or damaged by surgery, irradiation, infection (filariasis, tuberculosis, lymphogranuloma, actinomycosis, cat scratch fever), or tumor invasion, or as the result of an inflammatory process (snake or insect bite, chronic lymphangitis). Perhaps the most common worldwide cause is direct infestation of the lymph nodes by the parasite *Filaria bancrofti*, estimated to have been the source in 200 million documented cases of lymphedema [15, 28]. The occurrence of permanent lymphedema complicating other infections or inflammatory processes, however, is unusual.

The other common cause of this condition is regional axillary or groin lymph node resection during the treatment of malignant tumors. Approximately 10 to 15 percent of patients undergoing radical mastectomy develop significant postoperative arm swelling [20, 31]. In a study of 200 operable breast cancer patients, it was found that radiation to the axilla after radical node dissection significantly increased the risk of postmastectomy lymphedema in the ipsilateral extremity [40]. The use of radiotherapy as well as obesity and postmastectomy wound-healing problems cause an even higher incidence. The swelling rarely begins immediately, usually being delayed for approximately a year, particularly following irradiation. This delay is likely the result of the ongoing fibrotic process, which further constricts and obstructs lymphatic drainage. The swelling generally begins in the upper arm and in some patients can become massive.

## Differential Diagnosis

In the vast majority of patients the diagnosis of lymphedema can be made by history and physical examination. The gradual ascent of edema from the ankle proximally over a period of several months, unassociated with other symptoms, is characteristic. Classically, the swelling occurs in females at the time of the menarche or pregnancy. In other instances it can be traced to a preceding trauma, although whether this incident actually precipitates the lymphedema process is often not clear. In most patients, no apparent cause can be identified. Although unilateral extremity enlargement always raises the possibility of malignancy, lymphedema from this source is rather unusual and is almost always accompanied by numerous clinical signs pointing to the malignant process.

A frequent diagnostic problem is the determination of whether leg swelling is due to a lymphatic or venous etiology. This distinction, in all but a few patients, can be made based on clinical evidence. Chronic edema secondary to venous disease is usually due to incompetent valves, a condition that increases capillary pressure. As a result, capillary perfusion is decreased, and in time a characteristic dark, brawny edema occurs. When the problem is long-standing, ulceration of the skin results from the impaired perfusion and tissue anoxia. With lymphedema, however, capillary perfusion is unimpaired and ulceration rare; moreover, the deep brown discoloration typical of venous problems is unusual.

Left leg swelling (which is seen in 60 percent of lymphedema patients), has been attributed to obstruction of the left iliac vein produced by crossing the right iliac artery. This disorder has been termed the *iliac compression syndrome* and was proposed as an explanation of the lymphedema [33]. However, few of these patients demonstrate

any classic evidence of peripheral venous disease, and it is difficult to see how venous hypertension can be reflected as lymphedema without a high incidence of chronic skin changes and ulceration. Venography in such cases is useful but not always easily interpreted [15]. When *acute venous thrombosis* is a possible cause, Doppler findings are valuable [32].

After a period of bed rest, lymphedema typically resolves within several days, whereas venous edema tends to improve within hours. In difficult diagnostic situations, venography is generally more informative than lymphangiography and considerably easier and safer to perform. Indeed, lymphangiography is tedious, difficult, and not without hazard. Fairbairn et al. reported 16 fatalities among 16,000 studies [35]. In the authors' experience this method offers little information that is not available on clinical examination. Moreover, it is associated with numerous wound healing problems, and the lymphangiographic findings almost never influence management of the patient. In an effort to find other noninvasive techniques for the diagnosis of lymphedema, the role of computed tomography (CT) scans has been investigated in patients with swollen extremities. A characteristic "honeycomb" pattern is often seen in the subcutaneous compartment of lymphedematous extremities [37, 39].

More recently lymphoscintigraphy (using technetium 99-labeled antimony) has been effectively used as a means of making the diagnosis of lymphedema and as a test for the selection of patients for microvascular surgery [42]. The method is noninvasive, and qualitative scintigraphy can identify normal lymphatic patterns as well as large collateral vessels and dermal backflow. Quantitative scintigraphy or the rate of lymphatic clearance can accurately detect incipient lymphedema [44].

Lymphangiomas are localized endothelium-lined spaces that can appear in the extremity as soft tumors. They are not uncommon, and 90 percent appear before the second year of life [31]. Like congenital lymphedema and cystic hygromas, they are believed to be an inborn malformation of the lymphatic system. Although they can occur anywhere in the body, the hands, feet, and tongue are the most frequent locations. They do not spontaneously regress. Their localized nature, spongy nonpitting texture, and failure to resolve on bed rest distinguish them from lymphedema. Treatment is surgical, usually postponed until the child has grown to allow the anatomic extent of the tumor to be defined more easily. The rate of recurrence from inadequate excision is high [36].

*Lipedema*, a relatively rare condition, seen generally in women, is considered a lipodystrophy and is characterized by diffuse, symmetric, nonpitting enlargement of the subcutaneous tissue of the extremity. A weight-reduction regimen often has limited effectiveness, and surgery is helpful in selected cases.

An unusual entity, *yellow nail syndrome*, was first described in patients with lymphedema and yellow nails [41]. The triad of yellow dystrophic nails, primary lymphedema, and bilateral effusions is also associated with an increased incidence of maxillary sinusitis. One report of yellow nail syndrome included a refractory pericardial effusion [43]. The etiology of this disease remains obscure [34, 38].

## Medical Management

Most patients with lymphedema can be adequately managed without surgical intervention. Unfortunately, however, neither the medical nor the surgical approach can provide a cure, and it is therefore imperative that the patient completely understands the chronicity of this condition as well as the importance of *controlling the edema* and *preventing infection.*

Medical management can only attempt to improve lymphatic drainage by periodic elevation of the extremity, external compression, and the use of diuretics. Patient education

and cooperation is crucial. The avoidance of unnecessary standing for long periods, placement of 6-inch blocks to elevate the foot of the bed, and conscientious wearing of elastic stockings are important practices. The stockings must fit tightly and be measured to the individual patient after a period of bed rest, when the extremity is smallest in diameter. New stockings must be obtained every few months to maintain firm compression. Full-length stockings or the leotard type often prove inconvenient, and as a result they are discarded. A knee-length stocking in many patients is an excellent compromise because it is considerably easier to use.

Diuretics are often initially effective and in rare instances completely resolve the swelling, but the improvement is usually not permanent. To be most beneficial, they are taken intermittently, particularly during the premenstrual period. One of the longer-acting thiazides combined with a potassium-sparing diuretic given 3 or 4 days a week is recommended, but if it is not effective often combinations can be tried.

Benzopyrones have been shown to be effective for high-protein lymphedema. The benzopyrones promote proteolysis by enhancing macrophage phagocytic activity, thereby removing interstitial proteins [49]. Clinical trials have demonstrated that benzopyrones reduce lymphedema. They do not offer rapid relief but can slowly improve chronic high-protein edema [45, 50].

Often infection cannot be avoided. In most patients no predisposing injury can be identified. Others have fungal infections of the web space that precipitate skin breakdown and an ascending lymphangitis. Meticulous skin care and antifungal treatment frequently prove successful without additional measures. In patients with recurrent infectious episodes of unknown origin, prophylactic penicillin is the drug of choice in view of the fact that *Streptococcus* is the most common etiologic agent.

When the infection occurs, it must be treated early and aggressively. The patient is restricted to bed rest and the extremity elevated until the infection has resolved. This urgency is explained by the fact that the infection can be fulminant, and each inflammatory process exacerbates fibrosis. It must be emphasized that for patients with the chronic, incurable condition, education of the patient and support by the physician are perhaps the most significant features of management.

Mobilization of lymph fluid by external compression has been shown to be effective. Zelikovski et al. [51, 52] developed a high-pressure (100 mm Hg) short-cycle sleeve with multiple cells allowing a sequential pressure that forms proximal flow. Cycled pneumatic pumps designed to provide distal-to-proximal pressure gradients favoring lymph flow have also been used [47]. The results are better with early cases of swelling. Those patients with long-standing edema and significant fibrosis within the skin and subcutaneous tissue are resistant.

Limb hyperthermia as a treatment for lymphedema has been used for centuries and has been reported [46, 48]. An electric oven is used to heat the leg to approximately 41° to 42°C (1 hour each day for 20 days). After the treatment the leg is tightly wrapped in an elastic bandage. Good results in a series of 1000 patients have been reported, with the improvement attributed to lymphatic regeneration.

## Surgical Management

Surgical intervention is considered only after medical management has been attempted and failed. Functional impairment caused by inability to control the size of the extremity represents the predominant indication for surgery. Patients frequently complain of fatigue related to the weight of the swollen extremity. Edema can account for 10 pounds or more of additional weight. Despite the fact that cosmetic indications have been minimized in the past, it must be remembered that this condition frequently affects adoles-

**Table 52-1** *Surgical procedures*

*Physiologic operations*
  Lymphatic reconstruction
    Alloplastic implants (Teflon, Nylon)
    Microlymphatic grafts
    Lymph node–venous anastomosis
    Lymphatic–venous anastomosis
  Pedicle flap
    Local rotation
    Ilium bridge
    Buried dermis*
    Omentum*
*Excisional operations*
  Total subcutaneous excision and skin grafting
  Subcutaneous excision underneath flaps

*Procedures that also include significant excision of subcutaneous fat.

cent girls, and the associated physiologic problems must be considered. Finally, in some patients, regardless of conscientious medical management, recurrent lymphangitis cannot be controlled.

The frustration encountered in the surgical management of lymphedema is reflected in the numerous procedures described over the last 70 years. Several techniques based on divergent theoretical justification have been advocated. In general, these operations (Table 52-1) may be divided into two divergent categories: excisional and physiologic. The excisional procedures remove varying amounts of involved subcutaneous tissue and skin. The physiologic procedures attempt to reconstruct lymphatic drainage by introducing distant or local pedicles or by microvascular techniques. The dermal flap and omental transposition combine excisional and physiologic components.

As yet no operative procedure has restored normal lymphatic function, and significant swelling recurs after all of the currently available approaches. Because of the recurrence of edema the postoperative evaluation of any given procedure is often highly subjective. Indeed, we lack objective, reproducible standards by which we can assess a patient's progress and accurately judge operative results. Although circumferential measurements are frequently used to estimate the magnitude of swelling, they are subject to considerable variations. To be meaningful, the same measurement must be carefully reproduced on each occasion. Ideally, it is done in the afternoon after a full day's activity, utilizing a bone landmark for reference. As previously mentioned, comparatively small variations in extremity diameter can represent substantial changes in fluid accumulation and weight. A more accurate but cumbersome method of documenting changes in size is water volume displacement [61]. Several radioisotopes, particularly gold ($^{198}$Au)- and $^{132}$I-tagged albumin (RISHA) and $^{99}$Tc dextran have been used to quantify lymphatic function. In normal individuals approximately 80 percent of RISHA injected into the web space is cleared in 24 hours [78], but in those with lymphedema the percentage is approximately halved [13, 61, 80]. RISHA clearance has been used to document postoperative improvement in lymphatic function subsequent to the dermal flap procedure [13, 61, 71] and subcutaneous excision [80]. If the contralateral extremity is used as a control in patients with primary lymphedema, it is recommended that there be a high incidence of bilateral lymphatic abnormalities. Variables such as the volume of radioisotope injected, activity during the test, position of the extremity, and monitoring techniques (size of counter, time) must be rigidly controlled and standardized.

## Physiologic Operations
DIRECT LYMPHATIC RECONSTRUCTION
Perhaps one of the earliest procedures advocated for lymphedema was the subcutaneous implantation of silk threads (lymphangioplasty) advocated by Handley in 1908 [69]. A wide variety of other materials were subsequently used, but such techniques have proved totally unsuccessful because of the consistently high incidence of infection and extrusion [13, 18, 28, 70]. Theoretically, it is difficult to conceive how valveless channels

formed around a foreign body can drain lymph against gravity; nevertheless, this technique has been reproposed [100].

The intimate relation between the lymphatic and venous systems was used by Rivero et al. in 1967 when they surgically approximated a hemisectioned lymph node to the side of a vein [98]. Early results were encouraging, and this technique was repeated by others who also achieved initial patency [90, 96]. However, fibrous ingrowth eventually occluded the communication several months later [54].

O'Brien, who obtained limited success with microvascular repair of lymphatics in patients with postmastectomy edema [92], advocated a minimum of three lymphatic anastomoses. This approach is obviously the most direct method of lymphatic reconstruction, but long-term evaluation and increased experience are necessary.

Encouraging results have been reported, particularly concerning the treatment of postmastectomy lymphedema by the use of autologous lymphatic vessel grafts. After the microsurgical anastomosis of two collecting channels removed from another extremity, postoperative alleviation of swelling has been seen clinically and documented by radioisotope studies [53].

Satisfactory results have been reported in 80 percent of patients with microlymphaticovenous anastomoses to treat lower limb obstructive lymphedema [79]. However, these data are unconvincing to other investigators. First, the microlymphaticovenous approach had greater success in patients with minimal edema, the same patients who can usually be managed conservatively with satisfactory results [97]. Second, circumferential measurements are subject to variability owing to duration of dependency and wrapping of the extremity [87]. Lastly, there were concerns about methods of defining lymphatics for microlymphatic surgery [93] and how long anastomoses remain open [102]. Microlymphaticovenous anastomosis has also been used for lymphedema of the breast,

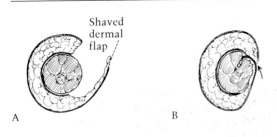

**Figure 52-1** Dermal flap. A. After excision of subcutaneous tissue. B. Buried in the muscle compartment.

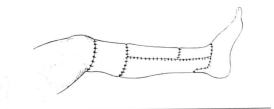

**Figure 52-2** Total subcutaneous excision followed by grafting.

scrotum, and female genitalia [74–76]. Advances have been reported with the microsurgical approach, including adipose venolymphatic transfers [95], harvesting a lymph collecting system as a composite graft [72], and tonometry [57] and lymphscintigraphy [103] as aids for microsurgery.

Basic research concerning lymphedema is encouraging with vein grafts [55, 105] and experimental models [58, 60]. However, the long-term success of microlymphatic repair depends on the patency of the anastomosis. In a study on the natural history of lymphovenous anastomoses, early anastomotic patency was excellent, but occlusion increased over the 8 months of the investigation [65].

PEDICLE FLAP RECONSTRUCTION

*Local rotation flaps* have been utilized [64, 104], but they have not been successful, probably because only the dermal lymphatic plexus is transferred. Kondoleon originally proposed the excision of deep muscle fascia so that the involved subcutaneous tissue would drain into the normal muscle compartment [80]. It was unsuccessful because of rapid fascial regrowth [94]. In 1962 Thompson introduced a procedure in which a deep-ithelialized *dermal flap* was buried in the muscle with the expectation of achieving a permanent lymphatic communication between the edematous subcutaneous tissue and uninvolved muscle compartment [106]

(Fig. 52-1). A favorable outcome of this operation for both primary and secondary forms of lymphedema has been reported [13, 28, 81]. Moreover, RISHA clearance studies have indicated postoperative improvement [13]. Although the success of this operation was attributed to the reconstructed lymphatic drainage within the dermal flaps, there has been no lymphangiographic documentation of function of this flap. The procedure is performed in two or occasionally three stages, and in each a substantial amount of subcutaneous tissue is excised (Fig. 52-1A). Almost identical improvement in RISHA clearance was noted after completion of subcutaneous and skin excision alone, suggesting that it is the excision of the subcutaneous tissue rather than the dermal flap that accounts for the improvement [80].

A pedicle of omentum has been employed to serve as a new conduit of lymphatic flow [67, 68] (Fig. 52-2). Although initial reports of this innovative procedure were encouraging, the long-term value and theoretical basis have been seriously questioned. Experimental studies have shown that no communication between the omentum and the extremity develops postoperatively [59]. Similar observations have been noted clinically at the time of reoperation, and the omentum was found to be surrounded by a smooth bursa-like sac [80]. Although the omentum is rich in lymphatics, its resorptive capacity is low [91]. In view of this finding and the fact that the omental lymphatics do not contain valves, it seems unlikely that substantial drainage could be achieved. Moreover, a high rate of postoperative complications after omental transposition has been reported [66].

In certain patients with lymphedema an unusual pattern of lymphatic occlusion in the iliac region has been identified by lymphangiography. Normal collecting channels are seen in the leg up to the level of the inguinal lymph node area. The proximal iliac lymphatics are reduced in number. With this comparatively rare entity, isotope scans clearly identify inguinal nodes. If contrast studies show patent distal lymphatics emptying into inguinal lymph nodes, alleviation of leg swelling has been reported utilizing an enteromesenteric flap. With this procedure a segment of ilium is removed with its mesentery intact. The mucosa is removed, and the ilium is then sutured to cover the inguinal lymph nodes after they have been transected. It is believed that lymph flow takes place between the raw surface of the lymph nodes and the ileal submucosa. Clinical experience has been limited but encouraging [77].

## Excisional Operation

### TOTAL SUBCUTANEOUS EXCISION

Originally described by Charles in 1912 [56] and commonly used since then, total subcutaneous excision is an extensive procedure that removes all of the skin, subcutaneous tissue (except in the foot and region overlying the calcaneal tendon), and deep fascia, covering the bare muscle with split- or full-thickness skin grafts (see Fig. 52-2). Although split-thickness grafts are technically easier and initially appear satisfactory, late scarring is marked and the grafts are likely to be injured easily, ulcerate frequently, and commonly develop a severe hyperkeratotic, weeping, chronically infected dermatitis.

On the other hand, full-thickness grafts taken from the excised tissue are considerably more durable [63, 83, 84], although it is admittedly a formidable technical challenge

to achieve a complete take of full-thickness grafts over such a large area. Moreover, if a problem with graft vascularization arises, the situation is exacerbated and morbidity is prolonged. Even when the grafts are successful, substantial scarring and chronic breakdown of these areas are not uncommon. With chronic, long-standing lymphedema, however, where there is a substantial element of fibrosis, this procedure may be the only technically feasible one available.

In some clinical situations, suction curettage has been suggested as a useful method for debulking lymphedematous limbs. Case reports have described the use of suction curettage as an adjunct to surgical management of primary and acquired lymphedema [82, 89]. It is difficult, however, to conceive how this method could be of significant value in the treatment of extremity edema of any magnitude without concomitant resection of the expanded skin envelope.

### STAGED SUBCUTANEOUS EXCISION UNDERNEATH FLAPS

Staged subcutaneous excision underneath flaps was first described by Sistrunk in 1918 [101] and later popularized by Homans [73]. In our opinion, this approach provides the most reasonable surgical compromise: It offers reliable improvement and a minimum of unfavorable postoperative complications. Improvement is directly related to the amount of skin and subcutaneous tissue removed as well as the personal care and attitude of each patient. The surgical procedure is presented to patients as a means of facilitating management of their lymphedema, not a cure [85]. During the operation as much subcutaneous tissue and skin are removed as possible while attempting to maintain skin flap viability and achieve primary wound healing [62, 85, 86]. An experience with 652 cases over 40 years demonstrated the safety and efficacy of this approach [99]. The following sections describe our preference with staged subcutaneous excision underneath flaps.

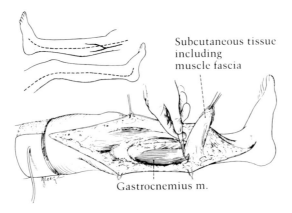

Subcutaneous tissue
including
muscle fascia

Gastrocnemius m.

*Figure 52-3* Subcutaneous excision on the medial aspect of the leg. Medial and lateral incisions are shown, and the area of subcutaneous excision is indicated by stippling.

*Preoperative Care*

All patients are placed at bed rest, and the extremity is elevated until the edema has subsided. Although this step can initially be done at home, the patient is admitted to the hospital 1 to 3 days preoperatively. A modified Thomas orthopedic splint suspended from an overhead frame may help patients with leg involvement. The rate of edema resolution can vary, depending on the chronicity of the condition and the amount of fibrous tissue present. While the patient is in bed, the extremity is washed daily. Preoperative antibiotics are not routinely used.

*Operative Technique*

The procedures are performed utilizing a pneumatic tourniquet placed as proximally as possible. In both leg and arm, more tissue can be removed from the medial than from the lateral aspect.

LEG. From a midmedial incision, flaps approximately 1.5 cm thick (2 cm in the thigh) are elevated anteriorly and posteriorly to the midsagittal plane of the calf (Fig. 52-3). The dissection is less extensive in the thigh and ankle. All subcutaneous tissue underneath the flap is removed. After excising the subcutaneous fat from the periosteum of the tibia, the deep fascia compartment of the calf is entered, affording a relatively avascular and easily developed plane of dissection.

Posteriorly, the sural nerve is identified and preserved. All of the attached subcutaneous fat and deep fascia along the medial aspect of the calf are removed. Dissection proceeds superiorly over the knee joint and inferiorly in the ankle region *above* the fascia, removing as much subcutaneous fat as possible. The flap is not developed beyond the anterior border of the malleolus. Because of the potential for avascular necrosis, flaps in the ankle are rarely longer than 6 cm. Substantial amounts of redundant skin can be excised (often 6 to 14 cm) (Fig. 52-4) after removal of subcutaneous fat (usually 450 to

*Figure 52-4* Closure after excision of redundant skin.

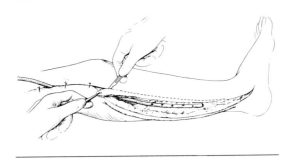

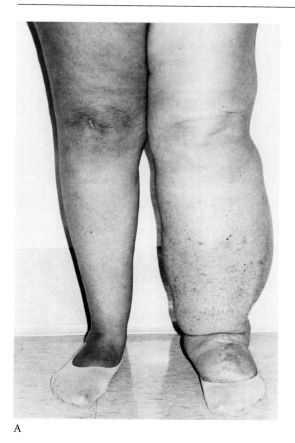

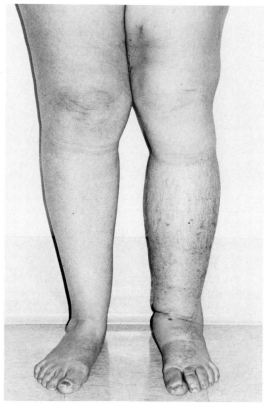

A

B

*Figure 52-5* A. *Legs of a 42-year-old woman with lymphedema of 18 years' duration after radical gross dissection. Two dermal flap procedures had been performed 5 years earlier. B. Patient's legs 1 year after lateral and medial skin and subcutaneous excision.*

900 gm). A rubber suction catheter is placed in the dependent portion of the posterior flap and is left in place a minimum of 5 days. Interrupted and continuous 4-0 nylon is employed for skin closure; no subcutaneous or dermal sutures are used. The extremity is immobilized by a gauze dressing reinforced with a posterior splint and is kept elevated. Sutures are removed on the eighth day and the wound secured by benzoin and tape. The patient is then measured for a form-fitting elastic stocking. Dependency of the leg is begun on the ninth day and ambulation by the eleventh postoperative day—but *only* when the leg is firmly wrapped.

The second stage is performed on the lateral aspect 2 to 3 months later. The operative technique is essentially the same, except that fascia is not removed and care is taken to avoid damage to the peroneal nerve or the sensory branches (superficial peroneal nerve) leading to the dorsum of the foot, which pierce the deep fascia approximately 4 to 6 cm above the extensor retinaculum of the ankle. Several months later specific areas of swelling in the ankle can be excised through separate incisions. The progress of a patient with lymphedema and who underwent this procedure is shown in Figure 52-5.

ARM. In postmastectomy patients medial excision is carried out from an incision extending from the distal ulna across the me-

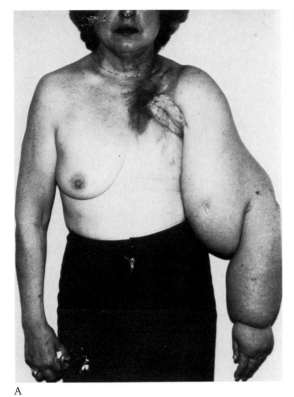

A

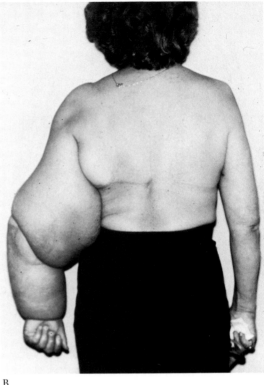

B

**Figure 52-6** *A, B. Arm of a 58-year-old woman 8 years after radical mastectomy.*
*C, D. Patient's arm 1 year after two-stage excisions.*

dial epicondyle through the posterior, medial upper arm. Flaps approximately 1 cm thick are elevated to the midsagittal aspect of the forearm and the dissection tapered distally and proximally. The deep fascia is left undisturbed. During lateral dissection the dorsal sensory branches of the ulnar and radial nerves are identified and preserved. Considerable amounts of fat can be excised from the upper arm. Flaps must be somewhat thicker in this area (approximately 1.5 to 3.0 cm); the ulnar nerve is identified in the region of the medial epicondyle and then traced proximally. Wide bands of redundant skin can be excised. If necessary, the tourniquet can be removed, the area prepped again, and the skin and subcutaneous tissue excised up to the axilla. A suction catheter is used for at least 3 days. The arm is immobilized and elevated for 5 days and there-

after can be placed in a sling. Otherwise, the postoperative management is similar to that described for the leg.

*Results After Skin and*
*Subcutaneous Excision*
Eighty-two operative procedures have been performed on 49 patients. Three postoperative complications related to ischemic necrosis of the flap have occurred, all of which healed by secondary intention and did not require further surgery. Although these patients have experienced varying degrees of decreased sensation (approximately 5 cm on either side of the line of incision), it has not

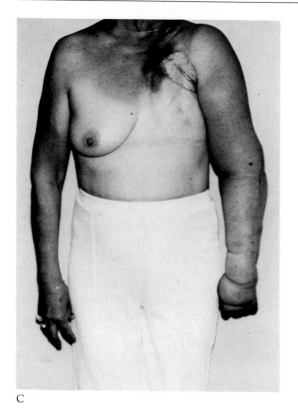

C

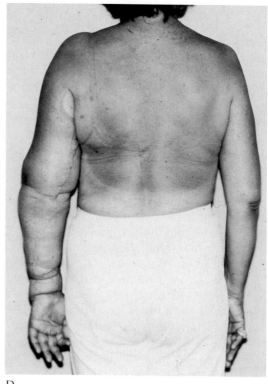

D

been a source of complaint. No alteration in hand or foot sensation has been observed. All patients have some recurrence of swelling. All patients wear elastic support stockings.

Sixty-five percent of patients have significant reduction in extremity size (range 30 to 60 percent reduction). Of the remaining group, 10 percent have had some improvement (10 to 30 percent reduction) that has lasted at least 2 years. The remainder have returned to preoperative swelling levels or continued to progress so that the extremity has enlarged. There seem little question that men have a significantly worse prognosis than women. The explanation for this difference is unclear.

The results of skin and subcutaneous excision for postmastectomy arm edema, however, have been much more varied. A sur-

gical approach is definitely indicated in patients with massive swelling. The postoperative improvement is usually significant, and function can be restored (Fig. 52-6). In ten patients surgically treated in this manner, arm volume was reduced 250 to 1200 ml, and the reduction has remained stable over a period of 1 to 6 years. In the remaining four patients arm swelling continued to become worse over the next 2 years despite the initial surgical reduction [86]. It has been observed that three of these patients with moderate swelling have had an increase in edema of the hand following skin and subcutaneous excision of the forearm and upper arm. Whether it is due to the surgical procedure or the natural progression of the disease is unclear. Generally speaking, however, staged skin and subcutaneous excision appears to have better results in the lower extremity than the arm, regardless of the etiology of the swelling.

*Postoperative Evaluation*

One year after surgery, a twofold increase in the rate of clearance of RISHA has been documented, suggesting that the excision of substantial amounts of subcutaneous tissue somehow improves lymphatic function [80]. The mechanism of this improvement remains unclear. Several possibilities exist: (1) Extensive surgical dissection may establish lymphaticovenous anastomoses during the process of healing. (2) The procedure may favorably alter the balance of lymph flow by reducing the amount of lymph-forming tissue while maintaining the dermal lymphatics. (3) The excision of substantial subcutaneous tissue and skin may result in external compression, effecting an increase in interstitial pressure (much like the effect of an elastic stocking), thus improving lymph flow.

Perhaps because there is always some recurrence of edema this operative approach was almost abandoned until recent years. Other, more theoretically appealing and innovative procedures, previously discussed, seem more attractive. Nevertheless, the discouraging fact remains that no procedure cures lymphedema; edema inevitably recurs after any of the currently available procedures. In our opinion, compared to all surgical methods of surgical management, skin and subcutaneous excision is the most reliable, consistently beneficial, uncomplicated means of managing the symptoms of lymphedema.

# References

ANATOMY AND PHYSIOLOGY

1. Acevedo, D. Motor control of the thoracic duct. *Am. J. Physiol.* 139:600, 1943.
2. Anson, B. J. *Atlas of Human Anatomy.* Philadelphia: Saunders, 1950.
3. Crockett, D. J. Lymphatic anatomy and lymphoedema. *Br. J. Plast. Surg.* 18:12, 1965.
4. Kinmonth, J. B., Taylor, G. W., Tracey, G. D., et al. Primary lymphedema: Clinical and lymphangiographic studies of a series of 107 patients in which the lower limbs were affected. *Br. J. Surg.* 45:1, 1957.
5. Larson, D. L. Deep lymphatic system of the lower extremity. *Am. J. Surg.* 2:217, 1967.
6. Malek, P., Belan, A., and Kocandrle, V. L. The superficial and deep lymphatic system of the lower extremities and their mutual relationship under physiological and pathological conditions. *J. Cardiovasc. Surg.* 5:686, 1964.
7. Ngu, V. A. Lymph drainage of the leg and its implications. *Clin. Radiol.* 15:197, 1964.
8. Rodbard, S., and Feldman, P. Functional anatomy of the lymphatic fluids and pathways. *Lymphology* 8:49, 1975.
9. Rusznyak, I. Recent experiments on the physiology and pathology of the lymphatic circulation. *Minerva Med.* 43:1468, 1954.
10. Sabin, F. R. The development of the Lymphatic System. In F. Keibel and F. P. Mall (eds.), *Manual of Human Embryology.* Vol. 2. Philadelphia: Lippincott, 1912. P. 709.
11. Selkurt, E. (ed.). *Physiology.* Boston: Little, Brown, 1966.
12. Taylor, A., and Gibson, H. Concentrating ability of lymphatic vessels. *Lymphology* 8:43, 1975.
13. Thompson, N. The surgical treatment of chronic lymphoedema of the extremities. *Surg. Clin. North Am.* 47:445, 1967.
14. Wang, G. Y., and Zhong, S. Z. Experimental study of lymphatic contractility and its clinical importance. *Ann. Plast. Surg.* 15:278, 1985.
15. Yoffey, J. M., and Courtice, F. C. *Lymphatics, Lymph and Lymphoid Tissue.* Cambridge: Harvard University Press, 1956. P. 1.

LYMPHEDEMA (PRIMARY AND ACQUIRED)

16. Buonocore, E., and Young, J. R. Lymphangiographic evaluation of lymphedema and lymphatic flow. *Am. J. Roentgenol. Radium Ther. Nucl. Med.* 95:751, 1965.
17. Calnan, J. Lymphoedema: The case of doubt. *Br. J. Plast. Surg.* 21:32, 1968.
18. Dale, A. The swollen leg. *Curr. Probl. Surg.* 140:1, 1973.
19. Ersek, R. A., Danese, C. A., and Howard, J. M. Hereditary congenital lymphedema (Milroy's disease). *Surgery* 50:1098, 1966.
20. Fitts, W. T., Keuhnelian, J. G., Ravdin, I. S.,

et al. Swelling of the arm after radical mastectomy. *Surgery* 35:460, 1954.

21. Gough, M. H. Primary lymphedema: Clinical and lymphangiographic studies. *Br. J. Surg.* 53:917, 1966.

22. Knight, K. R., Collopy, P. A., McCann, J. J., et al. Protein metabolism and fibrosis in experimental canine obstructive lymphedema. *J. Lab. Clin. Med.* 110:558, 1987.

23. Milroy, W. F. An undescribed variety of hereditary oedema. *N.Y. Med. J.* 56:505, 1892.

24. Pflug, J. J., and Calnan, J. S. The normal anatomy of the lymphatic system in the human leg. *Br. J. Surg.* 58:925, 1971.

25. Rooe, T. de. The value of lymphography in lymphedema. *Surg. Gynecol. Obstet.* 124:755, 1967.

26. Schirger, A., Harrison, E. G., and Janes, J. M. Idiopathic lymphedema: Review of 131 cases. *J.A.M.A.* 182:14, 1962.

27. Sordillo, P. P., Chapman, R., Hajdu, S. I., et al. Lymphangiosarcoma. *Cancer* 48:1674, 1981.

28. Stone, E. J., and Hugo, N. E. Lymphedema. *Surg. Gynecol. Obstet.* 135:625, 1972.

29. Taylor, G. W., Kinmonth, J. B., Rollinson, E., et al. Lymphatic circulation studied with radioactive plasma protein. *Br. Med. J.* 1:133, 1957.

30. Tomita, K., Yokogawa, A., Oda, Y., et al. Lymphangiosarcoma in postmastectomy lymphedema (Stewart-Treves syndrome): Ultrastructural and immunohistologic characteristics. *J. Surg. Oncol.* 38:275, 1988.

31. Treves, N. An evaluation of the etiological factors of lymphedema following radical mastectomy. *Cancer* 10:444, 1957.

## DIFFERENTIAL DIAGNOSIS

32. Barnes, R. W., Wu, K. K., and Hoak, J. C. Differentiation of superficial thrombophlebitis from lymphangitis by Doppler ultrasound. *Surg. Gynecol. Obstet.* 143:23, 1976.

33. Crockett, F. The iliac compression syndrome. *Br. J. Surg.* 52:391, 1967.

34. David. I., Crawford, F. A., Jr., Hendrix, G. H., et al. Thoracic surgical implications of the yellow nail syndrome. *J. Thorac. Cardiovasc. Surg.* 91:788, 1986.

35. Fairbairn, J. F., Juergens, J. L., and Spittell, J. A. *Peripheral Vascular Diseases* 4th ed. Philadelphia: Saunders, 1972.

36. Fonkalsrud, E. W. Surgical management of congenital malformations of the lymphatic system. *Am. J. Surg.* 1238:152, 1974.

37. Goltner, E., Gass, P., Haas, J. P., et al. The importance of volumetry, lymphscintigraphy and computer tomography in the diagnosis of brachial edema after mastectomy. *Lymphology* 21:134, 1988.

38. Gupta, A. K., Davies, G. M., and Haberman, H. F. Yellow nail syndrome. *Cutis* 37:371, 1986.

39. Hadjis, N. S., Carr, D. H., Banks, L., et al. The role of CT in the diagnosis of primary lymphedema of the lower limb. *A.J.R.* 144: 361, 1985.

40. Kissin, M. W., della Rovere, G. Q., Easton, D., et al. Risk of lymphoedema following the treatment of breast cancer. *Br. J. Surg.* 73:580, 1986.

41. Samman, P. D., and White, W. F. The "yellow nail" syndrome. *Br. J. Dermatol.* 76:153, 1964.

42. Vaqueiro, M., Gloviczki, P., Fisher, J., et al. Lymphscintigraphy in lymphedema: An aid to microsurgery. *J. Nucl. Med.* 27:1125, 1986.

43. Wakasa, M., Imaizumi, T., Suyama, A., et al. Yellow nail syndrome associated with chronic pericardial effusion. *Chest* 92:366, 1987.

44. Weissleder, H., and Weissleder, R. Lymphedema: Evaluation of qualitative and quantitative lymphscintigraphy in 238 patients. *Radiology* 167:729, 1988.

## MEDICAL THERAPY

45. Casley-Smith, J. R., and Casley-Smith, J. R. The pathophysiology of lymphedema and the action of benzo-pyrones in reducing it. *Lymphology* 21:190, 1988.

46. Chen, F. Y. Traditional oven heating for treatment of elephantiasis of the lower legs. *Chin. Surg. J.* 12:1, 1964.

47. Klein, M. J., Alexander, M. A., Wright, J. M., et al. Treatment of adult lower extremity lymphedema with the Wright linear pump: Statistical analysis of a clinical trial. *Arch. Phys. Med. Rehabil.* 69:202, 1988.

48. Lin, W. Y. Heating and bandage treatment for treating chronic lymphedema of the extremity. Unpublished report from the Department of Plastic and Reconstructive Surgery, The Ninth People's Hospital, Shanghai's Second Medical College.

49. Piller, N. B. Lymphedema, macrophages, and benzopyrones. *Lymphology* 13:109, 1980.

50. Piller, N. B., Morgan, R. G., and Casley-Smith, J. R. A double-blind, cross-over trial of O-(beta-hydroxyethyl)-rutosides (benzopyrones) in the treatment of lymphoedema of the arms and legs. *Br. J. Plast. Surg.* 41:20, 1988.

51. Richman, D. M., O'Donnell, T. F., and Zelikovski, A. Sequential pneumatic compression for lymphedema. *Arch. Surg.* 120:1116, 1985.

52. Zelikovski, A., Deutsch, A., and Reiss, R. The sequential pneumatic compression device in surgery for lymphedema of the limbs. *J. Cardiovasc. Surg.* 24:122, 1983.

SURGICAL THERAPY

53. Baumeister, R. G., Siuda, S., Bohmert, H., et al. A microsurgical method for reconstruction of interrupted lymphatic pathways: Autologous lymph-vessel transplantation for treatment of lymphedemas. *Scand. J. Plast. Reconstr. Surg.* 20:141, 1986.

54. Calnan, J. S., Reis, N. D., Rivero, O. R., et al. The natural history of lymph node-to-vein anastomosis. *Br. J. Plast. Surg.* 20:134, 1967.

55. Chang, T. S., Han, L. Y., and Hwang, W. Y. Venous versus lymphatic duct autotransplantation in the treatment of experimental lymphedema. *Ann. Plast. Surg.* 15:296, 1985.

56. Charles, R. H. *A System of Treatment.* Vol. 3. London: Churchill, 1912. P. 504.

57. Chen, H. C., O'Brien, B. M., Pribaz, J. J., et al. The use of tonometry in the assessment of upper extremity lymphoedema. *Br. J. Plast. Surg.* 41:399, 1988.

58. Chen, H. C., Pribaz, J. J., O'Brien, B. M., et al. Creation of distal canine limb lymphedema. *Plast. Reconstr. Surg.* 83:1022, 1989.

59. Danese, C. A., Papioannou, A. N., Morales, L. E., et al. Surgical approaches to lymphatic blocks. *Surgery* 56:821, 1968.

60. Das, S. K., Franklin, J. D., O'Brien, B. M., et al. A practical model of secondary lymphedema in dogs. *Plast. Reconstr. Surg.* 68:422, 1981.

61. Emmet, A. J., Barron, J. N., and Veall, N. The use of I 131 albumin tissue clearance measurements and other physiological tests for the clinical assessment of patients with lymphoedema. *Br. J. Plast. Surg.* 20:1, 1967.

62. Fonkalsrud, E. W., and Coulson, W. F. Management of congenital lymphedema in infants and children. *Ann. Surg.* 177:280, 1973.

63. Gibston, T., and Tough, J. S. A simplified one-stage operation for the correction of lymphedema of the leg. *Arch. Surg.* 71:809, 1955.

64. Gillies, H., and Fraser, F. R. The treatment of lymphoedema by plastic operation: A preliminary report. *Br. Med. J.* 1:96, 1935.

65. Gloviczki, P., Hollier, L. H., Nora, F. E., et al. The natural history of microsurgical lymphovenous anastomoses: An experimental study. *J. Vasc. Surg.* 4:148, 1986.

66. Goldsmith, H. S. Long term evaluation of omental transportation for chronic lymphedema. *Ann. Surg.* 189:847, 1984.

67. Goldsmith, H. S., and de los Santos, R. Omental transposition in primary lymphedema. *Surg. Gynecol. Obstet.* 125:607, 1967.

68. Goldsmith, H. S., de los Santos, R., and Beattie, E. J. Relief of chronic lymphedema by omental transposition. *Ann. Surg.* 166:572, 1967.

69. Handley, W. S. Lymphangioplasty: A new method for the relief of the brawny edema of breast cancer and for similar conditions of lymphatic oedema: preliminary note. *Lancet* 1:783, 1908.

70. Handley, W. S. Hunterian lectures on the surgery of the lymphatic system. *Br. Med. J.* 1:922, 1910.

71. Harvery, R. F. The use of I[131] labelled human serum albumin in the assessment of improved lymph flow following buried dermis flap operation in cases of postmastectomy lymphoedema of the arm. *Br. J. Radiol.* 42:260, 1969.

72. Ho, L. C. Y., Lai, M. F., Yeates, M., et al. Microlymphatic bypass in obstructive lymphoedema. *Br. J. Plast. Surg.* 41:475, 1988.

73. Homans, J. The treatment of elephantiasis of the legs: A preliminary report. *N. Engl. J. Med.* 215:1099, 1936.

74. Huang, G. K., Hu, R. Q., and Liu, Z. Microlymphaticovenous anastomoses for lymphedema of the breast. *Microsurgery* 6:32, 1985.

75. Huang, G. K., Hu, R. Q., Liu, Z. Z., et al. Microlymphaticovenous anastomosis for treating scrotal elephantiasis. *Microsurgery* 6:36, 1985.

76. Huang, G. K., Hu, R. Q., Shen, Y. L., et

al. Microlymphaticovenous anastomosis for lymphedema of external genitalia in females. *Surg. Gynecol. Obstet.* 162:429, 1986.

77. Hurst, P., Stewart, G., Kinmonth, J., et al. Long term results of the entero-mesenteric bridge operation in treatment of primary lymphoedema. *Br. J. Surg.* 72:272, 1985.

78. Ju, D. M. C., Blakemore, A., and Stevenson, T. W. A lymphatic function test. *Surg. Forum* 5:697, 1954.

79. Kang, H. G., Qi, H. R., Zhao, L. Z., et al. Microlymphaticovenous anastomosis in the treatment of lower limb obstructive lymphedema: Analysis of 91 cases. *Plast. Reconstr. Surg.* 76:671, 1985.

80. Kondoleon, E. Die Operative Behandlung der elephantiastichen Oedeme. *Zentralbl. Chir.* 39:1022, 1912.

81. Larson, D. L., Coers, C. R., Doyle, J. E., et al. Lymphedema of the lower extremity. *Plast. Reconstr. Surg.* 38:293, 1966.

82. Louton, R. B., and Terranova, W. A. The use of suction curettage as adjunct to the management of lymphedema. *Ann. Plast. Surg.* 22:354, 1989.

83. McCormack, R. M. Surgical treatment of postmastectomy lymphedema. *Plast. Reconstr. Surg.* 14:62, 1954.

84. McKee, D. M., and Edgerton, M. T. Surgical treatment of lymphedema of the lower extremities. *Plast. Reconstr. Surg.* 23:480, 1959.

85. Miller, T. A. Surgical management of lymphedema of the extremity. *Plast. Reconstr. Surg.* 56:633, 1975.

86. Miller, T. A. Surgical approach to lymphedema of the arm after mastectomy. *Am. J. Surg.* 148:152, 1984.

87. Miller, T. A. Invited discussion. *Plast. Reconstr. Surg.* 76:680, 1985.

88. Miller, T. A., Harper, J. D., and Longmire, W. P., Jr. The management of lymphedema by staged subcutaneous excision. *Surg. Gynecol. Obstet.* 136:1, 1973.

89. Nava, V. M., and Lawrence, W. T. Liposuction on a lymphedematous arm. *Ann. Plast. Surg.* 21:366, 1988.

90. Niclubowicz, J., Olszewski, W., and Sokolowski, J. Surgical lymphovenous shunts. *J. Cardiovasc. Surg.* 9:262, 1986.

91. Nylander, G., and Tjernberg, B. The lym-phatics of the greater omentum; an experimental study in the dog. *Lymphology* 2:3, 1969.

92. O'Brien, B. Replantation and reconstructive microvascula surgery. *Ann. R. Coll. Surg. Engl.* 58:87, 171, 1976.

93. O'Brien, B. M. Invited discussion. *Plast. Reconstr. Surg.* 76:682, 1985.

94. Peer, L. A., Shahgholi, M., Walker, J. D., Jr., et al. Modified operation for lymphedema of leg and arm. *Plast. Reconstr. Surg.* 14:347, 1954.

95. Pho, R. W. H., Bayon, P., and Tan, L. Adipose veno-lymphatic transfer for management of post-radiation lymphedema. *J. Reconstr. Microsurg.* 5:45, 1989.

96. Politowski, M., Bartkowski, S., and Dynowski, J. Treatment of lymphedema of the limbs of lymphatico-venous fistula. *Surgery* 66:639, 1969.

97. Puckett, C. L. Invited discussion. *Plast. Reconstr. Surg.* 76:678, 1985.

98. Rivero, O. R., Calnan, J. S., Reis, N. D., et al. Experimental peripheral lympho-venous communication. *Br. J. Plast. Surg.* 20:124, 1967.

99. Servelle, M. Surgical treatment of lymphedema: A report on 652 cases. *Surgery* 101:484, 1987.

100. Silver, D., and Puckett, C. Lymphangioplasty: A ten year evaluation. *Surgery* 80:748, 1976.

101. Sistrunk, W. E. Further experiences with the Kondoleon operation for elephantiasis. *J.A.M.A.* 71:800, 1918.

102. Slavin, S. A. Invited discussion. *Plast. Reconstr. Surg.* 76:684, 1985.

103. Smith, A. R., van Alphern, W. A., and van der Pompe, W. B. Lymphatic drainage in patients after replantation of extremities. *Plast. Reconstr. Surg.* 79:163, 1987.

104. Smith, J. W., and Conway, H. Selection of appropriate surgical procedures in lymphedema; introduction of hinged pedicle. *Plast. Reconstr. Surg.* 30:10, 1962.

105. Tang, H. Y., Zhu, J. K., Yu, G. Z., et al. Experimental observation of transplantation of vein graft to lymphatics. *Ann. Plast. Surg.* 15:285, 1985.

106. Thompson, N. Surgical treatment of chronic lymphoedema of the lower limb. *Br. Med. J.* 5319:1567, 1962.

# 53

Ricardo Baroudi

# Body Contour Surgery

Body contour surgery has become well accepted among physicians and patients owing to the progress of the surgical procedures, the minimal risk of anesthetics, and the natural changes in human tendencies. These three basic aspects present regional, ethnic, educational, religious, economic, and even political peculiarities that result in more or less receptivity in the medical and societal areas.

The tropical climate encourages outdoor life and exposure of the body. In addition, body distortions caused by weight variations, maternity, mild discipline to practice sports, and ethnic aspects are some of the factors that bring patients to specialists' offices as candidates for this type of surgery. These involvements were aided by the publicity in magazines, radios, television, and newspapers, making this surgery even more popular and acceptable. This chapter studies the technical procedures for the improvement of the body contour distortions.

Body contour surgery, also called torsoplasty by Gonzalez-Ulloa, involves surgery of the breasts, abdomen, buttocks, thighs, flanks, and arms, performed in one or more surgical stages. This surgical program depends on the age, health, and weight of the patient as well as the volume of tissue resection and the team's surgical qualifications.

Adequate hospital conditions and high-quality postoperative care complete the requirements for achieving good results for the patient.

The introduction of autotransfusion and liposuction to the routine plastic surgery armamentarium allows the performance of multiple procedures in a single surgical stage with no risk for the patient. Patients demonstrate gratifying postoperative recoveries and thereby motivate relatives and friends to become future candidates for this surgery.

## Types of Aesthetic Body Contour Problems

Problems that involve the aesthetic aspect of each region of the body contour are analyzed here to give a complete picture of the particular type of surgery required.

*1. Breasts:* Candidates for mammaplasty present problems of hypotrophic and hypertrophic breasts with all shapes, volumes, and asymmetries. Reduction, pexy, or augmentation are indicated after evaluating the proportions of the segments of the trunk, based on the patient's wishes and the specialist's best judgment.

*2. Abdomen:* Volume, shape, skin quality (elasticity, striae, flaccidity), scars due to

1319

previous surgery, and navel contour determine the selection of the procedure. It is important to consider that each case must be treated individually, according to the extent and nature of the problem.

**3.** *Flanks and Iliac Crest Roll:* These regions are affected by genetic factors or by natural fat deposits combined (or not) with flabbiness, resulting in contour problems.

**4.** *Buttocks:* The buttocks undergo distortions of shape, volume, and skin texture through the decades by weight variation, hormones, and genetic factors. The curve of the dorsal spine may also determine unaesthetic projections of the buttocks, which motivate some to submit to surgical improvement.

**5.** *Thighs:* The thighs present aesthetic problems when irregular fat deposits and flaccidity become visible. These aspects are more common in women with gynoid fat distribution, specifically in the upper-inner thigh region, the internal aspect of the knee, and the trochanteric area. Cellulite and skin flaccidity are irreversible conditions.

**6.** *Arms:* Similar to the upper-inner thigh, distortions of shape, volume, flabbiness, and fat deposits are commonly seen in this region. Physiotherapy, massage, and any medicine tried have proved to be inefficient. Surgery can be used to improve the upper arms.

### Skin Tissue Problems

Body contour surgery may be divided into pre- and postliposuction periods. Before liposuction was available traditional surgery was used for skin and fat resection, depending on the specific problem. When surgeons began to utilize liposuction, significant changes occurred in the surgical procedures and their indications. Traditional surgery became restrictive and has been replaced in a great number of cases by liposuction or is combined with it in the same or different surgical stages.

Patients who are candidates for body contouring surgery can be divided into four groups.

*Group I.* In this group the patients present with irregular fat deposits in one or more regions of the trunk. The skin is always firm, and there is no flabbiness or exaggerated volume. The patients are usually women under age 20 and are perfect candidates for liposuction. The results obtained are gratifying. Traditional surgery is not indicated for these cases.

*Group II.* Similar to group I, the fat deposits are not excessive but the skin is no longer firm. Liposuction is still highly recommended, and surgery is unnecessary. Liposuction is indicated in one or two surgical stages with at least 6 months between sessions. Removal of the fat must be conservative even if the results in the first stage are unsatisfactory. The natural retraction of the skin takes 2 to 3 months postoperatively. Within the limits of the skin's capability, a second stage may be indicated. When mild flaccidity becomes evident during the first stage, repeat liposuction on the same patient is avoided, as any attempt at a second liposuction will worsen the flaccidity, causing irregularity and unacceptable results.

Age is an important but not an absolute factor. The patients in group II are generally between 20 and 35 years old. In young women slightly over 20 years of age who have flaccidity and fat deposits, liposuction is contraindicated. Candidates for liposuction from groups I and II who have large localized fat volumes must be suctioned more critically in order to avoid complications such as hematoma, seroma, and contour irregularity.

*Group III.* In this group the patients have fat deposits combined with skin flaccidity. Surgery and liposuction should be performed in the same stage (or session). Traditional surgery makes the skin firm again, as in the group I and II patients. Then liposuction is used as a complementary procedure.

*Group IV.* Patients of this group have only skin flaccidity with minimal or no fat deposits. Traditional surgery alone is indicated. Liposuction cannot be used. Based on this classification, the selection of the surgical procedure becomes more objective, thereby avoiding secondary problems as much as possible.

## Surgery Planning

The surgical planning for body contouring surgery is based on the physical and psychological conditions of the patient and the surgical team's qualifications. These factors may be summarized as follows.

### AGE

Restrictions exist for patients over age 50; they are considered candidates for several body contouring procedures that may be performed at single sessions. The program is divided into two stages with at least 3 months between them. There may be exceptions, however, for those over age 50 who are in perfect health and require only moderate body contour alterations; these patients may be submitted to three or more surgical sessions without increasing the risk. Patients with flaccidity of the abdomen and flanks, breast ptosis (without hypertrophy), and skin flaccidity on the arms and upper-inner thighs can undergo all of these corrections at one surgical session if they are 50 to 55 years old. Extending the surgical time (estimated to be around 5 to 6 hours) is tolerable if the surgical team is well trained to reduce blood loss (and hence the risk).

### FLACCIDITY COMBINED WITH ADIPOSITY

Patients with flaccidity and adiposity require meticulous planning for pre-, intra-, and postoperative care. When the patient is over age 50, another surgical precaution is added. Patients must be informed that a surgical scale of priorities will be obeyed: In case unexpected problems occur during the surgery, once the main one has been performed, the remaining procedures are canceled for the time being. Some months later, the corrections may be concluded at a second surgical session with the patient in a better condition. The patient's health must

never be put at risk to complete a program of elective surgery. The patient must also be advised that a second surgical revision is part of the sculpturing program and that it takes place after some months when the tissues have returned to their normal condition. This plan is particularly used when the volume of the fat deposits and the skin flaccidity are extensive. It is prudent to explain these possibilities before the surgery so as to avoid problems with the doctor-patient relationship during the postoperative period.

### SURGICAL TEAM

The surgeon who assumes the responsibility for performing multiple corrections at a single surgical session must have in mind all problems that might interfere with the success of the surgery, as well as the limitations of the program. It is basic that the surgeon is qualified and has participated with other teams that have had experience with these multiple one-session surgeries. When one is a neophyte, too, it is important to start with only two corrections at a single session, gradually adding another and then another, thereby creating one's own systematization. The anesthesiologist must be well integrated into the surgeon's team. The other members of the surgical group must be trained under the surgeon's instructions to perform their job with a minimum of time and maximum efficiency.

In general, the teamwork is directed by the chief surgeon, accompanied by the anesthesiologist and his or her nurse, three assistant surgeons, two scrub nurses, and a room nurse. The same team must work together as much as possible, repeating the routine several times to make it a habit. The room nurse who remains with the team learns the requirements of the surgery and the group, and thereby avoids having to go out to fetch things required during the operation, avoiding unnecessary loss of time. These details may seem insignificant, but they are important to the surgical planning. When the combined procedures are programmed, as with any other type of surgery, the entire responsibility belongs to the chief surgeon.

Surgery on the two breasts done simultaneously—one side by the surgeon and the opposite by the assistant—is not recommended. Delegating surgical responsibility must be restricted. For breast surgery, all the surgical steps must be done by one surgeon.

The breast sutures, however, can be delegated to the assistant while the abdominoplasty stage is performed. This practice saves anesthetic and surgical time. Similarly, for the abdominoplasty the main surgical steps are done by the chief surgeon, leaving the final sutures to the assistant. There are situations where the surgeon finishes all abdominoplasty steps at the same time the assistant completes suturing the breast, including the nipple-areola complex positioning. Surgery time is thus reduced.

Upper-inner thigh and brachioplasty follow the same routine when combined with abdomen and breast sculpturing at the same surgical session. After finishing the mammaplasty and abdominoplasty, the upper arms and thighs are operated on. First, brachioplasty is performed through the previously demarcated skin, the resection and key stitches once again done by the chief surgeon. As he or she moves to the upper-inner thigh procedures, the assistant finishes the arm sutures. Synchronization of the surgical program must be precise, step by step.

When liposuction is included in the surgical program, it is left to the end. The skin, stretched by the traditional surgery, facilitates the procedure. The flaccid skin becomes firm after the resection and suture, and the complementary liposuction is more easily performed.

Finally, there is the clinical aspect of blood collections in the interstitial spaces of the subcutaneous tissue during the surgery. Consequently, distortions in the volume of the region and hemodynamic disequilibrium may be observed.

In summary, each surgeon has his or her own approach. The described procedure is influenced, of course, by the surgeon's personal experience but coincides in its basic aspects with the experience of all other specialists. Some peculiarities are different. The reader interested in body sculpturing surgery can absorb information from this chapter and combine it with the information from other specialists to form his or her own surgical "personality."

## *Technical Systematization*

Technical details relative to body contouring surgery—specifically to the breast and abdominoplasty—are not discussed here because of the limits of this chapter. Nevertheless, some specific points are presented.

### BREAST AND ABDOMINOPLASTY

For breast and abdominoplasty surgery the simplest team is comprised of the chief surgeon, one assistant physician, one scrub nurse, one anesthesiologist, and a room nurse. The patient is submitted to endotracheal anesthesia, and the surgery starts with the breast. Skin demarcation, reduction, mounting, and nipple-areola complex positioning are performed with the patient in a half-sitting position. After this stage is completed, the patient is returned to the supine position, and the abdominoplasty stage is initiated. At this time, a second surgical team is included (a second and even a third surgical assistant and another scrub nurse). They place the nipple-areola complex in its definitive position, and the suture is completed. Meanwhile, abdominoplasty is on its way. This protocol reduces the surgical time by as much as 1 hour. Mammaplasty and abdominoplasty can be performed within 3.0 to 3.5 hours.

For breast augmentation performed with abdominoplasty, the surgery is initiated with dissection of the breast pockets. After this procedure lap pads with saline are left inside, and abdominoplasty then begins.

## BREAST, ABDOMINOPLASTY, AND LIPOSUCTION

When liposuction is included in the program, the areas to be suctioned are marked with the patient in the standing position, before the anesthetic is given. The program starts with liposuction of the buttocks and sacral regions. The patient remains in a prone position for suction of these areas. If the trochanteric area and flanks are included in the program, they may also be suctioned at this stage.

If only trochanteric and flank liposuction is indicated, it may be performed at the end of the surgical program with the patient in the supine position.

Again, this procedure has variations according to the preference of the surgeon. Different procedures may produce similar results.

## BREAST, ABDOMEN, THIGHS, AND LIPOSUCTION

Inclusion of the thighs in the surgical program requires some study. Aesthetic thigh problems are characterized by skin flaccidity, fat deposits, or both. Each problem requires a specific procedure. In terms of the surgical planning, this stage is done after mammaplasty and abdominoplasty to minimize contamination.

## BREAST, ABDOMEN, UPPER ARMS, THIGHS, AND LIPOSUCTION

The surgical program for corrections of the breast, abdomen, upper arms, and thighs, including liposuction, follows the following steps.

**1.** All the liposuction procedures in the dorsal regions are done first with the patient in the prone position. After this step the patient is turned to the supine position, and the surgical areas for the breast, abdomen, and thighs are prepared. The upper arms remain out of the sterilized field until the end of the operation, giving the anesthesiologist a means of monitoring the patient.

**2.** The program starts with the breast surgery. The patient remains in a half-sitting position, with arms abducted. After breast mound and areola-nipple complex positioning, the abdominoplasty period is started. When breast augmentation is performed, saline pads remain in the pockets during the abdominoplasty period, after which the prosthesis is placed. Hemostasis is even better. When breast reduction or mammapexy is done, the second surgeon team completes work on the breast during the abdominoplasty period according to the already described routine.

**3.** The thigh and arm surgeries are now performed. Here some technical details must be noted. One of the arms is attached to a digital computer for heart monitoring and has an intravenous line for administering medication. The blood pressure cuff is placed on one of the legs to continue routine monitoring. Surgical areas on the thighs are prepared at the same time as for mammaplasty and abdominoplasty, and they remain covered with drapes until their surgery.

Surgery on the limbs starts with the upper arm. Technical details may be found in the literature. Upper arm (both arms) skin demarcations, dissections, resections, and key stitches are the responsibility of the chief surgeon. When the surgery is completed here, the surgeon moves to the upper-inner thigh while the other team sutures the arm (Fig. 53-1).

**4.** When necessary, liposuction in these regions can be done before or after the traditional surgery. Each case and the surgeon's attitude determine the performance.

## BREAST, ABDOMEN, THIGHS, ARMS, FLANKPLASTY, AND LIPOSUCTION

Planning is done such that surgical time, anesthesia, and surgical procedures are shortened as much as possible and there are no unnecessary manipulations. Such plans are made for all surgical sessions but especially for the combination of breast, abdomen, thighs, and arm sculpting plus flank-

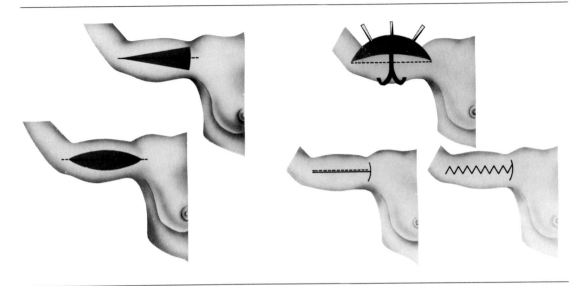

*Figure 53-1* A, B. Types of skin flabbiness combined (or not) with fat deposits localized in the upper arm. The dotted lines represent the inner brachial sulcus projection. The triangular and fusiform dark areas show the amount of tissue to be resected. The extension of the resections may go from the elbow to the armpit. C. After the skin incision and the necessary undermining, the flap is stretched and the skin resected. D, E. The sutures are performed at two levels. The final scar can be straight or in zigzag aspect. The skin excesses are compensated for and resected in the axillary region. Final positioning of the scar is over the projection of the inner brachial sulcus in order to obtain a better (hidden) configuration.

plasty and liposuction. Surgery starts with the patient in the prone position for liposuction of the sacral area, buttocks, flanks, knees, posterior areas of the upper-inner thigh, and trochanteric region. Flankplasty is also performed at this time. After these procedures are complete, the patient is turned to the supine position and the surgical areas prepared and sterilized accordingly. The flankplasty requires special planning when combined with surgery on the upper thighs and abdomen. Skin redundancies situated laterally on the abdominal and superior inguinal segments do not permit surgical conclusion of the flankplasty. Therefore these areas are closed with gauze pads to avoid contamination when the patient is turned to the supine position; the pads remain there during the mammaplasty and abdominoplasty.

Laterally, the incision on the abdomen joins with those on the flanks. Here the undermining, resection, and suturing are done to achieve a natural contour. When the incision of the abdomen and flank joins with that on the upper-inner thigh, there is an intersection of three skin edges that requires extra refinement to avoid irregular traction,

distortion, tension, and redundancy of the skin tissue.

Any complementary liposuction required may be done at this stage. Finally, brachioplasty is performed.

## Preoperative Care

The preoperative routine is similar to that for any surgical procedure where general or epidural anesthesia is indicated. Age, general health conditions, anesthetic period, and the extent of the surgery determine the risks, safety, and recovery of the patient. For patients in whom liposuction is estimated to be more than 1500 ml combined with abdomen and breast surgery, or even surgery on thighs and arms, autotransfusion (2 units) is indicated.

The surgical priorities are programmed in advance according to the patient's age. The operation starts with the patient's first priority. If during the following steps the patient's condition does not allow the operation to continue, the program is canceled after the main correction has been performed.

Monitors during the anesthetic period are part of the routine.

Patients are requested not to use aspirin or any anticoagulation drug, and it is strongly recommended that the patient stop smoking 2 weeks before surgery. The latter instruction is difficult for the smoker to follow, leaving the surgeon unsure if the patient has done so.

## Surgical Technique

Body contouring surgery can be performed at one or more surgical sessions, as already noted. One correction may be performed, or a combination may be done according to the conditions already discussed. Didactically, the procedures can be divided in the following categories.

### MAMMAPLASTY AND ABDOMINOPLASTY

Correction of problems with the breasts and abdomen are the most common procedures requested by patients. The causes of the disharmony of these regions are already known, and they do not need further discussion. The corrections may be done separately or in combination at one surgical session.

The surgery, performed under general anesthesia, starts with the breast. During the reduction or remodeling period, the patient remains in a supine, almost half-sitting, position. For breast augmentation, a subpectoral pocket is prepared, and meticulous hemostasis is established. The access

view is through a 3.5-cm skin incision in the inframammary sulcus. Saline lap pads are left in the pockets until the end of the abdominoplasty, which aids in hemostasis. At this time the prostheses are implanted.

The reduction mammaplasty may be performed by various techniques. In general, we use the Pontes (1981) procedures. Medial or lateral quadrantectomies can also be done according to the need. The mound of the new breast leaves an inverted T suture. All efforts are made to shorten the horizontal length of the scar. For certain hypertrophic breasts with no ptosis, the Cloutier (1979) technique is performed. Up to 30 percent breast reduction can be achieved through a 6-cm horizontal incision in the inframammary sulcus. The breast tissue is dissected at the muscular level and geometric trunk-of-cone-like glandular tissue in its base is resected. Within a few weeks the skin retracts to the definitive smaller volume but with the same shape. Resections of greater volume may produce ptosis and undesirable flabbiness.

While the breast is being sutured and the areola is being positioned, the abdominoplasty is performed. The operation is based on the procedure of Baroudi et al. (1974), although small variations have been introduced in the skin incision, leaving it lower at the pubic region than reported by Baroudi et al. and a bit higher laterally, near the anterosuperior iliac spine. This new positioning better hides the scar under today's swimming suits.

The systematization of these corrections saves a full hour of surgery time.

### MAMMAPLASTY, ABDOMINOPLASTY, AND LIPOSUCTION

Liposuction can be performed at the same surgical stage as the breast correction and the abdominoplasty. It is recommended that it be done at the end of the other procedures. The reverse can also be done, however (i.e., before the traditional surgeries), according to the surgeon's preference.

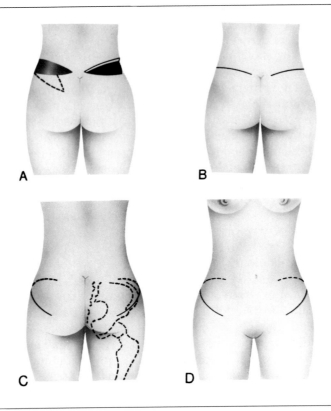

**Figure 53-2** *A, B. Posterior view of the skin excess demarcations for the flankplasty. Resection takes the fusiform aspect over the projection of the iliac bone, specifically from the anterosuperior iliac spine and along the posterior iliac crest. C, D. Posterior and anterior aspects of the final scar line.*

Liposuction in the superior quadrants of the breast after or even before the surgery helps the uniform reduction of volume, avoiding a more difficult surgical resection. Secondary problems of bulging epigastrium and flanks are commonly detected after traditional abdominoplasty. Liposuction of the epigastrium at the same surgical session with abdominoplasty is not recommended. Infraumbilical skin flap necrosis due to the loss of vessels that supply these region has been reported, and the incidence of hematomas and seromas is increased. Liposuction in the flank region at the same session as abdominoplasty has proved not to be dangerous. In fact, it helps improve the body contour and avoids secondary bulging flanks. It can be performed with the patient in the supine position.

Preaxillary fat deposits are easily removed by liposuction. As for other regions, liposuction can be performed at the end of the operation.

ABDOMEN AND FLANKPLASTY

Abdomen and flankplasty can be done at the same surgical session. These procedures are recommended to group III and IV patients in whom skin flaccidity is combined (or not) with localized fat deposits.

The flank demarcations are done with the patient in standing position, as the areas for surgical resection and liposuction can be better evaluated in this stance. The surgery starts with the patient in the prone position. The skin incisions have a fusiform-like aspect (Fig. 53-2A,B). The resections can be joined in the sacral region, as a V suture, opened cranially, or finished 3 to 6 cm from the intergluteal sulcus. The joining or not of the suture line depends on the skin redundancy over the sacral region (Fig. 53-2C,D).

The tissue resections go to the deep layer. Hemostasis must be meticulous and the sutures at three levels. Vicryl 2-0 stitches are placed in subcutaneous tissue to avoid deadspace; to leave no space for a seroma, 3-0 Vicryl stitches are placed in the entire dermis extension, and a running 3-0 Vicryl intracuticular suture is used for the final closure. Liposuction, when recommended, can be performed before the running suture is placed. Usually it is placed in the neighboring region above and below the suture.

The ideal final position of the suture is over the projection of the superoposterior iliac line and the upper part of the intergluteal sulcus (Fig. 53-3A–D); 1 to 3 cm above or below this position is acceptable. At the junction of the flanks and the abdomen, skin excess remains after the flankplasty. It is normal and does not interfere with the conclusion of the flank surgery. At this point the skin redundancies are covered by sterilized pads, and the patient is turned to the supine position.

The abdominoplasty demarcation and techniques are performed routinely. Two special cares must be noted: (1) The skin undermining the abdomen must be limited laterally. The vessels must not be severed, as they are important for skin flap preservation. (2) The junction between the flank and abdomen is treated with the necessary skin undermining and resections to eliminate the "dog ears." The final suturing is performed as shown in Figure 53-3F.

The previous liposuction, when the patient was in prone position, cannot be completed in the same or in different regions when in the supine position.

Breast reduction or augmentation, when combined with this program, is performed after the flank procedures and before the abdominoplasty. The breast surgery, done in almost a half-sitting position, may present higher anesthetic risk at the end of the surgical procedure than at the beginning.

THIGHS, FLANKS, AND LIPOSUCTION

Upper-inner thigh surgery combined with flankplasty is performed through an extensive fusiform skin tissue resection (Fig. 53-4). All the areas to be resected and subjected to liposuction are demarcated with the patient in the standing position.

Surgery starts with the flankplasty, according to the technique previously described (see Fig. 53-2). Liposuction is also done at this surgical step. The patient is then turned to the supine position for the thigh surgery. Here liposuction can be performed before or after tissue resection. For upper-inner thigh surgery the incision starts at the gluteal sulcus near its junction with the pudendal region. It goes along and parallel to all the extension of the labia majora, about 2 cm above the inner thigh sulcus. It continues parallel and 2 to 3 cm above the inguinal line until it joins the flank incision laterally. This inguinal incision line passes over the projection of the superoanterior iliac spine or a few centimeters below it.

Dissection of the skin excesses must be selective. The undermining is estimated using the previous demarcation through the finger-pinching maneuver done by the surgeon. Deadspace must always be avoided. The amount of resection is the amount undermined. Suturing is done at three levels: A deep suture with 2-0 Vicryl anchors the subcutaneous tissue and the dermis to the deep fascia and to the dermis at the upper edge of the incision. A 3-0 Vicryl stitch in the dermis and a final isolated 4-0 nylon stitch closes the skin. In cases where there is excess skin in the thigh, a triangular resection in the inner aspect is performed. The scar is about 5 to 7 cm, is almost vertical, and remains hidden.

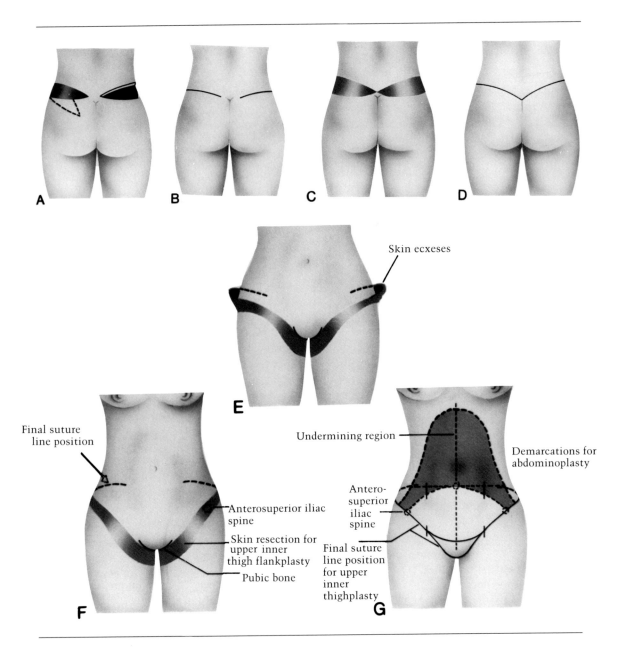

A

B

C

D

Skin ecxeses

E

Final suture
line position

Anterosuperior iliac
spine

Skin resection for
upper inner
thigh flankplasty

Pubic bone

F

Undermining region

Demarcations for
abdominoplasty

Antero-
superior
iliac
spine

Final suture
line position
for upper
inner
thighplasty

G

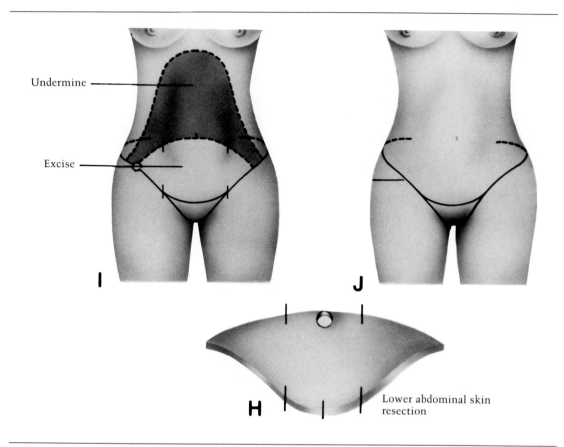

**Figure 53-3** *Abdomen, thigh, and flankplasty combined done at the same surgical session is programmed in the following steps. Surgery starts with the patient in the prone position for the flankplasty stage. A–D. Two optional skin resections and sutures. The final scars may or not may be joined with the opposite side, but they should remain over the projection of the iliac posterior crest (a few centimeters above or below it is acceptable). After closure with sutures and covering with bandages, the patient is turned to a supine position. E. Lateral excesses remain covered with pads. F. Upper-inner thigh surgery is then performed. Skin undermining, resection, and suture are done until the superior limits of the pubis are reached. G. The abdominoplasty step continues the procedure. Skin flap undermining must be economical laterally according to the shaded area. H. Aspect of the skin resected. I. The amount of skin undermined and resected is based on the routine abdominoplasty. J. Final scar line positioning after the three corrections have been performed.*

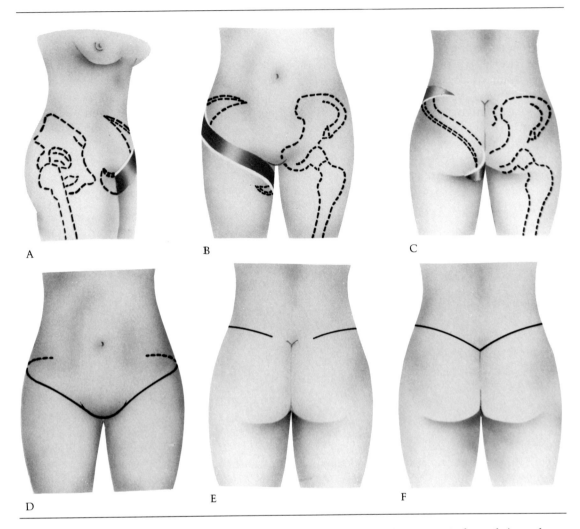

A

B

C

D

E

F

BREASTS, THIGHS, FLANKS,
ABDOMEN, AND LIPOSUCTION

Combined procedures such as that to repair breasts, thighs, flanks, and abdomen, as well as liposuction, requires special systematization from the surgical team in order to save time and provide better recovery for the patient (see Fig. 53-3).

The demarcations for repair of the flanks and thighs and for liposuction must be done with the patient in the standing position (see Fig. 53-4). The surgery starts with the patient in the prone position. Flankplasty and liposuction in the predetermined regions

*Figure 53-4* A–C. Aspects in lateral, frontal, and posterior views for the combined upper inner thigh and flankplasty. The skin resection takes an ellicoid form. D, E. Posteroanterior view of the final scar positioning. E. The suture and scar end 6 to 8 cm before reaching the intergluteal sulcus. F. Joining scars possibility. This situation may exist when skin excesses remain over the sacral region. A straight line in the junction is to be avoided. An open cranial V suture line position seems to be aesthetically better.

may be performed (specifically the flanks, sacral area, and buttocks). The patient is then turned to the supine position, and the breast surgery is done. Upper-inner thigh surgery and finally abdominoplasty follow. The junction points of the abdominoplasty, flanks, and thigh require special care. The dissection must be enough to resect and accommodate the skin for suturing, and there must be minimal tension in the suture to prevent dehiscence postoperatively. Narrowing the skin at the junction point must be avoided. The small skin strip sloughs easily. A rounded-edge skin flap is safer than the one with pointed edges. Even when care is exercised, there is frequently some small dehiscence and skin necrosis at this spot. Usually healing by secondary intention solves the problem. Finally, meticulous symmetry resection around the limits of the pubis is performed. Minimal distortions and tension determine if there is an unpleasant, unaesthetic effect in terms of scar positioning postoperatively.

## Postoperative Care

General and local postoperative precautions are evaluated together and separately. Antibiotic therapy, 1 gm of a third-generation cephalosporin, is given intravenously during operation and 1 gm intravenously every 6 hours for 4 to 5 days.

Autotransfusion is indicated for cases in which three or more corrections are combined with liposuction at the same session. No intensive postoperative therapy care has been necessary in our patients because of the basic attitude about canceling the final part of the surgical program if patient conditions became unstable or are out of control. No risks should exist for patients undergoing aesthetic plastic surgery. However, problems such as amnesia, mental depression, and mild mental confusion have been detected occasionally during the first 2 weeks postoperatively. They disappeared sponta-

neously, however, needing no special treatment. Lack of the ability to sleep is common and is corrected with sleeping pills. Local cares such as bandage changes, stitch removal, and use of local micropore tape do not demand any specific plan. Each surgeon has his or her own routine. Generally, however, some points must be emphasized.

**1.** Vacuum drains for abdominoplasty are highly recommended. They are left in place a minimum of 3 days or are removed when the amount of serum decreases to 40 ml in 24 hours.

**2.** For compression function, polyethylene sponges about 5 cm thick are tailored according to the size of the suctioned area. They are used for 48 to 72 hours during the postoperative period. They are fixed with micropore tape, and the patient wears an elastic girdle. Uniform, moderate continued pressure over the regions has been proved efficient and comfortable.

**3.** For breast reduction, abdominoplasty, and flank surgery, a Lycra girdle and a brassiere are used by the patient for 4 weeks postoperatively. When liposuction is performed only in the trunk, the girdle remains for only 10 days.

**4.** Patients are requested to stay 3 days in the hospital when abdominoplasty is performed. Regardless of whether it is combined with other procedures, this operation requires more time of hospitalization. After this time patients remain at home until the end of the first week. During the second week they may be more active: They may go to the doctor's office and remain some hours away from home in accordance to their wishes and their strength. After 14 days they are able to drive and perform their daily routine.

**5.** Moderate exercise is allowed after 8 weeks.

**6.** Outdoor activities, including swimming, are permitted after 4 weeks and direct sunbathing with exposure on the abdomen after 4 months. (Second degree burns in the infraumbilical regions have occurred with earlier exposure.)

## Complications

The complications associated with body contour surgery are varied in type and extent. Each surgical correction presents its own risk index, the limits of which may or may not be under the physician's control. Complications relative to the general patient conditions are treated accordingly and cannot be included within the limits of this chapter.

Local complications such as ecchymosis, necrosis, hematoma, dehiscence, and scar asymmetry are treated specifically. When one of these problems occurs, it must be considered as if it resulted from a single operation, not because of the multiple interventions that have been performed. If more than one of these complications occurs in several patients, the surgeon must recheck his or her routine.

## Comments

Body contour surgery is considered a multiple procedure in which several regions of the body are involved, with different skin textures, specific distortions, and different volumes of fat deposit, and in which unique patient-doctor relationships are involved. All these variations are combined with the natural limitations of the technical procedures, the scar quality, and the surgeon's qualifications. Based on these factors it became imperative to establish the following guidelines.

**1.** Never predict good results for a specific body part that is to be submitted to surgery without also explaining to the patient the complexity of the case.

**2.** For the extensive surgical program, the patient must be advised preoperatively that if something unpredictable occurs the other corrections will be canceled to avoid undue

risks or complications. A second, complementary surgical stage can later conclude the corrections left undone, when the patient is in good health.

**3.** Secondary revisions or refinements are considered part of the original surgical program and take place after a minimum of 3 months. Hence the second procedure is considered part of the previously agreed-on protocol and must not be considered a "claim" for better results from the patient.

**4.** It is fundamental to clarify all aspects before the surgery, rather than to say "sorry" during the postoperative period.

## Suggested Reading

Baroudi, R. Dermatolipectomy of the upper arm. *Clin. Plast. Surg.* 2:485, 1975.

Baroudi, R. Umbilicaplasty. *Clin. Plast. Surg.* 2:431, 1975.

Baroudi, R. Thigh Lift and Buttock-Lift. In E. H. Courtiss (ed.), *Aesthetic Surgery: Trouble—How to Avoid It and How to Treat It.* St. Louis: Mosby, 1978. P. 233.

Baroudi, R. Cuidados pós-operatórios locais e sistêmicos para lipoaspiração. In J. M. Avelar and Y. G. Illouz (eds.), *Lipoaspiração.* São Paulo: Hipócrates, 1984. P. 105.

Baroudi, R. Lipolysis Combined with Conventional Surgery. In G. P. Hetter (ed.), *Lipoplasty: The Theory and Practice of Blunt Suction Lipectomy.* Boston: Little, Brown, 1984.

Baroudi, R., Keppke, E. M., and Tozzi Netto, F. Abdominoplasty. *Plast. Reconstr. Surg.* 54:161, 1974.

Bozolla, A. R., et al. Mamoplastia em L. Contribuição pessoal. *Rev. Amrigs.*, Porto Alegre 263:207, 1982.

Cloutier, A. M. Volume reduction mammaplasty. Presented at the Seventh International Congress of Plastic Surgeons, São Paulo, Cartgraf, 1979.

Elbaz, J. S., and Verheecke, J. La cicatrice en L, dans les plasties mammaires. *Ann. Chir. Plast.* 17:283, 1972.

Erol, O. O., and Spira, M. A mastopexy technique for mild to moderate ptosis. *Plast. Reconstr. Surg.* 65:603, 1980.

Fournier, P. F., and Otteni, F. Traitement des Lipodystrophies Localisées par Aspiration: La Technique Sèche. In S. A. Maloine (ed.), *Chirurgie Esthétique*. Paris: Maloine, 1982. P. 59.

Gerrero-Santos, J. Brachioplasty. *Aesthetic Plast. Surg.* 3:1, 1979.

Gonzalez-Ulloa, M. Circular abdominoplasty with transposition of the umbilicus and aponeurotic technique. *Chirurgia* 27:394, 1959.

Gonzalez-Ulloa, M. Belt lipectomy. *Br. J. Plast. Surg.* 13:179, 1960.

Gonzalez-Ulloa, M. Torsoplasty. *Aesthetic Plast. Surg.* 357:3, 1979.

Grazer, F. M., and Klingbeil, J. R. *Body Image: A Surgical Perspective*. St. Louis: Mosby, 1980.

Illouz, Y. G. Une nouvelle technique pour les lipodystrophies localisées. *Rev. Chir. Esthétique Lang. Fr.* 6:3, 1980.

Kesselring, U. K., and Meyer, R. A suction curette for removal of excessive local deposits of subcutaneous fat. *Plast. Reconstr. Surg.* 62:305, 1978.

Lewis, J. R. The thigh lift. *J. Int. Coll. Surg.* 27:330, 1957.

Lewis, J. R. *Atlas of Aesthetic Surgery*. Boston: Little, Brown, 1973.

Lockwood, T. E. Fascial anchoring technique in medial thigh lift. *Plast. Reconstr. Surg.* 82:300, 1988.

Meyer, R., and Kesselring, K. U. Reduction mammaplasty with an L-shape suture line. *Plast. Reconstr. Surg.* 55:139, 1975.

Peixoto, G. Reduction mammaplasty: A personal technique. *Plast. Reconstr. Surg.* 65:217, 1980.

Pitanguy, I. Trochanteric lipodystrophy. *Plast. Reconstr. Surg.* 34:280, 1964.

Pitanguy, I. Surgical treatment of breast hypertrophy. *Br. J. Plast. Surg.* 20:78, 1967.

Planas, J. The crural meloplasty, for lifting of the thighs. *Clin. Plast. Surg.* 2:495, 1975.

Pontes, R. Reduction mammaplasty: Variation I and II. *Ann. Plast. Surg.* 6:437, 1981.

Regnault, P. Abdominal dermolipectomies. *Clin. Plast. Surg.* 2:411, 1975.

Regnault, P., and Daniel, R. K. *Aesthetic Plastic Surgery*. Boston: Little, Brown, 1984.

Somalo, M. Dermolipectomia circular del tronco. *Semin. Med.* 1:1435, 1940.

# VIII
## Genitalia

# 54

*Charles E. Horton*
*Richard Sadove*
*Charles J. Devine, Jr.*
*Bert Vorstman*

# Hypospadias, Epispadias, and Exstrophy of the Bladder

Hypospadias is a common anomaly. In the United States it is estimated to occur once in every 350 live male births. It is even more frequent in other parts of the world. It causes great concern to both the patient and the parents, who profess insecurity about the sexual potential of their child. In the past, hypospadias repairs were commonly associated with frequent complications. Many patients required multiple operations, and many "hypospadias cripples" [2–5, 11] were created. Because chordee persisted in a large number of cases after these early repairs it was thought that the abnormal tissue causing penile curvature regrew and recurred. This conclusion, however, is not true. Chordee reappeared after surgery because resection of the inelastic tissue was inadequate. Once tissue causing chordee is released and resected, the penis remains straight.

At the present time we prefer to operate on hypospadiac boys at age 1.5 to 2.0 years if the penis is of adequate size. We never recommend a staged procedure for any primary hypospadias repair [10]. Techniques today make it possible to offer a single operation before the age of memory recall so that the child can grow to adulthood without feeling inferior in any way regarding his sexuality.

Most hypospadias cases (90 percent) can be classified anatomically as distal, with the urethral meatus ending in the distal shaft or glans of the penis. Only 10 percent of all hypospadias cases are in the midshaft or proximal in the scrotum or perineum. Distal cases of hypospadias can be repaired with local tissue flaps, as there is inadequate skin in the prepuce for ventral shaft coverage. An aesthetic repair can be completed with an overall complication rate approaching 10 percent. Most of the complications are minor: fistulas, unsightly skin tags, diverticuli, meatal stenosis, or splashing or spraying of the urinary stream. These complications can be corrected easily after a one-stage operation and are no more difficult to correct than the same complications that occur even more commonly after staged surgery.

For more proximal cases, full-thickness skin graft urethroplasty or arterialized prepucial flap urethroplasty is the treatment of choice. With midshaft hypospadias when there is an abundant prepuce, the arterialized prepucial flap produces a good urethra with little torsion of the penis. When the hypospadias is more proximal, we prefer a full-thickness skin graft urethroplasty constructed from the prepuce. This graft allows resurfacing of the penis from the remaining shaft skin without twisting or devascularization of the dorsal skin, a complication that may arise when a long vascular prepucial pedicle has been developed. Refinements in hypospadias repair include the use of polydioxanone sutures (PDS) placed subcuticularly to build the urethra, the use of percutaneous suprapubic drainage in all except the most distal cases, and the use of Biocclusive dressing and cold compresses after surgery to minimize edema. The dressing is also transparent and allows visualization of the wound. The use of the microscope, or loupes, accentuates the meticulous repair necessary with hypospadias surgery and has decreased our complication rate. In one series of 50 consecutive hypospadias repairs, a 6 percent complication rate was recorded, including all types of complications [7]. The most common problem was a small pinpoint fistula, which was easily repaired at a second operation.

Earlier we refined our one-stage hypospadias technique and reported it elsewhere [12]. We also extended the use of the hypospadias technique to epispadias and pointed out that the urethral plate in epispadias was of deficient length, causing an upward curvature if the plate was not elongated. Since that time one-stage epispadias repairs have become standard, and the complication rate of this surgery does not surpass that of hypospadias repair even though the epispadias deformity is seen much less frequently.

Hypospadias repairs performed 25 years ago had little or no attention given to the aesthetic appearance of the penis after the completion of surgery. The surgical objectives at that time were simple: to correct the curvature associated with the hypospadias and to build a urethra to the subglanular location so that the penis could deposit sperm in the vagina and normal intercourse could occur. The timing of surgery was usually deferred until the patient developed sufficient penile growth to make the surgical repair easier. It usually required the patient to be of school age, and the hypospadias repairs were completed in two, three, or more stages. Psychological adjustment difficulties for both the patient and his parents were common.

In 1959 Horton and Devine presented a movie on one-stage hypospadias repair [11] and in 1961 reported this technique in the literature [4]. Our experience since that time has confirmed that one-stage repairs are reliable, and that the chordee of hypospadias does not recur [5]. Full-thickness grafts or flaps for urethroplasty increase in size at the rate of the normal growth increase of the patient. We also described for the first time the interposition of a flap in the new meatal opening to construct the urethra to the tip of the glans. Our operation is now universally accepted as a reliable one-stage repair for hypospadias. Since these techniques have been perfected, we have seen many older patients who have had obsolete hypospadias repairs where the meatus was constructed only to the subglanular position. These patients frequently request aesthetic surgery of the urethra to position the meatus in its normal central location in the glans in order to appear "normal."

With a heightened awareness of sexuality over the world, it is common now for women to know what a "normal" penis looks like. Men who are aesthetically abnormal *feel* abnormal and wish to be made normal. Homosexuals in particular wish to have a normal-appearing penis. It is now evident that older techniques, resulting in a penis suboptimal in appearance, are not acceptable.

## History of Hypospadias Repairs

The first skin graft urethroplasty was devised by Nové-Joserand. This technique consisted in the use of split-thickness grafts to fill a channel in the penis to build the urethra. The split-thickness graft required stenting for many months because of the inherent contracture of the split-thickness graft. Multiple stenoses and strictures occurred with this technique, and it was abandoned. It was later popularized by McIndoe [16], who recommended that the stent be left in place for 6 to 12 months to overcome the tendency for contracture. This technique has many complications and is not used for routine cases.

Thiersche and Duplay [6] were given credit for the first successful hypospadias repairs that were reproducible by others. Although J. P. Mettauer of Virginia reported the first successful hypospadias repair and "liberation of the tissues causing chordee," he did not have the use of catheters for urinary diversion, and his technique was not reproducible by others. Thiersche and Duplay performed a two-stage repair in which they first resected the tissue causing chordee and straightened the penis. The penile skin was closed, and months later the urethra was constructed by making longitudinal incisions down the ventral surface of the penis to tube a urethra, undermining the lateral skin flaps and covering the buried tube of skin. The deficiency of this operation is that it never adequately extended the urethra to the tip of the glans. In many cases adequate tissue for construction of the urethra and coverage of a new urethral tube was not present. This technique, however, was successfully reintroduced and popularized by Blair and Byars [1]. Byars was a meticulous surgeon and had great success with hypospadias surgery. This operation is probably the most common type of hypospadias repair reported in the literature up until one-stage repairs were popularized. Browne [2] modified this technique by not making the ventral strip of skin into a tube but simply leaving it as a strip of skin covered by the lateral skin flaps of the ventral surface of the penis. This ventral strip of skin then tubed itself with normal circumferential growth, and the urethra was formed. This simple technique gained popularity for hypospadias repair, but the complication rate was high; the operation has thus been largely abandoned by most hypospadias surgeons. All of these operations ended with a subglandar meatus.

A valuable technique for hypospadias repairs, introduced by Cecil [3] during the mid-1940s, considered the fact that adequate shaft skin was difficult to obtain in all cases. Therefore after the chordee was released and the penis straightened, at the second stage (6 months later) the urethra was constructed of tubed ventral penile skin by making parallel longitudinal incisions. An incision was then made in the scrotum, and the penis was sutured into the scrotal bed, suturing the scrotal skin to the lateral penile flaps. The penis was left in this position for 6 to 8 weeks while the new urethra was sutured and covered. At a third stage the scrotum was released from the penis, leaving normal vascularized scrotal skin present on the ventral surface of the penis to cover the neourethra. This technique is still useful for certain complicated hypospadias cripples; however, it has largely been abandoned as a primary form of hypospadias repair. It cannot be recommended because of the undesirable aesthetic appearance of the scrotal skin on the penis and because it is a three-stage operation with a high complication rate.

## Surgical Indications

For distal hypospadias repairs, a meatal advancement procedure is recommended. For hypospadias cases in which the urethra is subglandular, a "flip-flap" operation is utilized. If the meatus is adequate and there is no chordee, two parallel incisions can continue from the meatus to the neomeatus so that the flip flap can be sutured to this glans strip, thereby constructing the distal urethra. When chordee is present, transection of the urethral plate and excision of the underlying dysgenetic tissue is required. In such cases, a V-shaped midline glans flap is constructed. Lateral glans wings are closed over the new urethra, and prepucial skin is shifted from the dorsal surface to the ventral surface, covering the penile shaft. If the meatus is small, a meatotomy is performed and the midline V-shaped glans flap advanced into the meatus. After tissue causing chordee is resected, the flip flap is sutured to the midline glans flap to construct the urethra. The lateral glanular wings are used to cover the distal urethra. The prepuce is split and shifted ventrally for resurfacing. These three techniques ordinarily take care of 90 percent of all hypospadias cases. In more proximal cases, where the midline glans flap does not reach the native urethra without causing curvature, a new interposed urethra must be constructed to meet the glans flap.

In certain cases an arterialized vascular flap for urethroplasty works with great success. In other cases, a free full-thickness graft from the prepuce is more often our procedure of choice. Both techniques give approximately the same complication rate. Flap dissection may cause devascularization of the dorsal penile skin or result in tortuosity of the urethra and thus cause flow disturbances. For more proximal cases the flap may not have enough length. This flap is more difficult to construct and requires more operating time; it is also more prone to form diverticula.

The full-thickness graft urethroplasty allows greater freedom in resurfacing the penile shaft. Hairless flank skin for the neourethra in reoperative cases is also available. Redraping the skin for penile coverage is more easily performed and torsion of the penis more easily corrected.

## Release of Chordee

After the appropriate incisions for the type of hypospadias repair selected have been made and flaps elevated, all tissue causing curvature is removed from around the existing urethral meatus to underneath the glans.

After all inelastic fibrous tissue is resected, an artificial erection test is performed. If chordee remains despite this maneuver, further resection of dysgenetic tissue is required. Occasionally, a vertical cut down the midline of the penis between the two corporal bodies is recommended. Rarely, dorsal plication of the tunica is required.

## Preparation for Operation

Preoperative evaluation includes ultrasonography (to determine that the upper urinary system is normal) and standard preoperative blood tests and urinalysis. The patient is asked to take a tub bath with PhisoHex the night prior to surgery and is given prophylactic antibiotics. He is placed on the operating room table with the pelvis thrust upward. Urethroscopy is performed prior to the surgery to make certain there are no urinary tract anomalies such as a large verumontanum, urethral valves, or strictures. A traction suture is placed in the dorsal glans so that constant pressure may be placed on the penis, thereby reducing bleeding. The urethral meatus is calibrated to determine if stenosis is present, and the size of the normal urethra is determined.

## Specific Urethroplasty Techniques

The following cases are typical of the various one-stage hypospadias repairs that can be utilized for each specific anatomic entity.

### MEATAL ADVANCEMENT AND GLANSPLASTY

Meatal advancement and glansplasty is suitable for patients with distal glanular hypospadias. It cannot produce an adequate repair in subglanular cases.

After demonstrating that the penis is straight with an artificial erection, a circumcising incision is made (Fig. 54-1). Skin hooks are placed into the lateral edges of the glanular urethral groove and retracted laterally. This move raises a band of mucosa that is then incised longitudinally in the midline. This incision in the dorsal glanular wall of the urethra is then closed transversely with 6-0 chromic catgut. A skin hook is placed in the skin at the margin of the corona in the ventral midline. With traction distally, the edges of the glans are pulled forward and approximated in the midline with subcuticular interrupted 5-0 PDS sutures. The glans epithelium is closed with

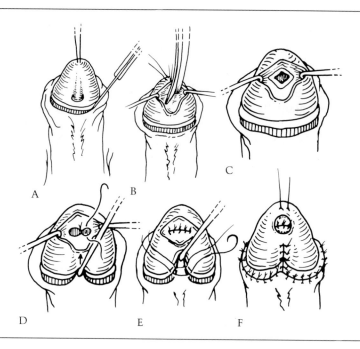

**Figure 54-1** *Meatal advancement and glansplasty. A. Circumcising incision. B. Cutting of the intraurethral transverse band. C, D. Closure of the longitudinal incision transversely. D, E. Approximation of the glans wings after partial mobilization and V-Y advancement rotation of the corporal heads. F. Completed glanular urethroplasty and reapproximated penile skin after excision of the dorsal prepucial hood.*

interrupted 6-0 chromic catgut. Redundant dorsal prepucial skin can be tailored for skin closure and reapproximated with interrupted 6-0 chromic catgut. Urinary diversion is not required. This procedure may be done in an outpatient setting; when done on an inpatient, the patient is sent home the following day after satisfactory voiding.

## SUBCORONAL HYPOSPADIAS WITHOUT CHORDEE
The second procedure is suitable for patients with subglanular hypospadias repair where there is no chordee and there is adequate meatus. A ventral penile flap based on the urethral meatus is used to construct the ven-

tral one-half of the neourethra (Fig. 54-2). Parallel incisions are extended from each side of the urethra to the tip of the glans to form the dorsal one-half of the urethra. A circumcising incision is made as marked. The lateral glans wings are dissected from the tips of the corpora. The midline strip of glans skin extends from the meatus to the tip of the glans, but it is not raised or dissected free from the glans. The flip flap is elevated, rotated, and secured to the end of the glans groove to advance the meatus to the tip of the glans. The edges of the flap are then sutured to the ventral glans strip using running 7-0 PDS sutures under loupe magnification to invert the epithelial edges. After this approximation, the anastomosis is tested with methylene blue-dyed saline to ensure that it is watertight. The glans is then reapproximated over the neourethra and secured with interrupted 5-0 PDS sutures. The glans skin is closed with interrupted 6-0 chromic catgut. The dorsal prepucial skin is then split and advanced ventrally for penile skin coverage. Redun-

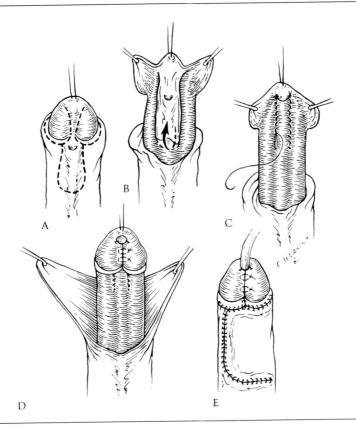

**Figure 54-2** *Flip flap without chordee.*
*A. Proposed incision marked out. Dorsal glans traction suture. B. Creation of ventral penile flaps and mobilization of glans wings from the corporal heads. C. Approximation of the flip flap to the dorsal skin bridge to advance the meatus to the glans tip. D. Approximation of the glans wings over the flip-flap urethroplasty. E. Excess dorsal penile skin is redraped ventrally with excision of redundant tissue. The W incision has been closed to rotate the hair-bearing skin superiorly and medially to normalize the escutcheon and provide extra skin to lengthen the dorsal surface of the penis.*

dant skin is excised. The penile skin flaps are reapproximated with interrupted 5-0 PDS in subcutaneous tissue, and the skin edges are approximated with interrupted 5-0 or 6-0 chromic catgut. A No. 8 French urethral "feeding tube catheter" is passed into the bladder and secured with the dorsal glans traction suture for 5 days, or a cysto-cath diversion is used. The penis is dressed with Biocclusive. Tub baths begin about the third postoperative day, and the bandage is removed on the sixth or seventh day.

## SUBCORONAL HYPOSPADIAS WITH CHORDEE

Yet another procedure is suitable for patients with subcoronal or distal shaft hypospadias with ventral chordee or a small meatus. It is difficult to fully resect underlying chordee on the ventral surface of the penis with the

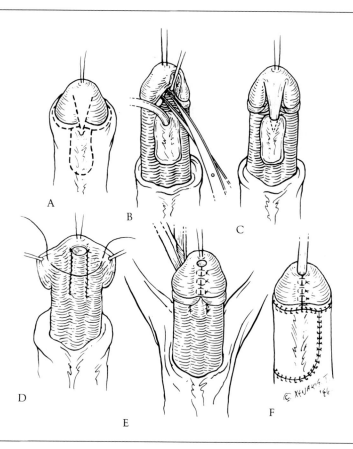

**Figure 54-3** *Flip flap with chordee. A. Proposed incision for the Horton-Devine flip-flap urethroplasty. B. Creation of a ventral penile flap with excision of dysgenetic tissue between the urethral meatus and the glans to correct chordee and mobilize the glans wings. A midline glans V-flap is created.*
*C. Approximation of the glans flap into a dorsal meatotomy. D. Approximation of the flip flap to the dorsal glans to advance the meatus to the glans tip. E. Approximation of glans wings over the flip-flap urethroplasty. Note the unfolding redundant dorsal prepucial skin and creation of Byar's flaps. F. Penile skin is redraped for ventral coverage.*

skin in place as described for the second technique. Therefore a different incision and flap elevation are required to allow access to the abnormal tissue. After insertion of a 5-0 silk dorsal glans traction suture, the incisions are marked on the penis (Fig. 54-3). An elliptical flip flap, as with the second technique, is designed proximal to the meatus on the ventral surface of the penis. A midline glans V-flap and a circumcising incision between the glans and the urethra are also marked. Incisions are made and the skin edges elevated. The glans V-flap is elevated and debulked, and the glans wings are dissected off the ends of the corpora. Exposure of the tunica of the corpora distal to the urethral meatus allows resection of dysgenetic tissue and correction of chordee. Penile straightness must then be confirmed with an artificial erection. A dorsal meatotomy is made in the native dorsal urethra and the end of the urethra fixed to the corpora. The midline glans flap is then advanced into the meatotomy and secured to the tunica with 5-0 chromic catgut sutures. The ventral penile flap is rotated and sutured to the distal edges of the glans wings with 5-0 chromic catgut. The edges of the flip flap are then secured to the midline glans flap with a running 7-0 PDS suture. Prepucial skin is used for coverage of the ventral penis.

## PERINEAL, SCROTAL, AND PROXIMAL SHAFT HYPOSPADIAS: TUBE GRAFT HYPOSPADIAS REPAIR (HORTON-DEVINE TECHNIQUE)

The procedure described below is suitable for proximal shaft, scrotal, and perineal urethral hypospadias. The incision circumscribes the native urethral meatus and is extended distally in the midline to meet a circumcising incision of the penis (Fig. 54-4). This maneuver allows exposure of the ventral penis and the native urethral meatus. All dysgenetic tissue is excised from the ventral surface of the corpora to correct the chordee. Penile straightness can then be checked with an artificial erection [14]. A full-thickness skin graft for the urethroplasty is obtained from unfolded prepucial skin. The appropriate dimensions can be determined with calipers. The skin can then be tubed over an appropriately sized stent using a running 7-0 PDS suture under loupe magnification, taking care to invert the mucosal edge into the lumen. The urethra is then brought out to the tip of the glans either by creating glans wings or coring through the glans and excising a central segment of glans tissue. If glans tissue is not excised during tunneling, meatal stenosis may arise unless a V-flap is constructed from the glans epithelium to be interposed into the circular anastomosis. The native urethral meatus is spatulated to allow a wide elliptical anastomosis of the native urethra to the tubed full-thickness skin graft urethra. This proximal

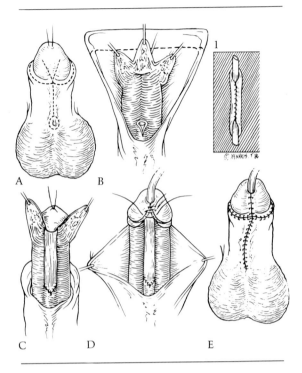

**Figure 54-4** *Full-thickness skin tube graft. A. Proposed incisions for a full-thickness tube graft urethroplasty. B. Resection of ventral dysgenetic fibrous tissue to correct chordee; the midline glans* **V***-flap and the glans wings have been created. C. The dorsal glans* **V***-flap has been secured to the ventral tunica, and the native urethral meatus has been spatulated. A tubed full-thickness skin graft has been anastomosed proximally to the spatulated native urethra and to the glans* **V***-flap. D, E. The glans wings have been reapproximated and the penile skin redraped.*

anastomosis is completed with interrupted 6-0 PDS sutures. The neourethra is then brought through the previously constructed tunnel in the glans and secured to the glans epithelium. The graft is also secured to the corpora along its length with several interrupted PDS sutures. The remaining dorsal prepucial skin is transferred ventrally for coverage of the penis. A small mini-vac drain is left in the wound for 24 hours. A No. 8 French stent is left in the neourethra for 5

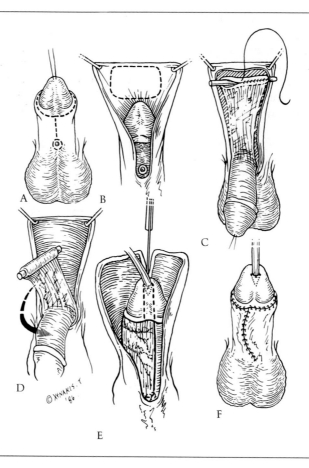

**Figure 54-5** *Vascularized prepucial flap.*
*A. Proposed incisions for a prepucial flap*
*urethroplasty have been marked out. B. Ventral*
*dysgenetic tissue has been excised to correct*
*chordee, and the prepucial flap has been*
*marked out on the inner surface of the dorsal*
*prepucial skin. C. The flap is tubularized over*
*an approximately sized sound with running 5-0*
*and 6-0 PDS sutures. The tubularized flap has*
*had a long pedicle mobilized. D, E. The flap is*
*swung ventrally. A tunnel is created in the*
*glans by excising a core of glans tissue. The flap*
*is approximated to the native urethra before*
*advancing it through the glans tunnel to secure*
*it distally. F. The dorsal penile skin is redraped*
*ventrally and sutured in such a way as to*
*counteract any penile torsion produced by the*
*prepucial flap.*

days, and a percutaneous suprapubic catheter is inserted for urinary drainage. The
penis is dressed with Biocclusive.

### PREPUCIAL ISLAND FLAP (HENDERER, STANDOLI, DUCKETT)

The procedure described here is used for
proximal hypospadias when the prepuce is
large and the rotation of an island of prepuce
does not cause torsion. Initially, chordee is
corrected, and penile straightness is confirmed on artificial erection. Attention is
then turned to the redundant dorsal prepucial skin in order to develop a flap for the
neourethra (Fig. 54-5). The prepuce is freed
from the penile shaft, and the length and
breadth of the tube for the neourethra is
marked on the inner surface of the prepuce.

Careful dissection is then performed to develop a vascular pedicle for this island flap. The vascular pedicle is dissected free from the dorsal penile skin until the flap can be easily moved to the underside of the penis. After complete dissection the adequacy of the blood supply to the flap and the residual dorsal penile skin can be tested with intravenous fluorescein. The neourethra can then be formed around an appropriately sized stent with a subcuticular PDS suture. A tunnel can be created in the glans for the distal neourethra, or glans flaps can be used. The proximal elliptical anastomosis is completed first. The chances of meatal stenosis can be minimized by excising a core of glans tissue from the tunnel or by use of a V-flap in the meatus. When the urethroplasty has been completed, residual dorsal penile skin is brought ventrally for skin coverage. A stent is left in the urethra for 5 days, and urine is drained via a percutaneous suprapubic catheter until the voiding trial 10 days later.

## Postoperative Care

After surgery the patient is treated with cold compresses to the area for the first 2 days. This method reduces edema and pain and keeps the area clean. In patients who have had a flip-flap repair, urinary diversion is achieved through use of a small feeding tube passed through the urethra into the bladder via a urethral stent, which is usually removed on the fifth postoperative day for a voiding trial. This catheter also acts as a stent. Patients who have had a suprapubic catheter inserted may also have a small Silastic urethral stent placed that is removed on the fifth postoperative day. When a tube graft or a prepucial flap has been constructed, urinary diversion is accomplished through a percutaneous suprapubic catheter. Depending on wound healing, this catheter is clamped on the tenth day for a voiding trial. If difficulties occur, the suprapubic tube is opened again for an additional 3 to 4

days to allow further healing. Occasionally we send patients home with a suprapubic tube in place for as long as 3 weeks if prolonged diversion seems necessary. At the end of 3 weeks we allow the patient to void even though a fistula may be present. We counsel that further surgery is probably going to be necessary in 6 months or more, when the inflammation has resolved. In many instances a small pinpoint fistula closes spontaneously.

After the voiding trial we ask the patient to be tubbed three times a day. The Bioocclusive dressing is removed easily on the sixth or seventh postoperative day. After stent removal or the voiding trial (or both), the mother is instructed to keep the meatus open with the nozzle of a tube of Neosporin ophthalmic ointment so that meatal crusting does not precipitate distal obstruction and cause inadvertent fistula formation while voiding.

## Hospitalization

For distal hypospadias cases the hospital stay can be short. For meatal advancement procedures an outpatient procedure or 1 to 2 days in the hospital may be desirable. For flip-flap cases, 5 or 6 days in the hospital are recommended. In more proximal cases we ordinarily keep the patient hospitalized for 10 days.

## Complications

Complications after hypospadias repair can be divided into two groups: those that occur immediately after the surgery during the postoperative phase, and those that occur late. Of those that occur early, bladder spasm, infection, wound dehiscence, and hematoma give the surgeon and the patient concern. If bladder spasms occur after surgery, opium suppositories, hot baths, and repositioning the catheter within the bladder are useful. Usually bladder spasms can be controlled with this therapy. Infection is controlled by the use of antibiotics pre- and postoperatively. Once an infection has been identified, the wound is cultured and appropriate antibiotics are selected.

Impending wound dehiscence is noted when the skin flaps become edematous and black and eschar formation occurs. We have found that it is not useful to resuture this type of skin on the penis, as the sutures cut through the tissues easily. We prefer to allow the patient to heal spontaneously and repair the dehisced wound 6 months later after scarring resolves and healthy tissue is seen adjacent to the damaged area. We have occasionally used a Montgomery-type strap bandage of Elastoplast to hold the edges together to keep tension from impending dehiscence.

Hematomas are troublesome in the penile area. The entire region is so vascular that straining at stool and ambulation may cause hematoma even after hemostasis appears to be adequate at surgery. If an acute hematoma occurs that jeopardizes a graft or the circulation of skin flaps, the patient is returned to the operating room and the hematoma evacuated. If the hematoma is minimal and does not seem to impair wound healing, it can be watched conservatively. It usually resolves. It is difficult to diagnose a hematoma because the skin of the penis becomes edematous and bruised immediately after surgery. It is better to err on the side of exploring the wound and evacuating the hematoma. The use of a pressure bandage of Biocclusive is important for preventing hematoma. The Biocclusive is clear, and the condition of the skin of the penis can be seen at all times. The Biocclusive keeps minimal pressure on the penis and helps prevent hematoma by compressing the vessels postoperatively. We also use cold compresses for 48 hours after the surgery, which causes vasoconstriction and reduces hematoma formation.

Late secondary complications after hypospadias repair consist in fistula, diverticulum, strictures, meatal stenosis, hair growth in the urethra, tortuosity of the new urethra causing an irregular urinary flow, and a retrusive meatus. These complications are best repaired 6 months after the hypospadias repair.

When a fistula is noted after surgery, we prefer to divert the urine from the urethra for another 2 weeks. This maneuver allows the fistula to heal if it is small. Most of the fistulas under 1 to 2 mm in size resolve spontaneously with this technique. Within 2 weeks the patient is allowed to pass urine normally. If the fistula remains, we wait 6 months for an elective fistula repair. The latter consists in first using the cystoscope to ensure that no valves or tortuosity of the urethra are present. It must be determined that no stricture or other problems are causing an impediment to flow that places stress on the wall of the urethra at the site of the fistula. Once it has been determined that the remainder of the urethra is normal, the fistula can be repaired easily by approximating the walls of the urethra after the fistula has been excised, if the fistula is small. If the fistula closure narrows the circumference of the urethra at the site of the repair, additional tissue must be placed in the urethra. It can be done by using a flap adjacent to the fistula (Duplay) so that epithelium from the wound edge is brought into the urethra.

If a diverticulum occurs, radiographic contrast studies demonstrate the site and size of the lesion. Urethroscopy and distention of the urethra demonstrate the problem at the operating table. An incision is made over the diverticulum, and a sound is placed in the urethra to allow tailoring of the urethra to a normal circumference. The urethra is repaired so that the size, for the entire length of the urethra, is symmetric.

If a stricture occurs in the urethra, the procedure for repair can be performed in one of two ways. A longitudinal flap is marked parallel and adjacent to the stricture that has as its base one side of the stricture. Its blood supply is from subcutaneous vessels adjacent to the stricture. The urethra stricture is incised well proximal and distal to ensure complete correction. The urethral edge adjacent to the flap is sutured to the ipsilateral edge of the penile shaft flap, taking care to preserve the subcutaneous circulation. The flap is then flipped over and the opposite flap edge sewed to the contralateral urethral edge. This flap of skin on a subcutaneous tissue mesentery can be utilized for strictures anywhere on the penile shaft where there is hairless skin. Skin containing hair follicles must not be used to repair the urethra. If this technique is prohibited because of inadequate subcutaneous circulation, excess adjacent scar tissue, or the presence of hair, the stricture is opened and a hairless full-thickness graft is placed in the defect to reconstruct the urethra to an adequate size.

Meatal stenosis is corrected using a triangular flap from the glans that is advanced in a Y-V procedure into the distal meatus. It is desirable to use this triangular dorsal flap rather than cutting the inferior edge of the meatus because by cutting the inferior edge of the meatus a hypospadias condition is accentuated by the surgeon. Most meatal strictures can be repaired by the triangular flap technique. If inadequate tissue is present in the glans to perform this technique, an incision can be made in the dorsal surface of the glans and a full-thickness patch of skin placed into the distal meatus to correct the stenosis.

When hair is causing difficulty in the urethra, the area of hair growth can be exposed surgically. If the hair follicles are not numerous, they can be electrocoagulated. This procedure usually takes care of the problem if hair growth is not luxuriant. If there is a great deal of hair growth, the pathologic portion of the urethra is excised and a new urethra formed with a full-thickness graft.

If tortuosity of the new urethra occurs, the excess skin and uroepithelium produce folds that cause eddies of the urinary stream. The excess tissue of the new urethra can simply be excised and the remaining urethra contoured into a lumen of normal size.

A retrusive meatus is present after certain hypospadias repairs, notably those of the Dennis-Browne, Thiersche, Duplay, Byars, and other techniques that do not attempt to bring the meatus to the tip. This retrusive meatus can be treated as distal hypospadias, and flip flaps and glans flaps may be used to reconstruct the meatus to the tip.

Aesthetic concern about the genital area is as important to patients and surgeons as for other areas of the body. Patients and parents are demanding that penile repairs leave the patient without evidence of deformity or previous abnormality. We believe that at one operation all patients with hypospadias can be offered straightening of the penis, a urethroplasty of adequate length so that the meatus ends in the midportion of the glans, and redraping of penile skin, which avoids ugly bulges, skin tags, and penile torsion. Our experience in genital surgery now totals more than 5000 cases. We have watched our patients grow through puberty to adulthood, and many have produced children. We believe it is essential that not only the function of the penis be restored but the aesthetic appearance in this reconstructive procedure be emphasized.

## Epispadias and Exstrophy of the Bladder

Epispadias and exstrophy of the bladder may be defined as congenital deformities of the external genitalia and bladder in which there is failure or blockage of normal development of the dorsal surface of the penis, abdomen, and anterior bladder wall. Although they are not completely understood embryologically, it is essential to consider these defects as varying degrees of a single disorder. It is not known whether the disorder results from a developmental arrest of the lower portion of the urogenital tract or because of an abnormal development of the cloacal membrane. Exstrophy rarely occurs in more than one member of a family, so the parents of children with this unfortunate anomaly can be reassured with some certainty that the chances of future offspring having this disorder are slight.

Exstrophy of the bladder with complete epispadias is the form of anomaly most commonly seen, occurring in approximately 1 per 30,000 births. It is three to four times more common in males. Probably 300 to 350 newborn infants with exstrophy are seen each year in the United States [9]. Complete epispadias of the penis or a bifid clitoris almost always accompanies exstrophy, but cases of exstrophy with a normal penis have been reported. Exstrophy of the bladder is seen four times more frequently than epispadias alone. The frequency is the same for males and females.

Even though the exstrophy is almost always complete, minor variations of an abdominal wall defect with a superior or inferior vesicle fissure may be seen. Simple layered closure of these defects is usually considered adequate treatment.

REPAIR OF EPISPADIAS

With epispadiac deformities distal to the bladder neck, urinary continence is not a problem. A cosmetically satisfactory and functional reconstruction is usually possible.

The distal epispadias problem is treated with the same technique as for the hypospadias problem located in the same anatomic position with the exception that the repair is reversed and the epispadias reconstruction is on the dorsal surface. For more proximal epispadias cases, a large prepuce is present on the ventral surface of the glans and can be used for the reconstruction. Patients with epispadias usually have a urethral plate that is deficient in length; therefore unless the urethral plate is divided and chordee released, the patient continues to have dorsal curvature (the reverse curvature from hypospadias).

In cases where the urethral meatus is on the penile shaft in a distal position, a flip-flap type of repair can be utilized. The flip flap is based on the urethral meatus. Excisions are made distal to the urethral meatus,

circumcising the glans to elevate the lateral skin. By incising distal to the meatus, the tissues causing chordee can be released adequately so that the penis dangles appropriately and chordee is not present with artificial erection. More severe epispadias cases (Fig. 54-6) have separate corporal bodies, and two artificial erection devices must be used to instill saline in each separate corporal body. In distal cases, one artificial erection device may suffice [13].

After chordee is corrected, a midline glanular flap and glanular wings are constructed. The flip flap is used to anastomose to the midline glanular flap, extending the urethra to the tip of the glans. The lateral glandar wings are then sutured over the urethra using 5-0 PDS suture subcutaneously and 6-0 chromic through the glans epithelium. The prepuce is divided in the midline and brought to the dorsal surface of the penis, where it can cover the dorsal defect. This operation is a simple reverse hypospadias repair. For more proximal cases of epispadias, when the midline glans flap cannot reach the epispadias meatus, a free full-thickness graft of prepucial skin is utilized similar to that used for the repair of proximal hypospadias previously described. Occasionally the prepuce of the epispadias patient is deficient in size, and adequate tissue appears difficult to obtain. We have also utilized the ventral surface of the penis and prepuce as a vascularized prepucial flap to swing to the dorsal side of the penis to reconstruct the urethral tube or to cover the skin deficit. The scrotum can be advanced anteriorly on the ventral surface of the penis to provide more skin to the area.

Epispadias that extends to the bladder neck with urinary incontinence can be repaired functionally by releasing the bladder from the symphysis pubis and resecting wedges of anterior bladder neck to elongate the urethra. This portion of the urethra is closed, and the surrounding tissue that contains sphincter muscle fibers is used to correct the sphincter urethral deformity. If the bladder size is not adequate, or if the ureters

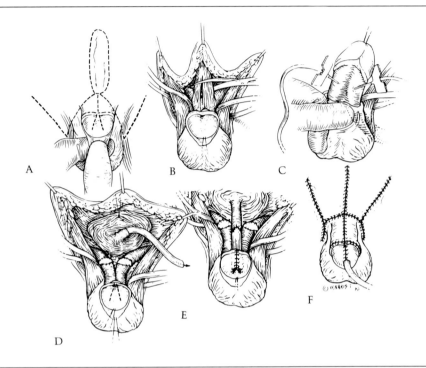

**Figure 54-6** *Exstrophy/epispadias. A. Proposed W-flaps have been marked out, including the ventral abdominal scar to be excised. B. Dysgenetic subcutaneous bands are divided and excised. The spermatic cord structures are identified on each side. C. Bilateral artificial erections are required to confirm a straight penis, as the corporal bodies usually do not communicate in patients with exstrophy/ epispadias. D. Further dissection has partially released the corporal bodies. In this case a previous urethroplasty has had to be transected to create a dangling penis. A catheter enters the proximal urethra and drains the bladder. Midline approximation of the ventral tunica produces outward rotation and straightening of the corpora; transverse incisions are placed in the dorsal aspects of the corpora at the site of maximum curvature to allow straightening. The defects created in the tunica albuginea are then repaired with separate dermal grafts or a single larger dermal graft. E. A tubed full-thickness skin graft has been anastomosed proximally to the spatulated native urethra and to the glans V-flap. F. The W incision has been closed to rotate the hair-bearing skin superiorly and medially to normalize the escutcheon and provide extra skin to lengthen the dorsal surface of the penis.*

are implanted in the bladder in a low position so that lower bladder muscle cannot be easily obtained without injuring the ureters, a replant of the ureters into a higher position must be performed. If the bladder capacity is inadequate, a colon augmentation may be necessary. A thorough work-up is necessary on these difficult incontinent patients.

Postoperative management is the same as for hypospadias.

REPAIR OF EXSTROPHY
OF THE BLADDER
Exstrophy of the bladder represents a more serious abnormality in which there is separation of the symphysis pubis and a defect in the abdominal wall. The anterior bladder wall is absent, and the bladder is everted. This abnormality may be accompanied by incompetence of the upper urinary tract. If this condition is not corrected, it results in infection, ureteral dilatation, renal destruction, and extensive pain. An occasional pa-

tient whose exstrophy has not been corrected has lived to adult life, but it is unusual. Carcinoma of the bladder frequently develops in older, untreated patients [8, 12].

The best treatment for exstrophy of the bladder remains controversial. There are two schools of thought: One advocates urinary diversion, with an ileal or colon conduit, excision of the bladder, and closure of the abdominal wall defect using local flaps of striated muscle, fascia, and skin. Some surgeons prefer placing the ureters in the sigmoid colon, thereby avoiding an abdominal stoma. Correction of the deformity of the external genitalia can be done at the same stage or later [20]. Other surgeons advocate functional closure of the bladder to attempt to provide some degree of continence without obstruction and without causing vesicoureteral reflux [15].

No method of treatment for this congenital anomaly is entirely satisfactory. Urinary diversion by ureterocolic anastomosis may provide continence, but a moderate percentage of patients with exstrophy of the bladder also have rectal incontinence (incontinence cannot be assessed in infants). Long-term results of this procedure have shown that it is not always satisfactory, even in those who are continent. Many die early from infection and its complications. Ileal or colon loop diversion is an alternative because it provides better protection to the kidneys, but it requires an external collection device. There is still strong feeling that sigmoid diversion is better tolerated in the young patient than in the older one. An isolated sigmoid loop diversion has been recommended. This method has the advantage that it can be replaced as the patient becomes older if the anal sphincter works adequately.

FUNCTIONAL CLOSURE OF
EXSTROPHY OF THE BLADDER
In recent years a "functional closure" for exstrophy of the bladder has become popular. Ideally, this procedure is done immedi-ately after birth. Bilateral iliac osteotomies to bring the symphysis pubis together at the midline, thereby reducing the size of the abdominal wall defect and simplifying the closure, are recommended by some authors; but we do not believe it is usually required [18]. The everted bladder is freed from its attachment to the abdominal wall, and the edges are approximated with a two-layer closure. The abdominal wall is closed in layers. Flaps of rectus muscle, rectus fascia, or both can be raised to provide anterior wall support. A catheter is left in as a suprapubic drain. Any deformities of the external genitalia are also repaired, or the external genitalia can be repaired at a second stage. Paired inguinal groin flaps as described by the authors help correct the shortness of skin and the deficiency of the escutcheon.

Vesicoureteral reflux is frequent in these reconstructed cases. It is often necessary to do an antireflux procedure either at the time of primary closure or later. Because of the distorted nature of the bladder wall and the irregularity of the mucosa, it is usually better to delay this procedure. If it is done at the primary stage, reimplanting the ureter is preferable to an intravesical reinforcing procedure. When the repair is carried out primarily, it is necessary to continue the suprapubic drainage for 6 to 8 weeks to avoid damage to the ureteral repair by increasing intravesical pressure.

Snyder [19] has reported a technique of dividing the sigmoid colon and attaching the distal segment to the posterior bladder wall to serve as a urinary receptacle. The defect of the anterior abdominal wall is closed in layers, and the epispadias is repaired. The intact anal sphincter provides voluntary control. Preservation of the normal ureterovesical junction decreases the possibility of recurrent complications of reflux. The distal end of the transected sigmoid colon is brought through the anal sphincter posterior to the normal anus, thus restoring fecal continence. Long-term results have not been as satisfactory as anticipated.

In all patients with exstrophy, the degree of continence to be expected depends on the sex of the patient. It is more unusual for male patients to become continent. Females have a better chance of being continent after functional closure. All patients frequently develop urinary tract infection and must be maintained on urinary antiseptics or antibiotics. If obstruction becomes a problem—with the sequelae of severe, uncontrollable infection and dilatation and destruction of the upper urinary tract—a diversionary procedure, usually with an ileal loop, is undertaken.

No current treatment of exstrophy of the bladder is giving good results in all patients. The immediate urinary diversionary procedures, with excision of the exstrophic bladder mucosa and repair of the abdominal defect and external genitalia, can give immediate good results, but the long-term results leave much to be desired. Functional repair of the bladder has improved but also has not proved to be the ideal solution. However, it now seems that this method may be the initial treatment of choice, particularly in females. If it fails, a urinary diversionary operation can be carried out. It must be emphasized that protection of renal function is the primary objective of treatment, and all other considerations are secondary [17].

# References

1. Blair, V. P., and Byars, L. T. Hypospadias and epispadias. *J. Urol.* 40:814, 1938.
2. Browne, D. An operation for hypospadias. *Proc. R. Soc. Med.* 42:466, 1949.
3. Cecil, A. B. Surgery of hypospadias and epispadias in the male. *J. Urol.* 27:507, 1932.
4. Devine, C. J., Jr., and Horton, C. E. A one stage hypospadias repair. *J. Urol.* 85:166, 1961.
5. Devine, C. J., Jr., Franz, J. P., and Horton, C. E. Evaluation and treatment of patients with failed hypospadias repair. *J. Urol.* Vol. 19, February 1978.
6. Duplay, S. Sur le traitement chirurgical de l'hypospadias et de l'epispadias. *Arch. Gen. Med.* 5:257, 1880.
7. Gilbert, D., Devine, C. J., Jr., Winslow, B. H., et al. Microsurgical hypospadias repair. *Plast. Reconstr. Surg.* 77:460, 1986.
8. Higgins, C. C. An evaluation of cystectomy: For exstrophy, for papillomatosis, and for carcinoma of the bladder. *J. Urol.* 80:279, 1958.
9. Hoffman, W. W., and Spence, H. M. Management of exstrophy of the bladder. *South. Med. J.* 58:436, 1965.
10. Horton, C. E. (ed.). *Plastic and Reconstructive Surgery of the Genital Area.* Boston: Little, Brown, 1973.
11. Horton, C. E., and Devine, C. J., Jr. One stage hypospadias repair. *Film by Eaton Laboratories, 1959.*
12. Horton, C. E., and Devine, C. J., Jr. Hypospadias and epispadias. *Clin. Symp. Ciba* 24:No. 3, 1972.
13. Horton, C. E., and Devine, C. J., Jr. Simulated erection of the penis with saline injection, a diagnostic maneuver. *Plast. Reconstr. Surg.* 59:670, 1977.
14. Horton, C. E., Devine, C. J., Jr., and Gilbert, D. A. Penile curvatures. *Plast. Reconstr. Surg.* 5:52, 1985.
15. Marshall, V. F., and Muecke, E. C. Variations in exstrophy of the bladder. *J. Urol.* 88:766, 1962.
16. McIndoe, A. The treatment of hypospadias. *Am. J. Surg.* 176, 1937.
17. Panel discussion: Anomalies of external genitalia in infancy and childhood. [H. M. Spencer, moderator; V. F. Marshall, discussant.] *J. Urol.* 93:1, 1965.
18. Shultz, W. G. Plastic repair of exstrophy of bladder combined with bilateral osteotomy of ilia. *J. Urol.* 79:453, 1958.
19. Snyder, C. C. A new therapeutic concept of the exstrophied bladder. *Plast. Reconstr. Surg.* 22:1, 1958.
20. Sweetser, T. H., Chisholm, T. C., Thompson, W. H., et al. Exstrophy of the urinary bladder: Its treatment by plastic surgery. *J. Urol.* 75:448, 1956.

# 55

# Correction of Male Impotence by Penile Implants

*Harvey Lash*
*David B. Apfelberg*
*Morton R. Maser*
*David N. White*

Because impotence in mankind is so common, efforts to correct malfunctions of the erectile-ejaculatory mechanisms have deluged the medical literature. Although in antiquity bizarre fertility rites and myriad external devices (some weird and others ingenious) preceded Hippocrates, we might view his statement that "business worries" and "female slovenliness" are the real causes of impotence as perhaps the earliest record of the psychological etiology, which until the 1980s was thought to be the major cause of impotence. Studies have challenged this view, and it is presently thought that in most cases the causes are indeed organic [19, 22].

Perhaps the knowledge that many animals have been provided with an os penis [40] stimulated clinical trials of autogenous implants, chiefly cartilage and bone, during the 1930s. As might now be predicted, warpage, resorption, and other difficulties severely limited their usefulness.

With the advent of well tolerated synthetic materials, new surgical avenues were opened, and in 1952 Goodwin and Scott [28] reported using acrylic for penile implants. In 1960 Loeffler and Sayegh reported two cases of a single acrylic rod placed deep to the tunica albuginea [39], and Beheri in the same year reported the use of double rods of polyethylene placed in the corpora.

With the advent of silicone, a material became available that not only was well tolerated by the body but also could be produced in any consistency ranging from a watery liquid to a hard rubber. Lash et al. reported the first silicone penile implant in 1964 [37], and the modern era of single rods, double rods, and inflatable implants was under way [3, 4, 35, 36].

## Physiology

Male sexual dysfunction may manifest in a variety of forms. Of them, only impotence is routinely amenable to surgical treatment. It is thus essential that the exact nature of the dysfunction be established prior to undertaking any form of therapy.

Clear definition of the psychological and physiologic etiologies of impotence is key to selecting the appropriate treatment and determining ultimate success. Because of the significant psychological overlay occurring in sexually related health problems, a definitive diagnosis is often not established purely on the basis of history and physical examination. Laboratory testing and multiple diagnostic modalities are presently avail-

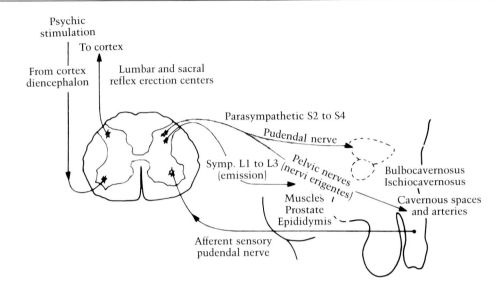

Psychic
stimulation

To cortex

From cortex
diencephalon

Lumbar and sacral
reflex erection centers

Parasympathetic S2 to S4

Pudendal nerve

Symp. L1 to L3
(emission)

*Pelvic nerves
(nervi erigentes)*

Bulbocavernosus
Ischiocavernosus

Muscles
Prostate
Epididymis

Cavernous spaces
and arteries

Afferent sensory
pudendal nerve

**Figure 55-1** *Neurologic component of the erectile-ejaculatory mechanism. (From H. Lash, D. B. Apfelberg, and M. R. Maser. Solid Penile Implants. In L. R. Rubin (ed.),* Biomaterials in Reconstructive Surgery. *St. Louis: Mosby, 1983.)*

able to assist in the clinical evaluation of these patients. Among the most promising are noninvasive methods of assessing penile vascular function [6]. Also included are Doppler determination of penile systolic pressures [1] and strain gauge measurement of nocturnal penile tumescence [14]. Additional testing is often needed to evaluate possible neurologic, endocrinologic, infectious, pharmacologic, and mechanical causes of impotence. Only after all medical and psychiatric possibilities have been considered should surgical treatment be entertained. The placement of a penile implant is but one of the methods. The development of microvascular surgery has introduced penile revascularization procedures and has been successful in selected cases [63]. Thus the clinician to whom the patient ultimately presents not only must establish an exacting diagnosis but must also carefully weigh the indications and anticipated results of the various forms of surgical treatment presently available.

A brief review of the erectile-ejaculatory mechanism illustrates its complexity [50, 53, 64] and the difficulty encountered when differentiating organic dysfunction from that of psychological origin (Fig. 55-1). Two neuropsychological mechanisms are involved in erection. One of these is "psychogenic" (mediated by thoracolumbar outflow through the hypogastric plexus at the T12–L1 levels) and another "reflexogenic" (arising via afferent nerve supply to the penis through the pudendal nerve and efferent parasympathetic fibers of the nervi erigentes at S2–S4). Function of the latter mechanism is illustrated by erections in patients with partial and complete cord transection.

Normally the cerebral mechanism augments the reflex mechanism via the accumulation in the cerebrum of multiple erotic stimuli. From this level impulses are transmitted through lateral spinal tracts to exit the cord in parasympathetic fibers at S2–S4. This outflow triggers the vascular changes necessary to initiate tumescence.

That both sympathetic and parasympathetic portions of the autonomic nervous system play a role in the physiology of erection is illustrated by the presence of both adrenergic and cholinergic fibers within the vessels supplying the corpora cavernosa. Either is capable of producing arteriolar dilatation and tumescence.

The ultimate result of these neurogenic factors is an increase in the rate of blood inflow to the corpora. This increase alone is sufficient to result in erection. Once thought essential to the initiation and maintenance of erection, venous obstruction exists only relative to the increased arterial inflow. Although not thought necessary for tumescence under normal circumstances, the exact role of venous obstruction remains controversial.

As tactile stimulation of the penis is carried through the cord to synapse with lumbar sympathetic fibers, peristalsis is initiated, emptying secretions within the vas deferens, seminal vesicles, and prostate into the prostatic urethra. Parasympathetic efferent discharge forces movement of semen through the pendulous urethra, resulting in ejaculation.

The neurophysiologic aspects of both erection and ejaculation are subject to neuroendocrine alterations. Changes within the pituitary-gonadal axis may result in decreased serum testosterone levels and impotence [61].

The problem of impotence must thus be evaluated in a multidisciplinary fashion. From a spectrum of possible etiologies, a clear path to successful treatment can be established.

## Tissue Reaction

Tolerance by body tissues of many materials presently used for implantation is excellent and in the case of silicone may be considered legendary, as often one fails to find even a giant cell reaction to this foreign body. Scars, however, form around all alloplastic implants, and research efforts to analyze and

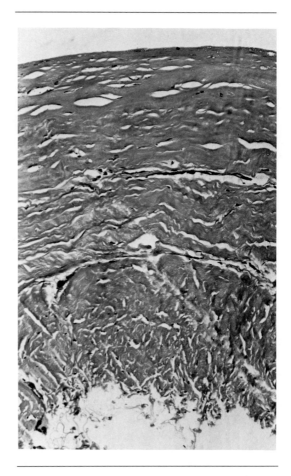

**Figure 55-2** *Microscopic view of thickened pseudocapsule surrounding a solid penile implant. Note the absence of any inflammatory reaction. (Courtesy of Dr. Michael P. Small.)*

explain the behavior of these capsules are legion. Reasons for gossamer versus thickened capsules in the same individual in similar locations (e.g., bilateral breast implants) remain elusive, as does the etiology of constriction, which may be unrelated to capsular thickness. Equally perplexing is the concept of "privileged sites," such as the subpectoral area where capsule constrictions are less common. The role played by bacteria, myofibroblasts, steroids, chemical irritants, blood, and trauma remains controversial. With solid penile implants, prob-

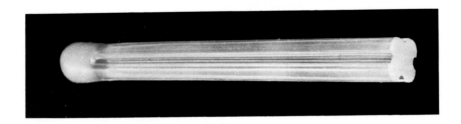

**Figure 55-3** *Current design of the single rod. The rounded distal end eliminates rotational orientation.*

lems with capsule formation are relatively unimportant and, paradoxically, in some instances may even be considered protective. Loeffler's observation that capsules seen several months to several years after implantation of solid silicone into the corpora cavernosa remain gossamer is borne out by the clinical evidence of patients with psychic impotence who more than 20 years after implantation can still achieve normal erection. Further corroboration was provided by Small, who described a clinically thickened pseudocapsule that did not interfere with cavernous function [59] (Fig. 55-2).

Capsular contractions do, however, become significant when one considers inflatable implants because, as might be anticipated, with this device function may be impaired. Furlow has reported this situation to be most notable in the reservoir area and less common in the corpora [23], indicating that the corpora, like the subpectoral area, might be considered a "privileged site."

## Implant Designs

Three varieties of implant are presently in use for the correction of impotence: the simple rod, the double rod, and the inflatable device.

### SIMPLE RODS

Initially made of cartilage or bone, later of acrylic, and presently of silicone, the simple rod retains its appeal in selected cases (Fig. 55-3). Placed through a dorsal incision, usually under local anesthesia, it is a simple sur-

gical procedure, and the device is relatively free of complications. Because the partition one sees in drawings that supposedly separates the corpora cavernosa is in reality almost nonexistent anteriorly, the rod can be centrally placed by incising the tunica albuginea dorsally, and the rod then simply "floats" between the corpora. Measured to extend from the corona to the pubis, it does not produce an erection but serves to prevent buckling in an otherwise flaccid organ. Thus intercourse is possible without an erection. In those individuals still capable of occasional erection, there has been no interference with this function, nor has the midline incision produced neurovascular problems. In clothing there is no discernible bulge, nor can it be detected during urination. Intercourse techniques, however, must be relearned because, in the absence of erection, thrusting must be somewhat limited to avoid disengagement, which then would require manual assistance for reinsertion. Most patients have readily adapted to these changes.

As might be anticipated, complications with this device have been relatively few. When first placed during the early 1960s fears of vascular compromise, prolonged edema, urinary blockage, and the rejection phenomenon failed to materialize. Erosion, however, was noted in several patients who were paraplegic and on external condom drainage. These patients remain the most difficult to implant [54], requiring special instructions about the avoidance of constricting rolls in their condom drains. If placed too anteriorly, the rod can erode through the fossa naviculare, necessitating its removal. However, in more than 150 patients the overall complication rate necessitating reoperation for any reason is less than 2 percent.

*Surgical Technique*

The placement of double rods and inflatable prostheses is well covered elsewhere [42, 52, 60] and is not discussed here. Our review is limited to the steps required to place the simple rod.

The patient is prepped and draped in the usual fashion. An adhering agent is placed on the glans penis, and four Steristrips are attached. Under traction to simulate the length of the penis in erection, the implant is measured from the proximal penile shaft to a point 1.5 cm proximal to the glans. The proximal portion of the implant is then cut to this length (Fig. 55-4A) and any sharp edge trimmed or removed with sandpaper (hand dermabrader). The midline of the dorsal penis is marked, and utilizing a ⅝-inch Penrose drain as a tourniquet, incision is begun 1 cm proximal to the glans and carried proximally 4 to 5 cm. Incision is then carried through Buck's fascia and the tunica albuginea into the corpora cavernosa, care being exercised to remain in the midline (Fig. 55-4B). No effort is made to retract the dorsal neurovascular structures. By blunt dissection immediately deep to the tunica albuginea a pocket is developed distal to the corona (Fig. 55-4C) and proximal to the penile base of sufficient size to admit the implant (Fig. 55-4D). The tourniquet may be temporarily released to facilitate insertion of the implant. With the implant in position the tourniquet may be reinstituted and closure obtained with 3-0 absorbable sutures in the tunica albuginea, 4-0 absorbable sutures in Buck's fascia, and 5-0 absorbable sutures in the skin. A xeroform dressing is held over the suture line by several Steristrips, which must not encompass more than one-half the circumference of the penis; a conforming roll is then placed, care being exercised to cover the entire glans (except for the meatus) with the prepuce fully forward. On the fourth postoperative day dressings are removed, and the patient is instructed in the use of an applicator stick moistened in hydrogen peroxide to clean the suture line and a thin application of bacitracin ointment after each voiding. Application of several loose turns of 2-inch conforming gauze roll protects the clothing. No effort is made to discourage erections in those patients still capable of erection; however, the patient is instructed to avoid intercourse for 6 weeks. In the absence of erections, intercourse techniques must be relearned, with greater reliance on rotation than thrust in order to avoid disengagement.

SOLID DOUBLE RODS

Although the simple rod enhanced penetration of the vaginal introitus without erection, the double rod produced, in most instances, a permanent erection that proved to be a mixed blessing. Initially reported by Beheri in Egypt [10] and subsequently by Morales et al. in the United States [49], a polyethylene rod was placed into each corpora through a dorsal incision in the distal penis. Subsequently, Small reported the use of silicone rods utilizing a perineal approach, achieving implantation via the crura. With the excellent body tolerance of silicone and the difficulties during the mid-1970s with inflatable prostheses, the Small-Carrion device gained considerable popularity (Fig. 55-5). Because the erection it produced was permanent, there were obvious difficulties with comfort and concealment when not in use. Efforts to overcome these problems resulted in modification of the original design. Loeffler in 1971 introduced a device consisting of a simple rod distally with a bifid hinged tail extending partially into the crura; it offered increased stability without a permanent erection. Finney [20, 21, 27] in 1977 utilized a

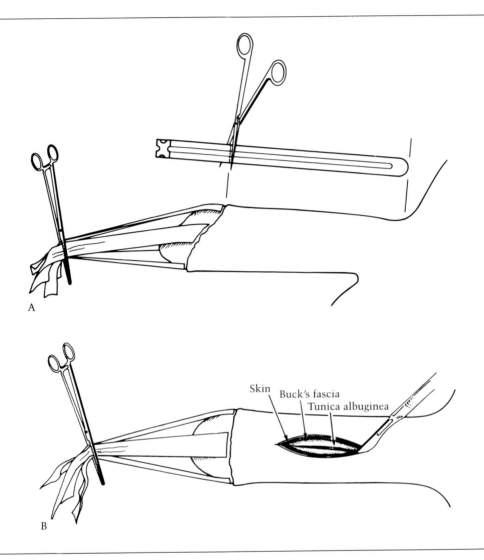

Skin   Buck's fascia
   Tunica albuginea

double rod that, though full length, employed a weakened area that when carefully positioned produced a hinge-like effect. Jonas and others placed metallic centers in the rods that could be manually bent [11, 34, 48, 55].

Complications with these rods, other than those attributable to permanent erection, consisted in proximal or distal perforations of the corpora or crura with the Hegar dilators employed for placing the rods, difficulty of determining proper size [7], erosion of the

**Figure 55-4** *A. The implant is measured from glans to pubis with the penis under mild traction. When fully extended to simulate erection, the implant should be approximately 1.5 cm less than the distance from glans to pubis. Note that the distal end of the implant is placed proximally against the pubis to facilitate measurements. B. Incision is carried through Buck's fascia and the tunica albuginea into the corpora. C. A pocket is developed distally by blunt dissection to the glans. D. The prosthesis is bent for insertion.*

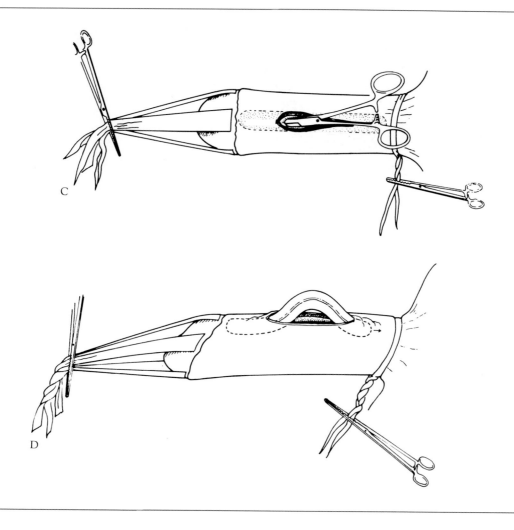

rods if they were too long, and a sliding forward of the glans over the distal implant if they were too short, producing what Small described as an SST (supersonic transport) deformity, stating that it could occur with as little as 0.5 cm of shortening [58]. Tawil et al. reported fracture of the wires in the Jonas type of implant after repeated bending [62]. Other problems included decreased sensation, persistent edema, paraphimosis, urinary retention, and urethral erosion [32]. Nevertheless, patient satisfaction with double rods, as is the case with all categories of penile implants [2, 9, 12, 13, 15, 18, 19, 25,

26, 29, 43, 56, 60], is reported to be high (89 to 95 percent).

INFLATABLE PROSTHESIS
It remains, of course, most appealing to closely mimic nature with a device that could produce penile tumescence on command and flaccidity when appropriate. In 1973 Scott et al. reported five cases in which an inflatable implant was introduced, consisting of paired inflatable cylinders placed in the corpora cavernosa, a scrotal pump to inflate and deflate these cylinders, and a reservoir placed in the prevesical space. These

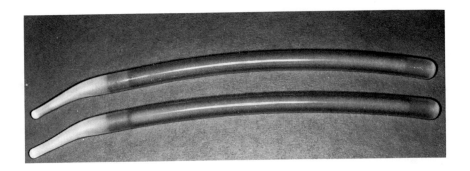

**Figure 55-5** *Small-Carrion double rods.*

parts were connected by a series of tubes and valves [57]. Initially, problems were legion, with a reported incidence of more than 40 percent requiring repeat exploration [5, 17]. In addition to the usual surgical difficulties [41], mechanical problems included cylinder leaks, buckling of tubes, pump malfunctions, and capsule constrictions in the reservoirs [8, 16, 22, 24, 31–33, 38, 44]. The surgical approach was cumbersome, and weakened areas in the tunica albuginea created ballooning with inflation of the clinders.

Many of these difficulties have been corrected [42, 51]. Improved surgical approach allows entry to the corpora, scrotum, and prevesical area by a single incision, which can be undertaken either via the scrotum [22, 47, 52] or suprapubically as modified by Furlow [24]. Teflon coating has reduced the incidence of cylinder leakage caused by wear of the tubing as it exits the cylinder, and an improved tubing design has reduced kinking. A revised pump facilitating easier cylinder deflation has been incorporated.

Other devices, as yet unproved by long follow-up, have been introduced in an effort to simplify both the surgery and the mechanics of inflatable implants [25, 45, 46]. One device (Hydroflex) consists of a tube in each corpora, a pump located behind the glans (which inflates the tubes), and a valve to return the fluid to an internal reservoir [30]. A single-rod inflatable implant (Lash designed), still in the experimental stage,

consists simply of a reservoir in the scrotum and a cylinder surrounding a centrally placed simple rod (Fig. 55-6). No pump is utilized. A single valve allows fluid to be transferred from reservoir to cylinder as needed by simply squeezing one or the other while the valve is compressed.

## Implant of Choice

Faced with the impotent patient whose medical options have been exhausted, one must consider which of the three types of implant is most appropriate. In the elderly and perhaps somewhat debilitated patient, the simple rod continues to have great appeal. The ease of implantation under local anesthesia during a 20- to 30-minute operation, with an implant that is nearly free of mechanical complication and practically undetectable when placed, must rank the simple rod as the implant of choice. Yet it does require, in most patients, relearning intercourse techniques, as no erection is produced.

The double rods, on the other hand, with their ability to produce erection, might be more readily accepted especially in the young individual, who can tolerate a more involved surgical approach with a somewhat higher rate of complications and who is willing to utilize some ingenuity in concealment. For the patient who seems highly motivated by the aesthetics of erection, rather than the

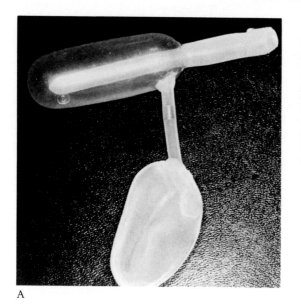
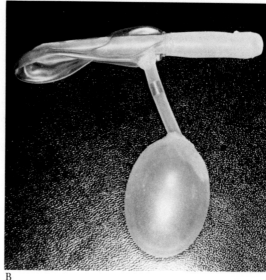

A                                    B

**Figure 55-6** *Single-rod inflatable implant.*
*A. Fluid is in the penile cylinder. B. Fluid is in*
*the scrotal reservoir.*

simple ability to function, and who is well
informed and willing to accept the possibility of a greater complication rate, the inflatable implant seems appropriate.

Our hope at present is that with continued
improvement in inflatable implant design
there will be less mechanical failure and easier surgical placement, so that this type of
device may ultimately be universally used.
While awaiting this ideal implant, we continue to favor, in most cases, the simple
rod, which permits successful and relatively
trouble-free intercourse.

## References

1. Abelson, D. Diagnostic value of the penile pulse and blood pressure: A Doppler study of impotence in diabetics. *J. Urol.* 113:636, 1975.
2. Ankenman, G. U., Sullivan, L. D., Wright, J. E., et al. Penile prosthesis for organic impotence. *Can. J. Surg.* 24:628, 1981.
3. Apfelberg, D. B., Maser, M. R., and Lash, H. Surgical management of impotence: Progress report. *Am. J. Surg.* 132:336, 1976.
4. Apfelberg, D. B., Maser, M. R., and Lash, H. The surgical treatment of erectile impotence. *Compr. Ther.* 2:6, 1976.
5. Apte, S. M., Gregory, J. G., and Purcell, M. H. The inflatable penile prosthesis, reoperation and patient satisfaction: A comparison of statistics obtained from patient record review with statistics obtained from intensive followup search. *J. Urol.* 131:894, 1984.
6. Bahlen, J. Sleep erection monitoring in the evaluation of male erectile failure. *Urol. Clin. North Am.* 8:119, 1981.
7. Barry, J. M. Prediction of semirigid penile prosthesis diameter from saline erection. *J. Urol.* 131:281, 1984.
8. Barry, J. M., Giesy, J. D., and McDuffie, R. Actuarial survivals of inflatable and flexible, hinged penile prostheses. *Urology* 20:605, 1982.
9. Beaser, R. S., Van der Hoek, C., Jacobson, A. M., et al. Experience with penile prostheses in the treatment of impotence in diabetic men. *J.A.M.A.* 248:943, 1982.
10. Beheri, G. E. The problem of impotence solved by a new surgical operation. *Kasr Aini J. Surg.* 1:50, 1960.
11. Benson, R. C., Jr., Barrett, D. M., and Patter-

son, D. E. The Jonas prosthesis—technical considerations and results. *J. Urol.* 130:920, 1983.

12. Beutler, L. E., Scott, F. B., Karacan, I., et al. Women's satisfaction with partners' penile implant: Inflatable vs. noninflatable prosthesis. *Urology* 24:552, 1984.

13. Blake, D. J., McCartney, C., Fried, F. A., et al. Psychiatric assessment of penile implant recipient: Preliminary study. *Urology* 21:252, 1983.

14. Britt, D. B., Kemmerer, W. T., and Robinson, J. R. Penile blood flow determination by mercury strain gauge plethysmography. *Invest. Urol.* 8:673, 1971.

15. Collins, S. F., Jr., and Kinder, B. N. Adjustment following surgical implantation of a penile prosthesis: A critical overview. *J. Sex Marital Ther.* 10:255, 1984.

16. Diokno, A. C. Asymmetric inflation of the penile cylinders: Etiology and management. *J. Urol.* 129:1127, 1983.

17. Fallon, B., Rosenberg, S., and Culp, D. A. Long-term followup in patients with an inflatable penile prosthesis. *J. Urol.* 132:270, 1984.

18. Farina, R., Cury, E., and Ackel, I. A. Surgical treatment of male impotence. *Aesthetic Plast. Surg.* 6:165, 1982.

19. Finan, B. F. The surgical management of erectile impotence. *J. Arkansas Med. Soc.* 81:417, 1985.

20. Finney, R. P. New hinged silicone penile implant. *J. Urol.* 118:585, 1977.

21. Finney, R. P. Finney flexirod prosthesis. *Urology* 23(5 spec. no.): 79, 1984.

22. Fishman, I. J., Scott, F. B., and Light, J. K. Experience with inflatable penile prosthesis. *Urology* 23(5 spec. no.):86, 1984.

23. Furlow, W. L. Personal communication, Rochester, Minnesota, 1980.

24. Furlow, W. L. The inflatable penile prosthesis: The case for the medical device data base. *J. Urol.* 135:72, 1985.

25. Furlow, W. L., and Barrett, D. M. Inflatable penile prosthesis: New device design and patient-partner satisfaction. *Urology* 24:559, 1984.

26. Gansai, M. P., Rivera, L. R., and Spence, C. R. Peyronie's plague: Excision and graft versus incision and stent. *J. Urol.* 127:55, 1982.

27. Gaur, D. D. Single implants in the treatment of erectile impotence. *J. Urol.* 126:745, 1981.

28. Goodwin, W. E., and Scott, W. W. Phalloplasty. *J. Urol.* 68:903, 1952.

29. Hollander, J. B., and Diokno, A. C. Success with penile prosthesis from patient's viewpoint. *Urology* 23:141, 1984.

30. Impotence Breakthrough: Breakthrough III, 1985.

31. Joseph, D., and Bruskewitz, R. C. Bilateral dislocation of rear tip extenders from the inflatable penile prosthesis. *J. Urol.* 128:1317, 1982.

32. Kaufman, J. J., Lindner, A., and Raz, S. Complications of penile prosthesis surgery for impotence. *J. Urol.* 128:1192, 1982.

33. Kossoff, J., Krane, R. J., and Naimark, A. Inflatable penile implant for impotence: Radiologic evaluation. *A.J.R.* 136:1109, 1981.

34. Krane, R. J., Freedberg, P. S., and Siroky, M. B. Jonas silicone-silver penile prosthesis: Initial experience in America. *J. Urol.* 126:475, 1981.

35. Lash, H. Silicone implant for impotence. *J. Urol.* 100:709, 1968.

36. Lash, H., Apfelberg, D. B., and Maser, M. R. Solid Penile Implants. In L. R. Rubin (ed.), *Biomaterials in Reconstructive Surgery.* St. Louis: Mosby, 1983. Pp. 936–945.

37. Lash, H., Zimmerman, D. C., and Loeffler, R. A. Silicone implantation inlay method. *Plast. Reconstr. Surg.* 34:75, 1964.

38. Leach, G. E., Shapiro, C. E., Hadley, R., and Raz, S. Erosion of inflatable penile prosthesis reservoir into bladder and bowel. *J. Urol.* 131:1177, 1984.

39. Loeffler, R. A., and Sayegh, E. S. Perforated acrylic implants in management of organic impotence. *J. Urol.* 84:559, 1960.

40. Loeffler, R. A., Sayegh, E. S., and Lash, H. The artificial os penis. *Plast. Reconstr. Surg.* 34:71, 1964.

41. Maatman, T. J., and Montague, D. K. Intracorporeal drainage after removal of infected penile prostheses. *Urology* 23:184, 1984.

42. Malloy, T. R., Mein, A. J., and Carpiniello, V. L. Revised surgical technique to improve survival of penile cylinders for the inflatable penile prosthesis. *J. Urol.* 130:1105, 1983.

43. Martin, L. M., and Montague, D. K. Ejaculatory incompetence following penile prosthesis implantation in men with primary psychogenic impotence. *Cleve. Clin. Q.* 49:93, 1982.

44. Merrill, D. C. Clinical experience with Scott inflatable penile prosthesis in 150 patients. *Urology* 22:371, 1983.

45. Merrill, D. C. Mentor inflatable penile prosthesis. *Urology* 22:504, 1983.

46. Merrill, D. C., and Javaheri, P. Mentor inflatable penile prosthesis: Preliminary clinical results in 30 patients. *Urology* 23(5 spec. no.):72, 1984.

47. Montague, D. K. Experience with semirigid rod and inflatable penile prostheses. *J. Urol.* 129:967, 1983.

48. Montague, D. K. Experience with Jonas malleable penile prosthesis. *Urology* 23(5 spec. no.):83, 1984.

49. Morales, P. A., Suarez, J. B., Delgado, J., et al. Penile implant for erectile impotence. *J. Urol.* 109:641, 1973.

50. Neuman, H. F., Northrup, J. D., and Devlin, J. Mechanism of human penile erection. *Invest. Urol.* 1:350, 1964.

51. Reed, H. M. Atraumatic color-coded mosquito clamps for inflatable penile prostheses. *Urology* 24:618, 1984.

52. Riemenschneider, H. W., Moon, S. G., Oliver, W. A., et al. Scrotal implantation of the inflatable penile prosthesis. *J. Urol.* 126:747, 1981.

53. Rivand, D. J. Anatomy, physiology, and neurophysiology of male sexual function. *Int. Papers Urol.* 5:219, 1982.

54. Rossier, A. B., and Fam, B. A. Indication and results of semirigid penile prostheses in spinal cord injury patients: Long-term followup. *J. Urol.* 131:59, 1984.

55. Rowe, P. H., and Royle, M. G. Use of Jonas silicon-silver prosthesis in erectile impotence. *J. R. Soc. Med.* 76:1019, 1983.

56. Schlamowitz, K. E., Beatler, L. E., Scott, F. B., et al. Reactions to the implantation of an inflatable penile prosthesis among psychogenically and organically impotent men. *J. Urol.* 129:295, 1983.

57. Scott, F. B., Bradley, W. E., and Timm, G. W. Management of erectile impotence: Use of implantable, inflatable prosthesis. *Urology* 2:80, 1973.

58. Small, M. P. Small-Carrion penile prosthesis: A new implant for management of impotence. *Mayo Clin. Proc.* 51:336, 1976.

59. Small, M. P. The Small-Carrion prosthesis. *Urol. Clin. North Am.* 5:549, 1978.

60. Small, M. P. Surgical treatment of impotence with Small-Carrion prosthesis: Preoperative, intraoperative, and postoperative considerations. *Urology* 23(spec. issue to May):93, 1984.

61. Spark, R. F., White, R. A., and Connolly, P. B. Impotence is not always psychogenic: New insights into hypothalamic-pituitary-gonadal dysfunction. *J.A.M.A.* 248:750, 1980.

62. Tawil, E., Hawatmeh, I. S., Apte, S., et al. Multiple fractures of the silver wire strands as a complication of the silicone-silver wire prosthesis. *J. Urol.* 132:762, 1984.

63. Virag, R. Revascularization of the penis. *Int. Papers Urol.* 5:219, 1982.

64. Weiss, H. D. The physiology of human penile erection. *Ann. Intern. Med.* 76:793, 1972.

# 56

*Donald R. Laub*
*Donald R. Laub, Jr.*
*Jeffrey Wisnicki*

# Injuries to the Male External Genitalia

Land mine explosions during war [45], torture, industrial "power takeoff" accidents, and self-mutilation are the more common etiologies for male genital injury. The general rules of priority applied to injuries of male genitalia are helpful for treatment.

1. Concomitant life-threatening injuries may delay diagnosis and treatment of the injuries to the genitalia and must be treated first.
2. The genital injury may be more threatening to the body image and psyche of the male patient than the more severe body trauma.
3. Urologic principles of scientific diagnostic tests and urinary diversion are helpful.
4. The general surgery and infectious disease disciplines contain knowledge with which the plastic surgeon is not generally conversant.

The anatomy of the penis and scrotum is fascinating, and knowledge of the muscle and fascia layers allows accurate localization of fistulas and trauma. The replantation of the penis or testis also requires special knowledge of physiology and anatomy.

The anatomy of the scrotum is diagrammed in Figure 56-1; it is a composite of the work of Netter, Pernkopf, Sobotta, Snell,

Thorek, and Spalteholz and highlights interesting clinical aspects. Scarpa's subcutaneous fascia of the abdomen extends to the scrotum and penis as dartos fascia, and it contains smooth muscle responsible for the scrotal rugae. The fact that Scarpa's fascia and dartos fascia contain distinct vasculature and that there is muscle in this layer in the scrotum suggests that it is homologous to the carnosus skin muscle of animals and to the platysma and subcutaneous muscu-loaponeurotic system (SMAS) of the human neck and face.

The external spermatic fascia is an extension of the external abdominal oblique muscle aponeurosis. Scrotal avulsion occurs commonly between this layer and dartos fascia in the areolar tissue (just as scalp avulsion occurs between galea and temporalis fascia). The resurfacing of avulsion with skin graft usually results in a good take, as it does in other areas where areolar tissue is the recipient site.

The next deeper layer, the cremasteric fascia and muscle, derives from internal oblique fascia and muscle; the internal spermatic fascia—the infundibuliform fascia—is the local form of the transversalis fascia. The tunica vaginalis is a peritoneum-like layer isolated from the intraabdominal contents when the testes descended from the

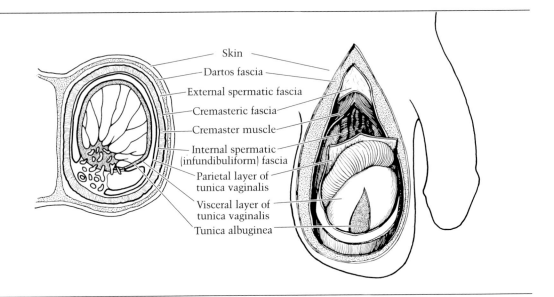

Skin
Dartos fascia
External spermatic fascia
Cremasteric fascia
Cremaster muscle
Internal spermatic (infundibuliform) fascia
Parietal layer of tunica vaginalis
Visceral layer of tunica vaginalis
Tunica albuginea

*Figure 56-1* *Anatomic layers of the scrotum. Avulsion of the scrotal skin usually occurs deep to dartos fascia.*

kidney area during intrauterine development. Hydrocele occurs in this sac. Indirect inguinal hernia may connect the peritoneum to the tunica vaginalis.

In placement of the testes in the scrotum, both teleologic reasoning and Culp's summary [6, 8] of the physiologic research indicate that the spermatogenic (and perhaps other) function of the testes is optimal at skin temperature rather than at internal body temperature. The above information is key to the decisions made regarding treatment options that are available for avulsion of the scrotum at this level.

1. The residual scrotal skin is contracted by the disrupted dartos muscle slips and appears deceptively inadequate in size but may be stretched to cover. Primary closure can be attempted even with some tension.
2. Immediate or delayed tissue expansion techniques must be kept in mind.
3. Skin grafting has enjoyed success [16, 31]. The areolar tissue, if sufficiently undamaged, nourishes a thick split-thickness graft. Innovative postoperative management techniques are useful to meet the challenge of the irregular, movable surface

[24]. Suturing the testes together prevents torsion of the testis and a bifid (female) postoperative appearance. Mesh grafting is of obvious benefit.

Because skin graft coverage has the disadvantages of vulnerability and contracture, [26] implanting the testes in the thighs as island flaps based on the spermatic cord may be indicated. The temperature of the deep thigh is 10°F higher than that of the scrotum, so the testes must be placed just below the dermis. Implantation of the two testes must also be at unequal heights, so that rubbing due to thigh motion does not occur.

Scrotal reconstruction can be done with bilateral thigh flaps (Fig. 56-2). The technique preserves sensation, but donor site defects may require tissue expansion for closure.

Peters and Bright advocated scrotal skin regeneration rather than reconstruction [35]. A 6-week regimen of human chorionic gonadotropin, 500 to 1000 units every other day, stimulates hypertrophy of the remaining scrotal skin. The testes can then be re-

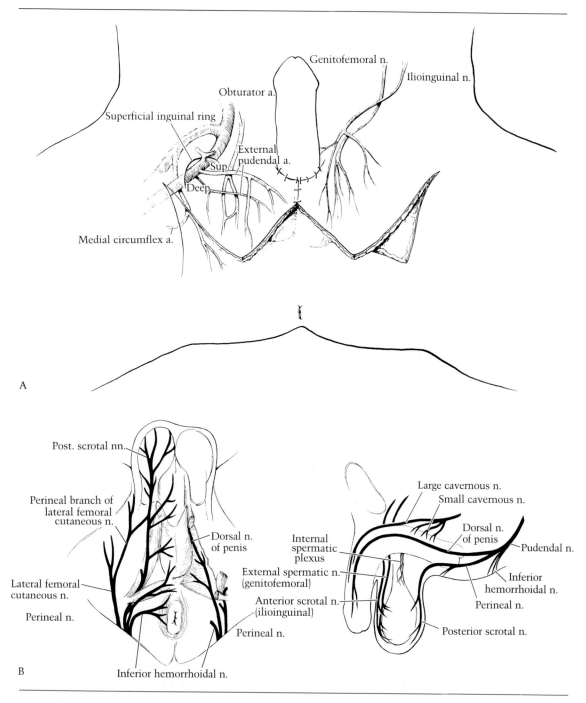

**Figure 56-2** *A. Suggestion regarding flaps for scrotal reconstruction, showing the arterial and nerve supplies. B. Nerves are severed; however, the rich and overlapping nature of the cutaneous nerves in this area is helpful.*

turned from the thigh into the enlarged scrotum.

Testicular replantation has met with some success [22], although the technical difficulty of distinguishing the distal testicular artery from the pampiniform veins has been reported [14]. In the nontraumatic setting, however, microvascular transfer has been successful for treatment of cryptorchidism (or even transplantation from one identical twin to another [1, 34]).

Testicular rupture from nonpenetrating scrotal trauma is uncommon because of the mobility afforded by the tunica vaginalis and the protection afforded by the tunica albuginea. After a kick to the groin, a motorcycle accident, or a contact-sports injury, the patient may present with severe pain, swelling, and scrotal ecchymosis. This patient is often misdiagnosed as having an isolated hematocele when in fact he has testicular rupture. Delay in surgical exploration in order to observe a presumptive hematocele may significantly reduce the possibility of testicular salvage [39]. The introduction of technetium 99 radionuclide scanning for blunt scrotal trauma has further refined diagnostic capabilities [27]. It has been suggested that those patients who have sustained testicular trauma but who have a normal scan do not require surgical exploration [19], but Cass's study [3] disputed this suggestion.

Penetrating injuries of the scrotum dictate a conservative approach. Testicular salvage may be effected with minimal debridement with an accent on the removal of necrotic testicular parenchyma but replacement of herniated tubules. The tunica albuginea must be closed, usually with absorbable suture material. If necessary, a dermal patch graft is helpful. The integrity of the spermatic cord, of course, must be assessed, and familiarity with the cross-sectional anatomy of that structure is essential. A drain is helpful because of the multiple vessels present in the areolar tissue.

The relative mobility of the testicles within the scrotal sack is partly attributed to the cremasteric muscular reflex, which causes retraction of the testicles themselves as well as their mobility within the tunica vaginalis. However, just as in injury to mobile intraperitoneal organs occurs, the mobile testicle may sustain a penetrating injury also.

## Injuries to the Penis

Physical examination after trauma to the penis must include a rectal examination to assess the bulbocavernosus reflex and to determine if blood is being expressed from the penile meatus, which may occur after a urethral injury. The rectal examination also determines the degree of contamination of the urinary tract with rectal bacteria.

Retrograde urethrography may diagnose loss of integrity of the urethra. "Corpus cavernosography" [10] may be helpful because it assesses the integrity of the tunica albuginea, which is the protective and functional sheath for the erectile bilateral corpus cavernosum. Passing a urethral catheter may convert a partial urethral laceration to a more complete one and therefore urinary diversion or assessment of the urinary system is preferably done via suprapubic catheterization.

Because of bleeding and the contamination that occurs with penetrating injuries of the penis, operative exploration and debridement are needed. Perioperative antibiotic coverage is obviously advocated. Debridement must be conservative, excising only obviously nonviable tissue. Unnecessary aggressiveness creates further hemorrhage within the corpora. Hemostasis in this area is difficult to achieve. Repair of Buck's fascia and tunica albuginea of the corpora is important for preventing subsequent penile deformity and loss of erectile function. If the extent of the defect in the corpora does not permit closure without angulation, the corpora are left open [38]. Delayed primary closure of the skin may be considered for a severe and highly contaminated injury; this principle was reinforced with the Vietnam experience. Ure-

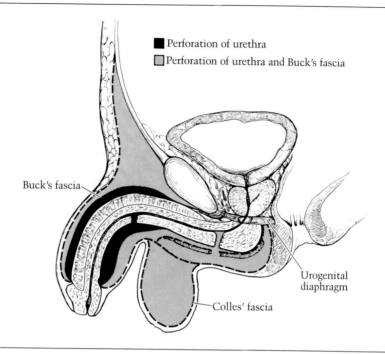

■ Perforation of urethra
□ Perforation of urethra and Buck's fascia

Buck's fascia

Urogenital
diaphragm

Colles' fascia

**Figure 56-3** *Extravasation of urine and hemorrhage from periurethral structures manifests according to the relation to Buck's fascia and Colles' fascia and the urogenital diaphragm.*

thral lacerations may be repaired primarily with fine chromic catgut sutures over a stent or catheter. Although the penile urethra permits surprising amounts of mobilization to achieve closure in cases where there is loss of small amounts of length, attempts at repair of extensive destruction usually result in stricture or fistula. Marsupialization of the urethra to the adjacent skin edges and delayed reconstruction have been recommended in these cases [38].

Iatrogenic instrumentation or catheterization may cause lacerations to the external meatus, partial urethral lacerations, or injury to the bulbous portion of the anterior urethra and the bladder neck. These injuries respond to catheter drainage alone for periods up to 1 month. More extensive injuries obviously require operative exposure for catheter placement, and repair can be done at that time [23]. For a short period of time the urinary urethral catheter serves as a stent, but after a few days it is a source of irritation—a foreign body that may promote bacterial contamination. During the healing process urinary diversion with perineal urethrostomy or a suprapubic catheter is more helpful than the urethral catheter.

The injury causing urethral extravasation of blood and urine may be located by physical examination if a working knowledge of the various fascial layers is known [35] (Fig. 56-3). If unrecognized extravasation of urine or internal bleeding persists, operative intervention for drainage, hemostasis, and appropriate urinary diversion may reverse an unrecognized life-threatening infection. Vacuum cleaner lacerations, insertion of foreign bodies into the urethra, silicone injections, and penile bites do occur and are regarded as "not uncommon" [5]. Risk of infection is of particular concern with bites because introduction of virulent organisms can lead to spreading infection and Fournier's gangrene.

## PENILE FRACTURE

Although relatively uncommon, penile fracture is interesting, and proper management is required to avoid late sequelae [11, 15, 30, 44]. Knowledge regarding the condition is needed to recognize and treat it. The injury typically is a consequence of external trauma to the erect penis, causing a tear in the tunica albuginea of one of the corpora. It may occur during intercourse. Rolling over in bed or other forceful injury are other etiologic mechanisms. The patient reports hearing a cracking sound, followed by flaccidity as blood extravasates from the corpora. Painful swelling, ecchymosis, and penile deviation rapidly ensue. Urethral rupture occurs in perhaps one-third of reported cases. It is in this instance that corpus cavernosography is useful. (Instill lidocaine with a 25-gauge needle into an area of the uninjured corpora cavernosa, followed by water-soluble contrast [10].) Fluoroscopy may reveal a filling defect and the extravasation as the opposite corpus fills by way of communicating channels across the midline [36]. Less than optimal sequelae of healing may occur if the lesion is treated conservatively with catheterization, elevation, and ice packs. If adequate facilities are available, penile deformity and impairment of erections may be avoided by surgical exploration, drainage of the hematoma, and repair of the corpora. It is recommended that the penile shaft be approached through either a circumferential coronal incision, undermining of the skin proximally, or a direct longitudinal incision over the injury if the site is localized easily [7]. The principles of repair are as discussed above: control of hemorrhage and restoration of the urethra and the corpora.

## ZIPPER INJURY

A zipper may entrap the penile prepuce between the fastener and the teeth, obviously an injury most commonly seen in pediatric patients. Treatment may involve partial circumcision or cutting of the median bar of the zipper fastener [13, 43].

## ISCHEMIA

Penile strangulation may be caused by hair, string, rings, rubber bands, or condoms, or it may be the result of an accident or intention, such as maintenance of erection or the prevention of enuresis [20]. There is an opportunity for a diagnosis of brilliance in the case of inadvertent penile encirclement with human hair. It is difficult to see the hair as it becomes buried in the skin and the resultant swelling. In fact, there may be epithelialization over the hair. Urethral transection, nerve injury, and distal necrosis have been reported [42]. Treatment is obvious, consisting in removal of the hair and repair of the damaged structure. Needless to say, knowledge of this type of injury and its diagnosis are the keys to proper treatment.

## AVULSION OF PENILE SKIN

Avulsion of penile skin is the classic injury referred to the plastic and reconstructive surgeon because treatment involves the principles of skin cover. Figure 56-4 shows that the skin of the penis is usually separated from Buck's fascia in a loose areolar plane occurring at this interval. Typically, there is minimal bleeding and not a great amount of damage to underlying structures. The injury is similar to avulsion of the scrotum in the areolar skin underneath dartos muscle [25] (see Fig. 56-1).

Penile skin avulsion is best treated with a split-thickness skin graft because the avulsed skin fares poorly when replaced as a graft [9]. The important points to remember are that the distal skin, even if it is in good condition, must be debrided to the corona level because prolonged distal edema commonly results secondary to disruption of the lymphatics that drain this tissue. Stretching the residual skin for coverage of the widely denuded shaft is not good practice, even though it has been recommended for the

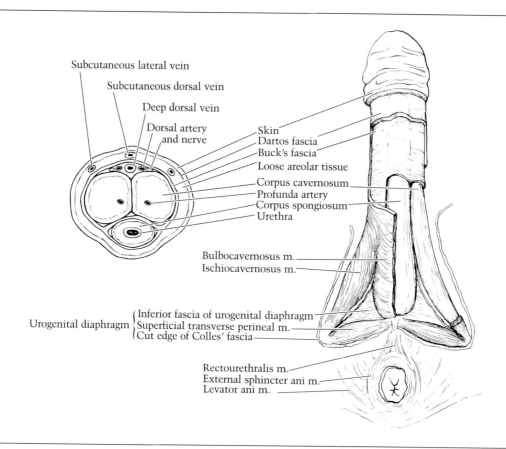

**Figure 56-4** *Penile anatomy. Avulsion classically occurs in the areolar tissue between the dartos and Buck's layers. Arteries are inside the corpora cavernosa and underneath Buck's fascia. Not shown is a significant arterial supply in the corpora spongiosum. The veins are superficial to and deep to Buck's layer. Note the dorsal nerves near the dorsal arteries. They branch from the internal pudendal nerves (see Figure 56-2B) and supply cutaneous innervation for most of the penis.*

scrotum. The necessity of the penis to enlarge for erection is the differential point. The recipient bed must be adequately prepared and the skin graft applied as a single sheet in an interdigitating fashion to minimize scar contracture in a longitudinal direction. Contact with viable tissue, immobilization, freedom from infection, and some pressure are achieved with a bolus dressing

left in place either for 10 to 14 days or, alternatively, removed within 48 to 72 hours and the wound treated using the exposure technique, utilizing a urethral catheter from an outrigger, such as a wire across the bed, to elevate the penis.

Other techniques of penile coverage include burial of the denuded shaft within the scrotum or use of a local flap. Skin grafting is the method of choice.

BURNS

Genital burns are usually not isolated but occur as a part of a larger, body surface burn. In respect to the penis, however, initial treatment must not neglect the escharotomy if a circumferential burn creates a constricting band [32]. Suprapubic catheter drainage is probably superior to the urethral

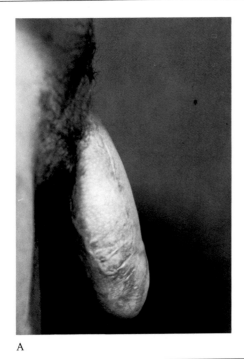

A

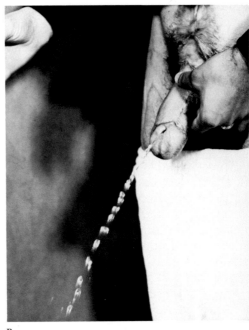

B

**Figure 56-5** *Postoperative composite phalloplasty showing a free flap of the forearm melded with the standard flap. A. Nine of these procedures have been performed, eight for transsexual surgery. B. One was done in a trauma patient, who now urinates forcefully and has fathered a child.*

Foley catheter drainage because it avoids the possibility of swelling [28, 29]. Topical antibacterials, conservative therapy with excision, and grafting as demarcation of the burn occurs may well be indicated. Contractures of the penile shaft are not uncommon late sequelae of burns and require the usual extensive release and split-thickness skin grafting [29], following the principles mentioned in the section above. All of these principles are of particular importance here: Contact of the graft with viable tissue, mild pressure, elevation, immobilization, freedom from hematoma, freedom from infection.

The electrical burn of the penis occurs as a result of either exit or entry of current. It occurs, for example, in young boys who have urinated on power lines or on electric train tracks [28].

## AMPUTATIONS
Psychological considerations are an integral part of the treatment program—for all inju-

ries of the penis but for amputations particularly. Patients are apprehensive about the appearance of the injured genitalia and suffer dramatic changes in self-image. Psychiatric consultation must be sought in all cases of self-emasculation, which is one of the most common etiologies of the penile amputation, occurring as a form of "focal suicide" [12, 40]. During the 1980s there was an epidemic of penile amputations performed by the wives of unfaithful husbands in Thailand [2]. A series of these patients were reported in whom deepithelialization or removal of the skin and burying the penis in surrounding vascular tissue was used to help bring a blood supply after anastomosis of the urethra and the corpora. This technique is recommended if an operating microscope is not available in the community or the patient cannot be rapidly transported to it (e.g., helicopter evacuation).

Knowledge of anatomy is important here. It is recommended that several arteries in the penis be repaired and a fewer number of veins. There is an artery in each corpora cavernosa and arteries in the two dorsal systems. The venous drainage concentrates more in the dorsal systems, and there are no veins in the corpora itself for anastomosis. The mechanical stabilization that must be accomplished initially involves the tunica albuginea of the corpora cavernosa, the urethra, and the surrounding corpora spongiosa; a catheter is essential. Dorsal nerves can be reanastomosed at this time as well [18] (see Fig. 56-4). The use of heparin is risky because of the vascularity of the region. Cold ischemia intervals of up to 15 hours have been reported with penile replantation [21].

## Total Phalloplasty

Reconstruction of the penis after traumatic loss or loss due to cancer surgery, or for microphallus or gender dysphoria, is a challenge undertaken during the 1980s. Much of the work done in this area has been outlined by Gilbert in articles, instructional courses, and lectures [17]. The armamentarium available is outlined in the phalloplasty section in Chapter 58. Many techniques are available, and the standard phalloplasty procedure has evolved from the experience of many [4, 33, 41]. A successful technique is outlined in Chapter 58 for a patient who had total loss of the penis when his penis was amputated by a tree shredder. He has since fathered a child with the use of the new penis, and he urinates via the neourethra within the phallus shown in Fig. 56-5.

Medical history is rich with reports of surgery of the external genitalia. As early as 5000 years ago the Ebers Papyrus described postoperative care of the circumcised penis.

Mutilation and castration was a common form of punishment and degradation, usually befalling an adulterer, a slave, or a prisoner of war [37]. Accidents, assault, and self-mutilation are more common injuries in recent times, and this chapter has dealt with the surgical experience of this century.

## References

1. Attaran, S. E., Hodges, C. V., Crary, L. S., et al. Homotransplants of the testis. *J. Urol.* 95:387, 1966.
2. Bhanganada, K., Chayavatana, T., Pongnumkul, C., et al. Surgical management of an epidemic of penile amputations in Siam. *Am. J. Surg.* 146:376, 1983.
3. Cass, A. S. Testicular trauma. *J. Urol.* 129:299, 1983.
4. Chang, T. S., and Hwang, W. Y. Forearm flap in one stage reconstruction of the penis. *Plast. Reconstr. Surg.* 74:251, 1984.
5. Citron, N. D., and Wade, P. J. Penile injuries from vacuum cleaners. *Br. Med. J.* 281:26, 1980.
6. Culp, D. A. Genital injuries—etiology and initial management. *Urol. Clin. North Am.* 4:143, 1977.
7. Culp, D. A. Penoscrotal Trauma. In J. R. Glenn (ed.), *Urologic Surgery.* Philadelphia: Lippincott, 1983. Pp. 813–820.
8. Culp, D. A., and Huffman, W. C. Temperature determination in the thigh with regard to burying the traumatically exposed testis. *J. Urol.* 76:436, 1956.
9. D'Alessio, E., Rossi, F., and d'Allesio, R. Reconstruction in traumatic avulsion of penile and scrotal skin. *Ann. Plast. Surg.* 9:120, 1982.
10. Datta, N. S. Corpus cavernosography in conditions other than Peyronie's disease. *J. Urol.* 118:588, 1977.
11. Denes, F. T., Netto, N. R., Jr., Srougi, M., et al. Traumatic rupture of the corpora cavernosa. *Int. Urol. Nephrol.* 9:317, 1977.
12. Evins, S. C., Whittle, T., and Rous, S. N. Self emasculation—review of the literature, report of a case and outline of the objectives of management. *J. Urol.* 118:775, 1977.
13. Flowerdew, R., Fishman, I. J., and Churchill, B. M. Management of penile zipper injury. *J. Urol.* 117:671, 1977.

14. Furnas, D. W., and McCraw, J. B. Resurfacing the genital area. *Clin. Plast. Surg.* 7:235, 1980.

15. Gannon, M. J., Butler, M. R., Kingdom, J. C. P., et al. Rupture of corpus cavernosum, the fractured penis. *Ir. Med. J.* 79:42, 1986.

16. Gibson, T. Avulsion of Penile and Scrotal Skin. II. In C. E. Horton (ed.), *Plastic and Reconstructive Surgery of the Genital Area.* Boston: Little, Brown, 1973. Pp. 463–466.

17. Gilbert, D. Instructional Course: Genital Reconstruction. Presented at the American Society of Plastic and Reconstructive Surgeons Meeting, Kansas City, 1985.

18. Gilbert, D., Horton, C., Terjes, J., et al. Phallic re-inervation via the internal pudendal nerve. *Plast. Surg. Forum* 2:39, 1986.

19. Gillenwater, J. Y., and Howards, S. S. (eds.). *Yearbook of Urology, 1983.* Chicago: Year Book, 1983. P. 183.

20. Haddad, F. S. Penile strangulation by human hair. *Urol. Int.* 37:375, 1982.

21. Henriksson, T. G., Hahne, V., et al. Microsurgical replantation of an amputated penis. *Scand. J. Urol. Nephrol.* 14:111, 1980.

22. Lin, S. D., Lai, C. S., and Su, P. Y. Replantation of the testis by microsurgical techniques. *Plast. Reconstr. Surg.* 76:620, 1985.

23. Malin, J. M., Jr., and Glenn, J. F. Rupture of the Urethra. In C. E. Horton (ed.), *Plastic and Reconstructive Surgery of the Genital Area.* Boston: Little, Brown, 1973. Pp. 533–541.

24. Mancharda, R. L., Singh, R., Keswani, R. K., et al. Traumatic avulsion of scrotum and penile skin. *Br. J. Plast. Surg.* 20:97, 1967.

25. Masters, F. W. Avulsion of Penile and Scrotal Skin. In C. E. Horton (ed.), *Plastic and Reconstructive Surgery of the Genital Area.* Boston: Little, Brown, 1973. Pp. 451–461.

26. Masters, F. W., and Robinson, D. W. The treatment of avulsions of the male genitalia. *J. Trauma* 8:430, 1968.

27. McConnell, J. D., Peters, P. C., and Lewis, S. E. Testicular rupture in blunt scrotal trauma—review of 15 cases with recent application of testicular scanning. *J. Urol.* 128:309, 1982.

28. McDougal, W. S., and Persky, L. Traumatic Injuries of the Genitourinary System. In *International Perspectives in Urology.* Vol. 1. Baltimore: Williams & Wilkins, 1981.

29. McDougal, W. S., Peterson, H. D., Pruitt, B. A., et al. The thermally injured perineum. *J. Urol.* 121:320, 1979.

30. Meares, E. M., Jr. Traumatic rupture of the corpus cavernosum. *J. Urol.* 105:407, 1971.

31. Millard, D. R. Scrotal construction and reconstruction. *Plast. Reconstr. Surg.* 33:10, 1966.

32. Muir, I. F. K., and Morgan, B. D. G. Burns of the Genitalia and Perineum. In C. E. Horton (ed.), *Plastic and Reconstructive Surgery of the Genital Area.* Boston: Little, Brown, 1973. Pp. 443–449.

33. Mukherjee, G. D. Reconstruction of penis with urethra from groin and mid-thigh flap. *J. Indian Med. Assoc.* 75:124, 1980.

34. O'Brien, B. M., Rao, V. K., MacLeod, A. M., et al. Microvascular testicular transfer. *Plast. Reconstr. Surg.* 71:87, 1983.

35. Peters, P. C., and Bright, T. C., III. Trauma to the Genitourinary System. In G. T. Shires (ed.), *Care of the Trauma Patient.* New York: McGraw-Hill, 1979. Pp. 349372.

36. Pliskow, R. J., and Ohme, R. K. Corpus cavernosography in acute "fracture" of the penis. *A.J.R.* 133:331, 1979.

37. Rogers, B. O. History of External Genital Surgery. In C. E. Horton (ed.), *Plastic and Reconstructive Surgery of the Genital Area.* Boston: Little, Brown, 1973. Pp. 3–47.

38. Salvatierra, O., Rigdon, W. O., Norris, D. M., et al. Vietnam experience with 252 urological war injuries. *J. Urol.* 101, 615, 1969.

39. Schuster, G. Traumatic rupture of the testicle and a review of the literature. *J. Urol.* 127:1194, 1982.

40. Strauch, B., Sharzer, L. A., Petro, J., et al. Replantation of amputated parts of the penis, nose, ear, and scalp. *Clin. Plast. Surg.* 10:115, 1983.

41. Sun, G. C., and Huang, J. J. One-stage reconstruction of the penis with composite iliac crest and lateral groin skin flap. *Plast. Surg. Hosp. Chin. Acad. Med. Sci.* 6:439, 1984.

42. Thomas, A. J., Jr., Timmons, J. W., and Perlmutter, A. D. Progressive penile amputation. *Urology* 9:42, 1977.

43. Uson, A. C., and Lattimer, J. Genitourinary Tract Injuries. In J. G. Randolph, M. M. Ravitch, K. J. Welch, et al. (eds.), *The Injured Child—Surgical Management.* Chicago: Year Book, 1979. Pp. 251–283.

44. Zenteno, S. Fracture of the penis. *Plast. Reconstr. Surg.* 52:669, 1973.

45. Zyblski, J. R. War Wounds. In C. E. Horton (ed.), *Plastic and Reconstructive Surgery of the Genital Area.* Boston: Little, Brown, 1973. Pp. 487–494.

# 57

*Donald R. Laub*
*Donald R. Laub, Jr.*

# Müllerian and Ectodermal Vaginal Agenesis

A woman born without a functioning vagina is deprived of both coitus and childbearing. The body image is disturbed, and the patient develops deep-seated doubts about her femininity. The resultant psychological discord may be reflected in all aspects of her life. In addition, a certain subgroup of patients develop severe physiologic derangements secondary to intact cyclic endometrial tissue.

Vaginal agenesis, by no means rare, is a frequent cause of primary amenorrhea [2]. The incidence of congenital absence of the vagina is usually stated to be 1 in 4000 to 5000 females [6, 12, 53]. Partial or complete absence of the vagina requiring surgical reconstruction may be part of several distinct syndromes.

In this chapter we discuss the relevant embryology of the female reproductive tract, the differential diagnosis of partial and complete vaginal absence, the work-up of such a patient, and the methods currently available for reconstruction.

## Embryology

To understand the possible etiologies of vaginal agenesis one must have a knowledge of the normal development of the genitourinary tract. At about 5 weeks' gestation sexually indifferent gonads begin to differentiate from the urogenital ridges. Differentiation into ovary or testis is determined by the sex chromosomes of the embryo. If the sex karyotype is XX, ovaries are formed; if the sex karyotype is XY, testes are formed. The mesonephroi are primitive excretory organs that join either the mesonephric or wolffian ducts. The ureter induces development of the metanephros, which will become the definitive adult kidney. The metanephros originally develops in the pelvis and later ascends to the adult position. The above information is helpful for understanding some of the renal anomalies associated with vaginal atresias.

If the embryo is female and hence has a primitive ovary, the absence of the two testicular-derived compounds (testosterone and müllerian inhibiting hormone) leads to growth and development of the müllerian ducts and regression of the wolffian ducts (which in the adult female are vestigially represented by the epoöphoron, the paraoöphoron, and Gartner's duct).

The solid cords of proliferating mesothelial cells that make up the müllerian ducts grow caudally and canalize. The two müllerian ducts fuse to form a single duct with two lumens. By 16 weeks' gestation, this septum disappears, forming a single uterus. The fallopian tubes are derived from the cephalic unfused portions of the müllerian ducts. At

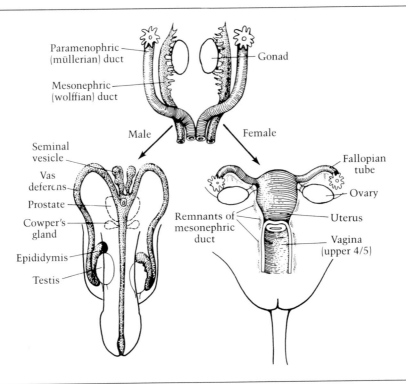

Paramenophric (müllerian) duct

Mesonephric (wolffian) duct

Gonad

Male

Female

Seminal vesicle

Vas deferens

Prostate

Cowper's gland

Epididymis

Testis

Fallopian tube

Ovary

Remnants of mesonephric duct

Uterus

Vagina (upper 4/5)

**Figure 57-1** *Each human starts embryologic development with four tubes: two müllerian and two wolffian. Without müllerian inhibiting factor or testosterone, all human embryos proceed to female development (right side of the figure). Male development is shown on the left. Mayer-Rokitansky-Kuster-Hauser syndrome is müllerian agenesis or absence of the highlighted structures in the right lower diagram (the usual vaginal atresia). Merch's association couples vaginal atresia with lumbar spine and renal anomalies, which are plausible associations from an embryologic point of view.*

8 weeks the paired sinovaginal bulbs form a solid cord—the vaginal plate—connecting the urogenital sinus to the fused müllerian ducts. This vaginal plate canalizes by 22 weeks to form the vagina [7] (Fig. 57-1).

It is conventionally taught in embryology [21, 27] that the müllerian ducts give origin to the tubes, uterus, cervix, and the proximal 70 to 80 percent of the vagina. The remaining distal external portion of the vagina is derived from the urogenital sinus. The junction of these two parts is represented by the hymen. Today, however, Koff's alternative hypothesis [56] seems to be favored. Here müllerian-derived tissues extend to the level of the hymen but are invaded and replaced by cells from the urogenital sinus up to the level of the external os. Thus, according to this hypothesis, the vagina consists of tissue derived from both müllerian and urogenital sinus origins. This theory helps to explain the condition of vaginal adenosis

and related adenocarcinoma found in girls who were exposed in utero to diethylstilbestrol. The adenosis extending for variable distances below the cervix is thought to represent rests of müllerian-derived lining that fail to be replaced by advancing lining derived from the urogenital sinus [98, 99].

In contrast, the external genitalia develop from a common genital eminence, which until the eighth week of fetal life, can differ-

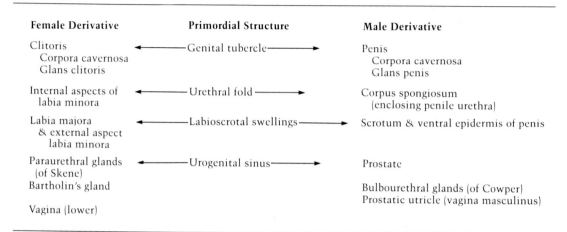

| Female Derivative | Primordial Structure | Male Derivative |
|---|---|---|
| Clitoris<br>  Corpora cavernosa<br>  Glans clitoris | ←——————Genital tubercle——————→ | Penis<br>  Corpora cavernosa<br>  Glans penis |
| Internal aspects of<br>  labia minora | ←——————Urethral fold ——————→ | Corpus spongiosum<br>  (enclosing penile urethra) |
| Labia majora<br>  & external aspect<br>  labia minora | ←——————Labioscrotal swellings——————→ | Scrotum & ventral epidermis of penis |
| Paraurethral glands<br>  (of Skene)<br>Bartholin's gland | ←——————Urogenital sinus——————→ | Prostate<br><br>Bulbourethral glands (of Cowper)<br>Prostatic utricle (vagina masculinus) |
| Vagina (lower) | | |

**Figure 57-2** *Male and female homologues in the external genitalia. The development of the external genitalia is different from that of the internal genitalia because male and female derive from the same primordial structures. All embryos develop female external anatomy unless male tissue receptors and 5-dihydrotestosterone are present. With vaginal atresia, all of these structures are normal. With ambiguous female genitalia or female pseudohermaphroditism, these structures have developed more toward male characteristics. See Figure 57-3 for an example: intrauterine male hormone effects on a female. In Figure 58-1 we have superimposed the homologous male and female nomenclature on the anatomy of a female adult driven with testosterone, thereby labeling external genitalia with both male and female words.*

entiate into the genitalia of either sex (Fig. 57-2). The development of male genitalia depends on androgens, most particularly dihydrotestosterone, a local metabolite of testosterone. Development of female genitalia occurs in the absence of androgenic influence.

## Congenital Absence of the Vagina—Müllerian Atresia

Congenital absence of the vagina is also known as the Mayer-Rokitansky-Kuster-Hauser syndrome [41, 60, 64, 83]. Patients with this disorder have a normal female karyotype or genotype, normal phenotype, and normal endocrine status. Patients present at the age of menarche or later because of amenorrhea, cryptomenorrhea, or the inability to accomplish intercourse. Rarely is this anomaly discovered at birth. The findings include a normal vulva with an absent vagina or a vagina that is represented by a shallow 1- to 2-cm dimple. The uterus and cervix are usually absent but are represented by bilateral non-canalized muscular bands. The ovaries are normal, and there is normal cyclic ovarian function as reflected by circulating hormone levels and ovulation. Therefore female breasts, pubic and axillary hair, and female body habitus develop normally [96].

The agenesis of müllerian duct tissue may be incomplete; in less than 10 percent of the patients functioning endometrial tissue is present. These patients present with hematometra, hematocolpos, monthly episodes of abdominal pain, and an increasing abdominal mass due to the accumulation of menstrual products. Patients have been reported to have presented with dyspareunia due to coitus per urethra [2, 95].

Dysgenesis may be as simple as a vaginal septum [75]. In cases of relatively complete uterine development, vaginal construction may salvage reproductive potential [8, 50,

52, 89], and pregnancy has been reported [66, 79, 90]. However, if the cervix is not competent, severe recurrent pelvic infections may result, and hysterectomy is indicated.

Development of the urinary tract is closely related to genital development; therefore it is not surprising that with vaginal atresia there is a high association of renal anomalies, ranging from 34 to 49 percent [22]. Skeletal abnormalities, most often lumbar spine malformations, occur in 10 to 15 percent of patients [38].

It appears that the occurrence of vaginal atresia is sporadic. Lischke and co-workers [61] have demonstrated a lack of concordance in a series of three pairs of monozygotic twins. Despite a report by Jones and Mermut [51] of a high incidence in a particular family, most authors believe that there is generally not a familial incidence, but that there is a multifactorial etiology. Furthermore, each müllerian duct is independent, and the ovarian, renal, and fallopian tube anomalies are often unilateral.

## Testicular Feminization Syndrome

Patients with the testicular feminization syndrome (also known as the androgen insensitivity syndrome) superficially resemble those with congenital absence of the vagina, but the two are really different, as the patients with testicular feminization syndrome are actually genetic males. Initial presentation is at puberty or thereafter because of primary amenorrhea. Examination reveals an individual with a normal female body habitus, normal female breast development, and normal external female genitalia. In most of the patients there is sparse development of axillary and pubic hair [32]. The vagina may be of variable length but ends in a blind pouch without a cervix. Often there are "bilateral inguinal hernias," which arouse the physician's suspicion regarding the possible presence of this syndrome in a female infant. Further evaluation shows an absence of internal female genitalia except for rudimentary anlage of müllerian structures, and the patients are therefore sterile. Intrabdominal or inguinal gonads are present in the form of testes. Histologic examination of these testes shows an absence of spermatogenesis but an increase in Leydig cells. Hormonal analysis reveals that the testes secrete both androgens and estrogens, and chromosomal analysis demonstrates a male karyotype. Unlike congenital absence of the vagina, testicular feminization syndrome has a high familial incidence [32]. Genetic transmission is apparently X-linked [39].

Currently, a deficiency in the androgen receptors and the resultant inability to concentrate androgens at the active sites in the cell nucleus is the most likely explanation for the testicular feminization syndrome. Thus the testes secrete normal amounts of androgens, but because the cells of the body are not able to respond to them no virilization takes place and the body develops a female phenotype in response to the testicular estrogens that are produced.

Those patients with testicular feminization syndrome who have markedly underdeveloped vaginas require surgical construction of a serviceable vagina. There is a relatively high incidence—as high as 33 percent according to Federman [20]—of malignant degeneration of the testes; therefore castration and hormone replacement are indicated.

However, it is argued [40] that puberty is best achieved with endogenous hormones and that malignant risk is small before age 20. Therefore removal of the testes is best delayed until after puberty. In either case, estrogen replacement is indicated to prevent menopause-like symptoms.

For the sake of completeness, note that there are several incomplete forms of testicular feminization syndrome (e.g., Reifenstein syndrome). The interested reader is referred to the articles by Glenn [32] and Dewhurst [16].

## Gonadal Dysgenesis

Patients with gonadal dysgenesis (Turner syndrome) are characterized by a female phenotype, an X0 karyotype, short stature, streak gonads, and various other congenital anomalies such as webbing of the neck and shortness of the fourth and fifth metacarpals. Despite the gonadal dysgenesis, these patients have female internal and external genitalia, although the genitalia remain infantile, and amenorrhea is the rule. Some of these patients have a cryptic vagina and require reconstruction to create a serviceable vagina. Various forms of mosaicism (the most common is X0/XX) may also exist; these patients generally have a high degree of feminization.

## Hermaphroditism and Other Intersexual Conditions

In the case of a child born with ambiguous genitalia, the vagina may not be apparent to the examining pediatrician, and the reconstructive surgeon may be consulted. She or he must be conversant with the material in the following section in order to work with a pediatric endocrinology colleague to effectively treat the child. Generally, a person's gender identity is still plastic at birth but is established by 18 to 30 months of age [70]. Therefore appropriate surgical and hormonal therapy must be instituted before 1 year of age to eliminate ambiguity in rearing, prevent later doubts of gender identity, and ensure normal adult sexual function.

## True Hermaphroditism

By definition, a true hermaphrodite has gonadal tissue of both sexes; it may be separate or combined as an ovotestis. Most true hermaphrodites have an XX karyotype.

Pseudohermaphroditism includes a variety of intersexual conditions involving ambiguous external genitalia but only one type of gonadal tissue.

## Male Pseudohermaphroditism

A child whose gonads are exclusively testes, but who is incompletely masculine, is a male pseudohermaphrodite. This condition can be caused by (1) tissue unresponsiveness to testosterone, i.e., testicular feminization; (2) lack of testosterone or dihydrotestosterone for various reasons; or (3) maternal ingestion of estrogens or progestins. The standard practice is to differentiate these etiologies by the response to exogenous testosterone or human chorionic gonadotropin. These tests also propitiously show the growth potential of the patient's phallus. The reconstructive surgeon can then participate in an enlightened manner in establishing the child's gender. For example, a negative testosterone response test in a neonate with a microphallus and perineal hypospadias would favor assignment of female gender, with early external genitalia reconstruction (discussed later in this chapter) and later vagina construction. On the other hand, a positive response would change one's viewpoint dramatically; the penis could be allowed to grow to adequate size by early release of chordee. Similarly, the traditional, wise advice that the male child who loses his penis as a result of complications of circumcision should be raised as a female may soon be challenged by advances in penis construction. These decisions are predicated on the attainment of normal adult sexual function, regardless of chromosomal or gonadal sex [58]. However, procreational function generally takes priority over intercourse function [31].

## Female Pseudohermaphroditism

A child with exclusively ovarian gonads and XX karyotype but masculinized external genitalia is a female pseudohermaphrodite. Because there are no testes to manufacture müllerian inhibiting factor, the internal structures are female. This condition can be caused by (1) maternal ingestion of androgens or progestins; or (2) adrenogenital syndrome.

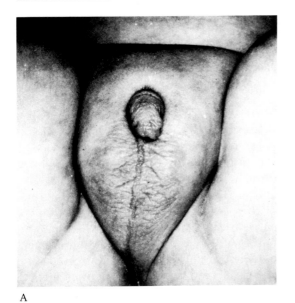

A

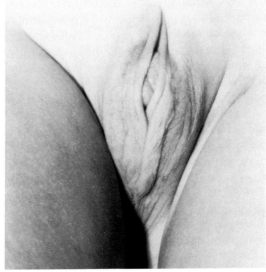

B

Iatrogenic virilization commonly occurs when a pregnant woman receives androgenic steroid therapy, e.g., danazol for endometriosis [86]; the woman is amenorrheic because of the steroid and does not notice she has become pregnant until later. By the time the medication can be discontinued, the fetus's genitalia has been virilized (Fig. 57-3).

The adrenogenital syndrome is due to a genetically determined defect in the metabolic pathway of cortisol synthesis [31, 53]. The resulting impaired cortisol production leads to overstimulation of the adrenal by ACTH, causing overproduction of adrenal androgens. In the female fetus it leads to virilization of the external genitalia, manifested by varying degrees of clitoral hypertrophy, labial fusion, and underdevelopment of the vagina. This condition is diagnosed shortly after birth because most forms of the syndrome are characterized by severe saltwasting, which may lead to severe dehydration and shock. Treatment is with adrenal steroids. These children should be raised as females; those who are more extensively virilized require corrective genital surgery that

*Figure 57-3* A. Ambiguous genitalia in a 9-month-old female infant who has normal müllerian-derived female internal genitalia (ovaries, tubes, uterus, upper third/vagina) but whose external genitalia were influenced in utero by the mother's ingestion of danazol for treatment of endometriosis. The urine came out the tip of the glans. The anatomy portrays female pseudohermaphroditism. B. Postoperative view 5 years later.

may include vaginal construction. Surgery is recommended during the first months of life unless there is a connection of the urethra to the vagina at a high level near the external female bladder sphincter. In this case vaginoplasty only is delayed for several years, although Jones and Scott would nevertheless operate early [53].

## History, Physical Examination, and Diagnostic Tests

It is complicated to differentiate definitively which intersex condition is involved when a child has ambiguous external genitalia [54]. However, the diagnosis among the conditions involving vaginal agenesis is relatively simple. Obviously, the first step is a good history. One must specifically inquire about possible maternal drug ingestion. A careful family history must be obtained, looking for similar conditions in family members. Monthly episodes of abdominal discomfort are highly significant.

A complete physical examination is done, with emphasis on the external genitalia, the distribution of body hair, evidence of secondary sex characteristics such as breast development, and the presence of abdominal or inguinal masses. The rectal examination reveals the presence or absence of derivatives of the müllerian system. Williams [106] has described a characteristic finding on rectal examination: The uterosacral ligaments can be palpated in front of the rectum continuously from one pelvic side to the other because there is no midline uterus or cervix.

Buccal smears are obtained for karyotyping; they are key to the differential between congenital absence of the vagina and testicular feminization syndrome. Hormone assays may be performed as needed. Because of the high association of renal tract anomalies, intravenous urography is mandatory; it may suggest that further studies such as cystoscopy, retrograde urography, or even lumbar spine examinations are needed. Sonography [63], laparoscopy, computed tomography, or magnetic resonance imaging examinations can elucidate the nature of the internal sex organs. As discussed earlier, hormone response tests may be indicated.

The information obtained from the history, physical examination, and diagnostic tests leads to the correct diagnosis in most cases. Only highly complicated cases require diagnostic laparotomy.

Capraro and Gallego [12] have stressed the importance of reinforcing the positive and normal aspects of the infant's condition. It must be emphasized that she will be able to marry and participate in sexual intercourse, and she may become a mother through adoption. In patients with testicular feminization syndrome, it is best to refer to the "go-nads" or "sex glands" rather than to "testes." Regarding body image, all these patients benefit from knowing that her surgeon, a professional, always regards her as *normal*— that the surgeon is opening up, rather than creating, the vagina.

## Treatment of Vaginal Agenesis

The history of attempts to form a vagina is a fascinating and colorful chapter in the history of medicine that begins in ancient times. The interested reader is referred to the excellent review by Goldwyn [35]. Our discussion here is limited to the methods that are in use today.

The various methods of vaginal construction are as follows.

| | |
|---|---|
| Dilation (a type of tissue expansion) | Frank technique; Broadbent |
| Dilation prior to full-thickness skin graft from introitus | Schaupp |
| Simple construction (dissect the cavity and await spontaneous reepithelialization) | Dupuytren's, Wharton's, or Yves' technique |
| Split-thickness skin graft | McIndoe or Counsellor |
| Full-thickness skin graft from abdomen | Horton |
| Mucosal graft | Wilfengseder |
| Groin flap | Huang |
| Labia majora | Williams technique |
| Labia minora | Huang, Chang, Sun, and Chung |
| Intestine | Baldwin technique |
| Rectosigmoid | Technique redescribed by author |
| Gracilis muscle and skin | McCraw, Dibbell |

Many methods are available for constructing a vagina [34, 62]. In general, the approaches to vaginal construction are as follows.

*1.* Hormonal stimulation of the atretic müllerian elements. (The gene splicing tech-

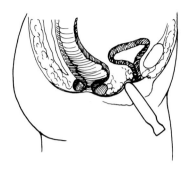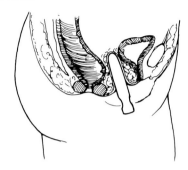

**Figure 57-4** *Frank-Wharton-Broadbent technique for nonsurgical (or presurgical) tissue expansion of the ectodermally derived external genital anatomy to substitute for the müllerian-derived vagina.*

nology for producing the tissue receptors is not yet available.)

2. Surgical transfer or substitution with another tissue.
3. Tissue expansion.
4. A combination of these techniques.

The authors favor No. 4.

The Frank technique [24, 25, 26, 27] has been reexplored, recorded, and recommended to us by Broadbent (Fig. 57-4). It can be considered a form of tissue expansion because it expands the lower one-fourth (or the urogenital sinus-derived) portion of the vagina to make up for the absent upper (müllerian derived) three-fourths of vagina. Graduated soft silicone dilators (McGhan Corporation, Goleta, CA) are used intermittently for several months.

The smallest dilator is used first, and the tip is applied to the vaginal dimple (see Fig. 57-4). The patient is instructed to apply pressure until mild discomfort is experienced. Pressure is alternately applied and released for 15 minutes twice daily. The size is progressively increased. (By the end of 2 months, all but one of the patients reported by Frank were using the largest dilator.) After 1 month's use of the largest dilator, the patient begins intercourse, and the use of a dilator is abandoned. These authors advocated that this method be tried first in all cases. If the method fails, operative construction may still be carried out. The tissue gained is an asset for the surgery [10, 11].

A bicycle seat with Lucite dilators has been devised by Ingram [48] (Faulkner Plastics, Tampa, FL). The tissue surrounding the vagina is movable and helps the expanded vaginal cavity seem even deeper. Teenage patients may be reluctant to try these devices, and the fundus may become thin enough to ulcerate with intercourse. In cases where the uterus is intact and the vagina absent, pregnancy has been reported after use of the dilation technique, utilizing surgery only to connect the cervix to the lower ascending segment. However, the usual situation is that the cervix of the isolated uterus is hypoplastic and lacks the functional ability to prevent ascending infection; hysterectomy to treat endometritis is the usual outcome. Cukier et al. [15] reported lining the endocervix with a skin graft to make it competent to resist infection.

Dissection of the cavity without surgical relining, but allowing for spontaneous epithelialization during a prolonged period of stent dilation, was described by Dupuytren himself in 1817 [19], Wharton in 1938 [100, 101], and Yves in 1974 [107]. The method seems incredulous and is contrary to our experience, but the reports are verified [84, 87, 97]. This technique may exploit epithelium present in the müllerian duct remnant [42]. The use of creams containing hydrocortisone to prevent granulation tissue formation and the use of topical estrogen to stimulate squamous epithelium may also be important to the (reported) success of this technique.

The McIndoe (and Counsellor, of course) technique is the classic skin graft vaginal construction [9, 14, 28, 66, 67]. Shrinkage and some stenosis occur in 25 percent of these cases, but shrinkage and stenosis do not occur if a good take is obtained initially and if motivated dilation is practiced religiously [74]. Verrucous cancer had been reported in these skin grafts [1, 18, 47, 49, 73, 80, 92].

A free graft of mucosa derived from resected (and discarded) intestine was reported by Wilfingseder of Innsbruck in 1974 [102].

The use of island pedicle groin flaps supplied by an axial pattern artery—the posterior labial artery or "the artery of Huang"—was described by Huang [44, 45] in Galveston during the 1980s and has been used by Leonard in Salt Lake City. These grafts are handy for secondary reconstruction and certainly are of use for neocolporrhaphy in gender dysphoria syndrome (Fig. 57-5).

The use of labia majora has been developed by Williams, of Oxford University, as a simple technique for patients with postradiation vaginal obliteration that does not involve the heavily irradiated field; it consists in suturing the labia majora together to form a cavity for intercourse [103–105].

The operation may be performed using local anesthesia. Dilators to enlarge the cavity and change its axis are aided by sexual intercourse. Williams stated that neither the patients nor their partners have complained about the slight misplacement of the new vagina, and he further stated that the patients are "often particularly successful at coitus" because of the sensibility of the tissue.

The viability of labia minora flaps depends on the surgeon's precise knowledge of their particular blood supply and the surgeon's ability to dissect the two leaves apart with the use of the microscope as described in a 1986 (brilliant) contribution by Hwang and colleagues in China [46].

The ilium, first used by Baldwin in 1904 [5, 6], was a (double) loop placed side-to-side and anastomosed to the perineum. Later a crushing clamp was applied to form a single lumen out of the two segments. Bleeding and paraumbilical pain with coitus, excessive secretion of mucus, ulcerative colitis [62], and prolapse were problems [55].

The lower portions of the colon, however, absorb fluid and do not secrete as much. Excess mucus is not a problem when the rectum or sigmoid is used. The rectum was used for constructing a vagina by Popov in Russia [76] and Schubert in Germany [85] in 1910 and 1911, respectively, via a posterior approach, resecting the coccyx. The original description of using the rectum for vaginal tissue was by the Russian Snegireff in 1892 [91] (apparently not using the posterior approach) and again by Franz in Pretoria in 1984 [26]. Franz used the middle and inferior hemorrhoidal system for the blood supply, and the segment is nourished for 8 to 10 cm above the peritoneal reflection. The segment reaches the vaginal introitus. It also may be considered a rectosigmoid segment and appears to produce results comparable to those of the authors. The sigmoid vaginostomy operation is practiced by Goligher [36, 37] and has been popular in Eastern Europe [3, 4, 29, 30]. Six hundred cases have been collected by Kung [59]. Sigmoid vaginostomy may have been the operation of choice in that area of the world and may be similar to the operation described here, but more skeletization of the blood supply is (or was) practiced by those surgeons. Shirodkar in Bombay [88] and Zangyl in Austria [108] reported sigmoid vaginostomy. The method we use may be different in that the segment is slightly lower than that used for the sigmoid vaginostomy and possibly has a more vigorous blood supply.

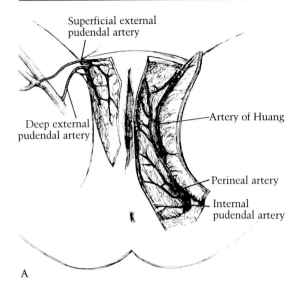

A

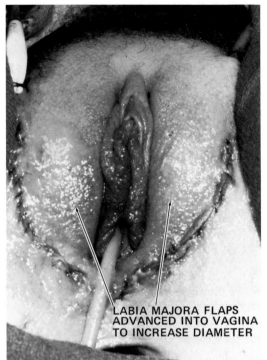

**LABIA MAJORA FLAPS
ADVANCED INTO VAGINA
TO INCREASE DIAMETER**

B

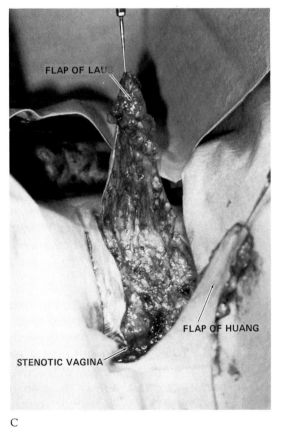

C

*Figure 57-5 A. On the patient's left is the axial flap described by Huang (University of Texas, Galveston) based on the internal pudendal to perineal labial scrotal artery system. The blood supply to the labial flap is shown on the patient's right side (our left). B. Postoperative views of a patient with vaginal stenosis in the most external 2 inches only. The anteriorly based labia majora flaps were used to resurface the distal vagina. The patient was a teenage girl who was previously operated on for "garden variety" vaginal atresia using rectosigmoid. Lateral incisions released the scar and approximately one-half of the thickness of the levator ani muscles. A large vein lies exactly in this area 1½ inches into the vagina and usually requires suture ligature. These flaps consist of relatively elastic skin and elongate well under moderate tension. C. Intraoperative view of the use of both the anteriorly based and posteriorly based flaps, which provide approximately 3.5 inches of added circumference. (Circumference equals πD; therefore 1 inch of diameter was added.) The patient had a vaginal stenosis, allowing admission of only the tip of the small finger. The function of the vagina was restored.*

Gracilis myocutaneous flaps are bulky when used for vaginal agenesis but are excellent when used for the defects following extirpative cancer surgery [65].

Some advantages [72] of rectosigmoid vaginostomy are apparent, but others are not as obvious [77–79].

1. Sensibility is retained in this colonic segment.
2. Natural lubrication is present, without excessive mucus production.
3. Vigorous arterial supply is maintained.
4. The malodor associated with skin placed in a body cavity is not present.
5. Long-term use of a stent is not necessary.
6. Skin graft donor site scarring is absent.
7. Examination reveals normal tactile feeling and visual qualities.
8. Carcinoma has been reported in seven studies of vaginal skin grafts and in one report on an intestinal transfer [82].

A technologic breakthrough, the stapling device, made this technique possible [56, 81, 93, 94]. Prior to introduction of the intestinal stapler, the low anterior resection was used and was much less secure [13]. The use of the stapling device has improved reliability dramatically [43, 71].

TECHNIQUE

A modified lithotomy position allows two teams to work simultaneously and thus significantly reduces the operating time. The perineal dissection opens up a cavity to the peritoneum. Simultaneously, a 15-cm segment of intestine is located and surgically isolated, based on the unpaired superior hemorrhoidal artery system from the inferior mesenteric, which branches from the aorta itself (Fig. 57-6). The segment is taken out of the gastrointestinal stream and moved only about 3 inches to its new vaginal position. Little mesentery, vascular, or nerve supply is disturbed. Recontinuity is established with the EEA stapling machine positioned via the anus. Because this intes-

tinal flap does not reach the perineum, skin flaps are necessary from adjacent labia majora, perineum, groin (or scrotal) areas, or preferably the dilated pouch. Figure 57-5 shows flaps that are occasionally used for the initial reconstruction.

A stent is used intermittently for 6 weeks to 6 months [33]. A frequency of twice per day for 20 minutes is adequate. A pneumatic inflatable stent (Mentor Corporation, Goleta, CA) is used for 10 days and then a silicone foam stent covered with a latex-rubber condom. (Precision Ocular Prosthetics, Redwood City, CA). Fashioning a larger colon circumference with darts, Z-plasty, or a bias cut is a must to decrease the incidence of circumferential contracture at the colon–skin anastomosis. Douching produces excess mucus production.

ANATOMY

The important clinical aspect of the anatomy is that the colon is interrupted at the level of the peritoneal reflection (or a little below), at a point where the inferior mesenteric (or superior rectal) artery and vein and their accompanying sympathetic and parasympathetic nerves are merging with another system: that of the middle rectal artery and vein. The middle rectal vessels are also accompanied by sympathetic and parasympathetic nerves. There is no significant interruption of arteries, veins, or nerves to either the remaining distal or proximal portions of intestine when this site of disconnection is selected. The ability of the brain to perceive vibration and to be able to discern gas from liquid or solid may be facilitated by the intact parasympathetic and sympathetic nerve pathways.

Surgery is undertaken at the time the patient wishes to become sexually active. Some patients request surgery because of feelings of inadequacy and the desire to be a "complete woman," even though they do not plan to become sexually active at the time of surgery. In most cases surgery is undertaken after age 16 and after full physical

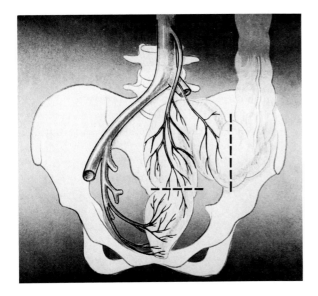

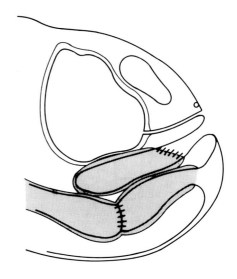

**Figure 57-6** *Use of the rectosigmoid colon from peritoneal reflection upward 15 cm on its vigorous arterial and nerve supply. The pedicle does not come all the way out to the perineum. The gastrointestinal stream is reconstituted with the EEA (end-to-end anastomosis) stapling device placed via the anus.*

growth. Regardless of the patient's age, she must be well motivated because it is necessary for her to use a vaginal stent postoperatively. Emotionally immature patients, in their early teens, may not easily sustain an operation of this magnitude.

## Surgery for Female With Ambiguous Genitalia

The operation for the female with ambiguous genitalia typically [17, 68] consists in converting the scrotum into both labia majora as well as the lateral aspect of the vaginal introitus, and converting the penis to a clitoris. Moreover, the skin of the penile shaft must be used to form the labia minora, the glans of the clitoris renamed the glans penis, and the male urinary meatus converted to the female urinary meatus. The müllerian portion of the vagina, i.e., the internal three-fourths of the vagina, is marsupialized and connected to skin flaps. Flaps of "scrotal" derivation are formed with a posterior base and are moved posteriorly and al-

lowed to form the labia majora and the lateral aspects or walls of the vaginal introitus (Fig. 57-7).

The ventral penile skin is brought down into the anterior vagina for coverage of a tissue deficit in this area, and it is also bundled up in the midline to simulate labia minora. This skin, of course, is erotically sensitive. The rationale is that these tissues are embryologically homologous; i.e., the penile shaft and labia minora are of the same derivation. The chordee is not released because it acts effectively to bring the penis into a more posterior, or clitoral, position. The glans is allowed to protrude through an aperture in the penis/labia minora flap. The corpora spongiosum, which is a tube of erectile tissue surrounding the urethra, is separated from the corpora spongiosum. The

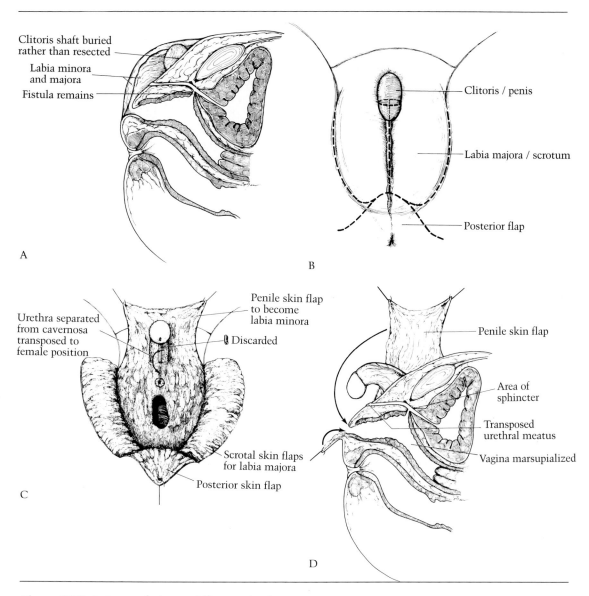

**Figure 57-7** *A. Internal view, midline sagittal. The U-V fistula was near the internal sphincter and not repaired in the small child. The knowledge of the structures named as homologous in Figure 57-2 (and Figure 58-1) was used to advantage when converting external genitalia back to female: penis to clitoris, ventral penis skin to labia minora, scrotum to labia majora. Postoperative view is shown in Figure 57-3B. B. The incision. C. The flaps from the front view. D. The flaps from a paramidline sagittal section.*

corpora spongiosum is liberated from a suspensory ligament connecting it to the posterior aspect of the pubic bone, a maneuver that allows the urinary channel to drop posteriorly into a more female position so that the urinary stream is in a downward direction in the sitting position. A penis reduction procedure is performed by resecting the greater portions of the shafts of the two corpora cavernosa after dissection and preservation of the large dorsal nerves and vessels. The two remaining segments of the cavernosa (tubes of erectile tissue contained in the tough albuginea) are reanastomosed end to end. This internal portion of the vagina is marsupialized and brought out to attach to skin of the labia majora and minora (i.e., penis and scrotal skin flaps) and a posterior flap. An attempt is made to break up the circumferential scar line with these flaps. The vagina is, of course, infantile, and it is not easy to predict if, with the stimulation at puberty, it will develop adequate function.

## Vaginal Stenosis

Another procedure may be necessary at puberty, e.g., release of the circumferential introital scar and resurfacing of the resultant defect with flaps from the labia or the groin. To release scars of vaginal stenosis, incisions are made in the lateral aspects, where there are fewer vital structures. Labia majora can be advanced 2 inches into the vagina, especially if they are more adult-sized ones (see Fig. 57-5B). These flaps retain their blood supply under the moderate tension that is necessary for their placement. They thus constitute a resource of banked tissue. The blood supply for the labia major is from the femoral "axis" via the deep external pudendal artery and the superficial external pudendal artery (see Fig. 57-5A).

If "pinpoint" stenosis is present, the labia major flaps may be used in addition to two other axial pattern flaps based posteriorly and running anteriorly in the groin crease, nourished by the artery of Huang (see Fig. 57-5C). Huang, at the University of Texas Medical Branch, Galveston, has contributed to our knowledge by elucidating an axial blood supply to the inguinal skin. The posterior labial (or posterior scrotal) artery derives from the perineal branches of the internal pudendal artery as it emerges from the pudendal canal. It surfaces in the ischiorectal fossa area, runs anteriorly, and supplies a large area of skin and subcutaneous tissue in the groin that can be carried as an island flap. The flap has been used to form the posterior one-half of a new vagina or for resurfacing indications. Note, however, that this vessel is sometimes interrupted during the course of exposure and dissection for a neovagina.

Effective procedures for stenosis of the more external portion of the vagina are included in this chapter because they are handy procedures to use to solve problems of dyspareunia secondary to an episiotomy scar, stenosis for lichen planus sclerosis et atrophica resistant to topical steroids, stenosis following a McIndoe type of split-thickness skin graft procedure, or female pseudohermaphroditism. These surgical methods, the preoperative preparation, and the postoperative management thus put to practical application a great many of the principles of plastic and reconstructive surgery.

## References

1. Abrenio, J. K., et al. Verrucous CA arising from an artificial vagina. *Obstet. Gynecol.* 50:185, 1977.
2. Akinkugbe, A. Vaginal atresia and cryptomenorrhea. *Obstet. Gynecol.* 46:317, 1975.
3. Alexandrov, M. S. *Berl. Ges. Gynakol Gebush.* 43:429, 1942.
4. Alexandrov, M. S. *Obrazovanie Iskustvennogo Ulagalishcha iz Sigmoidnoi Kishki.* [Formation of an artificial vagina from sigmoid colon.] Moscow: Mediz, 1955.
5. Baldwin, J. F. The formation of an artificial vagina by intestinal transplantation. *Ann. Surg.* 40:398, 1904.
6. Baldwin, J. F. Formation of an artificial vagina by intestinal transplantation. *Am. J. Obstet. Gynecol.* 56:636, 1907.
7. Baramki, T. A. Embryology of the urogenital system in man and genetic factors in intersex problems and transsexualism. *Clin. Plast. Surg.* 1:201, 1974.
8. Bates, G. W., and Wiser, W. L. A technique for uterine conservation in adolescents with vaginal agenesis and a functional uterus. *Obstet. Gynecol.* 66:290, 1985.

9. Blocker, T. G., Lewis, S. R., and Snyder, C. C. Plastic construction of an artificial vagina. *Plast. Reconstr. Surg.* 11:177, 1953.

10. Broadbent, T. R. Non-operative construction of the vagina: Two unusual cases. *Plast. Reconstr. Surg.* 73:117, 1984.

11. Broadbent, T. R., and Woolf, R. M. Congenital absence of the vagina: Reconstruction without operation. *Br. J. Plast. Surg.* 30:118, 1977.

12. Capraro, V. J., and Gallego, M. B. Vaginal agenesis. *Am. J. Obstet. Gynecol.* 124:98, 1976.

13. Cohn, I., and Nance F. C. The Colon and Rectum. In D. C. Sabastion Jr. (ed.), *Textbook of Surgery, The Biologic Basis of Modern Surgical Practice* (13th ed.). Philadelphia: Saunders, 1986.

14. Counseller, V. S., and Davis, C. F. Atresia of the vagina. *Obstet. Gynecol.* 40:835, 1968.

15. Cukier, J., Batzofin, J. H., Conner, J. S., et al. Genital tract reconstruction in a patient with congenital absence of the vagina and hypoplasia of the cervix. *Obstet. Gynecol.* 68:325, 1986.

16. Dewhurst, C. J. The aetiology and management of intersexuality. *Clin. Endocrinol. (Oxf.)* 4:625, 1975.

17. Donahoe, P. K., and Hendren, W. H. Perineal reconstruction in ambiguous genitalia infants raised as females. *Ann. Surg.* 200:363, 1984.

18. Duckler, L. Squamous cell carcinoma developing in an artificial vagina. *Obstet. Gynecol.* 40:35, 1972.

19. Dupuytren, G. Review Chiurgical de l'Hotel-Dieu. *Clin. Hop. de Laville.* L:3, 1827. Quoted by Marshall, H. K. *West. J. Surg.* 52:245, 1944.

20. Federman, D. D. *Abnormal Sexual Development: A Genetic and Endocrine Approach to Differential Diagnosis.* Philadelphia: Saunders, 1967.

21. Felix, W. The Development of the Urinogenital Organs. In F. Keibel and F. P. Mall (eds.), *Manual of Human Embryology.* Vol. 2. Philadelphia: Lippincott, 1912. Pp. 752–979.

22. Fore, S. R., Hammond, C. B., Partan, R. T., et al. Urologic and genital anomalies in patient with congenital absence of the vagina. *Obstet. Gynecol.* 46:410, 1975.

23. Frank, R. T. The formation of an artificial vagina without operation. *Am. J. Obstet. Gynecol.* 35:1053, 1938.

24. Frank, R. T. The formation of an artificial vagina without operation (intubation method). *N.Y.J. Med.* 40:1669, 1940.

25. Frank, R. T., and Geist, S. H. The formation of an artificial vagina by a new plastic technique. *Am. J. Obstet. Gynecol.* 14:712, 1927.

26. Franz. *Ann. R. Coll. Surg. Engl.* 66:223, 1984.

27. Frazer, J. E. *A Manual of Embryology: The Development of the Human Body.* London: Ballière, 1931.

28. Garcia, J., and Jones, H. W. The split thickness graft technique for vaginal agenesis. *Obstet. Gynecol.* 49:328, 1977.

29. Gigovsky, E. E. Scheidenbildung mit Hilfe endstandiger transplantation des mittleren Abschnittes des S-formiga Dickdamus zur Frage der Prioritat. *Zentralbl. Gynaekol.* 90:1684, 1968.

30. Gigovksy, E. E. Einschenkelige Kunstlicher sigmascheide. *Berl. Ges. Gynakol. Geburtsh.* 58:155, 1956 (abstract).

31. Gillenwater, J. Y. Intersex Problems: Diagnostic Aspects. In C. E. Horton (ed.), *Plastic and Reconstructive Surgery of the Genital Area.* Boston: Little, Brown, 1973.

32. Glenn, J. F. Testicular feminization syndrome. *Urology* 7:569, 1976.

33. Golditch, I. M. A modified mold in vaginal aplasia. *Am. J. Obstet. Gynecol.* 101:1135, 1968.

34. Golditch, I. M. Vaginal aplasia. *Surg. Gynecol. Obstet.* 129:361, 1969.

35. Goldwyn, R. M. History of attempts to form a vagina. *Plast. Reconstr. Surg.* 59:319, 1977.

36. Goligher, J. C. *Surgery of the Anus, Rectum and Colon.* (3rd ed.). London: Baillière, 1975. P. 28.

37. Goligher, J. C. The use of pedicled transplants of sigmoid or other parts of the intestinal tract for vaginal construction. *Ann. R. Coll. Surg. Engl.* 65(6):353, 1983.

38. Griffin, J. E., Edwards, C., Madden, J. D., et al. Congenital absence of the vagina: The Mayer-Rokitansky-Kuster-Hauser syndrome. *Ann. Intern. Med.* 85:224, 1976.

39. Grumback, M., and Conte, F. Disorders of Sex Differentiation. In R. Williams (ed.), *Textbook of Endocrinology.* Philadelphia: Saunders, 1981.

40. Hammond, C. B., and Addison, W. E. Agenesis of the Vagina. In D. Seraphin and N. Georgiade (eds.), *Pediatric Plastic Surgery.* St. Louis: Mosby, 1984.

41. Hauser, G. A., and Schreiner, W. E. Mayer-Rokitansky-Kuester syndrome: Rudimentary solid bipartite uterus with solid vagina. *Schweiz. Med. Wochenschr.* 91:381, 1961.

42. Herman, C. J., van Erp, A., Willemsen, W. N. P., et al. Artificial vaginas: Possible sources of epithelialization. *Hum. Pathol.* 13:1100, 1982.

43. Herrington, L. Discussion: Nance article. *Ann. Surg.* 189:598, 1979.

44. Huang, T. Use of anal artery groin skin flaps to construct a vagina. Presented to the 7th International Harry Benjamin Gender Dysphoria Association, Lake Tahoe, 1981.

45. Huang, T. Vaginoplasty with groin flaps. Presented to the American Association of Plastic Surgeons, Nashville, 1987.

46. Hwang, W., Chang, T., Sun, P., et al. Vaginal reconstruction using labia minor flaps in congenital total absence. *Ann. Plast. Surg.* 15:534, 1985.

47. Imrie, J. E. A., Kennedy, J. H., Holmes, J. D., et al. Intraepithelial neoplasia arising in an artificial vagina. *Br. J. Obstet. Gynaecol.* 93:886, 1986.

48. Ingram, J. The bicycle seat stool in the treatment of vaginal agenesis and stenosis: A preliminary report. *Am. J. Obstet. Gynecol.* 140:867, 1981.

49. Jackson, G. W. Primary carcinoma of an artificial vagina. *Obstet. Gynecol.* 14:534, 1959.

50. Jasoni, V. M., Tabanelli, S., Zannetti, G., et al. A rare case of absence of the vagina with the presence of functioning uterus: Surgical treatment. *Acta Eur. Fertil.* 15:137, 1984.

51. Jones, H. W., and Mermut, S. Familial occurrence of congenital absence of the vagina. *Am. J. Obstet. Gynecol.* 114:1100, 1972.

52. Jones, H. W., and Wheeless, C. R. Salvage of the reproductive potential of women with anomalous development of the müllerian ducts: 1868–1968–2068. *Obstet. Gynecol.* 104:348, 1968.

53. Jones, H. W., Jr., and Scott, W. W. *Hermaphroditism, Genital Anomalies and Related Endocrine Disorders* (2nd ed.). Baltimore: Williams & Wilkins, 1971.

54. Jost, A. Intersexuality. In H. W. Jones and W. W. Scott, (eds.), *Hermaphroditism, Genital Anomalies and Related Endocrine Disorders* (2nd ed.). Baltimore: Williams & Wilkins, 1971.

55. Judin, S. The Baldwin operation for the formation of an artificial vagina. *Surg. Gynecol. Obstet.* 44:530, 1927.

56. Kalinina, T. V. The Use of Apparatus PK25 and SK in the Clinic. In *Mechanical Sutures in Surgery of the Gastrointestinal Tract.* Moscow, 1964.

57. Koff, A. K. Development of the vagina in the human fetus. *Contrib. Embryol. Carnegie Inst.* 24:61, 1933.

58. Kramer, S. A., and Weinerth, J. L. Treatment of Ambiguous Genitalia. In D. Serafin and N. G. Georgiade (eds.), *Pediatric Plastic Surgery.* St. Louis: Mosby, 1984.

59. Kung, M. *Colpoporesis from the Colon.* Budapest: Akademai Kiado, 1975.

60. Kuster, H. Uterus bipartitus solidus rudimentarius cum vagina solida. *Zentralbl. Geb. Gynaekol.* 67:692, 1910.

61. Lischke, J., Curtis, C. H., and Lamb, D. J. Discordance of the vaginal agenesis in monozygotic terms. *Obstet. Gynecol.* 41:920, 1973.

62. Magrina, J. F., and Masterson, B. J. Vaginal reconstruction in gynecological oncology: A review of techniques. *Obstet. Gynecol. Surv.* 63:1, 1981.

63. Malini, S., Valdes, C., and Malinak, R. Sonographic diagnosis and classification of anomalies of the female genital tract. *J. Ultrasound Med.* 3:397, 1984.

64. Mayer, C. A. J. Uber Verdoppelungen des Uterus und ihre Arten, nebst Bemerkungen uber Hasenscharte und Wolfsrachen. *J. Chir. Aug.* 13:525, 1829.

65. McCraw, J. B., Massey, F. M., Shanklin, K. D., et al. Vaginal reconstruction with gracilis myocutaneous flaps. *Plast. Reconstr. Surg.* 58:176, 1976.

66. McIndoe, A. Treatment of congenital absence and obliterative conditions of the vagina. *Br. J. Plast. Surg.* 2:254, 1950.

67. McIndoe, A., and Bannister, J. B. An operation for the cure of congenital absence of the vagina. *J. Obstet. Gynecol. Br. Emp.* 45:490, 1938.

68. McKinnon, M., and Rayner, C. R. W. Phallic

urethra in an endocrine female and its surgical correction. *Plast. Reconstr. Surg.* 68:940, 1981.

69. Metz, A. A case of ulcerative colitis in vagina artificialis. *Gastroenterologia* 98:113, 1962.

70. Money, J., and Erhardt, A. A. *Man and Woman, Boy and Girl: The Differentiation and Dimorphism of Gender Identity from Conception to Maturity.* Baltimore: Johns Hopkins University Press, 1972.

71. Nance, F. C. New techniques of gastrointestinal anastomoses with the EEA stapler. *Ann. Surg.* 189:587, 1979.

72. Novak, F., Kos, L., and Pissko, F. The advantages of the artificial vagina derived from sigmoid colon. *Acta Obstet. Gynecol. Scand.* 57:95, 1978.

73. Obrenig, J. K., et al. Verrucous cancer arising from an artificial vagina. *Obstet. Gynecol.* 49:438, 1977.

74. Ortiz-Monasterio, F., Serrano, A., Barrera, G., et al. Congenital absence of the vagina—long term follow-up of 21 patients treated with skin grafts. *Plast. Reconstr. Surg.* 49:165, 1972.

75. Pinsonneault, O., and Goldstein, D. P. Obstructing malformations of the uterus and vagina. *Fertil. Steril.* 44:241, 1985.

76. Popoff, D. D. *Russk. Vrach. St. Petersburg* 60:1512, 1910.

77. Pratt, J. H. Sigmoidovaginostomy: A new method of obtaining satisfactory vaginal depth. *Am. J. Obstet. Gynecol.* 81:535, 1961.

78. Pratt, J. H. Vaginal atresia corrected by use of small and large bowel. *Clin. Obstet. Gynecol.* 15:639, 1972.

79. Pratt, J. H., and Smith, G. R. Vaginal reconstruction with a sigmoid loop. *Am. J. Obstet. Gynecol.* 96:31, 1966.

80. Ramming, K. Primary carcinoma in an artificial vagina. *Am. J. Surg.* 120:108, 1970.

81. Ravitch, M. M., and Steichen, F. M. A stapling instrument for end-to-end inverting anastomoses in the gastrointestinal tract. *Ann. Surg.* 189:791, 1979.

82. Ritchie, R. N. Primary carcinoma of the vagina following a Baldwin reconstruction operation for congenital absence of the vagina. *Am. J. Obstet. Gynecol.* 18:794, 1929.

83. Rokitansky, K. Uber die sogenannten Ver-

doppelungen des Uterus. *Med. Jahrb. Ost. Staat.* 26:39, 1838.

84. Rothman, D. The use of peritoneum in the construction of a vagina. *Obstet. Gynecol.* 40:835, 1972.

85. Schubert, G. Uber Scheidenbildung bei angeborenem Vaginaldefekt. *Zentralbl. Gynaekol.* 35:1017, 1911.

86. Schwartz, R. Ambiguous genitalia in a term female infant due to exposure to danazol in utero. *Am. J. Dis. Child.* 136:474, 1982.

87. Sheares, B. H. Congenital atresia of the vagina: A new technique for tunneling the space between bladder and rectum and construction of the vagina by a modified Wharton technique. *J. Obstet. Gynaecol. Br. Emp.* 67:24, 1960.

88. Shirodkar, V. N. *Contributions to Obstetrics and Gynecology.* Baltimore: Williams & Wilkins, 1960.

89. Singh, J., Lakshmi, and Devi, Y. Hysteroplasty and vaginoplasty for reconstruction of the uterus. *Int. J. Obstet. Gynecol.* 17:457, 1980.

90. Singh, J., and Lakshmi, D. Y. Pregnancy following surgical correction of nonfused müllerian bulbs and absent vagina. *Obstet. Gynecol.* 61:267, 1983.

91. Sneguireff, W. F. *Arch. de Tocal. et de Gynaek.* Paris, 1892. Cited by Baldwin [5].

92. Steffanoff, D. N. Late development of squamous carcinoma in a split skin graft lining the vagina. *Plast. Reconstr. Surg.* 51:454, 1973.

93. Steichen, F. M. The creation of autologous substitute organs with stapling instruments. *Am. J. Surg.* 134:659, 1977.

94. Steichen, F. M., and Ravitch, M. M. *Stapling in Surgery.* Chicago: Year Book, 1984.

95. Taneja, P. P., Heera, D., Gulati, S. M., et al. Urethral coitus in a case of vaginal agenesis. *Br. J. Urol.* 45:451, 1973.

96. Tarry, W. F., Duckett, J. W., and Stephens, F. D. The Mayer-Rokitansky syndrome: Pathogenesis, classification and management. *J. Urol.* 136:648, 1986.

97. Tozum, R. Homotransplantation of the amniotic membrane for the treatment of congenital absence of the vagina. *Int. J. Gynaecol. Obstet.* 14:553, 1976.

98. Ulfelder, H. Agenesis of the vagina. *Am. J.*

*Obstet. Gynecol.* 100:745, 1968.

99. Ulfelder, H., and Robboy, S. J. The embryologic development of the human vagina. *Am. J. Obstet. Gynecol.* 126:769, 1976.

100. Wharton, L. R. An improvement in the technique of constructing the vagina. *Am. J. Obstet. Gynecol.* 60:87, 1950.

101. Wharton, S. R. A simple method of constructing a vagina: Report of 4 cases. *Ann. Surg.* 107:842, 1938.

102. Wilfingseder, P. Panel discussion: vaginal reconstruction. Fifth International Congress of Plastic Surgery. Paris, 1974.

103. Williams, E. A. Congenital absence of the vagina: A simple operation for its relief. *J.*

*Obstet. Gynecol.* 71:511, 1964.

104. Williams, E. A. Vulva-vaginoplasty. *Proc. R. Soc. Med.* 63:1046, 1970.

105. Williams, E. A. A simple Method of Vaginal Construction. In M. L. Taymor and T. H. Grun, Jr. (eds.), *Progress in Gynecology.* Vol. 6. Orlando: Grune & Stratton, 1975.

106. Williams, E. A. Uterovaginal agenesis. *Ann. R. Coll. Surg. Engl.* 58:266, 1976.

107. Yves, J. Panel discussion: Vaginal construction. Fifth International Congress of Plastic Surgery, Paris, 1974.

108. Zangl, A. Die Sigmascheide: Tecknik und Ergebnisse. *Wien. Klin. Wochenschr.* 82:561, 1970.

# 58

## Gender Dysphoria Syndrome

*Donald R. Laub*
*Donald R. Laub, Jr.*
*Judy Van Maasdam*

I would like to remind everyone of an important fundamental fact—the difference between sex and gender. Sex is what you see. Gender is what you feel. Harmony between the two is essential for human happiness.—*Harry Benjamin, M.D., New York City, June 1976*

Gender confirmation surgery may be of benefit to a select group of patients.—*Milton Edgerton, 1985*

Plastic surgery is the application of surgical modalities to improve function and appearance, to enhance the dignity of those with great need, and to increase self-confidence with body image surgery [26]. These modalities catalyze an increase in patients' happiness and productivity. This chapter discusses perhaps the most dramatic and controversial example of the application of plastic surgery—the alteration of the sex of the body to meet the body image. Many workers today believe that an organic or somatic cause is present but is yet unidentified and that gender confirmation surgery is reconstructive surgery. Others believe that such profound alteration of a healthy body is being considered for a purely behavioral disorder. Many approach the work in this field as the ultimate application of aesthetic or cosmetic, palliative, self-improvement,

body image surgery. The surgeons who work in the field may find it disturbing, especially because it is uncertain in individual cases whether surgery is the treatment of choice. As with any rehabilitative surgical program, interdisciplinary teamwork is mandatory. Although the etiology of gender dysphoria syndrome is unclear, and therefore specific prevention and treatment are unknown, much can be done to palliate individuals with this form of disturbed behavior. The available data suggest that properly selected patients who participate in a well organized gender dysphoria rehabilitation program demonstrate significant improvements in life-style, social relationships, sense of self-esteem, body image, employment status, and sexual adjustment [22, 44, 55]. However, a rehabilitation program must give priority to the economic, social and psychological needs of the patient in addition to the anatomic requirements; surgery is only part of the program. It does little good to perform a technically perfect operation and still have a patient who is isolated from society, maladjusted, and receiving public assistance. A multidisciplinary approach is needed, and strict criteria must be met prior to any surgery if serious errors in patient selection are to be avoided. The guidelines published by the Harry Benjamin International Gender Dysphoria Association* [53, 75] are accepted by medical professionals, courts of law, insurance carriers, and malpractice insurance companies as the standards for clinical care.†

A dividend of gender dysphoria surgery is that the same surgical procedures may be adapted for use in patients who have suffered loss of either the vagina or the penis because of trauma, cancer, infection, or irradiation; the rehabilitation principles regarding patient management may be applied to many other plastic and cosmetic surgery patients.

## Historical Background

References to cross-gender behavior can be found in early Greek and Roman literature, and examples of cross-gender identification can be found among diverse cultural and racial groups [40]. Despite isolated reports of "sex conversion operations," during the 1930s, the interest of the lay public and the medical profession was not aroused until the well publicized story of Christine Jorgensen was reported by Hamburger and associates [42] in 1953. Interest in this phenomenon has existed since then.

Although the term *transsexual* was coined earlier by Caldwell [12], it was the pioneer sexologist Harry Benjamin who popularized the term and delineated the clinical aspects of transsexualism in his book *The Transsexual Phenomenon*. Benjamin [5] listed four characteristics: (1) a lifelong sense of being a member of the opposite sex; (2) gender behavior of the opposite sex and early, persistent cross-dressing without erotic feeling; (3) repugnance and disgust for one's genitalia without deriving pleasure

*The professional association that provides a forum for the exchange of knowledge between the workers of the disciplines involved in gender dysphoria.
†Available for $2.00 by writing the Executive Secretary, Harry Benjamin International Gender Dysphoria Association, Inc., 1515 El Camino Real, OBER Bldg. Palo Alto, CA 94306.

from them; and (4) disdain for homosexual behavior. Benjamin emphasized that the intensity of the motivation toward surgery was important prognostically.

In 1963 Edgerton, Jones, Knorr, and Money established the first gender identity clinic at Johns Hopkins University. It represented the first multidisciplinary attempt to study and treat disorders of gender identification. Subsequently, other groups were formed at major medical institutions across the United States. In 1969 Green and Money [40] published *Transsexualism and Sex Reassignment*, which was the first truly scientific book that dealt with this problem.

As more experience was gained by these groups, it became clear that not all of the patients who presented requesting sex change surgery conformed to the classic definition of transsexualism, although many patients had consciously or unconsciously developed congruous histories in their attempt to gain acceptance for surgery. Because it is not only the diagnostic subgroup but also the attainment of behavioral goals during the preoperative period that is important from a clinical point of view, Fisk in 1973 coined the generic description *gender dysphoria syndrome* [25].

## Differential Diagnosis

The gender dysphoria syndrome includes all patients who are so dissatisfied with their body that they demand gender-altering surgery. The syndrome includes the following diagnostic categories.

*1. Classic transsexualism.* It is estimated that only 15 to 20 percent of all patients with gender dysphoria fall into this category (the characteristics of this group have already been described by Benjamin).

*2. Gender dysphoria syndrome, former effeminate homosexuality.* Male patients in this category are sexually attracted to men and initially derive pleasure from their penis. With time, they gradually assume a more feminine life-style and evolve into seeking surgery as a means of avoiding the moral, financial, and social stigma of homosexuality. Furthermore, under hormonal therapy the penis becomes inactive as a source of pleasure. An analogous situation may exist for masculine lesbians.

**3.** *Gender dysphoria syndrome, former transvestitism.* Transvestites have been said to derive erotic stimulation from cross dressing, but we now know that they may merely enjoy cross dressing. They frequently possess an obsessive-compulsive, achieving personality. These men generally start out with a heterosexual orientation and are often married with children. Gradually some evolve into gender dysphoria for reasons similar to those of the previous group (gender dysphoria syndrome, former effeminate homosexuality). An analogous situation for genetic females may not exist.

**4.** *Gender dysphoria syndrome, psychosis.* Perhaps psychotic reaction with delusion regarding sexual identity is a more accurate designation. These patients are generally not surgical candidates but must be distinguished from those who develop psychosis as a reaction to the stress associated with gender dysphoria. It is a situation that is called "secondary transsexualism" and Bourgeois reported that it could be successfully treated by treating the primary condition (i.e., depression).

**5.** *Gender dysphoria syndrome, psychoneurotic sociopathy.* These patients are frank exhibitionists, and part of their motivation in seeking sex change is to obtain notoriety and publicity. They are generally poor surgical candidates.

**6.** *Gender dysphoria syndrome, inadequate and schizoid personality.* These individuals do not have a well developed sense of gender, and they request surgery in an attempt to minimize stress associated with functioning in society.

It is virtually impossible to obtain reliable statistics pertaining to the incidence of gender dysphoria syndrome. The incidence cited is that perhaps 7000 patients in the United States have been hormonally and surgically reassigned, and that 30,000 to 60,000 persons consider themselves candidates. In mid-1978 as many as 40 centers in the Western Hemisphere offered care that included surgery [75]. There have been centers that have discontinued work since then, and a few more low-profile treatment centers have become available in private practice.

## General Management

The plastic surgeon cannot manage this complex behavior disorder alone. Furthermore, the goal of a gender dysphoria program must be total rehabilitation of the patient, not just surgical change, which is only a small part of the rehabilitation program.

Just as not all patients who request aesthetic surgical procedures are appropriate candidates, similarly, surgery must not be performed at the demand of patients claiming to be transsexuals and desiring sex reassignment. Proper patient selection is paramount if the surgeon is to adhere to the basic tenet of *primum non nocere.* Many other disciplines must be brought into evaluation and therapy if these unfortunate people are to be truly helped. The treatment actually requires the family practitioner, psychiatrist, plastic surgeon (internist/endocrinologist), and gynecologist/urologist. Vital components of the program are provided by the social worker or psychologist, and the advice of an attorney is essential. Interaction with an insurance advisor, peer advisors, and the job supervisor/president of the company for which the patient works are also helpful.

At the present time, the plastic surgeon's pendulum has swung away from the field of genital reconstruction. As the cycle reverses, however, it is important to recall that most lawsuits in this field have involved surgeons who have had experience with only a few cases and particularly those who have not followed (or not been aware of) the strict guidelines for clinical practice as published by the Harry Benjamin Gender Dysphoria Association [53, 75]. A synopsis of these guidelines is as follows: (1) Prior to the initiation of genital or breast sex reassignment—augmentation mammoplasty, mastectomy (breast reduction), vaginoplasty, vaginectomy, phalloplasty, penectomy, castration, hysterectomy—the patient must be recommended and endorsed in writing to the surgeon by two clinical behavioral scientists competent in this area. One of these advocates must be at the doctoral level, and one of the two must have known the patient in a professional psychotherapeutic relationship for 6 months. (2) Most important, the patient must have been living successfully in the genetically other sex role for at least 1 year. (3) The two clinical behavioral scientists must establish the diagnosis by documenting that the specific symptoms for this condition were present in the patient for at least 2 years. (4) Furthermore, hormonal sex reassignment must precede surgical sex reassignment, as the hormonal effects (some irreversible) are both diagnostic and therapeutic. Surgeons must review the patient's history to check that the guidelines for the hormonal therapy are fulfilled: informed consent regarding possible undesirable effects and complications, monitoring of liver function, relevant blood chemistries, and periodic physical examination.

One important summary point is synoptic of the overall guidelines: Because surgery is not the treatment of the condition, but because the best treatment available is a rehabilitation program that includes surgery, surgery is more successful with a patient already enjoying success in the chosen sex and gender role. Surgery is less leveraged with existing success. Failure in life does not imply that lack of surgery is responsible for lack of success. The more self-rehabilitation that is accomplished preoperatively, the less the patient depends on surgery as the one and only key to solving the many problems. The surgeon is not only more responsible but safer if he or she is assured that the patient can negotiate successfully in the role: economically, psychologically, physically, socially, and sexually. Some degree of success in the previous gender is reassuring as well. The converse to the above criteria are the yellow danger flags: inability to hold a job in the new role without co-workers knowing; general unhappiness; inability to pass physically or to exhibit appropriate deportment; schizoid reclusive, loner behavior; workaholic with narrow social life; nonstandard, nonheterosexual, or no sexual desires.

Obviously, psychosis, psychopathic con artist personality, desire for notoriety or public relations exposure, perfectionism, narcissism (self-centered), flamboyancy, hysteria, penile eroticism, existing marriage in the sex of the anatomy, urgency, and manipulativeness regarding the date for surgery are as negative factors in this condition as these or similar factors are for aesthetic surgery.

## Etiology

The determination of sex is based on eight criteria, as shown in Table 58-1.

None of these factors has full control over the determination of the "true" sex. An ambiguity of the sexes according to the first five criteria is referred to by the term *intersexuality.* The latter three criteria correspond to the *gender identity problems* [58].

Sex-dimorphic differentiation of the brain occurs after differentiation of the genitalia. Gender role behavior and sexual orientation have parallels in animal behavior, but gender identity does not. These three categories have specific meaning in the nomenclature of the developing science of sex behavior. All three are generally grouped under sex-dimorphic behavior [58].

In mammals, we now know that sex-

**Table 58-1** *Criteria for determination of sex*

| Parameter | Time | Criteria |
|---|---|---|
| Chromosomal sex | Moment of conception | XX or XY chromosome |
| Gonads | 45 days | H-Y antigen |
| Internal genitalia | First 3 months | Testosterone + müllerian duct inhibitor |
| External genitalia | First 6 months | Tissue receptors, 5 dihydromethyl testosterone |
| Sex hormone patterns | Fetal life and up to menarche | Pulsatile FSH and LH vs. nonpulsatile |
| Pattern of behavior centers | Pre- or perinatally | Sex-dimorphic differentiation |
| Sex of assignment and rearing | Imprinting by the environment | Sex-dimorphic differentiation |
| Psychosexual differentiation | Lifelong | Gender identity |

*Key:* FSH = follicle-stimulating hormone; LH = luteinizing hormone.

dimorphic behavior* is regulated by brain systems that are organized during hormone-sensitive periods pre- or even perinatally. Actual structural changes in the hypothalmus, amygdala, and preoptic areas have been demonstrated to occur at pre- and perinatal times [58].

In the cat, rat, dog, and monkey, transsexual behavior can be produced by hormones given at birth (and in some instances later in life as well). In humans the hypothalamus differentiates during the second trimester, and we can consider this point the beginning of the critical period for sex differentiation into dimorphic behavior.

The human evidence obtained in both hypogonadal males, the syndrome of feminizing testes, and prenatally virilized girls (the fairly common adrenal hyperplasia cases) supports the idea that exposure to androgens before birth does play some role in programming a male gender role in later life. These hormonal factors are rarely decisive in the

human, and the changes are generally not great enough that they cannot be accommodated within the range of behavior accepted for a given gender [24, 60]. The most important element in the development of gender role is the assigned sex of rearing and the reinforcement that the early assignment receives during the period of infancy and early childhood. An important second factor in humans is the hormone (or replacement therapy) appropriate to the sex of rearing at the normal age of puberty [78]. Gender identity can be compared to acquisition of language in that the various experiences of growing up have great influence and are relatively well established at 2.5 years [58]. If this reinforcement is weak because of ambiguous attitudes in the parents, the outlook for attaining a normal gender identity during adult life is greatly diminished.

Later in life, the decision regarding to which sex a person belongs must take into consideration not only chromosomes, gonads, internal and external genitalia, and hormonal secretions but also the *behavioral* differentiation. In the human, one of the more important factors in respect to behavior is the sex of assignment and rearing, which may be discrepant to the other crite-

*Gender role behavior:* cultural differences in male and female behavior. *Sexual orientation:* erotic responsiveness to one sex or other. *Gender identity:* identification of an individual with one sex or another. *Sex dimorphia:* refers to the two forms of behavior: male versus female

ria. One must not forget that there is also some effect of androgens on behavior centers of the brain as we develop in utero [58].

Patients with gender dysphoria have no recognized abnormalities of chromosomes, external or internal anatomy, or adult hormonal patterns [27, 57]. Hypotheses as to the origin of this condition have generally fallen into two broad categories [55]: (1) the prenatal influence of sex hormones on the developing fetal nervous system and (2) postnatal social and psychological influences.

Evidence for the first category comes from experimental work with mammals and lower primates. The fact remains, however, that once gender identity has been established it is virtually impossible to change it. Attempts by psychiatrists to reverse adult transsexualism have been generally unsuccessful. Barlow and associates [3] have reported one case in which a young adult was successfully treated with behavior modification techniques. Kirkpatrick and Friedman [50] reported a few cases. Levine [56] has also reported that some patients have at least temporarily given up their desire for sex change surgery after intense psychotherapy, but he cautioned that these patients must not be considered cured. Hastings [43] has summarized the situation well:

Since the gender role seems to be laid down in indelible fashion during the first forty months of life, it is not surprising that attempts to change it in later life by whatever treatment modality have been found to be an exercise in futility. The only avenue of therapy, if one wishes to do anything to help these unfortunate people, seems to be that of the surgical route.

### Female to Male Change

Testerone administered to a female body causes profound changes.

1. Increase in blood pressure.
2. Weight gain; acne; increase in triglycerides and cholesterol, and probably coronary artery disease.
3. When coupled with smoking, weight gain, and living at a high altitude, an obstructive pulmonary disease occurs characterized by: (1) significantly decreased pulmonary compliance noted by the anesthesiologist; (2) bronchitis; and (3) significantly increased packed cell volume and hemoglobin.
4. Sleep apnea syndrome. This problem is logically explained by the enlarging effects of testosterone on the soft tissues of palate, tongue, and neck in the small female bony framework. Difficulty of anesthesia management (intubation of the trachea) is not uncommon.
5. Peliosis hepatica and liver function abnormality [6]. Testosterone and analogues are metabolized in the liver. Abnormal liver function tests are not uncommon, particularly when associated with other chemicals metabolized in the liver, e.g., alcohol. Peliosis hepatica is the formation of large cystic spaces in the liver associated with abuse of anabolic hormones by athletes. The condition also occurs with excess testosterone. It is detected by a liver scan, not liver function tests.
6. Increased libido.
7. Increased size of the clitoris, but no further differentiation of external genitalia toward male characteristics.
8. Hair growth on the skin of the face and body.
9. Android rather than gynecoid distribution of subcutaneous fat.
10. Some deepening of the voice.
11. Ovarian suppression without pituitary stimulation; cessation of menses; breast gland and duct decrease.
12. Personality changes chronologically associated with the hormone therapy, probably not entirely due to placebo or psychological effect.

Polycystic ovary syndrome is found in a high percentage of hormone-treated female-to-male transsexuals [29]. However, prior to the start of hormone therapy, female-to-male transsexuals have a higher than expected incidence of endocrine disorders, including polycystic ovarian disease [30]. Whether this finding has any relation to the etiology of gender dysphoria is not known.

Based on the above known alterations in pathophysiology, preoperative evaluation is therefore a history and physical examination with interest focused toward the following.

Blood pressure
Weight
Acne, as a source of postoperative wound infection
Bronchitis, sinusitis
Sleep apnea syndrome (deviated nasal septum; relatively large tongue, palate, hyoid)
Inguinal hernia
Liver nodules, liver size
Packed cell volume
Chest film, electrocardiogram
Liver function and blood fats

Thoughtful preoperative preparation insists on weight loss, decreased smoking, control of blood pressure, exercise program, control of acne, and decreased alcohol and substance intake. Standard practice is to give 200 mg of testosterone enanthate or propionate every 2 weeks intramuscularly. Testosterone given orally definitely produces more liver change than when given via the parenteral route. Two weeks after injection, the clinical and blood level is at the normal to subnormal threshold. Implanted slow-release testosterone has not been widely used.

PHALLOPLASTY

Surgery to find a solution to the problem of "no penis" falls into two broad divisions: procedures that utilize existing tissue and those that bring in new tissue. Metoidioplasty (Greek: *meta* = toward, *oidio* = male genitals, and *plasty* = to form) [52] utilizes existing tissue, and the surgery is based on the embryologic pattern. Male internal genitalia derive from the wolffian ducts, in contrast to the female's internal genitalia, which derive from the müllerian ducts. However, in regard to the *external* genitalia, the situation is different: Both male and female structures are derived from the same tissues. Therefore some rationale exists when considering the female external anatomy as "growth arrest" of male external anatomy. The labia minora (external surface) becomes the ventral penis shaft and the labia minora (internal aspect) the pendulous or spongiose urethra; the clitoris becomes the glans and dorsal penis; the bulbs of the vestibule become the corpora cavernosa penis. Rationale therefore exists for surgically changing the female external anatomy to the male counterparts. Testosterone enlarges the clitoris only to a certain size (Fig. 58-1A). Surgery attempts to complete the development onward into the male form by: (1) bringing the labia majora more posteriorly, fusing them in the midline, and filling them with testicular implants; and (2) moving the clitoris to the penile position more anteriorly by releasing the chordee and forming the ventral surface of the penis from the labia minora and the pendulous urethra from the labia minora internal surfaces (Fig. 58-1B–F).

At this stage in the development of the surgery, the authors have not yet attained the skill to provide urination and vaginal intromission. However, Bouman of Amsterdam has used the anterior vagina as a flap in a urethroplasty, and Durfee and Roland [19] extended the urinary channel. Erotic sensibility and good appearance (not size) are achieved.

Phalloplasty utilizing distant tissue transfer has been accomplished via various techniques. Each surgeon's contribution is an important entry in the "menu" of surgical alternatives available to the phalloplasty surgeon.

Not all of these methods have been used for the patients with gender dysphoria. They are included in the armamentarium here be-

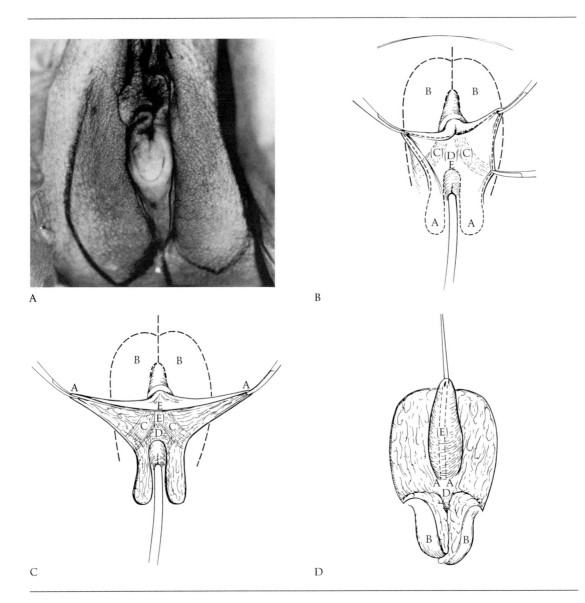

A

B

C

D

**Figure 58-1** *A. Preoperative photograph of a patient about to undergo metoidioplasty. The surgery is diagramed in B, C, and D. Dotted lines are incisions. (A = labia minora tissue; B = labia majora; C = corpora cavernosa; D = chordee.) The clitoris is circumscribed at its base; the chordee is released, allowing the clitoris/penis to move anteriorly 2 cm or more. The penis brings with it labia minora for a urethral tunnel and for surfacing the tissue-* *deficient posterior surface of the penis. Silicon gel testicular prostheses are placed in the new scrotum. A simultaneous or later colpectomy yields a flap of anterior vagina (Bouman) useful to cover the female urinary meatus and to turn the urinary stream in an anterior direction, bringing urethra toward the penile urethra. E, F. Two postoperative patients. (See Figure 57-2 for the homologous nature of the male and female external anatomy.)*

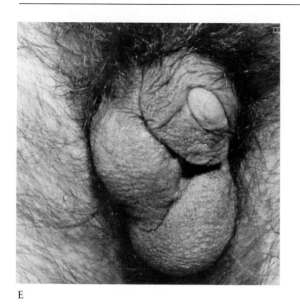

E

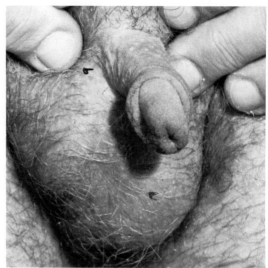

F

cause the innovative reconstruction surgeon must know about them.

*1.* In China, two methods of phalloplasty have been developed. Ti-Sheng Chang [13] in Shanghai formed a penis in one stage, using a large radial forearm flap to form the entire penis. He placed a costal cartilage graft as a stiffener.

*2.* Song [69, 70], in Beijing, has reported one-stage phalloplasties using low abdominal flaps, scrotal flaps, thigh flaps, and costal cartilage, as indicated for the particular case. Sensation and urination from the tip of the penis are features of this brilliant application of plastic surgery principles and modern knowledge of anatomy.

*3.* Puckett and colleagues [67, 68] perform a free flap phalloplasty in one stage utilizing the lateral groin flap of Macgregor. They place a Scott-Strauch inflatable prosthesis. It is done as a staged procedure.

*4.* Persoff [66] has contributed the concept of forming a urethra with less tendency for contraction from split-thickness skin

grafts on the deep superficial (Scarpa's) fascia of the groin flap.

*5.* Mukherjee [62], in Bombay, has used a seven-stage procedure utilizing groin and scrotal flaps for reconstructive phalloplasty in male burn victims. He reported great success with this technique.

*6.* Daverio [14], of Lausanne, has used the "Chinese flap" in gender dysphoria surgery. He, like the Chinese, brings three nerves from the forearm and utilizes a costal cartilage graft. The method is done simultaneously with hysterectomy and culpectomy, and vaginal mucosa is salvaged as a graft for the glans penis. He does not employ neurorrhaphy to the deep pudendal nerve but has reported early nerve regrowth to the midshaft of the penis.

*7.* Sun and Huang [72], at the plastic surgery hospital in Beijing, use the lateral groin flap in combination with a vascularized iliac crest bone graft.

*8.* Gilbert et al. [31, 32] and Horton et al. [47] employ a one-stage phalloplasty utilizing two arterialized flaps. The lateral brachial fasciocutaneous free flap, which forms the surface of the penis, is based on the radial collateral artery and includes the lateral brachial cutaneous nerve. This method fabricates the urethra from an inferior rectus abdominis musculocutaneous island flap. No skin grafting is required. Testing of sensation in the penis shaft—according to bulbocavernosus reflex, erogenous, vibratory, temperature, and two-point discrimination criteria—is reported positive.

**9.** Edgerton, Kenney, and colleagues [23] have devised a phalloplasty utilizing a long, well vascularized, full-thickness flap of the bladder for the urethral construction. The flap is brought out to the pendulous urethra in two stages. The donor tissue is closely related to the urethra, and the procedure appears reliable.

**10.** Slender ileum for urethra was reported in 1974 by Edgerton [20].

**11.** Historically, the tube pedicle was used for penile reconstruction by Borgas in Russia [8], Frumpkin in Germany [28], and Gilles and Harrison in England [35]; also of note in the development were the reports of Arneri [1], Morales et al. [61], Kaplan [49], and Boxer [10].

**12.** The gracilis muscle has been used as well by Dibbell [16], Orticochea [64], Hester et al. [46], and Greer and Johnston [41].

The authors have utilized two flaps in a composite form.

**1.** The radial forearm, or Chinese flap, is used a) to form the urethra because the relatively glabrous skin of the forearm prevents stone formation and hair balls, and b) to establish sensibility of the glans penis because the lateral cutaneous nerve of the forearm is contained in the forearm flap. The specialized nerve endings in this donor site are surprisingly "inexpensive." The details of the surgery are shown in Figure 58-2. To achieve sensibility for the glans and a urinary stream through a relatively glabrous skin-lined neourethra, and to obtain some ability for intromission, the Chinese, or radial forearm,

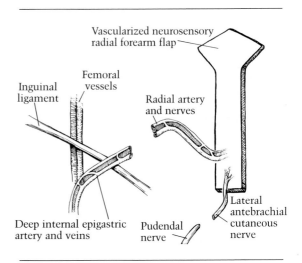

**Figure 58-2** *Details of microsurgery. The radial artery and its veins have alternatively been attached to the femoral artery and saphenous vein directly, instead of to the deep inferior epigastrics. The lateral antebrachial cutaneous nerve extends the (erotic) sensibility of the (clitoral) deep pudendal nerve to the glans penis. A portion of the glans was formed from distal forearm skin.*

flap is added to the "standard" flap. The ingredients for this composite and their respective functions are detailed in Table 58-2. Not all patients require the baculum or artificial stiffener.

**2.** The abdominal tube pedicle (midline, bipedicle, inside-out tube flap covered with a skin graft) adds appearance and bulk and provides a second tunnel for baculum placement [15, 63]. Figure 58-3 shows the stan-

**Table 58-2** *Details of phalloplasty procedure used by the authors*

| Materials | Use |
|---|---|
| Abdominal skin flap | Bulk |
| Chinese flap | Nerve and vessels; glabrous skin for the urethra |
| Split-thickness skin graft | Aesthetics of the shaft |
| Baculum | Stiffener |

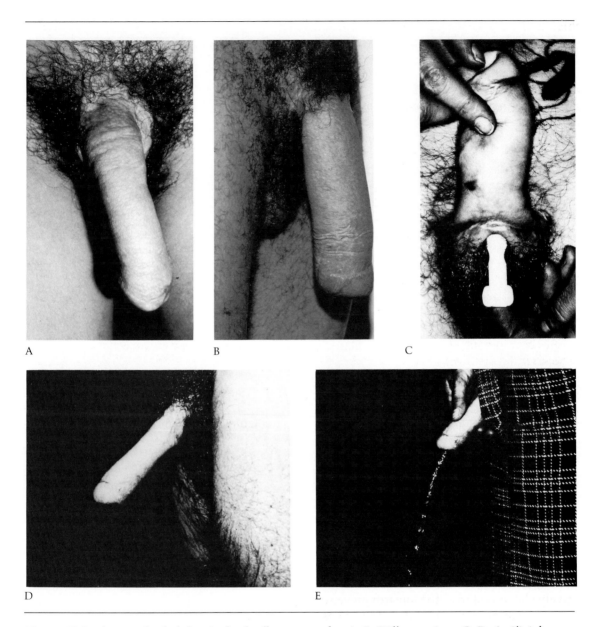

A          B          C

D          E

**Figure 58-3** *The standard abdominal tube flap is shown in all of these photographs. The important points to note are the variable size and the improved aesthetics afforded by the external surface formed by the thick split-thickness skin graft placed onto Scarpa's vascularized fascia and fed by the enlarged superficial external pudendal artery from the femoral axis. The flap is made in two stages, starting with a midline bipedicle inside the* tube. A, B. Different sizes. C, D. Artificial custom baculum stiffener, placed on an as-needed basis for intromission during intercourse. The pedicle is insensitive, but the baculum stimulates the erotic areas effectively. E. Urination via a urinary assist device. This custom device is external and is transmitting urine from the (female) urinary meatus into the tunnel of the phallus.

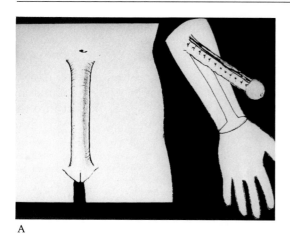

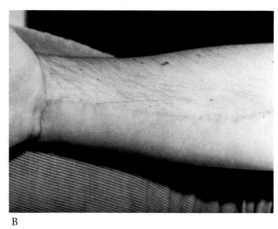

A

B

**Figure 58-4** *Composite tube. A. Donor tissues. B. Postoperative patient demonstrating a relatively inexpensive donor site scar that requires little or no anesthesia in the arm or hand.*

dard tube, and Figure 58-4 shows the composite tube donor sites [45, 54]. A postoperative example of the composite penis is shown in Figure 56-5.

Suction assisted lipoplasty may help reduce feminine subcutaneous contours and is an important adjunct. Augmentation rhinoplasty, "augmentation" mentoplasty, or genioplasty is occasionally requested. Body height-increasing procedures are usually not requested or practiced.

## Surgery for Male to Female Gender Dysphoria

In rehabilitation medicine—as in religion, modeling theory, and self-improvement programs—two schools of thought have polarized: *Accept yourself for what you are and build on it* versus *Take every advantage of medical science for self-improvement.* Abuse of the latter dictum means that the person does not make an effort himself relying on others to do *for* him. "Abuse" of the former, on the other hand, is to not take advantage of an operation that would significantly improve the quality of life. Obviously the compromise between the two seemingly divergent schools produces the best deci-

sions, particularly for application of body image change (aesthetic) surgery procedures in the male-to-female patient.

ELECTROLYSIS
A skilled electrologist can be of inestimable value for helping these patients rid themselves of beard and other unwanted hair. It ordinarily requires many sessions and causes the patient some pain, which may lead to the use of habituating drugs. It may also entail considerable expense.

HORMONAL SUPPORT
After cross-living and dressing, a manifestation of the intensity (see Benjamin) of the drive to change the body is the request for assistance in the hormone program. Female hormones given to the male body have many commonalities with female hormones given to postmenopausal or castrated females: The undesirable effects must be balanced against the desired effects. The undesirable effects—to be noted in the informed consent interaction with the patient—are the following.

1. Exposure to carcinogenic substances [73]
2. Exposure to hepatotoxin
3. Exposure to a substance reported to produce venous stasis (possible thromboembolism)
4. Temporary, but perhaps permanent, loss of testicular, hormonal, and procreation functions
5. Decrease in libido

In the case of the gender dysphoria patient, desired effects include (1) decreased penile eroticism, (2) breast enlargement, (3) some theoretical protection against coronary artery disease, (4) alteration of subcutaneous body fat distribution from android to gynecoid, (5) decrease in growth and amount of body hair, (6) a sense of self-satisfaction.

Fluid retention and alteration in personality are changes that are variably reported. Little change in bony structure toward the male pattern has been noted. Blood testosterone levels fall to a level below that of the normal male and above that of the normal female. Pituitary hormone, which stimulates the testes, is suppressed.

## AUGMENTATION MAMMAPLASTY

As in the female body substrate at puberty, female hormones produce a varying degree of mammary gland enlargement depending on the genetic programming for that organ. Biopsies show duct and stromal enhancement, similar to gynecomastia histopathology. The breasts should probably be "driven" by hormones for at least 2 years prior to consideration of augmentation mammaplasty. Evidence indicates that estrogen is the hormone more specific to the breast enlargement, but the progesterone increases the size of the areola and nipple. However, progesterone given cyclically offers some protection to the breast against mammary cancer, which has been reported in the transsexual. Some patients require additional augmentation, beyond the hormonal assistance.

Technical points regarding mammaplasty on the male body are as follows.

1. The chest is wider in the male, and the nipples are further apart; thus to achieve cleavage, broad-based wide implants are of help. Dissection of the pocket into the axilla is not helpful. Medial placement of small implants produces outward-looking nipples because the nipples are already laterally placed.
2. There is greater adherence of the breast to the pectoral fascia.
3. Submuscular augmentation has been more satisfactory in patients with a thin subcutaneous layer, e.g., pinch test less than 1.5 cm.
4. It is good medical practice to encourage periodic examination of the breasts for masses.

## FEMINIZATION OF FACIAL BONES

Ousterhout of San Francisco [65] contributed to plastic surgery knowledge when he pointed out the three characteristics used by physical anthropologists for differentiating the female from the male skull [33, 34, 71, 74].

1. The angle of the nasal bone takeoff from the forehead is more obtuse in the female (i.e., there is less of a dorsal hump).
2. The chin is more pointed in the female, broader in the male.
3. The forehead has clear-cut differences. The female has less supraorbital bossing, sometimes none at all. The male has a central midforehead flat area superior to the supraorbit, whereas the female has a continuous curve to the forehead profile.

Ousterhout has feminized the male forehead of transsexuals by sculpting the bone with the pineapple burr and rotary power equipment. He has achieved the gentle female roundness with methylmethacrylate augmentation onlay cranioplasty.

## RHINOPLASTY

Often a large, masculine-appearing nose (especially if there is a prominent dorsal hump) lessens the patient's ability to pass as a female. In these cases a rhinoplasty can improve the feminine body image. This procedure is often done during the cross-living period, prior to genital surgery, to aid the patient in being accepted as a female. It is interesting to note that not as much of the body image appears to be invested in the nose in these patients as in the genetic female requesting rhinoplasty.

## MENTOPLASTY

The patient with either a jutting or a square chin may benefit from sculpting the prominence to achieve a more feminine facial contour. It can be done conveniently through an intraoral approach, thereby leaving no external scars. The guidelines of Gonzales-Ulloa and Stevens [36] are used for shaping the profile. Horizontal osteotomies are becoming more common than implants.

## MALAR-CHEEKBONE ENLARGEMENT

With the field of plastic reconstructive surgery beginning to concentrate on alteration of the facial skeleton for aesthetic improvement (interface surgery), cheek bone enhancement by zygomatic-maxillary osteotomy and interposition of cranial bone graft, homologous irradiated cartilage, or synthetic material (Proplast or Interpore) can be of benefit to the gender patient, who in the past has all too often turned to silicone injection in this area.

## REDUCTION THYROID CHONDROPLASTY

A prominent "Adam's apple" due to the ala of the thyroid cartilage may be a source of concern for the patient and interfere with acceptance as female. The technique for chondroplasty is straightforward and has been described by Good [37] and Wolfort and Pany [77]. A horizontal neck incision is made in an inconspicuous natural crease that does not necessarily have to overlie the cartilage. Through this incision the thyroid cartilage is exposed after retraction of the strap muscles laterally. The mucosa of the larynx is gently teased away from the inner aspect of the offending cartilage, and subperiochondrial shaving of the cartilage is performed. This procedure can be performed on an outpatient basis. Rarely, patients are hoarse following the technique [12] because the vocal cords insert at this point of reduction.

Facelift, blepharoplasty, and many of the other aesthetic operations can provide more confidence in the female life.

## VOICE

Many patients have inquired about operations to raise the pitch of the voice. Donald at the University of California, Davis [17], has altered the insertion of the cords, but we are unaware of any popular procedure to accomplish voice change. Furthermore, with the aid of a voice coach many patients are able to modulate their voices to obtain a more pleasing pitch. Speech therapists also remind us that more than pitch is involved in feminine speech. Choice of words and other speech mannerisms are also important and can be cultivated by the patients.

## GENITALIA

Surgical transformation of male to female genitalia may take advantage of the fact that tissues are present locally for use in the formation of female external anatomy. Most procedures involve (1) high ligation of the spermatic cord (avoidance of any inguinal hernia) and orchiectomy; (2) excision of corpora cavernosa of the penis at the pubic symphysis; (3) use of the scrotum to form labia majora; (4) use of penile skin to form labia minora; (5) use of corpora spongiosum and urethra to provide sensitivity and a urinary conduit. Procedures vary with the tissue used for the vagina and the clitoris.

On a worldwide basis the most popular procedure for vaginal construction is penile inversion, as begun by Burou of Casablanca

[11] and perfected by Biber [7, 39] in the United States. Penile skin is actually inverted. This flap is pedicled by the widely undermined anterior abdominal wall, which is advanced posteriorly, moving the tissue from the penile to the vaginal position. Penile skin is amazing in terms of the amount of expansion that occurs when the dermis is thinned in the manner of full-thickness graft preparation. The curious anatomic point here is that the thinned skin of the distal one-third of the penis is thinned but remains viable, as a flap does. There may be a small capillary system in the penile skin; at least

it appears to be present macroscopically. Burou reported performing 1000 of these procedures and Biber more than 1500 [7]. Morbidity has decreased as their experience increased.

In the past, the McIndoe thick split-thickness skin graft procedure was popular with both this author [38, 55] and Forrester of Oklahoma. However, the donor site scar and the contractures associated with skin graft are obvious disadvantages, although several hundred well satisfied patients attest to its advantages when the technique is used with attention to detail [48].

The sigmoid vaginoplasty has been used for decades in Eastern Europe to treat vaginal atresia. The authors advocate rectosigmoid as the most natural vaginal substitute [51]. Figure 58-5 shows the typical external appearance of the authors' patients after surgery with various techniques.

At the 1987 Harry Benjamin International

*Figure 58-5 Postoperative views of the male to female perineum. Sexual climax in the postoperative gender confirmation patient is shown in the inset. Various techniques for vaginal construction have been used. The authors now prefer rectosigmoid colon and employ the end-to-end stapling device to reconstitute the intestine. The rectosigmoid has the most natural qualities of sensitivity and lubrication.*

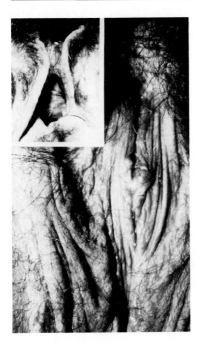 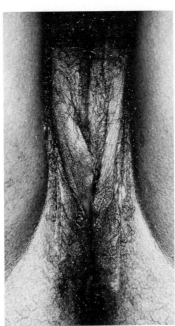 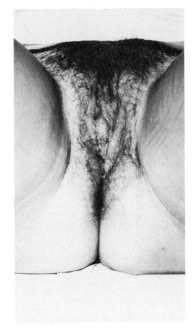

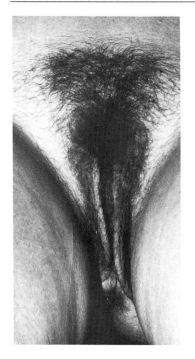
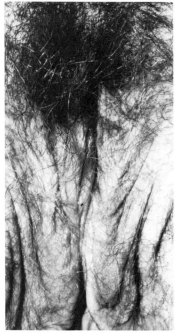
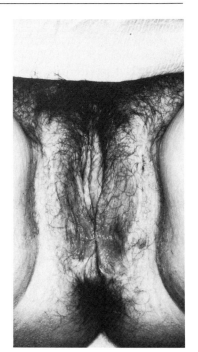

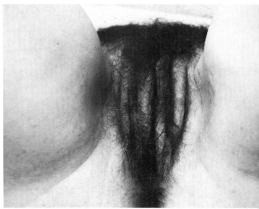

**Figure 58-5** (continued)

Gender Dysphoria Association meeting, two surgeons [18, 76] reported use of rectosigmoid in patients with gender dysphoria syndrome. These reports reinforced the author's enthusiasm for neocolporrhaphy with rectosigmoid colon. The technique exploits the safety of the stapling device to reconstitute the gastrointestinal tract. This technique is detailed in Chapter 57.

The Norfolk group used a full-thickness skin graft, closing the abdominal donor site in the manner of an abdominoplasty [31]. Barbosa used full-thickness penile skin grafts [2].

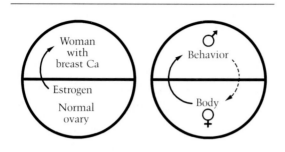

**Figure 58-6**  *The catholic "doctrine of the whole" may apply. See text for discussion.*

## Insurance: Legal and Moral Issues

Multiple references in the Bible regard cross dressing, and this activity is not condoned. Neither the Bible nor canon law refers to transsexualism and its treatment, which is a different condition from homosexuality and transvestitism.

Although the catholic doctrine regarding the destiny of body parts forbids removal of normal nonpathologic parts, the "doctrine of the whole" supersedes (Fig. 58-6). This doctrine states that, in the interest of the welfare of the whole organism, healthy parts may be removed; e.g., the normal ovary may be removed in the patient with breast cancer. The gender dysphoria patient has normal behavior and a normal body, but they are discordant. One part (in this case the body) may therefore be manipulated surgically in the interest of the welfare of the entire, or whole, organism. If the doctrine can be applied to a psychiatric condition or whether the pathology of gender dysphoria syndrome is somatic or psychiatric are questions to be answered as the field develops.

Legal issues are similar. The mayhem law is homologous to the doctrine of the destiny of normal parts but is again superseded by consideration of the greater good. If there are questions, the local district attorney can be helpful.

Insurance carriers may specifically exclude transsexual treatment as they do aesthetic surgery. 302.0 is the ICDA III code number for the diagnosis. Insurance companies and hospital boards are beginning to recognize the rehabilitative and economic benefits.

Legal name change and birth certificate amendments are accomplished according to the laws of the particular state.

The surgical methods, preoperative preparation, and postoperative management utilize a great many of the principles of plastic and reconstructive surgery.

## References

1. Arneri, V. Reconstruction of the male genitalia. In J. M. Converse (ed.), *Reconstructive Plastic Surgery.* Philadelphia: Saunders, 1977. P. 3902.
2. Barbosa, J. Surgery experience with large series of transsexual patients. Presented at the Harry Benjamin Fourth International Conference on Gender Identity, Stanford University, Palo Alto, 1975.
3. Barlow, D., Reynolds, J., and Agras, S. Gender identity change in a transsexual. *Arch. Gen. Psychiatry* 28:569, 1973.
4. Benjamin, H. *The Transsexual Phenomenon.* New York: Julian Press, 1966.
5. Benjamin, H. Honorary address to the Harry Benjamin International Gender Dysphoria Association Meeting, San Diego, 1976.
6. Bagheri, S. A., and Boyer, J. L. Peliosis hepatis associated with androgenic-anabolic steroid: A severe form of hepatic injury. *Ann. Intern. Med.* 81:610, 1974.
7. Biber, S. Harry Benjamin Fourth International Conference on Gender Identity, Stanford University, Palo Alto, 1975.
8. Borgas, N. A. Uber die Volle Plastiche Wiederherstellung eines zum Koitus Fastugen Penis (Peniplastic Totalis) *Zentrabl. Chir.* 63: 1271, 1936.
9. Bouman, J. Phalloplasty using existing tissue. Presented at the Harry Benjamin International Gender Dysphoria Association Meeting, Minneapolis, 1985.
10. Boxer, R. J. Reconstruction of the male external genitalia. *Surg. Gynecol. Obstet.* 141:939, 1975.

11. Burou, G. Male to female transformation. In *Proceedings of the Second Interdisciplinary Symposium on Gender Dysphoria Syndrome.* Palo Alto: Stanford University School of Medicine, 1973.

12. Caldwell, D. O. Psychopathis transsexualis. *Sexology* 16:274, 1949.

13. Chang, T-S., and Hwang, W-Y. Forearm flap in one-stage reconstruction of the penis. *Plast. Reconstr. Surg.* 74:251, 1984.

14. Daverio, P. One-stage reconstruction of the phallus. Presented at the Harry Benjamin International Gender Dysphoria Association Meeting, Minneapolis, 1985.

15. Davies, D. Reconstruction of the penis. Presented at the American Association of Plastic Surgeons Meeting, San Francisco, 1972.

16. Dibbell, D. G. *Gracilis and Anterior Rectus Muscle Flaps for Penis Reconstruction.* Videotape. Plastic Surgery Educational Foundation, Arlington Heights, Illinois.

17. Donald, P. J. Voice change in the transsexual. *Head Neck Surg.* 4:433, 1982.

18. Drogendijk, A. C. Construction of new vagina from sigmoid loop. Presented at the 10th Harry Benjamin International Gender Dysphoria Association Meeting, Amsterdam, 1987.

19. Durfee, R., and Roland, W. Penile substitution with clitoral enlargement and urethral transfer. In *Proceedings of the Second Interdisciplinary Symposium on Gender Dysphoria Syndrome.* Palo Alto: Stanford University School of Medicine, 1973.

20. Edgerton, M. The surgical treatment of male transsexuals. *Clin. Plast. Surg.* 1:285, 1974.

21. Edgerton, M. Presidential Address, Harry Benjamin International Gender Dysphoria Association Meeting, Minneapolis, 1985.

22. Edgerton, M. T. The role of surgery in the treatment of transsexualism. *Ann. Plast. Surg.* 13:473, 1984.

23. Edgerton, M. T., Gillenwater, J. W., Kenney, J. G., et al. The bladder flap for urethral reconstruction in total phalloplasty. *Plast. Reconstr. Surg.* 81:259, 1984.

24. Erhardt, A. The etiology of transsexualism. In *Proceedings of the Second Interdisciplinary Symposium on Gender Dysphoria Syndrome.* Palo Alto: Stanford University School of Medicine, 1973.

25. Fisk, N. Gender dysphoria syndrome—the how, why and what of a condition. In *Proceedings of the Second Interdisciplinary Symposium on Gender Dysphoria Syndrome.* Palo Alto: Stanford University School of Medicine, 1973.

26. Fredericks, S., Stark, R., Horton, C., et al. *The History of the Plastic Surgery Educational Foundation,* Plastic Surgery Educational Foundation, Arlington Heights, Illinois, 1983.

27. Friedman, R., Green, R., and Spitzer, R. Reassessment of homosexuality and transsexualism. *Annu. Rev. Med.* 27:57, 1976.

28. Frumpkin, A. P. Reconstruction of male genitalia. *Am. Rev. Soc. Med.* 2:14, 1944.

29. Futterweitz, W., and Deligdisch, L. Histopathological effects of exogenously administered testosterone in 19 female-to-male transsexuals. *J. Clin. Endocrinol. Metab.* 62:16, 1986.

30. Futterweitz, W., Weiss, R. A., and Fangerstrom, R. M. Endocrine evaluation of forty female-to-male transsexuals: Increased frequency of polycystic ovarian disease in female transsexualism. *Arch. Sex. Behav.* 15:69, 1986.

31. Gilbert, D. Instructional Course: Genital Reconstruction. American Society of Plastic and Reconstructive Surgeons Meeting, Kansas City, MO, 1985.

32. Gilbert, D., Horton, C., Terzis, J., et al. Phallic re-innervation via the internal pudendal nerve. *Plast. Surg. Forum* 2:39, 1986.

33. Giles, E. Sex determination by discriminant function analysis of the mandible. *Am. J. Physiol. Anthropol.* 22:129, 1964.

34. Giles, E., and Elliot, O. Sex determination by discriminant analysis of crania. *Am. J. Physiol. Anthropol.* 21:53, 1963.

35. Gilles, H. D., and Harrison, R. J. Congenital absence of the penis. *Br. J. Plast. Surg.* 1:8, 1948.

36. Gonzales-Ulloa, M., and Stevens, E. The role of chin correction in profileplasty. *Plast. Reconstr. Surg.* 41:477, 1968.

37. Good, R. Thyroid cartilage shaved. In *Proceedings of the Second Interdisciplinary Symposium on Gender Dysphoria Syndrome.* Palo Alto: Stanford University School of Medicine, 1973.

38. Govan, D., and Hentz, V. A surgical program and technique for male to female patients. In *Proceedings of the Second Interdisciplinary Symposium on Gender Dysphoria Syndrome.*

Palo Alto: Stanford University School of Medicine, 1973.

39. Granato, R. Surgical approach to male transsexuals. *Urology* 3:792, 1974.

40. Green, R., and Money, J. (eds.). *Transsexualism and Sex Reassignment*. Baltimore: Johns Hopkins University Press, 1969.

41. Greer, D. M., and Johnston, D. W. *One-Stage Penile Reconstruction.* Videotape. Plastic Surgery Educational Foundation, Arlington Heights, Illinois.

42. Hamburger, C., Sturup, J. K., and Dahl-Iverson, E. Transvestism: Hormonal, psychiatric and surgical treatment. *J.A.M.A.* 152:391, 1953.

43. Hastings, D. The surgical route. *Int. J. Psychoanal.* 9:273, 1970–1971.

44. Hastings, D. Post surgical adjustment of male transsexual patients. *Clin. Plast. Surg.* 1:325, 1974.

45. Hentz, V. R. The versatile forearm flap. Presented at the American Association of Plastic Surgery Meeting, San Diego, 1985.

46. Hester, T. R., Hill, H. L., and Jurkiewitz, M. J. One stage reconstruction of the penis. *Br. J. Plast. Surg.* 31:279, 1978.

47. Horton, C. E., Gilbert, D. A., Terzis, J. K., et al. A new technique for phallic reconstruction with sensation. Presented at the American Association of Plastic Surgery Meeting, San Diego, 1985.

48. Jayaram, D. Personal communication, 1977.

49. Kaplan, I. A rapid method for constructing a functional sensitive penis. *Br. J. Plast. Reconstr. Surg.* 24:342, 1971.

50. Kirkpatrick, M., and Friedman, C. Treatment of request for sex change surgery with psychotherapy. *Am. J. Psychiatry* 133:1194, 1976.

51. Laub, D. Repair of Female Genitalia. In B. Brent (ed.), *Artistry in Plastic Surgery*. St. Louis: Mosby, 1987.

52. Laub, D. R. Metoidioplasty. Presented to the Harry Benjamin International Gender Dysphoria Association Meeting, Bordeaux, France, 1982.

53. Laub, D. R. Invited comment to Edgerton, M. T. The role of surgery in the treatment of transsexualism. *Ann. Plast. Surg.* 13:476, 1984.

54. Laub, D. R. Phalloplasty with forearm flap. Presented at the Texas Plastic Surgery Society Annual Meeting, Dallas, 1986.

55. Laub, D. R., and Fisk, N. A rehabilitation program for gender dysphoria syndrome by surgical sex change. *Plast. Reconstr. Surg.* 53:388, 1974.

56. Levine, S. Case-Western Reserve University. Personal communication.

57. Meyer, J. Psychiatric considerations in the sexual reassignment of non-intersex individuals. *Clin. Plast. Surg.* 1:275, 1974.

58. Meyer-Bahlburg, H. F. L. Hormones and psychosexual differentiation: Implications for the treatment of intersexuality, homosexuality and transsexuality. *Clin. Endocrinol. Metab.* 11:681, 1982.

59. Money, J., and Ehrhardt, A. *Man and Woman, Boy and Girl*. Baltimore: Johns Hopkins University Press, 1972.

60. Money, J. Long-term psychological follow-up of intersexed patients. *Clin. Plast. Surg.* 1:271, 1974.

61. Morales, P. A., O'Conner, J. J., and Hotchkiss, R. S. Plastic reconstruction surgery of the penis. *Am. J. Surg.* 91:403, 1956.

62. Mukherjee, G. D. On reconstruction of the penis with urethra and a dorsal skin-lined socket for a removable prosthesis: A new approach. *Plast. Reconstr. Surg.* 69:377, 1982.

63. Noe, J., Birdsell, D., and Laub, D. The surgical construction of male genitalia for the female to male transsexual. *Plast. Reconstr. Surg.* 53:511, 1974.

64. Orticochea, M. A new method of total reconstruction of the penis. *Br. J. Plast. Surg.* 25:347, 1972.

65. Ousterhout, D. K. Feminization of the forehead: Contour changing to improve female aesthetics. Presented at the Facial Sculpture Symposium, Washington, D.C., 1984; and the American Society for Aesthetic Plastic Surgery, Boston, 1985.

66. Persoff, M. M. Groin flap phallus reconstruction with a new method of urethroplasty. *Ann. Plast. Surg.* 6:132, 1981.

67. Puckett, C. L., and Montie, J. E. Construction of the male genitalia in the transsexual, using a tubed groin flap for the penis and a hydraulic inflation device. *Plast. Reconstr. Surg.* 61:523, 1978.

68. Puckett, C. L., Reinisch, J. F., and Montie, J. E. Free flap phalloplasty. *J. Urol.* 128:294, 1982.

69. Song, R. Y. Reconstruction of the male genitalia. *Chin. Med.* 72:446, 1954.

70. Song, R. Y. Total reconstruction of the male genitalia. *Chin. Plast. Surg.* 9:97, 1982.

71. Stewart, T. D. *Essentials of Forensic Anthropology.* Springfield, IL: Thomas, 1979. P. 300.

72. Sun, G., and Huang, J. One-stage reconstruction of the penis with composite iliac crest and lateral groin flap. *Ann. Plast. Surg.* 15: 519, 1985.

73. Symmers, W. Carcinoma of the breast in transsexual individuals after surgical and hormonal interference with primary and secondary sex characteristics. *Br. Med. J.* 2:82, 1968.

74. Thieme, F. P., and Schull, W. J. Sex determination from the skeleton. *Hum. Biol.* 49:242, 1957.

75. Walker, P. A., Berger, J. C., Green, F., et al. (Founding Committee of the Harry Benjamin Gender Dysphoria Association). Standards of care: The hormonal and surgical sex reassignment of gender dysphoric persons. *Arch. Sex. Behav.* 14:75, 1985.

76. Wilson, N. The use of the rectosigmoid neocolporrhaphy in the treatment of late complications of vaginoplasty. Presented at the 10th Harry Benjamin International Gender Dysphoria Association Meeting, Amsterdam, 1987.

77. Wolfort, F., and Pany, R. Laryngeal chondroplasty for appearance. *Plast. Reconstr. Surg.* 56:371, 1975.

78. Yalom, I., Green, R., and Fisk, N. Prenatal exposure to female hormones: Effect on psychosocial development in boys. *Arch. Gen. Psychiatry* 28:554, 1973.

# Index

# Index